Larsen's Human Embryology

FOURTH EDITION

Gary C. Schoenwolf, Ph.D.

University of Utah School of Medicine
Salt Lake City, Utah

Steven B. Bleyl, M.D., Ph.D.

University of Utah School of Medicine
Salt Lake City, Utah

Philip R. Brauer, Ph.D.

Creighton University School of Medicine
Omaha, Nebraska

Philippa H. Francis-West, Ph.D.

King's College London Dental Institute
London, UK

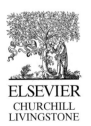

ELSEVIER
CHURCHILL
LIVINGSTONE

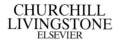

1600 John F. Kennedy Blvd.
Ste 1800
Philadelphia, PA 19103-2899

LARSEN'S HUMAN EMBRYOLOGY, 4TH EDITION   ISBN: 978-0-443-06811-9

Copyright © 2009 by Churchill Livingstone, an imprint of Elsevier Inc.

Notice

Knowledge and best practice in this field are constantly changing. As new research and experience broaden our knowledge, changes in practice, treatment and drug therapy may become necessary or appropriate. Readers are advised to check the most current information provided (i) on procedures featured or (ii) by the manufacturer of each product to be administered, to verify the recommended dose or formula, the method and duration of administration, and contraindications. It is the responsibility of the practitioner, relying on their own experience and knowledge of the patient, to make diagnoses, to determine dosages and the best treatment for each individual patient, and to take all appropriate safety precautions. To the fullest extent of the law, neither the Publisher nor the Authors assume any liability for any injury and/or damage to persons or property arising out of or related to any use of the material contained in this book.

The Publisher

Previous editions copyrighted 2001, 1997, 1993

Library of Congress Cataloging-in-Publication Data
Larsen's human embryology / Gary C. Schoenwolf . . . [et al.]. -- 4th ed.
    p. ; cm.
    Rev. ed. of: Human embryology / William J. Larsen. 3rd ed. c2001.
    Includes bibliographical references and index.
    ISBN 978-0-443-06811-9
1. Embryology, Human. I. Schoenwolf, Gary C. II. Larsen, William J. (William James). Human embryology. III. Title: Human embryology.
    [DNLM: 1. Embryology. 2. Embryonic Development. 3. Fetal Development. QS 604 L3345 2009]

    QM601.L37 2009
    612.6′4–dc22

                                                    2007025100

Acquisitions Editor: Madelene Hyde
Managing Editor: Rebecca Gruliow
Publishing Services Manager: Linda Van Pelt
Project Manager: Priscilla Crater
Design Direction: Lou Forgione

Printed in China

Last digit is the print number: 9   8   7   6   5   4   3   2

I proudly dedicate this edition to the memories of Fred Schoenwolf, Ray L. Watterson, Robert M. Sweeney, and Lucien Vakaet for their encouragement, guidance, training, and inspiration.

Gary C. Schoenwolf, Ph.D.

Content Experts

Kurt A. Albertine, Ph.D., University of Utah, USA

I. Santiago Alvarez, Ph.D., University of Extremadura, Spain

Laure Bally-Cuif, Ph.D., Institute of Developmental Genetics, Germany

Kate F. Barald, Ph.D., University of Michigan, USA

Edward Bersu, Ph.D., University of Wisconsin-Madison, USA

Arthur Brothman, Ph.D., University of Utah, USA

Janice L.B. Byrne, M.D., University of Utah, USA

Blanche Capel, Ph.D., Duke University Medical Center, USA

John C. Carey, M.D., University of Utah, USA

YiPing Chen, Ph.D., Tulane University, USA

Helena Edlund, Ph.D., Umea University, Sweden

Carol A. Erickson, Ph.D., University of California-Davis, USA

Donna M. Fekete, Ph.D., Purdue University, USA

Sabine Fuhrmann, Ph.D., University of Utah, USA

Richard P. Harvey, Ph.D., The Victor Chang Cardiac Research Institute, Australia

Brigid Hogan, Ph.D., Duke University, USA

Irene Hung, M.D., University of Utah, USA

Alexandra L. Joyner, Ph.D., HHMI and Skirball Institute of Biomolecular Medicine, USA

Gabrielle Kardon, Ph.D., University of Utah, USA

Margaret L. Kirby, Ph.D., Duke University, USA

Raj Ladher, Ph.D., RIKEN Centre for Developmental Biology, Japan

Andrew Lumsden, Ph.D., King's College London, UK

Suzanne L. Mansour, Ph.D., University of Utah, USA

Salvador Martinez, M.D., Ph.D., Universidad Miguel Hernandez, Spain

Anne Moon, M.D., Ph.D., University of Utah, USA

Bruce A. Morgan, Ph.D., Harvard Medical School, USA

L. Charles Murtaugh, Ph.D., University of Utah, USA

Harukazu Nakamura, Ph.D., Institute of Development, Aging and Cancer, Japan

José Xavier Neto, M.D., Ph.D., InCor, Brazil

Peter Nichol, M.D., University of Utah, USA

Marysia Placzek, Ph.D., University of Sheffield, UK

Olivier Pourquié, Ph.D., Stowers Institute for Medical Research, USA

Mahendra Rao, M.D., Ph.D., Invitrogen Corp., USA

Alan Rope, M.D., University of Utah, USA

Marian Ros, Ph.D., Universidad dc Cantabria, Spain

Raymond Runyan, Ph.D., University of Arizona, USA

Sheryl Scott, Ph.D., University of Utah, USA

Maya Sieber-Blum, Ph.D., Medical College of Wisconsin, USA

Cliff Tabin, Ph.D., Harvard Medical School, USA

Irma Thesleff, Ph.D., University of Helsinki, Finland

Paul Trainor, Ph.D., Stowers Institute for Medical Research, USA

Monica Vetter, Ph.D., University of Utah, USA

Michiko Watanabe, Ph.D., Case Western Reserve University School of Medicine, USA

David Winlaw, M.B.B.S., M.D., F.R.A.C.S., The Children's Hospital at Westmead, Australia

Gen Yamada, Ph.D., Kumamoto University, Japan

Kenneth S. Zaret, Ph.D., Fox Chase Cancer Center, USA

Preface

I am pleased and honored to lead the revision of the fourth edition of what I have entitled *Larsen's Human Embryology*, named in honor of William J. Larsen, Ph.D., the founding author of *Human Embryology*. Together with Drs. Bleyl (clinical author and editor of the "Clinical Taster" and "In the Clinic" sections), Brauer (author, revision of Chapters 12-15) and Francis-West (author, revision of Chapters 7, 8, 16-18), this edition has been extensively revised and largely rewritten. In addition to revising about half of the chapters (Introduction and Chapters 1-6 and 9-11), I have edited all chapters to enhance consistency of style and integration of content across topics. The third edition of *Human Embryology*, published in 2001, the year after Dr. Larsen's death, was completed by three of his colleagues: Lawrence S. Sherman, Ph.D., S. Steven Potter, Ph.D., and William J. Scott, Ph.D. The fact that this book is now in its fourth edition speaks not only of the vision, creativity and scholarship of Dr. Larsen, but also of the dedication and commitment of his colleagues to preserving his vision. I am particularly indebted to one of these colleagues, Dr. William J. Scott, who encouraged me to author the fourth edition. In this edition, I have built upon the solid foundation laid by Dr. Larsen and clearly expressed in the preface to the first edition: "to meet the needs of first-year medical students . . . and to offer them a glimpse of some of the exciting applications that are currently in use or on the horizon."

Since the publication of the third edition, much has been learned in the fields of developmental biology, genetics, reproductive biology, and the related fields of medical practice. This fourth edition has been extensively revised and rewritten to include these advances and to correct inaccuracies. In addition, many other changes have been made. These include the following:

- Addition of an Introduction. This section covers the reasons for studying human embryology, the various subdivisions of pregnancy (trimesters) and human embryogenesis (periods and phases), embryonic body axes and section planes, and how to learn more human embryology beyond that covered in the textbook. The Introduction should be read before reading subsequent chapters and referred to frequently as you read the rest of the text. This will help keep developmental events in temporal context. Chapter timelines provide more detailed guides to those developmental events discussed in each particular chapter.

- Reorganization of content into a more logical sequence. Some topics previously discussed in one chapter are now discussed in another chapter where they can be better integrated with other information to increase student understanding. As part of this, chapter order has been changed and some material has been grouped differently to form new chapters. Text headers have been simplified throughout the textbook to provide a clearer understanding of the flow of information discussed in each section.

- Integration of sections on mechanisms of development and clinical importance with the relevant descriptive embryology. These sections, entitled respectively, "In the Research Lab" and "In the Clinic," provide an immediate discussion of the importance of the descriptive embryology being covered at length in the preceding discussion. This juxtaposition helps students to understand not only what happens in human embryogenesis but also how it happens and why it is clinically significant. To meet the needs of a variety of course types and instructor goals, these sections are highlighted with color shading for easy reference. In some cases, a section entitled "In the Research Lab" may also discuss material more appropriately placed under the title "In the Clinic" and vice versa. This was done sometimes to provide better integration of mechanism and clinical relevance when it was logical to do so. This also serves to emphasize the role of the physician scientist and the need for the physician scientist to take information obtained from the bench (i.e., the lab) to the bedside (i.e., the patient) and vice versa, ultimately resulting in the translation of advances in basic science to improvements in the healthcare of children.

- Expansion of the number of chapters from 15 to 18. New Chapter 5 discusses principles of development and mechanisms underlying morphogenesis and dysmorphogenesis. In addition, this chapter describes the major signaling pathways controlling embryogenesis. It is designed to be read at any time, before or after any particular group of chapters. It is expected that students will refer to this chapter frequently throughout their study of the remaining chapters of the textbook. New Chapter 8 discusses development of the musculoskeletal system. By grouping material from several chapters into one chapter, students now can gain a better understanding of the development of the musculoskeletal system as a whole. New Chapter 17 covers development of the ear and eye. These sections were previously part of a chapter on development of the head and neck. As this chapter was previously overwhelming owing to the complexity of the head and neck region, it was reorganized and subdivided into two chapters to help students digest the complexity of the region.

- Enhancement of the previous illustrations, as well as the addition of over 400 new illustrations. Color schemes have been chosen to increase the vibrancy of the illustrations and to make it easier to discern important structures. New drawings have been added to illustrate new text sections, and new photographs have been included from the scientific and medical literature. Embryology is a visual science. To help students learn how to visualize embryos as they change their three-dimensional morphology over time requires many different types of illustrations and views of the developing embryo. Thus, our goal in adding new illustrations was to provide a range of types of illustrations and to add new visual perspectives to enhance student understanding.

- Addition of "Clinical Tasters" to the Introduction and to each chapter. A "Clinical Taster" differs from a case history or a clinical teaser in that its purpose is not to provide a clinical problem for the beginning student to solve. Rather, its goal is three-fold. First, to whet the student's appetite for the material discussed in that particular chapter (and hence the use of the word "taster" in the sense of an appetizer to enjoy before the main course of the meal). Second, to continue to emphasize the clinical importance of the descriptive human embryology that the students will study (a large part of which will involve the rote memorization of anatomical terms). And third, to provide a springboard for further discussion and self-directed (or group) learning using resources beyond the textbook (see Introduction for suggestions for further study). As such, the "Clinical Tasters" do not ask questions for the students to answer, and hence a list of answers is not provided, but each taster is further discussed and placed into context in the corresponding chapter. **Discussion of the tasters with your peers will be highly beneficial in gaining a deeper understanding of human embryology.**

- Focusing of references to mainly review articles published during the last 5 years. As discussed in the Introduction, there are several reasons for focusing on recent review articles. However, references from the previous edition remain helpful and provide an historical account of how particular areas of understanding of human embryology have evolved over time. **References from the third edition of this textbook, along with their PubMed listing when available, are posted on the textbook website to help you gain an appreciation of how this evolution has occurred.**

- Placing the Glossary online. This allows for better cross referencing and for terms to be looked up quicker than when using print. In addition, it reduces print costs, saving students money. **See the textbook website for the online Glossary.**

In closing, let me express my sincere hope that you will enjoy learning human embryology and that this textbook will serve as a helpful guide for your study.

I have enjoyed preparing the fourth edition; if it makes your study easier, your understanding greater, and grows your interest in human embryology, then I will have achieved my goal. If you would like to share your thoughts about this textbook, human embryology, or your experience in learning human embryology, please drop me a line (schoenwolf@neuro.utah.edu).

Gary C. Schoenwolf, Ph.D.

Acknowledgments

Without students there would be no need for text-books. Thus, the authors thank the many bright young students that we have been fortunate enough to interact with throughout our careers, as well as those students of the future, in eager anticipation of continuing fruitful and enjoyable interactions. For us as teachers, students have enriched our lives and have taught us at least as much, if not more, than we have taught them.

For this edition, we are especially grateful to the more than 40 content experts who were integral partners in the preparation of this fourth edition and who, like our students, have also taught us much. Each of the content experts read one or more chapters, offered numerous suggestions for revision and in some cases even provided new text and illustrations. We have pondered their many suggestions for revision but in the end, rightly or wrongly, we chose the particular direction to go. The authors share a captivation for the embryo and have sought to understand it fully, but of course we have not yet accomplished this objective; thus, our studies continue (we all have active research laboratories). Nevertheless, we took faith when writing this edition in a quote from one of the great scientific heroes, Viktor Hamburger: "Our real teacher has been and still is the embryo, who is, incidentally, the only teacher who is always right."

Finally, we must thank the many authors, colleagues, patients, and families of patients who provided figures for the textbook. Rather than acknowledging the source of each figure in its legend, we have clustered these acknowledgments into a "Credits" section. This was done not to hide contributions, but rather to focus the legends on what was most relevant to the student reading them.

Contents

In the research lab
In the clinic

*color coding indicates type
and title of boxes within text

Introduction

Summary   As you begin your study of **human embryology**, it's a good time to consider why knowledge of the subject will be important to your career. Human embryology is fascinating in itself and tells us about our own prenatal origins. It also sheds light on the **birth defects** that occur relatively frequently in human populations. So the study of both normal and abnormal human embryology tells us something about every human we will encounter throughout our lives. For those seeking a career in biology, medicine, or allied health sciences, there are many other reasons to learn human embryology, which include the following:

- Knowing human embryology provides a logical framework for understanding adult **anatomy**.
- Knowing human embryology provides a bridge between basic science (e.g., anatomy) and clinical science (e.g., obstetrics and pediatrics).
- Knowing human embryology allows the physician to accurately advise patients on many issues, such as **reproduction, birth defects, prenatal development, in vitro fertilization, stem cells**, and **cloning**.

Human pregnancy is subdivided in many ways to facilitate understanding of changes that occur in the developing organism over time. Prospective parents and physicians typically use **trimesters**: three-month periods (zero to three months, three to six months, and six to nine months) starting with the date of onset of the last menstrual period and ending at birth. Human embryologists use periods: **the period of the egg** (generally from fertilization to the end of the 3rd week), **the period of the embryo** (generally from the beginning of the 4th week to the end of the 8th week), and **the period of the fetus** (from the beginning of the 3rd month to birth).

Human embryologists also identify **phases of human embryogenesis**. Generally, six phases are recognized:

- **Gametogenesis**, the formation of the gametes, the egg and sperm
- **Fertilization**, the joining of the gametes to form the zygote
- **Cleavage**, a series of rapid cell divisions that result first in the formation of the morula, a solid ball of cells, and then in the formation of the blastocyst, a hollow ball of cells containing a central cavity
- **Gastrulation**, the rearrangement of cells into three primary germ layers: the ectoderm, mesoderm, and endoderm
- **Formation of the tube-within-a-tube body plan**, consisting of a cylindrically shaped embryonic body formed from an outer ectodermal tube (the future skin) and an inner endodermal tube (the gut tube)
- **Organogenesis**, the formation of organ rudiments and organ systems

During gastrulation, the three cardinal **body axes** are established. In the embryo and fetus, these three axes are called the **dorsal-ventral, cranial-caudal**, and **medial-lateral** axes. They are equivalent, respectively, to the **anterior-posterior, superior-inferior**, and **medial-lateral** axes of the adult.

Clinical Taster On a Monday morning you get a frantic call from a 22-year-old patient who is 3 months pregnant. That weekend, she witnessed a car accident in which two people were badly injured, and she can't get the images of their bloodied faces out of her mind. Her neighbor told her that viewing such a shocking event could traumatize her fetus and result in the birth of a "monster." Also, she remembers seeing a headline in a periodical at the checkout counter of the local grocery store, reporting the birth of a headless baby. The story reported that early in pregnancy the baby's mother watched a television program on the history of the guillotine, thereby traumatizing her fetus. Your patient wants to know whether seeing the accident could have traumatized her fetus in a similar fashion; if so, she says she wants to consider an abortion to prevent giving birth to a severely defective child. As her physician, she is calling you for advice.

You tell her that her neighbor is mistaken and that there is no medical evidence to support the idea that watching a disturbing television program or viewing a shocking event could traumatize her fetus, resulting in a severe birth defect such as the one she fears. She states that she is somewhat relieved by talking with you and agrees to continue her pregnancy. However, she admits that she still has some misgivings. You recognize that—depending on one's culture, education, and beliefs—legend and superstition can be as powerful to some as modern medicine. You continue to try to address her concerns and reduce her anxiety over the course of her remaining prenatal visits, which include normal ultrasound examinations. The last two trimesters of her pregnancy are uneventful, and at term she delivers a vibrant, healthy 7-pound 6-ounce baby girl.

Why Study Human Embryology?

Quite simply put, a good reason to study human embryology is that this topic is fascinating. All of us were once human embryos, so the study of human embryology is the study of our own prenatal origins and experience. Moreover, many of us are, or will someday be, parents and perhaps grandparents. Having a child or a grandchild is an awe-inspiring experience, which once again personalizes human development for each of us and piques our curiosity about its wonders. As teachers of human embryology, one of us now for more than a quarter century, we still find the subject to be utterly fascinating!

Human embryology does not always occur normally. Surprisingly, 3% to 4% of all live-born children will be diagnosed eventually (usually within the first two years) with a significant **malformation** (i.e., **birth defect**). Understanding why embryology goes awry and results in birth defects requires a thorough grasp of the molecular genetic, cellular, and tissue events underlying normal human embryology. Whether someone develops normally or not has a lifelong impact on that person, as well as on the person's family.

For a student pursuing a career in biology, medicine, or allied health sciences there are many other reasons to study human embryology.

- The best way to understand and remember human anatomy—microscopic anatomy, neuroanatomy, and gross anatomy—is to understand how tissues, organs, and the body as a whole are assembled from relatively simple rudiments. Knowing the embryology solidifies your knowledge of anatomy, and it also provides an explanation for the variation that you will observe in human anatomy.

- As you continue your studies and perhaps take courses such as human genetics, pathology, organ systems, and reproductive biology, and study disease processes and aging, your knowledge of human embryology will continue to benefit you. Cancer is now widely recognized as a disease involving mutations in genes controlling development and regulating key cellular events of development, such as division and death (apoptosis).

- Many of you will become medical practitioners. Embryology will serve to bridge your basic science and clinical science courses, particularly as you start your study of obstetrics and pediatrics. But perhaps more importantly, once you start your practice, your patients will have many questions about pregnancy and birth defects, and controversial and always newsworthy issues such as abortion, birth control, cryopreservation of gametes and embryos, reproductive and therapeutic cloning, in vitro fertilization, gamete and embryo donation, stem cells, and gestational surrogate mothers. Your knowledge of human embryology will allow you to provide scientifically accurate counsel, empowering your patients to make informed decisions based on current scientific understanding. Many of your patients will have reproductive concerns. As their physician, you will be their main source of reliable information.

- If you are a medical student, it is important for you to know that performing well on (and perhaps even passing) Step 1 National Boards involves a thorough knowledge of human embryology and the underlying developmental, molecular, and genetic principles and mechanisms. Both Drs. Larsen and Schoenwolf have served as Members, USMLE Step 1 Cell and Developmental Biology Test Material Development Committee, National Board of Medical Examiners (Dr. Schoenwolf joined the committee after Dr. Larsen's untimely death). Human embryology is an integral component of that examination. Moreover, because this textbook emphasizes clinical applications and developmental mechanisms (see "In the Clinic" and "In the Research Lab" sections, respectively, in each chapter), as well as descriptive aspects of development, studying human embryology and using this book also can have practical value.

- Finally, we think one of the best reasons to study human embryology is that it is a fun subject to learn. Although we now know a tremendous amount about how embryos develop, there are still many mysteries to unravel. Thus, human embryology is not a static subject; rather, our knowledge and understanding of human embryology is always evolving. As you study human embryology, be sure also to pay attention to the news—undoubtedly, advances in human embryology will be mentioned several times during the course of your study.

IN THE RESEARCH LAB

LINK BETWEEN DEVELOPMENT AND CANCER

The *Wnt* (*Wingless*; discussed in Ch. 5) family of secreted signaling molecules is one example of a signaling pathway that has multiple functions in the embryo and adult. In the embryo, *Wnt* signaling controls the specification of cell fate.

In the adult, *Wnt* signaling maintains homeostasis in self-renewing tissues. Mutation of members of the *Wnt* signaling pathway result in malignant transformation (i.e., **cancer**).

These multiple roles for *Wnt* signaling are best understood in the intestine (discussed in Ch. 14). Interestingly, the first hint that *Wnt* signaling was important in intestinal biology came from the finding in the early 1990s that the human **tumor suppressor gene**, *ADENOMATOUS POLYPOSIS COLI (APC)*—a component of the *Wnt* signaling pathway—was mutated in **colorectal cancer**. The mutation resulted in constitutively active *Wnt* signaling and the subsequent development of cancer. *APC* and colorectal cancers are also discussed in Chapter 14.

More recently, it has been shown that *Wnt* signaling plays important roles in gut development. First, formation of the endoderm during gastrulation (discussed in Chs. 2, 3) requires *Wnt* signaling (demonstrated by inactivating *β-Catenin* function, a component of the *Wnt* signaling pathway). Second, regional patterning of the gut and its folding to form the hindgut, and probably also the foregut, require *Wnt* signaling (demonstrated either by inactivating both *Tcf1* and *Tcf4* or *Apc*; *Tcf1* and *Tcf4* are two other components of the *Wnt* signaling pathway).

After the gut tube is formed it undergoes regional histogenesis. For example, within the small intestine, villi (finger-like projections) form, separated by invaginations called crypts, whereas within the colon (large intestine) crypts also form but villi are absent. The crypts consist of highly proliferative progenitor cells, with maturing cells moving out of the crypts to the surface epithelium of the gut tube. Normal proliferation of crypt cells requires continual stimulation of the *Wnt* pathway. Specifically, prevention of *Wnt* signaling (by inhibiting *Tcf4* or *β-Catenin*; or overexpressing a *Wnt* antagonist called *Dickkopf-1*) severely reduces crypt cell proliferation in both the fetal and adult intestine. Moreover, mutation of the negative regulator of *Wnt* signaling, *Apc*, results in hyperproliferation.

NOTE ABOUT GENE NAMES

Different naming conventions and font styles are often used to designate a gene, its mRNA, or its protein. Also, naming conventions are different for each animal model and in turn may differ from that used for humans. For example, the *Fibroblast growth factor 8* (*Fgf8*) gene in humans is designated as *FGF8*, its mRNA as *FGF8*, and its protein as FGF8. In mouse, the gene and its mRNA are designated as *Fgf8*, and its protein as FGF8. For the sake of simplicity, when this textbook refers to a gene, its transcript, or its protein, the name will be listed in italics, lower case, except for its first letter, which will be capitalized. When it is important to designate whether the name indicates a gene, mRNA, or protein, qualifiers will be added: the *Fgf8* gene, *Fgf8* transcript, or *Fgf8* protein, respectively. Although this is not strictly correct, it will make reading much easier for the student.

One exception to these rules will be when proteins are discussed in the context of their action in a process such as the menstrual cycle, rather than in a genomic/molecular genetic context. Thus, luteinizing hormone will be designated as luteinizing hormone (neither italicized nor with first letter capitalized) or by its abbreviation, LH. Another exception will be when mutations in human genes are discussed—generally the human nomenclature and style will be used.

Periods of Human Embryology

From a medical or prospective parent's viewpoint, human prenatal development is subdivided into three main intervals called the **1st, 2nd**, and **3rd trimesters**, each consisting of three-month periods. From an embryologist's viewpoint there are also three main subdivisions of human prenatal development, generally called the **period of the egg, period of the embryo**, and **period of the fetus**. The first period, the period of the egg or **ovum**, is generally considered to extend from the time of **fertilization** until formation of the **blastocyst** and **implantation** of the blastocyst into the uterine wall about one week after fertilization (Fig. Intro-1). The entire **conceptus** (i.e., the product of conception or fertilization) typically is called the *egg* during this period. The conceptus at the blastocyst stage has already differentiated to give rise to tissue destined to form the embryo proper, as well as other tissue that will form extraembryonic layers. During the period of the egg, human embryologists identify three stages of development: the **zygote** (formed at fertilization before the egg becomes multicellular), **morula** (formed after the zygote cleaves by mitosis giving rise to a cluster of multiple cells or blastomeres), and **blastocyst** (a large, fluid-filled central cavity that forms after the morula). The conceptus during this period may also be called the **pre-implantation embryo**, or more accurately the **preimplantation conceptus**. Thus, the period could also be called the period of the preimplantation

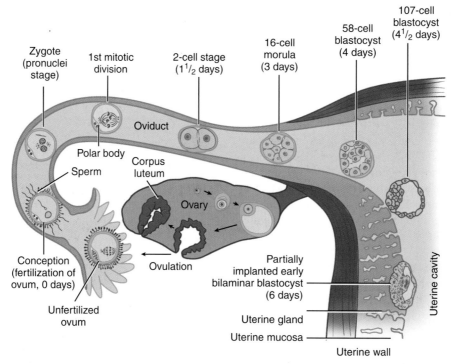

Figure Intro-1. The first week of prenatal development of the human.

embryo or preimplantation conceptus. The use of the terms *egg* or *embryo* for the conceptus at these stages is particularly helpful for those conducting in vitro fertilization (eggs/embryos are collected, eggs/embryos are washed, eggs/embryos are transplanted into the uterus—try saying these phrases quickly using "conceptuses" or "concepti"!). But in the strictest sense, *egg* (or *oocyte*) is the name of the female gamete before fertilization, so using the term *egg* to describe later stages can lead to confusion.

The exact beginning of the period of the embryo is poorly defined, and consequently there is no universal agreement about when the period begins. Some call the cleaving morula, or even the zygote, the *embryo*, so with this classification scheme the period of the embryo begins as early as immediately after fertilization or as late as three days after fertilization. Others use the term *embryo* only after the conceptus starts implanting into the uterine wall at the end of the 1st week of gestation or becomes fully implanted into the uterine wall at the end of the 2nd week of gestation. Still others use the term *embryo* only in the 4th week of gestation after the embryonic disc becomes three-dimensional and a typical tube-within-a-tube body plan is established. The period of the embryo could also be called the period of the *postimplantation embryo* or *postimplantation conceptus*, if these terms are restricted to stages after implantation occurs. In this textbook, the period of the embryo will be defined as beginning at the end of the 1st week of gestation, after implantation is initiated.

Despite the lack of agreement about when the period of the embryo begins, it is generally considered to end at the end of the 8th week of gestation (that is, at the end of the 2nd month after fertilization), after which the period of the fetus begins. This endpoint for the period of the embryo is arbitrary because there is no obvious major change in the embryo/fetus between the 8th and 9th week of gestation. The period of the fetus extends from the 9th week to birth and involves rapid growth of the fetus and functional maturation of its organ systems (discussed in Ch. 6). At birth, the baby or neonate breathes on its own, but development does not cease simply because birth has occurred. Although this textbook discusses only prenatal development, it is important remember that development is not just a prenatal experience; rather, development is a lifelong process, with aging and senescence involving further developmental events.

IN THE RESEARCH LAB

WHY DO WE AGE?

Animal models are playing an important role in understanding **aging** in humans. Using organisms as diverse as *Saccharomyces cerevisiae* (yeast), *Caenorhabditis elegans* (nematode worm), *Drosophila melanogaster* (fruitfly), and *Mus musculus* (mouse), the genetic pathways controlling aging are beginning to be elucidated. Animal models offer the key advantage that searches can be conducted for mutations that extend **life span**. These studies are relevant to humans; a locus recently identified on human chromosome 4 has been linked to exceptional longevity.

The following discussion is based mainly on what has been learned about aging in *C. elegans*, where the clearest picture has emerged, albeit still a very incomplete one. In *C. elegans*, four processes have been shown to affect life span, and it is likely that these four processes are at least partially interrelated and are at least partially conserved among species:

- Caloric restriction
- Signaling through the *Insulin/Igf-like1* pathway
- Germ line activity
- Signaling through the *Clk-1* pathway

Life span and the duration of good health can be extended by caloric restriction in all species, provided that the diet includes enough nutrition for routine maintenance of the body. However, although the value of caloric restriction has been known for more than a half century, the mechanism of its action remains unclear.

Puberty and menopause, two major postnatal developmental events, are controlled hormonally (discussed in Ch. 1). Thus, it is not surprising that aging, a more gradual postnatal developmental event, also seems to be regulated hormonally. In particular, it has been shown that the endocrine hormone *Insulin/Insulin-like growth factor 1* limits life span; thus, mutations in this signaling pathway extend life span. One way in which *Insulin/Igf-like1* hormone is regulated is through sensory neurons. Perturbations in *C. elegans* that decrease sensory perception extend life span (by up to 50%) by acting through this pathway. As surprising as it sounds, increased sensory perception leads to increased *Insulin/Igf-like1* hormone secretion and accelerated aging. The *Insulin/Igf-like1* pathway is likely also involved in regulating caloric intake.

The germ line (discussed in Ch. 1) can also regulate the rate of aging, perhaps to coordinate an animal's schedule of reproduction with its rate of aging. For example, strains of flies have been bred that produce offspring relatively late in life and have long life spans, whereas other strains have offspring at an earlier stage and are short lived. If germ cells are killed in the short-lived strain, its life span is extended. Oxidative damage also accelerates aging. *C. elegans* and fly mutants resistant to oxidative damage are long lived, whereas those mutations that increase oxidative damage are short lived. This has lead to the oxygen radical theory of aging, and hence, the shelves full of antioxidants in the health food section of grocery stores. Lending credence to this theory is the demonstration that mutation of the *p66^{shc}* gene in mice, which renders the mouse resistant to the action of oxygen radical generators, increases their life span by as much as 30%.

The final pathway involved in aging identified in *C. elegans* is the *Clk-1* pathway. This pathway regulates many processes in the worm such as cell division, and the rate of feeding and defecation. Mutations in the *Clk-1* pathway slow these processes and, in addition, lengthen life span by 15% to 30%. Ways in which this pathway may work include reducing the rate of oxidative damage and reducing caloric intake.

IN THE CLINIC

PROGERIA: PREMATURE AGING

In humans a severe form of **premature aging** occurs called Hutchinson-Gilford progeria syndrome (HGPS, typically called **progeria**, derived from the Greek words for early, *pro*, and old age, *geraios*). One in 4 to 8 million children are afflicted with progeria; they age at 5 to 10 times the normal rate. Although they usually appear normal at birth, afflicted children's growth rate slows and their appearance begins to change. Children with progeria often develop baldness, aged-looking skin, pinched noses, dwarfism, and small face and jaw (Fig. Intro-2). Their average life expectancy is 13 to 14 years, with death usually resulting from cardiovascular disease (heart attack or stroke).

In 2003 it was shown that the most common cause of progeria is a single base mutation in a gene that codes for LAMIN-A, a nuclear membrane protein. The mutation activates an aberrant cryptic splice site in *LAMIN-A* pre-RNA, leading to the synthesis of a truncated protein. The function of the full-length protein is not known, but cells from progeria patients have misshaped nuclear membranes, and it is speculated that tissues subjected to intense physical stress, such as those in the cardiovascular system, might undergo widespread cell death because of nuclear instability.

Using fibroblasts obtained from progeria patients, normal nuclear morphology (and several other critical cellular features) was restored by treating cells with a chemically

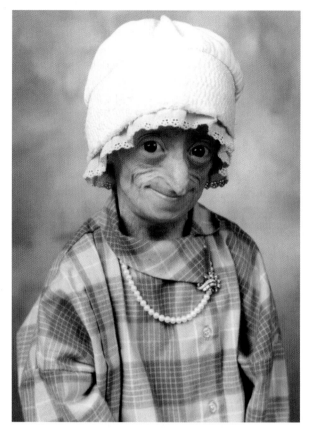

Figure Intro-2. Amy, a child with progeria, at age 16.

stable DNA oligonucleotide (short DNA sequence, called a morpholino, that cells cannot degrade) targeted to the activated cryptic splice site (to bind to the mutated site and prevent the splicing machinery from cutting in the wrong place). This approach thus provides proof of concept for the eventual correction of premature aging with **gene therapy** in children with progeria, an exciting possibility.

Phases of Human Embryology

Embryologists also subdivide human embryology into phases. These phases are introduced here to help you keep developmental events in context as you pursue your study of human embryology. Details of each of these phases are covered in subsequent chapters.

The first phase of human embryology is **gameto-genesis**. This process occurs in the gonads (ovaries and testes) of females and males and involves **meiosis.** In both females and males, the main purpose of meiosis is to establish a haploid cell, that is, a cell that contains half the number of chromosomes contained in typical body cells, such as skin cells. In addition to producing haploid cells, meiosis allows shuffling of genetic information to occur, increasing genetic diversity. In females, gametogenesis occurs in the ovaries and is called **oogenesis;** the final cells produced by oogenesis are the eggs or oocytes. In males, gametogenesis occurs in the testes and is called **spermato-genesis;** the final cells produced by spermatogenesis are the sperm or spermatozoa. Thus, as a result of gametogenesis, gametes undergo morphologic differentiation that allows the second phase of human embryology to occur.

The second phase of human embryology is **fertilization** (see Fig. Intro-1). This process occurs in one of the oviducts of the female after the egg has been ovulated and enters an oviduct, and sperm have been deposited in the vagina at coitus. Sperm move from the vagina into the uterus and finally into the oviducts, where, if an egg is encountered, fertilization can occur. One of the main purposes of fertilization is to restore the diploid number of chromosomes, that is, the normal number of chromosomes contained in typical body cells. Because the egg and sperm chromosomes are united in a single cell at fertilization, establishing a new cell called the **zygote**, fertilization also results in the production of a new cell having a unique genome, different from that of the cells of its mother or father. In addition to restoring the diploid number of chromosomes, another main purpose of fertilization is to activate the egg, allowing subsequent phases of human embryology to occur.

The third phase of human embryology is **cleavage** (see Fig. Intro-1). During cleavage the zygote divides by mitosis into two cells, each of which quickly divides into two more cells. The process continues to repeat itself, rapidly forming a solid ball of cells called a **morula**. Cleavage differs from the conventional cell division that occurs in many cell types throughout an organism's life in that during cleavage, each daughter cell formed by cleavage is roughly half the size of its parent cell. In contrast, after conventional cell division, cells grow roughly to parental cell size before undergoing the next round of division. A purpose of cleavage is to increase the **nucleocytoplasmic ratio**, that is, the volume of the nucleus compared to the volume of the cytoplasm. An egg, and subsequently a zygote, has a small nucleocytoplasmic ratio because it contains a single nucleus and a large amount of cytoplasm. With each cleavage the cytoplasm is partitioned as nuclei are replicated so that the nucleocytoplasmic ratio approaches that of a typical body cell. Another purpose of cleavage is to generate a multicellular embryo; the cells of the morula and subsequent **blastocyst** (the structure formed by hollowing out of the morula) are called **blastomeres**.

The fourth phase of human embryology is **gastrulation.** During gastrulation, cells undergo extensive movements relative to one another, changing their positions. This brings cells into contact with new neighbors and allows information to be passed among cells, ultimately changing their fates. A purpose of gastrulation is to establish primitive tissue layers, called **germ layers** (Fig. Intro-3). Three primary germ layers are formed, called the **endoderm, mesoderm**, and **ectoderm**. These germ layers give rise to tissues and organ rudiments during subsequent development. The three major axes of the embryo become identifiable during gastrulation: the **dorsal-ventral axis, cranial-caudal axis**, and **medial-lateral axis** (including the **left-right axis**).

The fifth phase of human embryology is **formation of the body plan**. Some consider this phase to be part of gastrulation, and others call this phase **morphogenesis**. Both of these viewpoints make sense: gastrulation continues during formation of the body plan, and formation of the body plan involves morphogenesis, that is, the generation of form. However, formation of the body plan also involves extensive folding of the embryo (see Fig. Intro-3). During gastrulation, the embryo consists of a flat two- or three-layered disc of cells (depending on its exact stage of development) that is positioned at the interface between two bubble-like structures: the **amnion** (and its enclosed, fluid-filled space, the *amniotic cavity*) and the **yolk sac** (and its enclosed, fluid-filled space, the *yolk sac cavity*). Near the perimeter of the embryonic disc, where the disc joins the amnion and yolk sac, folding begins. This is a complex process to visualize; it is covered in detail in Chapter 4. The purpose of this folding, called **body folding**, is to separate the embryo from its extraembryonic membranes (that is, amnion and yolk sac), except at the level of the future umbilical cord, and to convert the flat disc into a three-dimensional body plan, called the **tube-within-a-tube body plan** (see Fig. Intro-3). The tube-within-a-tube body plan consists of an

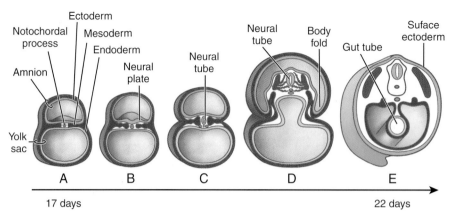

Figure Intro-3. Series of drawings of cross sections through the human embryo from 17 to 22 days of gestation. At the end of gastrulation (day 17), the conceptus consists of a trilaminar blastoderm that is composed of ectoderm, mesoderm, and endoderm, and is covered dorsally by amnion and ventrally by yolk sac in *A*. Body folding is well underway in *D* and is complete in *E*, establishing the tube-within-a-tube body plan (endodermal gut tube on the inside and ectodermal skin tube on the outside). For simplicity, the amnion and yolk sac are not shown in *E*. In *B*, the midline ectoderm has thickened as the neural plate, which folds to form the neural tube in *C*. The latter is not considered to be one of the two tubes of the tube-within-a-tube body plan because it is not formed by the body folds. For further details see Chapters 2 through 4.

outer tube (formed from the ectodermal germ layer) and an inner tube (formed from the endodermal germ layer), with the two tubes separated by the mesoderm. Additional tubes (such as the neural tube, the rudiment of the central nervous system, shown in Fig. Intro-3) form by secondary folding of other layers of the embryo (that is, these tubes are not formed by the action of the body folds), and they are not considered to be one of the two tubes contributing to the tube-within-a-tube body plan. In essence, with formation of the tube-within-a-tube, the embryo now has a distinctive embryo-like body shape, is protected from its outside environment by the outer tube (the primitive skin), and contains an inner tube (the primitive gut), separated by a primitive skeletal support (the mesoderm). With formation of the tube-within-a-tube body plan, the embryo now has a shape that more closely resembles that of the adult, and the three body axes are more evident (Fig. Intro-4).

After formation of the three primary germ layers, regional changes occur in each of these layers. One such change has already been mentioned, folding of part of the ectoderm to form the neural tube. Such changes establish organ rudiments. With the completion of formation of the body plan and the formation of organ rudiments, what remains to occur is the last phase of human embryology, the phase of **organogenesis**. During organogenesis, organ rudiments undergo growth and differentiation to form organs and organ systems. With continued growth and differentiation these organs and organ systems begin to function during intrauterine life. Some organs that begin to function in the fetus need to quickly adapt to another function at the time of birth. For example, as the fetus transitions from an aqueous intrauterine life to air breathing, the functioning of the lungs (and cardiovascular system) needs to be rapidly altered. How this transition occurs is discussed in Chapters 11 to 13.

Period of Egg and Embryo: Summary of Main Events

The period of the egg and embryo, collectively defined (as discussed earlier) as the first eight weeks following fertilization, is characterized by a large number of rapid changes. These changes are summarized in Table Intro-1. Also listed in the table, for selected days during each of the eight weeks of gestation, are the greatest length of the embryo, the number of somites, and the Carnegie stage. The latter is the most widely used stage series for human embryos. By providing a standardized set of criteria for accurate staging, it allows detailed comparisons to be made among different embryos in different collections around the world.

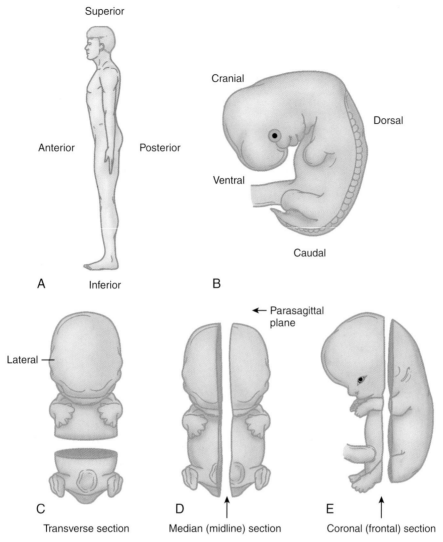

Superior

Cranial

Dorsal

Anterior   Posterior

Ventral

Caudal

A   Inferior   B

Lateral ―

Parasagittal plane

C   D   E
Transverse section   Median (midline) section   Coronal (frontal) section

Figure Intro-4. Body axes and section planes in the human adult and embryo. *A*, Lateral view of adult; *B*, Lateral view of 5-week human embryo; *C-D*, Ventral views of 6-week human embryos showing transverse (*C*) and sagittal (*D*) section planes. *E*, Lateral view of 6-week human embryo showing coronal (frontal) section plane.

Body Axes: Understanding Embryonic Coordinates

Understanding the structure of an embryo or fetus can be difficult and confusing, because embryos and fetuses are three-dimensional, complex objects that change their shape as they develop over time. As a metaphor, imagine examining an enlarged portion of a map without knowing the locations of north, south, east, and west. Without these coordinates, one could easily get lost trying to get from one landmark to another. Embryos and fetuses also have coordinates, and without understanding these coordinates, the study of embryos and fetuses can be perplexing. Moreover, because of our life experience, we often can use environmental clues to navigate from place to place during a journey, even if a compass or labeled map is not available. However, for most, the embryo or fetus is uncharted territory, and the lack of life experience prevents such navigation. Because we are all familiar with the shape of the adult human body, it is useful to begin with the coordinates of the adult

Table Intro–1 Timing of Human Development (Weeks 1 through 8)

Week	Day	Length (mm)[a]	Number of Somites	Carnegie Stage	Features (*Chapters in Which Features Are Discussed*)[b]
1	1	0.1-0.15	—	1	Fertilization (1)
	1.5-3	0.1-0.2	—	2	First cleavage divisions occur (2-16 cells) (1)
	4	0.1-0.2	—	3	Blastocyst is free in uterus (1)
	5-6	0.1-0.2	—	4	Blastocyst hatches and begins implanting (1, 2)
2	7-12	0.1-0.2	—	5	Blastocyst fully implanted (1, 2)
	13	0.2	—	6	Primary stem villi form (2); primitive streak develops (3)
3	16	0.4	—	7	Gastrulation commences; notochordal process forms (3)
	18	1-1.5	—	8	Neural plate and neural groove form (3, 4)
	20	1.5-2.5	1-3	9	Tail bud and first somites form (3); neuromeres form in presumptive brain vesicles (4, 9); primitive heart tube is forming (12); vasculature begins to develop in embryonic disc (13); otic pits form (17)
4	22	2-3.5	4-12	10	Neural folds begin to fuse; cranial end of embryo undergoes rapid flexion (4, 9); pulmonary primordium forms (11); myocardium forms and heart begins to pump (12); hepatic plate forms (14); first two pharyngeal arches and optic sulci begin to form (16)
	24	2.5-4.5	13-20	11	Primordial germ cells begin to migrate from wall of yolk sac (1, 15); cranial neuropore closes (4); oropharyngeal membrane ruptures (16); optic vesicles develop (17); *optic pits begin to form (17)*
	26	3-5	21-29	12	Caudal neuropore closes (4); cystic diverticulum and dorsal pancreatic bud form (14); urorectal septum begins to form (14, 15); upper limb buds form (18); pharyngeal arches 3 and 4 form (16)
	28	4-6	30+	13	Dorsal and ventral columns begin to differentiate in mantle layer of spinal cord and brain stem (9); septum primum begins to form in heart (12); spleen forms (14); ureteric buds form (14, 15); lower limb buds form (18); otic vesicles and lens placodes form (17); motor nuclei of cranial nerves form (9, 10)
5	32	5-7	—	14	Spinal nerves begin to sprout (10); semilunar valves begin to form in heart (12); lymphatics and coronary vessels form (13); greater and lesser stomach curvatures and primary intestinal loop form (14); metanephros begins to develop (15); lens pits invaginate into optic cups (17); endolymphatic appendage forms (17); secondary brain vesicles begin to form (9); cerebral hemispheres become visible (9)
	33	7-9	—	15	Atrioventricular valves and definitive pericardial cavity begin to form (12); cloacal folds and genital tubercle form (14, 15); hand plates develop (18); lens vesicles form (17); invagination of nasal pits occur and medial and lateral nasal processes form (16); sensory and parasympathetic cranial nerve ganglia begin to form (10); primary olfactory neurons send axons into telencephalon (10)
6	37	8-11	—	16	Muscular ventricular septum begins to form (12); gut tube lumen becomes occluded (14); major calyces of kidneys begin to form and kidneys begin to ascend (15); genital ridges form (15); foot plates develop (18); pigment forms in retinas (17); auricular hillocks develop (17)
	41	11-14	—	17	Bronchopulmonary segment primordia form (11); septum intermedium of heart is complete (12); subcardinal vein system forms (13); minor calyces of kidneys are forming (15); finger rays are distinct (18); nasolacrimal grooves form (16); cerebellum begins to form (9); melanocytes enter epidermis (7); dental laminae form (7)

Continued

Table Intro–1 Timing of Human Development (Weeks 1 through 8)—cont'd

Week	Day	Length (mm)[a]	Number of Somites	Carnegie Stage	Features (*Chapters in Which Features Are Discussed*)[b]
7	44	13-17	—	18	Skeletal ossification begins (8); Sertoli cells begin to differentiate in the male gonad (15); elbows and toe rays form (18); intermaxillary process and eyelids form (16); thalami of diencephalon expand (9); nipples and first hair follicles form (7)
	47	16-18	—	19	Septum primum fuses with septum intermedium in heart (12); urogenital membrane ruptures (15); trunk elongates and straightens (8)
8	50	18-22	—	20	Primary intestinal loop completes initial counterclockwise rotation (14); in males, müllerian ducts begin to regress and vasa deferentia begin to form (15); upper limbs bend at elbows (18)
	52	22-24	—	21	Pericardioperitoneal canals close (11); hands and feet rotate toward midline (18)
	54	23-28	—	22	Eyelids and auricles are more developed (17)
	56	27-31	—	23	Chorionic cavity is obliterated by the growth of the amniotic sac (6); definitive superior vena cava and major branches of the aortic arch are established (12); lumen of gut tube is almost completely recanalized (14); primary teeth are at cap stage (7)

[a] Length is the greatest length of embryo.
[b] Timing of some events will differ slightly in some embryos.

human before progressing to those of the embryo and fetus (see Fig. Intro-4).

The adult human standing erect with feet together and palms facing forward is said by anatomists to be in **anatomical position** (see Fig. Intro-4*A*). The head-feet axis represents the **superior-inferior axis**, with the head being **superior**, and the feet being **inferior**. From the midline of the body (i.e., an imaginary line drawn through the center of the superior-inferior axis) toward the right and left sides runs the **medial-lateral axis**, with the midline being the most **medial** level (but note that the exact midline is called the **median plane**), and the right and left sides being the most **lateral** levels. The **left-right axis** is part of the medial-lateral axis, defining differences (i.e., asymmetries) between the left and right sides of the body. From the front side of the body toward the back side of the body runs the **anterior-posterior axis**, with the front side being the **anterior** surface, and the back side being the **posterior** surface. Finally, in the adult the terms *proximal* and *distal* are used. **Proximal** refers to close to the center of the body, whereas **distal** refers to far from the center of the body. Thus one can define, for example, the **proximal-distal axis** of the upper limb, with the shoulder being at the **proximal** end of the upper limb and the fingers being at its **distal** end.

The human embryo and fetus have a similar set of axes, again defined based on adult **anatomical position** (see Fig. Intro-4*B*). The head-tail axis of the embryo is called the **cranial-caudal axis**, with the head end being the **cranial** end and the tail end being the **caudal** end. Sometimes this axis is referred to as the **rostral-caudal axis**, with the head end being the **rostral** end. The cranial-caudal axis can also be called the anterior-posterior axis, with the head end being the anterior end and the tail end being the posterior end. Anterior-posterior axis is often used in the developmental biology literature with animal models (especially four-legged ones), but because the anterior-posterior axis represents a totally different axis in the adult human (i.e., the front-back axis), its use with human embryos is discouraged; consequently, anterior-posterior axis will not used in this textbook to describe an *embryonic* axis. The axis extending from the midline to left and right sides in the embryo is called the **medial-lateral axis**, as it is in the adult. However, the axis extending from the back to the front is best called the **dorsal-ventral axis** in the embryo, with the back being **dorsal** and the front being **ventral**. It also can be called the anterior-posterior axis, as it is in the adult, although this is discouraged to prevent confusion as discussed above. Finally, embryos also have a **proximal-distal axis**, which is defined in the same way as in the adult.

Because human embryos and fetuses are opaque and have complex internal structures, as well as external structures, they are often studied as sets of serial sections (see Fig. Intro-4C-E). Throughout this book many sections are depicted. To understand these, it is important to know that **transverse (cross) sections** are cut perpendicularly with respect to the cranial-caudal axis of the body (i.e., within the **transverse plane**), so that a set of serial transverse sections progresses through the body in cranial-caudal (or caudal-cranial) sequence (see Fig. Intro-4C). **Sagittal sections** are cut in a plane that is parallel to the cranial-caudal or *long* axis of the body (i.e., the **longitudinal plane**), rather than in the transverse plane. These are oriented to cut through embryos or fetuses such that a midline (median) sagittal section (often called a **midsagittal section**) would separate the body into right and left halves (see Fig. Intro-4D). More lateral sagittal sections (often called **parasagittal sections**) are cut parallel to a midsagittal section but are displaced to the right or left of the midline. Serial sagittal sections can progress from the right side of the body to the midline (midsagittal) and continue to the left side (or they can progress in the opposite direction). One further set of sections is sometimes used, but less frequently: serial **coronal (or frontal) sections**. Like sagittal sections, coronal sections are cut in a plane parallel to the cranial-caudal or long axis of the body, but in contrast to sagittal sections, coronal sections are oriented 90 degrees with respect to sagittal sections (see Fig. Intro-4E). In other words, serial coronal sections can progress from the front (ventral) side of the embryo to its center (midcoronal) and then continue to the back (dorsal) side, or they can progress in the opposite direction. Hence, a midcoronal section would separate the body into ventral and dorsal halves.

Want to Learn More?

This textbook has been written to guide you in your study of human embryology, emphasizing important concepts, principles, and facts. In past editions of this textbook, a comprehensive list of references was included in each chapter to aid you in further study. We have chosen for this edition to list mainly key review articles published during the last five years (see "Suggested Readings" at the end of each chapter). This was done in part to keep the textbook from becoming too large and increasing its cost to students. But it was also done to serve as a more useful student guide to the current relevant scientific literature. Recently, there has been an explosion of journals publishing reviews in developmental biology, and most libraries throughout the world subscribe to review journals, providing easy access for students. By reading a few reviews, one can become quickly updated about a field. Also, by examining the references cited by these reviews, one can quickly find the most relevant primary literature for further detailed study.

With the advent of the worldwide web, how we find information has rapidly changed. In addition to going to the "Suggested Readings" in the text, if you wish to engage in further in-depth study or you want to find the very latest publications in the field (because of the delay in publication, the literature in any textbook is always at least one year out of date), online searches are the best approach. We have five suggestions for conducting these searches:

- Using key words in the textbook (i.e., those words indicated in bold type throughout the textbook and also listed in the index), go to Pubmed (www.pubmedcentral.nih.gov) and enter one or more keywords as search terms. This will identify many articles for you to consider.

- Using Pubmed, search under the names of authors of review articles listed in the "Suggested Readings." (Also consider using Google Scholar: www.scholar.google.com; Google Scholar ranks articles based on how many times an article by a particular author is cited—one indicator of its importance in the field.) Typically, the leaders in a particular area write review articles, and so this approach is likely to pull up many other articles on the same topic. Similarly, you can search under the names of other authors who are cited in the review articles.

- Again using Pubmed, scan the table of contents of recent issues of the main journals in the field by searching under journal title. In developmental biology, these include (in alphabetical order): *BiomedCentral Developmental Biology; Development; Development, Genes and Evolution; Developmental Biology; Developmental Cell; Developmental Dynamics; Differentiation; Evolution and Development; Genes and Development; Genesis, International Journal of Developmental Biology;* and *Mechanisms of Development* (as well as broader journals such as *Bioessays, Cell, Current Biology, Nature, Nature Genetics, Neuron, PNAS,* and *Science*). Many of these journals also publish review articles, which are particularly useful for beginning your study. In addition, scan the table of contents of recent issues of the review journals in the field; in developmental biology, these include *Annual Reviews of Cell and Developmental Biology, Current Opinion in Genetics and Development,* and *Current Topics in Developmental Biology.* Other useful review journals include the Trends series (for example, *Trends in Genetics*) and the Nature Reviews series *(Nature Reviews Neuroscience).*

- "Google" (www.google.com) keywords to find other information. For example, googling IVF (for in vitro fertilization) results in the listing of a number of interesting sites. However, unlike information obtained in journals, which is peer-reviewed by the scientific community to validate it, googled information may or may not be scientifically accurate, so it is important to verify googled information by checking it against the peer-reviewed journal literature.

- Seek out other useful websites and databases. For example, for genetic causes of birth defects in humans, go to the Online Mendelian Inheritance in Man (www.ncbi.nlm.nih.gov/sites/entrez?db=OMIM); for an extensive database of scanning electron micrographs of mouse embryos, go to Kathy Sulik's embryo images online (www.med.unc.edu/embryo_images); searching under topics such as "embryo" or "embryology" will locate many useful websites for further study.

Suggested Readings

Bienz M, Clevers H. 2000. Linking colorectal cancer to Wnt signaling. Cell 103:311-320.

Bijlsma MF, Spek CA, Peppelenbosch MP. 2004. Hedgehog: an unusual signal transducer. Bioessays 26:387-394.

Gems D, Partridge L. 2001. Insulin/IGF signalling and ageing: seeing the bigger picture. Curr Opin Genet Dev 11:287-292.

Gregorieff A, Clevers H. 2005. Wnt signaling in the intestinal epithelium: from endoderm to cancer. Genes Dev 19:877-890.

Guarente L, Kenyon C. 2000. Genetic pathways that regulate ageing in model organisms. Nature 408:255-262.

Hegele RA. 2000. The envelope, please: nuclear lamins and disease. Nat Med 6:136-137.

Hegele RA. 2003. Lamin mutations come of age. Nat Med 9:644-645.

Lefort K, Dotto GP. 2004. Notch signaling in the integrated control of keratinocyte growth/differentiation and tumor suppression. Semin Cancer Biol 14:374-386.

Lithgow GJ, Andersen JK. 2000. The real Dorian Gray mouse. Bioessays 22:410-413.

Massague J, Blain SW, Lo RS. 2000. TGFbeta signaling in growth control, cancer, and heritable disorders. Cell 103:295-309.

Moon RT, Kohn AD, De Ferrari GV, Kaykas A. 2004. WNT and beta-catenin signalling: diseases and therapies. Nat Rev Genet 5:691-701.

Olshansky SJ, Hayflick L, Carnes BA. 2002. No truth to the fountain of youth. Sci Am 286:92-95.

Peifer M, Polakis P. 2000. Wnt signaling in oncogenesis and embryogenesis–a look outside the nucleus. Science 287:1606-1609.

Perls T, Kunkel L, Puca A. 2002. The genetics of aging. Curr Opin Genet Dev 12:362-369.

Polakis P. 2000. Wnt signaling and cancer. Genes Dev 14:1837-1851.

Scaffidi P, Misteli T. 2005. Reversal of the cellular phenotype in the premature aging disease Hutchinson-Gilford progeria syndrome. Nat Med 11:440-445.

Taipale J, Beachy PA. 2001. The Hedgehog and Wnt signalling pathways in cancer. Nature 411:349-354.

van Noort M, Clevers H. 2002. TCF transcription factors, mediators of Wnt-signaling in development and cancer. Dev Biol 244:1-8.

Waite KA, Eng C. 2003. From developmental disorder to heritable cancer: it's all in the BMP/TGF-beta family. Nat Rev Genet 4:763-773.

Gametogenesis, Fertilization, and First Week

1

Summary A textbook of human embryology could begin at any of several points in the human life cycle. This textbook starts with a discussion of the origin of specialized cells called **primordial germ cells (PGCs)**. PGCs can be first identified within the wall of the **yolk sac**, one of the extraembryonic membranes, during the 4th to 6th weeks of gestation. These PGCs will give rise to the **germ line**, a series of cells that form the sex cells, or **gametes** (i.e., the **egg** and **sperm**). However, these gametes will not function to form the next generation for several decades (i.e., after the onset of **puberty**). Yet, remarkably, one of the first things that happens in the developing embryo is to set aside the germ line for the next generation. Similarly, the germ lines that gave rise to the developing embryo were established a generation earlier, when the embryo's father and mother were developing in utero (that is, when the embryo's maternal and paternal grandmothers were pregnant with the embryo's father and mother).

From the wall of the yolk sac, PGCs actively migrate between the 6th to 12th weeks of gestation to the dorsal body wall of the embryo, where they populate the developing gonads and differentiate into the gamete precursor cells called **spermatogonia** in the male and **oogonia** in the female. Like the normal somatic cells of the body, the spermatogonia and oogonia are **diploid**; that is, they each contain 23 pairs of chromosomes (for a total of 46 chromosomes each). When these cells eventually produce **gametes** by the process of **gametogenesis** (called **spermatogenesis** in the male and **oogenesis** in the female), they undergo **meiosis**, a sequence of two specialized cell divisions by which the number of chromosomes in the gametes is halved. The gametes thus contain 23 chromosomes (one of each pair) and are therefore **haploid**. The developing gametes also undergo cytoplasmic differentiation, resulting in the production of mature **spermatozoa** in the male and **definitive oocytes** in the female.

In the male, spermatogenesis takes place in the seminiferous tubules of the testes and does not occur until puberty. In contrast, in the female oogenesis is initiated during *fetal* life. Specifically, between the 3rd and 5th months of fetal life, oogonia initiate the first meiotic division, thereby becoming primary oocytes. However, the primary oocytes then quickly enter a state of meiotic arrest that persists until after puberty. After puberty, a few oocytes and their enclosing follicles resume development each month in response to the production of pituitary gonadotropic hormones. Usually, only one of these follicles matures fully and undergoes **ovulation** to release the enclosed oocyte, and the oocyte completes meiosis only if a spermatozoon fertilizes it. **Fertilization**, the uniting of the egg and sperm, takes place in the oviduct. After the oocyte finishes meiosis, the paternal and maternal chromosomes come together, resulting in the formation of a **zygote** containing a single diploid nucleus. Embryonic development is considered to begin at this point.

The newly formed embryo undergoes a series of cell divisions called **cleavage** as it travels down the oviduct toward the uterus. The cleavage divisions subdivide the zygote first into two cells, then into four, then into eight, and so on. These daughter cells do not grow between divisions, so the entire embryo remains the same size. Starting at the 8- to 16-cell stage, the cleaving embryo, or **morula**, differentiates into two groups of cells: a peripheral outer cell layer and a central **inner cell mass**. The outer cell layer, called the **trophoblast**, forms the fetal component of the placenta and associated extraembryonic membranes, whereas the inner cell mass, also called the **embryoblast**, gives rise to the embryo proper and associated extraembryonic membranes. By the 30-cell stage, the embryo begins to form a fluid-filled central cavity, the **blastocyst cavity**. By the 5th to 6th day of development, the embryo is a hollow ball of about 100 cells called a **blastocyst**. At this point, it enters the uterine cavity and begins to implant into the endometrial lining of the uterine wall.

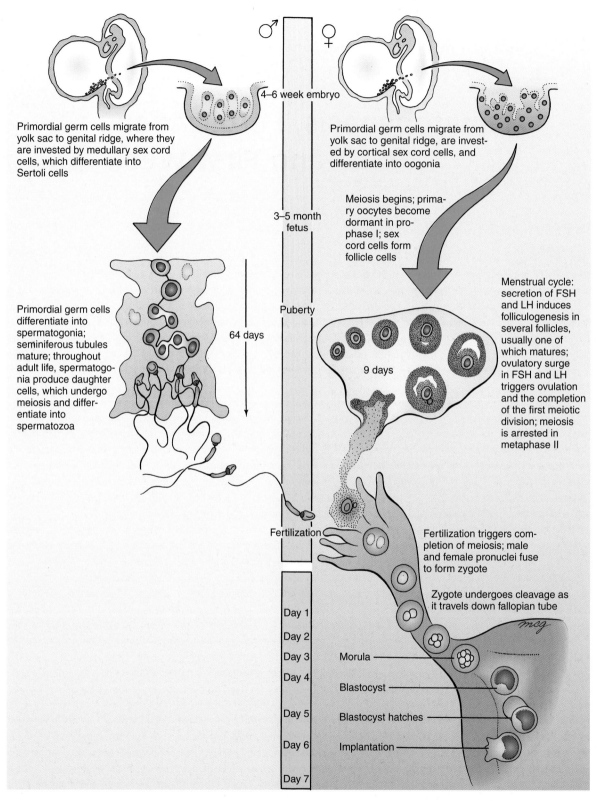

Primordial germ cells migrate from yolk sac to genital ridge, where they are invested by medullary sex cord cells, which differentiate into Sertoli cells

♂ 4–6 week embryo ♀

Primordial germ cells migrate from yolk sac to genital ridge, are invested by cortical sex cord cells, and differentiate into oogonia

3–5 month fetus

Meiosis begins; primary oocytes become dormant in prophase I; sex cord cells form follicle cells

Primordial germ cells differentiate into spermatogonia; seminiferous tubules mature; throughout adult life, spermatogonia produce daughter cells, which undergo meiosis and differentiate into spermatozoa

Puberty

64 days

9 days

Menstrual cycle: secretion of FSH and LH induces folliculogenesis in several follicles, usually one of which matures; ovulatory surge in FSH and LH triggers ovulation and the completion of the first meiotic division; meiosis is arrested in metaphase II

Fertilization

Fertilization triggers completion of meiosis; male and female pronuclei fuse to form zygote

Zygote undergoes cleavage as it travels down fallopian tube

Day 1

Day 2

Day 3   Morula

Day 4

Blastocyst

Day 5

Blastocyst hatches

Day 6

Implantation

Day 7

Time line. Gametogenesis and first week of development.

Clinical Taster A couple, both in their late 30s, is having difficulty conceiving a child. Early in their marriage about, 10 years ago, they used birth control pills and condoms thereafter, but they stopped using all forms of birth control more than 2 years ago. Despite this and having intercourse three or four times a week, a pregnancy has not resulted. On routine physical examination, both the man and woman seem to be in excellent health. The woman is an avid runner and competes in occasional marathons, and she has had regular periods since her menarche at age 13. The man had a varicocele, which was corrected when he was 19; the urologist who performed the surgery assured him that there would be no subsequent adverse affect on his fertility.

Because no obvious cause of their fertility problem is noted, the couple is referred to a local fertility clinic for specialized treatment. At the clinic, the man has a semen analysis. This reveals that his sperm count (60 million sperm per ejaculate), sperm mobility (vigorous motility and forward progression [i.e., straight swimming movement]), sperm morphology (70% with an oval head and a tail 7 to 15 times longer than the head), and semen volume (3.5 mL with a normal fructose level) are within the normal ranges. Semen viscosity and sperm agglutination are also normal. As a next step, a postcoital test is planned. Using the woman's recent menstrual history to estimate the time of her midcycle, and daily basal body temperature measurements and urine LH (luteinizing hormone) tests to predict ovulation, intercourse is timed for the evening of the day on which ovulation is expected to occur. The next morning, the woman undergoes a cervical examination. It is noted that the cervical mucus contains clumped and immotile sperm, suggesting a sperm-cervical mucus incompatibility.

Based on the results of the postcoital test, the couple decides to undergo **artificial insemination**. After five attempts in which the man's sperm are collected, washed, and injected into the uterus through a sterile catheter passed through the cervix, a pregnancy still has not resulted. The couple is discouraged and decides to take some time off to consider their options.

After considering adoption, gestational surrogacy, and remaining childless, the couple returns three months later and requests **IVF (in vitro fertilization)**. On the second of two very regimented attempts, the couple is delighted to learn that a pregnancy has resulted. A few weeks later Doppler ultrasound examination detects two fetal heart beats. This is confirmed two months later by ultrasonography. Early in the 9th month of gestation two healthy babies are delivered, a 6-pound 2-ounce girl and a 5-pound 14-ounce boy.

Primordial Germ Cells

Primordial Germ Cells Reside in Yolk Sac

Cells that give rise to **gametes** in both males and females can be identified during the 4th week of gestation within an extraembryonic membrane called the **yolk sac** (Fig. 1-1A). Based on studies in animal models, it is believed that these cells arise earlier in gestation, during the phase of gastrulation (discussed in Ch. 3). These cells are called **primordial germ cells (PGCs)**, and their lineage constitutes the **germ line**. PGCs can be recognized within the yolk sac and during their subsequent migration (see next paragraph) because of their distinctive pale cytoplasm and ovoid shape and because they specifically stain intensely with reagents that localize the enzyme alkaline phosphatase.

Primordial Germ Cells Migrate into Dorsal Body Wall

Between four and six weeks, PGCs migrate by ameboid movement from the yolk sac to the wall of the gut tube, and from the gut tube via the mesentery of the gut to the dorsal body wall (Fig. 1-1B). In the dorsal body wall, these cells come to rest on either side of the midline in the loose mesenchymal tissue just deep to the membranous lining of the coelomic cavity. Most of the PGCs populate the region of the body wall at the level that will form the gonads (discussed in Ch. 15). PGCs continue to multiply by mitosis during their migration. Some PGCs may become stranded during their migration, coming to rest at extragonadal sites. Occasionally, stray germ cells of this type may give rise to a type of tumor called a **teratoma** (Fig. 1-1C).

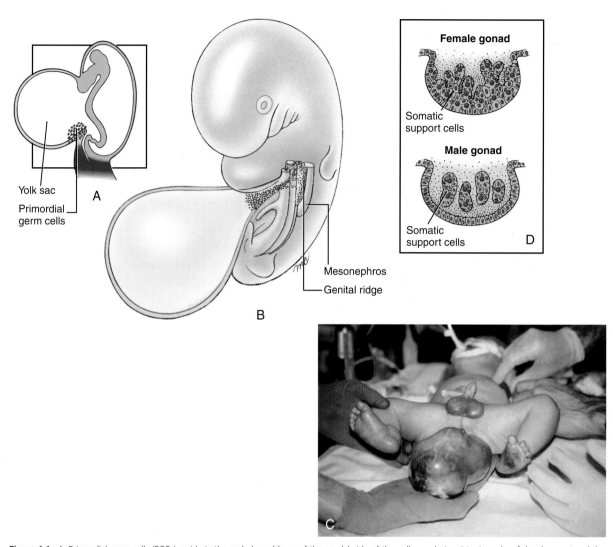

Yolk sac
Primordial germ cells
A

Mesonephros
Genital ridge
B

Female gonad
Somatic support cells

Male gonad
Somatic support cells
D

C

Figure 1-1. *A,* Primordial germ cells (PGCs) reside in the endodermal layer of the caudal side of the yolk sac during 4 to 6 weeks of development and then migrate to the dorsal body wall. *B,* Between 6 and 12 weeks, PGCs stimulate formation of the genital ridges. *C,* Infant with a large sacrococcygeal teratoma. *D,* Somatic support cells differentiate and invest PGCs. In females, somatic support cells become ovarian follicle cells; in males, somatic support cells become Sertoli cells of the seminiferous tubules.

IN THE CLINIC

TERATOMA FORMATION

Teratomas, tumors composed of tissues derived from all three germ layers, can be extragonadal or gonadal and are derived from PGCs. Sacrococcygeal teratomas are the most common tumors in newborns and occur in 1 in 20,000 to 70,000 births (see Fig. 1-1C). They occur four times more frequently in female newborns than in male newborns, and they represent about 3% of all childhood malignancies. Gonadal tumors are usually diagnosed after the onset of puberty. Both ovarian and testicular teratomas can form. The **pluripotency** (ability to form many cell types, not to be confused with **totipotency**, the ability to form *all* cell types) of teratomas is exhibited by their ability to give rise to a variety of definitive anatomic structures, including hair, teeth, pituitary gland, and even a fully formed eye.

Primordial Germ Cells Stimulate Formation of Gonads

Differentiation of the gonads is described in detail in Chapter 15. When PGCs arrive in the presumptive gonad region, they stimulate cells of the adjacent coelomic epithelium to proliferate and form **somatic support cells** (Fig. 1-1*D*; see also Fig. 15-16). Proliferation of the somatic support cells create a swelling just medial to each mesonephros (embryonic kidney) on both the right and left sides of the gut mesentery. These swellings, the **genital ridges**, represent the primitive gonads. Somatic support cells invest PGCs and give rise to tissues that will nourish and regulate development of maturing sex cells—**ovarian follicles** in the female and **Sertoli cells** of the **germinal epithelium (seminiferous epithelium)** of the **seminiferous tubules** in the male. Somatic support cells are essential for germ cell development within the gonad: if germ cells are not invested by somatic support cells, they degenerate. Conversely, if PGCs fail to arrive in the presumptive gonadal region, gonadal development is disrupted.

IN THE RESEARCH LAB

ORIGIN OF PGCs

Although the exact time and place of origin of PGCs in humans is unknown, cell tracing and other experiments in the mouse demonstrate that PGCs arise from the epiblast (one of the layers of the bilaminar and trilaminar blastoderm stages; discussed in Chs. 2, 3). During gastrulation, these cells move through the caudal part of the primitive streak and into the extraembryonic area. From there, they migrate to the gut wall and through the gut mesentery to the gonadal ridges, as in humans.

MOLECULAR REGULATION OF PGC DEVELOPMENT

Development of the germ line involves the sequential activation of genes that direct the initial induction, proliferation, survival, migration, and differentiation of PGCs. Animal models have been very useful for understanding these events and have been used to show that the function of many genes controlling PGC development are conserved across diverse organisms. However, mechanisms underlying the initial events of PGC formation in mammals seem to be very different from those of lower organisms.

In some model organisms, such as the fruitfly, worm, and frog, **maternal effect genes** (discussed in Ch. 5) are required for initiation of germ cell formation. Activation of these maternal genes regulates the segregation of the **germ plasm** (cytoplasm containing determinants of the germ line) to a specific region of the zygote so that it becomes incorporated during cleavage into a unique group of cells that will form the germ cell precursors.

The Drosophila *Vasa* gene is segregated to germ cells in this fashion. *Vasa* transcripts are expressed ubiquitously in the oocyte cytoplasm, but *Vasa* protein becomes specifically localized in the germ plasm. *Vasa* is an RNA-binding protein of the DEAD box family and its possible role is to bind mRNAs involved in germ line determination, such as *Oskar* and *Nanos*, and to control the onset of their translation. Vertebrate orthologs of *Vasa* exist, and in some vertebrates *Vasa* protein is expressed in germ cell precursors as they are forming (however, in mice, *Vasa* is expressed in germ cells only much later, after they have differentiated and are about to colonize the gonads).

In contrast to lower organisms, where germ cells are usually specified by the inheritance of maternal gene products, in the mouse and probably also in humans the germ line is induced. All cells of the mammalian morula are seemingly capable of forming pluripotent germ cells, but their capacity to do so becomes rapidly restricted first to the inner cell mass and then to the epiblast. Therefore, in mammals, the **initiation of germ line development** requires activation of genes that maintain pluripotency within the precursors that will form the germ line. One such gene encodes a POU domain transcription factor (*Oct4*, also called *Pou5f1*; transcription factors are discussed in Ch. 5). Its activity is present initially in all cells of the morula, but then only in the inner cell mass. It is then restricted to the epiblast, and finally it is expressed only in the presumptive germ cells themselves.

Further development of the germ line requires an inductive signal from the trophoblast (induction is discussed in Ch. 5). One such signal is *Bone morphogenetic protein 4* (*Bmp4*). In chimeric mouse embryos (mouse injection chimeras are discussed in Ch. 5) lacking *Bmp4* specifically within the trophoblast, PGCs, as well as the allantois (an extraembryonic membrane), fail to form. *Bmp4* induces expression of two germ–line specific genes in mice: *Fragilis* and *Stella*; however, their exact roles in PGC development are currently unknown.

Proliferation and survival of PGCs is ensured by the expression of **trophic factors** (factors that promote cell growth and survival) within the PGCs or within associated cells. A trophic factor expressed by PGCs and required for their early survival and proliferation is the RNA-binding protein *Tiar*. Another is a mouse ortholog of the Drosophila *Nanos* gene (*Nanos3*). Many other trophic factors seem to be required for the survival and proliferation of PGCs along their migratory pathway from the yolk sac to the gut and dorsal mesentery and then to the dorsal body wall. These include several factors expressed by tissues along the pathway, including the *c-Kit* ligand (*Stem cell factor* or *Steel factor*) and members of the *Interleukin/Lif* cytokine family (a cytokine is a regulatory protein released by cells of the immune system that acts as an intercellular mediator in the generation of an immune response). Study of *c-Kit* and *Steel* mutants has revealed that this signaling pathway suppresses **PGC apoptosis** (cell death) during migration. This finding provides an explanation for why PGCs that stray from their normal migratory path and come to rest in extragonadal sites usually (but not always; see above discussion of extragonadal teratomas) degenerate.

Other factors, including extracellular matrix proteins, must also be expressed by cells along the pathway to allow migration of PGCs and to direct their migration from the yolk sac to the gut and dorsal mesentery and then to the gonadal ridge (presumptive gonad) in the posterior body wall. *Tenascin C*, *β2 Integrin*, and *Laminin* all seem to be required for PGC migration. **Chemotropic signals** (i.e., attractive signals produced by the developing gonads) also seem to be involved to regulate PGC honing. One such factor is the chemokine (a type of cytokine) *Stromal cell-derived factor-1* (*Sdf1* or *Cxcl12*) and its receptor *Cxcr4*. PGC migration toward the gonad is disrupted in mouse or zebrafish embryos lacking the ligand or its receptor. In addition, *Sdf1* acts as a PGC survival factor.

Once PGCs arrive within the presumptive gonad, numerous genes must be expressed to **regulate the final differentiation of cells of the germ line**. Three new germ cell–specific genes are expressed shortly after PGCs enter the genital ridge (after which they are usually called **gonocytes**): *murine Vasa homolog* (*mVh*; the *Vasa* gene was discussed above), *Germ cell nuclear antigen 1* (*Gcna1*), and *Germ cell-less* (*Gcl1*). The last is expressed in the Drosophila germ line shortly after it is established, and it is named after the mutation in which the gene is inactivated and the germ line is lost.

Gametogenesis

Timing of Gametogenesis Is Different in Males and Females

In both males and females, PGCs undergo further mitotic divisions within the gonads and then commence **gametogenesis**, the process that converts them into mature male and female gametes (**spermatozoa** and **definitive oocytes**, respectively). However, timing of these processes differs in the two sexes (see Timeline; Fig. 1-3). In males, PGCs (usually now called **gonocytes**) remain dormant from the 6th week of embryonic development until puberty. At puberty, **seminiferous tubules** mature and PGCs differentiate into **spermatogonia**. Successive waves of spermatogonia undergo **meiosis** (the process by which the number of chromosomes in the sex cells is halved; see following section) and mature into spermatozoa. Spermatozoa are produced continuously from puberty until death.

In contrast in females, PGCs (again, usually now called **gonocytes**) undergo a few more mitotic divisions after they are invested by the somatic support cells. They then differentiate into **oogonia**, and by the 5th month of fetal development all oogonia begin meiosis, after which they are called **primary oocytes**. However, during an early phase of meiosis all sex cells enter a state of dormancy, and they remain in meiotic arrest as primary oocytes until sexual maturity. Starting at puberty, each month a few ovarian follicles resume development in response to the monthly surge of pituitary gonadotropic hormones, but usually only one primary oocyte matures into a **secondary oocyte** and is ovulated. This oocyte enters a second phase of meiotic arrest and does not actually complete meiosis unless it is fertilized. These monthly cycles continue until the onset of menopause at approximately 50 years of age. The process of gametogenesis in the male and female (called **spermatogenesis** and **oogenesis**, respectively) is discussed in detail later in this chapter.

IN THE RESEARCH LAB

WHY IS TIMING OF GAMETOGENESIS DIFFERENT IN MALES AND FEMALES?

Experiments in mouse embryos provide insight into why the timing of gametogenesis differs in males and females. Shortly after PGCs enter the genital ridge, they stop their migration and undergo two or three further rounds of mitosis and then enter a premeiotic stage during which they upregulate meiotic genes. In the male genital ridge, germ cells then reverse this process and arrest, but in the female genital ridge they enter meiotic prophase as primary oocytes and progress through meiosis until the diplotene stage, at which time they arrest. If male (XY) PGCs are transplanted into female (XX) embryos, the male PGCs follow the course just described for normal female

PGCs in females. Moreover, PGCs in female or male embryos that fail to reach the gonad also progress through meiosis as oocytes, regardless of their genotype. These two results suggest that all germ cells, regardless of their chromosome constitution, are programmed to develop as oocytes and that the timing of meiotic entry seems to be a cell-autonomous property rather than being induced. In contrast in males, the genital ridge prevents prenatal entry into meiosis. Experiments suggest that there is a **male meiosis inhibitor** and that this inhibitor is a diffusible signaling factor produced by Sertoli cells. Possible candidates for this factor include the protein *Prostaglandin D2* and the protein encoded by the *Tdl* gene (a gene showing sequence homology to antimicrobial proteins called *beta-Defensins*; *Prostaglandins* are synthesized from fatty acids and modulate several physiological functions such as blood pressure, smooth muscle contraction, and inflammation).

Meiosis Halves Number of Chromosomes and DNA Strands in Sex Cells

Although the timing of meiosis is very different in the male and female, the basic chromosomal events of the process are the same in the two sexes (Fig. 1-2). Like all normal somatic (nongerm) cells, PGCs contain 23 pairs of chromosomes, or a total of 46 chromosomes. One chromosome of each pair is obtained from the maternal gamete and the other from the paternal gamete. These chromosomes contain **deoxyribonucleic acid (DNA)**, which encodes information required for development and functioning of the organism. Of the total complement of 46 chromosomes, 22 pairs consist of matching, homologous chromosomes called **autosomes**. The remaining two chromosomes are called **sex chromosomes** because they determine the sex of the individual. There are two kinds of sex chromosome, X and Y. Individuals with one X chromosome and one Y chromosome (XY) are genetically male; individuals with two X chromosomes (XX) are genetically female. Nonetheless, one of the X chromosomes in the female genome is randomly inactivated, leaving only one active X chromosome in each cell (X-inactivation is discussed in Ch. 2). Mechanisms underlying sex determination are discussed further in Chapter 15.

Two designations that are often confused are the **ploidy** of a cell and its **N number**. *Ploidy* refers to the number of copies of each *chromosome* present in a cell nucleus, whereas the *N number* refers to the number of copies of each unique double-stranded *DNA molecule* in the nucleus. Each chromosome contains one or two molecules of DNA at different stages of the cell cycle (whether mitotic or meiotic), so the ploidy and N number of a cell do not always coincide. Somatic cells and PGCs have two copies of each kind of chromosome and hence are called **diploid**. Mature gametes, in contrast, have just one copy of each kind of chromosome and are called **haploid**. Haploid gametes with one DNA molecule per chromosome are said to be **1N**. In some stages of the cell cycle, diploid cells also have one DNA molecule per chromosome and hence are **2N**. However, during the earlier phases of meiosis or mitosis, each chromosome of a diploid cell has two molecules of DNA, and so the cell is **4N**.

Meiosis is a specialized process of cell division that occurs only in the germ line. Figure 1-2 compares mitosis (*A*) and meiosis (*B*). In **mitosis** (normal cell division), a diploid, 2N cell replicates its DNA (becoming diploid, 4N) and undergoes a single division to yield two diploid, 2N daughter cells. In meiosis, a diploid germ cell replicates its DNA (becoming diploid, 4N) and undergoes two successive, qualitatively different nuclear and cell divisions to yield four haploid, 1N offspring. In males, the cell divisions of meiosis are equal and yield four identical spermatozoa. However in females, the meiotic cell divisions are dramatically unequal and yield a single, massive, haploid definitive oocyte and three minute, nonfunctional, haploid **polar bodies**.

First Meiotic Division: DNA Replication and Recombination, Yielding Four Haploid, 2N Daughter Cells. The steps of meiosis are illustrated in Figure 1-2*B* and summarized in Table 1-1. The preliminary step in meiosis, as in mitosis, is the replication of each chromosomal DNA molecule; thus, the diploid cell is converted from 2N to 4N. This event marks the beginning of gametogenesis. In the female, the oogonium is now called a **primary oocyte**, and in the male, the spermatogonium is now called a **primary spermatocyte** (Fig. 1-3). Once the DNA replicates, each chromosome consists of two parallel strands or **chromatids** joined together at a structure called the **centromere**. Each chromatid contains a single DNA molecule (which is itself double stranded; don't confuse DNA double strands with the two chromatid strands composing each chromosome).

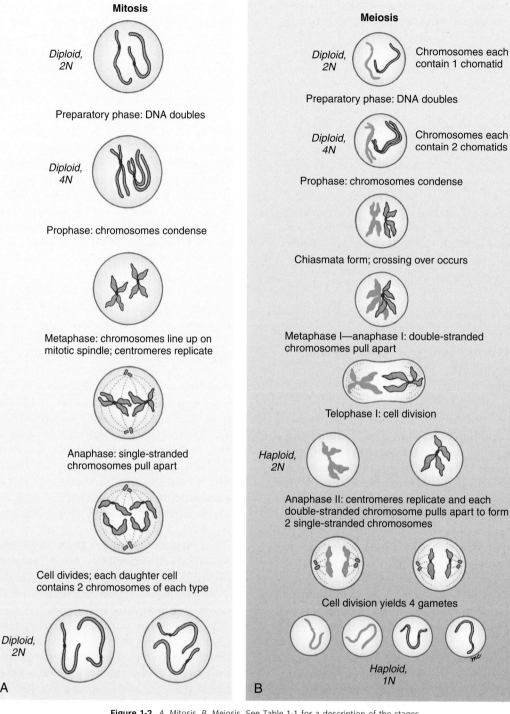

Figure 1-2. *A*, Mitosis. *B*, Meiosis. See Table 1-1 for a description of the stages.

Table 1-1 Events during Mitotic and Meiotic Cell Divisions in the Germ Line

Stage	Events	Name of Cell	Condition of Genome
Resting interval between mitotic cell divisions	Normal cellular metabolism occurs	♀ Oogonium	Diploid, 2N
		♂ Spermatogonium	
Mitosis			
Preparatory phase	DNA replication yields double-stranded chromosomes	♀ Oogonium	Diploid, 4N
		♂ Spermatogonium	
Prophase	Double-stranded chromosomes condense		
Metaphase	Chromosomes align along the equator; centromeres replicate		
Anaphase and telophase	Each double-stranded chromosome splits into 2 single-stranded chromosomes, one of which is distributed to each daughter nucleus		
Cytokinesis	Cell divides	♀ Oogonium	Diploid, 2N
		♂ Spermatogonium	
Meiosis I			
Preparatory phase	DNA replication yields double-stranded chromosomes	♀ Primary oocyte	Diploid, 4N
		♂ Primary spermatocyte	
Prophase	Double-stranded chromosomes condense; 2 chromosomes of each homologous pair align at the centromeres to form a 4-limbed chiasma; recombination by crossing over occurs		
Metaphase	Chromosomes align along the equator; *centromeres do not replicate*		
Anaphase and telophase	1 double-stranded chromosome of each homologous pair is distributed to each daughter cell		
Cytokinesis	Cell divides	♀ one secondary oocyte and the first polar body	Haploid, 2N
		♂ two secondary spermatocytes	
Meiosis II			
Prophase	*No DNA replication takes place during the second meiotic division*; double-stranded chromosomes condense		
Metaphase	Chromosomes align along the equator; *centromeres replicate*		
Anaphase and telophase	Each chromosome splits into 2 single-stranded chromosomes, one of which is distributed to each daughter nucleus		
Cytokinesis	Cell divides	♀ one definitive oocyte and three polar bodies	Haploid, 1N
		♂ four spermatids	

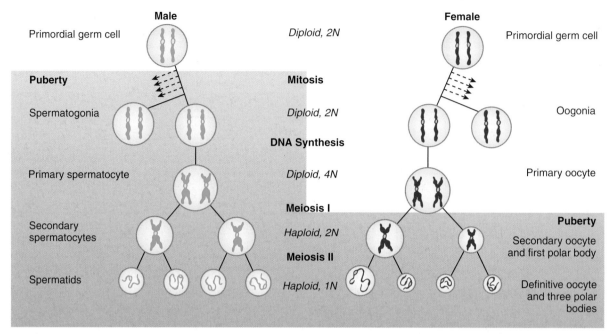

Figure 1-3. Nuclear maturation of germ cells in meiosis in the male and female. In the male, primordial germ cells (PGCs) remain dormant until puberty, when they differentiate into spermatogonia and commence mitosis. Throughout adulthood, spermatogonia produce primary spermatocytes, which undergo meiosis and spermatogenesis. Each primary spermatocyte yields four spermatozoa. In the female, PGCs differentiate into oogonia, which undergo mitosis and then commence meiosis as primary oocytes during fetal life. The primary oocytes remain arrested in prophase I until stimulated to resume meiosis during a menstrual cycle. If fertilization occurs, each primary oocyte yields one definitive oocyte and three polar bodies.

In the next step, called **prophase**, the chromosomes condense into compact, double-stranded structures (i.e., two chromatids joined by one centromere). During the late stages of prophase, the double-stranded chromosomes of each homologous pair match up, centromere to centromere, to form a joint structure called a **chiasma** (composed of four chromatids, two centromeres, and two chromosomes). Chiasma formation makes it possible for the two homologous chromosomes to exchange large segments of DNA by a process called **crossing over**. The resulting **recombination** of the genetic material on homologous maternal and paternal chromosomes is largely random and, therefore, increases the genetic variability of the future gametes. As mentioned earlier, the primary oocyte enters a phase of meiotic arrest during the first meiotic prophase.

During **metaphase**, the four-stranded chiasma structures are organized on the equator of a spindle apparatus similar to the one that forms during mitosis, and during **anaphase**, one double-stranded chromosome of each homologous pair is distributed to each of the two daughter nuclei. During the first meiotic division, the centromeres of the chromosomes do not replicate, and, therefore, the two chromatids of each chromosome remain together. The resulting daughter nuclei thus are haploid but 2N: they contain the same amount of DNA as the parent germ cell but half as many chromosomes. After the daughter nuclei form, the cell itself divides (undergoes **cytokinesis**). The first meiotic cell division produces two **secondary spermatocytes** in the male and a **secondary oocyte** and a **first polar body** in the female (see Fig. 1-3).

Second Meiotic Division: Double-Stranded Chromosomes Divide, Yielding Four Haploid, 1N Daughter Cells. No DNA replication occurs during the second meiotic division. The 23 double-stranded chromosomes condense during the second meiotic prophase and line up during the second meiotic metaphase. The chromosomal centromeres then replicate, and during anaphase, the double-stranded chromosomes pull apart into two single-stranded chromosomes, one of which is distributed to each of the daughter nuclei. In males, the second meiotic cell division produces two **definitive spermatocytes**, more commonly called **spermatids** (i.e., a total of four from each germ cell entering meiosis). In the female, the second meiotic cell division, like the first, is radically unequal, producing a large **definitive oocyte** and another diminutive polar body. The first polar body may simultaneously undergo a second meiotic division to produce a third polar body (see Fig. 1-3).

In the female, the oocyte enters a second phase of meiotic arrest during the second meiotic metaphase before replication of the centromeres. Meiosis does not resume unless the cell is fertilized.

Spermatogenesis

Now that meiosis has been described, it is possible to describe and compare the specific processes of spermatogenesis and oogenesis. At puberty, the testes begin to secrete greatly increased amounts of the steroid hormone **testosterone**. This hormone has a multitude of effects. In addition to stimulating development of many secondary sex characteristics, it triggers growth of the testes, maturation of seminiferous tubules, and commencement of spermatogenesis.

Under the influence of testosterone, Sertoli cells differentiate into a system of seminiferous tubules. The dormant PGCs resume development, divide several times by mitosis, and then differentiate into spermatogonia. These spermatogonia are located immediately under the basement membrane surrounding the seminiferous tubules, where they occupy pockets between Sertoli cells (Fig. 1-4A). Each spermatogonium is connected to the adjacent Sertoli cells by specialized membrane junctions (see next section). In addition, Sertoli cells are joined to each other by dense bands of intercellular membrane junctions that surround each Sertoli cell and thus isolate spermatogonia from the tubule lumen.

Male Germ Cells Are Translocated to Seminiferous Tubule Lumen during Spermatogenesis

Cells that will undergo spermatogenesis arise by mitosis from the spermatogonia. These cells are gradually translocated between the Sertoli cells from the basal to the luminal side of the seminiferous epithelium while spermatogenesis takes place (see Fig. 1-4A). During this migratory phase, primary spermatocytes pass without interruption through both meiotic divisions,

producing first two secondary spermatocytes and then four spermatids. The spermatids undergo dramatic changes that convert them into mature sperm while they complete their migration to the lumen. This process of sperm cell differentiation is called **spermiogenesis.**

Sertoli Cells Are Also Instrumental in Spermiogenesis

Sertoli cells participate intimately in the differentiation of the gametes. Maturing spermatocytes and spermatids are connected to surrounding Sertoli cells by intercellular junctions, typical of those found on epithelial cells, and unique cytoplasmic processes called **tubulobulbar complexes** that extend into the Sertoli cells. The cytoplasm of developing gametes shrinks dramatically during spermiogenesis; the tubulobulbar complexes are thought to provide a mechanism by which the excess cytoplasm is transferred to Sertoli cells. As cytoplasm is removed, spermatids undergo dramatic changes in shape and internal organization that transform them into spermatozoa. Finally, the last connections with Sertoli cells break, releasing the spermatozoa into the tubule lumen. This final step is called **spermiation**.

As shown in Figures 1-4B, C, a spermatozoon consists of a **head, midpiece**, and **tail**. The head contains the condensed nucleus and is capped by an apical vesicle filled with hydrolytic enzymes (e.g., acrosin, hyaluronidase, and neuraminidase). This vesicle, the **acrosome**, plays an essential role in fertilization. The midpiece contains large, helical mitochondria and generates energy for swimming. The long tail contains microtubules that form part of the propulsion system of the spermatozoon.

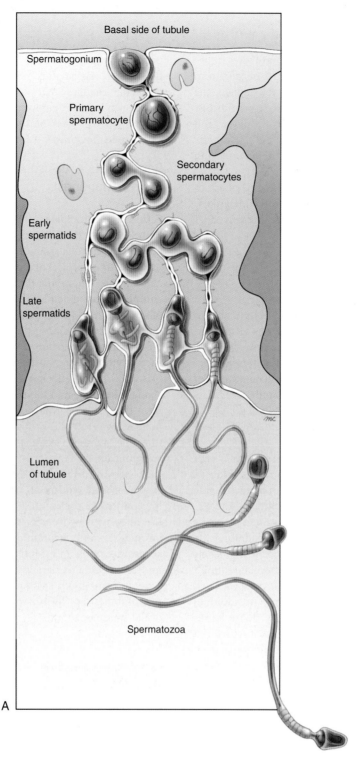

Figure 1-4. *A,* Schematic section through the wall of the seminiferous tubule. Spermatogonium just under the outer surface of the tubule wall (basal side) undergoes mitosis to produce daughter cells, which may either continue to divide by mitosis (thus renewing the spermatogonial stem cell population) or commence meiosis as primary spermatocytes. As spermatogenesis and spermiogenesis occur, the differentiating cell is translocated between adjacent Sertoli cells to the tubule lumen. Daughter spermatocytes and spermatids remain linked by cytoplasmic bridges. The entire clone of spermatogonia derived from each primordial germ cell is linked by cytoplasmic bridges.

Continued

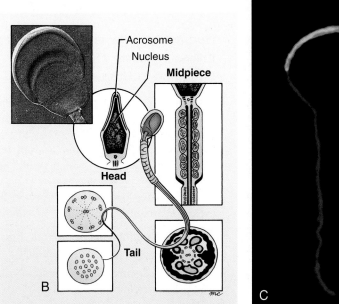

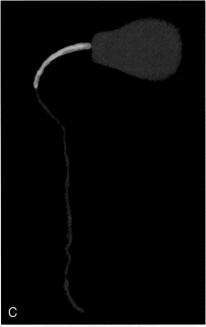

Figure 1-4, cont'd. *B,* Structure of the mature spermatozoon. The head contains the nucleus capped by the acrosome; the midpiece contains coiled mitochondria; the tail contains propulsive microtubules. The inset micrograph shows the head of a human sperm. *C,* Bull sperm labeled with fluorescent markers to reveal its nucleus (blue) in its head, mitochondria (green) in its midpiece, and microtubules (red) in its tail. The red labeling around the perimeter of the head is background labeling.

Continual Waves of Spermatogenesis Occur throughout Seminiferous Epithelium

Spermatogenesis takes place continuously from puberty to death. Gametes are produced in synchronous waves in each local area of the germinal epithelium, although the process is not synchronized throughout the seminiferous tubules. In many different mammals, the clone of spermatogonia, derived from each spermatogonial stem cell, populates a local area of the seminiferous tubules and displays synchronous spermatogenesis. That may be the case in humans as well. About four waves of synchronously differentiating cells can be observed in a given region of the human tubule epithelium at any time. Ultrastructural studies provide evidence that these waves of differentiating cells remain synchronized because of incomplete cytokinesis throughout the series of mitotic and meiotic divisions between the division of a spermatogonium and formation of spermatids. Instead of fully separating, daughter cells produced by these divisions remain connected by slender cytoplasmic bridges (see Fig. 1-4A) that could allow passage of small signaling molecules or metabolites.

In the human male, each cycle of spermatogenesis takes about 64 days. Spermatogonial mitosis occupies about 16 days, the first meiotic division takes about 8 days, the second meiotic division takes about 16 days, and spermiogenesis requires about 24 days.

Spermatozoa Undergo a Terminal Step of Functional Maturation Called Capacitation

During its journey from the seminiferous tubules to the ampulla of the oviduct, a sperm cell undergoes a process of functional maturation that prepares it to fertilize an oocyte. Sperm produced in the seminiferous tubules are stored in the lower part of the **epididymis,** a 15-to-20-foot long highly coiled duct connected to the **vas deferens** near its origin in the testis. During ejaculation, sperm are propelled through the vas deferens and urethra and are mixed with nourishing secretions from the **seminal vesicles, prostate**, and **bulbourethral glands** (these structures are further discussed in Ch. 15). As many as 300 million spermatozoa may be deposited in the vagina by a single ejaculation, but only a few hundred succeed in navigating through the cervix, uterus, and oviduct and into the expanded ampullar region. In the **ampulla** of the oviduct, sperm survive and retain their capacity to fertilize an oocyte for 1 to 3 days.

Capacitation, the final step of sperm maturation, consists mainly of changes in the acrosome that prepare it to release the enzymes required to penetrate the zona pellucida, a shell of glycoprotein surrounding the oocyte. Capacitation takes place within the female genital tract and is thought to require contact with secretions of the oviduct. Spermatozoa used in in vitro fertilization (IVF) procedures are artificially capacitated. Spermatozoa with defective acrosomes may be injected directly into oocytes to assist reproduction in humans (assisted reproduction technology, or ART, is discussed later in the chapter under **"In the Clinic"**).

Oogenesis

Primary Oocytes Form in Ovaries by Five Months of Fetal Life

As mentioned earlier, female germ cells undergo a series of mitotic divisions after they are invested by somatic support cells and then differentiate into oogonia (see Fig. 1-3). By 12 weeks of development, oogonia in the genital ridges enter the first meiotic prophase and then almost immediately become dormant. The nucleus of each of these dormant **primary oocytes**, containing the partially condensed prophase chromosomes, becomes very large and watery and is referred to as a **germinal vesicle**. The swollen condition of the germinal vesicle is thought to protect the oocyte's DNA during the long period of meiotic arrest.

A single-layered, squamous capsule of epithelial follicle cells derived from the somatic support cells tightly encloses each primary oocyte. This capsule and its enclosed primary oocyte constitute a **primordial follicle** (see Fig. 1-6). By 5 months, the number of primordial follicles in the ovaries peaks at about 7 million. Most of these follicles subsequently degenerate. By birth only 700,000 to 2 million remain, and by puberty, only about 400,000.

Hormones of Female Cycle Control Folliculogenesis, Ovulation, and Condition of Uterus

After reaching puberty, also called **menarche** in females, and until the woman enters **menopause** several decades later, monthly cycles in the secretion of hypothalamic, pituitary, and ovarian hormones control a **menstrual cycle**, which results each month in the production of a female gamete and a uterus primed to receive a fertilized embryo. Specifically, this 28-day cycle consists of:

- The monthly maturation of (usually) a single oocyte and its enclosing follicle
- The concurrent proliferation of the uterine endometrium
- The process of ovulation by which the oocyte is released from the ovary
- The continued development of the follicle into an endocrine corpus luteum
- The sloughing of the uterine endometrium and involution of the corpus luteum (unless a fertilized ovum implants in the uterus and begins to develop)

The menstrual cycle is considered to begin with menstruation (also called the menses), the shedding of the degenerated uterine endometrium from the previous cycle. On about the 5th day of the cycle (the 5th day after the beginning of menstruation), an increase in secretion by the hypothalamus of the brain of a small peptide hormone, gonadotropin-releasing hormone (GnRH), stimulates the pituitary gland to increase its secretion of two gonadotropic hormones (gonadotropins): follicle-stimulating hormone (FSH) and luteinizing hormone (LH) (Fig. 1-5). The rising levels of pituitary gonadotropins regulate later phases of folliculogenesis in the ovary and the proliferative phase in the uterine endometrium.

About Five to Twelve Primary Follicles Resume Development Each Month

Before a particular cycle, and independent of pituitary gonadotropins, the follicular epithelium of a small group of primordial follicles thickens, converting the single-layered follicular epithelium from a layer of

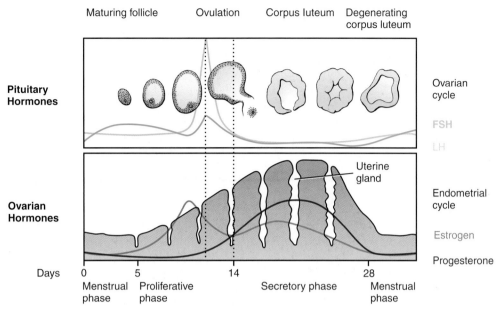

Figure 1-5. Ovarian, endometrial, and hormonal events of the menstrual cycle. Pituitary follicle-stimulating hormone (FSH) and luteinizing hormone (LH) directly control the ovarian cycle and also control production of estrogen and progesterone by responding follicles and corpus luteum of the ovary. These ovarian hormones in turn control the cycle of the uterine endometrium.

squamous cells to cuboidal cells (Fig. 1-6*A*). These follicles are now called **primary follicles**. The follicle cells and the oocyte jointly secrete a thin layer of acellular material, composed of only a few types of glycoprotein, onto the surface of the oocyte. Although this layer, the **zona pellucida**, appears to form a complete physical barrier between the follicle cells and oocyte (Figs. 1-6*B*, 1-7*A*), actually it is penetrated by thin extensions of follicle cells that are connected to the oocyte cell membrane by intercellular junctions (Fig. 1-7*B*). These extensions and their intercellular junctions remain intact until just before ovulation, and they probably convey both developmental signals and metabolic support to the oocyte. The follicular epithelium of five to twelve of these primary follicles then proliferates to form a multilayered capsule of follicle cells around the oocyte (see Fig. 1-6). The follicles are now called **growing follicles**. At this point, some of the growing follicles cease to develop and eventually degenerate, whereas a few continue to enlarge in response to rising levels of FSH, mainly by taking up fluid and developing a central fluid-filled cavity called the **antrum**. These follicles are called **antral** or **vesicular follicles**. At the same time, the connective tissue of the ovarian stroma surrounding each of these follicles differentiates into two layers, an inner layer called the **theca interna** and an outer layer called the **theca externa**. These two layers become vascularized, in contrast to the follicle cells, which do not.

Single Follicle Becomes Dominant and Remainder Degenerate

Eventually, one of the growing follicles gains primacy and continues to enlarge by absorbing fluid, whereas the remainder of the follicles recruited during the cycle degenerate (undergo **atresia**). The oocyte, surrounded by a small mass of follicle cells called the **cumulus oophorus**, increasingly projects into the expanding antrum but remains connected to the layer of follicle cells that lines the antral cavity and underlies the basement membrane of the follicle. This layer is called the **membrana granulosa**. The large, swollen follicle is now called a **mature vesicular follicle** or **mature graafian follicle** (see Fig. 1-6). At this point, the oocyte still has not resumed meiosis.

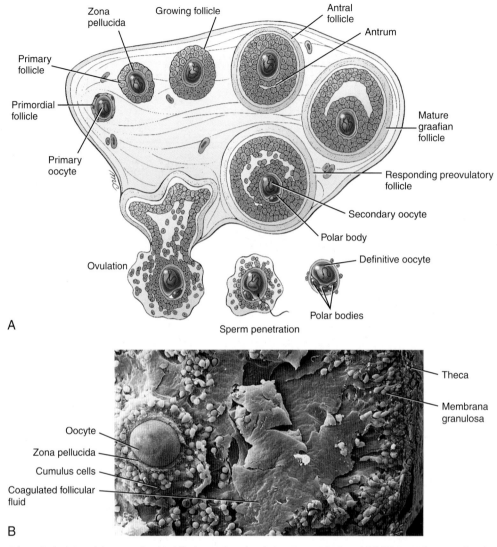

Figure 1-6. *A*, Schematic depiction of the ovary showing folliculogenesis and ovulation. Five to 12 primordial follicles initially respond to the rising levels of follicle-stimulating hormone (FSH) and luteinizing hormone (LH), but only one matures. In response to the ovulatory surge in LH and FSH, the oocyte of this mature graafian follicle resumes meiosis and ovulation occurs. Final steps of meiosis take place only if the released oocyte is penetrated by a sperm. *B*, Scanning electron micrograph of a preovulatory follicle.

Why Is Folliculogenesis Selectively Stimulated in Only a Few Follicles Each Month?

The reason why only five to twelve primordial follicles commence folliculogenesis each month—and why, of this group, all but one eventually degenerate—is not known. One possibility is that follicles become progressively more sensitive to the stimulating effects of FSH as they advance in development. Follicles that are slightly more advanced simply on a random basis would, therefore, respond more acutely to FSH and would be favored. Another possibility is that the selection process is regulated by a complex system of feedback between the pituitary and ovarian hormones and growth factors.

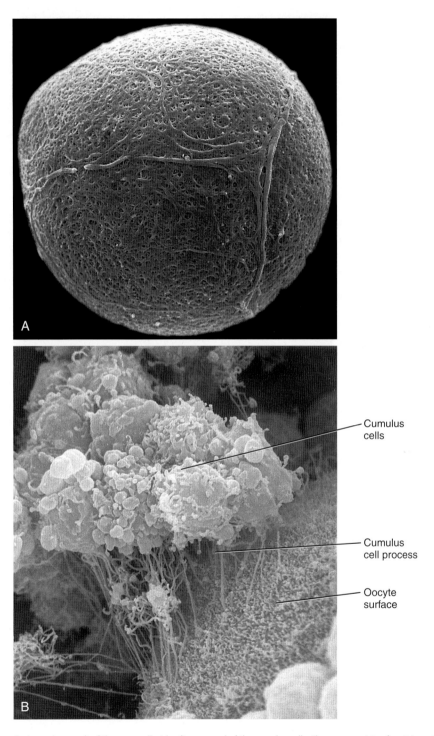

Figure 1-7. *A,* Scanning electron micrograph of the zona pellucida after removal of the cumulus cells. The zona consists of protein and mucopolysaccharide and forms a barrier that the sperm penetrates by means of its acrosomal enzymes. *B,* Scanning electron micrograph of the oocyte surface and cumulus oophorus, with the zona pellucida digested away. The cumulus cells maintain contact with the oocyte via thin cell processes that penetrate the zona pellucida and form intercellular junctions with the oocyte cell membrane.

IN THE CLINIC

CHROMOSOMAL ABNORMALITIES RESULT IN SPONTANEOUS ABORTION OR ABNORMAL DEVELOPMENT

It is estimated that one third of all conceptions in normal, healthy women abort spontaneously; approximately one fourth of these occur before pregnancy is detected. Chromosomal anomalies seem to cause about 40% to 50% of spontaneous abortions in those cases in which the conceptus has been recovered and examined. However, many chromosomal anomalies allow the fetus to survive to term. The resulting infants display nonrandom patterns of developmental abnormalities; that is, **syndromes**. One of these syndromes, Down syndrome, is discussed in the detail in the following section; others are discussed in detail in subsequent chapters.

MANY CHROMOSOMAL ANOMALIES ARISE DURING GAMETOGENESIS AND CLEAVAGE

Abnormal chromosomes can be produced in the germ line of either parent through an error in meiosis or fertilization, or can arise in the early embryo through an error in mitosis. Gametes or blastomeres that result from these events contain missing or extra chromosomes, or chromosomes with duplicated, deleted, or rearranged segments. Absence of a specific chromosome in a gamete that combines with a normal gamete to form a zygote results in a condition known as **monosomy** (because the zygote contains only one copy of the chromosome rather than the normal two). Conversely, the presence of two of the same kind of chromosome in one of the gametes that forms a zygote results in **trisomy**.

Down syndrome is a disorder most frequently caused by an error during meiosis. If the two copies of chromosome 21 fail to separate during the first or second meiotic anaphase of gametogenesis in either parent (a phenomenon called **nondisjunction**), half the resulting gametes will lack chromosome 21 altogether and the other half will have two copies (Fig. 1-8A). Embryos formed by fusion of a gamete-lacking chromosome 21 with a normal gamete are called **monosomy 21** embryos. These embryos die rapidly; monosomies of autosomal chromosomes are invariably fatal during early embryonic development. If, on the other hand, a gamete with two copies of chromosome 21 fuses with a normal gamete, the resulting **trisomy 21** embryo may survive (Fig. 1-8B). Trisomy 21 infants display the pattern of abnormalities described as **Down syndrome**. In addition to recognizable facial characteristics, mental retardation, and short stature, individuals with Down syndrome may exhibit congenital heart defects (atrioventricular septal defect is most common, that is, a failure to form both the atrial and ventricular septa; discussed in Ch. 12), hearing loss, duodenal obstruction, a propensity to develop leukemia, and immune system defects. Trisomy in most Down syndrome individuals is the result of nondisjunction in the mother, usually during the first meiotic division (75% to 80% of the cases). Identification of the extra chromosome as maternal or paternal in origin was originally based on karyotype analysis that compared banding patterns of the extra chromosome 21 with chromosome 21 of the mother and father. These early studies concluded that about 70% to 75% of Down syndrome cases occurred as a consequence of nondisjunction in the mother. However, by the late 1980s, more sensitive karyotype analysis increased this frequency to 80%, and by the early 1990s, an even more sensitive molecular technique (Southern blot analysis of DNA polymorphisms) provided evidence that as many as 90% to 95% of Down syndrome cases arise through nondisjunction in the maternal germ line. Consequently, it is now accepted that only about 5% of the cases of Down syndrome result from an error in spermatogenesis.

Occasionally, the extra chromosome 21 is lost from a subset of cells during cleavage. The resulting embryo develops as a **mosaic** of normal and trisomy 21 cells. Two percent to 5 percent of all individuals with Down syndrome are mosaics. These individuals may show a range of Down syndrome features depending on the abundance and location of abnormal cells. If nondisjunction occurs in the germ line, a seemingly normal individual could produce several Down syndrome offspring. Meiosis of a trisomic germ cell yields gametes with a normal single copy of the chromosome, as well as abnormal gametes with two copies, so normal offspring also can be produced.

Down syndrome does not always result from simple nondisjunction. Sometimes, a copy of chromosome 21 in a developing gamete becomes attached to the end of another chromosome, such as chromosome 14, during the first or second division of meiosis. This event is called a **translocation**. The zygote produced by fusion of such a gamete with a normal partner will have two normal copies of chromosome 21 plus an abnormal chromosome 14 carrying a third copy of chromosome 21 (Fig. 1-9). Two percent to five percent of all individuals with Down syndrome harbor such translocations.

Cases in which only a part of chromosome 21 is translocated have provided insight into which regions of chromosome 21 must be triplicated to produce specific aspects of Down syndrome, such as mental retardation, characteristic facial features, and cardiovascular defects. By determining which specific phenotypes occur in patients with Down syndrome having particular

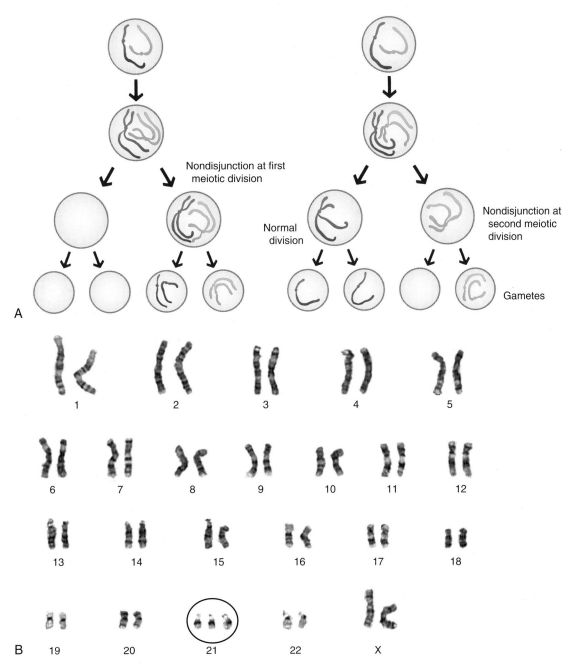

Figure 1-8. *A,* Mechanism of chromosomal nondisjunction in meiosis. Failure of homologous double-stranded chromosomes to separate before cytokinesis during the first meiotic division (left-hand panel) results in their distribution to only one of the secondary gonocytes (or first polar body). Failure of the two strands of a double-stranded chromosome to separate before cytokinesis during the second meiotic division (right-hand panel) results in their distribution to only one of the definitive gonocytes (or second polar body). *B,* Karyotype of a female with trisomy 21 (circled), causing Down syndrome.

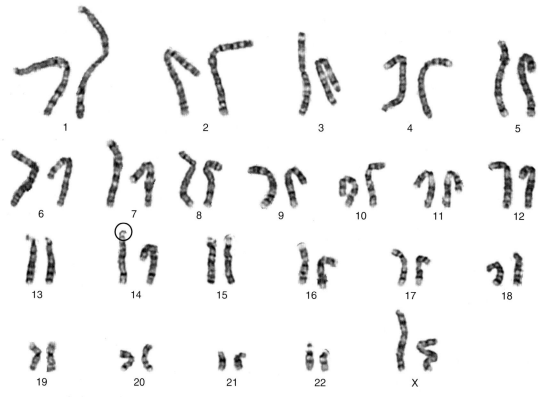

Figure 1-9. Karyotype of a female with Down syndrome caused by translocation of chromosome 21 onto chromosome 14 (circled).

translocated regions of chromosome 21, **Down syndrome candidate regions** on chromosome 21 have been identified. The completion of the sequencing of chromosome 21 (in May 2000) and the generation of transgenic mice (transgenic mice are discussed in Ch. 5) trisomic for these candidate regions is leading to the identification of those genes responsible for specific Down syndrome phenotypes in humans.

The incidence of Down syndrome increases significantly with the age of the mother but not with the age of the father. The risk of giving birth to a liveborn with Down syndrome at maternal age 30 is 1 in 900. The risk increases to 9 in 1000 by maternal age 40. However, it is not clear whether older women actually produce more oocytes with nondisjunction of chromosome 21 or whether the efficiency of spontaneously aborting trisomy 21 embryos decreases with age.

Trisomies of other autosomes (such as chromosomes 8, 9, 13, and 18) also produce recognizable syndromes of abnormal development, but these trisomies are present much less frequently in live births than is trisomy 21. Similarly, trisomies and monosomies of sex chromosomes

occur (for example, **Klinefelter** and **Turner** syndromes, two syndromes in which there are extra or decreased numbers of sex chromosomes, respectively; discussed in Ch. 15). **Triploid** or **tetraploid** embryos, in which multiple copies of the entire genome are present, can arise by errors in fertilization (discussed in Ch. 2).

Several other types of chromosome anomalies are produced at meiosis. In some cases, errors in meiosis result in deletion of just part of a chromosome or duplication of a small chromosome segment. The resulting anomalies are called **partial monosomy** and **partial trisomy**, respectively. Other errors that can occur during meiosis are **inversions** of chromosome segments and the formation of **ring chromosomes**.

CHROMOSOME ANALYSIS CAN DETERMINE PARENTAL SOURCE OF DEFECTIVE CHROMOSOME AND PROVIDES BASIS FOR DIAGNOSIS AND POSSIBLE TREATMENT

Genetic analysis of congenital defects is a very recent development. The normal human **karyotype** was not fully characterized until the late 1950s. Improved staining and culture conditions now allow high-resolution chromosome banding, increasing our ability to detect small deletions or duplications. Advances in molecular genetic techniques have led to a much finer analysis of DNA structure. As a result, it is possible to identify even smaller defects not evident with high-resolution banding. These techniques are used for both diagnosis and genetic counseling. Blood cells of a prospective parent can be checked for heritable chromosome anomalies, and embryonic cells obtained either from the amniotic fluid (**amniocentesis**) or from the chorionic villi (**chorionic villous sampling**) can be used to detect many disorders early in pregnancy (discussed in Ch. 6).

Three molecular approaches are used routinely for chromosomal analysis (Figs. 1-10, 1-11): fluorescence in situ hybridization (FISH), comparative genomic hybridization (CGH), and chromosome painting (whole chromosome painting and spectral karyotyping, or SKY). In all of these techniques, DNA probes linked to fluorescent dyes (fluorochromes, each of which emits a unique spectrum of light and is assigned a unique color by a computer) are used to probe specific loci on chromosomes. This is particularly useful for detecting changes in chromosome copy number (aneuploidy) or for characterizing chromosomal material involved in translocations.

Ovulation

Resumption of Meiosis and Ovulation Are Stimulated by an Ovulatory Surge in FSH and LH

On about day 13 or 14 of the menstrual cycle (at the end of the proliferative phase of the uterine endometrium), levels of FSH and LH suddenly rise very sharply (see Fig. 1-5). This **ovulatory surge** in pituitary gonadotropins stimulates the primary oocyte of the remaining mature graafian follicle to resume meiosis. This response can be observed visually about 15 hours after the beginning of the ovulatory surge, when the membrane of the swollen germinal vesicle (nucleus) of the oocyte breaks down (Fig 1-12A). By 20 hours, the chromosomes are lined up in metaphase. Cell division to form the secondary oocyte and first polar body rapidly ensues (Fig. 1-12B). The secondary oocyte promptly begins the second meiotic division but, about 3 hours before ovulation, is arrested at the second meiotic metaphase.

Cumulus Oophorus Expands in Response to Ovulatory Surge

As the germinal vesicle breaks down, the cumulus cells surrounding the oocyte lose their cell-to-cell connections and disaggregate. As a result, the oocyte and a mass of loose cumulus cells detach into the antral cavity. Over the next few hours, the cumulus cells secrete an abundant extracellular matrix, consisting mainly of hyaluronic acid, which causes the cumulus cell mass to expand severalfold. This process of **cumulus expansion** may play a role in several processes, including the regulation of meiotic progress and ovulation. In addition, the mass of matrix and entrapped cumulus cells that accompanies the ovulated oocyte may play roles in the transport of the oocyte in the oviduct, in fertilization, and in the early development of the zygote.

Ovulation Depends on Breakdown of the Follicle Wall

The process of **ovulation** (the expulsion of the secondary oocyte from the follicle) has been likened to an inflammatory response. The cascade of events that culminates in ovulation is thought to be initiated by the secretion of histamine and prostaglandins, well-known inflammatory mediators. Within a few hours after the ovulatory surge of FSH and LH, the follicle becomes more vascularized and is visibly pink and edematous in comparison with nonresponding follicles. The follicle is displaced to the surface of the ovary, where it forms a bulge (see Fig. 1-6A). As ovulation approaches, the projecting wall of the follicle begins to thin, resulting in formation of a small, nipple-shaped protrusion called the **stigma**. Finally, a combination of tension produced by smooth muscle cells in the follicle wall plus the release of collagen-degrading enzymes and other factors by fibroblasts in the region causes the follicle to rupture. Rupture of the follicle is not explosive: the oocyte, accompanied by a large number of investing cumulus cells bound in hyaluronic acid matrix, is slowly extruded onto the surface of the ovary. Ovulation occurs about 38 hours after the beginning of the ovulatory surge of FSH and LH.

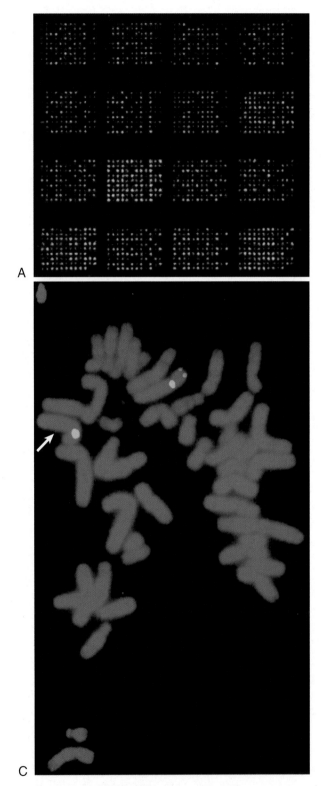

Figure 1–10. *For legend, see next page.*

Figure 1-10. Chromosomal deletions or duplications not apparent on high-resolution chromosome banding (karyotyping) can be detected using comparative genomic hybridization (CGH). This technology uses chip microarray (A) to compare fluorescently labeled DNA from a patient and a control. Two assays are run, swapping fluorescent dyes between the patient and control. The two assays are shown in B by the blue and red dots interconnected by lines. Each blue or red dot represents a different DNA probe, with multiple probes placed along the entire length of chromosome 4 (chromosome bands labeled at left). The patient has a deletion restricted to 4p16.2 (top). This is indicated by a deviation of the blue line (and multiple dots representing several telomeric probes) to the left, with reciprocal deviation of the red line to the right. The dashed lines indicate that there is a two-fold difference in copy number at this locus (center solid line represents a 1:1 ratio). C, The 4p16.2 deletion was verified using fluorescent in situ hybridization (FISH) on a metaphase chromosome spread. Green probe marks centromeres of the homologous chromosome 4 pair. Red probe marks the two sister chromatids of one 4p16.2; this region is deleted on the other chromosome 4 (arrow).

The sticky mass formed by the oocyte and cumulus is actively scraped off the surface of the ovary by the fimbriated mouth of the oviduct (Fig. 1-13). The cumulus-oocyte complex is then moved into the ampulla of the oviduct by the synchronized beating of cilia on the oviduct wall. Within the ampulla, the oocyte may remain viable for as long as 24 hours before it loses its capacity to be fertilized.

Ruptured Follicle Forms the Endocrine Corpus Luteum

After ovulation, membrane granulosa cells of the ruptured follicular wall begin to proliferate and give rise to the **luteal cells** of the **corpus luteum** (see Figs. 1-6 and 1-13). As described later, the corpus luteum is an endocrine structure that secretes steroid hormones to maintain the uterine endometrium in a condition ready to receive an embryo. If an embryo does not implant in the uterus, the corpus luteum degenerates after about 14 days and is converted to a scarlike structure called the **corpus albicans.**

Menstrual Cycle

Beginning on about day 5 of the menstrual cycle, the thecal and follicle cells of responding follicles secrete

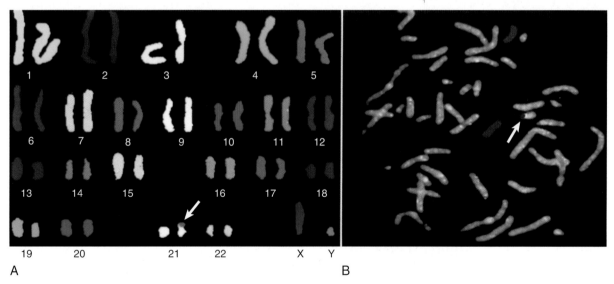

A   B

Figure 1-11. High-resolution chromosome banding occasionally detects complex chromosomal abnormalities where the origin of the deleted or duplicated chromosomal material is unknown. To identify such material, spectral karyotyping (SKY) can be used in which 24 combinatorially labeled chromosome painting probes are simultaneously hybridized (one probe for each of 22 chromosomes and probes for the X and Y chromosomes). A, Material attached to chromosome 21 was spectrally identified to be of chromosome 17 origin (arrow). B, This was verified using whole chromosome paint for chromosome 17 (red). The translocated chromosome 17 material is seen attached to chromosome 21 (arrow).

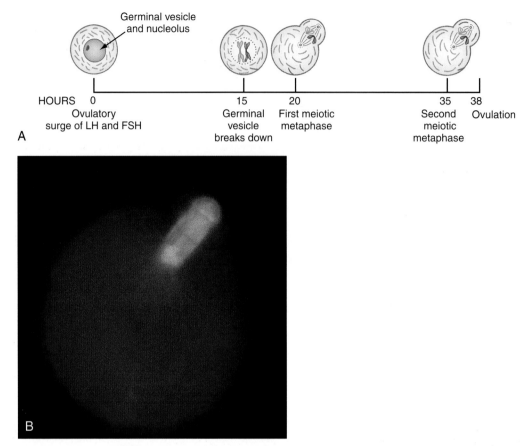

Figure 1-12. *A*, Timing of meiotic events during the ovarian cycle. *B*, Micrograph of preovulatory oocyte at the first meiotic metaphase. The cell is stained with fluorescent antibodies specific for the spindle proteins and shows the eccentric spindle apparatus and incipient first polar body.

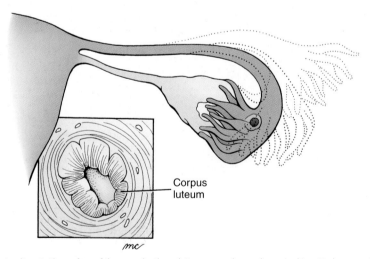

Figure 1-13. The ovulated oocyte clings to the surface of the ovary by the gelatinous cumulus oophorus and is actively scraped off by the fimbriated oviduct mouth. After ovulation, the membrana granulosa layer of the ruptured follicle proliferates to form the endocrine corpus luteum.

steroids called **estrogens**. These hormones in turn cause the endometrial lining of the uterus to proliferate and undergo remodeling. This **proliferative phase** begins at about day 5 of the cycle and is complete by day 14 (see Fig. 1-5).

After ovulation occurs, thecal cells in the wall of the corpus luteum continue to secrete estrogens, and **luteal cells** that differentiate from remaining follicle cells also begin to secrete high levels of a related steroid hormone, **progesterone**. Luteal progesterone stimulates the uterine endometrial layer to thicken further and to form convoluted glands and increased vasculature. Unless an embryo implants in the uterine lining, this **secretory phase** of endometrial differentiation lasts about 13 days (see Fig. 1-5). At that point (near the end of the menstrual cycle), the corpus luteum shrinks and levels of progesterone fall. The thickened endometrium, which is dependent on progesterone, degenerates and begins to slough. The 4- to 5-day **menstrual phase**, during which the endometrium is sloughed (along with about 35 mL of blood and the unfertilized oocyte), is by convention considered the start of the next cycle.

Fertilization

If viable spermatozoa encounter an ovulated oocyte in the ampulla of the oviduct, they surround it and begin forcing their way through the cumulus mass (Fig. 1-14A). In vitro evidence suggests that the ovulated follicle contains a currently unknown **sperm chemotropic factor** and that only capacitated sperm are able to respond to this factor by directed swimming toward the egg. Based on this, it might be said that the human sperm finds the human egg to be "attractive" (pun intended).

When a spermatozoon reaches the tough zona pellucida surrounding the oocyte, it binds in a species- (that is, human-) specific interaction with a glycoprotein sperm receptor molecule in the zona (ZP3, one of three glycoproteins composing the zona pellucida). Binding to ZP3 is mediated by a sperm surface protein called SED1. As a result of this binding, the acrosome is induced to release degradative enzymes that allow the sperm to penetrate the zona pellucida. When a spermatozoon successfully penetrates the zona pellucida and reaches the oocyte, the cell membranes of the two cells fuse {(Fig. 1-14B; see Fig. 1-14A)}. The egg tetraspanin (a 4-pass transmembrane protein), CD9, is required for this event, as is a sperm-specific

protein named IZUMO after the Japanese shrine to marriage. (IZUMO is a member of the immunoglobulin superfamily and as such is likely to be an adhesion molecule.) Other factors implicated in fusion are members of the ADAM superfamily (all 30 or so family members contain a disintegrin and a metalloprotease domain). FERTILINβ, also known as ADAM2, is present on the surface of mammalian sperm and interacts with an integrin (integrins are discussed in Ch. 5) on the egg surface. Membrane fusion immediately causes two events to occur: formation of a calcium wave that radiates over the surface of the egg from the point of sperm contact; and release of the contents of thousands of small **cortical granules**, located just beneath the oocyte cell membrane, into the **perivitelline space** between the oocyte and the zona pellucida. These two events alter the sperm receptor molecules, causing the zona to become impenetrable by additional spermatozoa. Therefore, these changes prevent **polyspermy** or the fertilization of the oocyte by more than one spermatozoon. Because a few hundred spermatozoa reach the vicinity of the egg, the need to block polyspermy is extremely important.

The fusion of the spermatozoon cell membrane with the oocyte membrane also causes the oocyte to resume meiosis. The oocyte completes the second meiotic metaphase and rapidly proceeds through anaphase, telophase, and cytokinesis, producing another polar body. Disregarding the presence of the sperm, the oocyte is now considered to be a **definitive oocyte** (considering only the oocyte's genome, it contains a haploid complement of chromosomes and a 1N quantity of DNA after completion of the second meiotic division). However, because the sperm has now penetrated the oocyte, the fertilized oocyte can also be called a **zygote** (from Greek *zugotos*, yoked). Although a single nucleus (surrounded by a nuclear membrane) containing both the oocyte's and sperm's chromosomes does not form in the zygote (see next paragraph and Figs. 1-14C, 1-15), taking into account both the oocyte's and sperm's genomes, the zygote contains a diploid complement of chromosomes and a 2N quantity of DNA.

After penetration of the oocyte by the sperm, the nuclei of the oocyte and sperm swell within the zygote and are called the **female** and **male pronuclei**, respectively (see Figs. 1-14C, 1-15). Their nuclear membranes quickly disappear as both maternal and

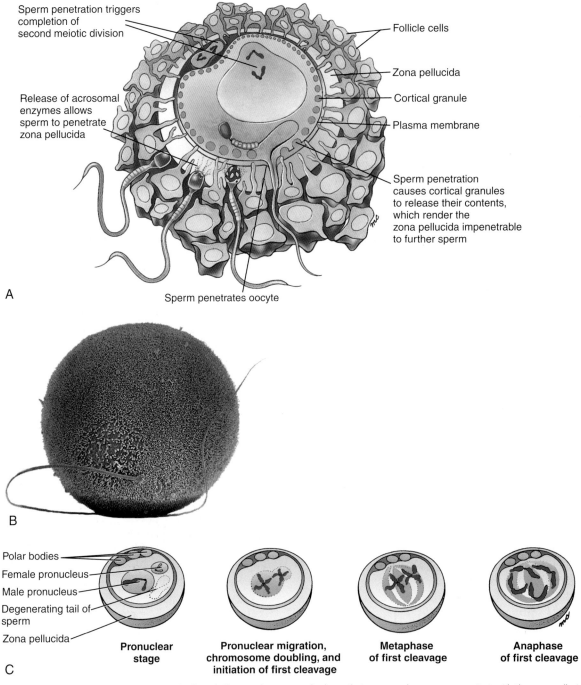

Figure 1-14. Fertilization. *A,* Spermatozoa wriggle through the cumulus mass and release their acrosomal enzymes on contact with the zona pellucida. Acrosomal enzymes dissolve the zona pellucida and allow sperm to reach the oocyte. Simultaneous with fusion of the membranes of the fertilizing sperm and oocyte, cortical granules of the oocyte release their contents, which causes the zona pellucida to become impenetrable to other sperm. Entry of the sperm nucleus into the cytoplasm stimulates the oocyte to complete the second meiotic division. *B,* Scanning electron micrograph showing a human sperm fusing with a hamster oocyte that has been enzymatically denuded of the zona pellucida. The ability of a man's sperm to penetrate a denuded hamster oocyte is often used as a clinical test of sperm activity. *C,* Early events in zygote development. After the oocyte completes meiosis, the female pronucleus and the larger male pronucleus approach each other as DNA is doubled in maternal and paternal chromosomes to initiate the first mitotic division. Pronuclear membranes then break down and maternal and paternal chromosomes assemble on the metaphase plate. Centromeres then replicate, and homologous chromosomes are distributed to the first two cells of the embryo.

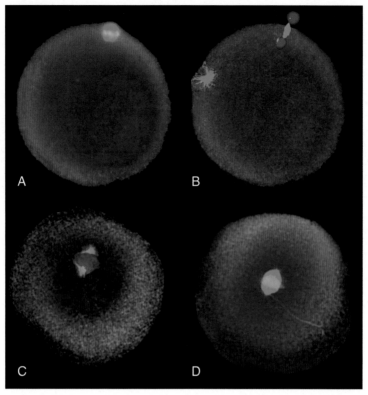

Figure 1-15. Fertilization of human eggs in vitro. *A,* The first meiotic division has occurred, forming the first polar body and secondary oocyte. *B,* The second meiotic division is completed after the sperm has entered the oocyte. This results in the formation of the second polar body and female pronucleus. The male pronucleus and microtubules condensing around it are located at the 9 o'clock position. *C,* The sperm centriole has split into two centrioles, which are organizing a spindle in association with the merged chromosomes from the male and female pronuclei. *D,* The sperm and egg chromosomes are aligned on the metaphase plate.

paternal chromosomes are replicated in preparation for the first cleavage (see next section).

Cleavage

Cleavage Subdivides Zygote without Increasing Its Size

Within 24 hours after fertilization, the zygote initiates a rapid series of mitotic cell divisions called **cleavage** (Fig. 1-16). These divisions are not accompanied by cell growth, so they subdivide the large zygote into many smaller daughter cells called **blastomeres**. The embryo as a whole does not increase in size during cleavage and remains enclosed in the zona pellucida. The first cleavage division divides the zygote to produce two daughter cells. The second division, which is complete at about 40 hours

after fertilization, produces four equal blastomeres. By 3 days, the embryo consists of 6 to 12 cells, and by 4 days, it consists of 16 to 32 cells. The embryo at this stage is called a **morula** (from Latin *morum,* mulberry).

Segregation of Blastomeres into Embryoblast and Trophoblast Precursors

The cells of the morula will give rise not only to the embryo proper and its associated extraembryonic membranes but also to part of the placenta and related structures. The cells that will follow these different developmental paths become segregated during cleavage. Starting at the 8-cell stage of development, the originally round and loosely adherent blastomeres begin to flatten, developing an inside-outside polarity that maximizes cell-to-cell contact among adjacent blastomeres (Fig. 1-17). As differential adhesion develops, the outer

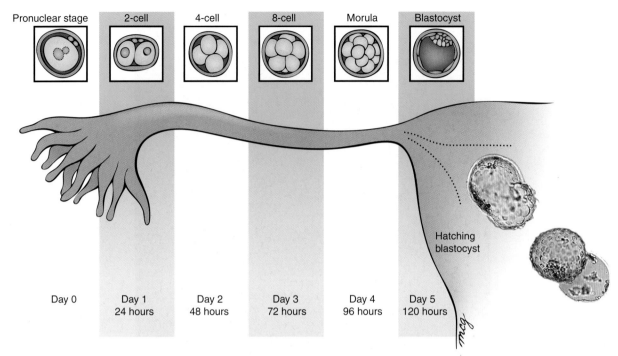

Figure 1-16. Cleavage and transport down the oviduct. Fertilization occurs in the ampulla of the oviduct. During the first 5 days, the zygote undergoes cleavage as it travels down the oviduct and enters the uterus. On day 5, the blastocyst hatches from the zona pellucida and is then able to implant in the uterine endometrium.

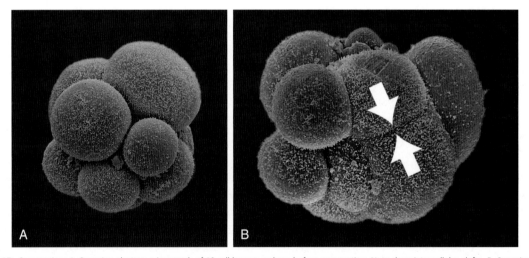

Figure 1-17. Compaction. *A,* Scanning electron micrograph of 10-cell human embryo before compaction. Note deep intercellular clefts. *B,* Scanning electron micrograph of 10-cell human embryo during process of compaction. Note absence of deep intercellular clefts between some of the blastomeres (arrows). The zona pellucida was mechanically removed from both embryos.

surfaces of the cells become convex and their inner surfaces become concave. This reorganization, called **compaction**, also involves changes in the blastomere cytoskeleton.

With compaction, some blastomeres segregate to the center of the morula and others to the outside. The centrally placed blastomeres are now called the **inner cell mass**, whereas the blastomeres at the periphery constitute the **trophoblast**. Because the inner cell mass gives rise to the embryo proper it is also called the **embryoblast**. The **trophoblast** is the primary source of the fetal component of the placenta (discussed in Ch. 2).

Morula Develops a Fluid-filled Cavity and Is Transformed into a Blastocyst

IN THE RESEARCH LAB

WHAT DETERMINES WHETHER A BLASTOMERE WILL FORM INNER CELL MASS OR TROPHOBLAST?

The "inside-outside" hypothesis explains the differentiation of blastomeres based on their position into either inner cell mass or trophoblast—more central cells of the morula become inner cell mass, and cells on the outside of the morula become trophoblast. But how does this differentiation occur? In the morula stage, two transcription factors (transcription factors are discussed in Ch. 5) are expressed uniformly throughout all blastomeres: *Oct4* (discussed earlier in the chapter) and *Nanog* (a homeobox-containing transcription factor). As the inner cell mass and trophoblast form, *Oct4* and *Nanog* expression is maintained in the inner cell mass, but both are turned off in the trophoblast. Loss-of-function experiments show that commitment of cells to the lineage of the inner cell mass requires the expression of these two transcription factors. Another transcription factor, *Cdx2* (like *Nanog*, also a homeobox-containing transcription factor), is expressed in the trophoblast as it is forming, as is the T box–containing transcription factor *Eomes* (also known as *Eomesodermin*). Loss-of-function experiments show that expression of these factors is required to downregulate expression of *Oct4* and *Nanog*. Collectively, these studies demonstrate that both expression of *Oct4* and *Nanog* in the inner cell mass and repression of expression of these two transcription factors in the trophoblast is required for the first overt differentiation event that occurs in the morula. Finally, the inner cell mass also expresses *Sox2*, an HMG box–containing factor highly related to SRY (discussed in Ch. 15). Experiments have shown that *Sox2/Oct4* regulate expression

of *Fgf4* protein in the inner cell mass, which is required for differentiation of the trophoblast. Thus, cell interactions occur between these two nascent populations of cells that are essential for specifying their fate.

By 4 days of development, the morula, consisting now of about 30 cells, begins to absorb fluid. Several processes seem to be involved. First, as the trophoblast differentiates it assembles into an epithelium in which adjacent cells are tightly adherent to one another. This adhesion results from the deposition on lateral cell surfaces of **E-CADHERIN**, a calcium-dependent cell adhesion molecule, and the formation of intercellular junctions, specifically, **tight junctions, gap junctions, adherens junctions**, and **desmosomes.** Second, forming trophoblast cells express a basally polarized membrane sodium/potassium ATPase (an energy-dependent ion-exchange pump), allowing them to transport and regulate the exchange of metabolites between the outside of the morula (i.e., the maternal environment of the oviduct) and the inside of the morula (i.e., toward the inner cell mass). The sodium/potassium ATPase pumps sodium into the interior of the morula, and water follows through osmosis to become blastocoelic fluid. As the hydrostatic pressure of the fluid increases, a large cavity called the **blastocyst cavity (blastocoel)** forms within the morula (see Fig. 1-16). The embryoblast cells (inner cell mass) then form a compact mass at one side of this cavity, and the trophoblast organizes into a thin, single-layered epithelium. The embryo is now called a **blastocyst**. The side of the blastocyst containing the inner cell mass is called the **embryonic pole** of the blastocyst, and the opposite side is called the **abembryonic pole.**

End of First Week: Initiating Implantation

Blastocyst Hatches from Zona Pellucida before Implanting

The morula reaches the uterus between 3 and 4 days of development. By day 5, the blastocyst hatches from the clear zona pellucida by enzymatically boring a hole in it and squeezing out (see Fig. 1-16). The blastocyst is now naked of all its original investments and can interact directly with the endometrium.

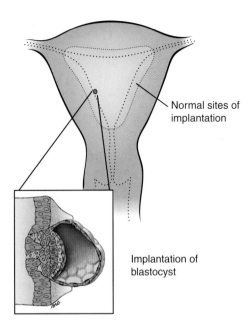

Normal sites of implantation

Implantation of blastocyst

Figure 1-18. Implantation. On about day 6.5 after fertilization, the trophoblast cells at the embryonic pole of the blastocyst proliferate to produce the syncytiotrophoblast, which is able to invade the uterine lining. The yellow area indicates normal sites of implantation in the uterine wall, and the enlargement shows the implanting blastocyst.

pregnancy). The corpus luteum continues to secrete sex steroids for 11 to 12 weeks of embryonic development, after which the placenta itself begins to secrete large amounts of progesterone and the corpus luteum slowly involutes, becoming a corpus albicans.

Implantation in Abnormal Site Results in Ectopic Pregnancy

Occasionally, a blastocyst implants in the peritoneal cavity, on the surface of the ovary, within the oviduct, or at an abnormal site in the uterus. The epithelium at these abnormal sites responds to the implanting blastocyst with increased vascularity and other supportive changes, so that the blastocyst is able to survive and commence development. These **ectopic pregnancies** often threaten the life of the mother because blood vessels that form at the abnormal site are apt to rupture as a result of growth of the embryo and placenta. Typically, ectopic pregnancy is revealed by symptoms of abdominal pain and/or vaginal bleeding. Drug (methyltrexate, which blocks rapid division) or surgical intervention is usually required to interrupt the pregnancy.

Very soon after arriving in the uterus, the blastocyst becomes tightly adherent to the uterine lining (Fig. 1-18). The adjacent cells of the endometrial stroma respond to its presence and to the progesterone secreted by the corpus luteum by differentiating into metabolically active, secretory cells called **decidual cells**. This response is called the **decidual reaction** (discussed in Ch. 6; see Fig. 6-2). The endometrial glands in the vicinity also enlarge, and the local uterine wall becomes more highly vascularized and edematous. It is thought that secretions of the decidual cells and endometrial glands include growth factors and metabolites that support growth of the implanting embryo.

The uterine lining is maintained in a favorable state and kept from sloughing partly by the progesterone secreted by the corpus luteum. In the absence of an implanted embryo, the corpus luteum normally degenerates after about 13 days. However, if an embryo implants, cells of the trophoblast produce the hormone **human chorionic gonadotropin (hCG)**, which supports the corpus luteum and thus maintains the supply of progesterone (**maternal recognition of**

IN THE CLINIC

CONTRACEPTION

Human Reproductive Efficiency Is Very High

An average couple who does not practice contraception and has intercourse twice a week (timed randomly with respect to ovulation) has a better than 50% chance of fertilizing any given oocyte. Because (as discussed above) about half of all embryos undergo spontaneous abortion, the chance that 1 month's intercourse will produce a term pregnancy is thus better than 25%. Healthy humans have astounding reproductive efficiency; it is not rare for couples who do not practice contraception to produce 10 to 20 offspring in a reproductive lifetime.

Contraception has played an important role in family planning for much of human history. Some of the oldest forms are simple **barrier contraceptives**, and these methods remain among the most frequently used today. Current contraceptive research focuses on developing strategies that interfere with many of the physiological mechanisms discussed earlier in this chapter that are required for successful conception.

Barrier Contraceptives Prevent Spermatozoa from Reaching Egg

One of the oldest types of contraceptive device is the **male condom**, originally made of animal bladders or sheep cecum and now made of latex rubber and often combined with a chemical spermicide. The male condom is fitted over the erect penis just before intercourse. The **female condom** is a polyurethane sheath that is inserted to completely line the vagina as well as the perineal area. Use of both the male and female condom can help prevent the spread of **sexually transmitted diseases (STDs)**. Other barrier devices, such as the **diaphragm** and **cervical cap**, are inserted into the vagina to cover the cervix and are usually used in conjunction with a spermicide. These must be fitted by a physician to determine the proper size. The **contraceptive sponge** is a spermicide-impregnated disc of polyurethane sponge that also blocks the cervix. Its advantage over the diaphragm and cervical cap is that the sponge does not need to be fitted by a physician because one size fits all.

Birth Control Pill Prevents Ovulation

Knowledge of the endocrine control of ovulation led to the introduction of the birth control pill ("the Pill") in the early 1960s. These early pills released a daily dose of estrogen, which inhibited ovulation by preventing secretion of the gonadotropic hormones FSH and LH from the pituitary. In modern pills, the estrogen dosage has been reduced, the progesterone analog **progestin** has been added, and the doses of estrogen and progestin are usually varied over a 21-day cycle. Although the normal function of progesterone is to support pregnancy through its effect on the endometrium, it also interferes with the release of FSH and LH, thus preventing ovulation. In addition, it prevents the cervical mucus from entering its midcycle phase of becoming thin and watery (which would allow spermatozoa to pass through it more readily) and the endometrium from thickening (in preparation for implantation), and it may also interfere with oocyte transport down the oviduct or with sperm capacitation.

Injected or Implanted Sources of Progesterone Deliver a Chronic Antiovulatory Dose

A **depot preparation** of medroxyprogesterone acetate (Depo-Provera) can be injected intramuscularly and will deliver antiovulatory levels of the hormone for 2 to 3 months. Alternatively, rods or capsules have been developed (Norplant or Implanon) that are implanted subdermally and release a synthetic form of progesterone (progestin) for a period of one to five years. Another alternative is the hormone patch (Ortho Evra), which can stay in place for a week, delivering both progesterone and estrogen transdermally. Other devices act by releasing the hormone into the female reproductive tract rather than the bloodstream. Progesterone-containing **intrauterine devices (IUDs)** emit low levels of progesterone for a period of 1 to 4 years. **Vaginal rings** are inserted and removed by the user and when in place around the cervix, release progestins continuously for 3 months.

Nonmedicated IUDs May Interfere with Conception through Effects on Both Sperm and Egg

The mechanism by which nonmedicated loop-shaped or T-shaped IUDs prevent conception when inserted in the uterus is unclear. Originally, they were thought to act by irritating the endometrium, resulting in an inflammatory reaction that prevented implantation of the conceptus. Because some people believe that preventing an embryo from implanting is an abortion (whereas others believe that an abortion involves removing an embryo that is already implanted), this potential mechanism of action creates ethical concerns for some people. It is now thought that IUDs act mainly by inhibiting sperm migration, ovum transport, and fertilization, rather than preventing implantation.

Antiprogesterone Compound RU-486 Is an Abortifacient

RU-486 (mifepristone) has potent antiprogesterone activity (its affinity for progesterone receptors is 5 times greater than that of endogenous progesterone) and may also stimulate prostaglandin synthesis. When taken within 8 weeks of the last menses, an adequate dose of RU-486 will initiate menstruation. If a conceptus is present, it will be sloughed along with the endometrial decidua. A large-scale French study in which RU-486 was administered along with a prostaglandin analog yielded an efficacy rate of 96%.

Sterilization Is Used by About One Third of American Couples

Sterilization of the male partner **(vasectomy)** or female partner **(ligation of the fallopian tubes)** is an effective method of contraception and is often chosen by people who do not want additional children. However, both methods involve surgery, and neither is reliably reversible.

How Effective is Contraception?

Sterilization and the use of hormonal contraceptives (such as the pill) have an annual pregnancy probability of from less than 1% to about 5%, whereas barrier contraception is less effective: the use of the male condom has an annual pregnancy probability of about 15%—equivalent to practicing the rhythm (natural family planning) method in which the couple practices abstinence in the days before, during, and after the expected time of ovulation; and the use of the diaphragm has an annual pregnancy probability of about

25%—equivalent to practicing the withdrawal method (coitus interruptus).

By 2020, about 16% of the world's population, or about 1.2 billion people, will enter their childbearing years, raising the issue that better contraceptive methods may need to be developed. Although new approaches are being tested, tough government regulations and concerns about liability and profitability (especially where the greatest demand for products will be in poor countries) is preventing most companies from striving to develop new contraceptive products. Contraceptive research had its heyday in the 1950s and 1960s, which resulted in a major breakthrough, the development of the birth control pill. However, similar breakthroughs have not occurred since, and contraceptive choices remain highly limited. For example, at the time the pill was introduced, men had only two choices for birth control: condoms and vasectomy. Some 50 years later, these are still the only choices.

ASSISTED REPRODUCTIVE TECHNOLOGY

About 1 in 6 couples have difficulty conceiving on their own. In about 30% of the cases the female is infertile, in about 30% the male is infertile, and in about 30% both the male and female are infertile. In another 10% of the cases whether the male or female (or both) is infertile is unknown. It is estimated that about 90% of the infertile couples can conceive with medical intervention. A variety of medical options are available to help couples conceive, including artificial insemination (AI) and hormonal therapies, which are the most common procedures. In vitro techniques also can be used to assist reproduction. These techniques are referred to as **assisted reproductive technology (ART)**, and they consist of **in vitro fertilization (IVF)** and **embryo transfer, intracytoplasmic sperm injection (ICSI), gamete intrafallopian transfer (GIFT)**, and **zygote intrafallopian transfer (ZIFT)**. Improved tissue culture techniques, including the use of defined culture media, have made it possible to maintain human gametes and cleavage-stage embryos outside the body. Gametes and embryos also can be successfully frozen **(cryopreserved)** and stored for later use, adding to the options for assisted reproduction.

Oocytes Can Be Fertilized In Vitro and Then Implanted in Uterus

The procedure of **in vitro fertilization (IVF)** and **embryo transfer** is widely used in cases in which scarring of the oviducts (a common consequence of pelvic inflammatory disease [PID], a serious complication of sexually transmitted diseases such as gonorrhea) prevents either the sperm from reaching the ampulla of the oviduct or the fertilized oocyte from passing to the uterus. In IVF, the woman's ovaries first are induced to **superovulate** (develop multiple mature follicles) by administration of an appropriate combination of hormones, usually human menopausal gonadotropin (hMG) or FSH, sometimes combined with clomiphene citrate—a drug that blocks the ability of hypothalamic cells to detect estrogen in the blood. In the presence of clomiphene citrate, hypothalamic cells respond to the perceived deficiency of estrogen by signaling the pituitary to release high levels of FSH, which stimulates follicles' growth and their secretion of estrogen. Once estrogen levels rise sufficiently, the pituitary gland rapidly releases LH, triggering maturation of oocytes. Sometimes to ensure that maturation of oocytes occurs, hCG is also given when follicles have attained optimal growth (determined by ultrasound examination of the ovaries and plasma estradiol concentration measurements).

Maturing oocytes are then harvested from the follicles, usually by using an ultrasonography-guided needle inserted via the vagina (transvaginal ultrasound–guided aspiration). Once retrieved, oocytes are allowed to mature in a culture medium to the second meiotic metaphase and are then fertilized with previously obtained and capacitated sperm (if obtained from the woman's partner, they are collected 2 hours before egg retrieval; if obtained from a sperm donor, they are obtained from a previously collected frozen aliquot). The resulting zygotes are allowed to develop in culture for about 48 hours and are then inserted (usually one or two) into the uterine cavity. IVF has increased our understanding of the earliest stages in human development, as embryos can be readily observed as they develop in vitro (Fig. 1-19).

Before the embryo is inserted into the uterine cavity, **assisted hatching** can be preformed in cases where the zona pellucida is tougher than normal and, consequently, make it more difficult for embryos to hatch. The zona pellucida ("shell") can be tougher in woman older than 40 or in younger woman who have a paucity of eggs. Assisted hatching involves making a small tear in the zona pellucida using acid tyrode solution, laser ablation, or mechanical means.

The first successful case of IVF occurred in 1978 with the birth of Louise Brown, the world's first "test-tube" baby. By the time of her 20th birthday, 300,000 IVF children had been born worldwide. By 2005, that number reached more than 1 million. On the average, IVF results in the delivery of a live baby in about 30% to 35% of the attempts (i.e., live births per egg retrieval; thus, to have 300,000 IVF children required about 1 million IVF conceptions). The success rate of IVF is remarkable considering that (as discussed above) for a normal healthy couple practicing unprotected intercourse, the successful pregnancy rate is about 25% per monthly cycle.

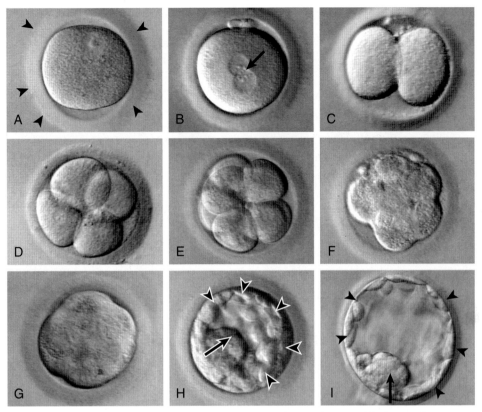

Figure 1-19. Human development in vitro. *A*, Ovulated secondary oocyte prior to introduction of sperm and fertilization. The oocyte containing its germinal vesicle is surrounded by the zona pellucida (arrowheads). *B*, Shortly after in vitro fertilization (IVF) the male and female pronuclei (arrow) have formed. *C*, Two-cell stage. *D*, Four-cell stage. *E*, Eight-cell stage. *F*, Morula initiating compaction. *G*, Compacted morula. *H*, Early blastocyst, with trophoblast (arrowheads) and inner cell mass (arrow). Hatching from the zona pellucida has not occurred. *I*, Hatched blastocyst, with trophoblast (arrowheads) and inner cell mass (arrow).

With IVF, preimplantation diagnosis of genetic conditions **(preimplantation genetic diagnosis, PGD)** can be performed using first or second polar bodies or blastomeres. These can be removed during IVF (Fig. 1-20), presumably without harm to further development, and then screened for aneuploidy or translocations with standard karyotypic analysis or FISH, and for mutations with techniques like the **polymerase chain reaction (PCR)**. PCR can be used to amplify DNA from a single cell, producing many copies for sequence analysis (eggs and embryos are stored until the diagnosis is made). Polar body diagnosis, unlike blastomere diagnosis, provides information about maternal contributions to the zygote but not paternal contributions, as polar bodies contain only maternal genes (i.e., they are formed by meiotic divisions of the oocyte). Hence, they are used only when the mother is at risk for transmitting a disease-causing mutation. If the mutation is found in a polar body, the assumption is made that the oocyte does *not* contain the mutation (if the rationale for this assumption is unclear, review meiosis). PGD offers the major advantage that it can be used to select only unaffected embryos for implanting, avoiding the later possibility of a selective termination of an affected pregnancy following prenatal diagnosis.

In cases in which a partner's spermatozoa are unable to penetrate the zona pellucida, a technique called **intracytoplasmic sperm injection (ICSI)** may be used. In this procedure, a single spermatozoon is selected under a microscope, aspirated into a needle, and injected into the oocyte cytoplasm (Fig. 1-21). In one recent study, children born after ICSI were twice as likely to have major congenital anomalies as children conceived naturally. Other risks for these children include an unbalanced chromosome complement (ICSI can damage the meiotic spindle,

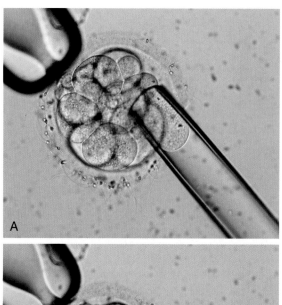

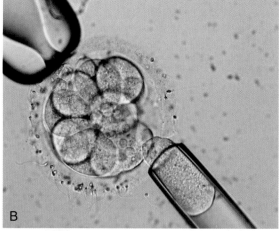

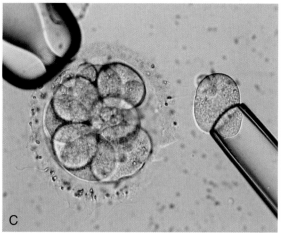

Figure 1-20. Human morula undergoing a blastomere biopsy. The temporal sequence is shown in order from top to bottom (*A-C*). The morula is held with a suction pipette and a hole is made in the zona pellucida. A micropipette is used to remove a selected blastomere by aspiration.

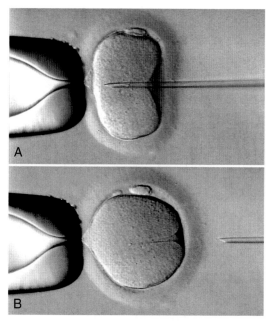

Figure 1-21. Intracytoplasmic sperm injection (ICSI). *A*, As the oocyte is held with a suction pipette, a micropipette, containing a single sperm, is used to penetrate the zona pellucida and oocyte. *B*, After pressure injection of the sperm, the micropipette is withdrawn, leaving a tract in the cytoplasm that soon disappears.

potentially leading to aneuploidy) and male infertility. Men with cystic fibrosis (CF), an autosomal recessive disease that affects breathing and digestion, also have congenital absence of the vas deferens and are, therefore, infertile. Using microsurgical epididymal sperm aspiration (MESA), sperm can be removed from the epididymis of CF men for use in IVF. However, such sperm are unable to fertilize an egg because they have not fully matured, a process that is completed during their passage through the epididymis and vas deferens. To overcome this problem ICSI can be used. The children born to fathers with CF using MESA and ICSI are normal CF carriers (to have CF, one must inherit a mutation in both the maternal and paternal chromosomes). Because absence of the vas deferens is associated with a mild form of CF that is otherwise asymptomatic, and tests for CF mutations detect only about 87% of the mutations, it is now recommended that both parents be genetically tested for CF mutations and appropriately counseled before using ICSI in cases in which the vas deferens is congenitally absent.

Gametes or Zygotes Can Be Introduced Directly into Ampulla of Oviduct

If the woman's oviduct is normal and the couple is infertile because of an innate deficiency in spermatozoon motility or for some other reason, a technique called **gamete intrafallopian transfer (GIFT)** is often used. Oocytes are harvested as described earlier and are then placed into a laparoscope catheter along with precapacitated spermatozoa. The oocytes and spermatozoa are introduced together directly into the ampulla of the oviduct, where fertilization takes place. Further development occurs by normal processes. In an alternative technique, **zygote intrafallopian transfer (ZIFT)**, the oocytes are fertilized in vitro, and only fertilized pronuclear zygotes are introduced into the ampulla.

ART in Perspective

In 1998 the following statistics were reported: in the United States, 60,000 births per year resulted from AI, 15,000 resulted from IVF, and at least 1,000 resulted from surrogacy arrangements (a couple arranges for another woman to carry their child to birth following IVF and implantation of an embryo in her uterine cavity). With about 4 million total births in the United States per year, the use of ART (IVF and IVF plus surrogacy) thus accounts for about 0.4% of all births in the United States. An infertile couple can choose to remain childless, undergo medical therapy including ART, or adopt a child. It was also reported in 1998 that only 30,000 healthy children were available for adoption in the United States. ART thus provides new opportunities for couples who choose not to be childless. ART is not without its risks, however: 37% of ART births are multiple as compared with 2% in the general population (risks associated with multiple births are discussed in Ch. 6), and ART increases pregnancy-related risks to woman, including preeclampsia, diabetes mellitus, bleeding, and anemia, as well as a possible risk of ovarian cancer owing to hormonal stimulation during ART. Moreover, ART-associated birth defects occur at a 1.4- to 2-fold higher rate than the overall rate of 3% to 4% of births in general.

Suggested Readings

Brinster RL. 2002. Germline stem cell transplantation and transgenesis. Science 296:2174-2176.

Cimini D, Degrassi F. 2005. Aneuploidy: a matter of bad connections. Trends Cell Biol 15:442-451.

Cooke HJ, Saunders PT. 2002. Mouse models of male infertility. Nat Rev Genet 3:790-801.

Eisenbach M, Tur-Kaspa I. 1999. Do human eggs attract spermatozoa? Bioessays 21:203-210.

Evans JP. 2001. Fertilin beta and other ADAMs as integrin ligands: insights into cell adhesion and fertilization. Bioessays 23:628-639.

Hackstein JH, Hochstenbach R, Pearson PL. 2000. Towards an understanding of the genetics of human male infertility: lessons from flies. Trends Genet 16:565-572.

Heard E. 2004. Recent advances in X-chromosome inactivation. Curr Opin Cell Biol 16:247-255.

Hemler ME. 2003. Tetraspanin proteins mediate cellular penetration, invasion, and fusion events and define a novel type of membrane microdomain. Annu Rev Cell Dev Biol 19:397-422.

Holden C. 2002. Research on contraception still in the doldrums. Science 296:2172-2173.

Inoue N, Ikawa M, Isotani A, Okabe M. 2005. The immunoglobulin superfamily protein Izumo is required for sperm to fuse with eggs. Nature 434:234-238.

ISLAT (Institute for Science Law, and Technology) Working Group. 1998. ART into science: regulation of fertility techniques. Science 281:651-652.

Johnson MH, Everitt BJ. 2000. Essential Reproduction. Oxford: Blackwell Science.

Jorde et al. 2006. Jorde LB, Carey JC, Bamshad MJ, White RL. 2006. Medical Genetics. 3rd. Edition, Updated Edition. St. Louis: Mosby.

Jungnickel MK, Sutton KA, Florman HM. 2003. In the beginning: lessons from fertilization in mice and worms. Cell 114:401-404.

Latham KE. 2005. X chromosome imprinting and inactivation in preimplantation mammalian embryos. Trends Genet 21:120-127.

Mader SS. 2005. Human Reproductive Biology. New York: McGraw Hill Higher Education.

Matzuk MM, Burns KH, Viveiros MM, Eppig JJ. 2002. Intercellular communication in the mammalian ovary: oocytes carry the conversation. Science 296:2178-2180.

McLaren A. 1998. Genetics and human reproduction. Trends Genet 14:427-431.

McLaren A. 2003. Primordial germ cells in the mouse. Dev Biol 262:1-15.

Pinon R. Jr. 2002. Biology of Human Reproduction. Sausalito, California: University Science Books p 535.

Primakoff P, Myles DG. 2002. Penetration, adhesion, and fusion in mammalian sperm-egg interaction. Science 296:2183-2185.

Raz E. 2003. Primordial germ-cell development: the zebrafish perspective. Nat Rev Genet 4:690-700.

Raz E. 2004. Guidance of primordial germ cell migration. Curr Opin Cell Biol 16:169-173.

Reeves RH, Baxter LL, Richtsmeier JT. 2001. Too much of a good thing: mechanisms of gene action in Down syndrome. Trends Genet 17:83-88.

Richards JS, Russell DL, Ochsner S, Espey LL. 2002. Ovulation: new dimensions and new regulators of the inflammatory-like response. Annu Rev Physiol 64:69-92.

Roberts RM, Ezashi T, Das P. 2004. Trophoblast gene expression: transcription factors in the specification of early trophoblast. Reprod Biol Endocrinol 2:47.

Runft LL, Jaffe LA, Mehlmann LM. 2002. Egg activation at fertilization: where it all begins. Dev Biol 245:237-254.

Saitou M, Barton SC, Surani MA. 2002. A molecular programme for the specification of germ cell fate in mice. Nature 418:293-300.

Schultz R, Williams C. 2005. Developmental biology: sperm-egg fusion unscrambled. Nature 434:152-153.

Schultz RM, Williams CJ. 2002. The science of ART. Science 296:2188-2190.

Shur BD, Ensslin MA, Rodeheffer C. 2004. SED1 function during mammalian sperm-egg adhesion. Curr Opin Cell Biol 16: 477-485.

Strich R. 2004. Meiotic DNA replication. Curr Top Dev Biol 61:29-60.

Strumpf D, Mao CA, Yamanaka Y, Ralston A, Chawengsaksophak K, Beck F, Rossant J. 2005. Cdx2 is required for correct cell fate specification and differentiation of trophectoderm in the mouse blastocyst. Development 132:2093-2102.

Tsuda M, Sasaoka Y, Kiso M, Abe K, Haraguchi S, Kobayashi S, Saga Y. 2003. Conserved role of nanos proteins in germ cell development. Science 301:1239-1241.

Warner CM, Brenner CA. 2001. Genetic regulation of preimplantation embryo survival. Curr Top Dev Biol 52:151-192.

Wylie C. 2000. Germ cells. Curr Opin Genet Dev 10:410-413.

Wylie C, Anderson R. 2002. Germ cells. Rossant J, Tam PPL, eds. Mouse Development. Patterning, Morphogenesis, and Organogenesis. San Diego: Academic Press pp 181-190.

Second Week: Becoming Bilaminar and Fully Implanting

2

Summary As discussed in the preceding chapter, the morula—formed by cleavage of the zygote—transforms during the 1st week into a blastocyst consisting of an inner cell mass, or embryoblast, and a trophoblast. At the beginning of the 2nd week, the embryoblast splits into two layers, the **epiblast** and the **hypoblast**, or **primitive endoderm**. A cavity, called the **amniotic cavity**, develops at the embryonic pole of the blastocyst between the epiblast and overlying trophoblast. It quickly becomes surrounded by a thin layer of cells derived from epiblast. This thin layer constitutes the lining of the **amnion**, one of the four **extraembryonic membranes**. The remainder of the epiblast and the hypoblast now constitute a **bilaminar embryonic disc**, or **bilaminar blastoderm**, lying between the amniotic cavity (dorsally) and the blastocyst cavity (ventrally). The cells of the embryonic disc develop into the **embryo proper** and also contribute to **extraembryonic membranes**. During the 2nd week, the hypoblast apparently send out two waves of migratory endodermal cells into the blastocyst cavity (blastocoel). The first of these waves forms the primary **yolk sac** (or the **exocoelomic membrane** or **Heuser's membrane**), and the second transforms the primary yolk sac into the secondary yolk sac.

In the middle of the 2nd week, the inner surface of the trophoblast and the outer surface of the amnion and yolk sac become lined by a new tissue, the **extraembryonic mesoderm**. A new cavity—the **extraembryonic coelom**, or **chorionic cavity**—develops as the extraembryonic mesoderm splits into two layers. With formation and splitting of the extraembryonic mesoderm, both the amnion and yolk sac (now sometimes called *definitive yolk sac*) become double-layered structures: amnion, consisting of ectoderm on the inside and mesoderm on the outside; and yolk sac, consisting of endoderm on the inside and mesoderm on the outside. In addition, the outer wall of the blastocyst is now called the **chorion**; like the amnion and yolk sac, it too contains a layer of mesoderm.

Meanwhile, implantation continues. The trophoblast differentiates into two layers: a cellular trophoblast, called the **cytotrophoblast**, and an expanding peripheral syncytial layer, the **syncytiotrophoblast**. These trophoblast layers contribute to the extraembryonic membranes, not to the embryo proper. The syncytiotrophoblast, cytotrophoblast, and associated extraembryonic mesoderm, together with the uterus, initiate formation of the **placenta**. During this process, the fetal tissues establish outgrowths, the **chorionic villi**, which extend into maternal **blood sinusoids**.

Many events occur in twos during the 2nd week. Thus, a "rule of twos" constitutes a handy mnemonic for remembering events of the 2nd week. During the 2nd week, the embryoblast splits into two layers, the epiblast and hypoblast. The trophoblast also gives rise to two tissues, the cytotrophoblast and syncytiotrophoblast. Two yolk sacs form, first the primary and then the secondary. Two new cavities form, the amniotic cavity and chorionic cavity. The extraembryonic mesoderm splits into the two layers that line the chorionic cavity, and the amnion, yolk sac, and chorion all become two-layered membranes.

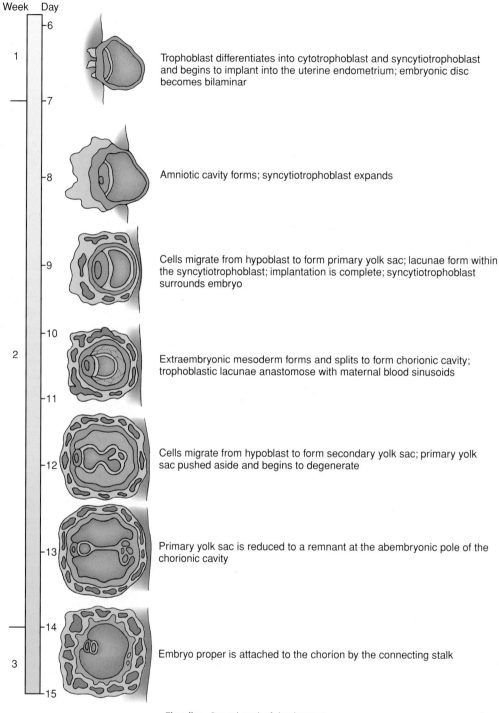

Week Day

1

6

Trophoblast differentiates into cytotrophoblast and syncytiotrophoblast and begins to implant into the uterine endometrium; embryonic disc becomes bilaminar

7

8

Amniotic cavity forms; syncytiotrophoblast expands

9

Cells migrate from hypoblast to form primary yolk sac; lacunae form within the syncytiotrophoblast; implantation is complete; syncytiotrophoblast surrounds embryo

2

10

Extraembryonic mesoderm forms and splits to form chorionic cavity; trophoblastic lacunae anastomose with maternal blood sinusoids

11

12

Cells migrate from hypoblast to form secondary yolk sac; primary yolk sac pushed aside and begins to degenerate

13

Primary yolk sac is reduced to a remnant at the abembryonic pole of the chorionic cavity

14

3

Embryo proper is attached to the chorion by the connecting stalk

15

Time line. Second week of development.

Clinical Taster   A 6-month old boy is referred by his primary care physician to University Hospital for genetic evaluation because of **failure to thrive**: both his weight-for-height and height-for-age fall below the third percentile for age as assessed using standard growth charts. His mother is 23 and his father is 29, and the boy is their first child. The woman became pregnant two months after stopping birth control (contraceptive sponge), and her pregnancy went smoothly with only a couple of weeks of mild morning sickness. She went into labor during the 39th week of gestation, but because labor progressed poorly and abnormal fetal heart rhythms were detected, her child was delivered by cesarean section 23 hours later.

At the child's 2-month well baby examination, his mother expressed concern that her baby didn't nurse well and seemed to have a weak cry. He also seemed not to move very much. On examination, the boy was somewhat small for his age and was hypotonic (had limp muscles). On a follow-up visit a few weeks later, the infant continued to show poor weight gain, and failure to thrive was diagnosed. To stimulate catch-up growth, the pediatrician recommended supplementing breast feeding with gavage feeding (feeding by tube) of high-calorie formula to achieve 150% of the caloric requirement for the boy's expected weight if it were at the 50th percentile.

Genetic testing occurred at 7 months. It revealed that the boy has a deletion of a portion of the long arm of chromosome 15, and he was diagnosed with **Prader-Willi syndrome**. The boy's parents are counseled about their son's prognosis and are given an information packet, which contains information about a local support group for parents of children with Prader-Willi syndrome. In meetings with the support group, they see other children of various ages with Prader-Willi, as well as their parents, and some children who are also said to have the same chromosomal deletion but who act very differently than their son. They are told that these children have a different syndrome called **Angelman syndrome**. Later, by searching the web, they find that both Prader-Willi syndrome and Angelman syndrome result from abnormalities in a process called **imprinting**, and that the difference in the two syndromes depends on whether the defect was inherited from the mother or father.

At 9 months of age, the boy is started on growth hormone replacement therapy, which has been shown to normalize height and increase lean muscle mass in children with Prader-Willi syndrome.

Becoming Fully Implanted

As described in Chapter 1, the blastocyst adheres to the uterine wall at the end of the first week. Contact with the uterine endometrium induces the trophoblast at the embryonic pole to proliferate. Some of these proliferating cells lose their cell membranes and coalesce to form a syncytium (a mass of cytoplasm containing numerous dispersed nuclei) called the **syncytiotrophoblast** (Fig. 2-1).

By contrast, the cells of the trophoblast that line the wall of the blastocyst retain their cell membranes and constitute the **cytotrophoblast**. The syncytiotrophoblast increases in volume throughout the 2nd week as cells detach from the proliferating cytotrophoblast at the embryonic pole and fuse with the syncytium (Figs. 2-2, 2-3).

Between days 6 and 9, the embryo becomes fully implanted in the endometrium. Proteolytic enzymes, including several metalloproteinases, are secreted by the cytotrophoblast to break down the extracellular matrix between the endometrial cells. Active finger-like processes extending from the syncytiotrophoblast then penetrate between the separating endometrial cells and pull the embryo into the endometrium of the uterine wall (see Figs. 2-1, 2-2). As implantation progresses, the expanding syncytiotrophoblast gradually envelops the blastocyst. By day 9, the syncytiotrophoblast blankets the entire blastocyst, except for a small region at the abembryonic pole (see Fig. 2-3). A plug of acellular material, called the **coagulation plug**, seals the small hole where the blastocyst implanted, temporarily marking this point in the endometrial epithelium.

IN THE RESEARCH LAB

WHAT REGULATES THE INITIAL PHASE OF IMPLANTATION: BLASTOCYST ADHERENCE TO THE UTERINE EPITHELIUM?

Prior to about 7 days postfertilization, both the blastocyst and the apical surface of the uterine epithelium are nonadhesive. Therefore, changes must occur in both the blastocyst and uterine epithelium to allow blastocyst attachment and the initiation of implantation.

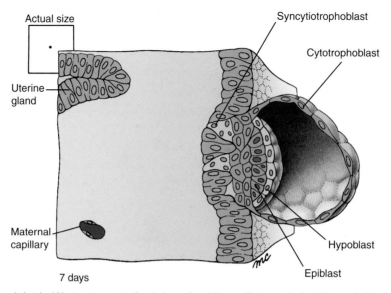

7 days

Figure 2-1. At 7 days, the newly hatched blastocyst contacts the uterine endometrium and begins to implant. The trophoblast at the embryonic pole of the blastocyst proliferates to form the invasive syncytiotrophoblast, which insinuates itself among the cells of the endometrium and begins to draw the blastocyst into the uterine wall. The embryonic disc is bilaminar, consisting of epiblast and hypoblast layers.

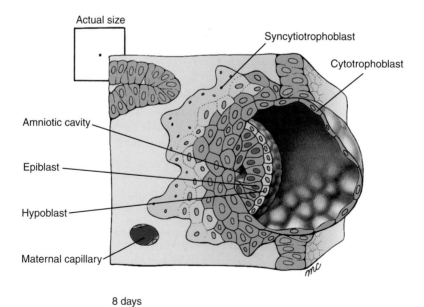

8 days

Figure 2-2. By 8 days, the amniotic cavity has formed within the epiblast. Implantation continues, and the growing syncytiotrophoblast expands to cover more of the blastocyst.

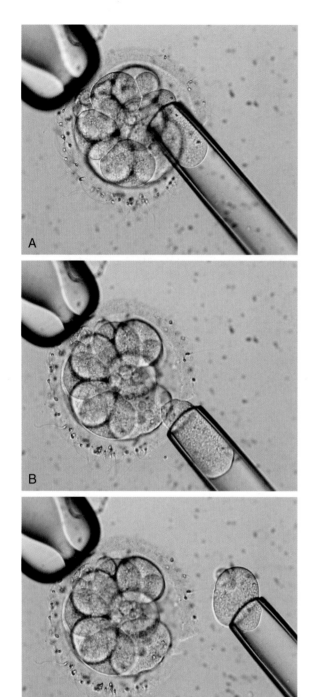

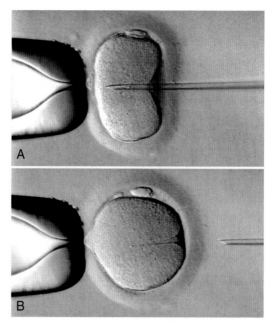

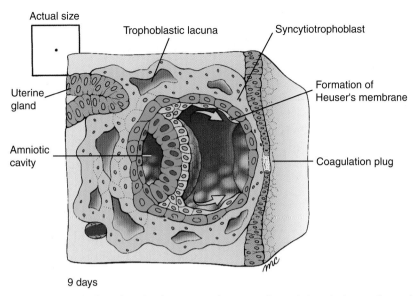

Actual size

Trophoblastic lacuna

Syncytiotrophoblast

Uterine gland

Formation of Heuser's membrane

Amniotic cavity

Coagulation plug

9 days

Figure 2-3. By 9 days, the embryo is completely implanted in the uterine endometrium. The amniotic cavity is expanding, and cells from the hypoblast have begun to migrate to form Heuser's membrane. Trophoblastic lacunae form in the syncytiotrophoblast, which now completely surrounds the embryo. The point of implantation is marked by a transient coagulation plug in the endometrial surface.

The uterus cycles through receptive and nonreceptive stages. As discussed in Chapter 1, entry into the receptive stage, during which implantation is possible, is controlled by estrogen and progesterone. As the uterus enters the receptive stage, its apical **glycocalyx** (a polysaccharide matrix surface coating of epithelial cells including—in the case of the uterine epithelium—abundant high–molecular-weight mucin glycoproteins) decreases in amount and negative charge. Moreover, apical **microvilli**, which are normally abundant, retract to establish a flattened surface in many areas of the epithelium, and large apical protrusions called **pinopodes** form.

The blastocyst undergoes a maturation from an attachment-incompetent stage to an attachment-competent stage. Although the presence of the nonadhesive zona pellucida prior to blastocyst hatching certainly prevents blastocyst attachment, experimental removal of the zona a few days earlier demonstrates that the blastocyst itself is still at the attachment-incompetent stage. As blastocysts mature to the attachment-competent stage, they express **Perlecan**, a **heparan sulfate proteoglycan**, on their surface. *Heparan sulfate proteoglycans* are known to have a high degree of specific binding to various extracellular matrix proteins and growth factor/cytokines, and thus could serve as attachment factors. A particularly intriguing finding, with respect to the role of *Perlecan* in attachment, is that the uterus at the time of implantation dramatically upregulates expression of **Heparin-binding Epidermal growth factor–like growth factor (Hb-Egf)** at implantation sites, presumably in response to blastocyst signaling. Studies have shown that binding of *Hb-Egf* to the blastocyst requires that the blastocyst expresses both the *Egf receptor* and *Heparan sulfate proteoglycan*. *Perlecan*-null mice do not exhibit defects in implantation, suggesting that *Perlecan* has functional redundancy with other *Heparan sulfate proteoglycans* that can substitute (or are compensatorily upregulated) in its absence.

In addition to *Heparan sulfate proteoglycans*, other factors possibly involved in adhesion include *Selectins* (a type of lectin—a sugar-binding protein), *αvß3* and *αvß5 Integrins* (transmembrane glycoproteins involved in adhesion and cell signaling; Ch. 5 provides more details), **metalloproteases** (enzymes that bind metal such as zinc and degrade proteins) and their inhibitors, **cytokines** (**Lif** and **Interleukin-11**) and a cell adhesion complex called **Trophinin-Tastin-Bystin**. Some of these latter factors (e.g., metalloproteases) play a role in trophoblast invasion of the endometrium in addition to possibly functioning in attachment.

WHY ISN'T CONCEPTUS REJECTED BY ITS MOTHER?

The conceptus, which expresses both maternal and paternal genes, can be considered as an allograft, that is, tissue transplanted from one member of a species to another member of the same species (such as from one human to another human). Allografts typically elicit an immune response in the host, resulting in rejection of the graft. In such a host-versus-graft reaction, peptides bound to major histocompatibility complex (MHC) molecules generate tissue alloantigens that are recognized by maternal T cells. Medawar proposed in 1953 three possibilities for why the developing conceptus is not rejected by its mother: fetal and maternal cells are physically separated from one another; the conceptus is antigenically immature; or the maternal immune system is suppressed or becomes tolerant to the conceptus during pregnancy.

It is likely that a combination of these possibilities prevents rejection of the conceptus. The trophoblast, which separates the actual tissues of the developing fetus from its mother, poorly expresses MHC molecules. Thus, the tissues are only partially separated and the conceptus is antigenically immature. However, there is evidence that maternal T cells are activated during pregnancy. Hence, because there is no complete cell-impermeable barrier between fetus and mother to prevent exposure of fetal alloantigens to maternal T cells (for example, fetal cells can be found in maternal blood during pregnancy, and maternal cells can be found in the fetus) and because fetal tissues are antigenic, it is likely that tolerogenic mechanisms block maternal T cell responses and prevent fetal rejection. The unique hormonal conditions of pregnancy that prepare the uterus for implantation and growth of the blastocyst apparently also induce tolerance. Such tolerance is specific for fetal antigens; for example, maternal antiviral immunity is not suppressed during pregnancy as shown in HIV+ women who do not suffer from AIDS-like disease during pregnancy.

One way in which tolerance to paternal antigens expressed by fetal tissue might occur is through the selective loss of maternal immune cells that respond to these antigens. For example, it has been proposed that maternal-activated T cells are induced to undergo apoptosis through the *Fas/Fasl* system. Trophoblast cells produce *Fasl*, a member of the *Tumor necrosis factor* (*Tnf*) and *Cd40* ligand family, which signals through the *Fas* receptor (also called *Cd95*, a membrane protein of the *Tnf* family). In support of this possibility, mice lacking functional *Fasl* display extensive leukocyte infiltrates at the placental-decidual interface, and deliver small litters.

In addition to a potential host-versus-graft reaction during pregnancy as just described, a graft-versus-host reaction could occur in which the fetus mounts an immune reaction against its mother. Why a graft-versus-host reaction

does not occur is unknown, but it is likely that the mother's immune system interacts with the conceptus either to prevent maturation of the fetus' immune system or to evoke tolerogenic mechanisms.

Embryoblast Reorganizes into Epiblast and Hypoblast

Even before implantation occurs, cells of the embryoblast begin to differentiate into two epithelial layers. By day 8, the embryoblast consists of a distinct external (or upper) layer of columnar cells, called the **epiblast**, and an internal (or lower) layer of cuboidal cells, called the **hypoblast**, or **primitive endoderm** (see Fig. 2-2). An extracellular basement membrane is laid down between the two layers as they become distinct. The resulting two-layered embryoblast is called the **bilaminar embryonic disc**, or **bilaminar blastoderm.** With formation of the bilaminar embryonic disc, the primitive **dorsal-ventral axis** of the embryo is defined (i.e., epiblast is dorsal, hypoblast is ventral).

IN THE RESEARCH LAB

INITIATING ENDODERM FORMATION

The hypoblast, or primitive endoderm, is the first layer to form from the inner cell mass. Studies mainly in Xenopus and zebrafish suggest that a series of factors initiate endoderm formation. These include a T-box–containing transcription factor (*VegT*), which activates *Nodal* (a member of the *Tgfβ* family of growth factors), which in turn induces expression of downstream transcriptional regulators (*Mixer*, a paired-homeobox–containing transcription factor; *Gata*, a zinc finger GATA-binding transcription factor). This in turn regulates expression of a relay of HMG-box–containing *Sox*-family transcription factors that ultimately result in the expression of *Sox17*, a critical factor in endoderm development.

The role of these genes in endoderm formation in mouse is less clear. Loss-of-function mutants of the mouse homolog of *VegT* (*Eomes*, also known as *Eomesodermin*) arrest very early in development, precluding analysis of their role in endoderm formation. *Nodal* loss-of-function mutants fail to form a primitive streak and node (discussed in Ch. 3), critical events in the genesis of not only endoderm but also mesoderm, so the exact role of *Nodal* in mouse endoderm formation is unclear. However, the use of a hypomorphic *Nodal* allele (i.e., a mutation in which *Nodal* expression is severely downregulated but not completely eliminated), as well as a *Cripto* loss-of-function mutation (*Cripto* is an essential cofactor required for *Nodal* signaling), provides more convincing evidence that *Nodal* signaling is required for endoderm formation. Additional loss-of-function mutations are consistent with a role for both *Mixer* and *Sox17* in mouse endoderm formation. Hence, in conclusion, it is likely that the same general cascade of factors initiate endoderm formation in all vertebrates.

Other loss-of-function studies in mouse suggest that at least four other transcription factors are required for endoderm formation and maintenance: *Gata6*, (a homeobox-containing transcription factor), *Hnf4* (a member of the steroid hormone *vHnf1* receptor family that functions as a ligand-activated transcriptional regulator), and *Foxa2* (a forkhead transcription factor previously known as *Hnf3β*). A regulatory hierarchy exists among some of these genes, with the first two factors (*Gata6* and *vHnf1*) regulating expression of *Hnf4*. *Foxa2* functions not only in formation of the endoderm but also in the formation of other lineages, such as the notochord and floor plate of the neural tube (discussed in Ch. 4). Interestingly, orthologs of these genes also function in endoderm formation in other organisms (e.g., the forkhead genes in Drosophila and the *Pha4* gene in *C. elegans* are orthologs of the *Hnf3* genes; *Serpent* in Drosophila and *End1* and *Elt2* in *C. elegans* are orthologs of *Gata* genes).

Development of Amniotic Cavity

The first new cavity to form during the 2nd week—the **amniotic cavity**—appears on day 8 as fluid begins to collect between cells of the epiblast and overlying trophoblast (see Fig. 2-2). A layer of epiblast cells expands toward the embryonic pole and differentiates into a thin membrane separating the new cavity from the cytotrophoblast. This membrane is the lining of the **amnion** (see Fig. 2-3), one of four extraembryonic membranes (i.e., amnion, chorion, yolk sac, and allantois; the first three are discussed below, and the allantois is discussed in later chapters). Although the amniotic cavity is at first smaller than the blastocyst cavity, it expands steadily. By the 8th week, the amnion encloses the entire embryo (discussed in Ch. 6).

Development of Yolk Sac and Chorionic Cavity

Proliferation of hypoblast cells, followed by two successive waves of cell migration, is believed to form the yolk sac membranes, which extend from the hypoblast into the blastocyst cavity. The first wave of migration begins on day 8 and forms the primary **yolk sac** (the **exocoelomic membrane**, or **Heuser's membrane**) {(Fig. 2-4; see Fig. 2-3)}. Simultaneously, the **extraembryonic mesoderm** forms, filling the remainder of the blastocyst cavity with loosely arranged cells (see Fig. 2-4). This early extraembryonic mesoderm is believed to originate in humans from the hypoblast/primary yolk sac, in contrast to the mouse embryo, where it arises from the caudal end of the incipient primitive streak; in addition, the trophoblast may contribute cells as well. By day 12, the primary yolk sac is displaced (and eventually degenerates) by the second wave of migrating hypoblast cells, which forms the secondary yolk sac (Figs. 2-5, 2-6). A new space—the **extraembryonic coelom**, or **chorionic cavity**—forms by splitting of the extraembryonic mesoderm into two layers. The extraembryonic coelom separates the embryo with its attached amnion and yolk sac from the outer wall of the blastocyst, now called the **chorion.** With splitting of the extraembryonic mesoderm into two layers, the amnion, yolk sac, and chorion all become two-layered structures, with the amnion and chorion being considered (based on comparative embryology) to consist of extraembryonic ectoderm and mesoderm, and the yolk sac, of extraembryonic endoderm and mesoderm. By day 13, the embryonic disc with its dorsal amnion and ventral yolk sac is suspended in the chorionic cavity solely by a thick stalk of extraembryonic mesoderm called the **connecting stalk** (see Fig. 2-6).

Traditionally, the *cavity* of the yolk sac has been labeled as yolk sac (or sometimes as the **exocoelomic cavity**) and its lining labeled as the exocoelomic membrane, or Heuser's membrane; this convention has been followed in this textbook. However, it should be remembered that, like the amnion, the yolk sac is an extraembryonic membrane that contains a cavity. Thus, the **definitive yolk sac**, formed after formation and splitting of the extraembryonic mesoderm, is a two-layered structure consisting of hypoblast-derived endoderm on the inside and mesoderm on the outside (examination of

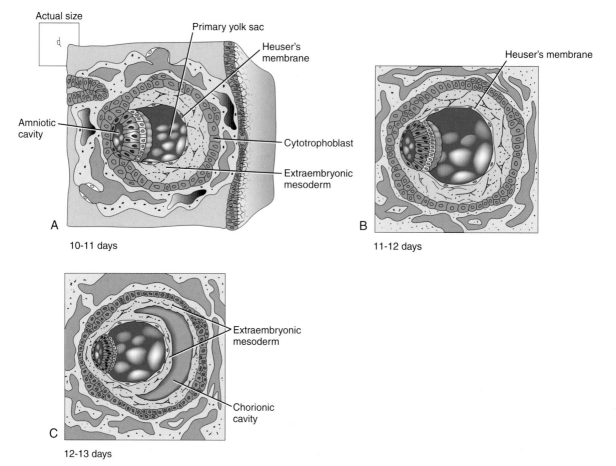

Figure 2-4. Extraembryonic mesoderm is formed in the middle of the 2nd week. *A,* On days 10 to 11, the space between Heuser's membrane and the cytotrophoblast becomes filled with loosely associated extraembryonic mesodermal cells. At the same time, the trophoblastic lacunae begin to anastomose with maternal capillaries and become filled with blood. *B,* On days 11 and 12, the extraembryonic mesoderm expands between the amnion and cytotropho-blast. *C,* By days 12 and 13, the extraembryonic mesoderm splits into two layers: one coating the outside of Heuser's membrane, and the other lining the inside of the cytotrophoblast. The space between the two layers is the chorionic cavity.

sections of the very few human embryos actually available for study at this stage makes it readily understandable why the origin of the yolk sac is uncertain; Fig. 2-7).

The definitive yolk sac remains a major structure associated with the developing embryo through the 4th week and performs important early functions. Extraembryonic mesoderm forming the outer layer of the yolk sac is a major site of **hematopoiesis** (blood formation; discussed in Ch. 13). Also, as described in Chapter 1, **primordial germ cells** can first be identified in humans in the wall of the yolk sac. After the 4th week, the yolk sac is rapidly overgrown by the developing embryonic disc. The yolk sac normally disappears before birth,

but on rare occasions it persists in the form of a digestive tract anomaly called **Meckel's diverticulum** (discussed in Ch. 14).

Uteroplacental Circulatory System Begins to Develop during Second Week

During the 1st week of development, the embryo obtains nutrients and eliminates wastes by simple diffusion. Rapid growth of the embryo makes a more efficient method of exchange imperative. This need is filled by the **uteroplacental circulation**—the system by which

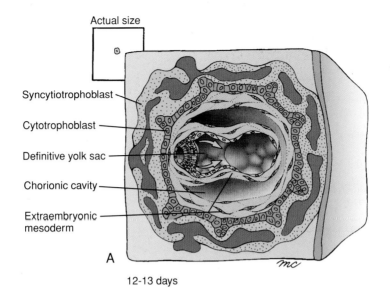

Actual size

Syncytiotrophoblast

Cytotrophoblast

Definitive yolk sac

Chorionic cavity

Extraembryonic mesoderm

A

12-13 days

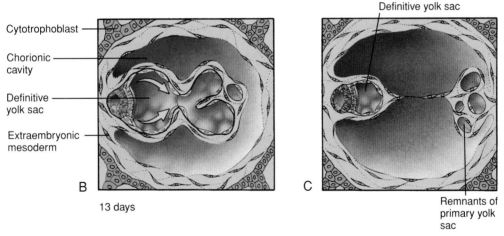

Cytotrophoblast

Chorionic cavity

Definitive yolk sac

Extraembryonic mesoderm

B

13 days

Definitive yolk sac

C

Remnants of primary yolk sac

Figure 2-5. *A*, On days 12 and 13, a second wave of migration of hypoblast cells produces a new membrane that migrates out over the inside of the extraembryonic mesoderm, pushing the primary yolk sac in front of it. This new layer becomes the endodermal lining of the secondary (definitive) yolk sac. *B, C*, As the definitive yolk sac develops on day 13, the primary yolk sac breaks up and is reduced to a collection of vesicles at the abembryonic end of the chorionic cavity.

maternal and fetal blood flowing through the **placenta** come into close proximity and exchange gases and metabolites by diffusion. This system begins to form on day 9 as vacuoles called **trophoblastic lacunae** open within the syncytiotrophoblast (see Fig. 2-3). Maternal capillaries near the syncytiotrophoblast then expand to form **maternal sinusoids** that rapidly anastomose with the trophoblastic lacunae

(see Figs. 2-4*A*, 2-8*A*). Between days 11 and 13, as these anastomoses continue to develop, the cytotrophoblast proliferates locally to form extensions that grow into the overlying syncytiotrophoblast (see Figs. 2-5*A*, 2-8*A*). The growth of these protrusions is thought to be induced by the underlying newly formed extraembryonic mesoderm. These extensions of cytotrophoblast grow out into the blood-filled lacunae, carrying

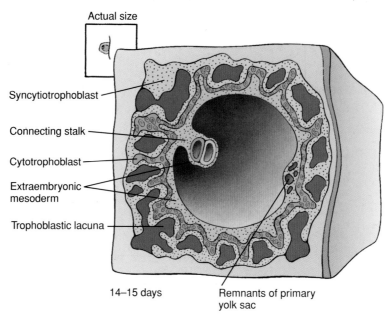

Actual size

Syncytiotrophoblast

Connecting stalk

Cytotrophoblast

Extraembryonic
mesoderm

Trophoblastic lacuna

14–15 days

Remnants of primary
yolk sac

Figure 2-6. By the end of the second week, the definitive yolk sac loses contact with the remnants of the primary yolk sac, and the bilaminar embryonic disc with its dorsal amnion and ventral yolk sac is suspended in the chorionic cavity by a thick connecting stalk.

with them a covering of syncytiotrophoblast. The resulting outgrowths are called **primary chorionic stem villi** (Fig. 2-8*A*).

It is not until day 16 that the extraembryonic mesoderm associated with the cytotrophoblast penetrates the core of the primary stem villi, thus transforming them into **secondary chorionic stem villi** (Fig. 2-8*B*). By the end of the 3rd week, this villous mesoderm has given rise to blood vessels that connect with the vessels forming in the embryo proper, thus establishing a working uteroplacental circulation (as discussed in Ch. 12, the primitive heart starts beating on day 22). Villi containing differentiated blood vessels are called **tertiary chorionic stem villi** (Fig. 2-8*C*). As can be seen from Figure 2-8*C*, the gases, nutrients, and wastes that diffuse between the maternal and fetal blood must cross four tissue layers:

- The endothelium of the villus capillaries
- The loose connective tissue in the core of the villus (extraembryonic mesoderm)
- A layer of cytotrophoblast
- A layer of syncytiotrophoblast

The endothelial lining of the maternal sinusoids does not invade the trophoblastic lacunae, so a maternal layer does not need to be crossed. Further differentiation of

the placenta and stem villi during fetal development is discussed in Chapter 6.

IN THE CLINIC

HYDATIDIFORM MOLES
Complete Hydatidiform Mole Is a Pregnancy without an Embryo

In a normal pregnancy, the embryoblast gives rise to the embryo, and the trophoblast gives rise to the fetal component of the placenta. However, in approximately 0.1% to 0.5% of pregnancies, the fetus is entirely missing, and the conceptus consists only of placental membranes. A conceptus of this type is called a **complete hydatidiform mole** (Fig. 2-9). Because the fetal vasculature that would normally drain the fluid taken up from the maternal circulation is absent, the placental villi of a complete mole are swollen and vesicular, resembling bunches of grapes ("hydatid" is from the Greek *hydatidos*, drop of water). Complete moles often abort early in pregnancy. If they do not abort, the physician may discover them because they result in vaginal bleeding, especially during the 6th to 16th weeks of pregnancy, and they often cause excessive nausea and vomiting (owing to elevated human chronic gonadotropin, hCG). Like normal trophoblastic tissue, moles

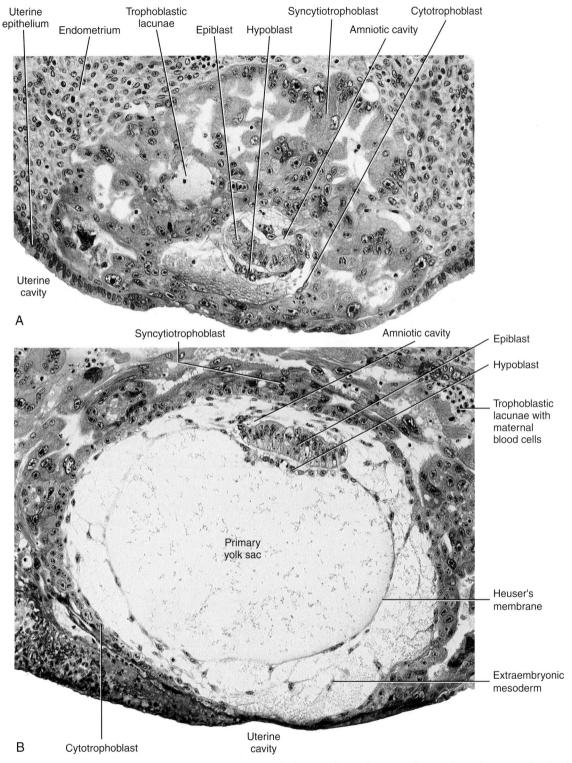

Figure 2-7. *A*, 9-day human embryo at the stage of amnion formation. *B*, 12-day human embryo with primary yolk sac. Both *A* and *B* are reproduced at about the same magnification, illustrating the rapid growth that occurs in the embryo in just 3 days.

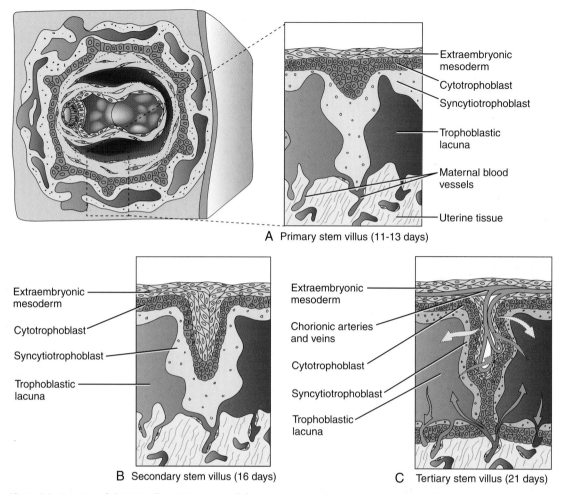

A Primary stem villus (11-13 days)

Extraembryonic mesoderm
Cytotrophoblast
Syncytiotrophoblast
Trophoblastic lacuna
Maternal blood vessels
Uterine tissue

Extraembryonic mesoderm
Cytotrophoblast
Syncytiotrophoblast
Trophoblastic lacuna

B Secondary stem villus (16 days)

Extraembryonic mesoderm
Chorionic arteries and veins
Cytotrophoblast
Syncytiotrophoblast
Trophoblastic lacuna

C Tertiary stem villus (21 days)

Figure 2-8. Formation of chorionic villi. *A*, Primary stem villi form on days 11 to 13 as cytotrophoblastic proliferations that bud into the overlying syncytio-trophoblast. *B*, By day 16, the extraembryonic mesoderm begins to proliferate and invade the center of each primary stem villus, transforming each into a secondary stem villus. *C*, By day 21, the mesodermal core differentiates into connective tissue and blood vessels, forming the tertiary stem villi.

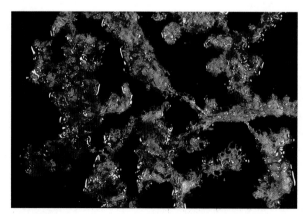

Figure 2-9. This complete, hydatidiform mole has been "dissected" to show the clear, swollen villi characteristic of these structures.

secrete hCG. Moles and mole remnants are readily diagnosed on the basis of an abnormally high level of plasma hCG.

Molar pregnancies are more common in women at the extremes of reproductive age: women in their early teenage or perimenopausal years have the highest risk. Also, the risk for molar pregnancy (including choriocarcinoma; discussed below), is up to 15 times higher for women of African or Asian ethnicity.

Definitive identification of hydatidiform moles requires cytogenetic analysis. Chromosome analysis has shown that even though the cells of a complete mole have a normal, diploid karyotype, all chromosomes are derived from the father. Further studies demonstrated that this situation usually arises in one of two ways (Fig. 2-10). Two spermatozoa may fertilize an oocyte that lacks (or loses) its own nucleus **(dispermic fertilization)**, and the two male pronuclei may then fuse to form a diploid nucleus. Alternatively, if a single spermatozoon inseminates an oocyte that lacks (or loses) its own nucleus **(monospermic fertilization)**, the resulting male pronucleus may undergo an initial mitosis (doubling its DNA) without cytokinesis (division of the single cell into two cells) to produce a diploid nucleus, which duplicates its DNA once again before the first

cleavage occurs. Complete moles produced by *dispermic* fertilization may have either a 46,XX or 46,XY karyotype. All complete moles produced by *monospermic* fertilization, in contrast, are 46,XX, because 46,YY zygotes lack essential genes located on the X chromosome and cannot develop. Karyotyping surveys show that most (90%) complete hydatidiform moles are 46,XX, indicating that monospermic fertilization is the dominant mode of production.

Rarely, complete moles can have chromosomes derived from both maternal and paternal chromosomes (biparental in origin). This occurs when imprinting of maternal genes is lost from the ovum (discussed in the following In the Research Lab under Genomic Imprinting), resulting in the functional equivalent of two paternal genomes. This type of complete mole is recurrent and is inherited as an autosomal recessive trait. A candidate region for this trait has been identified on the long arm of chromosome 19.

Partial Hydatidiform Moles Are Usually Triploid, with a Double Dose of Paternal Chromosomes, and Show Partial Development of an Embryo

In contrast to the complete hydatidiform mole, some evidence of embryonic development is usually found in **partial hydatidiform moles**. Even if no embryo remnant can

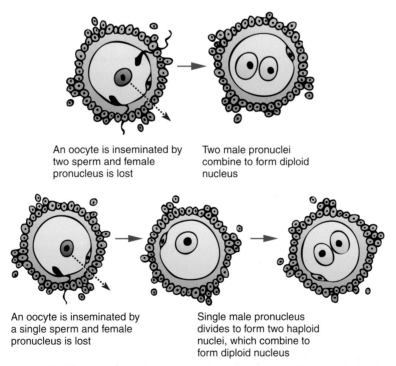

An oocyte is inseminated by two sperm and female pronucleus is lost

Two male pronuclei combine to form diploid nucleus

An oocyte is inseminated by a single sperm and female pronucleus is lost

Single male pronucleus divides to form two haploid nuclei, which combine to form diploid nucleus

Figure 2-10. Formation of complete hydatidiform mole. A complete mole is produced when an oocyte that has lost its female pronucleus acquires two male pronuclei. Two mechanisms are shown.

be found at the time the mole aborts or is delivered, the presence of typical nucleated embryonic erythroblasts in the molar villi, and the presence of fetal blood vessels, indicates that an embryo was present. On rare occasions, an abnormal fetus is delivered. The swollen villi that are the hallmark of a complete mole are present only in patches, and the clinical symptoms that indicate a molar pregnancy (discussed above) are usually milder and slower to develop than in the case of complete moles. Spontaneous abortion usually does not occur until the second trimester (4 to 6 months).

Karyotype analysis indicates that conceptuses of this type are usually triploid (69,XXX; 69,XXY; or 69,XYY), with two sets of chromosomes from the father. Studies have shown that these moles result from the insemination of an oocyte containing a female pronucleus by two spermatozoa or possibly by a single abnormal diploid sperm (Fig. 2-11).

Hydatidiform Moles Can Give Rise to Persistent Trophoblastic Disease or to Choriocarcinoma

Residual trophoblastic tissue remaining in the uterus after spontaneous abortion or surgical removal of a hydatidiform mole may give rise to a condition known as **persistent trophoblastic disease**, in which the mole remnant grows to form a tumor. Tumors arising from partial moles are usually benign. When tumors arising from complete moles become malignant, they may grow either as an **invasive mole** or as metastatic **choriocarcinoma**. Choriocarcinomas derived from moles are rare, occurring in 1 in 40,000 pregnancies. All forms of persistent mole, benign and malignant, secrete high levels of hCG.

Not long ago, the mortality rate for patients with invasive moles was about 60%, and the mortality for choriocarcinoma was approximately 100%. Today, surgery plus chemotherapy if needed has resulted in a cure rate for nonmetastatic and low-risk metastatic disease that approaches 100%, whereas the cure rate for high-risk metastatic disease is about 80% to 90%.

Cytogenetic analysis of hydatidiform moles supports the hypothesis (called the **genetic-conflict hypothesis**) that the paternal genetic complement is responsible for early development of the placenta and the maternal genetic complement is responsible for early development of the embryo. Experiments that both confirm this hypothesis and reveal molecular differences between the paternal and maternal chromosomes are discussed in the following section.

IN THE RESEARCH LAB

GENOMIC IMPRINTING
Maternal Chromosomes Regulate Embryoblast Development, and Paternal Chromosomes Regulate Trophoblast Development

As discussed in the preceding section, cytogenetic analyses of human hydatidiform moles suggest that the maternal and paternal genome complements play different roles in early development. These roles have been studied with mouse oocytes experimentally manipulated to contain either two male pronuclei (androgenotes) or two female pronuclei (gynogenotes). Oocytes of this type can be produced in several ways. Fertilized mouse oocytes can be removed from the ampulla of the oviduct at the pronuclear stage of development and held by light suction at the end of a glass pipette. Either the female pronucleus or the somewhat larger male pronucleus can then be removed with a very fine pipette and replaced with a pronucleus of the opposite type. Another technique involves removing the male or female pronucleus from a fertilized oocyte and then blocking cleavage with an appropriate blocking agent while a single mitosis takes place, thus producing a diploid zygote. Removing the female pronucleus from an unfertilized oocyte and fertilizing the

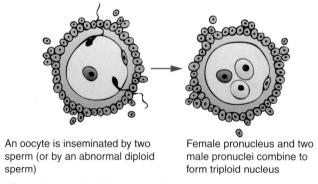

An oocyte is inseminated by two sperm (or by an abnormal diploid sperm)

Female pronucleus and two male pronuclei combine to form triploid nucleus

Figure 2-11. A partial hydatidiform mole is produced when a normal oocyte acquires two male pronuclei (or a diploid male pronucleus).

enucleated oocyte with an abnormal diploid sperm can also be used to produce oocytes with two male pronuclei.

When an experimental zygote containing two male pronuclei (possessing between them at least one X chromosome) is implanted into a pseudopregnant female mouse, it develops as trophoblast and gives rise to a mass of placental membranes resembling a human hydatidiform mole. Very rarely, an embryo forms and develops to a stage comparable to approximately the 3-week stage of human development. In contrast, zygotes containing two female pronuclei develop as small but recognizable embryos with reduced placental membranes. These gynogenic (or **parthenogenic;** both terms refer to development in the absence of fertilization, or in the absence of a male pronucleus) embryos never survive to term. It is important to emphasize that these developmental patterns do not depend on the sex chromosomes present in the zygote (XX or XY), but only on the sex of the parent from whom the genome is inherited.

Early Gene Expression and Genomic Imprinting

What mechanism underlies the independent expression of maternal and paternal genomes during early development? One way that this question was approached was by studying expression of a marker viral oncogene, the *Myc* oncogene, which was introduced into a line of *transgenic* mice (mice whose genome contains a foreign DNA sequence; discussed in Ch. 5). In theory, mice carrying this integrated transgene should express its gene product when appropriately stimulated. However, it was found that the gene product formed only when the gene had been inherited from the father, not when it had been inherited from the mother. Further investigation revealed an important difference between DNA of the male and female germ line cells: the DNA of the female germ line was more highly **methylated** (carries more methyl groups) than the DNA of the male germ line.

Further investigations were done with several different lines of transgenic mice carrying foreign transgenes at various locations in the genome. In cases where these transgenes showed a characteristic "male" or "female" degree of methylation, the pattern of methylation displayed in the somatic cells depended on the parent from which the gene had been inherited. Thus, a transgene showed the female pattern of methylation in the somatic cells of both sons and daughters if it was inherited from the mother. However, when one of these sons passed the gene to his offspring, their somatic cells showed the male pattern of methylation. The analogous reversal of methylation patterns also occurs when a grandfather's transgene is transmitted to grandchildren through a daughter.

Genomic imprinting is the process by which genes are imprinted, that is, marked so that rather than being expressed biallelically (i.e., from both maternal and paternal alleles contributed to the zygote during fertilization), they are expressed from only one allele in a parent-specific manner. One of the main ways that this marking occurs is through methylation of DNA. In addition to marking exogenously introduced transgenes as discussed above, methylation marks endogenous genes, particularly several genes implicated in regulation of intrauterine growth. About 80 imprinted genes have been identified and most are clustered. This allows groups of genes to be coordinately imprinted through specialized chromosomal regions called **imprinting centers**.

The first two imprinted endogenous genes to be discovered were *Igf2* (*Insulin-like growth factor 2*) and its receptor, *Igf2r*. Because of imprinting, the *Igf2* allele inherited from the father is expressed in the embryo and adult, whereas the allele inherited from the mother is silenced. By contrast, the *Igf2r* allele inherited from the mother is expressed, whereas the allele inherited from the father is silenced. Imprinting occurs only in viviparous mammals, that is mammals in which the fetus develops in utero (imprinting does not occur in egg-laying mammals). Imprinting is hypothesized to mediate a tug-of-war between maternal and paternal alleles. This hypothesis, the **genetic-conflict hypothesis** (or viviparity-driven conflict hypothesis), proposes that in polyandrous mammals (having multiple partners) there is a conflict between males and females over the allocation of maternal resources to offspring (in the hypothesis, the fetus is viewed as a parasite that competes with the mother and her future litters for resources). Fathers favor providing maximal resources for their offspring, at the expense of mothers and future offspring who may be fathered by other males. Mothers favor providing equal resources among all their litters. The outcome for this tug-of-war is that a compromise occurs in growth rate.

In support of the genetic-conflict hypothesis, loss-of-function mutations of mouse *Igf2* (a paternally expressed gene as discussed above) result in a 40% reduction in growth, whereas mutations in *Igf2r* result in oversized offspring. Further support comes for double mutants: loss of both *Igf2* and *Igf2* result in normal-sized mice.

The sites of DNA methylation during imprinting are often stretches of alternating cytosine and guanosine bases (so-called **CpG islands**; p indicates that C and G are joined by a phosphodiester bond). Because CpG islands can be located around gene promoters, methylation of CpG islands often leads to gene silencing or activation. Methylation imprints go through a life cycle (Fig. 2-12). In the embryo, imprinted

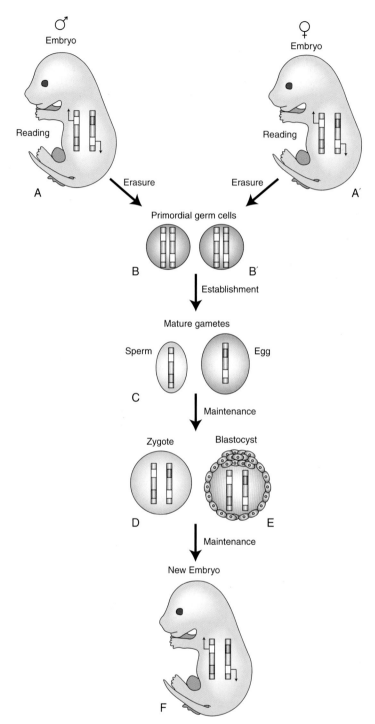

Figure 2-12. Three stages (erasure, establishment, and maintenance) in the life cycle of methylation imprints. *A, A'*, In the somatic (body) tissues of the embryo, imprinted genes are expressed from only one allele in a parent-specific manner. One chromosome pair is illustrated containing two imprinted genes (chromosome containing red mark was inherited from the mother, and blue mark from the father). In this example, methylated genes, indicated by the dark color, are silenced; therefore, the other allele of each gene is transcribed (arrows). *B, B'*, This pattern of genomic imprinting is erased in the embryo's primordial germ cells. *C*, Imprinting is established during gametogenesis (which begins in the embryo and is completed in the adult). *D, E, F*, From fertilization onward in development, imprinting is maintained.

genes are expressed in a parent-specific manner. But in primordial germ cells, imprints are erased. During gametogenesis, imprints are once again established, so that in the males undergoing spermatogenesis, the male-specific pattern is established (that is, the pattern of its father), whereas in females, the female-specific pattern is established (that is, the pattern of its mother). After fertilization, the parent-specific patterns are maintained in the new individual (except for in his or her primordial germ cells, where erasure once again occurs).

X INACTIVATION

To compensate for the presence of only one X chromosome in the cells of males (46,XY), one of the two active X chromosomes in each cell of the female blastocyst (46,XX) is stably inactivated (the process of **dosage compensation**). The inactivation is random with respect to the parental source of the X chromosome in the embryoblast (and is, therefore, not an example of imprinting), but only paternally derived X chromosomes are inactivated in the trophoblast (an example of imprinting). Inactivation of X chromosomes in female embryos requires expression of a specific X chromosome locus, the *Xist* (X inactive specific transcript gene) locus, which produces a large RNA, with no protein-coding capacity, that remains associated with ("coats") the chromosome. Moreover, the expression of *Xist* leads to the methylation of CpG islands at the 5' ends of the inactivated genes on this chromosome. The inactivated X chromosome also lacks histone H4 acetylation, and, ultimately, the chromosome condenses into a recognizable structure called a **Barr body**. Although this X chromosome remains inactive in all somatic cells of the female, inactivated X chromosomes in the oogonia of the female germ line are reactivated during early fetal life. Thus, the male zygote obtains a single active X chromosome from the mother, and the female zygote obtains two active X chromosomes, one from the mother and one from the father. Both of the X chromosomes in each cell of the early female embryo then remain active until one of them is again inactivated at the blastocyst stage (as discussed above).

IN THE CLINIC

X INACTIVATION AFFECTS INHERITANCE OF CONGENITAL DISEASE

One consequence of random X inactivation in female cells is that all females are **genetic mosaics**. Some cells express only the X-linked genes inherited from the mother, and some cells express only X-linked genes inherited from the father. Thus, in cases in which the female offspring inherits a *recessive* X-linked mutation from one parent and a wild-type allele from the other, she does not exhibit symptoms of the disease because of compensation by cells in her body that express the wild-type allele. This individual is called a **silent carrier**; she may transmit the disease to her sons (who inherit the X that carries the mutated gene). Examples of such X-linked recessive disease include **Duchenne muscular dystrophy** and **Simpson-Golabi-Behmel syndrome**. Duchenne muscular dystrophy results from a mutation in the gene encoding *DYSTROPHIN*. This mutation causes progressive dystrophy and degeneration of myofibers of skeletal or cardiac muscle, and mild mental retardation. Simpson-Golabi-Behmel syndrome results in some cases from a mutation in the gene for *GLYPICAN-3* gene. This mutation causes a protruding jaw, broad nasal bridge, short hands and fingers, heart defects, renal defects, and hypogonadism.

Offspring who inherit a *dominant* X-linked mutation from one parent exhibit some symptoms of the disease, regardless of their gender, because the expression of the wild-type allele in other cells cannot fully compensate. These include diseases such as **Goltz syndrome** (skin atrophy and skeletal malformations) and **incontinentia pigmenti** (spotty pigmentation); a gene has not been identified for either of these diseases.

GENOMIC IMPRINTING AFFECTS INHERITANCE OF CONGENITAL DISEASE

The pattern of inheritance of some human genetic disease is also dependent on **imprinting differences** in male and female *autosomes*. For example, deletions in a region of human chromosome 15 (15q11.2–q13) result in **Prader-Willi syndrome** when inherited from the father and **Angelman syndrome** when inherited from the mother. These two syndromes are characterized by vastly different symptoms. Symptoms of Prader-Willi syndrome include feeding problems in infancy and rapid weight gain in childhood, hypogonadism, and mild mental retardation. Symptoms of Angelman syndrome include developmental delay, speech and balance disorders, and a unique happy demeanor. Many imprinted genes are located in the 15q11.2–q13 region of chromosome 15, including the imprinting center (IC) that controls the imprinting of imprinted genes in the 15q11.2–q13 region. Most cases of Prader-Willi syndrome and Angelman syndrome result from large deletions in the 15q11.2–q13 region of chromosome 15. However, specific mutations of the IC in the paternally inherited chromosome cause Prader-Willi syndrome, whereas mutations of the maternal IC gene cause Angelman syndrome. A small percentage of the cases of Prader-Willi syndrome result from maternal uniparental disomy of chromosome 15, whereas a small percentage of the cases of Angelman syndrome result from paternal uniparental disomy of chromosome 15. **Uniparental disomy** is a condition in which both chromosomes of a given pair are inherited from the same parent.

The development of several congenital **overgrowth syndromes** also results from abnormal imprinting of human autosomes. For example, translocations, duplications, or mutations of human chromosome 11p15 may lead to altered expression of *INSULIN-LIKE GROWTH FACTOR* 2 *(Igf2)* and other genes causing **Beckwith Wiedemann syndrome**, a syndrome characterized by macrosomia (large body), renal abnormalities, and embryonal tumors. Disruption of normal imprinting may also lead to the development of cancers, including **renal (Wilms' tumor) colon**, and **cervical carcinoma**.

Suggested Readings

Ben-Porath I, Cedar H. 2000. Imprinting: focusing on the center. Curr Opin Genet Dev 10:550-554.

Brockdorff N. 1998. The role of Xist in X-inactivation. Curr Opin Genet Dev 8:328-333.

Carrel L, Willard HF. 2005. X-inactivation profile reveals extensive variability in X-linked gene expression in females. Nature 434:400-404.

Carson DD, Bagchi I, Dey SK, et al. 2000. Embryo implantation. Dev Biol 223:217-237.

Eakin GS, Behringer RR. 2004. Gastrulation in other mammals and humans. In: Stern CD, editor. Gastrulation. From Cells to Embryo. Cold Spring Harbor, New York: Cold Spring Harbor Laboratory Press. pp 275-287.

El-Maarri O, Seoud M, Coullin P, Herbiniaux U, et al. 2003. Maternal alleles acquiring paternal methylation patterns in biparental complete hydatidiform moles. Hum Mol Genet 12:1405-1413.

Fan JB, Surti U, Taillon-Miller P, et al. 2002. Paternal origins of complete hydatidiform moles proven by whole genome single-nucleotide polymorphism haplotyping. Genomics 79:58-62.

Grapin-Botton A, Constam D. 2004. Endoderm development. In: Stern CD, editor. Gastrulation. From Cells to Embryo. Cold Spring Harbor, New York: Cold Spring Harbor Laboratory Press. pp 433-448.

Gunter C. 2005. Genome biology: she moves in mysterious ways. Nature 434:279-280.

Huynh KD, Lee JT. 2005. X-chromosome inactivation: a hypothesis linking ontogeny and phylogeny. Nat Rev Genet 6:410-418.

Jiang Y, Lev-Lehman E, Bressler J, et al. 1999. Genetics of Angelman syndrome. Am J Hum Genet 65:1-6.

Jiang Y, Tsai TF, Bressler J, Beaudet AL. 1998. Imprinting in Angelman and Prader-Willi syndromes. Curr Opin Genet Dev 8:334-342.

Kanellopoulos-Langevin C, Caucheteux SM, Verbeke P, Ojcius DM. 2003. Tolerance of the fetus by the maternal immune system: role of inflammatory mediators at the feto-maternal interface. Reprod Biol Endocrinol 1:121.

Krugman SD, Dubowitz H. 2003. Failure to thrive. Am Fam Physician 68:879-884.

Mellor AL, Munn DH. 2000. Immunology at the maternal-fetal interface: lessons for T cell tolerance and suppression. Annu Rev Immunol 18:367-391.

Melton L. 2000. Womb wars. Sci Am 283:24-26.

Nicholls RD, Knepper JL. 2001. Genome organization, function, and imprinting in Prader-Willi and Angelman syndromes. Annu Rev Genomics Hum Genet 2:153-175.

Ohlsson R, Paldi A, Graves JA. 2001. Did genomic imprinting and X chromosome inactivation arise from stochastic expression? Trends Genet 17:136-141.

Paria BC, Reese J, Das SK, Dey SK. 2002. Deciphering the cross-talk of implantation: advances and challenges. Science 296:2185-2188.

Reik W, Lewis A. 2005. Co-evolution of X-chromosome inactivation and imprinting in mammals. Nat Rev Genet 6:403-410.

Reik W, Walter J. 2001. Genomic imprinting: parental influence on the genome. Nat Rev Genet 2:21-32.

Roberts RM, Ezashi T, Das P. 2004. Trophoblast gene expression: transcription factors in the specification of early trophoblast. Reprod Biol Endocrinol 2:47.

Rossant J, Cross JC. 2002. Extraembryonic lineages. In: Rossant J, Tam PPL, editors. Mouse Development. Patterning, Morphogenesis, and Organogenesis. San Diego: Academic Press. pp 155-180.

Rougeulle C, Avner P. 2004. The role of antisense transcription in the regulation of X-inactivation. Curr Top Dev Biol 63:61-89.

Shivdasani RA. 2002. Molecular regulation of vertebrate early endoderm development. Dev Biol 249:191-203.

Stainier DY. 2002. A glimpse into the molecular entrails of endoderm formation. Genes Dev 16:893-907.

Sutherland A. 2003. Mechanisms of implantation in the mouse: differentiation and functional importance of trophoblast giant cell behavior. Dev Biol 258:241-251.

Tam PPL, Kanai-Azuma M, Kanai Y. 2003. Early endoderm development in vertebrates: lineage differentiation and morphogenetic function. Curr Opin Genet Dev 13:393-400.

Tilghman SM. 1999. The sins of the fathers and mothers: genomic imprinting in mammalian development. Cell 96:185-193.

Vu TH, Hoffman AR. 2000. Comparative genomics sheds light on mechanisms of genomic imprinting. Genome Res 10:1660-1663.

Zeh DW, Zeh JA. 2000. Reproductive mode and speciation: the viviparity-driven conflict hypothesis. Bioessays 22:938-946.

Third Week: Becoming Trilaminar and Establishing Body Axes

3

Summary The first major event of the 3rd week, **gastrulation**, commences with the formation of a longitudinal midline structure, the **primitive streak**, in the epiblast near the caudal end of the bilaminar embryonic disc. The cranial end of the primitive streak is expanded as the **primitive node**; it contains a circular depression called the **primitive pit**, which is continuous caudally down the midline of the primitive streak with a trough-like depression called the **primitive groove**. The primitive pit and groove represent areas where cells are leaving the primitive streak and moving into the interior of the embryonic disc. Some of these cells invade the hypoblast, displacing the original hypoblast cells and replacing them with a layer of **definitive endoderm**. Others migrate bilaterally from the primitive streak and then cranially or laterally between endoderm and epiblast and coalesce to form the **intraembryonic mesoderm**. After gastrulation is complete, the epiblast is called the **ectoderm**. Thus, during gastrulation the three primary **germ layers** form: the ectoderm, mesoderm, and endoderm. Germ layers are the primitive building blocks for formation of **organ rudiments**.

Formation of the primitive streak also defines for the first time all major **body axes**. These consist of the **cranial-caudal** (or head-tail) axis, **dorsal-ventral** (or back-belly) **axis**, the **medial-lateral axis** and the **left-right axis**. Before the flat embryonic disc folds up into a three-dimensional tube-within-a-tube body plan, these axes remain incompletely delimited; their definitive form will be better understood after Chapter 4 is studied.

As gastrulation converts the bilaminar embryonic disc into a **trilaminar embryonic disc**, it brings subpopulations of cells into proximity so that they can undergo inductive interactions to pattern layers and specify new cell types. The first cells to move through the primitive streak and contribute to the intraembryonic mesoderm migrate bilaterally and cranially to form the **cardiogenic mesoderm**. Somewhat later in development, a longitudinal thick-walled tube of mesoderm extends cranially in the midline from the primitive node; this structure, the **notochordal process**, is the rudiment of the **notochord**. Migrating bilaterally from the primitive streak and then cranially, just lateral to the notochordal process, are cells that contribute to the **paraxial mesoderm**. In the future head region, paraxial mesoderm forms the **head mesoderm**. In the future trunk region, paraxial mesoderm forms the **somites**, a series of segmental blocklike mesodermal condensations. Two other areas of intraembryonic mesoderm form from the primitive streak during gastrulation: the **intermediate mesoderm** and **lateral plate mesoderm**. The intermediate mesoderm contributes to the urogenital system, and the lateral plate mesoderm contributes to the body wall and the wall of the gut (gastrointestinal system).

During gastrulation, a major inductive event occurs in the embryo: **neural induction**. In this process, the primitive node induces the overlying ectoderm to thicken as the **neural plate**, the earliest rudiment of the central nervous system. During subsequent development the neural plate will fold up into a **neural tube**. **Neural crest cells** arise from the lateral edges of the neural plate during formation of the neural tube. Also during subsequent development, the definitive endoderm will fold to form three subdivision of the primitive gut: **foregut**, **midgut**, and **hindgut**. The cranial midline endoderm, just cranial to the tip of the extending notochord, forms a thickened area called the **prechordal plate**. It contributes to the **oropharyngeal membrane** during later development and is an important signaling center for patterning the overlying neural plate. With the formation of endodermal, mesodermal, and ectodermal subdivisions during gastrulation, the stage is set by the end of the 3rd week for **formation of the tube-within-a-tube body plan** and subsequent **organogenesis**, the processes by which primitive organ rudiments are established and subsequently differentiated to form all major organ systems.

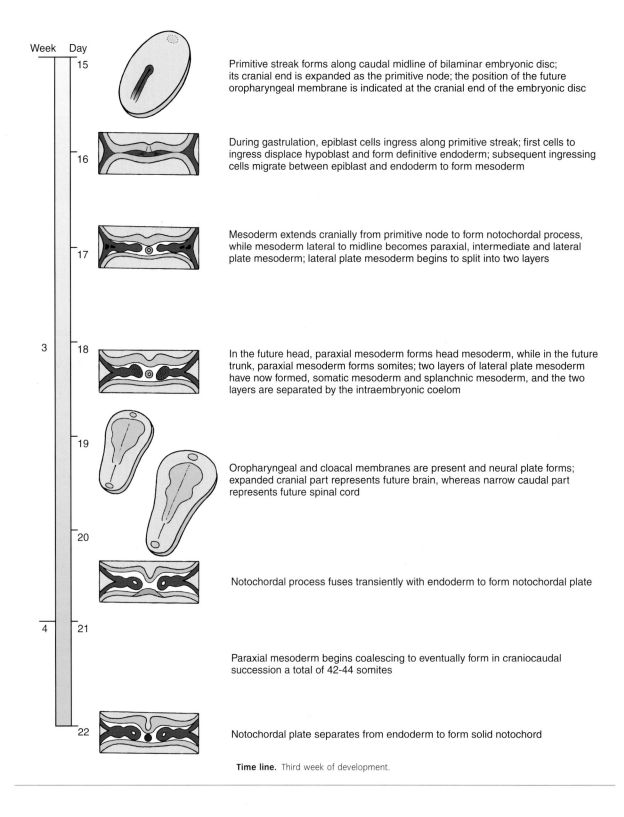

Week Day

15 Primitive streak forms along caudal midline of bilaminar embryonic disc; its cranial end is expanded as the primitive node; the position of the future oropharyngeal membrane is indicated at the cranial end of the embryonic disc

16 During gastrulation, epiblast cells ingress along primitive streak; first cells to ingress displace hypoblast and form definitive endoderm; subsequent ingressing cells migrate between epiblast and endoderm to form mesoderm

17 Mesoderm extends cranially from primitive node to form notochordal process, while mesoderm lateral to midline becomes paraxial, intermediate and lateral plate mesoderm; lateral plate mesoderm begins to split into two layers

3 18 In the future head, paraxial mesoderm forms head mesoderm, while in the future trunk, paraxial mesoderm forms somites; two layers of lateral plate mesoderm have now formed, somatic mesoderm and splanchnic mesoderm, and the two layers are separated by the intraembryonic coelom

19

Oropharyngeal and cloacal membranes are present and neural plate forms; expanded cranial part represents future brain, whereas narrow caudal part represents future spinal cord

20

Notochordal process fuses transiently with endoderm to form notochordal plate

4 21

Paraxial mesoderm begins coalescing to eventually form in craniocaudal succession a total of 42-44 somites

22 Notochordal plate separates from endoderm to form solid notochord

Time line. Third week of development.

Clinical Taster In 2004, a baby girl, Milagros Cerron, was born in Peru with a condition called **sirenomelia** (*siren* and *melos* are Greek, meaning "nymph limbs"). Because she is one of only three surviving children born with the "mermaid syndrome" (the oldest being 16 years old in 2005), her birth, first birthday, and surgery at 13 months of age received extensive press coverage.

Sirenomelia is a rare condition occurring in 1 in 70,000 births. Most babies born with sirenomelia die within a few days of birth with severe defects in vital organs. The most obvious defect in sirenomelia is a fusion of the two lower limbs in the midline (see fig. 3-18). In Milagros's case (her name is Spanish for miracles), her lower limbs were fused together from her thighs to her ankles, with her feet deviating from one another in a V-shaped pattern resembling a mermaid's tail. In the press, she is often referred to as "Peru's little mermaid." In addition to fused lower limbs, she was born with a deformed left kidney, a small right kidney that failed to ascend, and anomalies in her terminal digestive, urinary, and genital tracts. These anomalies have resulted in recurrent urinary tract infections.

For 3 months prior to her first surgery to separate her fused legs, saline-filled bags were inserted to stretch the skin to allow it to cover her legs once they were separated. She recovered quickly from surgery, and it is expected that she will need to undergo many other surgeries over the course of the next 15 years to correct her digestive, urinary, and reproductive organs.

Overview of Gastrulation: Forming Three Primary Germ Layers and Body Axes

Primitive Streak Forms at Beginning of Third Week and Marks Three Body Axes

On about day 15 of development, a thickening containing a midline groove forms along the midsagittal plane of the embryonic disc, which has now assumed an oval shape (Fig. 3-1). Over the course of the next day, this thickening, called the **primitive streak**, elongates to occupy about half the length of the embryonic disc, and the groove, called the **primitive groove**, becomes deeper and more defined. The cranial end of the primitive streak is expanded into a structure called the **primitive node**. It contains a depression, called the **primitive pit**, which is continuous caudally with the primitive groove.

Formation of the primitive streak heralds the beginning of **gastrulation**. During gastrulation, epiblast cells move toward the primitive streak, enter the primitive streak, and then migrate away from the primitive streak as individual cells. The movement of cells through the primitive streak and into the interior of the embryo is called **ingression**.

Formation of the primitive streak also defines all major **body axes**. The primitive streak forms in the caudal midline of the embryonic disc, thus defining the **cranial-caudal axis** and **medial-lateral axis**

(with the primitive streak forming in the midline, that is, most medially). Because formation of the primitive streak occurs in the midline, when the epiblast is viewed looking down at it from inside the amniotic cavity, what lies to the right of the primitive streak represents the right side of the embryo and what lies to the left represents its left side. Thus, formation of the primitive streak also defines the **left-right axis**. At the time of primitive streak formation, the future **dorsal-ventral axis** of the embryonic disc is roughly equivalent to its ectoderm-endoderm axis. Later, with body folding and formation of the tube-within-a-tube body plan (discussed in Ch. 4) the dorsal-ventral axis becomes better defined.

IN THE RESEARCH LAB

INDUCTION OF PRIMITIVE STREAK

Experiments in chick suggest that the primitive streak is induced by cell-cell interactions at the caudal end of the embryonic disc. Although the exact tissue interactions are disputed, it is clear that caudal (extraembryonic) tissues (either Koller's/Rauber's sickle or the caudal marginal zone) induce the adjacent epiblast to form primitive streak and that this process of induction continues as the extraembryonic endoderm migrates from caudal to cranial.

Misexpression studies (gain-of-function and loss-of-function; discussed in Ch. 5) in both mouse and chick suggest that *Tgfβ* and *Wnt1* family members induce the

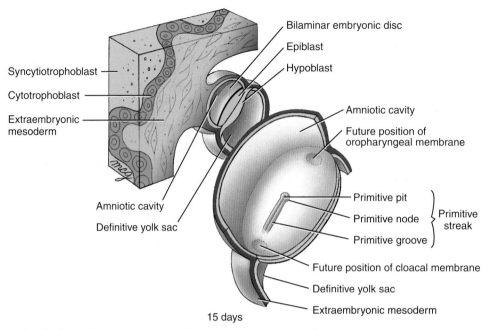

Syncytiotrophoblast

Cytotrophoblast

Extraembryonic mesoderm

Amniotic cavity

Definitive yolk sac

Bilaminar embryonic disc

Epiblast

Hypoblast

Amniotic cavity

Future position of oropharyngeal membrane

Primitive pit

Primitive node

Primitive groove

Primitive streak

Future position of cloacal membrane

Definitive yolk sac

Extraembryonic mesoderm

15 days

Figure 3-1. View of dorsal surface of bilaminar embryonic disc through sectioned amnion and yolk sac. Inset at upper left shows relation of the embryo to the wall of the chorionic cavity. The primitive streak, now 1 day old, occupies 50% of the length of the embryonic disc. The future positions of oropharyngeal and cloacal membranes are indicated.

primitive streak. In chick, *Vg1* (a *Tgfβ* family member) in conjunction with *Wnt8c*, induces the epiblast to express another *Tgfβ* family member, *Nodal*. *Nodal* in turn, along with *Fgf8* (and likely other *Fgfs*), induces epiblast cells to de-epithelialize and form primitive streak. Finally, inhibition of endogenous *Bmp* signaling (through its antagonist *Chordin*; discussed in Chs. 4, 5) also seems to be required for primitive streak formation.

In mouse, *Wnt3* and its downstream target *Brachyury* (a T-box containing transcription factor) are expressed in both the future cranial and caudal prestreak epiblast. During subsequent development, *Wnt3* is downregulated cranially, by signals from a specialized region of extraembryonic endoderm called the **anterior visceral endoderm**, and upregulated caudally (note: "anterior" in the mouse is equivalent to cranial in the human). Finally, expression of *Wnt3*, *Brachyury*, and *Nodal* becomes consolidated within the primitive streak. Loss-of-function mutations of genes expressed by the anterior visceral endoderm (e.g., *Cerl*, *Lefty1*—both inhibitors of *Tgfβ* and *Wnt* signaling) result in formation of extra primitive streaks. Moreover, embryos with loss-of-function mutations of *Nodal* (or its cofactor *Cripto*) fail to form a primitive streak. Further studies (using mouse chimeras; mouse injection chimeras are discussed in Ch. 5)

reveal that formation of the primitive streak involves signaling of *Tgfβ* family members from extraembryonic tissues (as in chick).

CELLULAR BASIS OF PRIMITIVE STREAK FORMATION

Studies in chick have revealed the cellular basis of primitive streak formation. Four major processes are involved: cell migration, oriented cell division, progressive delamination from the epiblast, and convergent extension. During formation of the primitive streak, cells are induced from the epiblast overlying a structure called Koller's sickle. As induction occurs, these cells delaminate from the epiblast and migrate cranially and medially. Analyses of labeled clones of cells show that cells are displaced mainly cranially as they undergo division, suggesting that their division plane is preferentially oriented. As extraembryonic endoderm migrates cranially, progressively more cranial epiblast cells along the midline are induced to delaminate, extending the cranial end of the primitive streak more cranially. Finally, cells within the forming streak merge medially and consequently the streak extends craniocaudally to accommodate the merging cells. Thus, convergent extension contributes to the later aspects of primitive streak formation and elongation.

ESTABLISHING LEFT-RIGHT AXIS

As discussed above, with formation of the primitive streak during gastrulation, the embryonic axes—cranial-caudal, dorsal-ventral, medial-lateral, and left-right—become defined. In mouse embryos, cranial patterning actually occurs prior to formation of the primitive streak, as a result of signaling from the anterior visceral endoderm (discussed in preceding section). Whether a similar signaling center exists in humans to provide early cranial patterning information is unknown. With formation of the primitive streak, and subsequently three primary germ layers, cell-cell interactions occur among the three layers, and within different subdivisions of these layers, to pattern the germ layers in both the cranial-caudal and dorsal-ventral planes. This patterning is discussed later in this chapter and in Chapter 4. Here, we discuss a third type of patterning, formation of the **left-right axis**, which begins at about the time that the primitive node forms at the cranial end of the primitive streak.

Handed asymmetry, as opposed to **mirror** (or **mirror-image**) **symmetry**, is the term that denotes anatomic differences on the left and right sides of the body. For example, in humans the gastrointestinal tract rotates during development so that the stomach is on the left and the liver is on the right. Also, the heart loops so that its apex points to the left, whereas its base is directed to the right. Furthermore, the right lung has three lobes and the left lung has two lobes. How is handed asymmetry initiated in the embryo?

Molecular Basis of Left-Right Asymmetry: A Simplified Scheme

Left-right asymmetry is established during gastrulation through cell-cell interactions centered at the primitive node (Fig. 3-2), or the homologous structure in animal models (e.g., embryonic shield in zebrafish, dorsal lip of the blastopore in Xenopus, Hensen's node in chick, and node in mouse). In chick, a secreted molecule, *Sonic hedgehog* (*Shh*), is expressed symmetrically in Hensen's node as it forms, but shortly thereafter expression of *Shh* becomes restricted to the left side. This is followed by left-sided expression of the *Tgfβ* family member, *Nodal* (both within the left side of the node and left lateral plate mesoderm; discussed in mesodermal divisions, below), and subsequently, by left-sided expression of a transcription factor, *Pitx2*. Gain-of-function experiments have revealed that *Shh* induces left-sided expression of *Nodal*, which in turn induces left-sided expression of *Pitx2*. *Pitx2* regulates the transcription of downstream targets (mostly unknown), presumably changing cell behaviors and resulting in asymmetric morphogenesis, leading to handed asymmetry.

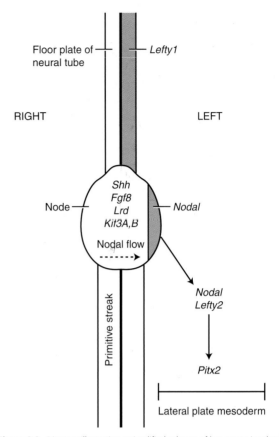

Figure 3-2. Diagram illustrating a simplified scheme of key genes involved in establishing left-right asymmetry. The primitive streak, node, and early floor plate of the neural tube are viewed from the ventral side. Motor proteins (*Lrd, Kif3A, B*) expressed by the node regulate leftward (dashed arrow) nodal flow. Secreted factors (*Shh, Fgf8, Nodal*) expressed by the node result in signaling to the lateral plate mesoderm, thereby resulting in asymmetric gene expression in the lateral plate mesoderm (e.g., *Nodal, Lefty2* in left lateral plate). This in turn results in expression of *Pitx2* in the left lateral plate and changes in cell behaviors that result in asymmetric morphogenesis. *Lefty1* is expressed in the left floor plate of the neural tube. It is believed to serve a barrier function, allowing information that specifies left and right sides to remain separate.

The scheme just outlined is a simplified version, as many molecules are known to be asymmetrically expressed at this time. However, this scheme includes the key players, and experiments, particularly in mouse, have shown that this pathway of key players is conserved. In addition to *Nodal*, two other *Tgfβ* family members, highly related to one another, show left-sided expression and play an essential role in establishing left-right asymmetry; they are appropriately named *Lefty1* and *Lefty2*. Moreover, *Fgf8*, secreted by the node, has been shown to play a role in left-right asymmetry, but this role differs in chick and in mouse: specifying right side in chick and left side in mouse. The precise role of *Shh* may also differ somewhat in chick and mouse (e.g., *Shh* is not asymmetrically expressed in mouse). Nevertheless, because mice containing *Shh* loss-of-function mutations exhibit laterality defects, it is clear that *Shh* acts in the left-right patterning of both species.

In the rare human disorder, **situs inversus viscerum totalis**, the handedness of all of the viscera is reversed. However, the reversal is rarely complete or exact, and errors in morphogenesis often produce subsidiary malformations such as the **malrotations of the midgut** (described below). More often, the different organ systems exhibit a discordance of sidedness, or **heterotaxy**. For example, the looping of the heart may be reversed (**dextrocardia;** discussed in Ch. 12), whereas lobulation of the lungs may be normal (three lobes on the right and two lobes on the left). More than 40 years ago, a mouse mutant was discovered that exhibits situs inversus, the *iv/iv* mouse (*iv* stands for *inversus viscerum*). The phenotype is inherited as an autosomal recessive single-gene trait (because it is a *recessive* mutation, its name is designated in lower case, the convention in mouse) and it has been mapped to chromosome 12. But only half the mice homozygous for the mutant *iv* allele exhibit situs inversus; the other half show normal left-right asymmetry (**situs solitus totalis**). Thus, the gene product of the wild-type locus seems to be an essential component of the mechanism that *biases* the development of handed asymmetry in the correct direction, and thus determines the correct handedness or **situs** of the viscera. If this gene product is absent or defective (as in the *iv/iv* mouse), normal or inverted situs is apparently adopted at random.

The cloning of the *iv* mutation provided interesting clues that led to better understanding of the early stages of left-right development. The *iv* mutation occurs in a dynein gene designated *Left-right dynein*, or *Lrd*. Dyneins are molecular motors composed of heavy and intermediate polypeptide chains. Dyneins use energy from ATP hydrolysis to move cargo towards the minus end of microtubules, or cause bending of cilia and flagella by creating a sliding force between microtubules. Thus, there are two kinds of dyneins, cytoplasmic and axonemal. The sequence of the *Lrd* gene suggests that it encodes an axonemal dynein, but the functions of the two kinds of dyneins are probably not completely independent of one another, as suggested from mouse loss-of-function mutations (in which mutations in single motor proteins affect both ciliary action and intracellular transport).

This connection between dynein and laterality in mice was reminiscent of a previous connection between dynein and laterality made in humans. Patients with **Kartagener syndrome** have inverted laterality as well as immotile respiratory cilia and sperm flagella. They often exhibit male infertility and chronic respiratory tract infections. Kartagener syndrome patients have mutations in *DYNEIN* genes (both heavy and intermediate chain mutations have been identified), as well as deficiencies in their ciliary DYNEIN arms (DYNEINS form arm-like projections that interconnect the outer microtubule doublets, as viewed ultrastructurally in electron micrographs). Kartagener syndrome is discussed further in Chapters 11 and 12.

Nodal Flow Model

In gastrulating mouse embryos, expression of the *Lrd* gene is restricted to the node, an important organizer region (discussed below). The cells of the node each contain a single cilium, called a **monocilium** (Fig. 3-3). The monocilia of the central nodal cells are motile, in contrast to the peripheral nodal cells. The central cilia rotate in a vortical fashion and generate a leftward flow of fluid across the node (as demonstrated by the displacement of fluorescent beads across the node). Based on this finding, and the experimental reversal of flow in cultured embryos, the **nodal flow model** of left-right development was proposed (note: nodal in the model refers to the node and should not be confused with the gene named *Nodal*). According to the original formulation of the model, the leftward movement of fluid across the node generates an asymmetric distribution of an unknown **morphogen**, that is, a diffusible protein that affects tissue development based on its concentration. The resulting left-right morphogen concentration gradient is believed to break symmetry and initiate left-right development. Several candidate proteins have been proposed for this morphogen including *Nodal*, *Shh*, *Fgf8*, retinoic acid, *Bmp*, and *Gdf1* (*Growth and differentiation factor 1*). Whether the primitive node of humans contains monocilia (and if it does, whether some are motile) is unknown, however, nodal monocilia have been identified in several species.

Loss-of-function experiments in mice provide compelling support for the nodal flow model. Mice mutant for either kinesin gene *Kif3A* or *Kif3B* have nodal cells without cilia and altered left-right development. Kinesins are functionally similar to dyneins in that they generate motive force along microtubules (although generally in the opposite direction). These results indicate the *Kif3A* and *Kif3B* genes are required for node cilia assembly and suggest the cilia, in turn, are necessary for normal left-right development.

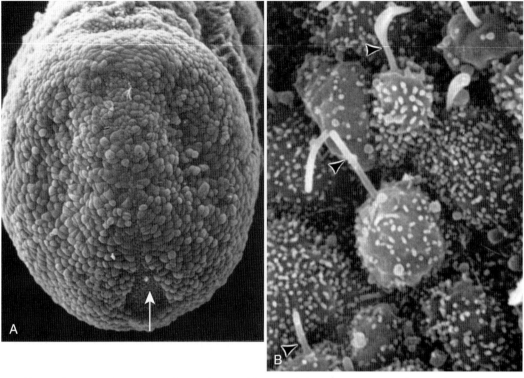

Figure 3-3. Nodal monocilia. *A*, Gastrulating mouse embryonic disc viewed from its endodermal surface. Arrow marks the node. *B*, Enlargement of nodal cilia (arrowheads).

In addition, mice with a mutation in the *Lrd* gene have immotile nodal cilia. This shows that not just the presence but the movement of the nodal cilia is critically important for normal left-right development, again consistent with the nodal flow model.

Variations on the Nodal Flow Model

Three major variations on the nodal flow model have been proposed. In the first variation, it has been proposed that motor proteins involved in establishing left-right asymmetry might function intracellularly within the node (to transport cargo that carries left-right patterning information) rather than extracellularly across the node. Thus, ciliary motility per se, may or may not be relevant for establishing left-right asymmetry, and may merely be marking another relevant intracellular event. In the second variation, additional studies of the mouse node have led to the formulation of the **mechanosensory model**, in which it is proposed that motile cilia drive nodal fluid flow, which in turn activates a **calcium flux** on the left side of the node, rather than transporting a morphogen (Fig. 3-4). In support of this model, both the centrally located motile cilia and peripherally located immotile cilia of the node contain

a cation channel protein called *Polycystein2*, which is the product of the *Polycystic kidney disease type 2* gene, *Pkd2*. By contrast, only motile cilia express the *Lrd* protein. Imaging of calcium levels (using a fluorescent reporter dye and confocal microscopy) revealed that asymmetric calcium signaling appears at the left margin of the node coincident with the onset of nodal flow. Thus, the immotile cilia act as mechanosensors to detect fluid flow. In the third variation, also based on additional studies of the mouse node, a new mode of extracellular transport was discovered in which so-called **nodal vesicular parcels (NVP)**, membrane-sheathed vesicles that carry morphogens, are moved across the node by nodal flow to establish a left-right gradient of morphogens (Fig. 3-5). These parcels contain two known morphogens, *Shh* and retinoic acid, and their leftward transport elicits a calcium flux on the left side of the node, in support of the mechanosensory model. Secretion of NVPs is triggered by *Fgf* signaling, as is calcium flux on the left side of the node. Thus, the last variation of the nodal flow model provides support for both chemical and mechanical extracellular signal transduction across the node.

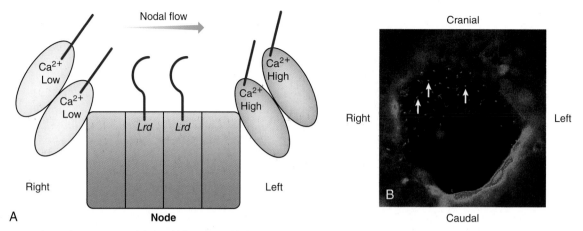

Figure 3-4. The mechanosensory model of nodal flow. *A,* Model showing that nodal flow, generated by motile monocilia in cells expressing *Lrd,* stimulates calcium flux in cells containing nonmotile cilia that sense flow on the left side. *B,* Mouse node viewed from its endodermal side showing calcium signaling predominantly at the left side of the node. Arrows indicate motile cilia expressing *Lrd* fused with a fluorescent reporter gene.

Ordering Genes in a Genetic Hierarchy

The order of genes in a genetic program is often determined by examining gene expression patterns in mutants. For example, if gene A activates gene B, which activates gene C in a program, then mutation of gene B would alter the expression of gene C but not gene A. In this manner, the *Lrd* gene was shown to occupy a high-level position in the genetic hierarchy of left-right development. In *Lrd* loss-of-function mutants, the expression patterns of *Nodal, Lefty1, Lefty2,* and *Pitx2* are all altered, indicating that they are downstream of *Lrd.* The expression of *Nodal,* for example, is randomized in mice with an *Lrd* loss-of-function mutation. One fourth of these mutant embryos show normal *Nodal* expression only on the left, one fourth show reversed expression only on the right, one fourth show expression on both sides, and one fourth show expression on neither side.

IN THE CLINIC

DEVELOPMENT IN ANIMAL MODELS VERSUS HUMANS

As discussed earlier in the chapter, the homeobox-containing gene *Pitx2* is downstream of *Nodal* and *Lefty2* in the genetic program of left-right development. *Pitx2,* like *Nodal* and *Lefty2,* is expressed on the left side, and it seems to be an effector gene, with its expression persisting later in development, during organogenesis. In mice homozygous for *Pitx2* loss-of-function mutations, laterality defects occur. One striking defect observed is right lung isomerism (two right lungs). Normally, the two lungs of the mouse are quite distinct, with the left lung having a single lobe, and the right lung having four lobes. However, in the *Pitx2* mutant, both lungs have four lobes. On the left side, in the absence of *Pitx2* expression, a right lung develops. Mice heterozygous for *Pitx2* mutations are apparently normal.

To date, homozygous mutations of the *PITX2* gene have not been identified in humans, so the potential role of this gene in human laterality defects has not been confirmed. However, haploinsufficiency (one wild-type and one mutant allele) of the *PITX2* gene in humans has been identified. It results in **Rieger syndrome**, a condition in which defects form in both eyes and teeth, but laterality defects are absent.

An important lesson to be learned from this example is that animal models, although extremely useful for understanding the normal function of genes in a particular species, may or may not develop in *exactly* the same way as does the human embryo. Thus, when making comparisons using multiple animal models, it is important to identify highly conserved events (morphogenetic processes, gene expression patterns, etc.) across species; such conserved events are more likely to function also during human development. But as Rieger syndrome illustrates, caution must be exercised when extrapolating data from animal models to humans. This problem is certainly not unique to embryology, and will be encountered many times in the study of human biology and medicine, perhaps most commonly in drug development and testing where animal models are heavily used.

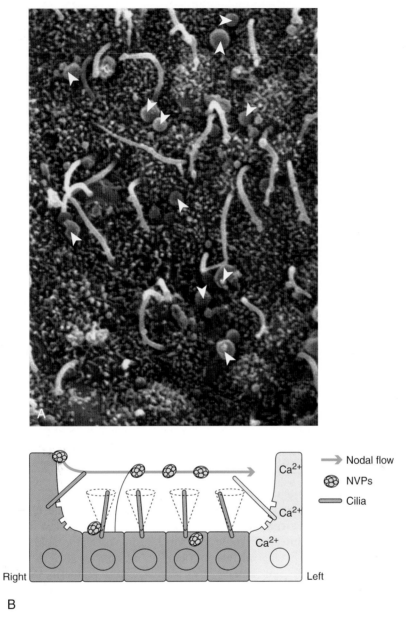

Figure 3-5. *A*, Scanning electron micrograph showing mouse node monocilia and nodal vesicular parcels (arrowheads). *B*, Model showing the transport of nodal vesicular parcels by motile cilia and the stimulation of calcium signaling (blue) at the left side of the node by nonmotile cilia.

Formation of Definitive Endoderm

On day 16, epiblast cells lateral to the primitive streak begin to move into the primitive streak where they undergo an **epithelial-to-mesenchymal transformation (EMT)**. An **epithelium** consists of a sheet of regularly shaped (often cuboidal) cells tightly interconnected to one another at their lateral cell surfaces; a **mesenchyme** consists of much more irregularly shaped (often stellate) and loosely connected cells. During EMT, epiblast cells often elongate and become flask or bottle shaped (see Fig. 3-6), detaching from their neighbors as they extend footlike processes called **pseudopodia** (as well as thinner processes called **filopodia** and flattened processes called **lamellipodia**), which allow them to migrate through the primitive streak into the space between the epiblast and hypoblast (or into the hypoblast itself). This collective movement of cells through the primitive streak and into the interior of the embryo to form the three primary germ layers constitutes **gastrulation**. The first ingressing epiblast cells invade the hypoblast and displace its cells, so that the hypoblast eventually is completely replaced by a new layer of cells, the **definitive endoderm** (Fig. 3-6A). Definitive endoderm gives rise to the lining of the future gut and gut derivatives.

Formation of Intraembryonic Mesoderm

Starting on day 16, some epiblast cells migrating through the primitive streak diverge into the space between epiblast and nascent definitive endoderm to form a third germ layer, the **intraembryonic mesoderm** (Figs. 3-6B; C, 3-7). These cells migrate bilaterally from the primitive streak and initially form a loose mat of cells between epiblast and endoderm. Shortly thereafter the mat reorganizes to form four main subdivisions of intraembryonic mesoderm: **cardiogenic mesoderm, paraxial mesoderm, intermediate mesoderm** (also called **nephrotome**), and **lateral plate mesoderm**. In addition, a fifth population of mesodermal cells migrates cranially from the primitive node in the midline to form a thick-walled midline tube called the **notochordal process**.

During the 3rd week of development, two faint depressions form in the ectoderm, one at the cranial end of the embryo overlying the prechordal plate and the other at the caudal end behind the primitive streak. Late in the 3rd week, the ectoderm in these areas fuses tightly with the underlying endoderm, excluding the mesoderm and forming bilaminar membranes. The cranial membrane is called the **oropharyngeal membrane**, and the caudal membrane is the **cloacal membrane**. The oropharyngeal and cloacal membranes later become the blind ends of the gut tube. The oropharyngeal membrane breaks down in the 4th week to form the opening to the oral cavity, whereas the cloacal membrane disintegrates later, in the 7th week, to form the openings of the anus and the urinary and genital tracts (discussed in Chs. 14 and 15).

Formation of Ectoderm

Once formation of the definitive endoderm and intraembryonic mesoderm is complete, epiblast cells no longer move toward and ingress through the primitive streak. The remaining epiblast now constitutes the **ectoderm**, which quickly differentiates into the central **neural plate** and peripheral **surface ectoderm**. However, the embryo develops in cranial-to-caudal sequence, so that once epiblast is no longer present cranially, for some time it will still be present caudally where cells continue to move into the primitive streak and undergo ingression (Fig. 3-8). Eventually, the process of gastrulation is complete. At that time, formation of the three definitive germ layers of the **trilaminar embryonic disc**—the ectoderm, mesoderm, and definitive endoderm—will be complete throughout the disc. Thus, all three germ layers derive from epiblast during gastrulation (note: some textbooks call the epiblast the *primitive ectoderm*, but because epiblast gives rise to mesoderm and endoderm as well as ectoderm, the term *epiblast* is a more appropriate one).

Morphogenetic changes (i.e., shape-generating events) occur in each of these germ layers to form the primitive organ rudiments. Thus, we often speak of ectodermal, mesodermal, and endoderm derivatives. In reality very few organ rudiments form from only one germ layer; rather two or more layers often collaborate (for example, the gut tube is derived from endoderm and mesoderm). The formation of organ rudiments during the formation of the tube-within-a-tube body plan (Ch. 4) is followed by the transformation of organ rudiments into organ systems, that is, the process of **organogenesis**; organogenesis is the major topic of most of the remaining chapters of this textbook.

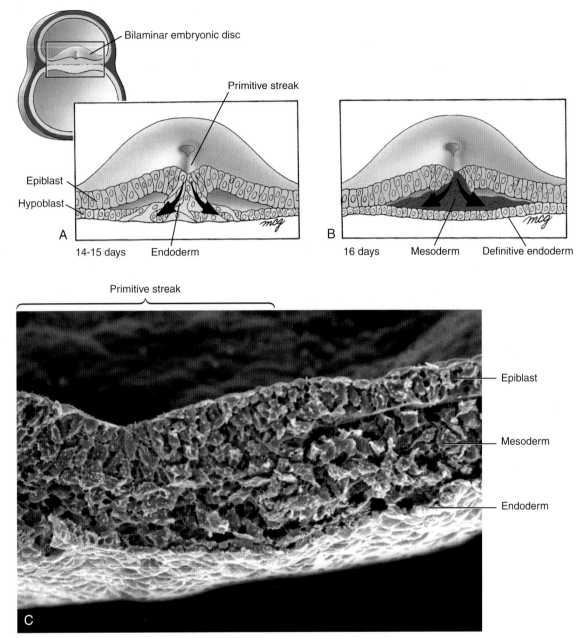

Figure 3-6. Embryonic discs sectioned through the region of primitive streak, showing ingression of epiblast cells during gastrulation. *A,* On days 14 and 15, ingressing epiblast cells displace hypoblast and form definitive endoderm. *B,* Epiblast that ingresses on day 16 migrates between endoderm and epiblast layers to form intraembryonic mesoderm. *C,* Scanning electron micrograph of a cross section through the chick primitive streak.

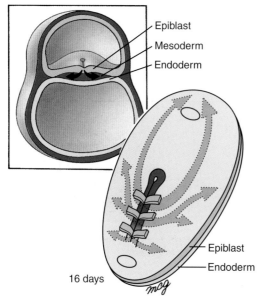

Epiblast
Mesoderm
Endoderm

Epiblast
Endoderm
16 days

Figure 3-7. Paths of migration of mesoderm during gastrulation. Cells of the primitive node migrate cranially in the midline to form the notochordal process (not shown; occurs later). Cells that ingress more caudally through the primitive streak migrate to form the mesoderm lying on either side of the midline. The most cranially migrating of these cells form the cardiogenic mesoderm, which moves cranial to the future position of the oropharyngeal membrane (cranial oval structure). The more laterally migrating of these cells form the paraxial, intermediate, and lateral plate mesoderm.

IN THE RESEARCH LAB

CELLULAR BASIS OF GASTRULATION

The cellular basis of gastrulation has been studied in a large variety of animal models. During gastrulation, cells undergo four types of coordinated group movements, called **morphogenetic movements**: epiboly (spreading of an epithelial sheet), **emboly** (internalization), **convergence** (movement toward the midline), and **extension** (lengthening in the cranial-caudal plane). The last two movements occur in conjunction with one another as a coordinated movement, and are called **convergent extension**. Thus, convergent extension involves cell rearrangement to narrow the medial-lateral extent of a population of cells, and concomitantly increase its cranial-caudal extent. Morphogenetic movements are each generated by a combination of **changes in cell behaviors**. These behaviors include **changes in cell shape, size, position, and number**. These changes are often associated with **changes in cell-to-cell** or **cell-to-extracellular matrix adhesion**.

Changes in cell shape involve cell flattening (from columnar or cuboidal to squamous), cell elongation or shortening (from cuboidal to columnar or from columnar to cuboidal), and cell wedging (from columnar to wedge shaped). Changes in cell size involve either an increase in cell volume (**growth**) or a decrease. Changes in cell position involve the active (i.e., **migration**) or passive displacement of

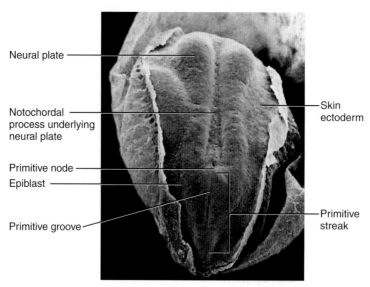

Neural plate

Notochordal process underlying neural plate

Primitive node
Epiblast

Primitive groove

Skin ectoderm

Primitive streak

Figure 3-8. Scanning electron micrograph of a Macaque embryo comparable to a 19-day human embryo showing the ectodermal surface of a trilaminar embryonic disc (cranial end at top). Even though the neural plate and surface ectoderm are well formed throughout the cranial two thirds of the embryo, a regressing primitive streak and flanking epiblast are still present caudally.

cells from one region of an embryo to another, and changes in cell number involve either an increase (**mitosis**) or decrease (**apoptosis**, also called **programmed cell death**).

Both epiboly and emboly are involved in human gastrulation as cells move toward, into, and through the primitive streak. Epiboly involves the spreading of a sheet of cells, generally on the surface of an embryo. Epiblast cells undergo epiboly to move toward and into the primitive streak. Emboly involves the movement of cells into the interior of an embryo and is also called **internalization**. Emboly can involve the movement of individual cells or sheets of cells. Movement of cells through the primitive streak and into the interior involves a type of emboly called **ingression**—the internalization of individual cells undergoing an epithelial-to-mesenchymal transformation (EMT).

EMT involves changes in both **cell-to-cell adhesion** and **cell shape**, with the latter mediated by changes in the **cytoskeleton**. During EMT, epiblast cells within the primitive streak shift their predominant adhesive activity from cell-to-cell to cell-to-substratum (basement membranes and extracellular matrix). One gene responsible for repressing epithelial characteristics in the mesenchymal cells of the streak is *Snail*, a zinc-finger transcription factor. Under its influence, expression of certain cell-to-cell adhesion molecules such as *E-Cadherin* cease, whereas expression of cytoskeletal proteins such as *Vimentin* is induced. In addition, the cytoskeleton is altered by expression of members of the *Rho* family of GTPases such as *RhoA* and *Rac1*. These are required to regulate actin organization and the development of lamellipodia of gastrulating cells within the primitive streak. When GTPases are disrupted, cells accumulate and die within the space between epiblast and hypoblast. Similarly, loss-of-function mutations of a variety of adhesion and cytoskeletal molecules disrupt EMT. These include *N-Cadherin*, a cell-cell adhesion molecule, and *β-Catenin*, a cytoplasmic component of the *Cadherin/Catenin* adhesion complex, as well as *Afadin*, an actin filament-binding protein. In addition to changes in adhesion and cytoskeleton, *Fgf* signaling plays a role in EMT. In loss-of-function mutations of *Fibroblast growth factor receptor 1* (*Fgfr1*), involuting cells lose their ability to ingress, and, as a consequence, accumulate within the primitive streak.

ESTABLISHING MEDIAL-LATERAL SUBDIVISIONS OF MESODERM

Before discussing formation of the mesoderm and its medial-lateral subdivisions, it is important to understand two areas of the early embryo that exert inductive influences across the embryo: the **Nieuwkoop center** and the **organizer** (often called the Spemann-Mangold organizer). The Nieuwkoop center is an early-forming organizing center that induces the organizer. The organizer in turn sends out signals to pattern the newly formed mesoderm into its medial-lateral subdivisions. These two signaling centers were first discovered in amphibians, but homologous centers exist in all vertebrate embryos. The Nieuwkoop center is not structurally distinct; rather it is defined by location in the early embryo and by its ability to induce the organizer. With molecular characterization of the Nieuwkoop center, gene expression patterns are also used to identify it. In contrast to the Nieuwkoop center, the organizer is structurally distinct; it consists of the dorsal lip of the blastopore in amphibians, the embryonic shield in fish, Hensen's node in chick, the node in mouse, and the primitive node in humans. It also can be defined by its position in the early embryo, its ability to induce and pattern an embryonic axis (discussed later in the chapter), and gene expression patterns.

As discussed earlier in the chapter, the mesoderm, after it moves between the endoderm and ectoderm, quickly subdivides into several medial-lateral subdivisions. How are these subdivisions established? Experiments originally conducted in amphibian embryos suggest that gradients of secreted growth factors (i.e., **morphogens**) induce the mesodermal subdivisions. Because the early amphibian embryo is spherical rather than flat like the human embryo, formation of the medial-lateral subdivisions of the mesoderm is often referred to as dorsal-ventral patterning, with the most dorsal mesodermal subdivision being notochord, and the most ventral being lateral plate mesoderm (Fig. 3-9). Thus, to understand medial-lateral patterning of mesodermal subdivisions in the human embryo, it must be understood that dorsal mesoderm of the amphibian is equivalent to medial mesoderm of the human, and ventral mesoderm of the amphibian is equivalent to lateral mesoderm of the human. With formation of the body folds and establishment of the three-dimensional tube-within-a-tube body plan (discussed in Ch. 4), the mesoderm that was originally most medial in the human (notochord) becomes the most dorsal mesoderm, and the mesoderm that was originally lateral in the human (lateral plate mesoderm) becomes the most ventral mesoderm.

Gradients involved in mesodermal patterning involve synergistic interactions between both dorsalizing factors and ventralizing factors. **Dorsalizing factors** include the protein products of the *Noggin*, *Chordin*, *Nodal*, *Follistatin*, and *Cerberus* genes, whereas *Bmps* and *Wnts* act as **ventralizing factors**. These dorsalizing factors are secreted by the organizer and its derivatives (the notochord and floor plate of the neural tube), and they act by antagonizing *Bmp* and/or *Wnt* signaling. Thus, each mesodermal subdivision is

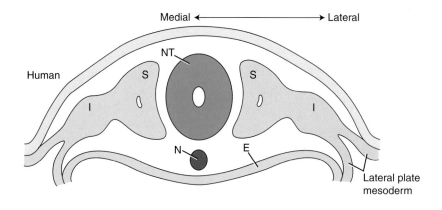

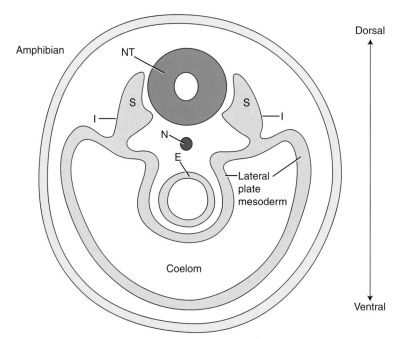

Figure 3-9. Diagrammatic cross-sectional views showing that the medial-lateral axis of the mesodermal subdivisions (N, notochord; S, somite; I, intermediate mesoderm) of a flat embryo like that of the early human (embryonic disc) is equivalent to the dorsal-ventral axis of the same mesodermal subdivisions in tubular amphibian embryos. NT, neural tube; E, endoderm.

patterned by the specific level of *Bmp* and *Wnt* signaling that occurs in that subdivision, based on its position in relation to the organizer. In the presence of low *Bmp* and *Wnt* signaling, notochord forms; in the presence of high *Bmp* and *Wnt* signaling, lateral plate mesoderm forms. *Bmp* and *Wnt* signaling in the somites is attenuated with respect to that occurring in the lateral plate mesoderm, but enhanced relative to that occurring in the notochord. As one example, over expression of *Bmps* or *Wnt* ventralizes the mesoderm and suppresses formation of the notochord, whereas over expression of *Bmp* or *Wnt* antagonists (e.g., *Cerberus*) induces ectopic notochords.

Loss-of-function experiments in mouse have identified transcription factors involved in the specification of intraembryonic mesoderm. For example, with loss of *Foxa2* (a forkhead transcription factor previously known as *Hnf3β*) function, the node is not maintained as a distinct structure, and the notochord subsequently fails to form. Moreover, loss of *Tbx6* function (a T-box–containing transcription factor gene closely related to the prototypical T-box gene *Brachyury*) is required for the formation of paraxial mesoderm (i.e., somites). Thus, in addition to gradients of diffusible factors controlling specification of intraembryonic mesoderm, expression of transcription factors is required for differentiation and maintenance of cell fate.

Specifics of Gastrulation: Moving Cells to New Locations and Making Organ Rudiments That Undergo Inductive Interactions

Fates of Epiblast Cells Depends on Their Site of Origin

Fate mapping and **cell lineage studies** in animal models have revealed the sites of origin of epiblast cells that give rise to various subdivisions of the ectoderm, endoderm, and mesoderm. In fate mapping, groups of cells are marked in some manner (often with fluorescent dyes) and then followed over time. In cell lineage studies, individual cells are marked (often genetically with reporter genes), rather than groups of cells, and their descendants are then

followed over time. Both techniques allow construction of **prospective fate maps** (Fig. 3-10), diagrams that show the locations of prospective groups of cells prior to the onset of gastrulation. Prospective fate maps show that cells of different germ layers and different subdivisions within germ layers are partially segregated from one another in the epiblast and primitive streak, although there is usually overlap between adjacent groups of cells. Prospective fate maps reveal only what groups of cells in a particular region of the epiblast (or primitive streak) form during normal development. They reveal nothing about whether these cells are committed to a particular fate or are still **pluripotent**—that is, innately capable of developing into almost any cell type of the organism. Experiments have shown that most cells within the epiblast and primitive streak are indeed pluripotent and that their fates are specified by cell-cell interactions that occur during their migration, or shortly after they arrive at their final destination. Thus, during gastrulation, the **prospective potency** of a group of epiblast cells, that is, what they are capable of forming at a particular stage of development, is typically far greater than their **prospective fate**, that is, what they are destined to form during normal development based on their place of origin.

Gastrulation involves a highly choreographed series of movements that occur over time (see Fig. 3-10). Beginning at the early primitive streak stage (see Fig. 3-10*A*), **prospective gut (definitive) endoderm** moves from the epiblast surrounding the cranial half of the primitive streak into the primitive streak. It then migrates into the hypoblast to displace that layer and to form a new layer of **definitive endoderm**. This process of endoderm formation occurs as late as the fully elongated primitive streak stage. Additionally at the early primitive streak stage, **prospective prechordal plate** within the cranial end of the primitive streak is ingressing in the cranial midline to form **prechordal plate**. The prechordal plate is one of the most misunderstood structures in human embryology. Experiments in chick and mouse provide strong evidence that the prechordal plate arises from the cranial end of the streak and intercalates into the endodermal layer, where it forms a thickening. The prechordal plate (some textbooks refer to it as *prochordal plate*) contributes to the **oropharyngeal membrane**, a two-layered membrane (ectoderm and endoderm) that ruptures to form the **mouth** opening. In addition, it forms an important signaling center involved in patterning the cranial end of

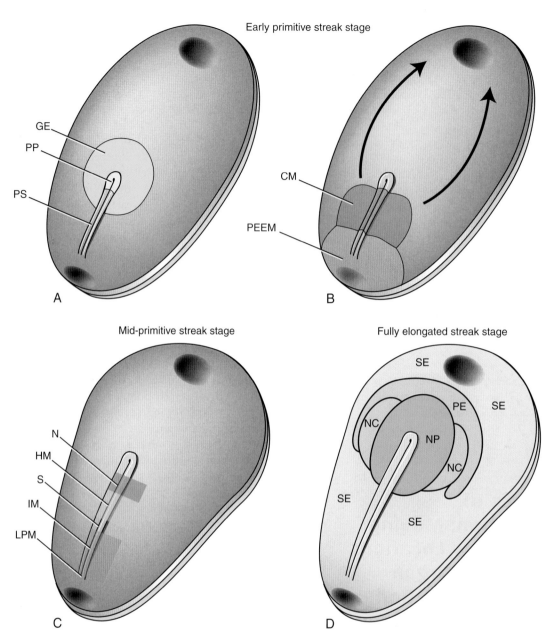

Early primitive streak stage

GE
PP
PS

A

CM

PEEM

B

Mid-primitive streak stage

N
HM
S
IM
LPM

C

Fully elongated streak stage

SE
PE
SE
NC
NP
NC
SE
SE

D

Figure 3-10. Prospective fate maps of the epiblast (based on data obtained from both chick and mouse embryos), showing the regions of epiblast that ingress through the primitive streak and form the major subdivisions of the trilaminar embryonic disc. *A,* Early primitive streak stage showing locations of prospective gut endoderm (GE) in epiblast and prospective prechordal plate (PP) in the cranial end of the primitive streak (PS; dark outline in subsequent figures). Oval at the cranial end of the epiblast (in all figures) indicates the location of the future oropharyngeal membrane; caudal oval indicates future cloacal membrane. *B,* Early primitive streak stage showing locations of prospective cardiogenic mesoderm (CM) and prospective extraembryonic mesoderm (PEEM) in epiblast and primitive streak. Arrows indicate the directions of migration of the cardiogenic mesoderm. *C,* Midprimitive streak stage showing locations of prospective mesoderm in epiblast and primitive streak. These include prospective notochord (N), head mesoderm (HM), somites (S), intermediate mesoderm (IM), and lateral plate mesoderm (LPM). *D,* Fully elongated primitive streak stage showing locations of the neural plate (NP), surface ectoderm (SE), neural crest cells (NC), and placodal ectoderm (PE) after cells in the cranial half of the embryonic disc have completed their ingression into the primitive streak. Some epiblast still remains caudally at this stage, where cells are still moving into and ingressing through the primitive streak.

the neural tube (future forebrain; discussed in Ch. 4). Finally, evidence from animal models suggests that part of the prechordal plate undergoes an **epithelial-to-mesenchymal transformation** to form head mesenchyme cells that eventually reside in the cranial midline beneath the forebrain, just cranial to the notochord. Because the prechordal plate forms both mesodermal (part of head mesenchyme) and endodermal (part of oropharyngeal membrane) derivatives, it is often considered to be a **mesendodermal** structure.

Formation of the mesoderm also begins during the early primitive streak stage (see Fig. 3-10*B*). **Prospective cardiogenic mesoderm** from the epiblast moves into the middle part of the primitive streak and then migrates cranially to form **cardiogenic mesoderm** flanking the oropharyngeal membrane. **Prospective extraembryonic mesoderm** moves from the epiblast into the caudal end of the primitive streak to contribute to the **extraembryonic mesoderm** of the amnion, yolk sac, and allantois (discussed in Ch. 6).

At the midprimitive streak stage (see Fig. 3-10*C*), **prospective notochord** migrates cranially in the midline to form the **notochordal process**. More caudally, and in cranial-to-caudal succession, **prospective head mesoderm** in the epiblast moves into and through the primitive streak to form the **head mesoderm; prospective somites** in the epiblast move into and through the primitive streak to form the **somites; prospective intermediate mesoderm** moves into and through the primitive streak to form **intermediate mesoderm;** and **prospective lateral plate mesoderm** moves into and through the primitive streak to form **lateral plate mesoderm.** Collectively, the prospective head mesoderm and prospective somites constitute the **paraxial mesoderm.**

At the fully elongated primitive streak stage, when the primitive streak has reached its maximal length and has not yet initiated its regression (see Fig. 3-10*D*), movement of epiblast cells into the primitive streak is completed, except adjacent to the caudal end of the primitive streak. Thus, most of the epiblast now consists of **ectoderm**. The **prospective neural plate** is located cranial and lateral to the cranial end of the primitive streak. **Prospective neural crest cells**, a migratory population of ectodermal cells (discussed in Ch. 4), flank the lateral sides of the neural plate. The **prospective placodal ectoderm**, a horse-shoe–shaped area that forms sensory placodes (discussed in Ch. 4), lies peripheral to the craniolateral

borders of the neural plate, and the **prospective surface ectoderm** constitutes the remaining areas of the ectoderm. At this stage, only the neural plate and surface ectoderm can be distinguished from one another when the ectoderm is viewed with scanning electron microscopy (see Fig. 3-8).

Notochord Is Formed in Multiple Steps

Formation of the notochord begins with cranial midline extension from the primitive node of a hollow tube, the **notochordal process**. This tube grows in length as primitive node cells are added to its proximal end, concomitant with regression of the primitive streak (Fig. 3-11).

When the notochordal process is completely formed, on about day 20, several morphogenetic transformations are believed to take place to convert it from a hollow tube, to a flattened plate, to a solid rod (summarized in Fig. 3-12). First, the ventral floor of the tube fuses with the underlying endoderm and the two layers break down, leaving behind the flattened **notochordal plate (Fig. 3**-12*A*, *B*). At the level of the primitive pit, the yolk sac cavity now transiently communicates with the amniotic cavity through an opening called the **neurenteric canal** (see Fig. 3-12*B*). The **notochordal plate** then completely detaches from the endoderm and its free ends fuse as it rolls up into the mesoderm-containing space between ectoderm and endoderm, changing as it does so into a solid rod called the **notochord** (see Fig. 3-12*C*). Because the notochord derives from the primitive node and because it ends up in the mesodermal layer, it is considered to be a mesodermal derivative.

During later development, the rudiments of the vertebral bodies coalesce around the notochord, and it is commonly stated that the notochord forms the nucleus pulposus at the center of the vertebral discs. Certainly, this is true in the embryo, the fetus, and young children. However, in early childhood the nucleus pulposus cells of notochordal origin degenerate and are replaced by adjacent mesodermal cells. Thus, the notochord does not contribute to the bony elements of the spinal column. Rather, the notochord plays important inductive and patterning roles in early development (discussed in Ch. 4) and is also involved in induction of the vertebral bodies (discussed in Ch. 8).

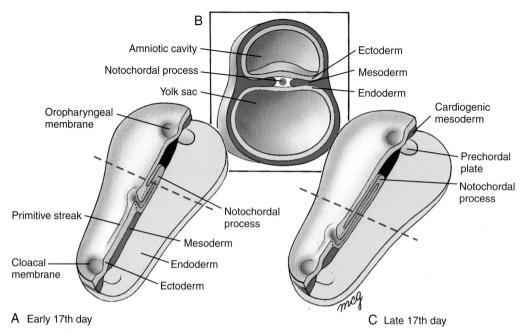

Figure 3-11. Formation of the notochordal process. *A, C,* Stages showing hollow notochordal process growing cranially from the primitive node. Note changes in relative length of the notochordal process and primitive streak as the embryo grows. Also note fusion of ectoderm and endoderm in the oropharyngeal and cloacal membranes. *B,* Cross section of the embryonic disc at the level indicated by the dotted lines.

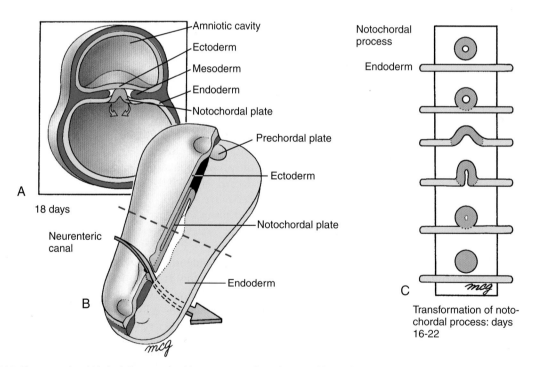

Figure 3-12. The process by which the hollow notochordal process is transformed into a solid notochord between days 16 and 22. *A, B,* First, the ventral wall of the notochordal process fuses with the endoderm and the two layers break down, leaving behind the flattened notochordal plate. As shown in *B,* this process commences at the caudal end of the notochordal process and proceeds cranially (the dotted line marks the level of *A*). An open neurenteric canal is briefly created between the amniotic cavity and the yolk sac cavity. *C,* Series of events by which the notochordal process becomes the notochordal plate and then the notochord.

CELLULAR BASIS OF CONVERGENT EXTENSION

In addition to epiboly and emboly, discussed earlier in the chapter, convergent extension plays a role during gastrulation. In particular, formation of the notochordal plate involves convergent extension—the coordinated narrowing of a cluster of node-derived cells in the medial-lateral plane and concomitant lengthening in the cranial-caudal plane as the notochordal plate forms. Detailed studies of the process in amphibian embryos have revealed that convergent extension of the notochord is driven by **cell-to-cell intercalation**, that is, the medial-lateral interdigitation of cells. As a metaphor, imagine four lanes of traffic merging into two lanes. If each lane contains 5 cars, to accommodate all 20 cars in 2 lanes each lane would need, on the average, to double its length (and the number of cars it contains) as the number of lanes is halved.

In other words, there would be a concomitant increase in the length of the column of cars, as the width of the merging traffic column was decreased.

Amphibians differ from birds and mammals in that early development of amphibians involves virtually no growth, whereas in birds and mammals, extensive growth occurs. Studies of notochord elongation in birds and mammals have revealed that, in addition to convergent extension generated by cell-to-cell intercalation, **oriented cell division** plays a role in convergent extension. Thus, mitotic division planes (i.e., metaphase plates) are positioned in dividing notochordal cells to separate daughter cells preferentially in the cranial-caudal plane, rather than in the medial-lateral plane. Modeling studies suggest that about half of the convergent extension that occurs in notochordal formation in birds and mammals is driven by cell-to-cell intercalation, whereas the other half is driven by oriented cell division.

Paraxial Mesoderm Differs in Head and Trunk

The mesoderm that begins ingressing through the middle part of the primitive streak in midprimitive streak stage embryos gives rise to the paraxial mesoderm that immediately flanks the notochord. In the future head region, this mesoderm forms bands of cells that remain unsegmented as the **head mesoderm** (Fig. 3-13A). The mesoderm becomes more dispersed with development to loosely fill the developing head as the **head mesenchyme**. Later, once neural crest cells start to migrate (discussed in Ch. 4), the head mesenchyme becomes supplemented with **neural crest cells**. Thus, the head mesenchyme is derived from both head mesoderm and ectodermal neural crest cells (and in the most cranial midline, from the prechordal plate, as discussed earlier in the chapter).

The head mesoderm eventually gives rise to the striated muscles of the face, jaw, and throat. As described in Chapter 16, these muscles differentiate within the segmental pharyngeal arches, which develop on either side of the pharynx. The pharyngeal arches are central elements in the development of the neck and face.

In the future trunk region, the paraxial mesoderm also forms bands of cells, but these bands soon segment into **somites**, blocklike condensations of mesoderm (Figs. 3-13B, 3-14, 3-15). The first pair of

somites forms on about day 20 at the head-trunk border. The remainder form in cranial-caudal progression at a rate of about 3 or 4 a day, finishing on about day 30. Approximately 42 to 44 pairs of somites form, flanking the notochord from the occipital (skull base) region to the tip of the embryonic tail. However, the caudalmost several somites eventually disappear, giving a final count of approximately 37 pairs.

Somites give rise to most of the axial skeleton, including the vertebral column and part of the occipital bone of the skull; to the voluntary musculature of the neck, body wall, and limbs; and to the dermis of the neck. Thus, formation and segmentation of somites are of major importance in organization of the body structure.

The first four pairs of somites form in the occipital region. These somites contribute to the development of the occipital part of the skull; to the bones that form around the nose, eyes, and inner ears; to the extrinsic ocular muscles; and to muscles of the tongue (discussed in Ch. 16). The next eight pairs of somites form in the presumptive **cervical** region. The most cranial cervical somites also contribute to the occipital bone, and others form the cervical vertebrae and associated muscles, as well as part of the dermis of the neck (discussed Ch. 8). The next 12 pairs, the **thoracic somites**, form thoracic vertebrae; the musculature and bones of the thoracic wall; the thoracic dermis; and part of the abdominal wall. Cells from cervical and thoracic

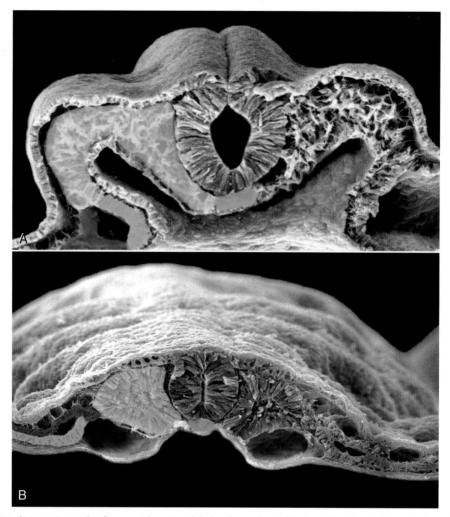

Figure 3-13. Scanning electron micrographs of transversely sectioned chick embryos showing the head (*A*) and trunk (*B*) neural tube and subdivisions of the mesoderm (colored on left side, but uncolored on right side): notochord (green), paraxial mesoderm (yellow), intermediate mesoderm (red), and lateral plate mesoderm consisting of somatic mesoderm (purple) and splanchnic mesoderm (blue). In the head, the lateral plate mesoderm (sometimes called lateral mesoderm) is equivalent to the cardiogenic mesoderm. The splanchnic layer forms the heart wall, and the somatic layer forms part of the lining of the pericardial cavity.

somites also invade the upper limb buds to form the limb musculature (discussed in Ch. 18).

Caudal to the thoracic somites, the five **lumbar somites** form the abdominal dermis, abdominal muscles, and lumbar vertebrae, and the five **sacral somites** form the sacrum with its associated dermis and musculature. Cells from lumbar somites invade the lower limb buds to form the limb musculature. Finally, the three or so **coccygeal somites** that remain after degeneration of the caudalmost somites form the coccyx.

IN THE RESEARCH LAB

MOLECULAR MECHANISM OF SOMITOGENESIS

Somites form rhythmically from the trunk and tail paraxial mesoderm—often referred to as the **presomitic mesoderm**—through the process of **segmentation**. Segmentation involves the formation of serially repeated, functionally equivalent units or **segments**, and segmentation is a common process occurring throughout much of the animal kingdom. Invertebrates and vertebrates seem to have developed somewhat different developmental strategies for

Cranial

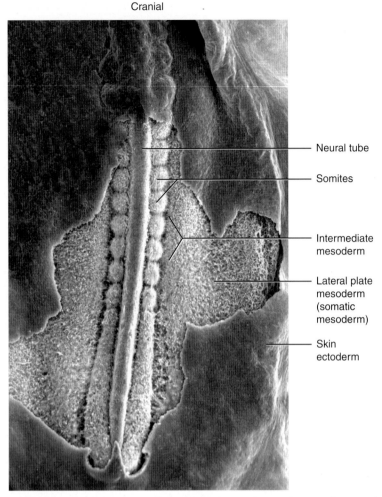

— Neural tube

— Somites

— Intermediate
mesoderm

— Lateral plate
mesoderm
(somatic
mesoderm)

— Skin
ectoderm

Figure 3-14. Scanning electron micrograph of the trunk region of a chick embryo with the surface ectoderm partially removed to show the underlying neural tube and mesoderm (cranial is toward the top). Note the somites and, more caudally, the paraxial mesoderm that has not yet segmented. Lateral to the somites the mesoderm has subdivided into the intermediate and lateral plate mesoderm (somatic mesoderm, the layer just deep to the surface ectoderm, is visible).

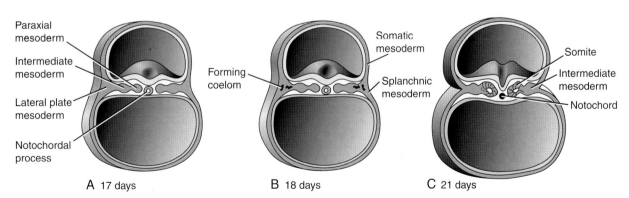

Paraxial
mesoderm

Intermediate
mesoderm

Lateral plate
mesoderm

Notochordal
process

Forming
coelom

Somatic
mesoderm

Splanchnic
mesoderm

Somite

Intermediate
mesoderm

Notochord

A 17 days   B 18 days   C 21 days

Figure 3-15. Sections through embryos at 17 to 21 days of gestation showing the differentiation of the mesoderm on either side of the midline. *A*, On day 17, the mesoderm has begun to differentiate into paraxial, intermediate, and lateral plate mesoderm. *B*, On day 18, the lateral plate begins to split to form intraembryonic coelom and somatic and splanchnic mesoderm. *C*, On day 21, the notochord, somites, and intermediate mesoderm are well formed and splitting of the lateral plate mesoderm is complete.

segmentation. In Drosophila, for example, the entire blastoderm segments all at once, whereas during somitogenesis in vertebrates, segmentation occurs in a cranial-to-caudal wave. As a metaphor to visualize the difference between invertebrate and vertebrate segmentation, think of a bread-slicing machine in which the entire loaf of bread is sliced into "segments" all at the same time, as compared to using a bread knife to slice a loaf into segments beginning at one end of the loaf and progressing slice by slice to the other end.

A breakthrough in our understanding of somitogenesis came with the discovery that certain genes, particularly those in the *Notch* signaling pathway (discussed in Ch. 5), cycle in their expression in the presomitic mesoderm in concert with somitogenesis (Fig. 3-16). Specifically, expression of members of the *Notch* family (such as *Lunatic fringe*) spreads through the presomitic mesoderm in caudal-to-cranial sequence in a cycle that is synchronized with formation of each pair of somites. Thus, at a given axial level of presomitic mesoderm, cyclic gene expression seems to turn on and off when

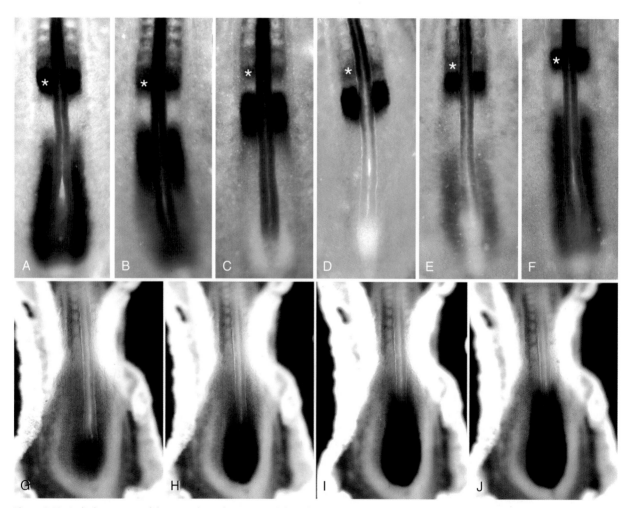

Figure 3-16. Cyclical expression of the gene *Lunatic fringe; A-F* and the *Fgf8* protein gradient (*G-J*) during somitogenesis in the caudal region of the chick embryo (cranial is toward the top of each figure). *A-F*, Time course over the 90-minute cycle of somite pair formation. Note the wave of *Lunatic fringe* mRNA expression moving from caudal-to-cranial (*A-E*) in the unsegmented paraxial mesoderm, and into the last pair of newly formed somites (*F*). *G-H*, Increasing time of exposure of an antibody to *Fgf8* protein. With a short exposure time to the antibody (*G*), only the tail bud and most caudal segmental plate labels, indicating that a high concentration of protein is present in this region. With longer exposures (*H-J*), increasingly more cranial areas of segmental plate are labeled, demonstrating a caudal-to-cranial concentration gradient. Asterisk, level of last somite pair.

examined with in situ hybridization as each pair of somites form. Cycling can be very rapid, occurring every 90 minutes in chick and every 20 minutes (at 25° C) in zebrafish, the exact time it takes to from a new pair of somites in these organisms.

A number of years before cyclic genes were identified in the presomitic mesoderm, a model was proposed to explain somitogenesis. According to this model, called the **clock and wavefront model**, formation of somites involves an oscillator, the so-called **segmentation clock**, whose periodic signal is used to specify somite boundaries at progressively more caudal levels where the signal coincides in both time and space with a traveling threshold level of expression of another signaling molecule (Fig. 3-17). The segmentation clock controls expression of cyclic genes, the first of which to be identified was the *Hairy1* gene, an ortholog of the Drosophila segmentation gene *Hairy* and a member of the *Notch* family. Many other members of the *Notch* family are now known to be part of the segmentation clock and *Wnt* signaling also plays a role, such that the clockwork of the oscillator apparently involves a series of negative feedback loops between *Notch* and *Wnt* signaling. Thus, this interaction establishes the rhythm of the clock and consequently the rhythm of somitogenesis.

Spacing of the somites is achieved by controlling the positioning of somite boundaries along the cranial-caudal axis using the wavefront. The wavefront is generated by a gradient of *Fgf8*, which is transcribed in the tail bud as the embryo undergoes cranial-caudal elongation. As cells migrate out of the tail bud into the presomitic mesoderm (discussed in Ch. 4), transcription of *Fgf8* stops. Moreover, *Fgf8* progressively decays over time in the cranial-caudally elongating presomitic mesoderm such that a concentration gradient of *Fgf8* protein is established that is low cranially and high caudally in the presomitic mesoderm (see Fig. 3-16). This gradient is further refined by a gradient of retinoic acid that extends caudally from the previously formed somites into the presomitic mesoderm. The retinoic acid gradient antagonizes *Fgf8* signaling in the cranial presomitic mesoderm and activates somitic genes such as the *Mesp* genes (bHLH transcription factors), the earliest-expressed somitic genes. As expression of cycling genes crosses the threshold-level point in the presomitic mesoderm, a region called the **determination** or **maturation wavefront**, the caudal boundary of a new pair of somites is specified. This is followed by new gene expression—as well as by changes in cell shape, position, and adhesion—all of which results in formation of somites.

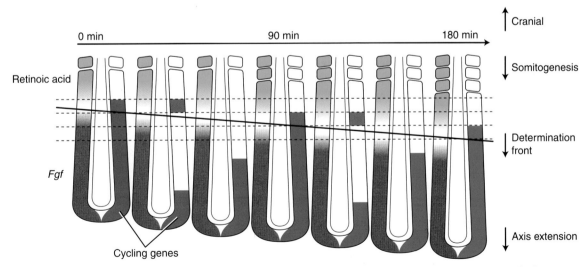

Figure 3-17. The molecular basis of the clock and wavefront model. Diagrams of the caudal end of chick embryos during two rounds of somitogenesis. Retinoic acid (blue) and *Fgf8* (gray) gradients move caudally as the embryo elongates (axis extension) during somitogenesis. In chick, a somite pair forms every 90 minutes, which constitutes the length of the clock cycle. Expression of cycling genes (red) extends from caudal to cranial, and when expression of these genes spreads cranially to cross the threshold level of *Fgf8* signaling (called the determination wavefront; diagonal line), somites are established (indicated by expression of *Mesp* genes; purple).

The clock and wavefront model is supported by several experiments. For example, implantation of beads coated with *Fgf8* protein into the cranial presomitic mesoderm of chick embryos prevents activation of their segmentation program. Furthermore, loss-of-function mutations in mouse cycling genes result in segmentation anomalies, including misplaced somitic boundaries and malformations of the vertebral column and ribs. Similarly, mutations in *NOTCH* signaling family in humans result in segmentation defects. Specifically, mutation of the *NOTCH* pathway ligand *DELTA-LIKE3* gene results in an autosomal recessive condition called **spondylocostal dysostosis syndrome** (Jarcho-Levin syndrome), a condition in which abnormal segmentation of the vertebral column and ribs occurs. Moreover, **Alagille syndrome**, which includes segmentation defects, results from mutations of the *NOTCH* pathway ligand *JAGGED1* or the *NOTCH* receptor *NOTCH2* (*Alagille syndrome is also mentioned in Chs. 5 and 12 to 14*).

Intermediate and Lateral Plate Mesoderm Form Only in Trunk

In addition to the notochord and paraxial mesoderm, both of which form in the head and trunk, two other subdivisions of mesoderm form in the trunk only: **intermediate mesoderm** and **lateral plate mesoderm** (see Figs. 3-13*B*, 3-14, 3-15). The mesoderm lying immediately lateral to each somite also segments and forms a small cylindric condensation, the **intermediate mesoderm.** The **intermediate mesoderm** produces the urinary system and parts of the genital system (discussed in Ch. 15). Lateral to the intermediate mesoderm, the mesoderm remains unsegmented and forms a flattened sheet, the **lateral plate mesoderm.** Starting on day 17, the **lateral plate mesoderm** splits into two layers: a ventral layer associated with the endoderm and a dorsal layer associated with the ectoderm (see Figs. 3-13*B*, 3-15*B, C*). The layer adjacent to the endoderm gives rise to the mesothelial covering of the visceral organs (viscera), and well as part of the wall of the viscera; hence, it is called the **splanchnic mesoderm** (from the Greek *splanchnon*, viscera). The layer adjacent to the ectoderm gives rise to the inner lining of the body wall and to parts of the limbs; hence, it is called the **somatic mesoderm** (from the Greek *soma*, body). Because the splanchnic mesoderm and adjacent endoderm act together to form structures, they are collectively called the **splanchnopleure.** Similarly, the somatic mesoderm and adjacent ectoderm act together

to form structures; they are collectively called the **somatopleure**.

IN THE CLINIC

ABNORMAL GASTRULATION LEADS TO CAUDAL DYSPLASIA

Caudal dysplasia, also called c**audal regression syndrome, caudal agenesis**, or **sacral agenesis**, is characterized by varying degrees of (1) flexion, inversion, and lateral rotation of the lower extremities; (2) anomalies of lumbar and sacral vertebrae; (3) imperforate anus; (4) agenesis of the kidneys and urinary tract; and (5) agenesis of the internal genital organs except for the gonads. In extreme cases, the deficiency in caudal development leads to fusion of the lower limb buds during early development, resulting in a "mermaid-like" habitus called **sirenomelia** (Fig. 3-18; also see Clinical Taster for this chapter).

In some individuals, caudal malformations are associated with more cranial abnormalities. One of these associations is called the **VATER association** because it includes some or all of the following anomalies: vertebral defects, anal atresia, tracheal-esophageal fistula (discussed in Ch. 11), and renal defects and radial forearm anomalies. An extension of this association, the **VACTERL association**, also includes cardiovascular anomalies with renal and limb defects. A number of other syndromes may be related to these associations.

Although the anomalies found in these associations are diverse, it is believed that they all arise from defects resulting from abnormal growth and migration during gastrulation. Mesodermal structures formed during the 3rd and 4th weeks participate in the development of most of the structures involved in caudal dysplasia and associated malformations. For example, the sacral and coccygeal vertebrae form from structures called **sclerotomes** that develop from the sacral and caudal somites (discussed in Ch. 4). The intermediate mesoderm differentiates into kidneys in response to induction by the ingrowing mesoderm ureteric buds (discussed in Ch. 15). Imperforate anus may result from the improper migration of caudal mesodermal in relation to the forming anal membrane (discussed in Ch. 14), whereas tracheoesophageal fistulas may be caused by defective interaction between the endodermal foregut anlage and mesoderm (discussed in Ch. 11). Radial forearm malformations apparently result from anomalous migration and differentiation of lateral plate mesoderm (discussed in Ch. 18).

In animal models, caudal dysplasia can be induced by both environmental factors and mutations. For example, *Insulin*, when injected into the chick egg during gastrulation,

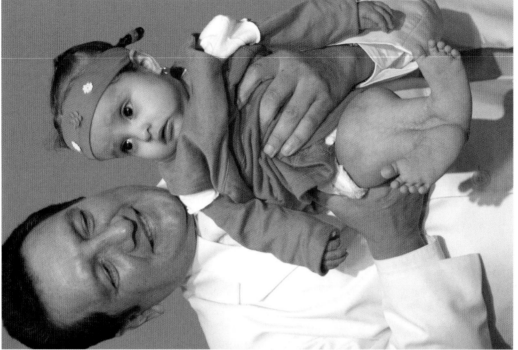

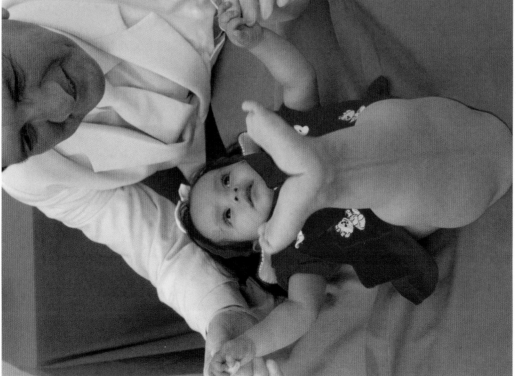

Figure 3-18. Sirenomelia. Severe reduction of caudal structures has resulted in fusion of the lower limb buds. Shown is Milagros Cerron at about 1 year of age with her physician.

causes caudal dysplasia, thereby acting as a **teratogen**—a substance that causes malformation of the embryo or fetus (**teratogenesis** is further discussed in Chs. 5 and 6). Similar defects are also observed in mice with mutations in the *Brachyury* gene, a T-box–containing transcription factor expressed throughout the primitive streak during gastrulation (Fig. 3-19). Analysis of such mice indicates that the mutation interferes with gastrulation by preventing the normal ingression of epiblast cells through the primitive streak, thus providing insight into how widespread mesodermal anomalies could result in humans with caudal dysplasia. In humans, caudal dysplasia is a common manifestation of **maternal (gestational) diabetes** with elevated INSULIN levels (discussed in Ch. 6).

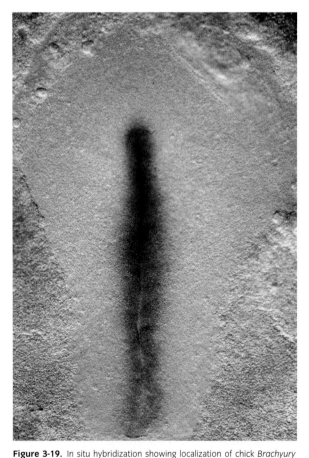

Figure 3-19. In situ hybridization showing localization of chick *Brachyury* mRNA, a T-box–containing transcription factor, which is expressed throughout the primitive streak.

Formation of Neural Plate

The first event in development of the future central nervous system is the formation on day 18 of a thickened **neural plate** in the ectoderm just cranial to the **primitive node** (Figs. 3-20, 3-21, 3-22). Formation of the neural plate is induced by the primitive node, the human equivalent of the **organizer** discussed early in the chapter. Thus, the process of neural plate formation is called **neural induction**. As a result of neural induction, ectodermal cells differentiate into a thick plate of pseudostratified, columnar **neuroepithelial cells (neuroectoderm)**. The neural plate forms first at the cranial end of the embryo and then differentiates in a cranial-to-caudal direction. As described in Chapter 4, the neural plate folds during the 4th week to form a neural tube, the precursor of the central nervous system. The lateral lips of the neural plate also give rise to an extremely important population of cells, **neural crest cells**, which detach during formation of the neural tube and migrate in the embryo to form a variety of structures.

The neural plate is broad cranially and tapered caudally. The expanded cranial portion gives rise to **brain**. Even at this very early stage of differentiation, the presumptive brain is visibly divided into three regions: the future **forebrain, midbrain**, and **hindbrain** (see Figs. 3-20, 3-21). The narrower caudal portion of the neural plate (continuous cranially with the hindbrain) gives rise to the **spinal cord**. Eventually, this level of the developing nervous system will be flanked by somites. The notochord lies in the midline just deep to the neural plate. It extends cranially from the primitive node to end near the future juncture between the forebrain and midbrain.

IN THE RESEARCH LAB

NEURAL INDUCTION

As in dorsal-ventral patterning of the mesoderm, induction of the neural plate also involves the secretion of antagonists by the **organizer** to inhibit signaling. Recall that the **Nieuwkoop center** induces the organizer, which patterns the mesoderm in the dorsal-ventral plane. In addition, the organizer induces the **neural plate**. Although the location of the **Nieuwkoop center** is well established in amphibians, its location is birds and mammals remains uncertain.

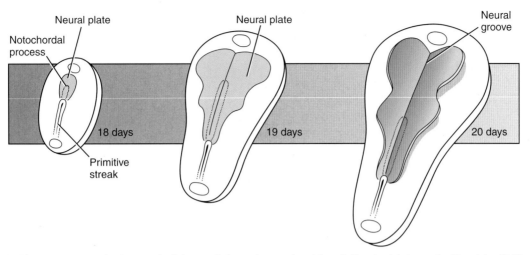

Figure 3-20. Schematic sequence showing growth of the neural plate and regression of the primitive streak between day 18 and day 20. The primitive streak shortens only slightly, but it occupies a progressively smaller proportion of the length of the embryonic disc as the neural plate and embryonic disc grow.

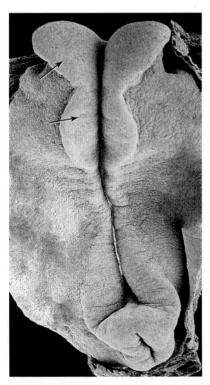

Figure 3-21. Scanning electron micrograph of a Macaque embryo comparable to a 20-day human embryo. The neural plate is clearly visible, and the expansions that will become the major subdivisions of the brain are apparent (arrows). Only a small region of the primitive streak remains. The primitive streak will disappear on day 25.

Nevertheless, loss-of-function experiments in mouse suggest that similar molecules induce the organizer in both lower and higher vertebrates. These include members of the *Tgfβ* (e.g., *Nodal*) and *Wnt* families.

The **organizer** has the amazing capacity to induce an entire secondary embryonic axis if grafted to an ectopic site of another embryo (Fig. 3-23*A*). This phenomenon was first discovered in the 1920s by Hilde Mangold and Hans Spemann, who were working with amphibian embryos. More than one dozen molecules are secreted by the organizer, and many of these, especially *Chordin* (discussed earlier in the chapter), have the capacity to induce secondary axes when ectopically expressed. In addition to secreted factors, the organizer expresses about 10 transcription factors. Ectopic expression of some of these, such as *Goosecoid*, also induces secondary axes (Fig. 3-23*B*).

The organizer induces neural plate by antagonizing the *Bmp* signaling pathway. In the presence of *Bmp* signaling, ectoderm forms **surface ectoderm**, but when *Bmp* signaling is inhibited, ectoderm forms **neural plate**. *Bmp* signaling is antagonized by the secretion of *Bmp* antagonists (discussed earlier in the chapter) such as *Noggin*, *Chordin*, *Nodal*, *Follistatin*, and *Cerberus*, all of which bind *Bmp* in the extracellular space and prevent *Bmp* binding to its receptors.

In addition to antagonizing the *Bmp* signaling pathway, the organizer induces neural plate by secreting other growth factors such as *Fgf8* and members of the *Igf* (*Insulin-like*

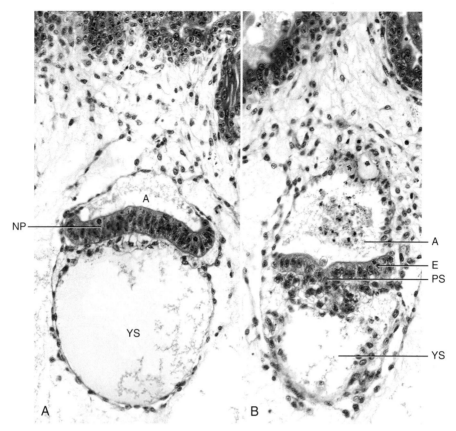

Figure 3-22. Cross sections through early human embryos. *A*, Level of neural plate (NP). Note yolk sac cavity (YS) and amniotic cavity (A). *B*, Level of primitive streak (PS). Note that the epiblast (E) is not as thickened as is the neural plate.

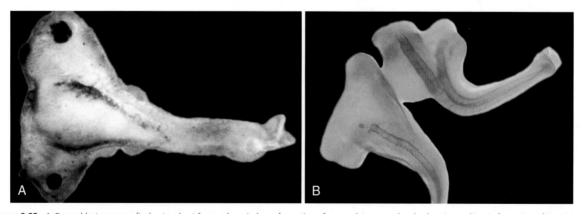

Figure 3-23. *A*, Donor blastopore grafted onto a host frog embryo induces formation of a complete secondary body axis resulting in formation of "conjoined" twins. *B*, A frog embryo was irradiated with ultraviolet light to abolish "organizer" activity, and then two blastomeres were injected with *Goosecoid* mRNA resulting in induction of two embryonic axes.

growth factor) family. Interesting, the *Fgf*, *Igf*, and *Bmp* pathways intersect at a common point during neural induction: *Smad1* phosphorylation. Both *Fgf/Igf* and *Bmp* signaling result in *Smad1* phosphorylation, although at different sites. Phosphorylation as a result of *Fgf/Igf* signaling causes inhibition of *Smad1* activity, whereas phosphorylation as a result of *Bmp* signaling causes stimulation of *Smad1* activity. Consequently, the combined effect of *Fgf/Igf* signaling (inhibition of *Smad1* activity) and antagonism of *Bmp* signaling (nonstimulation of *Smad1* activity) results in a low level of *Smad1* activity and neural induction.

HEAD, TRUNK, AND TAIL ORGANIZERS

Once the primitive streak has formed, it will give rise to endoderm and mesoderm of three distinct regions of the body: head, trunk, and tail. Neural induction results in the formation of the neural plate, and as discussed in Chapter 4, neurulation subsequently converts the neural plate into a neural tube. The latter is quickly regionalized along the cranial-caudal axis into forebrain, midbrain, hindbrain, and spinal cord. Similarly, the mesoderm is regionalized along the cranial-caudal axis (e.g., unsegmented head paraxial mesoderm vs. segmented trunk paraxial mesoderm). How does this regionalization occur?

Our understanding of cranial-caudal patterning comes from a large series of experiments in four vertebrate models: Xenopus, zebrafish, chick, and mouse. Thus cranial-caudal patterning of the embryo is typically called *anterior-posterior patterning* because the cranial-caudal axis of human embryos is equivalent to the anterior-posterior axis of vertebrate embryo models (discussed in Introduction). In some of the vertebrate embryo models, separate **organizing centers** exist to pattern different levels of the cranial-caudal axis. For example, in mouse the head is patterned by the **head organizer**, also known as the **anterior visceral endoderm (AVE)**, a specialized region of extraembryonic endoderm (discussed earlier in the chapter), whereas the **node** functions as a **trunk organizer**. In zebrafish, a separate **tail organizer** has been identified called the **ventral margin**. In other vertebrate models, these organizers seem to be combined, at least partly, in the classic organizer. For example, in chick, the cranial end of the primitive streak first contains cells that pattern the head and later contains cells that pattern the trunk and tail. Thus, the organizer in chick is a dynamic structure in which cell populations contained within it change over time, and as a result of this change in populations, changes occur in the molecules secreted by the organizer that act to pattern the overlying neural plate in the cranial-caudal axis.

Regardless of where the signals originate during cranial-caudal patterning, comparison of results from gain-of-function and loss-of-function experiments in all four vertebrate models (discussed above) has revealed that mechanisms of head, trunk, and tail patterning are highly conserved among species. Formation of all three levels of the body involve a common theme: **combinatorial signaling**, in which the amount expressed of three signaling molecules varies at different levels. The signaling molecules consist of *Wnts*, *Bmps*, and *Nodal*.

Formation of the **head** requires inhibition of *Wnt* and *Bmp* signaling. Thus, the head organizer, be it a separate signaling center or part of the organizer itself depending on the organism, secretes *Wnt* and *Bmp* signaling antagonists. Loss-of-function of these inhibitors results in loss of head structures. For example, loss-of-function in mouse of the *Wnt* signaling inhibitor *Dickkopf1*, which is expressed by the AVE, results in loss of the most cranial part of the head (Fig. 3-24A). In addition to factors secreted by the AVE, transcription factors are required for head development. One of these is the homeobox-containing gene *Lim-1* (Fig 3-24B). Similar experiments suggest that *Nodal* signaling plays little if any direct role in patterning of the head.

Formation of the trunk, in contrast to that of the head, requires both *Wnt* and *Nodal* signaling, as well as inhibition of *Bmp* signaling. Similarly, formation of the tail requires both *Wnt* and *Nodal* signaling, but in contrast to that of the trunk, formation of the tail also requires *Bmp* signaling.

Primary versus Secondary Body Development

Gastrulation Ends with Formation of Tail Bud

On day 16, the primitive streak spans about half the length of the embryo. However, as gastrulation proceeds the primitive streak regresses caudally, becoming gradually shorter. By day 22, the primitive streak represents about 10% to 20% of the embryo's length, and by day 26, it seems to disappear. However, on about day 20, remnants of the primitive streak swell to produce a caudal midline mass of mesoderm called the **tail bud** or **caudal eminence**, which will give rise to the most caudal structures of the body. Formation of the tail bud provides a reservoir of cells that allows the embryo to extend caudally during formation of its rudimentary and transient tail. In particular, the tail bud contributes cells to the caudal end

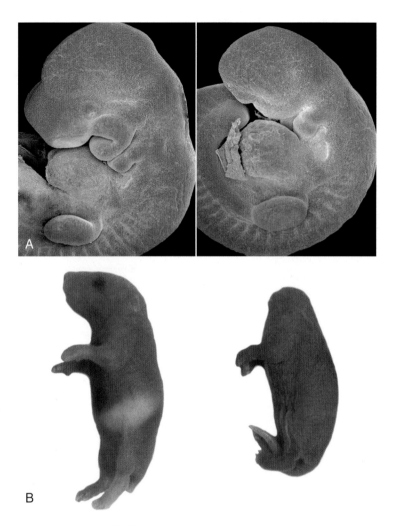

Figure 3-24. "Headless" mice. *A*, Loss-of-function of *Dickkopf1*, a secreted antagonist of *Wnt* signaling, causes loss of the most cranial end of the head in mice (shown on right; left, wild-type control mouse). *B*, Similarly, loss-of-function of the homeobox-containing gene *Lim-1* results in a more dramatic loss (shown on right; left), wild-type control mouse).

of the **neural tube** and **neural crest cells** (sacral and coccygeal), as well as the caudal **somites**. By contrast, the **notochord** of the tail extends into this region from more cranial levels, rather than forming from the tail bud, and may serve a role in organizing and patterning caudal organ rudiments.

Gastrulation occurs during a period of development called **primary body development**. During primary body development, the primitive streak gives rise to the three primary germ layers, which subsequently assemble into organ rudiments. Formation of the rudimentary tail occurs after gastrulation is complete,

during a period of development called **secondary body development**. In contrast to primary body development, secondary body development involves the direct formation of organ rudiments from the tail bud without the prior formation of distinct germ layers.

Suggested Readings

Adams DS, Levin M. 2004. Early patterning of the left/right axis. In: Stern CD, editor. Gastrulation. From Cells to Embryo. Cold Spring Harbor, New York: Cold Spring Harbor Laboratory Press. pp 403-417.

Ang S-L, Behringer RR. 2002. Anterior-posterior patterning of the mouse body axis at gastrulation. In: Rossant J, Tam PPL, editors. Mouse Development. Patterning, Morphogenesis, and Organogenesis. San Diego: Academic Press. pp 37-53.

Bessho Y, Kageyama R. 2003. Oscillations, clocks and segmentation. Curr Opin Genet Dev 13:379-384.

Burdine RD, Schier AF. 2000. Conserved and divergent mechanisms in left-right axis formation. Genes Dev 14:763-776.

Callebaut M. 2005. Origin, fate and function of the components of the avian germ disc region and early blastoderm: role of ooplasmic determinants. Dev Dyn 233:1194-1216.

Capdevila J, Vogan KJ, Tabin CJ, Izpisua Belmonte JC. 2000. Mechanisms of left-right determination in vertebrates. Cell 101:9-21.

Casey B, Hackett BP. 2000. Left-right axis malformations in man and mouse. Curr Opin Genet Dev 10:257-261.

Ciruna B, Rossant J. 2001. FGF signaling regulates mesoderm cell fate specification and morphogenetic movement at the primitive streak. Dev Cell 1:37-49.

Cohen MM Jr. 2001. Asymmetry: molecular, biologic, embryopathic, and clinical perspectives. Am J Med Genet 101:292-314.

Cooke J. 2004. Developmental mechanism and evolutionary origin of vertebrate left/right asymmetries. Biol Rev Camb Philos Soc 79:377-407.

Cooke J. 2004. The evolutionary origins and significance of vertebrate left-right organisation. Bioessays 26:413-421.

Dawid IB. 2004. Organizing the vertebrate embryo. PLoS Biol 2:E127.

De Robertis EM, Kuroda H. 2004. Dorsal-ventral patterning and neural induction in Xenopus embryos. Annu Rev Cell Dev Biol 20:285-308.

De Robertis EM, Larrain J, Oelgeschlager M, Wessely O. 2000. The establishment of Spemann's organizer and patterning of the vertebrate embryo. Nat Rev Genet 1:171-181.

de Souza FS, Niehrs C. 2000. Anterior endoderm and head induction in early vertebrate embryos. Cell Tissue Res 300:207-217.

Dubrulle J, Pourquie O. 2002. From head to tail: links between the segmentation clock and antero-posterior patterning of the embryo. Curr Opin Genet Dev 12:519-523.

Dubrulle J, Pourquie O. 2004. Coupling segmentation to axis formation. Development 131:5783-5793.

Eakin GS, Behringer RR. 2004. Gastrulation in other mammals and humans. In: Stern CD, editor. Gastrulation. From Cells to Embryo. Cold Spring Harbor, New York: Cold Spring Harbor Laboratory Press. pp 275-287.

Essner JJ, Vogan KJ, Wagner MK, Tabin CJ, Yost HJ, Brueckner M. 2002. Conserved function for embryonic nodal cilia. Nature 418:37-38.

Fraser SE, Stern CD. 2004. Early rostrocaudal patterning of the mesoderm and neural plate. Cold Spring Harbor: Cold Spring Harbor Laboratory Press. pp 389-401.

Gossler A, Tam PPL. 2002. Somitogenesis: Segmentation of the paraxial mesoderm and the delineation of tissue compartments. In: Rossant J, Tam PPL, editors. Mouse Development. Patterning, Morphogenesis, and Organogenesis. San Diego: Academic Press. pp 127-149.

Grapin-Botton A, Constam D. 2004. Endoderm development. In: Stern CD, editor. Gastrulation. From Cells to Embryo. Cold Spring Harbor, New York: Cold Spring Harbor Laboratory Press. pp 433-448.

Halpern ME, Liang JO, Gamse JT. 2003. Leaning to the left: laterality in the zebrafish forebrain. Trends Neurosci 26:308-313.

Hamada H. 2002. Left-Right Asymmetry. In: Rossant J, Tam PPL, editors. Mouse Development. Patterning, Morphogenesis, and Organogenesis. San Diego: Academic Press. pp 55-73.

Harland R. 2000. Neural induction. Curr Opin Genet Dev 10:357-362.

Harland R. 2004. Dorsoventral patterning of the mesoderm. In: Stern CD, editor. Gastrulation. From Cells to Embryo. Cold Spring Harbor, New York: Cold Spring Harbor Laboratory Press. pp 373-388.

Ip YT, Gridley T. 2002. Cell movements during gastrulation: snail dependent and independent pathways. Curr Opin Genet Dev 12:423-429.

Juan H, Hamada H. 2001. Roles of nodal-lefty regulatory loops in embryonic patterning of vertebrates. Genes Cells 6:923-930.

Keller R. 2005. Cell migration during gastrulation. Curr Opin Cell Biol 17:533-541.

Keller R, Davidson L. 2004. Cell movements of gastrulation. In: Stern CD, editor. Gastrulation. From Cells to Embryo. Cold Spring Harbor, New York: Cold Spring Harbor Laboratory Press. pp 291-304.

Kiefer JC. 2005. The somite segmentation clock: it takes a licking and keeps on ticking. Dev Dyn 232:519-523.

Kimelman D, Bjornson C. 2004. Vertebrate mesoderm induction. In: Stern CD, editor. Gastrulation. From Cells to Embryo. Cold Spring Harbor, New York: Cold Spring Harbor Laboratory Press. pp 363-372.

Kourakis MJ, Smith WC. 2005. Did the first chordates organize without the organizer? Trends Genet 21:506-510.

Kuroda H, Fuentealba L, Ikeda A. 2005. Default neural induction: neuralization of dissociated Xenopus cells is mediated by Ras/MAPK activation. Genes Dev 19:1022-1027.

Ladher R, Schoenwolf GC. 2005. Making a neural tube: Neural induction and neurulation. In: Rao MS, Jacobson M, editors. Developmental Neurobiology, 4th ed. New York: Kluwer Academic/Plenum Pub. pp 1-39.

Levin M. 2003. Motor protein control of ion flux is an early step in embryonic left-right asymmetry. Bioessays 25:1002-1010.

Levin M. 2005. Left-right asymmetry in embryonic development: a comprehensive review. Mech Dev 122:3-25.

Lohnes D. 2003. The Cdx1 homeodomain protein: an integrator of posterior signaling in the mouse. Bioessays 25:971-980.

Marshall WF, Nonaka S. 2006. Cilia: tuning in to the cell's antenna. Curr Biol 16:R604-R614.

Martindale MQ. 2005. The evolution of metazoan axial properties. Nat Rev Genet 6:917-927.

McGrath J, Brueckner M. 2003. Cilia are at the heart of vertebrate left-right asymmetry. Curr Opin Genet Dev 13:385-392.

McGrath J, Somlo S, Makova S, et al. 2003. Two populations of node monocilia initiate left-right asymmetry in the mouse. Cell 114:61-73.

Mercola M, Levin M. 2001. Left-right asymmetry determination in vertebrates. Annu Rev Cell Dev Biol 17:779-805.

Mikawa T, Poh AM, Kelly KA, et al. 2004. Induction and patterning of the primitive streak, an organizing center of gastrulation in the amniote. Dev Dyn 229:422-432.

Mlodzik M. 2002. Planar cell polarization: do the same mechanisms regulate Drosophila tissue polarity and vertebrate gastrulation? Trends Genet 18:564-571.

Montero JA, Heisenberg CP. 2004. Gastrulation dynamics: cells move into focus. Trends Cell Biol 14:620-627.

Mukhopadhyay M, Shtrom S, Rodriguez-Esteban C, et al. 2001. Dickkopf1 is required for embryonic head induction and limb morphogenesis in the mouse. Dev Cell 1:423-434.

Munoz-Sanjuan I, Brivanlou AH. 2001. Early posterior/ventral fate specification in the vertebrate embryo. Dev Biol 237:1-17.

Munoz-Sanjuan I, Brivanlou AH. 2002. Neural induction, the default model and embryonic stem cells. Nat Rev Neurosci 3:271-280.

Myers DC, Sepich DS, Solnica-Krezel L. 2002. Convergence and extension in vertebrate gastrulae: cell movements according to or in search of identity? Trends Genet 18:447-455.

Niehrs C. 2004. Regionally specific induction by the Spemann-Mangold organizer. Nat Rev Genet 5:425-434.

Nikolaidou KK, Barrett K. 2005. Getting to know your neighbours; a new mechanism for cell intercalation. Trends Genet 21:70-73.

Okada Y, Takeda S, Tanaka Y, Belmonte JC, Hirokawa N. 2005. Mechanism of nodal flow: a conserved symmetry breaking event in left-right axis determination. Cell 121:633-644.

Pourquie O. 2000. Segmentation of the paraxial mesoderm and vertebrate somitogenesis. Curr Top Dev Biol 47:81-105.

Pourquie O. 2001. The vertebrate segmentation clock. J Anat 199:169-175.

Pourquie O. 2001. Vertebrate somitogenesis. Annu Rev Cell Dev Biol 17:311-350.

Pourquie O. 2003. The segmentation clock: converting embryonic time into spatial pattern. Science 301:328-330.

Pourquie O. 2003. Vertebrate somitogenesis: a novel paradigm for animal segmentation? Int J Dev Biol 47:597-603.

Pourquie O. 2004. The chick embryo: a leading model in somitogenesis studies. Mech Dev 121:1069-1079.

Pourquie O, Kusumi K. 2001. When body segmentation goes wrong. Clin Genet 60:409-416.

Raya A, Belmonte JC. 2004. Sequential transfer of left-right information during vertebrate embryo development. Curr Opin Genet Dev 14:575-581.

Raya A, Izpisua Belmonte JC. 2004. Unveiling the establishment of left-right asymmetry in the chick embryo. Mech Dev 121:1043-1054.

Rida PC, Le Minh N, Jiang YJ. 2004. A Notch feeling of somite segmentation and beyond. Dev Biol 265:2-22.

Rossant J, Tam PP. 2004. Emerging asymmetry and embryonic patterning in early mouse development. Dev Cell 7:155-164.

Saga Y, Takeda H. 2001. The making of the somite: molecular events in vertebrate segmentation. Nat Rev Genet 2:835-845.

Sasai Y. 2001. Regulation of neural determination by evolutionarily conserved signals: anti-BMP factors and what next? Curr Opin Neurobiol 11:22-26.

Schier AF. 2001. Axis formation and patterning in zebrafish. Curr Opin Genet Dev 11:393-404.

Schier AF. 2003. Nodal signaling in vertebrate development. Annu Rev Cell Dev Biol 19:589-621.

Schneider H, Brueckner M. 2000. Of mice and men: dissecting the genetic pathway that controls left-right asymmetry in mice and humans. Am J Med Genet 97:258-270.

Solnica-Krezel L. 2005. Conserved patterns of cell movements during vertebrate gastrulation. Curr Biol 15:R213-R228.

Stemple DL. 2005. Structure and function of the notochord: an essential organ for chordate development. Development 132:2503-2512.

Stern CD. 2004. Gastrulation in the chick. In: Stern CD, editor. Gastrulation. From Cells to Embryo. Cold Spring Harbor, New York: Cold Spring Harbor Laboratory Press. pp 219-232.

Supp DM, Potter SS, Brueckner M. 2000. Molecular motors: the driving force behind mammalian left-right development. Trends Cell Biol 10:41-45.

Tam PPL, Gad JM. 2004. Gastrulation in the mouse embryo. In: Stern CD, editor. Gastrulation. From Cells to Embryo. Cold Spring Harbor: Spring Harbor Laboratory Press. pp 233-262.

Tanaka Y, Okada Y, Hirokawa N. 2005. FGF-induced vesicular release of Sonic hedgehog and retinoic acid in leftward nodal flow is critical for left-right determination. Nature 435:172-177.

Wallingford JB, Fraser SE, Harland RM. 2002. Convergent extension: the molecular control of polarized cell movement during embryonic development. Dev 2:695-706.

Weaver C, Kimelman D. 2004. Move it or lose it: axis specification in Xenopus. Development 131:3491-3499.

Wilson SI, Edlund T. 2001. Neural induction: toward a unifying mechanism. Nat Neurosci 4 Suppl:1161-1168.

Wright CV. 2001. Mechanisms of left-right asymmetry: what's right and what's left? Dev Cell 1:179-186.

Yost HJ. 2001. Establishment of left-right asymmetry. Int Rev Cytol 203:357-381.

Yost HJ. 2003. Left-right asymmetry: nodal cilia make and catch a wave. Curr Biol 13:R808-R809.

Fourth Week: Forming the Embryo

4

Summary During the 4th week, the tissue layers laid down in the 3rd week differentiate to form the primordia of most of the major organ systems of the body. Simultaneously, the embryonic disc undergoes a process of folding that creates the basic vertebrate body form, called the **tube-within-a-tube body plan**. The main force responsible for embryonic folding is the differential growth of different portions of the embryo. The embryonic disc grows vigorously during the 4th week, particularly in length, whereas the growth of the yolk sac stagnates. Because the outer rim of the embryonic endoderm is attached to the yolk sac, the expanding disc bulges into a convex shape. Folding commences in the cranial and lateral regions of the embryo on day 22 and in the caudal region on day 23. As a result of folding, the cranial, lateral, and caudal edges of the embryonic disc are brought together along the ventral midline. The endodermal, mesodermal, and ectodermal layers of the embryonic disc each fuse to the corresponding layer on the opposite side, thus creating a tubular **three-dimensional body form**. The process of midline fusion transforms the flat embryonic endoderm into a **gut tube**. Initially, the gut consists of cranial and caudal blind-ending tubes—the **foregut** and **hindgut**, respectively—separated by the future **midgut**, which remains open to the yolk sac. As the lateral edges of the various embryonic disc layers continue to join together along the ventral midline, the midgut is progressively converted into a tube, and the yolk sac neck correspondingly is reduced to a slender **vitelline duct**. When the edges of the ectoderm fuse along the ventral midline, the space formed within the lateral plate mesoderm is enclosed in the embryo and becomes the **intraembryonic coelom**. The lateral plate mesoderm gives rise to the **serous membranes** that line the coelom—the **somatic mesoderm** coating the inner surface of the body wall and the **splanchnic mesoderm** ensheathing the gut tube.

Neurulation converts the neural plate to a hollow **neural tube** covered by **surface ectoderm**. The neural tube then begins to differentiate into the **brain** and **spinal cord**. Even before the end of the 4th week, the major regions of the brain—the **forebrain**, **midbrain**, and **hindbrain**—become apparent, and neurons and glia begin to differentiate from the neuroepithelium of the neural tube. As neurulation occurs, a special population of cells, **neural crest cells**, detach from the lateral lips of the neural folds and migrate to numerous locations in the body, where they differentiate to form a wide range of structures and cell types.

Somites continue to segregate from the paraxial mesoderm in cranial-caudal progression until day 30. Meanwhile, beginning in the cervical region, the somites subdivide into three kinds of mesodermal primordium: **myotomes, dermatomes**, and **sclerotomes**. The myotomes develop into the segmental musculature of the back and the ventrolateral body wall, and give rise to cells that migrate into the limb buds to form the **limb musculature**; the dermatomes contribute to the dermis of the neck and trunk; and the sclerotomes give rise to the vertebral bodies and vertebral arches, and also contribute to the base of the skull.

Weeks Days

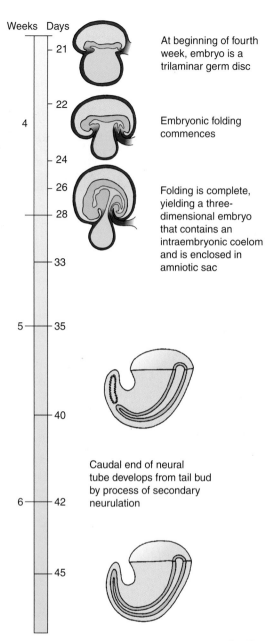

At beginning of fourth week, embryo is a trilaminar germ disc

Embryonic folding commences

Folding is complete, yielding a three-dimensional embryo that contains an intraembryonic coelom and is enclosed in amniotic sac

Neurulation begins

Cranial neuropore closes

Caudal neuropore closes and primitive streak disappears

Caudal end of neural tube develops from tail bud by process of secondary neurulation

Neural crest begins to migrate, commencing in cervical region

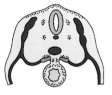

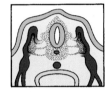

Sclerotome cells surround neural tube and notochord

Time line. Fourth week of development.

Clinical Taster A 20-year-old university sophomore is surprised to learn that his 19-year-old girl friend is pregnant. They have been having sex for only three months and have timed intercourse using the **rhythm method** of **birth control**, at least most of the time. On their first visit to student health services, they are told that the pregnancy is now in the 8th week and all seems normal. They decide to wait two months until spring break, when they will visit with their families who live in neighboring towns, to inform them about the pregnancy.

Although both sets of parents are shocked by the news, they are supportive and arrange an immediate appointment with an obstetrician. Ultrasound examination reveals that the fetus is growing normally. However, a mass of bowel is detected protruding from the ventral (anterior) body wall into the amniotic cavity. The diagnosis of **gastroschisis** is made (see Fig. 4-3B). On a follow-up visit, the young mother-to-be is very anxious. She's concerned that perhaps she did something to cause her baby to have gastroschisis. The doctor assures her that this is not the case, and that sometimes developmental events just go awry, resulting in birth defects.

The couple decides to return to school to complete the semester and then to move back home, where they can receive more intensive prenatal care. Beginning at 30 weeks of gestation, weekly ultrasounds are scheduled to examine the thickness of the bowel wall. Based on evidence that the wall is beginning to thicken and thus becoming damaged by exposure to the amniotic fluid, a cesarean section is scheduled at 35 weeks. At delivery, a three-centimeter opening in the abdominal wall is noted to the right of the baby's umbilicus, with multiple loops of protruding bowel. The newborn baby is taken immediately to surgery to return the bowel to the abdominal cavity and to repair the body wall defect. Although a relatively common birth defect, the cause of gastroschisis remains unknown.

Tube-within-a-Tube Body Plan Arises through Body Folding

At the end of the 3rd week, the embryo is a flat, ovoid, trilaminar disc. During the 4th week it grows rapidly, particularly in length, and undergoes a process of folding that generates the recognizable vertebrate body form (Figs. 4-1, 4-2). Although some active remodeling of tissue layers takes place, including localized changes in cell shape within the **body folds**, the main force responsible for embryonic folding is the differential growth of various embryonic structures. During the 4th week, the embryonic disc and amnion grow vigorously, but the yolk sac hardly grows at all. Because the yolk sac is attached to the ventral rim of the embryonic disc, the expanding disc balloons into a three-dimensional, somewhat cylindrical shape. The developing notochord, neural tube, and somites stiffen the dorsal axis of the embryo; therefore, most of the folding is concentrated in the thin, flexible outer rim of the disc. The cranial, caudal, and lateral margins of the disc fold completely under the dorsal axial structures and give rise to the ventral surface of the body. The areas of folding are referred to as the **cranial (head), caudal (tail)**, and **lateral body folds**, respectively. The cranial and caudal folds are best viewed in midsagittal sections

(see Fig. 4-1A-C; arrows in B), and the paired lateral body folds are best viewed in cross sections (see Fig. 4-1D, E; arrows in D). Although in sections these folds have different names, it is important to realize that these folds become continuous with one another as a ring of tissue at the position of the future umbilicus.

As described in Chapter 3, the cranial rim of the embryonic disc—the thin area located cranial to the neural plate—contains the oropharyngeal membrane, which represents the future mouth of the embryo. Cranial to the oropharyngeal membrane, a second important structure has begun to appear: the horseshoe-shaped **cardiogenic area**, which will give rise to the heart (discussed in Ch. 12). Cranial to the cardiogenic area, a third important structure forms: the **septum transversum**. This structure appears on day 22 as a thickened bar of mesoderm; it lies just caudal to the cranial margin of the embryonic disc. The septum transversum forms the initial partition separating the coelom into thoracic and abdominal cavities and gives rise to part of the diaphragm and the ventral mesentery of the stomach and duodenum (discussed in Chs. 11, 14).

Forward growth of the neural plate causes the thin cranial rim of the disc to fold under, forming the ventral surface of the future face, neck, and chest. This process translocates the oropharyngeal membrane to the region of the future mouth and also

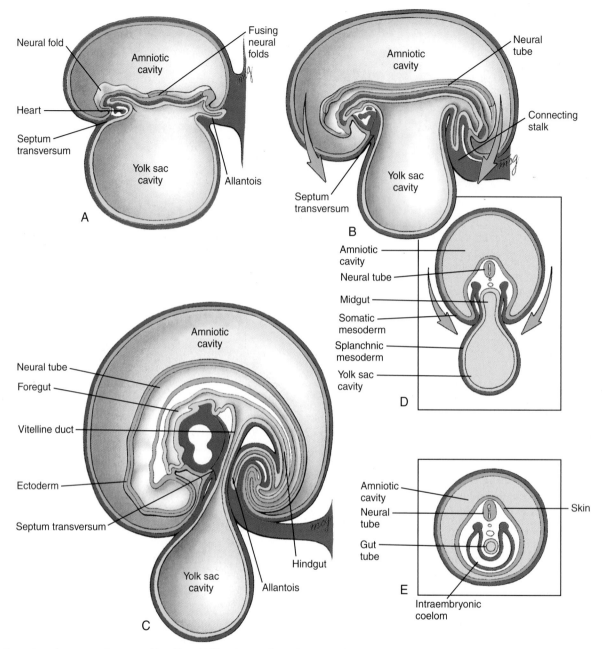

Figure 4-1. The process of craniocaudal and lateral folding that transforms the embryo from a flat embryonic disc to a three-dimensional tube-within-a-tube body plan. As folding occurs, the embryo grows more rapidly than the yolk sac, the cavity of which remains continuous with the developing gut tube through the narrowing vitelline duct. *A-E*, The septum transversum forms cranial to the cardiogenic area in the embryonic disc (*A*), and both it and the cardiogenic area are translocated to the future thoracic region through the folding of the cranial end of the embryo (*B, C*). The allantois and connecting stalk combine with the yolk sac and vitelline duct through the folding of the caudal end of the embryo. Fusion of the ectoderm, mesoderm, future coelomic cavities, and endoderm from opposite sides is prevented in the immediate vicinity of the vitelline duct (*D*) but not in the more cranial and caudal regions (*E*). The outer ectodermal (skin) and inner endodermal (gut) tubes of the tube-within-a-tube body plan are formed by body folding (*E*).

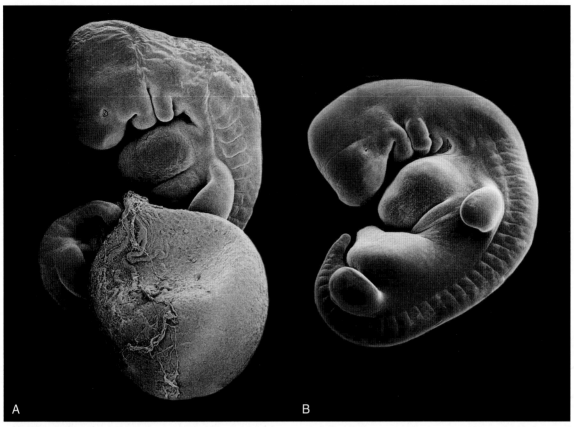

Figure 4-2. *A,* The form of this embryo is characteristic of that of a 4-week human embryo just subsequent to body folding. Note the relatively large yolk sac. *B,* The yolk sac has been removed in this 5-week embryo.

carries the cardiogenic area and septum transversum toward the future chest (see Fig. 4-1*A-C*).

Starting on about day 23, a similar process of folding commences in the caudal region of the embryo as the rapidly lengthening neural tube and somites overgrow the caudal rim of the yolk sac. Because of the relative stiffness of these dorsal axial structures, the thin caudal rim of the embryonic disc, containing the cloacal membrane, folds under and becomes part of the ventral surface of the embryo (see Fig. 4-1*A-C*). When the caudal rim of the disc folds under the body, the connecting stalk (which connects the caudal end of the embryonic disc to the developing placenta) is carried cranially until it merges with the neck of the yolk sac, which has begun to lengthen and constrict (see Figs. 4-1, 4-2). The root of the **connecting stalk** contains a slender endodermal hindgut diverticulum called the **allantois** (see Fig. 4-1*A-C*). The fate of the allantois is discussed in Chapter 15.

Simultaneously with cranial-caudal body folding, the right and left sides of the embryonic disc flex sharply ventrally, constricting and narrowing the neck of the yolk sac (see Fig. 4-1*D*). At the head and tail ends of the embryo, these lateral edges of the embryonic disc make contact with each other and then zip up toward the site of the future **umbilicus**. When the edges meet, the ectodermal, mesodermal, and endodermal layers on each side fuse with the corresponding layers on the other side (see Fig. 4-1*D, E*). As a result, the ectoderm of the original embryonic disc covers the entire surface of the three-dimensional embryo except for the future **umbilical region**, where the yolk sac and connecting stalk emerge. The ectoderm, along with contributions from the dermatomes, lateral plate mesoderm, and neural crest cells, will eventually form the skin (discussed in Ch. 7).

The endoderm of the trilaminar embryonic disc is destined to give rise to the lining of the gastrointestinal tract. When the cranial, caudal, and lateral edges of the embryo meet and fuse, the cranial and caudal portions of the endoderm are converted into blind-ending tubes—the future **foregut** and **hindgut**. At first, the central **midgut** region remains broadly open to the yolk sac (see Fig. 4-1A-D). However, as the gut tube forms, the neck of the yolk sac is gradually constricted, reducing its communication with the midgut. By the end of the 6th week, the gut tube is fully formed and the neck of the yolk sac has been reduced to a slim stalk called the **vitelline duct** (see Fig. 4-1C). The cranial end of the foregut is capped by the oropharyngeal membrane, which ruptures at the end of the 4th week to form the mouth. The caudal end of the hindgut is capped by the cloacal membrane, which ruptures during the 7th week to form the orifices of the anus and urogenital system (discussed in Chs. 14, 15).

As described in Chapter 3, the lateral plate mesoderm splits into two layers: the **somatic mesoderm**, which adheres to the ectoderm, and the **splanchnic meso-derm**, which adheres to the endoderm. The space between these layers is originally open to the chorionic cavity. However, when the folds of the embryo fuse along the ventral midline, this space is enclosed within the embryo and becomes the **intraembryonic coelom** (see Fig. 4-1E). The **serous membranes** lining this cav-ity form from the two layers of the lateral plate meso-derm: the inside of the body wall is lined with the somatic mesoderm, and the visceral organs derived from the gut tube are invested by splanchnic mesoderm.

As a result of body folding, the **tube-within-a-tube body plan** is established (see Fig. 4-1E). This plan consists of an embryo body design composed of two main tubes: an outer ectodermal tube forming the skin and an inner endodermal tube forming the gut. The space between the two tubes is filled mainly with mesoderm, the lateral plate mesodermal part of which splits to form the body cavity, or **coelom**. The neural tube, derived from the outer ectodermal tube, becomes internalized during the process of neurulation (discussed below).

IN THE CLINIC

ANTERIOR BODY WALL DEFECTS

Failure of the anterior (ventral) body wall to form properly during body folding or subsequent development results in anterior body wall defects. The most common of these include **omphalocele** and **gastroschisis**, which when grouped together occur in 1 in 2,500 live births. In both these defects, a portion of the gastrointestinal system herniates beyond the anterior body wall. However, in omphalocele, the bowel is membrane covered, in contrast to gastroschisis, in which the bowel protrudes through the body wall (Fig. 4-3). Anterior body wall defects can also occur in the thoracic wall. In this case, the heart can be exposed on the surface resulting in **ectopia cordis** (about 5 in 1 million live births). In the extremely rare **pentalogy of Cantrell**, considered an anterior body wall defect, five major anomalies occur together: 1) midline abdominal wall defect, 2) anterior diaphragmatic hernia, 3) cleft sternum, 4) pericardial defect, and 5) intracardiac defects such as a ventricular septal defect. In **prune belly syndrome (Eagle-Barrett syndrome)**, the anterior body wall closes, the

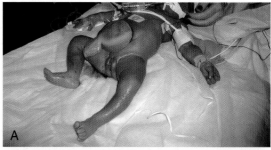

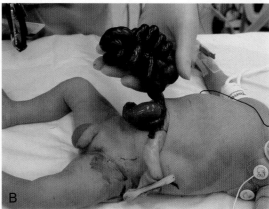

Figure 4-3. Omphalocele (A) and gastroschisis (B) in neonates. Note that in omphalocele the herniated bowel is contained within a membranous sac (part of the umbilical cord). However, in gastroschisis the bowel herniates through an opening in the body wall, typically to the right of the umbilical cord (the umbilical cord is clamped just proximal to its level of transection) and is not contained within a membranous sac.

abdomen becomes distended by bladder outlet obstruction, and the abdominal muscles fail to develop. Consequently, there is a marked wrinkling of the anterior abdominal wall. This syndrome occurs almost exclusively in males and is also associated with undescended testicles, suggesting a complex etiology. **Limb-body wall complex (LBWC; amniotic band syndrome)** also involves a complex etiology and in some cases may result from rupture of the amnion and constriction of limbs by fibrous amniotic bands (hence its alternative name, although not all cases of LBWC exhibit amniotic bands). In addition to limb defects (discussed in Ch. 18) and sometimes craniofacial defects (discussed in Ch. 16) and exencephaly or encephalocele (discussed later in chapter), anterior body wall defects such as omphalocele or gastroschisis are present in LBWC.

Neurulation: Establishing the Neural Tube, the Rudiment of the Central Nervous System

As discussed in Chapter 3, by the end of the 3rd week, the neural plate consists of a broad cranial portion that will give rise to the brain and a narrow caudal portion that will give rise to the spinal cord (see Figs. 3-20, 3-21). On day 22 (eight pairs of somites), the narrow caudal portion of the neural plate—the future spinal cord—represents only about 25% of the length of the neural plate. However, as somites continue to be added, the spinal cord region lengthens faster than the more cranial neural plate. By day 23 or 24 (12 and 20 pairs of somites, respectively), the future spinal cord occupies about 50% of the length of the neural plate, and by day 26 (25 pairs of somites), it occupies about 60%. The rapid lengthening of the neural plate during this period is driven by **convergent extension** (discussed in Ch. 3) of the **neuroepithelium** and underlying tissues.

Formation of the neural tube occurs during the process of **neurulation** (Fig. 4-4). Neurulation involves four main events: formation of the neural plate, shaping of the neural plate, bending of the neural plate, and closure of the neural groove (Fig. 4-5). Formation of the neural plate was discussed in Chapter 3 under the topic of neural induction.

The main morphogenetic change that occurs during formation of the neural plate is the apicobasal elongation of ectodermal cells to form the thickened, single-layered neural plate (see Fig. 4-5A, B). Shaping of the neural plate involves the process of convergent extension, discussed in the preceding paragraph. During shaping, the neural plate narrows in the transverse plane and lengthens in the longitudinal plane. Because the neural plate is initially broader cranially than caudally and convergent extension occurs at a greater rate in the future spinal cord level of the neural plate than in the future brain level, the future brain level of the neural plate remains much broader than the future spinal cord level.

Bending of the neural plate involves formation of **neural folds** at the lateral edges of the neural plate, consisting of both **neuroepithelium** and adjacent **surface ectoderm** (see Fig. 4-5C). During bending, the neural folds elevate dorsally by rotating around a central pivot point overlying the notochord called the **median hinge point**. The groove delimited by the bending neural plate is called the **neural groove**. Bending around the median hinge point resembles the closing of the leaves of a book. Because the neural plate/groove at the future brain level is much broader than that at the future spinal cord level, additional hinge points form in the brain neural plate to bring the neural folds together in the dorsal midline. These hinge points, called the **dorsolateral hinge points**, allow the neural folds in the future brain level to converge medially toward one another (see Fig. 4-5D, E). As a result of bending, the paired neural folds are brought into apposition in the dorsal midline.

Closure of the neural groove involves the adhesion of the neural folds to one another and the subsequent rearrangement of cells within the folds to form two separate epithelial layers: the **roof plate of the neural tube** and the overlying **surface ectoderm**. Forming in the interface between these epithelial layers are **neural crest cells** (see Fig. 4-5F). These arise from the neural folds by undergoing an **epithelial-to-mesenchymal transformation (EMT);** neural crest cells are discussed later in the chapter. In humans, closure of the neural groove begins on day 22 at the future occipital and cervical region (i.e., adjacent to the four occipital somites and first cervical somite) of the neural tube (see Fig. 4-4). From this level, closure progresses both cranially and caudally, eventually closing the **cranial** and **caudal neuropores**, respectively, on day 24 and day 26.

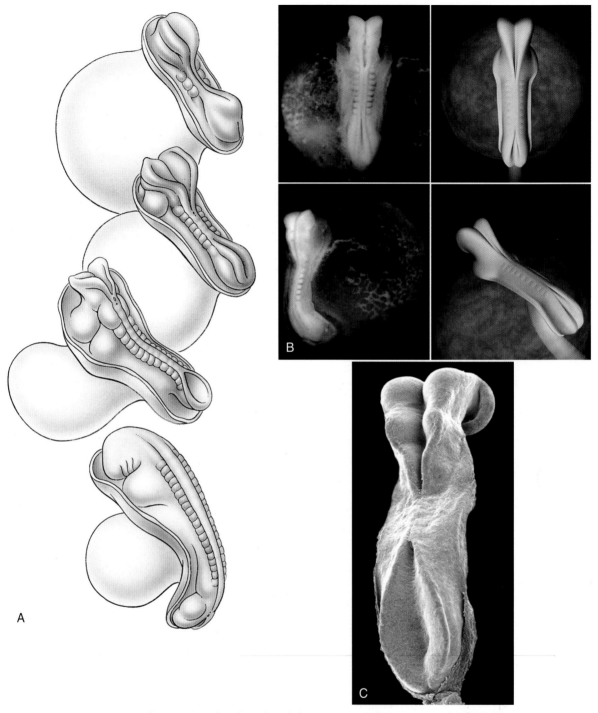

Figure 4-4. Neurulation. *A,* Drawings of human embryos from day 21 through days 24 to 25 (top to bottom, respectively). The lateral edges of the neural folds first begin to fuse in the occipitocervical region on day 22, leaving the cranial and caudal neuropores open at each end. The neural tube lengthens as it zips up both cranially and caudally, and the neuropores become progressively smaller. The cranial neuropore closes on day 24, and the caudal neuropore closes on day 26. *B,* Photographs of human embryos from the dorsal (top) or lateral (bottom) side and comparable computer-generated images. *C,* Scanning electron micrograph of a mouse embryo comparable to a day 21 or day 22 human embryo. The cranial and caudal neuropores are both open.

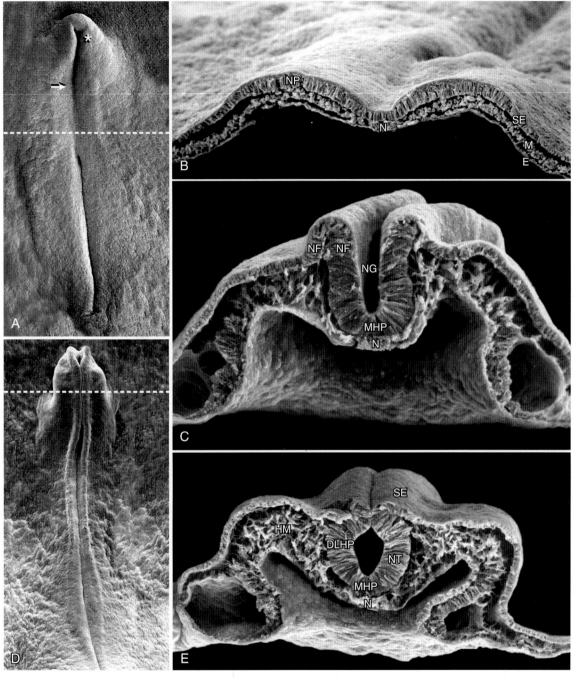

Figure 4-5. Neurulation in the chick. *A,* Dorsal view showing that neurulation occurs in cranial-to-caudal sequence such that at the level of the line in *A,* the neural plate is forming. More cranially (arrow), the neural plate is shaping, and still more cranially the neural plate is bending (asterisk) and a neural groove and paired neural folds have formed. *B,* Level of the forming neural plate (NP) at level of line in *A.* E, endoderm; SE, surface ectoderm; M, mesoderm; N, notochord. *C,* Transverse section through neural groove (future midbrain level) at a stage midway between *A* and *D.* MHP, median hinge point; N, notochord; NF, neural fold; NG, neural groove. *D,* Dorsal view during closure of the neural groove. In contrast to humans, the neural groove in chick first closes at the future midbrain level (rather than at the occipitocervical level) and then progresses cranially and caudally to close, respectively, the small cranial neuropore and elongated caudal neuropore/neural groove. Line indicates level of transverse section in *E. E,* Transverse section through the incipient neural tube (NT). DLHP, dorsolateral hinge point; HM, head mesoderm; N, notochord; MHP, median hinge point; SE, surface ectoderm.

Continued

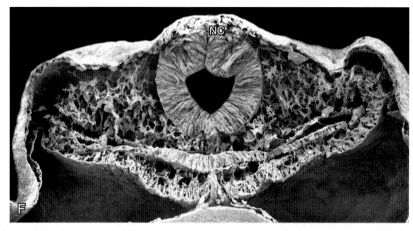

Figure 4-5, cont'd. F, Transverse section showing a slightly later stage in neurulation than shown in E. Neural crest cells (NC) are beginning to form and emigrate from the fusing neural folds.

IN THE RESEARCH LAB

MECHANISMS OF NEURULATION
Tissue and Cellular Events

Neurulation, in particular shaping and bending of the neural plate, involves a number of different forces that act in concert. These forces are generated by changes in cell behavior, particularly changes in cell shape, position, and number. Some of these forces are generated within the neural plate itself, whereas other forces are generated in surrounding tissues. Forces arising within the neural plate are called **intrinsic neurulation forces**, as opposed to those arising outside the neural plate, which are called **extrinsic neurulation forces**.

The cellular basis of neurulation has been mechanistically examined most thoroughly in chick embryos (see Fig. 4-5). Although shaping and bending of the neural plate occur simultaneously, to understand their mechanisms it is best to consider them separately. As discussed earlier in this chapter, shaping involves **convergent extension**, that is, a transverse narrowing and longitudinal lengthening. In addition, the neural plate thickens apicobasally during shaping as its cells get taller (i.e., change shape to high columnar), continuing the process of cell elongation initiated during neural plate formation. Apicobasal elongation requires the presence of paraxial microtubules, that is, microtubules oriented along (parallel to) the apicobasal axis of the cell. **Cell elongation** not only contributes to neural plate thickening but also to its narrowing, because as cells get taller they reduce their diameters to maintain their size (this would also reduce the length of the neural plate, but this is compensated for by cell rearrangement and oriented cell division; discussed below). However, the major factor that narrows the neural plate is not cell elongation. Rather it is **cell rearrangement** (also called **cell intercalation**). During cell rearrangement, cells move from lateral to medial within the neural plate, thereby narrowing the neural plate and stacking up in the cranial-caudal plane, increasing the length of the neural plate. Moreover, **cell division** occurs rapidly during neurulation, such that the neural plate continues to grow during shaping and bending. Many of these cell divisions are oriented to place daughter cells into the length of the neural plate rather than into its width, resulting in cranial-caudal extension of the neural plate. Thus, shaping of the neural plate involves changes in cell shape, position, and number within the neural plate. Experiments have shown that shaping is largely autonomous to the neural plate, that is, *intrinsic* forces drive neural plate shaping.

As discussed earlier in this chapter, bending of the neural plate involves the formation of hinge points. The **median hinge point** forms at all craniocaudal levels of the bending neural plate, whereas the **dorsolateral hinge points** form at future brain levels where the neural plate is much broader than it is more caudally. Hinge points involve localized regions where neuroepithelial cells change their shape from column-like to wedge like and where the wedge-shaped cells become firmly attached to an adjacent structure through the deposition of extracellular matrix. Thus, the median hinge point cells of the neural plate are firmly attached to the underlying **notochord**, and the dorsolateral hinge point cells of the neural plate on each side are firmly attached to the adjacent surface ectoderm of the **neural folds**. Cell wedging within the hinge points is generated by both apical constriction and basal expansion. The apices of neuroepithelial cells contain a circumferential ring of microfilaments whose contraction leads to apical narrowing. In addition, bases of neuroepithelial cells simultaneously expand as the nucleus moves basally. Recall that neuroepithelial cells are dividing throughout neurulation. As these elongated cells divide, their nuclei undergo a to-and-fro movement called **interkinetic nuclear migration**. During the G1/S phase of the cell cycle, nuclei move basally. After DNA synthesis is completed during the S phase, nuclei move apically and cells then round up at the apex of the neuroepithelium where mitosis **(cytokinesis)** occurs. After division, cells elongate once again and their nuclei move basally. During wedging, the cell cycle of neuroepithelial cells is prolonged so that cells spend more time in G and S phases, and consequently, more time with their bases expanded, because each neuroepithelial cell is very narrow except at the level where the nuclei resides. Thus, basally expanded neuroepithelial cells are wedge shaped.

Historically, most studies on neurulation have focused on changes in neuroepithelial cell shapes (i.e., wedging), which generate intrinsic forces for neurulation. But more recent studies have shown that **extrinsic forces** are both sufficient and necessary for neurulation. These studies have revealed that tissues lateral to the neural plate (surface ectoderm and mesoderm) generate extrinsic forces for bending of the neural plate. Like intrinsic forces acting during shaping, these extrinsic forces are generated by changes in cell behavior and also involve changes in cell shape, position, and number. Lateral tissues, like the neural plate, also undergo convergent extension driven by both oriented cell division and cell rearrangement. This results in their medial expansion, which pushes the neural folds, resulting in their elevation and convergence toward the dorsal midline. Lateral cells also exhibit changes in cell shape that contribute to medial expansion. For example, surface ectodermal cells transform from cuboidal to squamous (i.e., they flatten), increasing their surface area.

The cellular basis of neural groove closure, specifically fusion of the neural folds, is poorly understood. Some studies suggest that apical extracellular adhesive coats are involved, but their molecular nature remains uncharacterized. In addition, cell rearrangements occur as epithelial sheets (i.e., neural folds) fuse and then reorganize into new epithelial (i.e., roof of neural tube and overlying surface ectoderm) and mesenchymal (i.e., neural crest cells) structures. However, precisely how cells accomplish these feats remains largely unstudied.

Molecular Mechanisms

The molecular basis of neurulation is now beginning to receive study. Almost 200 mutations in mouse have been shown to result in defective neurulation and, consequently, to result in **neural tube defects (NTDs)**; thus, these mutations provide insight into which genes are involved in both normal and abnormal neurulation. Because neurulation is driven by changes in cell behavior, it is not surprising that mutation of

cytoskeletal, extracellular matrix/cell adhesion, cell cycle, and cell death genes results in NTDs. Neurulation is a highly choreographed morphogenetic event that must be precisely timed and coordinated across multiple tissues. This presumably involves signaling among tissues. It is the hope of studies using mouse mutations that such signaling pathways will be identified, ultimately leading to an understanding of the molecular basis of neurulation and the formation of NTDs in both animal models and ultimately in humans.

Planar-cell polarity pathway and convergent extension. As discussed early in this chapter and in Chapter 3, convergent extension plays a major role in vertebrate gastrulation and neurulation. Recent studies have revealed that convergent extension is regulated by the *Wnt* signaling pathway. During development, epithelial sheets become polarized not only apicobasally but also within the plane of the epithelium itself. In Drosophila, the **planar cell polarity (PCP) pathway** functions in this latter polarization of the epithelium. Thus, for example, the orientation of wing hairs is established by the PCP pathway. In vertebrates, the PCP pathway is required for proper orientation of stereociliary bundles in the outer hair cells of the mouse inner ear (discussed in Ch. 17), and for convergent extension during gastrulation and neurulation. How are the PCP and *Wnt* signaling pathways related?

The Drosophila PCP pathway consists of a several core proteins that collectively act to convert an extracellular polarity cue into specific changes in the cytoskeleton. These core proteins are now known to be components of the *Wnt* signaling pathway, and orthologs of several of the Drosophila components are conserved in vertebrates. Thus, convergent extension during gastrulation and neurulation is blocked in loss-of-function mutations of the cytoplasmic protein *Dishevelled* in Xenopus and its two orthologs in mouse (*Dishevelled 1 and 2*). As discussed in Chapter 5, *Wnt* signaling involves both a so-called canonical *Wnt* pathway and noncanonical *Wnt* pathways. The PCP pathway utilizes the noncanonical pathway in which certain *Wnts*, such as *Wnt 11*, bind to their receptors (known as *Frizzleds*). Several other proteins, including *Dishevelled*, must interact in this pathway for proper signaling, and consequently, for proper convergent extension, to occur. In addition to double *Dishevelled 1 and 2* mutants, four other mouse mutants exhibit convergent extension defects: *circletail*, *crash*, *spin cycle*, and *loop-tail*. *Loop-tail* mice have a mutation in the ortholog of the *Strabismus/Van Gogh* gene, which encodes a transmembrane protein that interacts with *Dishevelled*. Both *crash* and *spin cycle* mice have a mutation in the ortholog of the Drosophila protocadherin *Flamingo* gene, called *Celsr1*. In Drosophila, *Flamingo* is required for PCP signaling. *Circletail* mice have a mutation in the ortholog of the Drosophila *Scribble* gene. *Scribble* interacts with *Strabismus*. Thus, obtaining an understanding of the PCP pathway in Drosophila has had a surprising result—a better understanding also of vertebrate gastrulation and neurulation, and potentially, a better understanding of how NTDs form in humans.

Actin-binding proteins and apical constriction

Several actin-associated proteins when genetically ablated in mice result in NTDs. One of these, the actin-binding protein *Shroom*, has received considerable study. Over expression of *Shroom* in cultured epithelial cells is sufficient to cause apical constriction. *Shroom* causes apical constriction by altering the distribution of F-actin to the apical side of epithelial cells and regulating the formation of a contractile actomyosin network associated with apical intercellular junctions. When *Shroom* is inactivated in Xenopus embryos, hinge point formation is drastically altered and neural tube closure fails to occur, providing further evidence for a role of cell shape changes in generating intrinsic forces important for neurulation.

DORSAL-VENTRAL PATTERNING OF THE NEURAL TUBE

As the neural tube is forming, it receives signals from adjacent tissues that result in its patterning in the dorsal-ventral axis. Three tissues provide patterning signals: surface ectoderm, paraxial mesoderm, and notochord. Thus, these signals originate dorsally, laterally, and ventrally, respectively (Fig. 4-6).

Ventral signals are the best understood. Several microsurgical experiments in which notochords were removed (extirpated) from the ventral midline or transplanted adjacent to the lateral wall of the neural tube revealed that the notochord was both sufficient and necessary for formation of the **median hinge point**, and subsequently for the **floor plate** of the neural tube (the floor plate derives from the median hinge point during subsequent development). Using loss-of-function and gain-of-function experiments mainly in chick and mouse, it was shown that *Sonic hedgehog* (*Shh*), secreted initially by the notochord, was the signal that induced the median hinge point and floor plate. As the floor plate is induced it also secretes *Shh* (Fig. 4-7), which in turn induces **neurons** in the ventral neural tube (e.g., motoneurons in the ventral spinal cord; discussed in Ch. 9). *Shh* acts as a **morphogen**, such that high concentrations induce ventral neurons, lower concentrations induce more intermediate neurons, and the lowest concentrations induce more dorsal neurons.

In addition to producing a ventral-to-dorsal concentration gradient of *Shh* within the neural tube, the notochord also produces a ventral-to-dorsal concentration gradient of *Chordin*, a *Bmp* antagonist. The *Chordin* gradient interacts with a dorsal-to-ventral concentration gradient of *Bmp* produced by the surface ectoderm. Because *Chordin* blocks *Bmp* signaling, *Bmp* signaling is robust dorsally (where *Chordin* concentration is weak or absent and *Bmp* concentration is high) and weak or absent ventrally (where *Chordin* concentration is high and *Bmp* concentration is weak or absent). A high level of *Bmp* signaling dorsally, along with *Wnt* signaling by the surface ectoderm, results in the induction of **neural crest cells** and the **roof plate of the neural tube**.

The paraxial mesoderm lying adjacent to the lateral walls of the neural tube also provides patterning signals but these are the least understood. Among the secreted factors produced by the paraxial mesoderm are *Fgfs*, such as *Fgf8*. Both gain-of-function and loss-of-function experiments in Xenopus provide support for a role for paraxial mesoderm and *Fgfs* in neural crest cell induction.

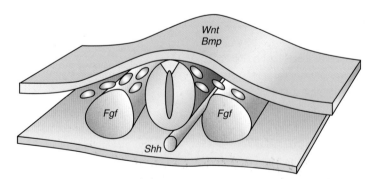

Figure 4-6. Diagram showing factors involved in dorsal-ventral patterning of the neural tube. The neural tube is dorsalized by surface ectoderm, which secretes both orthologs of the Drosophila , *Wingless* family (*Wnts*) and *Bone morphogenetic proteins* (*Bmps*), resulting in formation of the roof plate of the neural tube and neural crest cells. The neural tube is ventralized by the notochord, which induces the floor plate of the neural tube through the secretion of *Sonic hedgehog* (*Shh*). Subsequently, both the notochord and floor plate secrete *Shh*. Additional patterning signals are provided by the somites (Fibroblast *growth factors* or *Fgfs*).

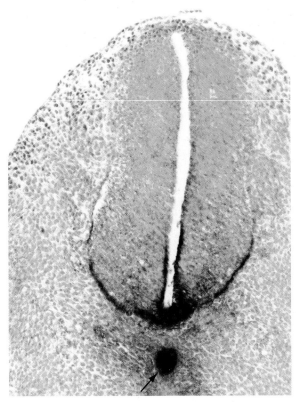

Figure 4-7. Expression of *Sonic hedgehog* (*Shh*) protein (dark brown) in the 11- to 11.5-day postcoitum mouse notochord and overlying floor plate of the neural tube.

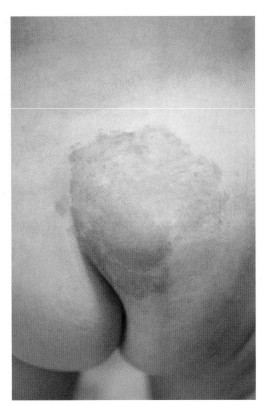

Figure 4-8. Lumbosacral spina bifida occulta in a newborn with associated lipoma and angioma.

IN THE CLINIC

NEURAL TUBE DEFECTS (NTDS)

Neural tube defects (NTDs) result when **neurulation** fails to occur normally. Thus, these defects arise during weeks 3 to 4 of gestation and can be open to the surface or covered with skin. Open NTDs are the most severe. They range from total **dysraphism**, called **craniorachischisis**, in which the entire length of the neural tube opens onto the surface of the head and back, to localized dysraphism, such as lumbosacral **myeloschisis**, in which only the lowermost region of the spinal cord is open. Myeloschisis is commonly referred to as **spina bifida aperta** (meaning the spinal cord is open to the body surface), because bifid vertebral spines are also present. Total dysraphism of the brain, with normal formation of the spinal cord, is called **cranioschisis** or **anencephaly**. Infants with anencephaly lack a functional forebrain (cerebrum) and fail to gain consciousness; most do not survive more than a few hours after birth. Skin-covered NTDs can be present at both the spinal cord and brain levels (Fig. 4-8, 4-9; also see Fig. 4-12*A*). In the spinal cord, skin-covered

NTDs are referred to as **spina bifida occulta** (meaning the defect is hidden); they occur in about 2% of the population. Typically, the location of spina bifida occulta is marked externally on the back by a tuft of hair, pigmented nevus (mole), angioma (port-wine colored birth mark of the skin), lipoma (a skin doming caused by an underlying mass of fatty tissue), or dimple. In the brain, skin-covered NTDs are called **encephaloceles**, with brain tissue protruding through the skull (Fig. 4-10; see Fig. 4-9). Large encephaloceles can severely affect neurologic function and threaten survival.

NTDs encompass a wide variety of malformations with a number of specific names. The most common open NTD is a type of spina bifida in which the neural tube and its surrounding membranes **(dura mater** and **arachnoid)** protrude from the vertebral canal, forming a fluid-filled sac or **cele**. This type of defect is called a **myelomeningocele** (Figs. 4-11, 4-12*C*). Less frequently, the membranes protrude into the sac but the spinal cord does not. This defect is called a **meningocele** (Fig. 4-12*B*).

Open NTDs occur in about 0.1% of all live births. Approximately 4000 pregnancies are affected by open NTDs

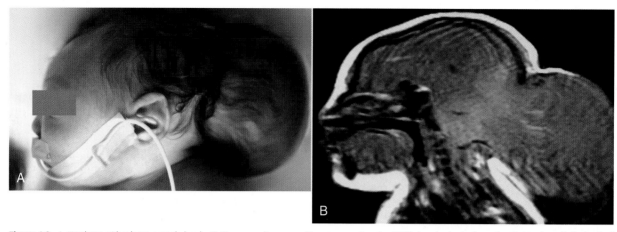

Figure 4-9. *A*, Newborn with a large encephalocele. *B*, Corresponding magnetic resonance imaging (MRI) showing brain tissue herniating through the back of the skull into a cele.

each year in the United States and in these cases, as many as 50% of the fetuses are electively aborted. Approximately 500,000 infants with spina bifida aperta are born worldwide each year. The early detection of NTDs in utero has improved greatly since the advent of **maternal serum alpha-fetoprotein** (MSAFP) screening after 12 weeks of gestation. If elevated levels of alpha-fetoprotein are detected in maternal serum, two other tests can be conducted: **ultrasound examination** of the fetal spine and head, and **amniocentesis** (discussed in Ch. 6); the latter procedure is used to sample and measure levels of alpha-fetoprotein contained in amniotic fluid. Alpha-fetoprotein is produced by the fetal liver and excreted by the fetal kidneys into the amniotic fluid; eventually, it is absorbed into the maternal blood stream. Alpha-fetoprotein levels are elevated in pregnancies affected by NTDs (and by ventral body wall defects such as **gastroschisis**) and are lower in pregnancies affected by **Down syndrome** (or other chromosomal anomalies), but why alpha-fetoprotein levels are altered in these conditions is unclear.

NTDs can result in serious health problems that require lifelong management. For example, the spinal cord and

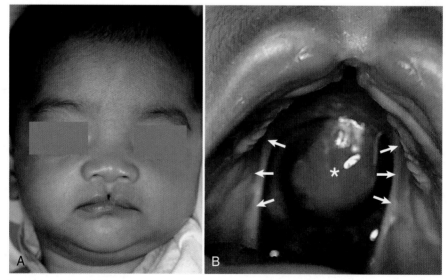

Figure 4-10. *A*, Newborn with a midline cleft lip. *B*, Examination of the oral cavity revealed the presence of a cleft palate (arrows mark nonfused palatal shelves) and an encephalocele (asterisk) herniating into the nasal cavity.

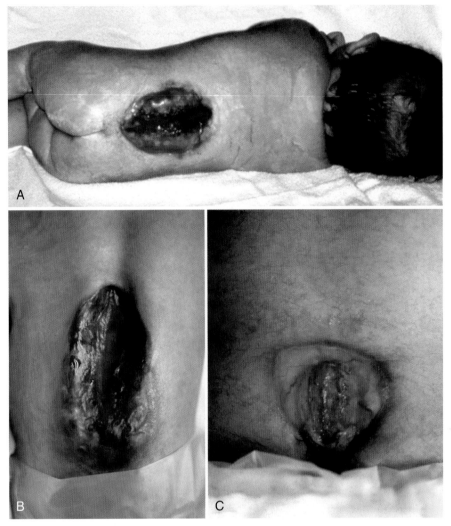

Figure 4-11. Three newborns with myelomenigoceles. *A, B,* The myelomenigoceles extend from the thoracic to lumbosacral level. Note the location of the split vertebral elements to the left of the lesion in *B. C,* The myelomenigocele is localized to the lumbosacral level. In *B* and *C,* the infant's diapers (bottom of each illustration) are shown for orientation.

spinal nerves affected by a myelomeningocele fail to develop normally, resulting in dysfunction of pelvic organs and lower limbs. In general, higher and larger defects result in more neurologic deficit than lower and smaller defects. In as many as 90% of the infants with myelomeningocele, **hydrocephalus** develops (commonly referred to as water on the brain). This occurs because the myelomeningocele is associated for unknown reasons with an abnormality at the base of the brain called **Arnold-Chiari malformation.** This malformation disrupts the normal drainage of cerebrospinal fluid (CSF) from the brain ventricles to the subarachnoid space surrounding the spinal cord. This in turn increases the volume and pressure of CSF in the cerebral ventricles, causing their enlargement at the expense of more peripheral brain tissue. Hydrocephalus is usually controlled by implanting a shunt—an inert, flexible plastic tube about one eighth of an inch thick and containing a unidirectional flow valve—into the lateral ventricles to allow fluid to drain into a body cavity (typically the abdominal cavity) where it can be resorbed. Another complication of NTDs is a **tethered spinal cord,** a condition in which the lower end of the spinal cord is attached to the skin as a result of an open or closed NTD.

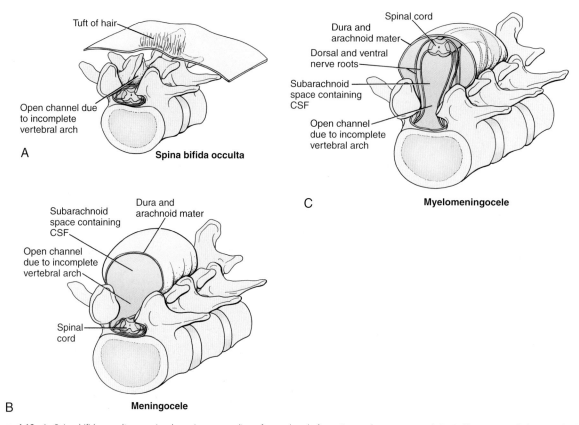

Figure 4-12. *A,* Spina bifida occulta may involve minor anomalies of neural arch formation and may not result in malformations of the neural tube. This condition often occurs in the midsacral region and may be indicated by a small dimple, tuft of hair, lipoma, or nevus overlying the defective vertebra. More extensive malformation of neural arches occurs in conjunction with formation of a cele. This cele is called a *meningocele* if it includes dura and arachnoid only (*B*) or a *myelomeningocele* if it contains a portion of the spinal cord and associated spinal nerves as well as meninges (*C*). CSF, cerebrospinal fluid.

As the child grows and his/her vertebral column elongates, the restricted cord is stretched and damaged, resulting in neurological deficit. It is important to identify tethered cords and to surgically untether them before such neurologic damage occurs, as this damage is not reversible. In infants with skin-covered NTDs, the presence of a tethered cord would not be evident. However, as discussed earlier in this section, infants born with a hairy tuft, pigmented nevus, angioma, lipoma, or dimple—so called **neurocutaneous signatures**—in the lumbosacral region might have an underlying NTD. Thus, these infants should be examined with magnetic resonance imaging (MRI) to identify tethered cords associated with a closed NTD so that the cord can be untethered before neurologic damage occurs.

NTDs have no single genetic or teratogenic cause and are believed to be multifactorial, that is, to arise from the interaction of both genetic and environmental factors. About 95% of the babies with NTDs are born to parents with no family history of these disorders. However, if one child in the family has an NTD, the risk of a recurrence in any subsequent pregnancy rises to about 1 in 40, and if two children are affected, the incidence rises to 1 in 20, strongly suggesting a genetic predisposition. The frequency of NTDs also varies by race, again suggesting a genetic predisposition. For example, in the United States as a whole the frequency of NTDs is approximately 0.1%, but the frequency of NTDs is 0.035% among African Americans. In contrast, the frequency of NTDs in some parts of India and in Ireland is on the order of 1.1%.

Teratogens that induce NTDs in animals and humans have also been identified, opening the possibility that some human NTDs may be caused by environmental toxins or nutritional deficiencies. For example, studies on experimental animals have implicated retinoic acid, *Insulin,* and high plasma glucose in the formation of NTDs. Factors implicated in the induction of NTDs in humans include the antiepileptic drug **valproic acid, maternal diabetes**, and **hyperthermia**.

Folate acid (vitamin B9) supplementation (400 micrograms of synthetic folic acid per day in a prenatal multivitamin) can reduce the incidence of NTDs by up to 75%. However, in a 2000 Gallup poll, only 13% of the women of child-bearing age in the United States were aware of this fact. If a mother has had a previous child with spina bifida, it is recommended that she take a prenatal multivitamin with a 10-fold higher concentration of folic acid (that is, 4 milligrams). The role of folic acid in developmental processes is complex, including the regulation of DNA synthesis, mitosis, protein synthesis, and DNA methylation, so the actual mechanism(s) by which folic acid supplementation prevents NTDs (and likely other birth defects) remains unclear.

Secondary Neurulation

As discussed in Chapter 3, gastrulation ends with formation of the tail bud. And as discussed earlier in this chapter, the neural tube develops through the process of neurulation. Neurulation is completed with closure of the caudal neuropore at about the level of somite 31. Yet in the fetus, the neural tube extends caudal to this level into the sacral and coccygeal levels. This is because the level of the closing caudal neuropore is merged with the forming tail bud, and the latter undergoes morphogenesis to form the most caudal extent of the neural tube. Formation of the neural tube from the tail bud is called **secondary neurulation**, as opposed to *neurulation* (or **primary neurulation**), which involves formation of the neural tube from the neural plate, as discussed earlier in the chapter.

Experimental studies have shown that the caudal levels of the neural tube, neural crest cells, and somites develop from the tail bud (Figs. 4-13, 4-14). Secondary neurulation involves the condensation of central tail bud cells into a solid mass called the **medullary cord**. Subsequently, the medullary cord undergoes cavitation to form a lumen, which quickly merges with the neural canal of the more cranial neural tube. Neural crest cells then arise from the roof of the neural tube and undergo migration to form the caudal spinal ganglia. Lateral tail bud cells undergo segmentation to form the caudal somites, and as mentioned in Chapter 3, the caudal end of the notochord grows into the sacral, coccygeal, and tail regions. Secondary neurulation is completed by about 8 weeks of development.

Cranial-Caudal Regionalization of the Neural Tube

Shortly after the neural tube forms, it becomes subdivided in the cranial-caudal axis into **forebrain, midbrain, hindbrain**, and **spinal cord**. Concomitantly, the embryo becomes C-shaped through the process of body folding and flexure of the neural tube. Thus, by the end of the 1st month of development, the

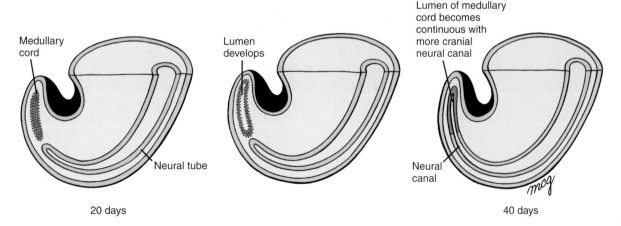

Figure 4-13. Secondary neurulation in humans. Formation of the caudal neural tube occurs by secondary neurulation. During this process, the tail bud gives rise to the medullary cord, which subsequently cavitates to form a lumen. At the end of the 6th week, this lumen merges with the neural canal of the more rostral neural tube.

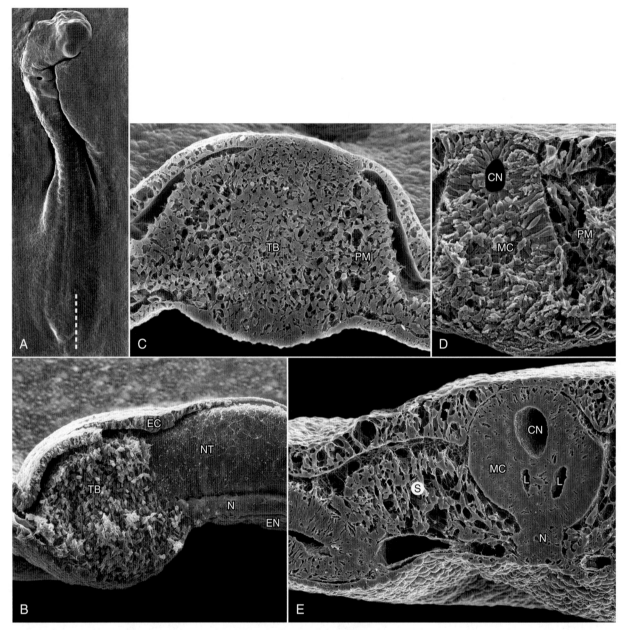

Figure 4-14. Secondary neurulation in chick as shown in scanning electron micrographs. *A*, Surface view of a chick embryo shortly after closure of the caudal neuropore. Line indicates level of the slice shown in *B*. *B*, Parasagittal slice at the level shown in *A*. The lateral wall of the caudal end of the closed neural tube (NT) is shown, as is the notochord (N) and underlying endoderm (EN). Also shown are the tail bud (TB) and overlying ectoderm (EC). *C*, Transverse slice through the tail bud (TB). Also shown is the paraxial mesoderm (PM) that will form the most caudal somites. *D*, Slightly later stage than shown in *C* of a transverse slice through the medullary cord (MC), which in the chick is partially overlapped by the caudal neuropore (CN) formed during primary neurulation. Also shown is the paraxial mesoderm (PM). *E*, Slightly later stage than shown in *D* of a transverse slice through the cavitating medullary cord (MC). CN, caudal neuropore; L, lumina formed in the medullary cord by cavitation; N, caudal rudiment of the notochord; S, somite.

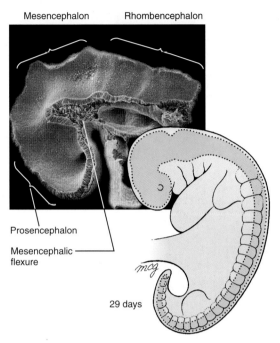

Mesencephalon   Rhombencephalon

Prosencephalon

Mesencephalic flexure

mcg

29 days

Figure 4-15. The anlage of the central nervous system, the neural tube, is formed by the end of the 4th week. Even at this early stage, the primary vesicles of the bend can be identified. Note the sharp ventral bend in the neural tube, the mesencephalic flexure, which separates the prosencephalon from the mesencephalon.

embryonic body is well formed and the basic body plan is well established (Fig. 4-15). Midsagittal sections through the cranial end of the embryo at this stage reveal the forebrain (also called **prosencephalon**), midbrain (also called **mesencephalon**), and hindbrain (also called **rhombencephalon**). The sharp flexure separating the prosencephalon and mesencephalon is the **mesencephalic flexure**. Further development of the neural tube and its cranial-caudal regionalization is discussed in Chapter 9.

Neural Crest Cells

Neural Crest Cells Originate During Neurulation

Neural crest cells are a unique population of cells that arise from the dorsal part of the forming neural tube during neurulation. These cells undergo an **epithelial-to-mesenchymal transformation** as they detach from the neural tube (Fig. 4-16). Subsequently, they migrate to many specific locations

in the body, where they differentiate into a remarkable variety of structures.

Neural crest cells differentiate first in the mesencephalic zone of the future brain. These cranial or cephalic neural crest cells associated with the developing brain begin to detach and migrate before closure of the cranial neuropore, even while the **neural folds** are fusing in the dorsal midline. In the spinal cord portion of the neural tube, the neural crest cells detach after the neural folds have fused. Neural crest cells at the very caudal end of the neural tube are formed from the **medullary cord** after the caudal neuropore closes on day 26. Thus, detachment and migration of the neural crest cells occur in a craniocaudal wave, from the mesencephalon to the caudal end of the spinal neural tube.

IN THE RESEARCH LAB

EPITHELIAL-TO-MESENCHYMAL TRANSFORMATION (EMT)

Formation of neural crest cells involves an epithelial-to-mesenchymal transformation (EMT) not unlike that occurring as cells undergo ingression through the primitive streak (discussed in Ch. 3). Consequently, some of the same molecular players function in both events. Separation of the neural crest from the neural folds or neural tube is referred to as **delamination** of neural crest cells. Three key factors are known to promote neural crest cell delamination: *FoxD3*, a winged-helix transcription factor; *Slug*, a zinc-finger transcription factor; and *Bmp2/4*. Over expression of *FoxD3* promotes delamination of neural crest cells at all axial levels, showing that it is sufficient by itself for delamination. *FoxD3* promotes delamination without upregulating the expression of *Slug* (or *RhoB*; discussed momentarily), suggesting that *FoxD3* acts in parallel with (not upstream or downstream of) the other factors. *Slug* over expression also promotes neural crest cell delamination, but only in the cranial region, not in the trunk region. Why *Slug* is only active cranially in inducing neural crest cell delamination is unknown, but this experiment does show that *Slug* is sufficient by itself to promote cranial neural crest cell delamination. *Bmp* signaling is required for delamination of neural crest cells, as over expression of the *Bmp* antagonist, *Noggin*, blocks delamination. *Bmp* signaling in forming neural crest cells is regulated by the adjacent paraxial mesoderm. As a result of *Bmp* signaling, *RhoB*, a small GTP-binding protein implicated in assembly of the actin cytoskeleton, is expressed by neural crest cells. Changes in the cytoskeleton are likely required for both change in cell shape, which accompanies an epithelial-to-mesenchymal transformation, and subsequent neural crest cell migration.

4

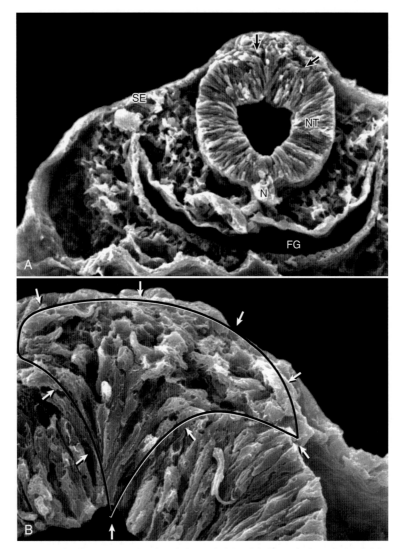

Figure 4-16. Scanning electron micrographs of a transverse slice through the newly formed chick neural tube at the level of the midbrain. *B* is an enlargement of the neural crest cell–forming region of *A*. NT, neural tube; SE, surface ectoderm; N, notochord; FG, foregut; arrows and outlined region demarcate forming and migrating neural crest cells.

Neural Crest Cells Undergo Extensive Migration along Well-Defined Pathways

Migration of neural crest cells from various craniocaudal levels of the neural folds and roof of the neural tube have been mapped by cell tracing studies in animal models. These studies reveal that neural crest cells undergo extensive migration throughout the body and subsequently differentiate into a large number of different cell types. Migration occurs along well-defined pathways or routes (Fig. 4-17). The route that particular neural crest cells take and where they stop migrating along this route determines in part what type of cell they will form. In addition, cranial (brain) and more caudal (spinal cord) neural crest cells give rise to some identical cell types (such as neurons), but also some different cells types (e.g., only cranial neural crest cells form cartilage and bone). The differentiation of neural crest cells is discussed in more detail in later chapters (e.g., Chs. 10, 12, 14, and 16).

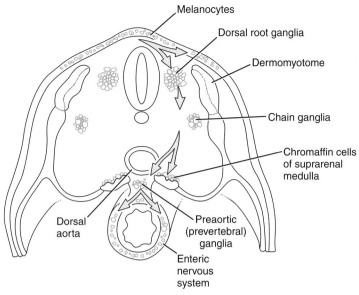

Figure 4–17. Neural crest cell migratory routes.

IN THE RESEARCH LAB

WHAT LOCAL FACTORS GUIDE MIGRATION OF NEURAL CREST CELLS?

Pathways of neural crest cell migration are established by **extracellular matrix molecules** that can be permissive for migration, and hence determine the path, as well as inhibitory for migration, thereby determining the boundaries of the paths. For example, neural crest cells migrate only through the cranial half of the somite and fail to enter the caudal half; in so doing, they establish the segmental patterning of the peripheral nervous system (discussed in Ch. 10). Probably no one individual molecule determines the pathway. **Permissive molecules** in the cranial somite include the basement membrane proteins *Tenascin*, *Fibronectin*, *Laminin*, and *Collagen*, to name a few. **Inhibitory molecules** found in the caudal somite include *Proteoglycans*, *PNA-binding molecules* (i.e., molecules that specifically bind the lectin *Peanut agglutinin*), *F-Spondin* (a secreted protein produced by the floor plate of the neural tube), and *Ephrins* (membrane-bound proteins that interact with *Eph* tyrosine kinases; *Ephs* and *Ephrins* are discussed in Ch. 5). Besides permissive molecules, there are also **chemotactic molecules** that attract neural crest cells and **negative chemotactic molecules** that repulse the crest from a distance. *Gdnf* (Glial cell line-derived neurotropic factor) and *Neuregulin* are examples of the former, whereas *Semaphorins* and *Slits* are examples of the latter (discussed further in Ch. 10). Several approaches have allowed us to determine what cues guide the crest. These include the use of mouse mutants (discussed in next section), in vitro studies to directly determine migratory ability on the extracellular matrix or chemotactic responses, and perturbation studies in the embryo. Determining which molecules guide the crest has been difficult because of molecular redundancy.

Recently, we have learned that not all subpopulations of neural crest cells respond the same way to these local signals. For example, neural crest cells that will become neurons or glial cells are inhibited by *Ephrins*, whereas melanoblasts (cells derived from neural crest cells that differentiate into melanocytes, that is, pigment cells) are stimulated to migrate on *Ephrins*. Thus, melanoblasts are able to migrate into pathways where neurons and glial cells cannot go. Similarly, trunk neural crest cells are repulsed by *Slit*, which is expressed in the gut mesenchyme and keeps them out of the gut, whereas vagal neural crest cells do not possess the receptor for *Slit* and, therefore, are able to migrate into the gut to form the **enteric nervous system** (discussed later in this chapter and in Ch. 10). Increasingly, we are discovering that different subpopulations of neural crest cells are specified early in their migration and respond differentially to cues in the microenvironment.

MUTANTS PROVIDE INFORMATION ABOUT MECHANISMS OF NEURAL CREST CELL MIGRATION AND DEVELOPMENTAL RESTRICTION

Several mouse mutants characterized by defects of neural crest cell development have been described. Some of these mutations affect the proliferative activity of neural crest cell stem cell populations, whereas others are characterized by regional defects in pigmentation, innervation of the gut, or defects in the development of cranial neural crest cells.

An interesting series of mouse mutants that affect neural crest cell migration are called *white-spotting* and *steel* mutants. The *white-spotting* locus is a proto-oncogene that encodes a *c-Kit Tyrosine kinase receptor* (*c-Kit receptor*), whereas the *steel* locus encodes the ligand for this receptor, *c-Kit* ligand. As expected, mutations of either gene produce a similar spectrum of anomalies, specifically involving migrating embryonic stem cells. For example, in severe mutations of either of these loci, **primordial germ cells** fail to populate the gonads, resulting in sterility (discussed in Ch. 15), and **hematopoietic stem cells** fail to migrate from the yolk sac into the liver, resulting in severe deficiencies of blood formation (discussed in Ch. 13). Less severe mutations may result in differential male or female sterility and selective loss of specific hematopoietic progenitors. In addition to disruptions of germ cell and blood cell development, these mutants also display a spectrum of pigmentation defects suggesting an effect on another population of migrating embryonic cells, the neural crest cell precursors of the melanocytes.

It seems likely that *c-Kit* ligand is a trophic factor and that it is required for survival of premelanocytes rather than for their early differentiation and migration. It has been suggested that *c-Kit* ligand may regulate the expression of *c-Kit* receptor by melanocyte precursors of neural crest cells and that *c-Kit* ligand and *c-Kit* receptor together then regulate the adhesion of these cells to the extracellular matrix. Thus, it seems that *c-Kit* ligand must be expressed by cells along the melanocyte migration route and at its ultimate target, whereas the *c-Kit* receptor must be expressed by the premelanocytes themselves. A **soluble form** of the *c-Kit* ligand is apparently required for early survival of premelanocytes in a **migration staging area** between the somite, surface ectoderm, and neural tube. In contrast, expression of a **membrane-associated form** of *c-Kit* ligand seems to be required for the later survival of the premelanocytes within the dermis.

A staggering array of additional genes affecting specific mechanisms of neural crest cell differentiation, migration, and survival in mice have been described within the last few years. The *patch* mutation affects the alpha subunit of the *Platelet-derived growth factor* (*Pdgf$_{2\alpha}$*) disrupting the development of non-neuronal derivatives of neural crest cells. Null mutations of genes encoding Retinoic acid receptor proteins results in defects of heart outflow tract septation (discussed in Ch. 12; septation of the outflow tract requires the presence of neural crest cells, as discussed below). Mice harboring the *kreisler* mutation exhibit wide-ranging craniofacial defects attributed to abnormal expression of several *Hox* genes and consequent disruption of neural crest cell development. Therefore, *Hox* genes apparently play pivotal roles in the signaling cascades that regulate differentiation and migration of cranial neural crest cells (discussed in Ch. 16).

Neural Crest Cells Have Many Diverse Derivatives

Neural crest cells are traditionally grouped into four cranial-caudal subdivisions based on their specific regional contributions to structures of the embryo (Fig. 4-18): cranial (caudal forebrain to the level of rhombomere 6 of the myelencephalon; rhombomeres are discussed in Ch. 9); vagal (level of somites 1 to 7; the cranial part of the vagal level overlaps the caudal part of the cranial level, as the first few somites form adjacent to the rhombencephalon, not the spinal cord); trunk (level of somites 8 to 28); and sacral/lumbosacral (level caudal to somite 28). Each of these subdivisions is discussed below.

Cranial neural crest cells. Neural crest cells from the caudal prosencephalon (forebrain) and mesencephalon (midbrain) regions give rise to the parasympathetic ganglion of cranial nerve III, a portion of the connective tissue around the developing eyes and optic nerves, the muscles of the iris and ciliary body, and part of the cornea of the eye; they also contribute, along with head mesoderm, to the head mesenchyme cranial to the level of the mesencephalon (discussed in Chs. 10 and 16).

Neural crest cells from the mesencephalon and rhombencephalon (hindbrain) regions also give rise to structures in the developing **pharyngeal arches** of the head and neck (discussed in Ch. 16). These structures include cartilaginous elements and several bones of the nose, face, middle ear, and neck. The mesencephalon and rhombencephalon neural crest cells form the dermis, smooth muscle, and fat of the face and ventral neck, and the odontoblasts of the developing teeth. Neural crest cells arising from the caudalmost rhombencephalon contribute, along with

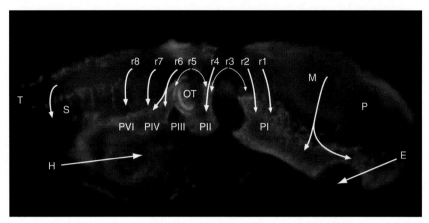

Figure 4-18. The head of a chick embryo labeled (red) with a specific neural crest cell antibody (HNK-1). Arrows show migratory routes of neural crest cells. P, prosencephalon; E, eye; M, mesencephalon; OT, otic vesicle; R, rhombencephalon; T, trunk (spinal cord level); S, somite; H, heart.; r1-r8, rhombomers 1-8; PI-PVI, pharyngeal arches I to IV, and VI.

vagal neural crest cells (discussed later), to the **parafollicular cells of the thyroid**.

The rhombencephalic neural crest cells also contribute to some of the cranial nerve ganglia. Specifically, rhombencephalic neural crest cells give rise to some neurons and all glial cells in the sensory ganglia of cranial nerves V, VII, IX, and X (Fig. 4-19). The remaining neurons in the sensory ganglia of cranial nerves V, VII, IX, and X arise from small ectodermal placodes, called **epibranchial** or **epipharyngeal placodes**. The special sensory nerves, associated glia, and ganglia (when present) also arise from placodes (discussed in Chs. 16, 17): Cranial nerve I (olfactory) arises from the **olfactory placode**; cranial nerve II (optic) arises from the **optic cup** (the distal end of which thickens as the placode-like rudiment of the neural retina); and cranial nerve VIII (vestibulocochlear nerve) and the vestibulocochlear ganglion arises from the **otic placode**.

The rhombencephalic neural crest cells also give rise to the cranial component of the parasympathetic division of the autonomic nervous system (discussed further below). Specifically, rhombencephalic neural crest cells give rise to all neurons (called postganglionic neurons; preganglionic neurons arise in the ventral wall of the neural tube, as discussed in Chs. 9, 10) and glial cells in the parasympathetic ganglia of cranial nerves VII, IX, and X. Thus, in conjunction with the neural crest cells derived from the caudal prosencephalon and mesencephalon (that give rise to the parasympathetic ganglia of cranial nerve III), the entire cranial component of the parasympathetic division of the autonomic nervous system is formed from cranial neural crest cells.

Cranial neural crest cells as a group also give rise to other cell types that populate the head and neck. These include the pia mater and arachnoid—the inner and middle of the three meninges—of the occipital region; the dura mater, the outermost layer of the three meninges, arises largely or exclusively from head (paraxial) mesoderm. In addition, some cranial neural crest cells invade the surface ectoderm as they migrate away from the neural tube to form the melanocytes (pigment cells) of the skin of the head and neck.

Vagal neural crest cells. Neural cells originating from the vagal region have three major contributions. Some of these neural crest cells migrate into the cranial pole of the developing heart, where they contribute to the septum (aorticopulmonary) that forms to partition the outflow tract of the heart (discussed in Ch. 12). Other vagal neural crest cells migrate more distally into the gut wall mesenchyme to form neurons, constituting the enteric nervous system, that innervate all regions of the gut tube from the esophagus to the rectum (discussed later and in Ch 14). Still other vagal neural crest cells migrate with those from the caudal rhombencephalon (discussed earlier) to the pharyngeal pouches, where they contribute to the **parafollicular cells of the thyroid** (discussed in Ch. 16).

Trunk neural crest cells. The peripheral nervous system of the neck, trunk, and limbs includes the following four types of peripheral neurons: the peripheral sensory neurons, the cell bodies of which reside in the dorsal root ganglia; the sympathetic and

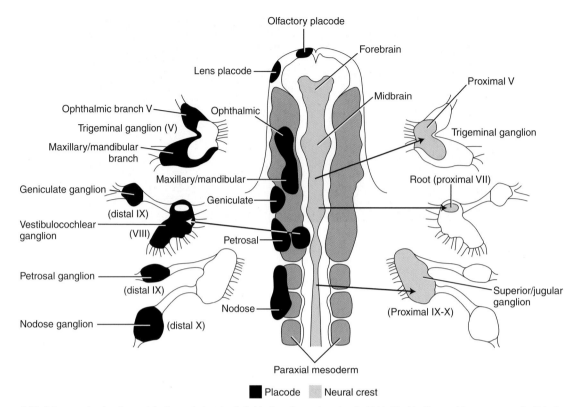

Figure 4-19. Fate map showing the contributions of placodes (left; black) and neural crest cells (right; blue) to the cranial sensory ganglia. Note in ganglia derived from both neural crest cells and epipharyngeal placodes that the proximal (most dorsal) ganglia (and neuron cell bodies) are derived from neural crest cells. The distal (most ventral) ganglia (and neuron cell bodies) are derived from placodes. Glial cells in both the proximal and distal ganglia of mixed origin are derived exclusively from neural crest cells. The special sensory nerves and associated glia (and ganglia when present) are derived from other placodes, namely, the olfactory and otic placodes and the optic cup (derived from a portion of the forebrain adjacent to the lens placode).

parasympathetic autonomic peripheral motoneurons, the cell bodies of which reside, respectively, in the sympathetic and parasympathetic ganglia; and the enteric neurons, considered a third subdivision of the autonomic nervous system. All four types of peripheral neurons, plus their associated glia, are derived from neural crest cells. The following paragraphs describe the origin of these structures; their subsequent development is discussed in Chapter 10.

Some of the neural crest cells arising from the trunk neural tube aggregate lateral to the neural tube, where they form small clumps in register with the somites (Fig. 4-20; see Fig. 4-17). These clumps then differentiate into the segmental **dorsal root ganglia** of the spinal nerves, which house the sensory neurons that conduct impulses to the spinal cord from end organs in the viscera, body wall, and extremities. Fate mapping experiments demonstrate that most cells in each ganglion are derived from the neural tube at the corresponding level, although many originate from neural crest cells at adjacent cranial and caudal levels.

A pair of dorsal root ganglia develops at every segmental level except the 1st cervical and the 2nd and 3rd coccygeal levels (see Fig. 4-20). Thus, there are 7 pairs of cervical, 12 pairs of thoracic, 5 pairs of lumbar, 5 pairs of sacral, and 1 pair of coccygeal dorsal root ganglia. The most cranial pair of cervical dorsal root ganglia (adjacent to the 2nd cervical somite) forms on day 28, and the others form in craniocaudal succession over the next few days.

Some trunk neural crest cells migrate to a zone just ventral to the future dorsal root ganglia, where they form a series of condensations that develop into the **chain ganglia** of the **sympathetic division of the autonomic nervous system** (see Figs. 4-17, 4-20). In the thoracic, lumbar, and sacral regions, one pair of chain ganglia forms in register with each pair of somites. However, in the cervical region, only three larger chain ganglia

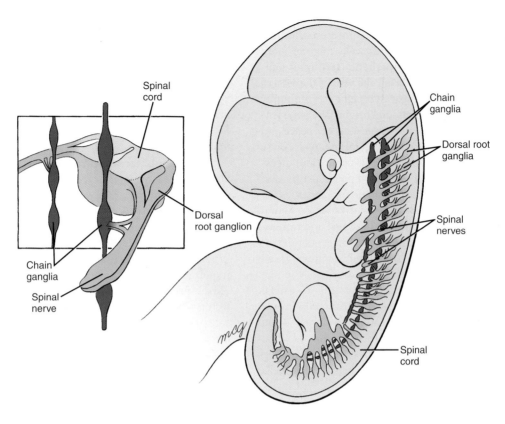

Figure 4-20. Neural crest cells form two types of segmental ganglia along almost the entire length of the spinal cord: dorsal root ganglia and chain ganglia.

develop, and the coccygeal region has only a single chain ganglion, which forms at the first coccygeal level. Fate mapping experiments indicate that the neural crest cells that give rise to the cervical chain ganglia originate along the cervical neural tube, whereas the thoracic, lumbar, and sacral ganglia are formed by crest cells from these corresponding levels of the neural tube.

The neurons that develop in the chain ganglia become the peripheral (postganglionic) neurons of the **sympathetic division of the autonomic nervous system**. The sympathetic division provides autonomic motor innervation to the viscera and exerts control over involuntary functions such as heartbeat, glandular secretions, and intestinal movements. The sympathetic division is activated during conditions of "fight or flight," and this system consists of two-neuron pathways: the viscera are innervated by axons from the peripheral sympathetic neurons (whose cell bodies develop in the chain ganglia, or other ganglia described in the next paragraph), which in turn receive axons from central sympathetic motoneurons arising in the spinal cord. These central sympathetic motoneurons are located at

all 12 thoracic levels and at the first 3 lumbar levels. For that reason, the sympathetic division (central and peripheral) is called a **thoracolumbar system**.

Not all peripheral (postganglionic) sympathetic neurons are located in the chain ganglia. The peripheral ganglia of some specialized sympathetic pathways develop from neural crest cells that congregate next to major branches of the dorsal aorta (see Fig. 4-17; discussed in Ch. 10). For example, one pair of these **prevertebral** or **preaortic ganglia** forms at the base of the celiac artery. Other, more diffuse ganglia develop in association with the superior mesenteric artery, the renal arteries, and the inferior mesenteric artery. These are formed by thoracic and lumbar neural crest cells.

The **parasympathetic division of the autonomic nervous system** innervates the same structures as does the sympathetic division of the autonomic nervous system. It also consists of two-neuron (peripheral and central) pathways. Peripheral (postganglionic) parasympathetic neurons arise from neural crest cells that form ganglia. As discussed above, some of these ganglia are associated with four cranial nerves: III, VII, IX, and

X. Other of these ganglia arise from neural crest cells originating from the lumbosacral neural crest cells (discussed below). These neural crest cells migrate more distally to form the **parasympathetic (terminal) ganglia**, typically located near or on the wall of the viscera they innervate. Thus, the parasympathetic autonomic nervous system has a craniosacral origin. The parasympathetic division is active during periods of "peace and relaxation" and stimulates the visceral organs to carry out their routine functions of housekeeping and digestion; thus, the function of the parasympathetic division is opposite to that of the sympathetic division.

The **enteric nervous system** is derived from neural crest cells originating from both the vagal and lumbosacral regions. As discussed above, the vagal neural crest cells migrate into the wall of the gut tube to innervate all regions of the gut tube from the esophagus to the rectum. They invade the gut tube in a cranial-to-caudal wave. Similarly, lumbosacral neural crest cells invade the gut tube, but do so in a caudal-to-cranial wave. Thus, the terminal part of the gut has a dual innervation, with its enteric nervous system originating from both vagal and lumbosacral neural crest cells (Fig. 4-21).

In addition to forming neurons and glia, trunk neural crest cells form a variety of other cell types. These include the inner and middle meningeal coverings of the spinal cord (the pia mater and arachnoid mater); Schwann cells, which form the myelin sheaths (neurilemma) of peripheral nerves; and neurosecretory chromaffin cells of the suprarenal medulla. Like cranial neural crest cells, trunk neural crest cells invade the surface ectoderm as they migrate away from the neural tube to form the melanocytes of the skin of the trunk and limbs.

Sacral/lumbosacral neural crest cells. As discussed above, in the most inferior regions of the gut, the enteric nervous system has a dual origin: Some enteric neurons arise from the vagal neural crest cells, whereas others arise from the lumbosacral neural crest cells. These caudal neural crest cells apparently arise from both the primary and secondary portions of the neural tube. Their importance in gut innervation is exemplified by Hirschsprung disease (congenital megacolon), which results when lumbosacral neural crest cells fail to innervate the terminal portion of the colon, resulting in impaired gut motility (Hirschsprung disease is discussed in Ch. 14).

As discussed above, neural crest cells form a diversity of cell types. Many of the major derivatives of the cranial and trunk neural crest cells are summarized in Figure 4-22. Other contributions to derivatives of the

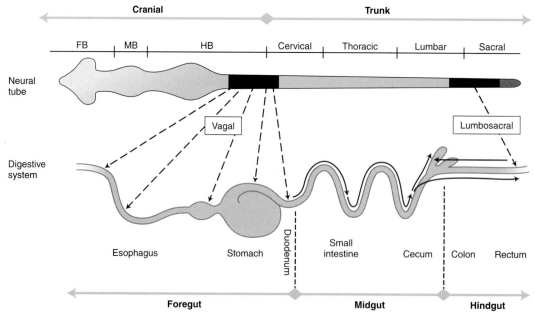

Figure 4-21. Neural crest cells invade the developing gut in two waves to form the enteric nervous system. The entire length of the gut receives contributions from vagal neural crest cells, which invade the gut in a cranial-to-caudal sequence. The terminal (caudal) part of the gut is also invaded by lumbosacral neural crest cells, which colonize the gut in a caudal-to-cranial sequence.

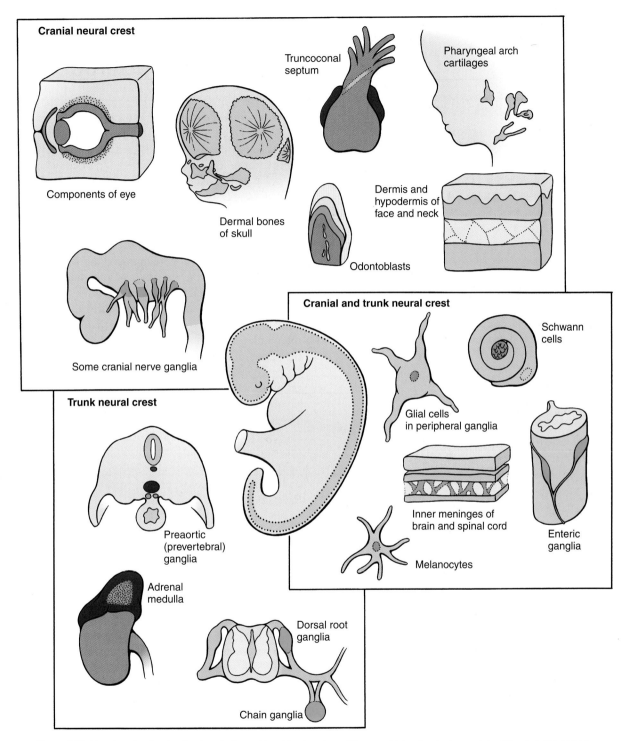

Figure 4-22. Neural crest cells migrating from both cranial and trunk regions of the neural tube give rise to a variety of tissues in the embryo.

pharyngeal pouches and associated structures are covered in Chapter 16.

SURVIVAL AND DIFFERENTIATION OF PERIPHERAL NEURONS

Experimental studies have shown that the survival and differentiation of peripheral neurons requires the presence of small growth factors called **neurotrophins**. For dorsal root ganglion cells, these include *Nerve growth factor* (*Ngf*), *Neurotrophin-3* (*Nt-3*), and *Brain-derived growth factor* (*Bdnf*), secreted by the neural tube and the dermomyotome subdivision of the somite (discussed later in the chapter). Thus, the dorsal root ganglia are virtually absent in mice lacking the *Ngf*, *Ngf receptor*, or *Nt-3* genes. Similarly, survival and differentiation of the sympathetic chain ganglion cells depends on *Ngf* and *Nt-3*, as well as on growth factors such as *Insulin-like growth factor* (*Igf*).

NEURAL CREST CELL DISEASE: NEUROCRISTOPATHIES

Because neural crest cells contribute to a large diversity of structures, abnormal development of neural crest cells can affect many different organ systems. Such defects of neural crest cell development are known as **neurocristopathies**, that is, pathologies associated with neural crest cell derivatives. These occur in conditions such as **neurofibromatosis** (Von Recklinghausen disease; e.g., peripheral nerve tumors), **Charcot-Marie-Tooth** (a chronic demyelinating disease of peripheral nerve, especially the peroneal nerve), **Waardenburg type I and II** and **albinism** (pigmentation defects), **pheochromocytoma** (tumors of the chromaffin cells of the suprarenal medulla), and **Hirschsprung disease** (congenital megacolon; absence of innervation of the terminal part of the colon), as well as in syndromes such as **CHARGE** (*c*oloboma of the eye, *h*eart defects, *a*tresia of the choanae, *r*etarded growth and development, *g*enital and urinary anomalies and *e*ar anomalies and hearing loss), and **22q11.2 deletion syndrome** (also known as **DiGeorge** or **velocardiofacial syndrome**) that affect development of the craniofacial and cardiovascular systems. Each of these neurocristopathies is discussed in the appropriate chapter covering development of the affected organ system.

Somite Differentiation: Forming Dermatome, Myotome, and Sclerotome

As discussed in Chapter 3, the paraxial mesoderm of the trunk undergoes segmentation to form the epithelial somites (Fig. 4-23). Shortly thereafter, each somite reorganizes into two subdivisions, the epithelial **dermomyotome** (sometimes spelled, "dermamyotome" in the literature) and mesenchymal **sclerotome** (Fig. 4-24). Thus, formation of the sclerotome, like ingression of cells through the primitive streak and formation of neural crest cells, is another example of an **epithelial-to-mesenchymal transformation**.

During subsequent development, the **sclerotomes** will develop into the vertebrae. Note that the ventral portion of the sclerotome surrounds the notochord; this portion of the sclerotome will form the vertebral body. More dorsally, the sclerotome flanks the neural tube and will eventually expand dorsal to it to form the vertebral arch.

The dermomyotome later subdivides into the **dermatome**, which lies beneath the surface ectoderm, and **myotome**, immediately subjacent to the dermatome. The dermatome contributes to the **dermis of the skin** throughout the trunk. The **myotome** forms the **epaxial** (dorsal) and **hypaxial** (ventrolateral) **muscles** of the body wall. In addition, after formation of the limb buds, myotome cells migrate into the developing limbs to form the **limb muscles**.

INDUCTIVE INTERACTIONS UNDERLIE FORMATION OF SOMITE SUBDIVISIONS

Experiments involving tissue transplantation and ablation have shown that structures adjacent to the developing somites are responsible for patterning the somites into their subdivisions. Signals from the notochord induce sclerotome, whereas signals from the dorsal neural tube, surface ectoderm, and adjacent lateral plate (and intermediate) mesoderm induce and pattern the dermomyotome (Fig. 4-25). More recent molecular genetic experiments have begun to elucidate the molecules mediating these signaling interactions. Notochord (and subsequently the floor plate of the neural tube) secretes *Sonic hedgehog* (*Shh*), which along with *Noggin* (a *Bmp* inhibitor), also secreted by the

Somite　　　　　　　　Neural tube

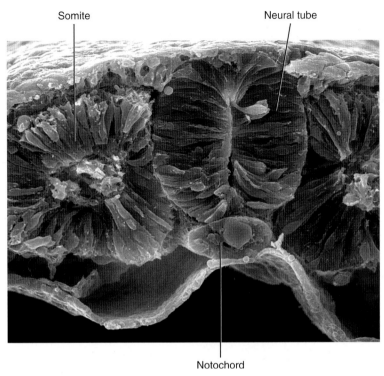

Notochord

Figure 4-23. Scanning electron micrograph of a transversely sectioned chick embryo showing the neural tube and underlying notochord and adjacent newly formed epithelial somite on one side.

Dermomyotome

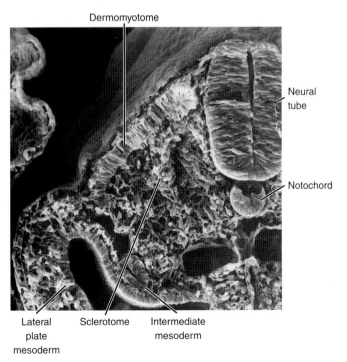

Neural tube

Notochord

Lateral plate mesoderm　　Sclerotome　　Intermediate mesoderm

Figure 4-24. Scanning electron micrograph of a transversely sectioned chick embryo showing the neural tube and underlying notochord and adjacent somite on one side subdivided into dermomyotome and sclerotome. Also note the intermediate mesoderm and lateral plate mesoderm.

notochord, is required for induction and maintenance of the sclerotome; specifically, these factors are required for the expression of *Pax1*, a paired-box transcription factor. *Pax1* is mutated in several of the *undulated* mouse mutants, characterized by vertebral body and vertebral disc defects. In the *Shh* null mouse, vertebrae do not form, in part due to increased cell death. Dorsal neural tube and surface ectoderm produce various *Wnts*, which induce dermomyotome (*Wnt1, -3a,* and *Wnt4, -6,* respectively); formation of the dermomyotome is marked by the expression of another paired-box transcription factor, *Pax3*. *Pax3* is needed for development of both the dermomyotome and myotome. *Wnt6* signaling from the ectoderm also maintains the epithelial characteristics of the dermomyotome. In addition, long-range *Shh* signaling is needed for the initial specification of the epaxial (defined and discussed below) part of the dermomyotome.

As the dermomyotome is forming, it is further patterned by a gradient of *Bmp4* signaling. This gradient is established by the secretion of *Bmp4* by the lateral plate mesoderm, and the secretion of *Noggin* by the dorsal neural tube and notochord. *Noggin*, a *Bmp* inhibitor, attenuates *Bmp* signaling. Thus a gradient of *Bmp* signaling occurs across the dermomyotome, resulting in the subsequent patterning of cells in this anlage. Further development of the somites and its subdivisions, including myogenesis, skeletogenesis, and resegmentation, is discussed in Ch. 8.

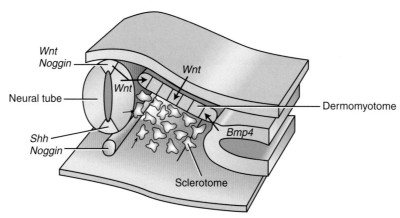

Figure 4-25. Inductive interactions involved in formation of somite subdivisions.

IN THE CLINIC

SPINAL ANOMALIES

A number of spinal defects are caused by abnormal formation of the sclerotomes and neural tube. Defective formation of vertebral bodies on one side of the body may result in a severe congenital **scoliosis** (lateral bending of the spinal column), which may require surgical correction. Open neural tube defects of the spinal cord (discussed earlier in the chapter) also result in an open spine in which the vertebral arches fail to form properly and form a spinelike bony protuberance on either side of the open spinal cord. Hence, the use of the term **spina bifida** as the common name for such defects.

Suggested Readings

Aybar MJ, Mayor R. 2002. Early induction of neural crest cells: lessons learned from frog, fish and chick. Curr Opin Genet Dev 12:452-458.

Baker C. 2005. Neural crest and cranial ectodermal placodes. In: Rao MS, Jacobson M, editors. Developmental Neurobiology. New York: Kluwer Academic/Plenum Pubs. pp 67-127.

Barrallo-Gimeno A, Nieto MA. 2005. The Snail genes as inducers of cell movement and survival: implications in development and cancer. Development 132:3151-3161.

Basch ML, Garcia-Castro MI, Bronner-Fraser M. 2004. Molecular mechanisms of neural crest induction. Birth Defects Res C Embryo Today 72:109-123.

Borycki AG, Emerson CP, Jr. 2000. Multiple tissue interactions and signal transduction pathways control somite myogenesis. Curr Top Dev Biol 48:165-224.

4

Boyles AL, Hammock P, Speer MC. 2005. Candidate gene analysis in human neural tube defects. Am J Med Genet C Semin Med Genet 135:9-23.

Brand-Saberi B, Christ B. 2000. Evolution and development of distinct cell lineages derived from somites. Curr Top Dev Biol 48:1-42.

Brent AE, Tabin CJ. 2002. Developmental regulation of somite derivatives: muscle, cartilage and tendon. Curr Opin Genet Dev 12:548-557.

Brewer S, Williams T. 2004. Finally, a sense of closure? Animal models of human ventral body wall defects. Bioessays 26:1307-1321.

Colas JF, Schoenwolf GC. 2001. Towards a cellular and molecular understanding of neurulation. Dev Dyn 221:117-145.

Copp AJ, Greene ND, Murdoch JN. 2003. Dishevelled: linking convergent extension with neural tube closure. Trends Neurosci 26:453-455.

Dockter JL. 2000. Sclerotome induction and differentiation. Curr Top Dev Biol 48:77-127.

Farlie PG, McKeown SJ, Newgreen DF. 2004. The neural crest: basic biology and clinical relationships in the craniofacial and enteric nervous systems. Birth Defects Res C Embryo Today 72:173-189.

Gammill LS, Bronner-Fraser M. 2003. Neural crest specification: migrating into genomics. Nat Rev Neurosci 4:795-805.

Garcia-Castro MI, Marcelle C, Bronner-Fraser M. 2002. Ectodermal Wnt function as a neural crest inducer. Science 297:848-851.

Graham A. 2003. The neural crest. Curr Biol 13:R381-R384.

Greene ND, Copp AJ. 2005. Mouse models of neural tube defects: investigating preventive mechanisms. Am J Med Genet C Semin Med Genet 135:31-41.

Haigo SL, Hildebrand JD, Harland RM, Wallingford JB. 2003. Shroom induces apical constriction and is required for hingepoint formation during neural tube closure. Curr Biol 13:2125-2137.

Hildebrand JD. 2005. Shroom regulates epithelial cell shape via the apical positioning of an actomyosin network. J Cell Sci 118:5191-5203.

Hildebrand JD, Soriano P. 1999. Shroom, a PDZ domain-containing actin-binding protein, is required for neural tube morphogenesis in mice. Cell 99:485-497.

Honein MA, Paulozzi LJ, Mathews TJ, et al. 2001. Impact of folic acid fortification of the US food supply on the occurrence of neural tube defects. JAMA 285:2981-2986.

Huang X, Saint-Jeannet JP. 2004. Induction of the neural crest and the opportunities of life on the edge. Dev Biol 275:1-11.

Iulianella A, Melton KR, Trainor PA. 2003. Somitogenesis: breaking new boundaries. Neuron 40:11-14.

Kalcheim C, Burstyn-Cohen T. 2005. Early stages of neural crest ontogeny: formation and regulation of cell delamination. Int J Dev Biol 49:105-116.

Kiefer JC. 2005. Planar cell polarity: heading in the right direction. Dev Dyn 233:695-700.

Klein TJ, Mlodzik M. 2005. Planar cell polarization: an emerging model points in the right direction. Annu Rev Cell Dev Biol 21:155-176.

Knecht AK, Bronner-Fraser M. 2002. Induction of the neural crest: a multigene process. Nat Rev Genet 3:453-461.

Kuan CY, Tannahill D, Cook GM, Keynes RJ. 2004. Somite polarity and segmental patterning of the peripheral nervous system. Mech Dev 121:1055-1068.

Kulesa P, Ellies DL, Trainor PA. 2004. Comparative analysis of neural crest cell death, migration, and function during vertebrate embryogenesis. Dev Dyn 229:14-29.

LaBonne C. 2002. Vertebrate development: wnt signals at the crest. Curr Biol 12:R743-R744.

Ladher R, Schoenwolf GC. 2005. Making a neural tube: Neural induction and neurulation. In: Rao MS, Jacobson M, editors. Developmental Neurobiology. New York: Kluwer Academic/ Plenum Pubs. pp 1-39.

Lee KJ, Jessell TM. 1999. The specification of dorsal cell fates in the vertebrate central nervous system. Annu Rev Neurosci 22:261-294.

Liu A, Niswander LA. 2005. Signalling in development: Bone morphogenetic protein signalling and vertebrate nervous system development. Nat Rev Neurosci 6:945-954.

Lynch SA. 2005. Non-multifactorial neural tube defects. Am J Med Genet C Semin Med Genet 135:69-76.

Marti E, Bovolenta P. 2002. Sonic hedgehog in CNS development: one signal, multiple outputs. Trends Neurosci 25:89-96.

Mills JL, England L. 2001. Food fortification to prevent neural tube defects: is it working? JAMA 285:3022-3023.

Mitchell LE. 2005. Epidemiology of neural tube defects. Am J Med Genet C Semin Med Genet 135:88-94.

Monsoro-Burq AH. 2005. Sclerotome development and morphogenesis: when experimental embryology meets genetics. Int J Dev Biol 49:301-308.

Morales AV, Barbas JA, Nieto MA. 2005. How to become neural crest: from segregation to delamination. Semin Cell Dev Biol 16:655-662.

Nieto MA. 2001. The early steps of neural crest development. Mech Dev 105:27-35.

Nieto MA. 2002. The snail superfamily of zinc-finger transcription factors. Nat Rev Mol Cell Biol 3:155-166.

O'Rahilly R, Muller F. 2002. The two sites of fusion of the neural folds and the two neuropores in the human embryo. Teratology 65:162-170.

Patten I, Placzek M. 2002. Opponent activities of Shh and BMP signaling during floor plate induction in vivo. Curr Biol 12:47-52.

Placzek M, Briscoe J. 2005. The floor plate: multiple cells, multiple signals. Nat Rev Neurosci 6:230-240.

Saburi S, McNeill H. 2005. Organising cells into tissues: new roles for cell adhesion molecules in planar cell polarity. Curr Opin Cell Biol 17:482-488.

Stockdale FE, Nikovits W, Jr., Christ B. 2000. Molecular and cellular biology of avian somite development. Dev Dyn 219:304-321.

Strahle U, Lam CS, Ertzer R, Rastegar S. 2004. Vertebrate floor-plate specification: variations on common themes. Trends Genet 20:155-162.

Taneyhill LA, Bronner-Fraser M. 2005. Dynamic alterations in gene expression after Wnt-mediated induction of avian neural crest. Mol Biol Cell 16:5283-5293.

Torban E, Kor C, Gros P. 2004. Van Gogh-like2 (Strabismus) and its role in planar cell polarity and convergent extension in vertebrates. Trends Genet 20:570-577.

Ueno N, Greene ND. 2003. Planar cell polarity genes and neural tube closure. Birth Defects Res C Embryo Today 69:318-324.

van der Put NM, van Straaten HW, Trijbels FJ, Blom HJ. 2001. Folate, homocysteine and neural tube defects: an overview. Exp Biol Med (Maywood) 226:243-270.

Wu J, Saint-Jeannet JP, Klein PS. 2003. Wnt-frizzled signaling in neural crest formation. Trends Neurosci 26:40-45.

Yanfeng W, Saint-Jeannet JP, Klein PS. 2003. Wnt-frizzled signaling in the induction and differentiation of the neural crest. Bioessays 25:317-325.

Principles and Mechanisms of Morphogenesis and Dysmorphogenesis

5

Summary Formation of the embryo and its parts involves **morphogenesis**, a form-shaping process controlled by fundamental **cell behaviors** that result in **differential growth.** Perturbation of differential growth due to a **genetic mutation, teratogen** exposure, or a combination of the two processes results in **dysmorphogenesis** and the formation of structural **birth defects**. Structural birth defects involve both **malformations**—involving perturbation of developmental events directly involved in forming a particular structure—and **deformation**—involving perturbation of a developing structure indirectly owing to mechanical forces. Malformation can involve single organs or body parts or a constellation of organs or body parts. In the latter case, if a single cause is involved, the condition constitutes a **syndrome**. To understand how development occurs requires the use of **animal models** in which experiments can be conducted. Because developmental mechanisms are conserved across species, the use of animal models provides insight into how normal development of the human embryo occurs and how development can be perturbed by genetic mutation or environmental insult, resulting in birth defects. The tool kit for the developmental biologist's experiments is vast, including techniques derived from the fields of **cell biology, molecular biology**, and **genetics**, combined with the classical approaches of **cut-and-paste experimental embryology**. Manipulation of the **mouse genome** has been a particularly fruitful approach for understanding how genes function during development and for developing models for human disease and birth defects. Using experimental approaches, a small number of highly conserved **signaling pathways** have been identified. These pathways are used repeatedly and in various combinations throughout embryonic development. Tools originally used to study mouse embryos have been adapted for use in human embryos. This has resulted in advances in reproductive technologies such as IVF (discussed in Ch. 1) and recently in the development of **stem cells**—cells that could be used potentially to regenerate diseased or damaged organs.

Principles of Morphogenesis and Dysmorphogenesis

Having described the initial steps in embryogenesis in Chapters 1 to 4, it is appropriate to pause to lay down the basic groundwork for understanding the concepts of the normal and abnormal embryology that are discussed in later chapters. Moreover, because these concepts have been formulated using animal models for experimental studies, it is important to understand the attributes each of these models provide for understanding human development. Finally, experimental techniques are described to provide an understanding of how experiments are conducted in the field, and signaling pathways are discussed to place molecules that control developmental events into context.

As discussed in preceding chapters, the initially flat three-layered embryonic disc undergoes **morphogenesis** to form a three-dimensional embryo with a tube-within-a-tube body plan and the beginnings of rudiments that will form all of the adult organs and systems. In this chapter, we consider how morphogenesis occurs and how morphogenesis goes awry during the formation of **birth defects**. Morphogenesis results from **differential growth**. Differential growth is driven by a small number of fundamental **cellular behaviors** such as changes in cell shape, size, position, number, and

Clinical Taster A first-year pediatrics fellow in medical genetics is on full-time service for the month of May. Early in the month, she is asked to consult on an infant with cleft lip and palate and possible brain abnormalities that were identified on prenatal ultrasound. Review of the prenatal and postnatal history is significant only for an abnormal ultrasound during the 24th week of gestation that showed dilation and possible fusion of the lateral ventricles of the brain, and for premature birth at 32 weeks after the onset of preterm labor. The family history seems negative at first, but on further discussion the fellow elicits a history of a single central incisor in the patient's father. The physical exam shows microcephaly (small head), ocular hypotelorism (closely spaced eyes), a flat nasal bridge, and bilateral **cleft lip** and **cleft palate** (Fig. 5-1A). Magnetic resonance imaging (MRI) of the brain shows fusion of the left and right frontal lobes and partial fusion of the parietal lobes characteristic of semilobar **holoprosencephaly**. Genetic testing discovers a deleterious mutation in the **SONIC HEDGEHOG (SHH)** gene in both the patient and her father.

Near the end of the month, the fellow is called to the nursery to examine a newborn with limb anomalies. She finds an otherwise healthy, full-term girl with **polydactyly** (extra-digits) of both hands and feet occurring on the thumb and great toe side (preaxial; Fig. 5-1B). Chromosome analysis shows a translocation involving chromosomes 5 and 7, with the chromosome 7 breakpoint occurring distant from the SHH gene, but in a region known to affect SHH expression in the limb. Disruption of these regulatory elements is known to cause preaxial polydactyly.

The fellow is impressed with the variability of manifestations caused by different defects in the same gene (SHH), with one mutation causing brain and face abnormalities and another causing limb defects.

adhesivity. If these behaviors are perturbed during embryogenesis, by a genetic mutation, environmental insult (i.e., a **teratogen**), or a combination of the two, differential growth is abnormal and **dysmorphogenesis** results with the formation of a structural birth defect.

Dysmorphogenesis can result from both **malformation** and **deformation**. Malformations consist of primary morphologic defects in an organ or body part resulting from abnormal developmental events that are *directly* involved in the development of that organ or body part. For example, failure of the neural groove to close results in a malformation called a neural tube defect. Similarly, failure of the digits to fully separate results in syndactyly, that is, fusion of the digits.

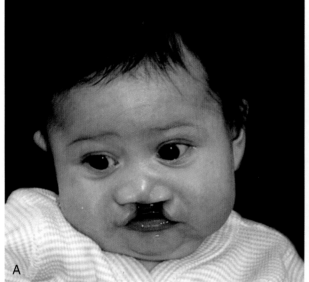
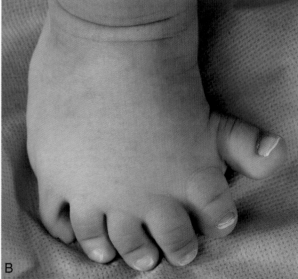

Figure 5-1. Mutations in the *SONIC HEDGEHOG (SHH)* gene have multiple manifestations. *A,* Infant with bilateral cleft lip and facial findings associated with holoprosencephaly. *B,* Foot of an infant with preaxial polydactyly.

Deformations consist of secondary morphologic defects that are imposed upon an organ or body part owing to mechanical forces; that is, deformations affect the development of an organ or body part *indirectly*. For example, if insufficient amniotic fluid forms (i.e., oligo-hydramnios), deformation of the feet can occur due to mechanical constraints, resulting in club foot. Dysmorphogenesis can occur in an isolated organ or body part or can occur as a pattern of multiple primary malformations with a single cause. In the latter case, the condition is referred to as a **syndrome**. Common examples, discussed elsewhere in the text, include Down syndrome (trisomy 21) and 22q11.2 deletion syndrome, two syndromes that result from genetic mutations.

Other syndromes can result from teratogen exposure. A common example is **fetal alcohol syndrome**, also known as **fetal alcohol spectrum disorder**. This disorder affects 2 in 1000 live-born infants (Fig. 5-2). Consumption of amounts of alcohol as low as 80g per day (i.e., between two and three shots of a grain liquor such as rum) during the 1st month of pregnancy can cause significant defects, and it has been suggested that even a single binge may be teratogenic. Common components of the disorder include defects of brain and face development, namely, microcephaly (small head), short palpebral fissures (eye openings), epicanthal folds (folds over eye lids), a low nasal bridge with a short nose, flat midface, minor external ear anomalies, and jaw anomalies including a thin upper lip with indistinct philtrum and micrognathia (small jaw). Chronic consumption of even quite small amounts of alcohol later in pregnancy can result in other, less-destructive effects, such as some degree of growth retardation and minor physical defects.

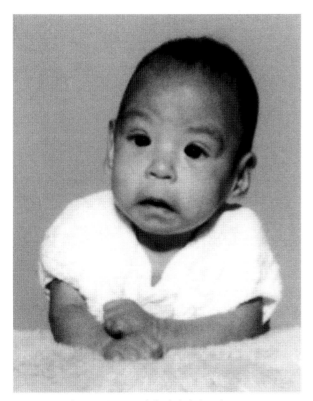

Figure 5–2. Boy with fetal alcohol syndrome.

Animal Models

The aim of research in developmental biology/embryology is to understand how development occurs at the tissue, cellular, and molecular levels. This aim speaks largely to our innate curiosity to understand nature and how it works. An additional aim is to understand how normal development can go awry, resulting in birth defects, particularly in humans. Understanding how both normal and abnormal development occur could lead to ways to detect (diagnose), prevent, and cure birth defects. Thus, this aim speaks to our desire to prevent and relieve human suffering.

Although the only perfect organism for studying how the human embryo develops is the human embryo, **animal models** provide useful surrogates because of the principle that **developmental mechanisms are highly conserved** from organism to organism (Fig. 5-3). Six animal models have been particularly useful for deciphering mechanisms and principles of embryogenesis: two invertebrates and four vertebrates. These models provide complementary information, which, when assembled across animal models, provide considerable insight into how the human embryo develops. All of these models are practical to obtain, use, and maintain in the laboratory, and all can be acquired and used throughout the year (i.e., they are not seasonal breeders). The main unique strengths of each of these organisms for understanding mechanisms of development are discussed below.

Drosophila

The developing field of genetics was greatly enhanced in the early 20th century using *Drosophila melanogaster*, the common fruitfly. Thus, the first studies to merge the burgeoning fields of genetics and

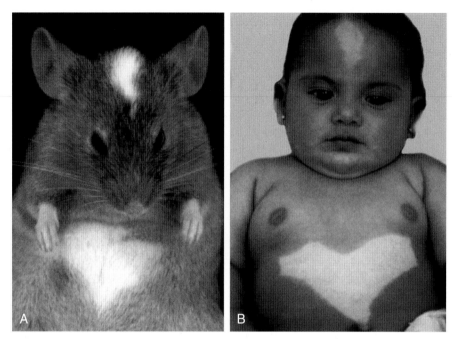

Figure 5-3. Animal models for disease can precisely phenocopy human diseases. *A*, Mouse with a mutation in the *c-Kit* gene shows pigmentation deficits on the forehead and chest. *B*, Child with a mutation in the *c-Kit* gene, a condition known as piebaldism, shows pigmentation deficits that are similar to those shown by the mouse model.

developmental biology utilized Drosophila. Drosophila offers several advantages for understanding mechanisms of development. Through saturation mutagenesis using chemicals such as EMS (ethyl methane sulfonate) and subsequent screening to identify unique phenotypes, mutations have been identified in virtually every gene (Drosophila has 13,639 predicted genes). This powerful process of using random mutations in unknown genes to identify perturbed developmental events (i.e., thereby resulting in **phenotypes**), followed by identification and cloning of the mutated gene, is referred to as the **forward genetic approach**.

The life cycle of Drosophila is relatively short (about 9 days; Fig. 5-4); thus, new generations can be bred very quickly (that is, Drosophila is genetically amenable). Embryogenesis also occurs very rapidly, with embryogenesis being completed and the first larval stage forming about 1 day after fertilization. After formation of a series of larval stages, a pupa forms, which subsequently metamorphoses into the adult fruitfly.

Several techniques have been developed for gene over expression or under expression in Drosophila, allowing experimental analyses of gene function during development. Also, a web site (Flybase) has been developed to disseminate information on Drosophila as a model system (www.flybase.bio. indiana.edu).

A surprising finding of the genomic era has been the realization that the genomes of fruitflies and humans are highly similar. Orthologs of about 60% of the genes expressed during Drosophila embryogenesis have been identified in other animal models, as well as in humans, although total gene number in humans is about double that in Drosophila (it is estimated that humans have 20,000 to 25,000 genes). Vertebrates, including humans, typically have multiple family members orthologous to each identified Drosophila gene. Thus, for example, in Drosophila there is one *Fgf* gene (*Branchless*) and one *Fgf receptor* (*Breathless*), whereas in mammals there are 22 *Fgf* genes and 4 *Fgf receptor* genes (*Fgfs* and *Fgf receptors* are discussed later in this chapter; *Branchless* and *Breathless* are discussed in the "In the Research Lab" section of Ch. 11).

Caenorhabditis elegans

The nematode worm, *Caenorhabditis elegans*, shares many of the features that make Drosophila an outstanding model system for understanding mechanisms

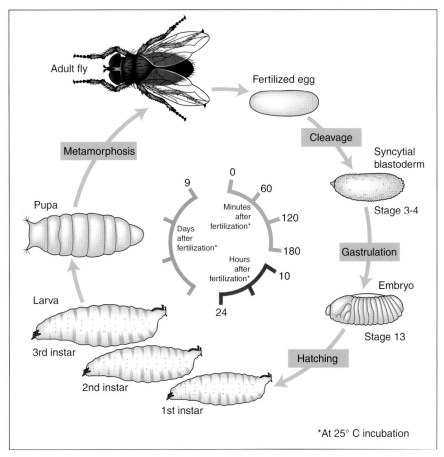

Figure 5-4. The life cycle of Drosophila.

of development. Like Drosophila, *C. elegans* has a short life cycle of 3 to 4 days and a short period of embryogenesis—going from fertilization to hatching (as a worm) in about 1 day (Fig. 5-5). Chemical mutagenesis has also been used in *C. elegans* to generate a series of mutants that have greatly advanced the field (that is, using the forward genetic approach), particularly leading to an understanding of mechanisms underlying programmed cell death or **apoptosis**, and gene misexpression techniques are well developed (including feeding worms RNAi to knock down gene expression; RNAi is discussed later in the chapter). Also, a web site (Wormbase) has been developed to disseminate information on *C. elegans* as a model system (elegans.swmed.edu).

In addition to having many attributes shared with Drosophila, the *C. elegans* embryo is transparent. This, along with a relatively small number of cells generated during development (the adult worm is composed of only about 1000 cells, and cell number is

essentially invariant between individuals), has allowed investigators to map out the complete **cell lineage** of *C. elegans* by watching cells as they divide, change position, and differentiate during embryogenesis. As a result of such study, the origin and fate of every cell in the *C. elegans* embryo is known, including 131 cells whose normal fate in development is to die (undergo apoptosis). The *C. elegans* genome contains 20,000 predicted genes.

Zebrafish

The zebrafish model, *Danio rerio*, enables the use of mutagenesis and phenotype screening to study directly *vertebrate* development. Using ENU (*N*-ethyl-*N*-nitrosourea) mutagenesis, mutant embryos can be identified and studied developmentally, and more than 8000 mutations have been identified using the forward genetic approach. Such study is greatly facilitated by the fact that zebrafish embryos, like *C. elegans* embryos, are

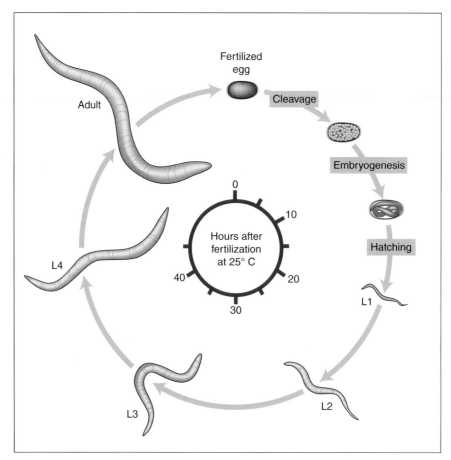

Figure 5-5. The life cycle of *C. elegans*.

transparent, so internal structures can be readily visualized without the need in many cases for histologic study. Also, like the other model systems discussed so far, zebrafish embryos develop rapidly, progressing from fertilization to free swimming fry in about 2 days, and fish reach sexual maturity in about 3 months (Fig. 5-6).

The cells (blastomeres) of cleaving zebrafish embryos are relatively large and can be injected with lineage tracers or RNAs for gene misexpression studies. Morpholinos (discussed later in the chapter) can be injected to knock down gene expression, and can also be injected in mutant embryos to study the combined effects of loss of function of multiple genes. In addition, transgenic approaches, including generating gene knock ins and knock outs (discussed later in the chapter), have been recently developed in zebrafish. The zebrafish genome has been sequenced and it is estimated to contain 30,000 to 60,000 genes (genome duplications have occurred during zebrafish evolution). A web site, Zfin, has been established to

disseminate information on zebrafish as a model system (www.Zfin.org).

Xenopus Laevis

The field of experimental embryology began in the 19th century with the use of amphibian—frog and salamander—embryos. However, during the last few decades *Xenopus laevis*, the South African clawed toad, has become the amphibian of choice for developmental biologists. Amphibian embryos readily tolerate microsurgical manipulation, so-called cutting-and-pasting experimental embryology (discussed later in the chapter). In addition, because cells (blastomeres) of cleaving embryos are relatively large, as they are in zebrafish, they can be injected with lineage tracers. In fact, probably the most precise **fate maps** produced to date using this approach are for *X. laevis*. *X. laevis*, like the models already discussed, develops relatively rapidly, progressing from the fertilized egg to the tadpole

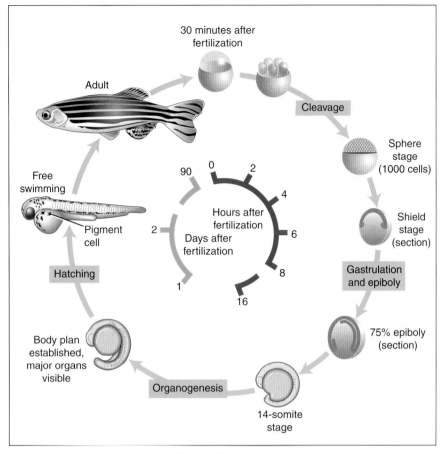

Figure 5-6. The life cycle of zebrafish.

in about 4 days (Fig. 5-7). The tadpole undergoes metamorphosis to form the adult terrestrial form, which becomes sexually mature in about 2 months.

Because genome duplication has occurred in *X. laevis*, this species is tetraploid. This fact makes it difficult to use *X. laevis* for gene manipulation studies. However, another species of Xenopus, *X. tropicalis*, is diploid, and it has been possible to use this species to generate **transgenic animals**, that is, animals in which the genome has be modified using molecular genetic techniques. Sequencing of the *X. tropicalis* genome has been completed recently, greatly enhancing the value of Xenopus as a model system. A web site, Xenbase, has been developed to disseminate information on the Xenopus model (www.xenbase.org).

Chick

Chick, or *Gallus gallus domesticus*, embryos, like Xenopus embryos, can be readily manipulated

microsurgically during development. Because the chick is a warm-blooded organism (as is the human) and because it can be so readily manipulated during development, it has become over the last several decades the favored workhorse for studies utilizing cut-and-paste experimental embryology approaches. One particularly fruitful approach has been to construct quail-chick transplantation chimeras (Fig. 5-8). In this approach, a small piece of tissue, say dorsal neural tube, is removed from a chick host embryo and replaced with a comparable piece from a donor quail embryo. By using histologic staining to reveal differences in nuclear heterochromatin at the end of the experiment, or more recently by using chick- or quail-specific antibodies, the fate of the transplanted cells can be followed, creating prospective fate maps (discussed in Ch. 3). This approach has been used extensively to determine the fates of neural crest cells arising from different cranial-caudal levels along the entire extent of the neural tube (discussed in Ch. 4). Although currently the chicken is not used extensively for genetic studies, it

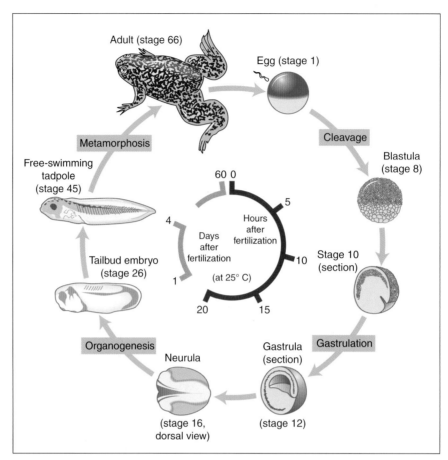

Figure 5-7. The life cycle of Xenopus.

was a popular model for such studies early in the 20th century, primarily for studies in agricultural colleges and poultry science departments. Many developmental mutants were collected, and some of these are still available today for study. As compared to the other models discussed earlier in the chapter, development of the chick embryo is relatively slow, taking about 21 days from fertilization to hatching, and birds reach sexually maturity 3 to 4 months after hatching (Fig. 5-9).

The chicken genome has been sequenced, enhancing the use of this organism for understanding molecular mechanisms of development. It is estimated that the chicken genome contains about 25,000 genes. Techniques have been developed recently for: over expressing proteins locally at specific times during chick development (e.g., using small beads coated with growth factors, injecting engineered viruses, or injecting transfected cells); over expressing genes using whole-embryo electroporation (or techniques such as sonoporation and lipofection) to target plasmids expressing the gene of interest to desired tissues in the chick embryo; and RNAi or morpholinos (discussed later in the chapter) to knock down gene expression (typically, introduced through whole-embryo electroporation). Useful web sites have been developed to disseminate information, especially genomic information and gene expression patterns, on the chick model (e.g., see www.ncbi.nlm.nih.gov).

Mouse

The laboratory mouse, *Mus musculus*, was originally used for genetic studies, and hundreds of naturally occurring mutations have been identified and are available for study. Sexual maturity is reached in 1 to 2 months after birth, facilitating the breeding of

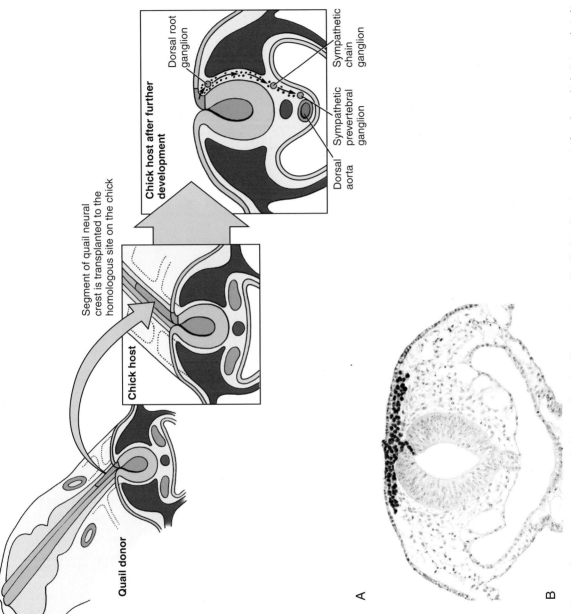

Figure 5-8. Quail-chick transplantation chimeras. *A*, To generate quail-chick transplantation chimeras as pioneered by Nicole Le Douarin, a segment of quail neural tube is transplanted to the same position in a chick embryo of the same age. After the graft has healed, quail neural crest cells migrate to their normal targets, where they are easily distinguished from chick cells by using an anti–quail antibody (*B*).

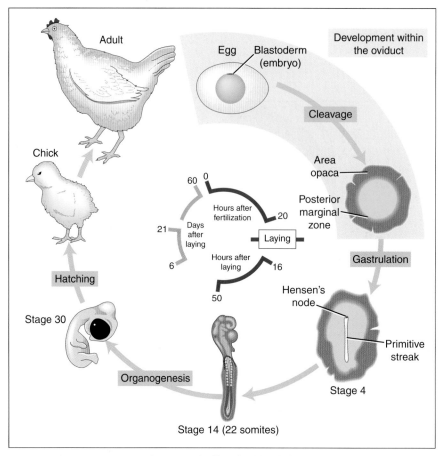

Figure 5-9. The life cycle of the chick.

mutant animals (Fig. 5-10). The time of gestation of the mouse is similar to that of the chick, ranging from 19 to 21 days after fertilization.

The main strength of the mouse model is the availability of techniques to make **transgenic mice** (discussed later in the chapter). Using homologous recombination, it is possible to inactivate (knock out) any gene of interest or to replace one gene with another (knock in). About 30% of the mouse genes have been knocked out by this approach. In contrast to the forward genetic approach used in Drosophila, *C. elegans*, and zebrafish, the so-called **reverse genetic approach** used in mouse starts with a *known* gene and mutates it to determine its function during development. In a variation of this approach using *conditional* transgenics, it is now possible to use tissue specific promoters to drive expression of a transgene (including reporter genes) in specific tissues (or to knock out

the gene in specific tissues only), enhancing the precision of the experiment. The mouse genome has been sequenced and is predicted to contain about 30,000 genes. Useful web sites include: www.jaxmice.jax.org and www.ensembl.org/Mus_musculus.

Experimental Techniques

Understanding how normal and abnormal development occurs requires a detailed understanding of *what* happens during development—that is, a detailed understanding of **descriptive embryology**. However, descriptive embryology alone cannot reveal *how* development occurs. Descriptive embryology provides a catalog of developmental events, which when carefully studied and reflected upon, can lead to the formulation of **hypotheses** about how a developmental

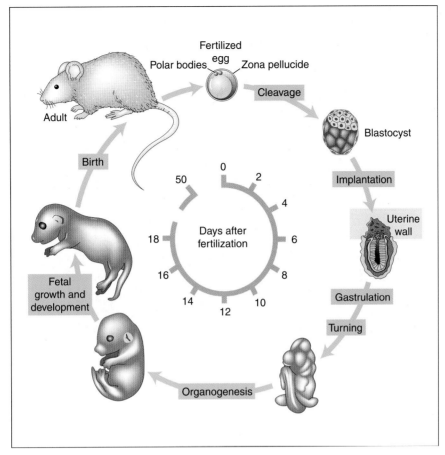

Figure 5-10. The life cycle of the mouse.

event occurs. The investigator then designs and conducts tests of the formulated hypotheses. Hypotheses are tested through a series of **experiments** (specific manipulations that usually perturb a developmental process) as compared to **controls** (nonspecific manipulations used to ensure that results obtained from particular manipulations are specific and not artifactual). Through this approach hypotheses are refuted, modified, or supported (never truly proven to be correct, but often proven to be incorrect). The cycle continues as new hypotheses are crafted, based on additional data obtained through experiments, leading to new experimental tests of their veracity.

Conducting experiments on developing model embryos constitutes the science of **experimental embryology**. Classically, experimental embryology has been used to define the tissue and cellular basis of development through a series of microsurgical manipulations. More recently, experimental embryology has merged with cell biology, molecular biology,

and genetics, allowing investigators to define the molecular-genetic basis of development.

Classical Experimental Embryology

Classical experimental embryology involves three basic techniques often referred to as cutting, pasting, and painting (Figs. 5-11, 5-12). These kinds of experiments address the question of whether a tissue or cell is **sufficient** and/or **necessary (required)** for a particular developmental event to occur. In a typical approach, a developmental biologist might ask: What is the origin of the cells that give rise to a particular region of ectoderm that forms the lens of the eye? To determine this, the ectoderm might be fate mapped at the gastrula stage by applying fluorescent dyes to its surface (that is, painting) and then following the movement of patches of labeled cells over time. This would not only fate map the prospective lens ectodermal cells, but would also reveal what tissues the prospective lens cells potentially

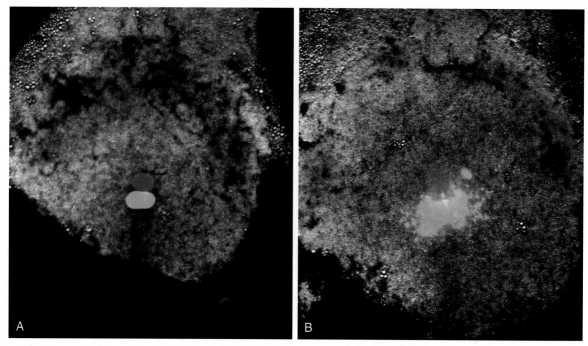

Figure 5-11. The use of fluorescent dyes to fate map cells (i.e., painting) of the primitive streak during gastrulation. Two dyes were injected into the primitive streak. *A*, Immediately after injection. *B*, 5 hours after injection. Cells are now leaving the primitive streak (ingressing) to form endoderm and mesoderm.

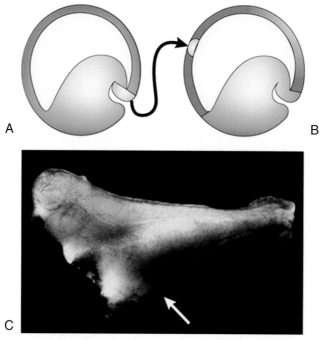

Figure 5-12. Classical cut-and-paste experimental embryology. *A*, Removal (i.e., cutting) of the dorsal lip of the blastopore of an amphibian embryo. *B*, Grafting (i.e., pasting) of the dorsal lip to the future belly ectoderm of another embryo. *C*, A secondary embryo (arrow) is induced from the belly ectoderm by the dorsal lip of the blastopore.

interact with (because they come in close proximity to them) during their movement to form the lens. As a second step, the prospective lens cells might be removed (extirpated or ablated; that is, cutting) to ask whether adjacent cells could grow back, replace them, and form a lens. If so, this would suggest that the fate of lens cells is not a result of their lineage, but perhaps requires some instructive information from adjacent tissues. As another test of this, a patch of ectoderm that is not fated to form lens could be removed (cutting) from a host embryo (perhaps a chick embryo) and replaced (pasting) with a patch from a donor embryo (perhaps a quail embryo) that is fated to form lens. Also, the converse experiment could be done: a patch of ectoderm fated to form lens could be removed (cutting) from a host embryo and replaced (pasting) with a patch from a donor embryo that is not fated to form lens. If in both cases the transplanted patch of ectoderm changed its fate, this would again suggest that the fate of lens cells is not a result of their lineage, but perhaps requires some instructive information from adjacent tissues. By repeating these experiments at different times in development, it would be possible to determine approximately when signaling might occur between adjacent tissues to establish ectodermal cell fate as lens. A third step could also be taken. Tissues adjacent to the prospective lens cells could be extirpated (cutting) to ask if the lens can form in their absence. If not, this would again suggest that lens cell fate requires some instructive information from adjacent tissues, that is, that the adjacent tissues are *necessary* for acquiring lens cell fate. But the gold standard in experimental embryology is to go one step further to take the adjacent tissue and transplant it beneath other ectoderm that never forms a lens in normal development and ask: Can the transplanted tissue **induce** a lens? If so, then the experiment has revealed that the adjacent tissue is *sufficient* for conferring lens cell fate.

The situation just described is a common one in development in which one tissue acts upon another to change its fate. This process is called **induction**. It requires at least two tissues: an **inducing tissue** and a **responding tissue**. It also requires that the responding tissue be capable of responding to the inducing tissue by changing its fate. This ability is called **competence**, and it is a property that is lost over time. Thus, using the example above, transplanting tissue beneath *gastrula* ectoderm may induce a lens from cells that would never form lens in normal development. However, repeating the experiment at the

neurula stage may fail to induce a lens because the ectoderm may no longer be competent to be induced.

In recent years is has become clear that **inductive interactions**, as well as so-called **suppressive interactions** that prevent a tissue from forming its "default" tissue type (e.g., *Bmps* prevent surface ectoderm from forming its default fate, neural ectoderm; discussed in Ch. 4), depend on the secretion of small growth factors from the inducing tissue, where they bind to specific receptors present on the surface of the responding tissue. The families of growth factors involved and the cascades of signaling events evoked in the responding tissue are discussed later in this chapter.

Visualizing Gene Expression

Techniques have been developed to reveal patterns of gene expression in developing embryos. For relatively young (and small) embryos, these techniques can be done on intact whole embryos (so-called *whole mounts*). If more tissue detail is required, such embryos can be subsequently serially sectioned and studied histologically. Although more labor intensive for older embryos, in which penetration of reagents can be a problem, tissue first can be sectioned and then labeled as sections (rather than as whole mounts) to reveal patterns of gene expression. Two techniques are used, one to visualize patterns of protein expression—immunohistochemistry—and one to visualize patterns of RNA expression—in situ hybridization.

Both these techniques can be used on untreated (control) embryos to describe normal patterns of gene expression over time. Also, they can be used in experimental studies, often to visualize markers of specific tissue types. Using the example discussed above, specific lens markers might be used to demonstrate that the induced ectoderm was truly forming lens and not some other ectodermal structure having a similar morphology (e.g., otic placode, the early ectodermal rudiment that forms the inner ear; discussed in Ch. 17).

Immunohistochemistry. Immunohistochemistry is used to show patterns of protein expression (Fig. 5-13). The main limitation for this technique is that it requires a specific antibody to identify the protein the investigator is interested in visualizing. Assuming that a specific antibody is available, one typical procedure (there are many variations) is to fix embryos to preserve them, treat them with detergents to make small holes

5

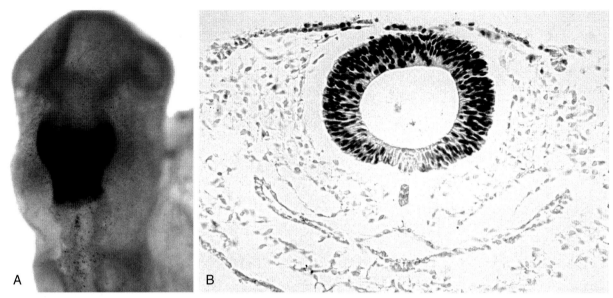

Figure 5-13. The use of specific antibodies and immunocytochemistry to label specific groups of cells. *A*, Head of a chick embryo after labeling with an antibody to *Engrailed-2*, a transcription factor produced in cells of the future midbrain/rostral hindbrain (so-called isthmus region). *B*, A transverse section through the midbrain shows labeling in the nuclei of most of the cells of the midbrain region (except those cells in the floor plate overlying the notochord). A few cells in the surface ectoderm overlying the midbrain are also labeled.

in cell membranes that facilitate reagent penetration, treat with the specific antibody (for example, an antibody to *Sonic hedgehog* protein; often a rabbit IgG-type antibody), and then to use a secondary antibody made against the first antibody (assuming the first or so-called *primary antibody* is a rabbit IgG, the second might be a goat anti–rabbit IgG). The secondary antibody is coupled to a marker such as peroxidase (revealed through a subsequent color reaction).

In situ hybridization. In situ hybridization is used to show patterns of RNA expression (Fig. 5-14). The approach is similar to that used in immunohistochemistry, beginning with fixation and detergent treatment. Embryos are then hybridized with a specific RNA probe (so-called riboprobe) that is complementary to the mRNA of interest (i.e., an anti-sense riboprobe). When the riboprobe is prepared, it is labeled with digoxigenin, a small antigenic molecule obtained from the *digitalis* plant. After hybridization and washing to remove unbound riboprobe, digoxigenin (DIG) can be detected essentially as described above for immunohistochemistry by using an anti–DIG antibody.

When examining results from in situ hybridization, it is important to keep in mind two caveats. First, although some RNAs function in the embryo without

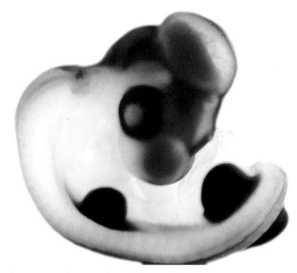

Figure 5-14. The use of specific riboprobes and in situ hybridization to label specific groups of cells. Whole chick embryo labeled with a probe for *Lmx1*, a transcription factor. Labeling occurs in several areas of the embryo including much of the brain and limb buds. Interestingly, only the dorsal sides of the limb buds label, not their ventral sides (the ventral sides are not visible in the view shown). The eye, which also appears labeled in this photo, is not labeled by the probe (it appears dark because it contains pigmentation).

being translated into protein (e.g., micro-RNAs), for many genes, translation of its RNA into protein is required for function. For example, *Sonic hedgehog* RNA does not function unless it is translated into *Sonic hedgehog* protein. Typically, expression of RNA is used to infer function of the translated protein, but this may not be a valid inference because RNAs can be transcribed at a particular time in development without being translated. Second, RNAs mark cells transcribing a particular gene, but if the translated protein is secreted and diffuses, it may act at some distance from where its RNA is transcribed. Thus, the site of expression of RNA does not necessarily correspond to the site of the protein's function.

Manipulation of Gene Expression

A powerful approach in developmental biology is to misexpress genes in developing embryos, that is, either to ectopically (over) express genes or block their expression (or function). Ectopically expressing genes in an embryo is the molecular equivalent of classical **pasting experimental embryology**, and often the question that is asked is, Is the gene of interest *sufficient* to cause some particular developmental event to occur (Fig. 5-15)? Knocking a gene down or out is the molecular equivalent of classical **cutting experimental embryology**, and often the question that is asked is, Is the gene of interest *necessary* for some particular developmental event to occur? The differences and similarities between classical experimental embryology and molecular experimental embryology are illustrated in Figures 5-12 and 5-15 using a specific example: induction of a secondary embryo through transplantation of the dorsal lip of the blastopore of the frog embryo (the organizer; discussed in Ch. 3), or ectopic over expression of molecules secreted by the organizer. Many techniques have been developed for gene misexpression. These techniques take advantage of the unique experimental attributes that each of the model systems offer. Because **gene targeting** in the mouse is considered the premier approach for gene manipulation by many developmental biologists, the following section emphasizes gene manipulation in this model system.

Manipulation of the mouse genome. Over the last several years, a number of powerful molecular-genetic techniques have been developed to manipulate the mouse genome. Several lines of research have coalesced to yield techniques that make it possible to insert specific DNA sequences into their correct locations in the mouse genome, a process called

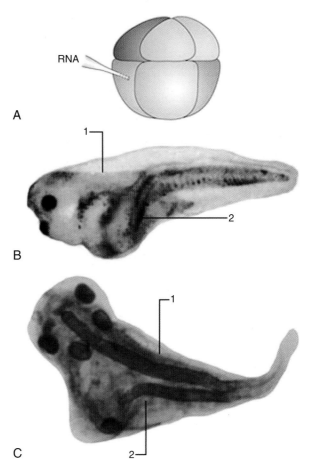

Figure 5-15. The molecular equivalent of cut-and-paste embryology. *A*, A ventral blastomere of a Xenopus early embryo is injected with an RNA encoding a protein normally expressed specifically within the dorsal lip of the blastopore. *B, C* (lateral and dorsal views, respectively), After further development a secondary embryo (2) is induced by the ectopically (i.e., pasted) expressed gene. 1, primary embryo.

gene targeting. These techniques give researchers the power to alter and manipulate the genome and to investigate the function of any gene of interest. Disabling specific normal genes (by *knocking out* the desired gene), or replacing a normal gene with a mutated gene (by *knocking in* the mutated gene in place of the normal gene) can create animal models of human genetic diseases. Moreover, the ability to correct defective genes lays the groundwork for developing techniques to cure genetic disorders.

A **transgenic mouse** is a mouse whose genome has been altered by the integration of donor DNA sequences. The most direct way to create a transgenic mouse is to inject many copies of the donor DNA

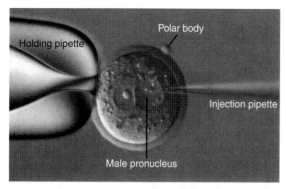

Figure 5-16. A procedure used to make a transgenic mouse. An egg is held in place using a suction (holding) pipette and DNA is injected into the male pronucleus, the larger of the two nuclei, just after fertilization has occurred.

sequence into the male pronucleus of a fertilized egg; the male pronucleus is used because it is larger than the female pronucleus (Fig. 5-16). The injected DNA sometimes integrates stably into the host chromosomes, and in many cases the donor gene is expressed. In a pioneering experiment, for example, a zinc-dependent rat growth hormone gene was introduced into the genome of a series of mice. When zinc was added to the drinking water to induce the expression of the rat growth hormone gene, these transgenic mice grew at twice the rate of control animals.

Although a simple method, the injection of DNA into the male pronucleus of the fertilized egg does not target the donor gene to a specific location in the host genome. However, targeting can be accomplished by inserting donor DNA into cells obtained from the inner cell mass of the blastocyst, and the rare cells in which the donor DNA has integrated correctly are identified and used to create a special type of transgenic animal called an **injection chimera**. In this approach, blastocysts are obtained from the oviducts of fertilized mice and are grown on a layer of fibroblasts in a culture dish. Culturing causes a cluster of cells from the inner cell mass to erupt from the blastocyst. These inner cell mass clusters are harvested and subcultured to produce stable lines of **embryonic stem (ES) cells** that are **totipotent** (able to give rise to any tissue in the body).

Donor DNA sequences can be introduced into cultured ES cells by a technique called **electroporation**, in which a suspension of ES cells is mixed with many copies of the donor DNA and subjected to an electric current. The current facilitates the movement of the donor DNA through the cell membrane, allowing the

DNA to enter the nucleus. In a tiny fraction of these cells, the introduced DNA is incorporated into the desired target site on the genome by **homologous recombination**. Appropriate marker genes and screening techniques are used to isolate and subculture these rare "targeted" cells.

If introduced DNA sequences are mutated to block transcription of the targeted gene, the gene is said to be **knocked out.** Also, the allele containing the mutated sequence (or ultimately the transgenic mouse containing the mutated sequence; see next paragraph) is said to be **null** for the particular gene.

To create transgenic mice containing the new DNA, groups of 8 to 12 targeted ES cells are injected into the cavity of normal mouse blastocysts, where they combine with the inner cell mass and participate in the formation of the embryo (Fig. 5-17). The resulting blastocysts (called **chimeras** because they are composed of cells from two different sources) are then implanted in the uterus of a pseudopregnant mouse, where they develop normally. Depending on their location in the embryonic disc, the ES cells may contribute to any tissue of the chimeric mouse. When they contribute to the germ line, the donor genes can be passed on to the offspring. Dominant donor genes may be expressed in the immediate offspring; if the donor genes are recessive (as they usually are), an inbreeding program is used to produce a homozygous strain that can express the gene.

It is not uncommon in gene knock out studies in mice to have mice born that seem to be normal despite the lack of what the scientist would have predicted (based, for example, on patterns of gene expression) to be a critical developmental gene. There are three likely reasons for such an outcome. First, many scientists believe that a mouse cannot be "normal" if it lacks any particular gene—that is, they believe that if the mouse were fully and appropriately tested, some defect (anatomic, biochemical, physiologic, or behavioral) would be found. In other words, they believe that a subtle defect is present that could be easily overlooked unless appropriately tested. Second, because gene duplication has occurred during vertebrate development, such that critical developmental control genes in Drosophila are represented by multiple family members in mouse, **gene redundancy** exists. Thus, for example, in the absence of, say, one of the *Hox* genes, the animal seems normal because a second (or third) redundant *Hox* gene, which is still expressed, has an overlapping function with the knocked-out gene. Third, in the absence of expression of one

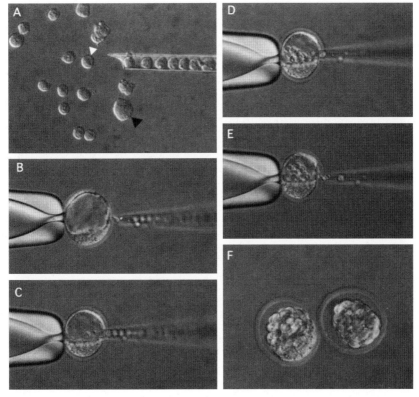

Figure 5-17. A procedure used to make chimeric mice. *A,* Blastocysts are dissociated into individual blastomeres, or, alternatively, embryonic stem (ES) cells derived the inner cell mass are collected using a pipette. *B-E,* Using a suction pipette to hold a blastocyst, the collected cells are injected into the blastocele. *F,* Injected cells intermix randomly with both inner cell mass and trophoblast cells, and later newly reorganized blastocysts are formed. These are injected into the uterine horns of pseudopregnant females, where they implant and undergo normal development.

gene, the expression of another gene can be upregulated. Thus, **compensation** can occur. Despite these possibilities, mice harboring knocked-out genes often have very obvious developmental defects that allow investigators to gain an understanding of the role(s) of the knocked-out gene in development.

Conditional transgenic mice can also be engineered such that the mutated (knocked-out) or inserted (knocked-in) gene is expressed only in particular tissues or only at desired times in development. This is important because, for example, a gene such as an *Fgf* family member that is required for gastrulation and subsequently for ear development might die during gastrulation; hence its role in ear development (which occurs a couple of days later) could not be studied. There are two approaches to this problem. First, by using **tissue-specific promoters** and the **cre-lox system**, the gene of interest could be specifically knocked out only in the ear-forming region, not in the primitive streak. Second, by using **inducible promoters** and the **cre-lox system**, the time at which the gene is knocked out could be delayed until gastrulation has occurred but before ear development has been initiated.

In the first approach, the gene of interest is flanked in a targeting vector with so-called *loxP* sites, and transgenic mice are produced as described above. A second group of transgenic mice are engineered in which a promoter is used to drive the expression of *cre* recombinase to the tissue of interest. (*Cre* recombinase is a site-specific recombinase derived from phage; in an alternative procedure, *Flp* recombinase derived from yeast is used when the gene of interest is flanked with the so-called *FRT sequence.*) The two groups of transgenic mice are bred, and during development the tissue-specific promoter drives expression of *cre* recombinase at the appropriate times and in the appropriate tissues during development. *Cre* recombinase acts on the *loxP* sites flanking the gene of interest, which is then excised, preventing its expression only in the tissue of interest (i.e., there is precise spatial control of gene inactivation).

In the second approach, an inducible promoter is used to drive *cre* recombinase, and the gene of interest is knocked out only in the presence of an exogenously applied reagent such as the anti–breast cancer drug Tamoxifen or the antibiotic tetracycline. Thus, at the desired time in gestation, pregnant mice are injected in their peritoneal (abdominal) cavity with Tamoxifen, which quickly diffuses to the uterine horns containing the developing embryos and activates the inducible promoter. The gene of interest is excised, through expression of *cre* recombinase, providing precise temporal control of gene inactivation.

The *cre*-lox system also has been used with ROSA26 transgenic mice, that is, mice that express the reporter gene *lacZ* in all of their tissues during development (*lacZ* encodes the enzyme beta galactosidase, whose activity can be readily detected with a colorimetric reaction). However, because expression of the *lacZ* gene is blocked by the presence of a *loxP*-flanked "stop" DNA fragment that prevents transcription and translation of the *lacZ* gene, *lacZ* is expressed only in the presence of *cre*. By breeding mice containing a tissue-specific promoter driving *cre* with ROSA26 mice, cells and their descendents expressing the gene of interest will be labeled, allowing them to be followed over time to map cell **lineage**. Thus, this approach is the molecular genetic equivalent of painting used for fate mapping studies.

Manipulation of gene expression in other models. A common approach in zebrafish and Xenopus embryos is to generate **transient transgenic animals** by injecting early blastomeres with desired DNA constructs (recently, as discussed above, techniques also have been developed in both Xenopus [*tropicalis*] and zebrafish to generate transgenic lines of animals). Using this method, genes can be ectopically expressed in embryonic tissues derived from the lineages of the injected cell. Alternatively, cells can be injected with **morpholinos** (stabilized antisense RNA) or **RNAi** (interfering, double-stranded RNA). Both of these approaches knock *down* gene expression, rather than completely blocking it.

Recently, these approaches have been applied to chick embryos, and sometimes mouse embryos, to generate transient transgenic animals. Because chick and mouse embryos have relatively small cells, these cells cannot be injected as can the cells of early zebrafish and Xenopus embryos. Instead, genes are introduced into cells using engineered viruses or through **whole-embryo electroporation** (or other techniques such as sonoporation and lipofection). Fundamentally, whole-embryo electroporation is the same as the process used to electroporate cells in culture (discussed above). Whole-embryo electroporation allows an investigator to spatially and temporally target a DNA sequence to a particular tissue at a particular time in development and to study its effects when over expressed (sequences consist of full-length gene) or knocked down (sequences consist of antisense, morpholino, or RNAi, specifically designed to knock down the gene of interest).

Another important approach, utilized very effectively to study growth factor signaling especially in Xenopus, is to inject **dominant negative receptors** (Fig. 5-18). These are engineered growth factor receptors that contain the ligand-binding extracellular domain, which binds the growth factor but lack the intracellular domain necessary for signaling (i.e., they are truncated). When present in excess in the extracellular space (or bound to cell surfaces in excess), dominant negative receptors bind to secreted growth factors, preventing them from binding to intact receptors, thus blocking signaling.

Signaling Pathways

Human embryos, like those of animal models, are progressively patterned during embryogenesis largely through **cell-cell interactions**. These interactions are a form of **intercellular communication** that is mediated by the secretion of soluble signaling molecules that diffuse within the extracellular environment to reach adjacent cells. The **cascades of signals** that cells receive during development determine their fate. Thus, early-acting regulatory genes initiate development of groups of cells by inducing expression of other "downstream" genes. The activities of these genes then induce the expression of yet additional genes, and so on, until the genes that encode the actual structural and functional characteristics of specific cells and tissues of the embryo are activated. A relatively small number of signaling pathways (fewer than 20) act in these cascades. Many of these signaling pathways were first identified in Drosophila. Subsequently, families of orthologs of the genes encoding these signaling pathways were identified in vertebrates. Before the major signaling pathways involved in vertebrate development are addressed, the general scheme of signaling pathways acting in Drosphilia development will be discussed.

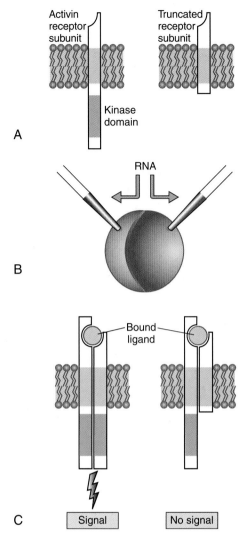

A

B

C

Figure 5-18. The molecular equivalent of cut-and-paste experimental embryology. *A,* In this example, truncated *Activin* receptors lacking the intercellular signaling domain are engineered. *B,* RNA encoding the truncated (dominant negative) receptor is injected into a blastomere of an early Xenopus embryo. *C,* Because injected message for the truncated receptor is far in excess of endogenous message for the wild-type receptor, most receptors upon receptor dimerization have one or two truncated subunits and thus cannot signal.

Patterning the Drosophila Embryo: A Major Entry Point into Understanding Human Development

In Drosophila, a signaling cascade is initiated by genes expressed before fertilization, the so-called **maternal effect genes** (Fig. 5-19). Because they are expressed before fertilization, paternal genes are not involved. The maternal effect genes encode signals that establish the axes of the embryo, namely, the anterior-posterior axis (cranial-caudal axis in humans), and the dorsal-ventral axis. In Drosophila, maternal effect genes encode protiens that impart differences to subregions of the oocyte, zygote, and early embryo along the respective axes, including **growth factors** and **transcription factors**. Although such localized **cytoplasmic determinants** are important in development of Drosophila and some vertebrates (such as Xenopus), most evidence suggests that the mammalian oocyte cytoplasm is relatively homogeneous in composition and that maternal effect genes play little or no role in early patterning.

During early embryonic development, the expression of maternal effect genes is superseded by a class of genes called **zygotic genes** (see Fig. 5-19). These genes are called *zygotic* because they are expressed after fertilization and involve both maternally and paternally inherited genes. In Drosophila, there are four classes of zygotic genes, which act in establishing the basic anterior-posterior body plan: **gap genes, pair-rule genes, segment polarity genes**, and **homeotic selector genes**. The maternal effect genes regulate the expression of the gap genes, which in turn regulate the expression of the pair-rule genes, which in turn regulate the expression of the segment polarity genes. These genes specify the specific segments. The segment polarity genes regulate the expression of the homeotic selector genes, which provide regional identity to the different segments.

Although the cascade of expression and regulation of zygotic genes is much more varied in vertebrates, orthologs of all classes of Drosophila zygotic genes function during vertebrate patterning. Thus, our understanding of the molecular-genetic basis of patterning in Drosophila has provided a major entry point in understanding development of vertebrates, including humans. In general, vertebrate orthologs of Drosophila patterning genes constitute two types of molecules: secreted factors that act as **signaling molecules** and **transcription factors**. Transcription factors switch other genes on or off by binding to regulatory regions of their DNA. Several transcription factors containing nucleotide sequences related to the pair-rule, segment polarity, and homeotic selector genes of Drosophila have been identified in mammals, and as is the case in Drosophila, some of these mammalian orthologs also play a role in segmentation. For example, segmentation of the mammalian hindbrain

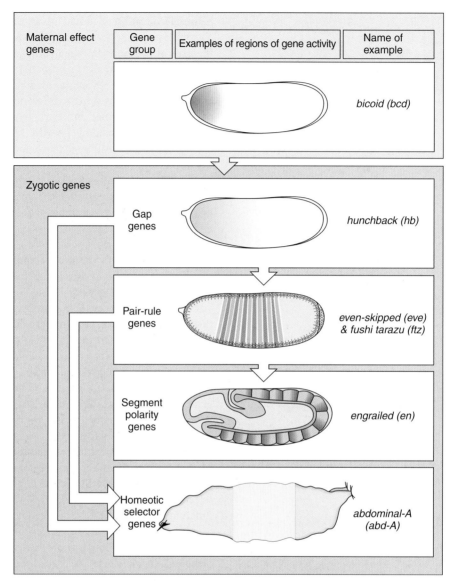

Figure 5-19. Genes underlying Drosophila early patterning. These consists of both maternal effect genes and four types of zygotic genes: gap genes, pair-rule genes, segment polarity genes, and homeotic selector genes.

(discussed in Chs. 9, 10, and 16), the pharyngeal arches of the head and neck region (discussed in Ch. 16), and the somites of the trunk (discussed in Ch. 4) is regulated at least in part by these genes.

One important and well-studied group of mammalian orthologs of the homeotic selector genes of Drosophila contains a highly conserved 183–base pair region of DNA called the **homeobox**, which encodes the 61–amino acid **homeodomain.** The homeodomain recognizes and binds to specific DNA sequences of other genes. Therefore, these encoded proteins function as transcription factors that regulate the activity of many "downstream" genes and as a consequence are often referred to as **master control genes**. A special subset of Drosophila homeotic selector genes are organized in two clusters on chromosome 3 and are collectively called the **homeotic complex**, or **HOM-C** (Fig. 5-20). A common ancestor of this complex was duplicated once, and then each resulting complex was duplicated again during the evolution of mammals. The four complexes of homeobox genes in mammals are called *Hox* **genes**.

In Drosophila, mutations of homeotic selector genes often result in remarkable transformations of

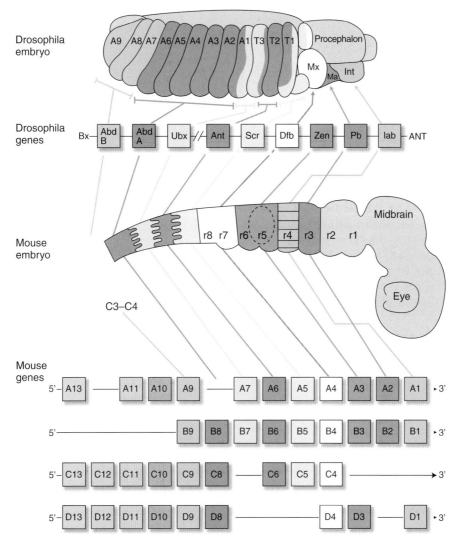

Figure 5-20. Alignment of the four vertebrate Hox complexes with the Drosophila homeotic complex.

body parts. A mutation resulting in misexpression of the *Antennapedia* gene during development, for example, causes cells that would normally form antennae to instead develop into legs, which now protrude from the head. Similarly, a mutation in the *Ultrabithorax* gene results in homeotic transformation of the 3rd thoracic segment into an additional second thoracic segment, giving a fruitfly with four wings instead of the normal two.

The Drosophila HOM-C and mammalian *Hox* genes have been extremely well conserved during evolution at the levels of clustered organization, sequence, expression, and function. Although the mammalian *Hox* genes have been individually altered through

evolution, they retain significant sequence homology to the insect HOM-C genes. The order of the *Hox* genes in the mammalian clusters parallels that observed in the Drosophila HOM-C. The amino acid sequences of the encoded homeodomains of the Drosophila genes and their mammalian orthologs, or corresponding genes, are often greater than 90% identical. In addition, in both mammals and fruitflies, these genes exhibit the property of colinearity, with the position of a gene within the cluster reflecting its expression domain in the developing embryo. As shown in Figure 5-20, genes located in more 5' positions within clusters are expressed in more caudal regions of the embryo.

Transgenic fruitflies, carrying experimentally added genes, have been used to demonstrate an unexpected level of functional conservation between the Drosophila HOM-C and mammalian *Hox* genes. For example, misexpression of the mammalian ortholog of the *Antennapedia* gene in the developing fruitfly also causes homeotic transformation of antennae into legs. This suggests that both the Drosophila and mammalian genes are capable of recognizing the same downstream gene targets and initiating the same genetic cascade. It is interesting to note that misexpression of either the Drosophila *Antennapedia* gene or the corresponding mammalian gene results in the formation of ectopic Drosophila legs and not mammalian legs. This is because, within the genetic context of the fruitfly, the downstream target genes are only capable of programming the development of a fruitfly leg.

Patterning the Vertebrate Embryo

As discussed in the previous section, patterning of the vertebrate embryo occurs through signaling cascades generated by families of orthologs of genes involved in Drosophila patterning. A general scheme for how such patterning occurs is shown in Figure 5-21. An inducer cell (in vertebrates, typically a group of cells rather than a single cell) secretes a small signaling molecule, or **growth factor**. This factor diffuses through the extracellular matrix to a responding cell (in vertebrates, again, typically a group of cells rather than a single cell), where it binds to a **receptor** on the cell's surface. Binding activates (often through **phosphylation** of intracellular proteins) an intracellular signaling cascade (a series of **signal transduction proteins**) that ultimately results in the movement of transcription factors into the nucleus, where they bind to specific regions of DNA and alter transcription. This in turn can result in cell differentiation to form a specific cell type. Often, altered transcription leads to the secretion of new growth factors that modify the fate of other cells or provide feedback to regulate the secretion of growth factors from the inducing cell.

Below, some of the major signaling pathways known to play specific roles in vertebrate development (and discussed in more detail in the appropriate chapters) will be briefly discussed. A hallmark of each of these pathways is their complexity. The purpose of this section is to help you place the major players into context so that you will have a more global understanding of signaling as you encounter specific members of these pathways (e.g., *Sonic hedgehog*) in various chapters. Each of the signaling pathways has been

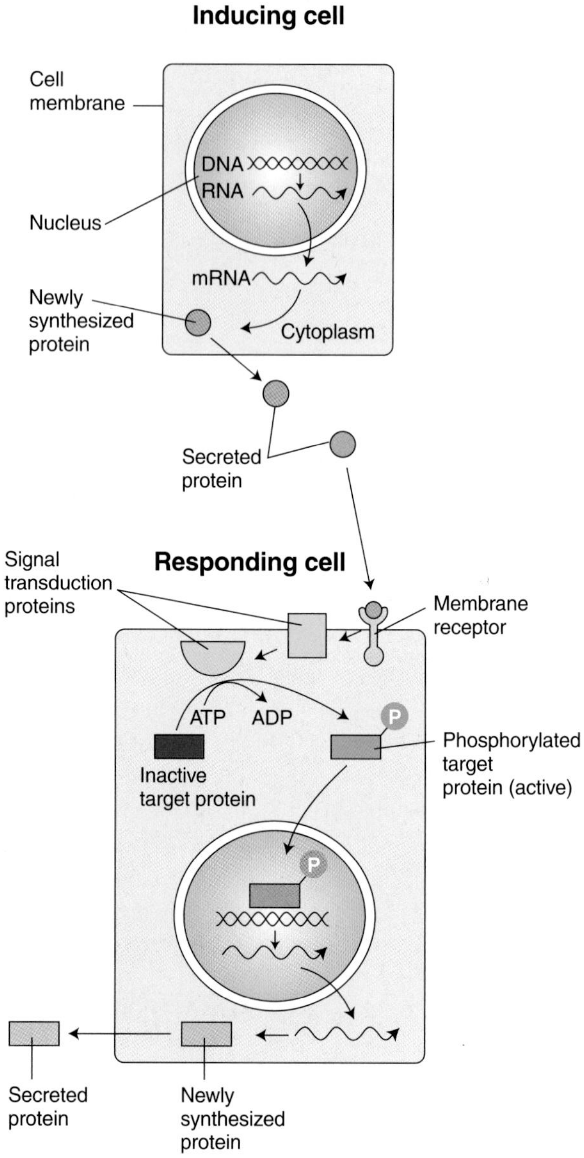

Figure 5-21. A generic cascade of signal transduction. Inducing cells influence their neighbors by secreting small proteins (growth factors) that diffuse to adjacent cells (responding cells) and bind to their membrane receptors. This initiates an intracellular signaling cascade through a series of signal transduction proteins and phosphorylation events. Phosphorylated proteins enter the nucleus, where they alter gene expression, leading to the synthesis of new proteins.

greatly simplified to cover only the key players discussed elsewhere in the textbook. Seven major signaling pathways will be discussed: *Wnt* signaling, *Hedgehog* signaling, *TGFβ* signaling, *Tyrosine kinase* signaling, *Notch* signaling, *Integrin* signaling, and retinoic acid signaling. In addition, the relationships among cell adhesion molecules, *Integrins*, and the cytoskeleton will be briefly discussed. The wide range of developmental processes regulated by signaling pathways is reflected by the wide range of developmental disorders that result from mutations in these pathways. Examples of such disorders are listed below.

***Wnt* signaling**. Vertebrate *Wnts* are orthologs of Drosophila *Wingless*, a segment polarity gene. *Wnts* are secreted by cells into the extracellular milieu and bind to *Wnt* receptors (*Frizzleds;* seven-pass transmembrane receptors) on the surfaces of other cells. In mammals, there are 19 *Wnts* and 10 *Frizzled* receptors.

Binding of a *Wnt* to a *Frizzled* receptor initiates an intracellular signaling cascade involving three pathways: the **canonical *Wnt* pathway**, the planar cell polarity pathway (discussed in Ch. 4), and the calcium-signaling pathway. The canonical pathway is the best studied and will be the only one discussed here (Fig. 5-22); it requires the coreceptor *Lrp5/6* (*LDL receptor-related* proteins 5/6). In the canonical *Wnt* pathway, in the *absence* of *Wnts*, cytoplasmic

β-Catenin (a component of the *Cadherin/Catenin* adhesion complex) interacts with a complex of proteins, including *Axin* (product of the mouse gene *Fused* that regulates axis development), *Apc* (*Adenomatous polyposis coli*), and *Gsk3* (a serine threonine kinase). This interaction results in the proteolysis of *β-Catenin* and no *Wnt* signaling.

However, in the presence of *Wnts* and their binding to a *Frizzled/Lrp5/6* complex, a signal is transduced to Dishevelled (*Dsh*) and *Axin* that prevents degradation of *β-Catenin*. *β-Catenin* accumulates in the cytoplasm and diffuses to the nucleus, where it binds to the transcriptional corepressors *Tcf/Lef*. This binding de-represses the expression of *Wnt*-responsive genes, resulting in new transcription and *Wnt* signaling.

In addition to binding *Frizzled* receptors, *Wnts* can bind to soluble extracellular proteins called *sFrps* (*secreted Frizzled-like proteins*). When they do so, they are no longer able to bind to *Frizzled* receptors. Thus, *sFrps* act as naturally occurring inhibitors of *Wnt* signaling. *Dickkopfs* are other extracellular proteins that antagonize *Wnt* signaling (specifically, the

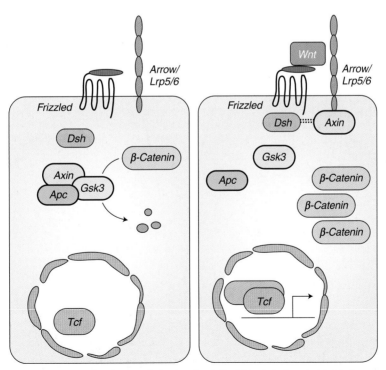

Figure 5-22. Canonical *Wnt* signaling pathway. In the absence of *Wnt* signaling (left), *β-Catenin* is degraded, but in the presence of *Wnt* signaling (right), *β-Catenin* accumulates and enters the nucleus, where in partnership with *Tcf/Lef*, gene expression is altered (i.e., *Wnt* target genes are activated). Arrow in nucleus indicates transcription.

canonical *Wnt* pathway). They do so not by binding *Wnts* but by binding *Lrp5/6*.

Defects in *Wnt* signaling that result in human disorders include cancers (*APC*, *β-CATENIN, AXIN1, -2*), osteoarthritis of the hips (*FRIZZLEDB1*), retinopathy (*FRIZZLED4*), autosomal recessive tetra-amelia (absence of all four limbs; *WNT3*) bone and eye disorders (*LRP5*), and genitourinary anomalies (*WNT4*).

***Hedgehog* signaling**. Three orthologs of the Drosophila *Hedgehog* gene are expressed in mammals: *Sonic hedgehog, Indian hedgehog,* and *Desert hedgehog.* In addition to these three hedgehog genes, zebrafish express two other hedgehog genes called *Echidna hedgehog* and *Tiggywinkle hedgehog. Sonic hedgehog* (*Shh*) signaling is discussed below because of its role in the development of a number of different systems in the vertebrate embryo, and because more is known

about *Shh's* role in signaling during development than is known about any other member of the *hedgehog* family (Fig. 5-23).

Shh is translated as a 45 kDa precursor protein, which is subsequently cleaved in the cytoplasm into a 20 kDa N-terminal signaling domain and a 25 kDa C-terminal catalytic domain. As these domains form, cholesterol binds to the 20 kDa domain, a process important for the subsequent secretion and signaling activity of *Shh* protein. After secretion into the extracellular milieu, the 20 kDa domain binds to a transmembrane receptor called *Patched*. In the absence of *Shh* protein, *Patched* interacts with another transmembrane signaling protein, *Smoothened*, that inhibits *Smoothened* signaling. In the absence of *Shh* signaling this inhibition represses the expression of *Smoothened* target genes. But in the presence of *Shh* protein *Smoothened* is no longer inhibited and an intracellular

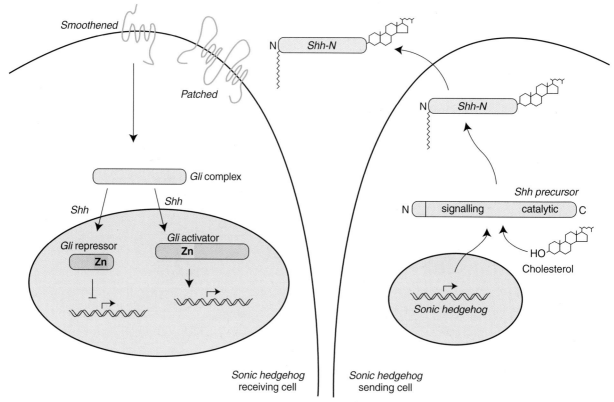

Figure 5-23. *Sonic hedgehog* signaling pathway. The *Sonic hedgehog* sending cell synthesizes a precursor molecule that is cleaved into N- and C-terminal fragment, and Cholesterol is added to the N-terminal fragment. The N-terminal fragment after secretion binds to *Patched* on the *Sonic hedgehog* receiving cell. This binding activates a signaling cascade involving *Smoothened* (which in the absence of the N-terminal fragment binding is inhibited by *Patched*) and a zinc (Zn) containing *Gli* complex. Both *Gli* repressors and activators exist, and their relative amounts control which target genes are expressed in the presence and absence of *Sonic hedgehog* signaling.

signaling cascade is initiated that results in transcriptional activation of target genes. Interestingly, *Smoothened* signaling in mammals involves three proteins (called *Gli* proteins) that function as either transcriptional activators or repressors. These proteins are orthologs of the Drosophila *Ci*, or *Cubitus interruptus* protein. In vertebrates, the combination of *Gli* proteins expressed in a cell as a result of *Shh* signaling determines the fate of that cell.

Defects in *SONIC* signaling that result in human disorders include cancers (*PATCHED*); midline defects, including **holoprosencephaly** (*SHH, GLI2, -3,* and *PATCHED*); **polydactyly** (duplicated digits; *SHH, GLI2, -3,* and *PATCHED*); craniofacial defects and **tracheoesophageal fistula** (*GLI3*); and gonadal dysgenesis (*DESERT HEDGEHOG*).

***Tgfβ* signaling**. The *Tgfβ* superfamily is a large family of proteins that signals through receptors having a cytoplasmic serine/threonine kinase domain. The best-known Drosophila member is the protein *Decapentaplegic*. Many members of this family play important roles in vertebrate development, such as the *Bone morphogenetic proteins* (*Bmps*), *Activin, Vg1,* and *Nodal*. In addition, several inhibitors of *Bmp* signaling are expressed in early development and are involved in important events such as neural induction and establishment of left-right asymmetry, as discussed in Ch. 3. These include *Chordin, Noggin, Follistatin, Lefty,* and *Cerberus*.

Bmp signaling has been studied in detail (Fig. 5-24). A signaling cascade is initiated when a particular *Bmp* (several *Bmps* have been identified) binds within the extracellular milieu to a transmembrane *Bmp* receptor (*Bmpr*). The latter consists of hetero- and homodimers of what are known as Type I and Type II *Tgfβ* receptors. Binding in turn results in phosphorylation of another family of nine proteins called the *Smads* (orthologs of the Drosophila *Mad*, or *Mothers against Decapentalegic*, protein). Phosphorylated *Smads* then enter the nucleus, where they act either as transcriptional coactivators or corepressors. Defects in *Tgfβ* signaling that result in human disorders include cancer and pulmonary hypertension (*BMPR2*) and a wide range of vascular and skeletal disorders (*NOGGIN, TGFβ1, TGFβ RECEPTORS,* and a *TGFβ*-binding protein called *ENDOGLIN*).

***Tyrosine kinase* signaling**. Several families of growth factors bind to receptors that have a cytoplasmic Tyrosine kinase domain. These include the *Fibroblast growth factors* (*Fgfs*), *Epidermal growth factor* (*Egf*), *Insulin-like growth factors* (*Igfs*), *Platelet-derived growth factors* (*Pdgf*), *Hepatocyte Growth Factor/Scatter factor* (*Hgf/Sf*), *Vascular endothelial growth factor* (*Vegf*), and *Ephrins*. In addition, *Steel* (*Stem cell factor*) signals through the Tyrosine kinase c-Kit receptor and functions in the migration of melanoblasts (see Fig. 5-3; discussed in Chs. 4, 7). Because of the complexity of the *Tyrosine kinase* family, only *Fgfs* (Fig. 5-25) and *Ephrins* will be discussed here as examples of growth factors that signal through receptors with a *Tyrosine kinase* domain.

In mammals the *Fgfs* consist of 22 family members (numbered 1 to 23, with species differences in the presence or absence of *Fgf15* and *Fgf19*). *Fgf* ligands bind to *Fgf receptors* (*Fgfrs*), numbered 1 to 4, numbers 1 to 3 of which undergo alternative splicing to each form two isoforms, resulting in a total of seven *Fgfrs*. The presence of *Heparin sulfate proteoglycan* is

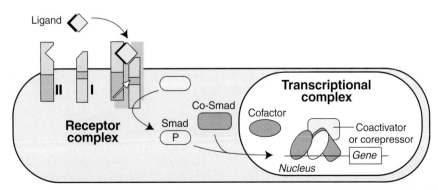

Figure 5-24. *Tgfβ* signaling pathway. Ligand binding activates receptor dimerization and phosphorylation of *Smads*. Phosphylated *Smads*, along with *Co-Smads*, translocate to the nucleus to alter target gene expression.

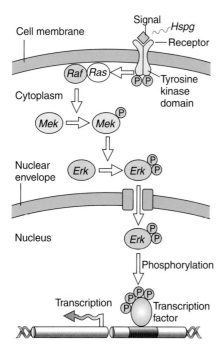

Figure 5-25. *Fgf* signaling pathway. *Fgfs* bind to *Fgf receptors* aided by presentation of the ligand by *Heparin sulfate proteoglycan (Hspg)*. This activates *Ras* as well as a phosphylation cascade that sequentially phosphylates *Raf*, *Mek*, and *Erk*. Phosphylated *Erk* translocates to the nucleus, where it regulates target gene expression.

required for presentation of the ligand to the receptor and subsequent binding. Binding induces hetero- or homodimerization of the receptor and activation of the small GTPase *Ras*. Binding also initiates a phosphorylation cascade, known as an *Erk/Mapk* (*Extracellular signal–regulated kinase/Mitogen–activated protein kinase*) cascade, in which three kinases are sequentially phosphorylated: *Mapk kinase kinase* (*Mapkkk*—also called *Raf*); *Mapk kinase* (*Mapkk*—also called *Mek*); and *Map kinase* (also called *Erk*). Phosphylated *Erk* translocates to the nucleus to phosphorylate and activates transcription factors, thereby regulating cell survival, growth, and differentiation. *Fgf* signaling induces the expression of *Sprouty* (at least four family members in mammals), an intracellular inhibitor of *Fgf* signaling that establishes a regulatory feedback loop limiting the amount of *Fgf* signaling.

Defects in *Fgf* signaling result in disorders in humans that affect the skeletal system particularly and involve mutations in three of the four *FGF RECEPTORS*. Some of the more frequent mutations include **Pfeiffer syndrome** (*FGFR1* or *FGFR2*

mutation; results in craniosynostosis with limb defects), **Apert syndrome** (*FGFR2* mutation; results in **craniosynostosis** and severe fusion of digits—**syndactyly**), **Crouzon syndrome** (*FGFR2* mutation; results in **craniosynostosis** without limb defects), **Thanatophoric dysplasia** (*FGFR3* mutation; results in severe skeletal dysplasia and is usually lethal at birth), and achondroplasia (*FGFR3* mutation; results in **dwarfism**).

Ephrins are a family of proteins that bind to the so-called *Eph* receptors. The "Eph" name is derived from the cell line from which the first member of the family was isolated—the erythropoietin-producing human hepatocellular carcinoma line. The "Ephrin" name is derived from Eph family receptor interacting proteins. Both *Ephrins* and *Eph* receptors are classified into A and B subgroups consisting of *Ephrins A1* to *A5, B1* to *B3*, and *Ephs A1* to *A8, B1* to *B6*. Both the type A and B *Eph* receptors consist of an extracellular ligand-binding domain, a transmembrane domain, and an intracellular *Tyrosine kinase* domain. Thus, they are similar to other *Tyrosine kinase* receptors. However, the *Ephrin* ligands that bind to these receptors differ from other ligands that bind to *Tyrosine kinase* receptors, such as the *Fgfs*, in that instead of being secreted into the extracellular milieu, they remain bound to the cell surface that produces them. Type A *Ephrins* are attached to the cell surface by a GPI (glycosylphosphatidylinositol) link, whereas type B *Ephrins* span the cell membrane. Thus, signaling occurs only between immediately adjacent cells.

Another important difference with *Ephrin* signaling is that it occurs bidirectionally. That is, binding of the ligand to the receptor not only results in a signaling cascade within the cell containing the *Eph* receptor, but also signaling is activated upon binding to the *Eph* receptor in the cell containing the *Ephrin*.

One human disorder that results from defects in *EPHRIN* signaling is **craniofrontonasal dysplasia syndrome**. This syndrome involves a mutation in *EPHRIN-B1*. Although this mutation affects the development of bones in the skull and face, multiple other defects occur such as umbilical hernia; genitourinary anomalies; skin, nail, and hair anomalies; and developmental delay.

Notch signaling. Like *Ephrin* signaling, *Notch* signaling can occur only between closely associated cells (Fig. 5-26). *Notch* proteins (numbered 1 to 4 in mammals) consist of transmembrane receptors containing an extracellular domain with *Egf-like* repeats for ligand binding and an intracellular domain rich with *Ankyrin*

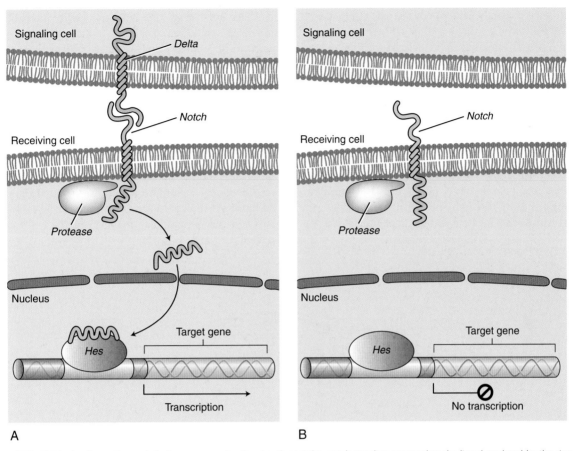

Figure 5-26. *Notch* signaling pathway. *A,* In the presence of a ligand such as *Delta, Notch* signaling occurs when the ligand produced by the signaling cell binds to a *Notch* receptor on an adjacent cell. Binding activates a protease that cleaves off a portion of the *Notch* receptor, which in turn translocates to the nucleus, where it regulates target gene expression in partnership with *Hes. B,* In the absence of a ligand such as *Delta, Notch* signaling does not occur and target genes are not regulated.

repeats for intracellular signaling. Ligands for *Notch* receptors, like the *Ephrins,* are not secreted into the extracellular milieu; rather, they consist of transmembrane proteins of the DSL family of proteins, named for the ligands *Delta* and *Serrate* from Drosophila (consisting of multiple *Delta* and *Jagged* genes in vertebrates), and *Lag2* from *C. elegans.* Although these ligands are transmembrane proteins, their extracellular domain can be cleaved by proteases (such as the protease *Kuzbanian*), allowing diffusion to adjacent cells.

Notch signaling is regulated extracellularly through actions that modify *Notch* and its ligands. In mammals, three *Glycosyltransferases* with whimsical names regulate *Notch* signaling: *Lunatic fringe, Manic fringe,* and *Radical fringe.*

Binding of *Delta* or *Jagged/Serrate* ligands to *Notch* receptors initiates *Notch* signaling. Through proteolysis, the intracellular domain of *Notch* is cleaved and migrates to the nucleus, where it interacts with *Hes* proteins (orthologs of Drosophila *Hairy* and *Enhancer of split* proteins) and/or *Hes-related* proteins (*Hesr*). This complex regulates the expression of basic helix-loop-helix (bHLH) transcriptional repressors.

One human disorder that results from defects in *NOTCH* signaling is **Alagille syndrome** (also called **arteriohepatic dysplasia**). This syndrome, caused by mutation of the *JAGGED1* or *NOTCH2* genes, affects the skeletal, cardiovascular, and gastrointestinal systems (Alagille syndrome is also mentioned in Chs. 3 and 12 to 14). Another human skeletal disorder associated with defective *NOTCH* signaling is **spondylocostal dysostosis** (*DELTA-3, LUNATIC FRINGE*; discussed in Ch. 8). Mutations in the *NOTCH* signaling are associated with the development of cancer; namely, a *NOTCH1* mutation is the cause of more than 50% of the cases of T-cell acute lymphoblastic leukemia.

Integrin **signaling.** Spaces between tissue layers and between cells within tissue layers are filled with a rich extracellular matrix. This matrix consists of a number of proteins. Epithelia are lined by basement membranes. These consist largely of *Collagens* (especially *type IV*), *Laminin*, and *Fibronectin*. A number of large complex proteoglycans are more broadly distributed within and across tissue spaces. These include *Syndecan*, *Perlecan*, *Heparan sulfate*, and *Chondroitin sulfate*.

Cells adhere to one another using intercellular junctions, such as gap and tight junctions, and calcium-dependent and calcium-independent **cell adhesion molecules.** The calcium-dependent adhesion molecules consist of the *Cadherins*, such as *N-Cadherin (Neural Cadherin)*, *E-Cadherin (Epithelial Cadherin)*, and *P-Cadherin (Placental Cadherin)*. The calcium-independent adhesion molecules consist of the *CAMs*—e.g., *N-Cam (Neural-Cell adhesion molecule)*; *V-Cam (Vascular-Cell adhesion molecule)*; and *Pe-Cam (Platelet-endothelial–Cell adhesion molecule)*. Cells also adhere to their matrix. This adhesion involves *Integrins*, which provide a link between the extracellular matrix and the cells' cytoskeletal network.

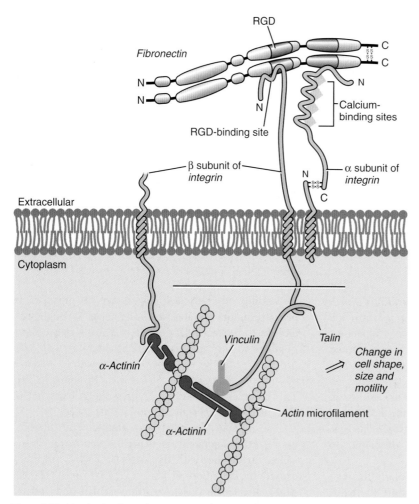

Figure 5-27. *Integrin* signaling pathway. *Integrins* form critical transmembrane links between extracellular matrix molecules such as *Fibronectin* and the intracellular *Actin* cytoskeleton (microfilaments). RGD, argine-glycine-asparate.

The *Integrins* consist of noncovalently linked heterodimers of alpha and beta transmembrane subunits (Fig. 5-27). At least 15 alpha subunits and 8 beta subunits exist, but all combinations of the 23 subunits apparently do not exist. Collectively, the two heterodimers of each *Integrin* form a binding domain for ligands contained in basement membrane molecules such as *Laminin* or *Fibronectin*. One such domain is the RGD sequence (arginine-glycine-aspartate). Upon binding of this domain to its ligand, signaling is transduced to cytoplasmic **microfilaments** via linker proteins such as *alpha-Actinin*, *Vinculin*, and *Talin*. This signaling leads to cytoskeletal rearrangements that in turn lead to changes in cell shape, size, and motility.

Defects in *Integrin* signaling result in human disorders that affect skin and connective tissues. These include **epidermolysis bullosa** (blistering skin) with **pyloric atresia** (*INTEGRINß4*) and cancers of the gut, breast, and female reproductive organs.

Retinoic acid signaling. Retinoic acid is a powerful regulator of early development that is believed to act in a concentration-dependent manner to determine cell fate. Because it diffuses through the extracellular milieu, with its concentration decreasing with distance from its tissue of synthesis, a concentration gradient can form across an early organ rudiment such as the limb bud. This gradient is believed to provide **positional information** to cells, establishing different cell fates in different areas of an organ rudiment. Thus, retinoic acid is considered to be a **morphogen**—a diffusible substance that determines cell fate during development in a concentration-dependent manner.

Retinoic acid is derived from Vitamin A (retinol). Retinol passes through the cell membrane from the extracellular milieu and binds to cytoplasmic-binding proteins called the *Cellular retinol-binding proteins (CRBPs)* (Fig. 5-28). Within the cytoplasm, retinol is enzymatically converted (by *Retinol dehydrogenases)* to retinal and then to retinoic acid (by *Retinaldehyde dehydrogenases)*. Retinoic acid quickly binds to other binding proteins in the cytoplasm, the *Cellular retinoic acid-binding proteins (Crabps)*. Retinoic acid is then released from the *Crabps* and enters the nucleus, where it binds to the *Retinoic acid receptors (RARs)*. These receptors are related to the steroid and thyroid

5

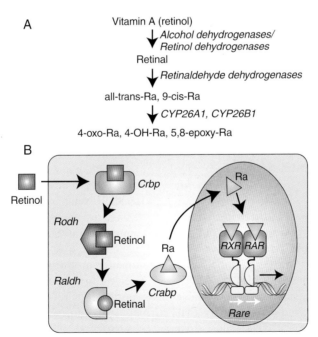

Figure 5-28. Retinoic acid (Ra) signaling pathway. *A*, Vitamin A or Retinol undergoes metabolism to its biologically active form, Retinoic acid (all-trans). This metabolism is mediated by a series of enzymes such as *Retinol dehydrogenase (Rodh)* and *Retinaldehyde dehydrogenase (Raldh)*. *B*, Retinol is transported during its metabolism in the cytoplasm by a binding protein, *Crbp*. Retinoic acid is transported to the nucleus by another binding protein *Crabp*, where it binds to receptors (*RXR* and *RAR*). This results in activation of *Retinoic acid response elements (Rare)* and regulation of target gene expression.

hormone receptors. A second group of receptors, the *Retinoid X receptors (RXRs)*, is less understood. Both the *RARs* and *RXRs* exist as three isoforms: the alpha, beta, and gamma isoforms.

RARs, like the steroid and thyroid hormone receptors, are ligand-dependent transcription factors. Upon ligand binding in the nucleus, *RARs* bind to a *Retinoic acid response element (Rare)* within gene promoters, thereby regulating the expression of target genes. Several hundred genes are known to be regulated by Retinoic acid signaling.

Retinoic acid signaling can be perturbed in humans by environmental and pharmacologic agents. **Accutane**, a drug taken orally for treatment of severe acne, causes both craniofacial and limb anomalies in offspring when used by mothers during pregnancy.

Embryonic Stem Cells and Cloning

Techniques discussed earlier in this chapter to manipulate and study mouse development have been modified for use in humans, particularly for overcoming reproductive problems. As discussed in Chapter 1, human eggs and sperm are now routinely manipulated during in vitro fertilization. Other techniques used in mouse can also be modified for use in humans. For example, **mouse embryonic stem cells** (called **ES cells**), derived from the inner cell mass of the mouse blastocyst, can be grown and then transplanted into tissues (such as the pancreas of diabetic mice) or manipulated genetically to form transgenic animals. Similarly, human ES cells can be derived from the inner cell mass of the human blastocyst. Such cells are potentially valuable for replacing tissues in people suffering from various diseases such as heart disease, juvenile diabetes, Alzheimer's, and Parkinson's disease, as well as from spinal cord injuries and resulting paralysis. Although proven to be at least partially effective in animal models, the potential value of human ES cells has not been determined. By definition, **stem cells** are cells that can self-renew under appropriate conditions and produce daughters that can differentiate into multiple cell types. Thus, stem cells are **totipotent** (i.e., capable of forming all cell types) or **pluripotent** (i.e., capable of forming many but not all cell types). One example of an adult stem cell (from the bulge of the hair follicle) is discussed in the first "In the Research Lab" section of Chapter 10.

Many articles are published each year in the general press regarding the "cloning of humans." Two types of cloning are distinguished: **therapeutic cloning** and **reproductive cloning**. Cloning, which has been accomplished in several plant and animal species, refers to the production of one or more individual organisms that are genetically identical to the original organism (genes can also be cloned). Both therapeutic and reproductive cloning use an unfertilized egg of the species of choice (say a mouse) and involve the process of **somatic cell nuclear transfer**. In this process, the female pronucleus is removed from the egg (usually by using a suction pipette) and then replaced with a diploid nucleus obtained from a donor cell obtained from an adult animal. In some cases such eggs go on to develop blastocysts. In *therapeutic* cloning, ES cells are derived from the inner cell mass of such a blastocyst and then transplanted into a tissue of the donor adult to replace a defective cell type (such as beta cells of the pancreatic islets in a diabetic mouse). Because the nucleus used for somatic cell nuclear transfer was obtained from the same animal that receives the ES cells, both the cells and the animal are genetically identical, eliminating the problem of tissue rejection.

In contrast, in *reproductive* cloning, in which the blastocyst is used to make ES cells, the blastocyst is transplanted into the uterus of the *donor* animal (thus, only female donors can be used). If normal embryogenesis then ensues, a **clone** will be delivered, that is, an offspring genetically identical to its mother. The most famous clone to date is the sheep **Dolly**, born in 1995.

Cloning of humans is a highly controversial topic. In the United States under the current administration at the time of this writing, human therapeutic cloning can be attempted only in private institutions that do not receive funding from the National Institutes of Health. Human reproductive cloning has been condemned by the worldwide biomedical and scientific community as ethically unacceptable. However, the public-at-large is fascinated with the possibility of human reproductive cloning, based on the publicity received by a couple of completely undocumented reports of reproductive cloning in humans and the popularity of fictional novels based on this scenario.

Suggested Readings

Anderson KV. 2000. Finding the genes that direct mammalian development: ENU mutagenesis in the mouse. Trends Genet 16:99-102.

Anderson KV, Ingham PW. 2003. The transformation of the model organism: a decade of developmental genetics. Nat Genet 33 Suppl:285-293.

Arnaout MA, Goodman SL, Xiong JP. 2002. Coming to grips with integrin binding to ligands. Curr Opin Cell Biol 14:641-651.

Arnaout MA, Mahalingam B, Xiong JP. 2005. Integrin structure, allostery, and bidirectional signaling. Annu Rev Cell Dev Biol 21:381-410.

Attisano L, Wrana JL. 2000. Smads as transcriptional co-modulators. Curr Opin Cell Biol 12:235-243.

Bahls C, Weitzman J, Gallagher R. 2003. Model Organisms. The Scientist 17 (Suppl 1):1-40.

Balda MS, Matter K. 2003. Epithelial cell adhesion and the regulation of gene expression. Trends Cell Biol 13:310-318.

Bale AE. 2002. Hedgehog signaling and human disease. Annu Rev Genomics Hum Genet 3:47-65.

Balemans W, Van Hul W. 2002. Extracellular regulation of BMP signaling in vertebrates: a cocktail of modulators. Dev Biol 250:231-250.

Beachy PA, Karhadkar SS, Berman DM. 2004. Tissue repair and stem cell renewal in carcinogenesis. Nature 432:324-331.

Bejsovec A. 2005. Wnt pathway activation: new relations and locations. Cell 120:11-14.

Betsholtz C. 2003. Biology of platelet-derived growth factors in development. Birth Defects Res C Embryo Today 69:272-285.

Betsholtz C, Karlsson L, Lindahl P. 2001. Developmental roles of platelet-derived growth factors. Bioessays 23:494-507.

Bhalla US. 2004. Models of cell signaling pathways. Curr Opin Genet Dev 14:375-381.

Biesecker LG. 2005. Mapping phenotypes to language: a proposal to organize and standardize the clinical descriptions of malformations. Clin Genet 68:320-326.

Bijlsma MF, Spek CA, Peppelenbosch MP. 2004. Hedgehog: an unusual signal transducer. Bioessays 26:387-394.

Blobel CP. 2005. ADAMs: key components in EGFR signalling and development. Nat Rev Mol Cell Biol 6:32-43.

Bogdan S, Klambt C. 2001. Epidermal growth factor receptor signaling. Curr Biol 11:R292-R295.

Bokel C, Brown NH. 2002. Integrins in development: moving on, responding to, and sticking to the extracellular matrix. Dev Cell 3:311-321.

Bornstein P, Sage EH. 2002. Matricellular proteins: extracellular modulators of cell function. Curr Opin Cell Biol 14:608-616.

Braga VM. 2002. Cell-cell adhesion and signalling. Curr Opin Cell Biol 14:546-556.

Bray S. 2000. Notch. Curr Biol 10:R433-R435.

Brembeck FH, Rosario M, Birchmeier W. 2006. Balancing cell adhesion and Wnt signaling, the key role of beta-catenin. Curr Opin Genet Dev 16:51-59.

Brown EJ. 2002. Integrin-associated proteins. Curr Opin Cell Biol 14:603-607.

Caestecker M. 2004. The transforming growth factor-beta superfamily of receptors. Cytokine Growth Factor Rev 15:1-11.

Capecchi MR. 2000. Choose your target. Nat Genet 26:159-161.

Carpenter G. 2000. The EGF receptor: a nexus for trafficking and signaling. Bioessays 22:697-707.

Chang L, Karin M. 2001. Mammalian MAP kinase signalling cascades. Nature 410:37-40.

Cibelli JB, Lanza RP, West MD, Ezzell C. 2002. The first human cloned embryo. Sci Am 286:44-51.

Cooper MK, Wassif CA, Krakowiak PA, et al. 2003. A defective response to Hedgehog signaling in disorders of cholesterol biosynthesis. Nat Genet 33:508-513.

Corbit KC, Aanstad P, Singla V, et al. 2005. Vertebrate Smoothened functions at the primary cilium. Nature 437:1018-1021.

Couchman JR. 2003. Syndecans: proteoglycan regulators of cell-surface microdomains?. Nat Rev Mol Cell Biol 4:926-937.

Coumoul X, Deng CX. 2003. Roles of FGF receptors in mammalian development and congenital diseases. Birth Defects Res C Embryo Today 69:286-304.

Cowan CA, Henkemeyer M. 2002. Ephrins in reverse, park and drive. Trends Cell Biol 12:339-346.

Cutforth T, Harrison CJ. 2002. Ephs and ephrins close ranks. Trends Neurosci 25:332-334.

Czirok A, Zamir EA, Filla MB, et al. 2006. Extracellular matrix macroassembly dynamics in early vertebrate embryos. Curr Top Dev Biol 73:237-258.

Damsky CH, Ilic D. 2002. Integrin signaling: it's where the action is. Curr Opin Cell Biol 14:594-602.

Danen EH, Sonnenberg A. 2003. Integrins in regulation of tissue development and function. J Pathol 200:471-480.

Davis RJ. 2000. Signal transduction by the JNK group of MAP kinases. Cell 103:239-252.

Davy A, Soriano P. 2005. Ephrin signaling in vivo: look both ways. Dev Dyn 232:1-10.

DeArcangelis A, Georges-Labouesse E. 2000. Integrin and ECM functions: roles in vertebrate development. Trends Genet 16:389-395.

Derynck R, Zhang YE. 2003. Smad-dependent and Smad-independent pathways in TGF-beta family signalling. Nature 425:577-584.

Drescher U. 2002. Eph family functions from an evolutionary perspective. Curr Opin Genet Dev 12:397-402.

Duester G. 2000. Families of retinoid dehydrogenases regulating vitamin A function: production of visual pigment and retinoic acid. Eur J Biochem 267:4315-4324.

Dupont J, Holzenberger M. 2003. Biology of insulin-like growth factors in development. Birth Defects Res C Embryo Today 69:257-271.

Eswarakumar VP, Lax I, Schlessinger J. 2005. Cellular signaling by fibroblast growth factor receptors. Cytokine Growth Factor Rev 16:139-149.

Feng XH, Derynck R. 2005. Specificity and versatility in tgf-beta signaling through Smads. Annu Rev Cell Dev Biol 21:659-693.

ffrench-Constant C, Colognato H. 2004. Integrins: versatile integrators of extracellular signals. Trends Cell Biol 14:678-686.

Fukata M, Kaibuchi K. 2001. Rho-family GTPases in cadherin-mediated cell-cell adhesion. Nat Rev Mol Cell Biol 2:887-897.

Geiger B, Bershadsky A, Pankov R, Yamada KM. 2001. Transmembrane crosstalk between the extracellular matrix—cytoskeleton crosstalk. Nat Rev Mol Cell Biol 2:793-805.

Germino GG. 2005. Linking cilia to Wnts. Nat Genet 37:455-457.

Ginsberg MH, Partridge A, Shattil SJ. 2005. Integrin regulation. Curr Opin Cell Biol 17:509-516.

Glass DAII, Karsenty G. 2006. Molecular bases of the regulation of bone remodeling by the canonical Wnt signaling pathway. Curr Top Dev Biol 73:43-84.

Goetz JA, Suber LM, Zeng X, Robbins DJ. 2002. Sonic Hedgehog as a mediator of long-range signaling. Bioessays 24:157-165.

Gooding JM, Yap KL, Ikura M. 2004. The cadherin-catenin complex as a focal point of cell adhesion and signalling: new insights from three-dimensional structures. Bioessays 26:497-511.

Gumbiner BM. 2005. Regulation of cadherin-mediated adhesion in morphogenesis. Nat Rev Mol Cell Biol 6:622-634.

5

Guo W, Giancotti FG. 2004. Integrin signalling during tumour progression. Nat Rev Mol Cell Biol 5:816-826.

Hacker U, Nybakken K, Perrimon N. 2005. Heparan sulphate proteoglycans: the sweet side of development. Nat Rev Mol Cell Biol 6:530-541.

Haines N, Irvine KD. 2003. Glycosylation regulates Notch signalling. Nat Rev Mol Cell Biol 4:786-797.

He X. 2003. A Wnt-Wnt situation. Dev Cell 4:791-797.

He X, Semenov M, Tamai K, Zeng X. 2004. LDL receptor-related proteins 5 and 6 in Wnt/beta-catenin signaling: arrows point the way. Development 131:1663-1677.

Henig RM. 2003. Pandora. Sci Am 288:62-67.

Henkemeyer M, Frisen J. 2001. Eph receptors tingle the spine. Neuron 31:876-877.

Himanen JP, Nikolov DB. 2003. Eph signaling: a structural view. Trends Neurosci 26:46-51.

Hoch RV, Soriano P. 2003. Roles of PDGF in animal development. Development 130:4769-4784.

Holmberg J, Frisen J. 2002. Ephrins are not only unattractive. Trends Neurosci 25:239-243.

Hood JD, Cheresh DA. 2002. Role of integrins in cell invasion and migration. Nat Rev Cancer 2:91-100.

Hooper JE, Scott MP. 2005. Communicating with Hedgehogs. Nat Rev Mol Cell Biol 6:306-317.

Imondi R, Thomas JB. 2003. Neuroscience. The ups and downs of Wnt signaling. Science 302:1903-1904.

Ingham PW, Placzek M. 2006. Orchestrating ontogenesis: variations on a theme by sonic hedgehog. Nat Rev Genet 7:841-850.

Iozzo RV. 2005. Basement membrane proteoglycans: from cellar to ceiling. Nat Rev Mol Cell Biol 6:646-656.

Janssens K, ten Dijke, P Janssens, et al. 2005. Transforming growth factor-beta1 to the bone. Endocr Rev 26:743-774.

Jones WM, Bejsovec A. 2003. Wingless signaling: an axin to grind. Curr Biol 13:R479-R481.

Jorde LB, Carey JC, Bamshad MJ, White RL. 2006. Medical Genetics 3rd edition. St. Louis: Mosby.

Juliano RL, Dixit VR, Kang H, et al. 2005. Epigenetic manipulation of gene expression: a toolkit for cell biologists. J Cell Biol 169:847-857.

Justice NJ, Jan YN. 2002. Variations on the Notch pathway in neural development. Curr Opin Neurobiol 12:64-70.

Kadesch T. 2000. Notch signaling: a dance of proteins changing partners. Exp Cell Res 260:1-8.

Kalb C, Rosenberg D. 2004. Stem cell division. Newsweek 144:42-47.

Kalderon D. 2002. Similarities between the Hedgehog and Wnt signaling pathways. Trends Cell Biol 12:523-531.

Keller G. 2005. Embryonic stem cell differentiation: emergence of a new era in biology and medicine. Genes Dev 19:1129-1155.

Kim HJ, Bar-Sagi D. 2004. Modulation of signalling by Sprouty: a developing story. Nat Rev Mol Cell Biol 5:441-450.

Kinbara K, Goldfinger LE, Hansen M, et al. 2003. Ras GTPases: integrins' friends or foes? Nat Rev Mol Cell Biol 4:767-776.

Klambt C. 2000. EGF receptor signalling: the importance of presentation. Curr Biol 10:R388-R391.

Klein R. 2001. Excitatory Eph receptors and adhesive ephrin ligands. Curr Opin Cell Biol 13:196-203.

Knoll B, Drescher U. 2002. Ephrin-As as receptors in topographic projections. Trends Neurosci 25:145-149.

Kramer KL, Yost HJ. 2003. Heparan sulfate core proteins in cell-cell signaling. Annu Rev Genet 37:461-484.

Kullander K, Klein R. 2002. Mechanisms and functions of Eph and ephrin signalling. Nat Rev Mol Cell Biol 3:475-486.

Larsen M, Tremblay ML, Yamada KM. 2003. Phosphatases in cell-matrix adhesion and migration. Nat Rev Mol Cell Biol 4:700-711.

Lewandoski M. 2001. Conditional control of gene expression in the mouse. Nat Rev Genet 2:743-755.

Lin X. 2004. Functions of heparan sulfate proteoglycans in cell signaling during development. Development 131:6009-6021.

Logan CY, Nusse R. 2004. The Wnt signaling pathway in development and disease. Annu Rev Cell Dev Biol 20:781-810.

Lonai P. 2005. Fibroblast growth factor signaling and the function and assembly of basement membranes. Curr Top Dev Biol 66:37-64.

Louvi A, Artavanis-Tsakonas S. 2006. Notch signalling in vertebrate neural development. Nat Rev Neurosci 7:93-102.

Maden M. 2002. Retinoid signalling in the development of the central nervous system. Nat Rev Neurosci 3:843-853.

Mason I. 2003. Fibroblast growth factors. Curr Biol 13:R346.

Massague J. 2000. How cells read TGF-beta signals. Nat Rev Mol Cell Biol 1:169-178.

Massague J, Chen YG. 2000. Controlling TGF-beta signaling. Genes Dev 14:627-644.

McLaren A. 2000. Cloning: pathways to a pluripotent future. Science 288:1775-1780.

McMahon AP, Ingham PW, Tabin CJ. 2003. Developmental roles and clinical significance of hedgehog signaling. Curr Top Dev Biol 53:1-114.

Miner JH, Yurchenco PD. 2004. Laminin functions in tissue morphogenesis. Annu Rev Cell Dev Biol 20:255-284.

Minucci S, Ozato K. 1996. Retinoid receptors in transcriptional regulation. Curr Opin Genet Dev 6:567-574.

Moon RT, Kohn AD, De Ferrari GV, Kaykas A. 2004. WNT and beta-catenin signalling: diseases and therapies. Nat Rev Genet 5:691-701.

Mullor JL, Sanchez P, Altaba AR. 2002. Pathways and consequences: Hedgehog signaling in human disease. Trends Cell Biol 12:562-569.

Nagy A, Gertsenstein M, Vintersten K, Behringer R. 2003. Manipulating the Mouse Embryo A Laboratory Manual. New York: Cold Spring Harbor.

Nelson WJ, Nusse R. 2004. Convergence of Wnt, beta-catenin, and cadherin pathways. Science 303:1483-1487.

Nusse R. 2003. Wnts and Hedgehogs: lipid-modified proteins and similarities in signaling mechanisms at the cell surface. Development 130:5297-5305.

Nusse R. 2005. Cell biology: relays at the membrane. Nature 438:747-749.

Nusse R. 2006. The Wnt homepage. http://www.stanford.edu/~rnusse/wntwindow.html..

Nybakken K, Perrimon N. 2002. Hedgehog signal transduction: recent findings. Curr Opin Genet Dev 12:503-511.

Ornitz DM. 2000. FGFs, heparan sulfate and FGFRs: complex interactions essential for development. Bioessays 22:108-112.

Ornitz DM, Itoh N. 2001. Fibroblast growth factors. Genome Biol 2:REVIEWS3005.

Palmer A, Klein R. 2003. Multiple roles of ephrins in morphogenesis, neuronal networking, and brain function. Genes Dev 17:1429-1450.

Panakova D, Sprong H, Marois E, Thiele C, Eaton S. 2005. Lipoprotein particles are required for Hedgehog and Wingless signalling. Nature 435:58-65.

Pasquale EB. 2005. Eph receptor signalling casts a wide net on cell behaviour. Nat Rev Mol Cell Biol 6:462-475.

Popovici C, Roubin R, Coulier F, Birnbaum D. 2005. An evolutionary history of the FGF superfamily. Bioessays 27:849-857.

Povelones M, Nusse R. 2002. Wnt signalling sees spots. Nat Cell Biol 4:E249-E250.

Raymond CS, Soriano P. 2006. Engineering mutations: Deconstructing the mouse gene by gene. Dev Dyn 235:2424-2436.

Reya T, Clevers H. 2005. Wnt signalling in stem cells and cancer. Nature 434:843-850.

Schier AF. 2003. Nodal signaling in vertebrate development. Annu Rev Cell Dev Biol 19:589-621.

Schoenwolf GC. 2001. Cutting, pasting and painting: experimental embryology and neural development. Nat Rev Neurosci 2: 763-771.

Seto ES, Bellen HJ. 2004. The ins and outs of Wingless signaling. Trends Cell Biol 14:45-53.

Sewell W, Kusumi K. 2007. Genetic analysis of molecular oscillators in mammalian somitogenesis: clues for studies of human vertebral disorders. Birth Defects Res C Embryo Today 81:111-120.

Shi Y. 2001. Structural insights on Smad function in TGFbeta signaling. Bioessays 23:223-232.

Shi Y, Massague J. 2003. Mechanisms of TGF-beta signaling from cell membrane to the nucleus. Cell 113:685-700.

Shifley ET, Cole SE. 2007. The vertebrate segmentation clock and its role in skeletal birth defects. Birth Defects Res C Embryo Today 81:121-133.

Smith AG. 2001. Embryo-derived stem cells: of mice and men. Annu Rev Cell Dev Biol 17:435-462.

Souchelnytskyi S, Moustakas A, Heldin CH. 2002. TGF-beta signaling from a three-dimensional perspective: insight into selection of partners. Trends Cell Biol 12:304-307.

Spagnoli FM, Hemmati-Brivanlou A. 2006. Guiding embryonic stem cells towards differentiation: lessons from molecular embryology. Curr Opin Genet Dev 16:469-475.

Sparrow DB, Chapman G, Turnpenny PD, Dunwoodie SL. 2007. Disruption of the somitic molecular clock causes abnormal vertebral segmentation. Birth Defects Res C Embryo Today 81:93-110.

Strutt D. 2003. Frizzled signalling and cell polarisation in Drosophila and vertebrates. Development 130:4501-4513.

Talbot WS, Hopkins N. 2000. Zebrafish mutations and functional analysis of the vertebrate genome. Genes Dev 14:755-762.

Tam PP, Rossant J. 2003. Mouse embryonic chimeras: tools for studying mammalian development. Development 130:6155-6163.

Taniguchi CM, Emanuelli B, Kahn CR. 2006. Critical nodes in signalling pathways: insights into insulin action. Nat Rev Mol Cell Biol 7:85-96.

Tepass U, Truong K, Godt D, et al. 2000. Cadherins in embryonic and neural morphogenesis. Nat Rev Mol Cell Biol 1:91-100.

Thiery JP. 2003. Cell adhesion in development: a complex signaling network. Curr Opin Genet Dev 13:365-371.

Timpl R, Sasaki T, Kostka G, Chu ML. 2003. Fibulins: a versatile family of extracellular matrix proteins. Nat Rev Mol Cell Biol 4:479-489.

Tolwinski NS, Wieschaus E. 2004. Rethinking WNT signaling. Trends Genet 20:177-181.

Tomari Y, Zamore PD. 2005. Perspective: machines for RNAi. Genes Dev 19:517-529.

Turnbull J, Powell A, Guimond S. 2001. Heparan sulfate: decoding a dynamic multifunctional cell regulator. Trends Cell Biol 11:75-82.

van Es JH, Barker N, Clevers H. 2003. You Wnt some, you lose some: oncogenes in the Wnt signaling pathway. Curr Opin Genet Dev 13:28-33.

Vats A, Bielby RC, Tolley NS, Nerem R, Polak JM. 2005. Stem cells. Lancet 366:592-602.

Veeman MT, Axelrod JD, Moon RT. 2003. A second canon. Functions and mechanisms of beta-catenin-independent Wnt signaling. Dev Cell 5:367-377.

von Bubnoff A, Cho KW. 2001. Intracellular BMP signaling regulation in vertebrates: pathway or network? Dev Biol 239:1-14.

Wang HY, Malbon CC. 2003. Wnt signaling, Ca2+, and cyclic GMP: visualizing Frizzled functions. Science 300:1529-1530.

Wedlich D. 2002. The polarising role of cell adhesion molecules in early development. Curr Opin Cell Biol 14:563-568.

Weitzman JB. 2000. Quick guide. Jnk. Curr Biol 10:R290.

Weston CR, Lambright DG, Davis RJ. 2002. Signal transduction. MAP kinase signaling specificity. Science 296:2345-2347.

Wheelock MJ, Johnson KR. 2003. Cadherins as modulators of cellular phenotype. Annu Rev Cell Dev Biol 19:207-235.

White MF. 2003. Insulin signaling in health and disease. Science 302:1710-1711.

Whitman M. 2001. Nodal signaling in early vertebrate embryos: themes and variations. Dev Cell 1:605-617.

Wight TN. 2002. Versican: a versatile extracellular matrix proteoglycan in cell biology. Curr Opin Cell Biol 14:617-623.

Wolpert L. 2002. Principles of Development. New York: Oxford University Press.

Wrana JL. 2000. Regulation of Smad activity. Cell 100:189-192.

Xia Y, Karin M. 2004. The control of cell motility and epithelial morphogenesis by Jun kinases. Trends Cell Biol 14:94-101.

Yagi T, Takeichi M. 2000. Cadherin superfamily genes: functions, genomic organization, and neurologic diversity. Genes Dev 14: 1169-1180.

Fetal Development and the Fetus as Patient

6

Summary   The gestation period of humans from fertilization to birth is usually 266 days, or 38 weeks. As discussed in the Introduction, the **embryonic period**, during which most of the major organ systems are formed, ends at the end of the 8th week of gestation. The remainder of gestation constitutes the **fetal period**, which is devoted mainly to the maturation of organ systems and to growth. For convenience, the 9-month gestation period is divided into three 3-month **trimesters**. It is not yet possible to keep alive fetuses born before 22 weeks. Fetuses born between 22 to 28 weeks have progressively increasing survival rates (from about 15% at 22 weeks to 90% at 28 weeks), but up to one third of these have significant morbidity that affects their long-term survival.

Both the embryo during weeks 3 to 8 and the fetus receive nutrients and eliminate their metabolic wastes via the **placenta**, an organ that has both maternal and fetal components. The mature placenta consists of a mass of feathery fetal **villi** that project into an **intervillous space** lined with fetal syncytiotrophoblast and filled with maternal blood. The fetal blood in the villus vessels exchanges materials with the maternal blood across the villus wall. However, exchange of nutrients is not the only function of the placenta; the organ also secretes a plethora of hormones, including the sex steroids that maintain pregnancy. Maternal antibodies cross the placenta to enter the fetus, where they provide protection against fetal and neonatal infections. Unfortunately, teratogenic compounds and some microorganisms also cross the placenta. The placenta grows along with the fetus; at birth it weighs about one sixth as much as the fetus.

Development of the placenta begins when the implanting blastocyst induces the **decidual reaction** in the maternal endometrium, causing the endometrium to become a nutrient-packed, highly vascular tissue called the **decidua**. By the second month, the growing embryo begins to bulge into the uterine lumen. The protruding side of the embryo is covered with a thin capsule of decidua called the **decidua capsularis**, which later disintegrates as the fetus fills the womb. The decidua underlying the embedded **embryonic** pole of the embryo—the pole at which the embryonic disc and connecting stalk are attached—is called the **decidua basalis**, which forms the maternal face of the developing placenta. The remainder of the maternal decidua is called the **decidua parietalis**.

The **umbilical cord** forms as a result of body folding. During this process the amnion, which initially arises from the dorsal margin of the embryonic disc ectoderm, is carried ventrally to enclose the entire embryo, taking origin from the **umbilical ring** surrounding the roots of the vitelline duct and connecting stalk. The amnion also expands until it fills the chorionic space and fuses with the chorion. As the amnion expands, it encloses the connecting stalk and yolk sac neck in a sheath of amniotic membrane. This composite structure becomes the umbilical cord.

As described in Chapter 2, the intervillous space of the placenta originates as lacunae within the syncytiotrophoblast, which anastomose with maternal capillaries and become filled with maternal blood at about 10 weeks. **Stem villi** grow from the fetal chorion into these spaces. Each villus has a core of extraembryonic mesoderm containing blood vessels and a two-layered outer skin of cytotrophoblast and syncytiotrophoblast. Villi originally cover the entire chorion, but by the end of the 3rd month they are restricted to the area of the embryonic pole, which becomes the site of the mature placenta. This part of the chorion is called the **chorion frondosum;** the remaining, smooth chorion is the **chorion laeve**. The villi continue to grow and branch throughout gestation. The intervillous space is subdivided into 15 to 25 partially separated compartments, called **cotyledons**, by wedge-like walls of tissue called **placental septae** that grow inward from the maternal face of the placenta.

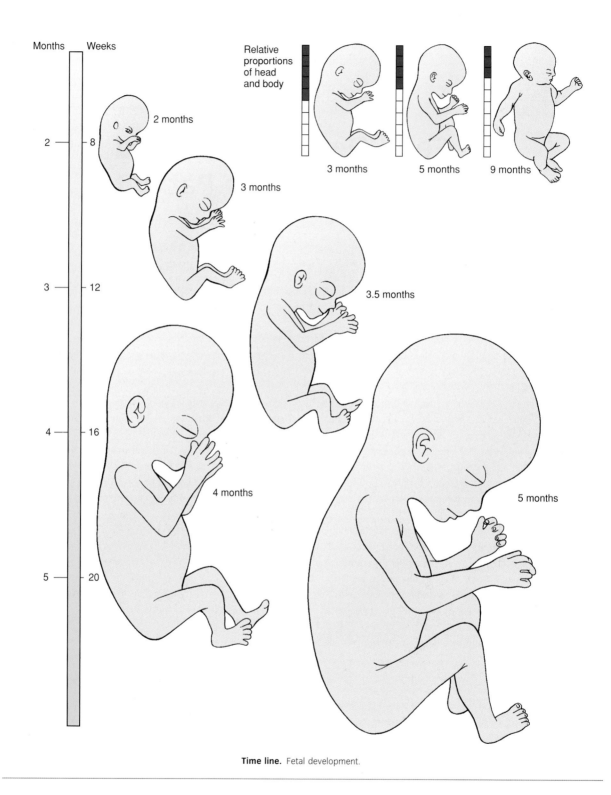

Time line. Fetal development.

Human twins formed by the splitting of a single early embryo (monozygotic twins) may share fetal membranes to varying degrees. In contrast, twins formed by the fertilization of two oocytes (dizygotic twins) always implant separately and develop independent sets of fetal membranes. Sharing of membranes can have negative consequences when vascular connections between the two placentas exist. Although rare, this can result in vascular compromise of one fetus and the subsequent loss of that fetus, or even both fetuses.

Advances in analyzing fetal products in maternal serum, the safety and sophistication of techniques for sampling fetal tissues, and the use of novel imaging techniques to examine the fetus are rapidly providing new approaches to the prenatal diagnosis and treatment of congenital disorders. The increasing ability to diagnose and treat diseases in utero and in very premature infants raises ethical and legal questions that require thoughtful debate. Questions of this nature have always arisen at the forefront of new medical techniques. What is somewhat unusual in this case is the extreme speed with which both our understanding of developmental biology and our clinical practice are advancing, and the fact that decisions about and solutions to the resulting medical questions affect a new category of patient: the unborn fetus. The study and treatment of the fetus constitutes the field of **prenatal pediatrics**, or **fetology**.

6

Clinical Taster   A young couple is seen for a routine midgestational (week 20) **ultrasound** during their first pregnancy. The ultrasonographer is showing the couple their child, a boy, when she pauses. After a couple of minutes, she says that there may be "abnormalities," so she will ask the doctor to take a look. After reviewing the scans, the perinatalogist (an obstetric subspecialist who provides care for the mother and fetus in higher-risk pregnancies) comes in and explains that the fetus has **oligohydramnios** (too little amniotic fluid), **hydronephrosis** (dilated ureters and kidneys), and **megacystis** (dilated bladder). She states her suspicion that the boy has bladder outlet obstruction due to a condition called **posterior urethral valves**. She tells them this is an abnormality of the urethra that prevents normal urine excretion and causes the urine to back up into bladder, ureters, and kidneys. She says that this backup can damage the kidneys, and the lack of amniotic fluid can prevent the lungs from developing normally. The parents are warned that if nothing is done, this defect will likely be fatal at the time of birth due to respiratory failure.

An **amniocentesis** is performed for subsequent chromosome analysis that shows a normal 46,XY karyotype, and in a second ultrasound no other structural abnormalities are found. The couple is referred to a center with expertise in **fetal surgery** for correcting posterior urethral valves. After weighing the risks of surgery against the likelihood of postnatal death from **pulmonary hypoplasia**, the couple elects to undergo placement of a vesicoamniotic catheter (which shunts urine from the bladder to the amniotic cavity) at 22 weeks gestation. The procedure goes well and follow-up ultrasound shows decompression of the bladder and urinary collecting system. The pregnancy is followed closely for signs of shunt malfunction, infection, amniotic fluid leakage, and preterm labor. The boy is delivered at 36 weeks of gestation, and surgery is done to create a vesicostomy (opening from the bladder to the abdominal wall), with urinary reconstruction surgery planned in the future.

During Fetal Period, Embryonic Organ Systems Mature and Fetus Grows

The preceding chapters have focused on the **embryonic period**, the period during which the organs and systems of the body are formed (Fig. 6-1A). The succeeding **fetal period**, from 8 weeks to birth at about 38 weeks, is devoted to the maturation of these organ systems and to growth (Fig. 6-1B; Table 6-1). The fetus grows from 14 g at the beginning of the fetal period (end of the 2nd month) to about 3500 g at birth, a 250-fold increase. Most of this weight is added in the 3rd trimester (7 to 9 months), although the fetus grows in length mainly in the 2nd trimester (4 to 6 months). The growth of the fetus is accompanied by drastic changes in proportion: at 9 weeks, the head of the fetus represents about half its **crown-rump length** (the "sitting height" of the fetus), whereas at birth it represents about one fourth the crown-rump length.

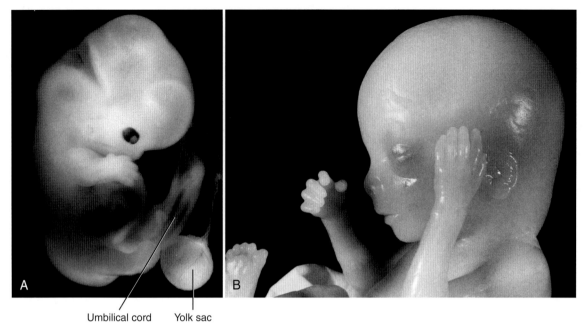

Umbilical cord   Yolk sac

Figure 6-1. Images of human embryos. *A*, Embryo at about 7 weeks of gestation showing the umbilical cord and yolk sac. *B*, Head of a fetus at about 16 weeks of gestation.

Although all organ systems are present by 8 weeks, few of them are functional. The most prominent exceptions are the heart and blood vessels, which begin to circulate blood during the 4th week. Even so, the reconfiguration of the fetal circulatory system described in Chapter 13 is not complete until 3 months. The sensory systems also lag. For example, the auditory ossicles are not free to vibrate until just before birth, and although the neural retina of the eye differentiates during the 3rd and 4th months, the eyelids remain closed until 5 to 7 months, and the eyes cannot focus properly until several weeks after birth.

A number of organs do not finish maturing until after birth. The most obvious example is the reproductive system and associated sexual characteristics, which, as in most animals, do not finish developing until the individual is old enough to be likely to reproduce successfully. In humans, a relatively large number of other organs are also immature at birth. This accounts for the prolonged helpless infancy of humans as compared with many mammals. The most slowly maturing organ of humans, and the one that largely sets the pace of infancy and childhood, is the brain. The cerebrum and cerebellum are both quite immature at birth.

Development of Placenta

As the blastocyst implants, it stimulates a response in the uterine endometrium called the **decidual reaction**. The cells of the endometrial **stroma** (the fleshy layer of endometrial tissue that underlies the endometrial epithelium lining the uterine cavity) accumulate lipid and glycogen and are then called **decidual cells**.

Table 6-1 Fetal growth

Gestational Age (Completed Months of Development)	Approximate CR Length (cm/in)	Approximate Weight/mass (g/oz)
2	5.5/2	14/0.5
3	12/4.5	100/3.5
4	16.5/6.5	300/10.5
	Approximate CH Length (cm/in)	Approximate Weight/mass (g/lb)
5	30/12	600/1.3
6	37.5/15	1000/2.2
7	42.5/16.5	1700/3.8
8	47/18.5	2600/5.8
9	51/20	3500/7.5

The stroma thickens and becomes more highly vascularized, and the endometrium as a whole is then called the **decidua**.

Late in the embryonic period, the **abembryonic** side of the growing embryo (the side opposite to the **embryonic** pole, where the embryonic disc and connecting stalk attach) begins to bulge into the uterine cavity (Fig. 6-2). This protruding portion of the embryo is covered by a thin capsule of endometrium called the **decidua capsularis**. The embedded embryonic pole of the embryo is underlain by a zone of decidua called the **decidua basalis**, which will participate in forming the mature placenta. The remaining areas of decidua are called the **decidua parietalis**. In the 3rd month, as the growing fetus begins to fill the womb, the decidua capsularis is pressed against the decidua parietalis, and in the 5th and 6th months the decidua capsularis disintegrates. By this time, the placenta is fully formed and has distinct fetal and maternal surfaces (Fig. 6-3).

As described in Chapter 2, development of the uteroplacental circulatory system begins late in the 2nd week as cavities called **trophoblastic lacunae** form in the syncytiotrophoblast of the chorion and anastomose with maternal capillaries. At the end of the 3rd week, fetal blood vessels begin to form in the connecting stalk and extraembryonic mesoderm. Meanwhile, the extraembryonic mesoderm lining the chorionic cavity proliferates to form **tertiary stem villi** that project into the trophoblastic lacunae that become blood-filled after 10 weeks. By the end of the 4th week, tertiary stem villi cover the entire chorion. Hypoxia, or lower tissue oxygen content in the decidua, is critical for normal trophoblast invasion.

As the embryo begins to bulge into the uterine lumen during the 2nd month, the villi on the protruding abembryonic side of the chorion disappear (see Fig. 6-2). This region of the chorion is now called the **smooth chorion**, or **chorion laeve**, whereas the portion of the chorion associated with the decidua basalis retains its villi and is called the **chorion frondosum** (from Latin *frondosus*, leafy).

The placental villi continue to grow during most of the remainder of gestation. Starting in the 9th week, the tertiary stem villi lengthen by the formation of terminal **mesenchymal villi**, which originate as sprouts of syncytiotrophoblast (**trophoblastic sprouts**) similar in cross section to primary stem villi (Fig. 6-4). These terminal extensions of the tertiary stem villi, called **immature intermediate villi**, reach their maximum length in the 16th week. The cells of the cytotrophoblastic layer become more dispersed in these villi, leaving gaps in that layer of the villus wall.

Starting near the end of the 2nd trimester, the tertiary stem villi also form numerous slender side branches called **mature intermediate villi**. The first-formed mature intermediate villi finish forming by week 32 and then begin to produce small, nodule-like secondary branches called **terminal villi**. These terminal villi complete the structure of the **placental villous tree**. It has been suggested that the terminal villi are formed not by active outgrowth of the syncytiotrophoblast but rather by coiled and folded villous capillaries that bulge against the villus wall.

Because the **intervillous space** into which the villi project is formed from trophoblastic lacunae that grow and coalesce, it is lined on both sides with syncytiotrophoblast (see Fig. 6-4). The maternal face of the placenta, called the **basal plate**, consists of this syncytiotrophoblast lining plus a supporting layer of decidua basalis. On the fetal side, the layers of the chorion form the **chorionic plate** of the placenta.

During the 4th and 5th months, wedge-like walls of decidual tissue called **placental (decidual) septa** grow into the intervillous space from the maternal side of the placenta, separating the villi into 15 to 25 groups called **cotyledons** (see Figs. 6-3*B*, 6-4). Because the placental septa do not fuse with the chorionic plate, maternal blood can flow freely from one cotyledon to another.

Development of Umbilical Cord

As discussed in Chapter 4, **body folding** separates the forming embryo from its **extraembryonic membranes**. As this process occurs and the embryo grows, the amnion keeps pace, expanding until it encloses the entire embryo except for the umbilical area, where the connecting stalk and yolk sac emerge (Fig. 6-5). Between the 4th and 8th weeks, an increase in the production of amniotic fluid causes the amnion to swell until it completely takes over the chorionic space (Fig. 6-6). When the amnion contacts the chorion, the layers of extraembryonic mesoderm covering the two membranes fuse loosely. Thus, the chorionic cavity disappears except for a few rudimentary vesicles.

After embryonic folding is complete, the amnion takes origin from the **umbilical ring** surrounding the

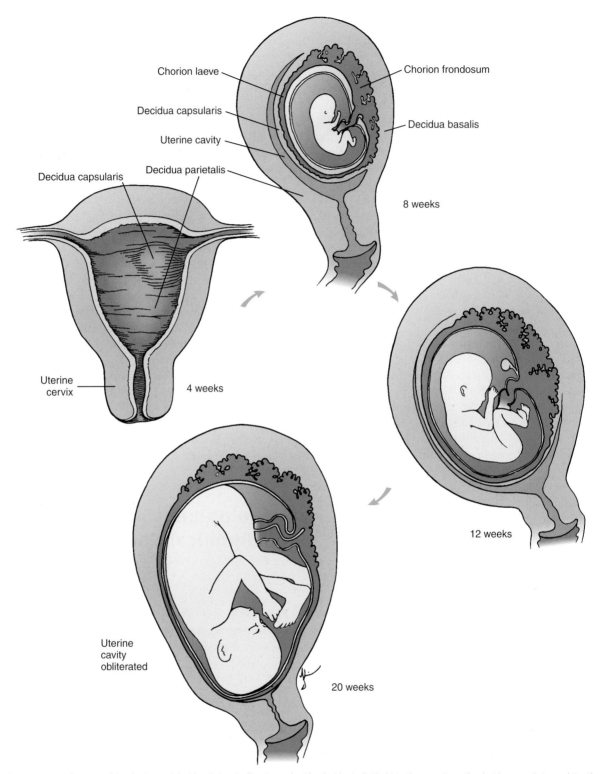

Figure 6-2. Development of the chorion and decidua during the first 5 months. The decidua is divided into three portions: the decidua capsularis overlying the growing conceptus, the decidua basalis underlying the placenta, and the decidua parietalis lining the remainder of the uterus. Note that the original uterine cavity is obliterated by 20 weeks owing to the growth of the fetus and expansion of the amnion cavity.

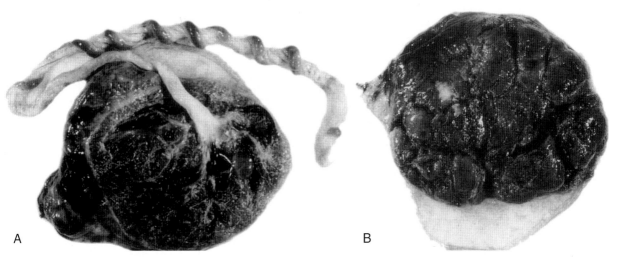

Figure 6-3. *A*, Fetal side of the mature placenta with attached umbilical cord; *B*, Maternal side of the mature placenta showing several cotyledons.

roots of the vitelline duct and connecting stalk. Therefore, the progressive expansion of the amnion creates a tube of amniotic membrane that encloses the connecting stalk and the vitelline duct. This composite structure is now called the **umbilical cord** (see Figs. 6-1*A*, 6-3*A*). As the umbilical cord lengthens, the vitelline duct narrows and the pear-shaped body of the yolk sac remains within the umbilical sheath. Normally, both the yolk sac and the vitelline duct disappear by birth.

The main function of the umbilical cord is to circulate blood between the embryo and the placenta. Umbilical arteries and veins develop in the connecting stalk to perform this function (discussed in Ch. 13). The expanded amnion creates a roomy, weightless chamber in which the fetus can grow and develop freely. If the supply of amniotic fluid is inadequate (the condition known as **oligohydramnios**), the abnormally small amniotic cavity may restrict fetal growth, which may result in severe malformations and **pulmonary hypoplasia** (discussed in the "Clinical Taster" for this chapter).

Exchange of Substances between Maternal and Fetal Blood in Placenta

Maternal blood enters the intervillous spaces of the placenta through about 100 **spiral arteries**, bathes the villi, and leaves again via **endometrial veins**. The placenta contains approximately 150 mL of maternal blood, and this volume is replaced about 3 or 4 times per minute. Nutrients and oxygen pass from the maternal blood across the cell layers of the villus into the fetal blood, and waste products such as carbon dioxide, urea, uric acid, and bilirubin (a breakdown product of hemoglobin) reciprocally pass from the fetal blood to the maternal blood.

Maternal proteins are endocytosed and degraded by the trophoblast unless bound to receptors (e.g., *IgG, Transcobalamin II*). Antibodies cross the placenta to enter the fetal circulation, and in this way the mother gives the fetus limited passive immunity against a variety of infections, such as diphtheria and measles. These antibodies persist in the infant's blood for several months after birth, guarding the infant against infectious diseases until its own immune system matures.

Erythroblastosis Fetalis

There is one fairly common instance in which the transfer of antibodies from the mother to the fetus is not beneficial: when the antibodies are directed against an Rh factor on the fetal red blood cells and cause hemolysis (dissolution) of the fetal red blood cells. The **Rh factors** are a group of genetically determined surface molecules that are present on the plasma membrane of red blood cells in most, but not all, individuals. Individuals whose blood cells carry an Rh factor are **Rh+**; individuals whose blood cells lack

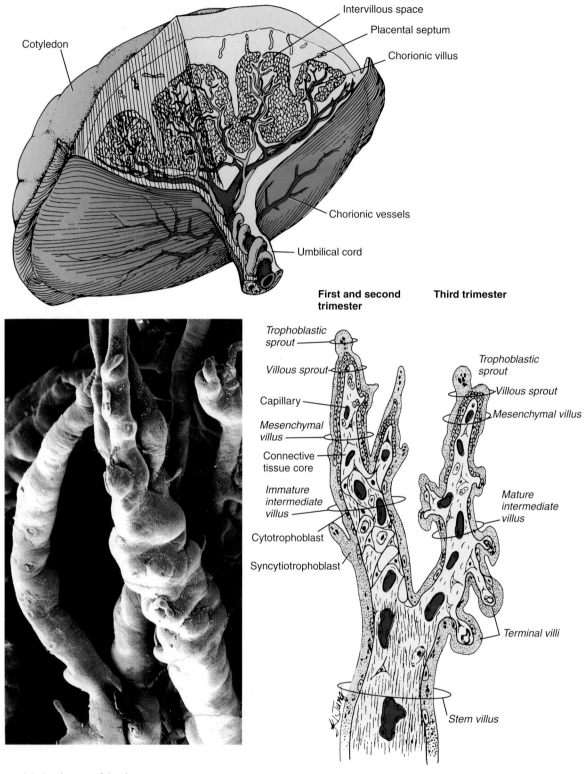

Figure 6-4. Development of the placenta.

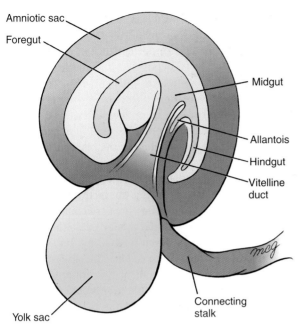

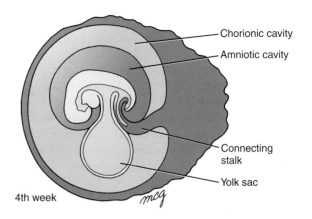

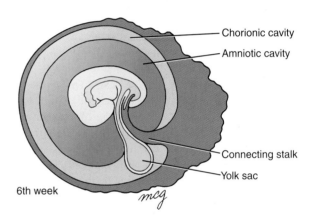

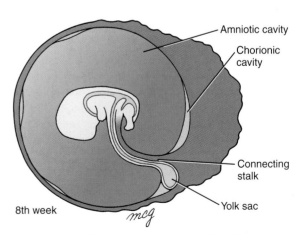

Figure 6-5. Genesis of the umbilical cord. The folding of the embryo and expansion of the amniotic cavity bring the connecting stalk and yolk sac together to form the umbilical cord. As the amnion continues to grow, a layer of amniotic membrane gradually encloses the umbilical cord.

Figure 6-6. The rapidly expanding amniotic cavity fills with fluid and obliterates the chorionic cavity between weeks 4 and 8.

one are **Rh-**. Rh factors provoke a strong immune response in Rh- individuals. If an Rh- mother carries an Rh+ fetus and fetal blood leaks into the maternal circulation, the mother will manufacture antibodies against the fetal red blood cells. Significant leaks of fetal blood across the placenta into the maternal circulation normally occur only at birth, so the resulting antibodies do not form in time to harm the fetus that first induces them. However, if the same mother bears a second Rh+ fetus, her anti-Rh antibodies can cross the placenta and destroy fetal red blood cells, causing anemia in the fetus and newborn. This condition is called **hemolytic disease of the newborn** or **erythroblastosis fetalis**. The latter name comes from the fact that the destruction of red blood cells stimulates a compensatory production of large numbers of immature nucleated fetal red blood cells called **erythroblasts**. Another, sometimes fatal, consequence of the disease is **hydrops fetalis**—the accumulation of water in the fetus. Moreover, the destruction of red blood cells releases large amounts of bilirubin (a breakdown product of hemoglobin) into the fetal circulation. This substance can be deposited in the developing brain, leading to cerebral damage and, in some cases, to death.

The effects of erythroblastosis fetalis can be prevented by giving transfusions of Rh- blood to the fetus in utero and to the newborn, so that the maternal antibodies find fewer cells to destroy. A more economical preventive approach is to administer anti-Rh antibodies (RhoGam) to the Rh- mother immediately after the birth of each Rh+ baby. These antibodies destroy the fetal Rh+ red blood cells in her circulation before they stimulate her own immune system, preventing her from manufacturing anti-Rh antibodies.

Placenta Allows Passage of Some Viral and Bacterial Pathogens

Although the placenta is fairly impermeable to microorganisms, a number of viruses and bacteria can cross it and infect the fetus. Because the fetus has no functioning immune system and relies solely on maternal antibodies for protection, it is often inept at fighting infections. Therefore, a disease that is mild in the mother may damage or kill the fetus. The types of viruses that can cross the placenta and infect the fetus can be remembered by using the acronym TORCH: **toxoplasma virus** (a virus that can be transmitted to humans from cat litter and soil), **other** viruses such as **parvovirus** (a virus that causes rashes in school-aged children; the canine form of this virus does not infect humans) and **varicella-zoster virus** (the agent of varicella or chickenpox), **rubella virus** (the agent of rubella or German measles), **cytomegalovirus** (infection with this virus in adults and children may be asymptomatic), and **herpes simplex virus** (the virus that causes canker sores and genital warts).

Cytomegalovirus causes one of the most common viral infections of the fetus. If this virus infects the embryo early in development, it may induce abortion; infection occurring later may cause a wide range of congenital abnormalities, including blindness, microcephaly (small head), hearing loss, and mental retardation.

One bacterium that has recently come to unpleasant prominence as a cause of congenital infections in American children is *Treponema pallidum*, the agent of **syphilis**. Congenital syphilis can result in fetal anomalies or death.

HIV Can Be Transmitted across Placenta during Parturition or in Breast Milk

Human immunodeficiency virus (HIV) is the agent of **acquired immune deficiency syndrome (AIDS)** and related syndromes. This virus can sometimes cross the placenta from an infected mother to infect the unborn fetus. It is important to note that 25% to 40% of babies are HIV positive if their mothers are HIV positive and untreated with anti-HIV therapies; with appropriate treatment (discussed in next paragraph) this number can be as low as 1%. The difference in transmission rate of 25% to 40% in untreated pregnancies is related to whether the placenta has specific coreceptors for specific strains of HIV and whether the placenta expresses active virus. HIV is commonly transmitted during the birth process or in the mother's milk during breast-feeding. Infants infected perinatally with HIV may seem healthy at birth, but they usually develop AIDS by the time that they are 3 years old. As in adults, the disease slowly destroys a crucial component of the immune system and leaves the infant vulnerable to repeated infections. Parotid gland infections, diarrhea, bronchitis, and chronic middle ear infections are common in infants with AIDS. Pneumonia caused by the protozoan *Pneumocystis carinii*, a characteristic infection of adults with AIDS, is a particularly alarming symptom in infants: the mean survival time of infants diagnosed with AIDS and *Pneumocystis carinii* pneumonia is 1 to 3 months. HIV-1 infection is also correlated with an increased rate of low birthweight, intrauterine fetal death, and preterm birth.

In 2005 it was estimated that more than 40 million people worldwide were infected with HIV. According to the Centers for Disease Control and Prevention, through approximately 1984 (roughly when the AIDS epidemic began in the United States) to 1993 a total of about 15,000 HIV-infected children were born to HIV-positive women in the United States (about 6,000 to 7,000 HIV-infected women give birth each year in the United States). From 1984 to 1992, the number of babies born with AIDS increased each year, but between 1992 and 1996 the number of such babies declined by 43%. This reduction occurred because of a number of factors including enhanced prenatal care, HIV testing before or during pregnancy, and administration of antiretroviral drugs such as zidovudine (ZDV) to HIV-positive women during pregnancy and at delivery, as well as treatment of babies born to HIV-positive women with the same drugs postnatally.

Teratogens Cross Placenta

Teratogens are environmental (i.e., nongenetic) substances that are capable of causing a **birth defect** when embryos or fetuses are exposed at critical times in development to sufficiently high doses (concentrations). The study of the role of environmental factors in disrupting development is known by the unfortunate name of **teratology**, which literally means the study of (developmental) monsters. A number of **principles of teratology** have emerged, but here only three are discussed because of their direct relevance to human birth defects.

The first principle of teratology that we will discuss is that an embryonic structure is usually susceptible to teratogens only during specific **critical sensitive periods**, which usually correspond to periods of active differentiation and morphogenesis. Thus, a potent teratogen may have no effect on the development of an embryonic structure if it is administered before or after the critical period during which that structure is susceptible to its action. The timeline illustrations at the beginning of the chapters in this book generally define the sensitive periods of the corresponding tissues and organ systems. Because the major events of organogenesis take place during the first 8 weeks of development, that is the period during which the fetus is most vulnerable to teratogens. A second principle of teratology is that an embryonic structure is susceptible to a critical **dose** of teratogen during its specific critical sensitive period. Thus, in teratologic studies a **dose-response curve** is constructed for a suspected teratogen in which lowest dose has no effect and the highest dose is lethal to the embryo. A third principle of teratology is that susceptibility to a teratogen depends on the **genetic constitution** of the developing embryo or fetus. For example, if two embryos of the same age are exposed to the same dose of teratogen, one may develop severe cardiac malformations whereas the other may remain unaffected. The molecular basis for this difference in susceptibility might, for instance, be a genetic difference in the rate at which the enzyme systems of the two embryos detoxify the teratogen. Thus, there is a **gene-environmental interaction** underlying susceptibility to birth defects that varies from embryo to embryo.

It is not always easy to identify a compound as a teratogen. Two approaches are used: **epidemiologic studies**, which attempt to relate antenatal exposure to a suspect compound with the occurrence of various congenital anomalies in humans (so-called retrospective studies); and studies in which the compound is administered to pregnant **experimental animals** and the offspring are checked for abnormalities (so-called prospective studies). However, it is often difficult to gather enough epidemiologic data to yield a clear result, and findings from animal studies are not necessarily applicable to humans. These difficulties are compounded by the fact that most congenital anomalies are multifactorial in etiology, that is, their pathogenesis depends on the genetic makeup of the individual (third principle of teratology discussed in preceding paragraph), as well as on exposure to the teratogen (i.e., dose; second principle of teratology discussed in preceding paragraph). Finally, malformations of a given structure can usually be caused only during the critical period (first principle of teratology discussed in preceding paragraph).

Many therapeutic drugs are known to be teratogenic; these include retinoids (vitamin A and analogs), the anticoagulant warfarin, the anticonvulsants valproic acid and phenytoin, and a number of chemotherapeutic agents used to treat cancer. Most teratogenic drugs exert their main effects during the embryonic period. Although, as stated above, most care must be exercised in administering certain anesthetics and other drugs even late in pregnancy or at term, because they may endanger the health of the fetus.

Some recreational drugs are also teratogenic; these include tobacco, alcohol, and cocaine. The manifestations of fetal alcohol syndrome are described in Chapter 5. Cocaine, used by alarming numbers of pregnant women (the drug affected 300,000 to 400,000 newborns in 1990 in the United States), readily crosses the placenta and may cause addiction in the developing fetus. In some of the major cities of the United States, as many as 20% of babies are born to mothers who abuse cocaine. Unfortunately, fetal cocaine addiction may have permanent effects on the individual, although studies suggest that early intervention with intensive emotional and educational support in the first few years of life may be helpful.

Pregnant women who use cocaine have higher frequencies of fetal morbidity (disease) and mortality (death) than pregnant women who do not. Cocaine use is associated not only with low birthweight but also with some specific developmental anomalies, including infarction of the cerebral cortex and a variety of cardiovascular malformations. However, it is often difficult to isolate cocaine as the teratogen responsible for a given effect, because women who use cocaine often use other drugs as well, including marijuana, alcohol, tobacco, and heroin.

Children of cocaine-abusing mothers may be born premature as well as addicted: cocaine-using mothers have a very high frequency of **preterm labor**.

6

Preterm labor occurs in 25% of women who test positive for cocaine on a urine test at admission to the hospital for labor and delivery but in only 8% of women who do not test positive for cocaine at admission. Two mechanisms have been proposed by which cocaine could cause preterm labor: cocaine, a potent constrictor of blood vessels, may cause abruption of the placental membranes (premature separation of the placenta from the uterus) by partly shutting off the flow of blood to the placenta; or as there is evidence that cocaine directly affects the contractility of the uterine myometrium (muscle layer), it perhaps makes the myometrium hypersensitive to signals that initiate labor.

Intrauterine Growth Restriction

Intrauterine growth restriction (IUGR), often called **small for gestational age (SGA)**, is a condition in which fetal growth in markedly retarded. IUGR carries a higher risk of perinatal mortality and morbidity, so IUGR is a life-threatening birth defect. A newborn is considered to be SGA if he/she weighs less than 2500 grams at term or falls below the 10th percentile for gestational age. There are many causes for IUGR, including teratogen exposure such as congenital viral or bacterial infections, fetal chromosomal anomalies (e.g., Down syndrome), maternal factors (such as **preeclampsia**, a condition affecting about 5% of pregnancies characterized by high blood pressure and protein in

the urine), and placental factors (such as **placenta previa**, or "low-lying" placenta, a condition in which the blastocyst implants near the uterine cervix and the placenta covers part of the opening of the cervix). Unlike many other birth defects discussed throughout the book, IUGR is a birth defect that involves the entire fetus, rather than just one organ or organ system.

Maternal Diabetes and Obesity

Both maternal diabetes and maternal obesity during pregnancy constitute risk factors for birth defects of the fetus. Thus, the health of the mother and the resulting maternal environment impacts development of the fetus (Fig. 6-7). Approximately 1:200 women of childbearing age have diabetes before pregnancy (preexisting diabetes) and another 2% to 5% develop diabetes during pregnancy (gestational diabetes). Women with preexisting diabetes are 3 to 4 times more likely to have a child with a major birth defect than are nondiabetic women. Such defects are widespread and include neural tube defects and heart defects. Women with gestational diabetes usually do not have an increased frequency of children with birth defects. However, if diabetes in either group is poorly managed during pregnancy, there is an increased risk of delivering a very large baby (greater than 10 pounds). Such babies may have an increased risk for obesity and diabetes in later life.

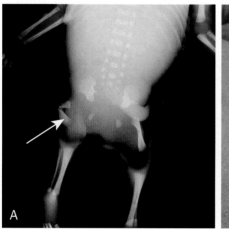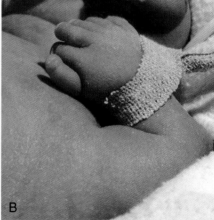

Figure 6-7. Birth defects in infants born to diabetic mothers exhibiting diabetic embryopathy. *A*, X-ray showing abnormal lower limbs in a stillborn fetus. Note the disrupted pelvis and small and bent (arrow) femurs. *B*, Photo showing preaxial polydactyly in the hand of an infant.

Maternal obesity (defined in the United States as a body mass index greater than 30 kg/meter squared) is also a risk factor for birth defects. Fetuses born to obese women are 2 to 3.5 times more likely than those born to average-weight women to have neural tube defects, heart defects, and omphalocele.

Placenta Produces Several Important Hormones

The placenta is an extremely prolific producer of hormones. Two of its major products are the steroid hormones **progesterone** and **estrogen**, which are responsible for maintaining the pregnant state and preventing spontaneous abortion or preterm labor. As discussed in Chapter 1, the corpus luteum produces progesterone and estrogen during the 1st weeks of pregnancy. However, by the 11th week the corpus luteum degenerates and the placenta assumes its role.

During the first 2 months of pregnancy, the syncytiotrophoblast of the placenta produces the glycoprotein hormone **human chorionic gonadotropin (hCG)**, which supports the secretory activity of the corpus luteum. Because this hormone is produced only by fetal tissue and is excreted in the mother's urine, it is used as the basis for pregnancy tests. However, it is also produced abundantly by hydatidiform moles (see the In the Clinic section of Ch. 2), and persistence of the hormone beyond 2 months of gestation may indicate a molar pregnancy.

The placenta produces an extremely wide range of other protein hormones, including, to name a few, human placental lactogen (hPL), human chorionic thyrotropin, human chorionic corticotropin, insulin-like growth factors, prolactin, relaxin, corticotropin-releasing hormone, and endothelin. Interestingly, hPL converts the mother from being principally a carbohydrate user to being a fatty acid user, thus sparing carbohydrates for the conceptus.

In addition to protein hormones, placental membranes synthesize **prostaglandins**, a family of compounds derived from fatty acids, which perform a range of functions in various tissues of the body. Placental prostaglandins seem to be intimately involved in the maintenance of pregnancy and onset of labor. The signal that initiates labor seems to be a reduction in the ratio of progesterone to estrogen, but the effect of this signal may be mediated by an elevation in the levels of prostaglandins produced by the placenta.

Production and Resorption of Amniotic Fluid

As described in Chapter 4 and in this chapter, embryonic folding transforms the amnion from a small bubble on the dorsal side of the embryonic disc to a sac that completely encloses the embryo. By the 8th week, the expanding amniotic sac completely fills the old chorionic cavity and fuses with the chorion. The expansion of the amnion is due mainly to an increase in the amount of **amniotic fluid**. The volume of amniotic fluid increases through the 7th month and then decreases somewhat in the last 2 months. At birth the volume of amniotic fluid is typically about 1 L.

Amniotic fluid, which is very similar to blood plasma in composition, is initially produced by transport of fluid across the amniotic membrane itself. After about 16 weeks, fetal urine also makes an important contribution to the amniotic fluid. If the fetus does not excrete urine—either because of bilateral **renal agenesis** (absence of both kidneys; discussed in Ch. 15) or because the lower urinary tract is obstructed (**posterior urethral valves**; discussed in Clinical Taster this chapter and in Ch. 15)—the volume of amniotic fluid will be too low (the condition called **oligohydramnios**), and the amniotic cavity in consequence will be too small. A small amniotic cavity can cramp the growth of the fetus (resulting in deformations; discussed in Ch. 5) and cause various congenital malformations, notably pulmonary hypoplasia (discussed in "Clinical Taster" this chapter and in Ch. 11).

Because amniotic fluid is constantly produced, it must also be constantly resorbed. This is accomplished mainly by the fetal gut, which absorbs the fluid drunk by the fetus. Excess fluid is then returned to the maternal circulation via the placenta. Malformations that make it impossible for the fetus to drink—for example, esophageal atresia or anencephaly (discussed in Chs. 4 and 14)—result in an overabundance of amniotic fluid, a condition called **hydramnios** or **polyhydramnios**.

Twinning

Twinning occurs naturally (that is, excluding ART, in which as described in Ch. 1, multiple blastocysts routinely are introduced into the uterus) in about 3% of the births. Twins that form by the splitting of a single original embryo are called **monozygotic**, or **identical**, twins; this type of twinning occurs infrequently (i.e., about 0.4% naturally). These twins share an identical genetic makeup and, therefore, look alike as they grow up. In contrast, **dizygotic** (i.e., **fraternal**) twins arise from separate oocytes produced during the same menstrual cycle. This type of twinning is by far the more frequent (averages about 1.2% but increases with maternal age from 0.3% at age 20 to 1.4% at ages 35 to 40; it seems to have a genetic basis). Dizygotic twin embryos implant separately and develop separate fetal membranes (amnion, chorion, and placenta). Monozygotic twins, in contrast, may share none, some, or all of their fetal membranes, depending on how late in development the original embryo splits to form twins.

If the splitting occurs during cleavage—for example, if the two blastomeres produced by the first cleavage division become separated—the monozygotic twin blastomeres will implant separately, like dizygotic twin blastomeres, and will not share fetal membranes (Fig. 6-8). Alternatively, if the twins are formed by splitting of the inner cell mass within the blastocyst, they will occupy the same chorion but will be enclosed by separate amnions and will use separate placentae, each placenta developing around the connecting stalk of its respective embryo. Finally, if the twins are formed by splitting of a bilaminar embryonic disc, they will occupy the same amnion. In rare cases, such twins may not fully separate, resulting in the birth of **conjoined twins** (Fig. 6-9).

Because fetal membranes fuse when they are forced together by the growth of the fetus, it may not be immediately obvious whether the membranous septum separating a pair of twins represents just amniotic membranes (meaning that the twins share a chorion) or fused amnions and chorions (meaning that the twins originally did not share fetal membranes). The clue is the thickness and opacity of the septum: amniotic membranes are thin and almost transparent, whereas chorionic membranes are thicker and somewhat opaque.

In twin pregnancies, anastomoses can form between vessels supplying the two placentae. This shared circulation usually poses no problem, but if one twin dies late in gestation or if the blood pressure of one twin drops significantly, the remaining twin is at risk. If one twin dies, the other twin may be killed by an **embolism** (blocked blood vessel) caused by bits of tissue that break off in the dead twin and enter the shared circulation. If the blood pressure of one twin falls sharply, the other twin may suffer heart failure as its heart attempts to fill both circulatory systems at once.

Two other serious complications can occur when vessels are shared between placentae: **twin-twin transfusion syndrome (TTTS)** and **twin-reversed arterial perfusion (TRAP sequence).** In TTTS (occurs in 10% to 20% of all monochorionic, diamniotic twins and is responsible for about 15% of all perinatal deaths in twins), vascular anastomoses occur between vessels in the two placentae that result in unbalanced blood flow between the twins. One twin, the so-called donor twin, exhibits oligohydramnios and growth restriction, whereas the other, the so-called recipient twin, exhibits polyhydramnios and cardiac enlargement and eventually cardiac failure. In TRAP sequence (incidence of about 1 in 35,000 births), one twin, the so-called pump twin, provides all of the blood flow to a second acardiac/acephalic twin through placental vascular anastomoses. Because of the additional stress placed on the pump twin's heart, cardiac failure and the pump twin's subsequent demise occur in 50% to 75% of the cases (the acardiac twin cannot survive without the pump twin, and it dies either with death of the pump twin or at birth).

In the past, the only treatment for these situations was to wait until the healthy twin was old enough to have a chance of surviving outside the womb and then to perform a cesarean section. However, surgical techniques are being developed that may provide in utero treatment of these serious conditions.

Prenatal Diagnosis Assesses Health of Unborn

The study and treatment of the fetus constitutes the field of **prenatal pediatrics** or **fetology.** Four diagnostic techniques have revolutionized the diagnosis of fetal malformations and genetic diseases and have lead to new treatments. These are **maternal serum screening, ultrasonography, amniocentesis,** and **chorionic villus sampling.**

Maternal Serum Screening

Current **maternal serum screenings** are of two types: the *triple* screen and the *quadruple* screen. These screens are sometimes referred to as the MSAFP+ screen, as they measure maternal serum *alpha-Fetoprotein* plus other serum components. In the triple screen, in addition to measuring serum levels of **alpha-Fetoprotein** (**AFP**), a protein produced

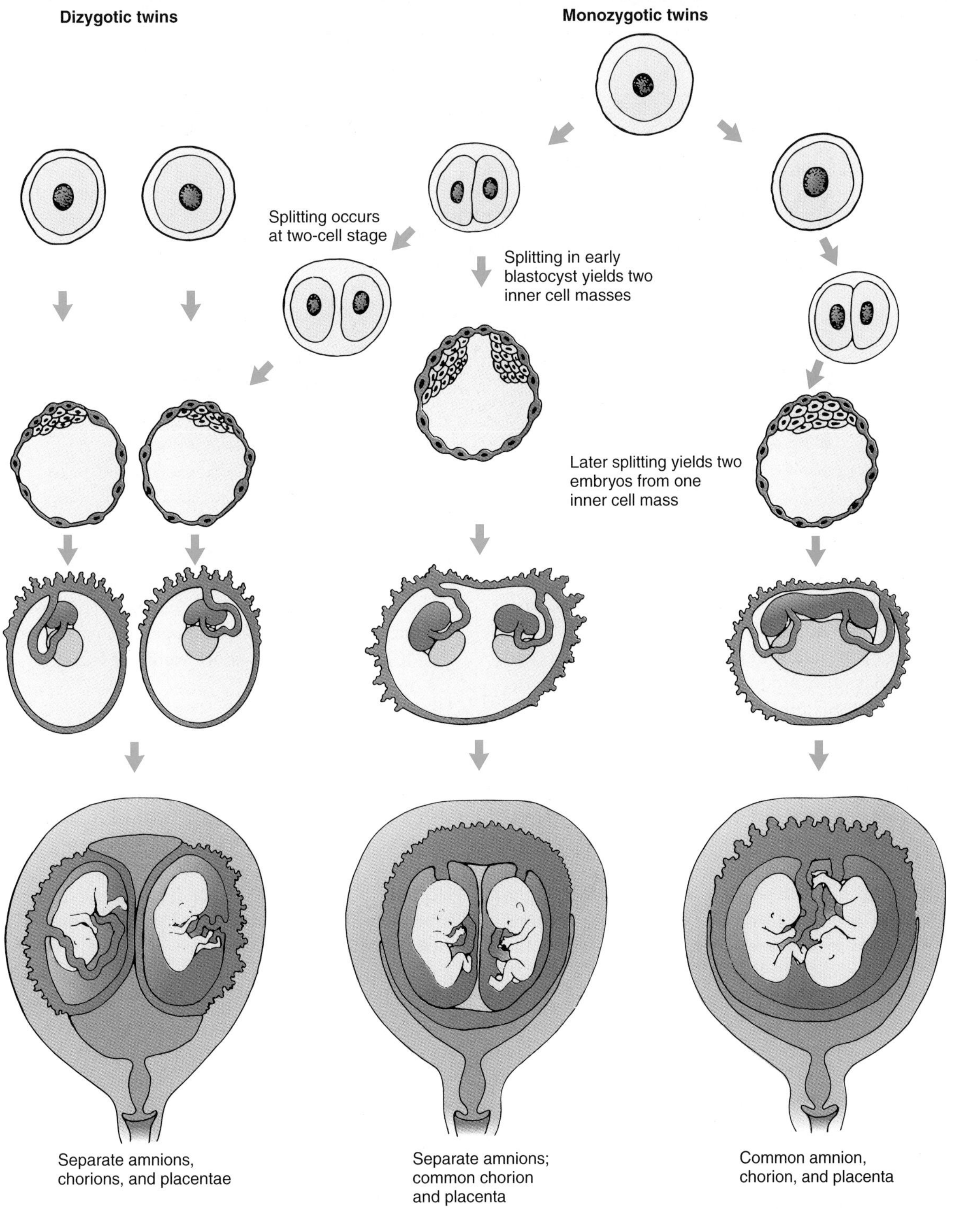

Dizygotic twins

Monozygotic twins

Splitting occurs at two-cell stage

Splitting in early blastocyst yields two inner cell masses

Later splitting yields two embryos from one inner cell mass

6

Separate amnions, chorions, and placentae

Separate amnions; common chorion and placenta

Common amnion, chorion, and placenta

Figure 6-8. Fetal membrane development in various types of twins. The degree to which monozygotic twins share placental membranes depends on the stage of development at which the originally single embryo separates: if the splitting occurs at the two-cell stage of cleavage, the twins will develop as separately as dizygotic twins; if the splitting yields a blastocyst with two inner cell masses, then the embryos will share a single chorion and placenta but occupy separate amnions; if the splitting occurs after the formation of the inner cell mass, the embryos will occupy a single amnion.

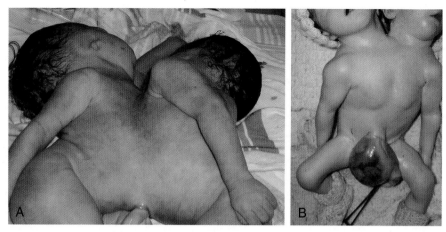

Figure 6-9. Conjoined twins. *A,* Joined front to front. *B,* Joined side to side; note the presence of an omphalocele.

by the fetal liver whose level steadily increases during pregnancy, two other serum components are measured: **human chorionic gonadotropin (hCG)**, produced by the placenta, with levels peaking at about 14 weeks of gestation and dropping thereafter; and **estriol (uE3)**, also produced by the placenta. In the quadruple screen, *Inhibin-A* is measured in addition to the other three serum components. *Inhibin-A* is produced by the fetus and placenta. These screens are most often done in combination with ultrasonography examination of the fetus (Figs. 6-10, 6-11, 6-12)

The levels of these serum components can suggest the presence of a fetus with **Down syndrome** or a birth defect such as a **neural tube defect.** For example, AFP levels are high (when compared to normal levels at the same week of gestation) when the mother is carrying a fetus with a neural tube defect. When carrying a fetus with Down syndrome, maternal serum hCG and inhibin-A levels are elevated, and estriol levels are low.

The maternal serum screen is not a "test" that diagnoses a birth defect; it only indicates the possibility of some types of birth defects. If abnormal results are obtained, the maternal serum screen is followed by other diagnosis procedures, including some of those described in the following paragraphs. It is important to point out to parents that the maternal serum screen has a high false-positive rate. Thus, a risk of this screen is that it can lead to unnecessary worrying by the parents. It has been estimated that the quadruple screen detects more than 80% of the fetuses with Down syndrome. However, high levels of serum *AFP*, when assessed at 16 to 18 weeks of gestation when the test is most accurate for predicting the presence of a fetus with a neural tube defect, are correlated with the presence of a fetus with a neural tube defect in only 1 in 16 to 1 in 33 cases. Thus, without further testing such as ultrasonography, parents might decide unknowingly to abort a normal fetus.

Ultrasonography

In **ultrasonography**, the inside of the body is scanned with a beam of ultrasound (sound with a frequency of 3 to 10 MHz), and a computer is used to analyze the pattern of returning echoes. Because tissues of different density reflect sound differently, revealing tissue interfaces, the pattern of echoes can be used to decipher the inner structure of the body. The quality of the images yielded by ultrasonography has rapidly improved, and it is now possible to visualize the structure of the developing fetus and to identify many malformations. Ultrasonography is also now used to guide the needles or catheters used for amniocentesis and chorionic villus sampling (amniocentesis and chorionic villus sampling are described later in the chapter). These procedures were formerly performed unguided, with a higher consequent risk of piercing the fetus. There is no evidence that ultrasound is harmful to the fetus.

Various types of "display modes," or ways of analyzing and displaying ultrasound data, are used, each with particular advantages. **B-mode** ultrasonography shows an image **(sonogram)** of the anatomy of a two-dimensional plane of scanning and can be performed in real time (see Fig. 6-10). Recently, it has become possible to use this type of ultrasonography with advanced equipment to obtain three-dimensional sonograms (see Fig. 6-11) and "four-dimensional"

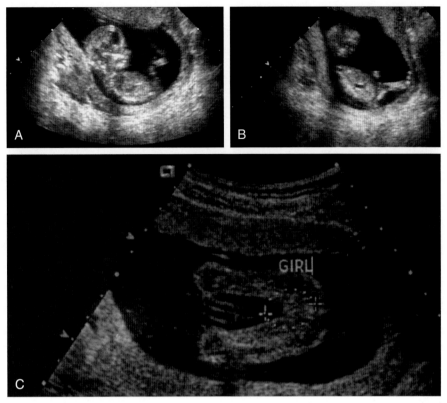

Figure 6-10. Sonograms. *A, B,* Fetus at 12 weeks of gestation. The images taken just a few seconds apart show that the fetus is constantly shifting positions in the amniotic cavity. With ultrasonography, this movement can be viewed in real time and the entire three-dimensional extent of the fetus and placenta can be examined. *C,* Fetus at 18 weeks of gestation. Image shows that the fetus is a girl.

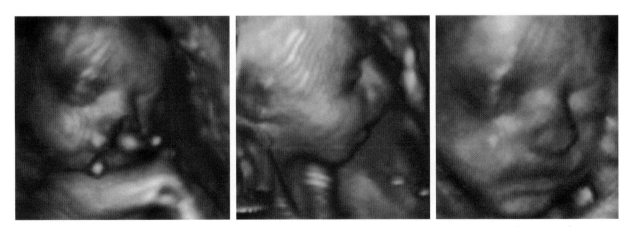

Figure 6-11. Three-dimensional sonograms of different fetuses showing state-of-the-art imaging of three-dimensional morphology.

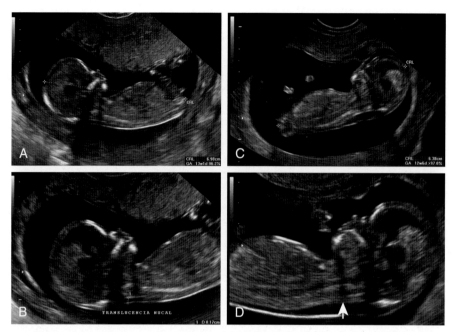

Figure 6-12. Sonograms of fetuses showing the area measured during nuchal translucency screening. *A, B,* Overview and enlargement in a fetus with a measurement in the normal range; the points of the electronic caliper are indicated by small plus signs in B (just above the letters "uc" in translucenia). *C, D,* Overview and enlargement in a fetus with a measurement that suggests Down syndrome. Arrow indicates enlarged Nuchal translucency.

sonograms (i.e., movies of sequential images that show movement). **M-mode** ultrasonography shows the changes in position of a structure such as a heart valve with time. **Doppler ultrasonography** yields flow information and can be used to study the pattern of flow within the heart and developing blood vessels. The miniaturization of ultrasound electronics has led to the development of **endosonography**, in which a miniature ultrasound probe is inserted into a body orifice such as the vagina and is thus brought close to the structure of interest, permitting a higher-resolution image.

Real-time B-mode ultrasonography is the type most often used to examine the fetus (see Fig. 6-10). A wide variety of fetal anomalies can be seen and diagnosed by this technique, including craniofacial defects, limb anomalies, diaphragmatic hernias, caudal dysgenesis syndromes, teratomas, spina bifida, and renal agenesis. Abnormalities of the fetal heart and heart beat can be analyzed using **fetal echocardiography**, a more detailed ultrasonography of the heart performed by a pediatric cardiologist. Ultrasonography can also be used to measure the thickness of the clear area at the back of the neck (i.e., **nuchal region**), a procedure known as **nuchal translucency screening** (see Fig. 6-12). Fetuses with **Down syndrome**, other

chromosomal anomalies, and major heart anomalies accumulate fluid in the back of their neck during the first trimester. Thus, the thickness of the clear area provides an indication of the likelihood that such a congenital anomaly is present.

Amniocentesis

In **amniocentesis** amniotic fluid is aspirated from the amniotic cavity (usually between 14 and 16 weeks gestation) through a needle inserted via the abdominal wall (Fig. 6-13) and is examined for various clues to fetal disease. Amniotic fluid contains metabolic byproducts of the fetus as well as cells sloughed from the fetus (possibly the lungs) and amniotic membrane. The protein α-**Fetoprotein**, for example, is a useful indicator. Elevated levels of this protein may indicate the presence of an open neural tube defect, such as anencephaly, or other open defects such as gastroschisis. Fetal cells in the amniotic fluid can be cultured and karyotyped to determine the sex of the fetus and to detect chromosomal anomalies. Other molecular-genetic techniques can be used to screen the genome for the presence or absence of specific mutations that cause heritable diseases (discussed in Ch. 1). Amniocentesis has limitations early in gestation, both

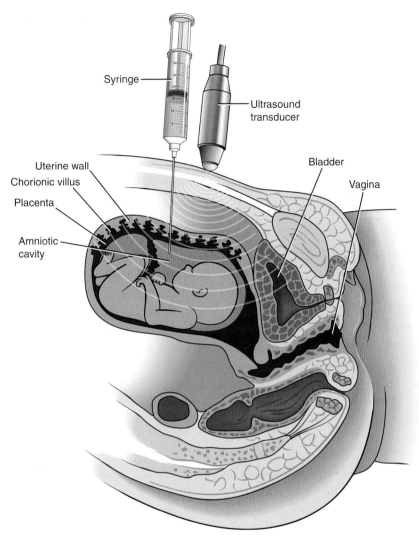

Figure 6-13. Schematic illustration of amniocentesis.

because it is difficult to perform when the volume of amniotic fluid is small and because a small sample may not yield enough cells for analysis. Later in pregnancy, amniocentesis is used to assess fetal lung maturity and Rh sensitization, and to test for fetal infection.

Chorionic Villus Sampling

In chorionic villus sampling (CVS), a small sample of tissue (10 to 40 mg) is removed from the chorion by a catheter inserted through the cervix or with a needle inserted through the abdominal wall (Fig. 6-14) under ultrasound guidance. This tissue may be directly karyotyped or karyotyped after culture.

Chorionic villus sampling can be performed early in gestation (10 to 12 weeks) and yields enough tissue for many kinds of molecular-genetic analyses. Because placental tissue is examined directly, amniotic AFP cannot be measured by using CVS. The technique is also complicated by the fact that in 1 to 2% of cases the results of CVS are ambiguous due to chromosomal mosaicism (mosaicism is discussed in an "In the Clinic" of Ch. 1). This can be due to a mosaic fetus or because the placental chromosome complement differs from that of the fetus—a phenomenon called confined placental mosaicism. Such abnormal CVS results must be confirmed by amniocentesis.

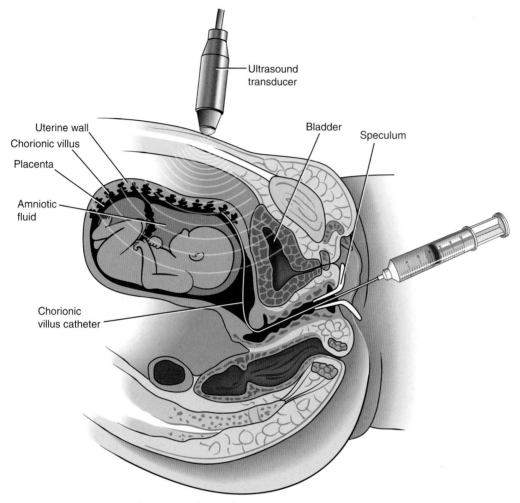

Figure 6-14. Schematic illustration of chorionic villus sampling.

Treating Fetus in Utero

If amniocentesis or chorionic villus sampling reveals that a fetus has a significant genetic anomaly, should the fetus be aborted? If ultrasonography shows a malformation serious enough to kill or deform the fetus, should corrective fetal surgery be attempted? What if fetal surgery might result in a cosmetic improvement, for example, a better repair of a cleft lip with little or no scarring? The answers to these questions involve many factors, including (1) the risk to the mother of continuing the pregnancy, (2) the availability of surgeons and resources for fetal surgery, (3) the risk of the operation to the fetus and the mother, (4) the severity of the anomaly or disease, (5) the advantage of correcting the defect in utero instead of after birth, and

(6) the ethical, moral, and religious beliefs of the families involved. Thus, there are no easy answers to these complex questions, and acquiring answers will require input from both the individuals involved and society as a whole.

Over the past 20 years, several approaches have been attempted to treat the fetus in utero, potentially lessening the impact of birth defects diagnosed prenatally. These treatments are of two broad types: **surgical intervention** and **drug intervention**.

Surgical intervention has been used to treat **congenital diaphragmatic hernia, spina bifida (myelomeningocele), hydrocephalus** (enlargement of the brain ventricles due to blockage of the flow of cerebrospinal fluid; corrected with shunts inserted either in utero or usually postnatally), **thoracic cysts** (e.g., **congenital** cystic adenomatoid malformation—a multicystic mass of pulmonary tissue that causes lung compression and resulting hypoplasia), **sacrococcygeal teratomas** (enormous tumors that require such a large blood flow that fetal heart failure can occur), vascular issues threatening fetal life in **twin** pregnancies (e.g., **twin-twin transfusion syndrome and TRAP sequence**), and **urinary tract obstructions** (e.g., **posterior urethral valves**). These surgical procedures have had variable success. For example, **congenital diaphragmatic hernias** that would result in pulmonary

hypoplasia have been corrected by opening the uterus, restoring the herniated viscera to the abdominal cavity, and repairing the fetal diaphragm (Fig. 6-15). However, based on clinical trials involving multiple cases and surgical centers, no survival benefit of fetal surgery over postnatal surgery has been found, so postnatal repair remains the accepted treatment. **Posterior urethral valves** (constriction of the lower urinary tract that prevents the urine produced by the kidneys from escaping) results in oligohydramnios and consequent fetal malformations, including pulmonary hypoplasia and

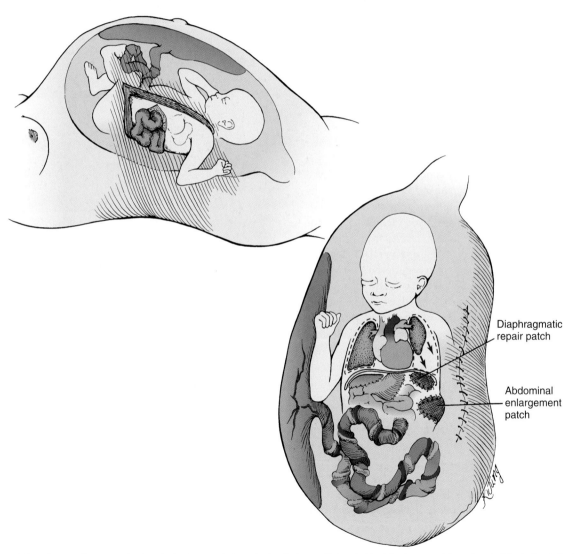

Diaphragmatic repair patch

Abdominal enlargement patch

Figure 6-15. Schematic illustration showing the in utero surgical repair of a diaphragmatic hernia. The fetus is exposed through an incision in the abdominal and uterine walls (brown, v-shaped area). The fetal viscera are retracted from the left pleural cavity, and the hole in the diaphragm is repaired with a Gore-Tex patch. The left lung now has room to grow normally. Because the fetal abdominal cavity is too small for the restored viscera, a second Gore-Tex enlargement patch is placed in the fetal abdominal wall.

defects of the face and limbs (discussed in "Clinical Taster" this chapter and in Ch. 15). The condition also damages the developing kidneys because of the backpressure of urine in the kidney tubules. Repair of the obstruction may prevent these problems and is now occurring more frequently. The efficacy of most of the other in utero surgical treatments is largely unknown, mainly because they have not been rigorously studied in a sufficiently large population, although some multicenter clinical trials are underway.

Drug intervention has been used to prevent **neural tube defects** and to treat **congenital adrenal** (suprarenal) **hyperplasia**, **methylmalonic acidemia**, and **multiple carboxylase deficiency**. Drugs can also help prevent **congenital heart block** (a problem in the conduction system of the fetal heart that can result in a slow heart rate and, eventually, heart failure). As discussed in Chapter 4, **prenatal folic acid supplementation** has been shown to prevent as many as two thirds of the expected cases of neural tube defects. Like folic acid supplementation, treatment of fetal disease involves treating the mother with substances that cross the placenta. In fetal congenital adrenal (suprarenal) hyperplasia (CAH), the mother is treated during her pregnancy with the potent corticosteroid **dexamethasone**. CAH is caused by a deficiency in the enzyme 21-hydroxylase, which results in a reduction of cortisol production by the suprarenal cortex and accumulation of 17-hydroxyprogesterone. This in turn results in suprarenal hyperplasia and excess production of suprarenal androgens (these are negatively regulated by the presence of cortisol). In female fetuses with CAH, external genitalia are masculinized (e.g., enlargement of the clitoris and fusion of the labia; Fig. 6-16; also discussed in Ch. 15). Female CAH fetuses are born with normal genitalia following appropriate maternal treatment with dexamethasone.

Dexamethasone is also being used to treat congenital heart block, especially in mothers with **lupus.** Lupus is a chronic inflammation caused by an autoimmune disease. Maternal antibodies present in lupus can affect the fetal cardiac conduction system and result in heart block (as discussed in this chapter, maternal antibodies can cross the placental). In addition, these antibodies can cause neonatal lupus. A clinical trial is currently underway to determine the efficacy of prenatal dexamethasone treatment in improving heart function and general health of newborns with neonatal lupus. Fetal drug therapy is also used to treat **heart arrhythmias** in fetuses. Drugs such as **digoxin** and

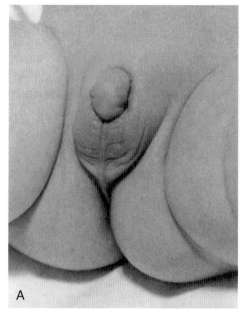

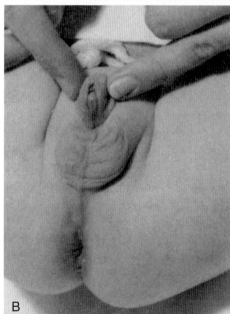

Figure 6-16. External genitalia in a newborn XX individual with congenital adrenal (suprarenal) hyperplasia. *A*, The clitoris is enlarged and the labia are partially fused as a scrotum-like structure. *B*, The urethral meatus is visible at the base of the enlarged clitoris.

propranolol, both of which cross the placenta, are given to the mother to treat arrhythmia in her unborn fetus.

Like CAH, methylmalonic acidemia and multiple carboxylase deficiency, involve deficiencies in fetal enzymes. In some types of methylmalonic acidemia, there is a deficiency of vitamin B_{12}, a coenzyme required for the conversion of methylmalonyl coenzyme A to succinyl coenzyme A. This deficiency results in increased methylmalonic acid excretion in maternal urine. Treatment involves maternal intravenous administration of **cyanocobalamin**, which markedly raises maternal serum B_{12} levels and presumably increases the amount of B_{12} available to the fetus. In multiple carboxylase deficiency there is a deficiency of the enzyme **biotinidase**. Unless treated, multiple carboxylase deficiency results in neonatal death from acidosis. Treatment involves maternal administration of the vitamin **biotin**, which readily crosses the placenta.

Fetal Cord Blood and Stem Cells

It may be feasible to apply the technique of gene therapy to correct some of the human genetic blood diseases in utero by using a procedure called **fetal liver transplant**. In preliminary trials, this procedure was used to treat fetuses that were diagnosed with diseases that severely cripple the white blood cells of the immune system (such as the disease suffered by the "boy in the bubble") or with **thalassemia** (a blood disease caused by a genetic error that prevents the synthesis of a protein involved in the production of hemoglobin). In these cases, cells from the fetal liver (i.e., the first major hematopoietic organ, as discussed in Ch. 13) were obtained from normal aborted fetuses and were infused via an ultrasound-guided needle into the umbilical vein of the affected fetus. These cells successfully colonized the liver of the developing fetus and proceeded to manufacture the missing protein, alleviating the disease. It is possible to transplant cells from one fetus to another because the immature fetal immune system does not reject foreign tissue. It is also possible to use umbilical cord blood for transplants such as these because this is an excellent source of hematopoietic stem cells.

For some disorders it may be advantageous to use gene therapy to correct an infant's own cells. For example, the infant's own umbilical cord may provide cells that can be appropriately transfected with genes, grown up, and reintroduced without rejection. The collection and storage of fetal cells from umbilical cords is called **cord blood banking**. Advantages of

the use of cord blood (compared with bone marrow or fetal liver) include (1) lack of discomfort during collection, (2) high recovery of viable **stem cells**, (3) rapid expansion of stem cells in culture, (4) high rate of recovery of viable stem cells after **cryopreservation**, (5) reduced graft vs host disease, and (6) efficiency of transfection with "corrected" genes. Umbilical cord blood has already been used in many human patients to treat diseases potentially curable with bone marrow transplants, including **severe combined immunodeficiency.**

The availability of cord blood banking has added another decision to the parenting process: Should we decide to bank cord blood in the event that my child needs it later—for example, to provide stem cells if he/she develops leukemia? And if so, should it be banked in a private or public repository. The former can be costly but guarantees that an exact genetic match will be available if the child ever needs the cells. The latter can be free and provides access to the cells to anyone who needs them if they are a genetic match. However, these cells will unlikely be available to the donor years later, so having an exact genetic match available is unlikely. Both cord blood-banking companies and the Academy of Pediatrics provide further information on the subject for parents' consideration (google under "cord blood banking").

Suggested Readings

Adzick NS, Walsh DS. 2003. Myelomeningocele: prenatal diagnosis, pathophysiology and management. Semin Pediatr Surg 12:168-174.

Agarwal SK, Fisk NM. 2001. In utero therapy for lower urinary tract obstruction. Prenat Diagn 21:970-976.

Anderson JL, Waller DK, Canfield MA, et al. 2005. Maternal obesity, gestational diabetes, and central nervous system birth defects. Epidemiology 16:87-92.

Askanase AD, Friedman DM, Copel J, et al. 2002. Spectrum and progression of conduction abnormalities in infants born to mothers with anti-SSA/Ro-SSB/La antibodies. Lupus 11:145-151.

Banek CS, Hecher K, Hackeloer BJ, Bartmann P. 2003. Long-term neurodevelopmental outcome after intrauterine laser treatment for severe twin-twin transfusion syndrome. Am J Obstet Gynecol 188:876-880.

Buyon JP, Clancy RM. 2003. Neonatal lupus syndromes. Curr Opin Rheumatol 15:535-541.

Buyon JP, Clancy RM. 2003. Neonatal lupus: review of proposed pathogenesis and clinical data from the US-based Research Registry for Neonatal Lupus. Autoimmunity 36:41-50.

Buyon JP, Clancy RM. 2005. Autoantibody-associated congenital heart block: TGFbeta and the road to scar. Autoimmun Rev 4:1-7.

Buyon JP, Rupel A, Clancy RM. 2004. Neonatal lupus syndromes. Lupus 13:705-712.

Cortes RA, Farmer DL. 2004. Recent advances in fetal surgery. Semin Perinatol 28:199-211.

Crombleholme TM, Coleman B, Hedrick H, et al. 2002. Cystic adenomatoid malformation volume ratio predicts outcome in prenatally diagnosed cystic adenomatoid malformation of the lung. J Pediatr Surg 37:331-338.

Crombleholme TM, Johnson MP. 2003. Fetoscopic surgery. Clin Obstet Gynecol 46:76-91.

Dickinson JE, Duncombe GJ, Evans SF, et al. 2005. The long term neurologic outcome of children from pregnancies complicated by twin-to-twin transfusion syndrome. Bjog 112:63-68.

Dickinson JE, Evans SF. 2000. Obstetric and perinatal outcomes from the Australian and New Zealand twin-twin transfusion syndrome registry. Am J Obstet Gynecol 182:706-712.

Duncombe GJ, Dickinson JE, Evans SF. 2003. Perinatal characteristics and outcomes of pregnancies complicated by twin-twin transfusion syndrome. Obstet Gynecol 101:1190-1196.

Evans MI. 2006. Stem cell therapy: moving towards reality. Am J Obstet Gynecol 194:662-663.

Evans MI, Britt DW. 2005. Fetal reduction. Semin Perinatol 29:321-329.

Evans MI, Krivchenia EL. 2001. Principles of screening. Clin Perinatol 28:273-278, vii.

Evans MI, Wapner RJ. 2001. Future directions. Clin Perinatol 28: 477-480, xi-x.

Evans MI, Wapner RJ. 2005. Invasive prenatal diagnostic procedures 2005. Semin Perinatol 29:215-218.

Evans MI, Harrison MR, Flake AW, Johnson MP. 2002. Fetal therapy. Best Pract Res Clin Obstet Gynaecol 16:671-683.

Evans MI, Krivchenia EL, Yaron Y. 2002. Screening. Best Pract Res Clin Obstet Gynaecol 16:645-657.

Evans MI, O'Brien JE, Dvorin E, et al. 2001. Second-trimester biochemical screening. Clin Perinatol 28:289-301.

Evans MI, Pryde PG, Reichler A, et al. 1993. Fetal drug therapy. West J Med 159:325-332.

Farmer D. 2003. Fetal surgery. BMJ 326:461-462.

Farmer DL, von Koch CS, Peacock WJ, et al. 2003. In utero repair of myelomeningocele: experimental pathophysiology, initial clinical experience, and outcomes. Arch Surg 138:872-878.

Feldman B, Hassan S, Kramer RL, et al. 1999. Amnioinfusion in the evaluation of fetal obstructive uropathy: the effect of antibiotic prophylaxis on complication rates. Fetal Diagn Ther 14:172-175.

Feldstein VA, Machin GA, Albanese CT, et al. 2000. Twin-twin transfusion syndrome: the 'Select' procedure. Fetal Diagn Ther 15:257-261.

Fisk NM, Galea P. 2004. Twin-twin transfusion—as good as it gets? N Engl J Med 351:182-184.

Gardiner HM, Taylor MJ, Karatza A, et al. 2003. Twin-twin transfusion syndrome: the influence of intrauterine laser photocoagulation on arterial distensibility in childhood. Circulation 107:1906-1911.

Golombeck K, Ball RH, Lee H, et al. 2006. Maternal morbidity after maternal-fetal surgery. Am J Obstet Gynecol 194:834-839.

Graf JL, Paek BW, Albanese CT, et al. 2000. Successful resuscitation during fetal surgery. J Pediatr Surg 35:1388-1389.

Harkness UF, Crombleholme TM. 2005. Twin-twin transfusion syndrome: where do we go from here? Semin Perinatol 29: 296-304.

Hedrick HL, Crombleholme TM, Flake AW, et al. 2004. Right congenital diaphragmatic hernia: Prenatal assessment and outcome. J Pediatr Surg 39:319-323; discussion 319–323.

Hedrick HL, Flake AW, Crombleholme TM, et al. 2004. Sacrococcygeal teratoma: prenatal assessment, fetal intervention, and outcome. J Pediatr Surg 39:430-438; discussion 430-438.

Herberg U, Gross W, Bartmann P, et al. 2006. Long term cardiac follow up of severe twin to twin transfusion syndrome after intrauterine laser coagulation. Heart 92:95-100.

Johnson JR, Rossi KQ, O'Shaughnessy RW. 2001. Amnioreduction versus septostomy in twin-twin transfusion syndrome. Am J Obstet Gynecol 185:1044-1047.

Karatza AA, Wolfenden JL, Taylor MJ, et al. 2002. Influence of twin-twin transfusion syndrome on fetal cardiovascular structure and function: prospective case-control study of 136 monochorionic twin pregnancies. Heart 88:271-277.

Keller RL, Hawgood S, Neuhaus JM, et al. 2004. Infant pulmonary function in a randomized trial of fetal tracheal occlusion for severe congenital diaphragmatic hernia. Pediatr Res 56:818-825.

Keswani SG, Crombleholme TM, Rychik J, et al. 2005. Impact of continuous intraoperative monitoring on outcomes in open fetal surgery. Fetal Diagn Ther 20:316-320.

Keswani SG, Johnson MP, Adzick NS, et al. 2003. In utero limb salvage: fetoscopic release of amniotic bands for threatened limb amputation. J Pediatr Surg 38:848-851.

Lim FY, Crombleholme TM, Hedrick HL, et al. 2003. Congenital high airway obstruction syndrome: natural history and management. J Pediatr Surg 38:940-945.

Lopriore E, Nagel HT, Vandenbussche FP, Walther FJ. 2003. Long-term neurodevelopmental outcome in twin-to-twin transfusion syndrome. Am J Obstet Gynecol 189:1314-1319.

Mackenzie TC, Crombleholme TM, Johnson MP, et al. 2002. The natural history of prenatally diagnosed conjoined twins. J Pediatr Surg 37:303-309.

Mari G, Detti L, Oz U, Abuhamad AZ. 2000. Long-term outcome in twin-twin transfusion syndrome treated with serial aggressive amnioreduction. Am J Obstet Gynecol 183:211-217.

Mari G, Roberts A, Detti L, et al. 2001. Perinatal morbidity and mortality rates in severe twin-twin transfusion syndrome: results of the International Amnioreduction Registry. Am J Obstet Gynecol 185:708-715.

Martinez-Frias ML, Frias JP, Bermejo E, et al. 2005. Pre-gestational maternal body mass index predicts an increased risk of congenital malformations in infants of mothers with gestational diabetes. Diabet Med 22:775-781.

Moise KJJr., Dorman K, Lamvu G, et al. 2005. A randomized trial of amnioreduction versus septostomy in the treatment of twin-twin transfusion syndrome. Am J Obstet Gynecol 193:701-707.

Pacheco-Alvarez D, Solorzano-Vargas RS, Gravel RA, et al. 2004. Paradoxical regulation of biotin utilization in brain and liver and implications for inherited multiple carboxylase deficiency. J Biol Chem 279:52312-52318.

Paek B, Goldberg JD, Albanese CT. 2003. Prenatal diagnosis. World J Surg 27:27-37.

Quintero RA, Chmait R, Dickinson J, et al. 2006. OP05.06: Quasi-randomized multicenter international clinical trial of amniocentesis versus laser therapy for stage III-IV twin-twin transfusion syndrome. Ultrasound Obstet Gynecol 28:450.

Quintero RA, Dickinson JE, Morales WJ, et al. 2003. Stage-based treatment of twin-twin transfusion syndrome. Am J Obstet Gynecol 188:1333-1340.

Rintoul NE, Sutton LN, Hubbard AM, et al. 2002. A new look at myelomeningoceles: functional level, vertebral level, shunting, and the implications for fetal intervention. Pediatrics 109:409-413.

Sanchis A, Cervero L, Bataller A, et al. 2005. Genetic syndromes mimic congenital infections. J Pediatr 146:701-705.

Santer R, Muhle H, Suormala T, et al. 2003. Partial response to biotin therapy in a patient with holocarboxylase synthetase deficiency: clinical, biochemical, and molecular genetic aspects. Mol Genet Metab 79:160-166.

Sbragia L, Paek BW, Feldstein VA, et al. 2001. Outcome of prenatally diagnosed solid fetal tumors. J Pediatr Surg 36:1244-1247.

Senat MV, Deprest J, Boulvain M, et al. 2004. Endoscopic laser surgery versus serial amnioreduction for severe twin-to-twin transfusion syndrome. N Engl J Med 351:136-144.

Sutcliffe AG, Sebire NJ, Pigott AJ, et al. 2001. Outcome for children born after in utero laser ablation therapy for severe twin-to-twin transfusion syndrome. Bjog 108:1246-1250.

Tan TY, Sepulveda W. 2003. Acardiac twin: a systematic review of minimally invasive treatment modalities. Ultrasound Obstet Gynecol 22:409-419.

Tsao K, Feldstein VA, Albanese CT, et al. 2002. Selective reduction of acardiac twin by radiofrequency ablation. Am J Obstet Gynecol 187:635-640.

Tsao K, Hawgood S, Vu L, et al. 2003. Resolution of hydrops fetalis in congenital cystic adenomatoid malformation after prenatal steroid therapy. J Pediatr Surg 38:508-510.

Walsh DS, Adzick NS. 2000. Fetal surgical intervention. Am J Perinatol 17:277-283.

Walsh DS, Adzick NS, Sutton LN, Johnson MP. 2001. The rationale for in utero repair of myelomeningocele. Fetal Diagn Ther 16:312-322.

Watkins ML, Rasmussen SA, Honein MA, et al. 2003. Maternal obesity and risk for birth defects. Pediatrics 111:1152-1158.

Woodward PJ, Kennedy A, Sohaey R, et al. 2005. Diagnostic Imaging Obstetrics. Salt Lake City, Utah: Amirsys.

6

Development of the Skin and Its Derivatives

7

Summary   The skin, or integument, consists of two layers: the **epidermis** and the **dermis**. The epidermis is formed mainly by the embryonic surface ectoderm, although it is also colonized by **melanocytes** (pigment cells) from neural crest cells and by **Langerhans cells**, which are immune cells of bone marrow origin. In addition, it contains pressure-sensing **Merkel cells**, which are derived from neural crest cells. The dermis of the trunk is a mesodermal tissue. The ventral dermis is derived mainly from the somatic layer of the lateral plate mesoderm, whereas the dorsal dermis is derived from the dermatome subdivision of the somites. The dermis of the head forms mostly from neural crest cells (discussed in Ch. 16).

After neurulation, the ectoderm, originally a single-cell layer thick, proliferates to produce an outer layer of simple squamous epithelium called the **periderm**. The inner layer of proliferating cells is now called the **basal layer**. In the 11th week, the basal layer produces a new **intermediate layer** between itself and the periderm. The basal layer is now called the **stratum germinativum**; this layer will continue to produce the epidermis throughout life. By the 21st week, the intermediate layer is replaced by the definitive three layers of the outer epidermis: the inner **stratum spinosum**, the middle **stratum granulosum**, and the outer **stratum corneum**, or **horny layer**. The cells of these layers are called **keratinocytes** because they contain the *Keratin* proteins characteristic of the epidermis. The layers of the epidermis represent a maturation series: keratinocytes produced by the stratum germinativum differentiate as they pass outward to form the two intermediate layers and the flattened, dead, *Keratin*-filled mature keratinocytes of the horny layer, which are finally sloughed from the surface of the skin. As the definitive epidermis develops, the overlying periderm is gradually shed into the amniotic fluid.

The dermis contains most of the tissues and structures of the skin, including blood vessels, nerves, muscle bundles, and most of the sensory structures. The superficial layer of the dermis develops projections called **dermal papillae**, which interdigitate with downward projections of the epidermis called **epidermal ridges**.

A number of specialized structures develop within the skin, including hair, nails, and a variety of epidermal glands. **Hair follicles** originate as rod-like downgrowths of the stratum germinativum into the dermis. The club-shaped base of each hair follicle is indented by a hillock of dermis called the **dermal papilla**, and the hair shaft is produced by the **germinal matrix** of ectoderm that overlies the dermal papilla. The various types of epidermal glands also arise as diverticula of the epidermis. Some bud from the neck of a hair follicle; others bud directly downward from the stratum germinativum. The four principal types of epidermal glands are the **sebaceous glands**, which secrete the oily sebum that lubricates the skin and hair; the **apocrine glands**, found in the axillae, pubic region, and other specific areas of skin that secrete odorous substances; the **sweat glands;** and the **mammary glands**. The primordia of the nails arise at the distal tips of the digits and then migrate around to the dorsal side. The nail plate grows from a specialized stratum germinativum located in the **nail fold** of epidermis that overlaps the proximal end of the nail primordium.

Tooth development also occurs in conjunction with development of the skin. The first sign of tooth development is the formation of a U-shaped epidermal ridge called the **dental lamina** along the crest of the upper and lower jaws. Twenty dental lamina downgrowths, which induce condensation of the underlying neural crest cell-derived mesenchyme, together form the **tooth buds** of the primary (deciduous) teeth. The secondary, permanent teeth are formed by secondary tooth buds that sprout from the primary buds. Soon after each tooth bud forms, its mesenchymal component forms a hillock-like **dental papilla** that indents the

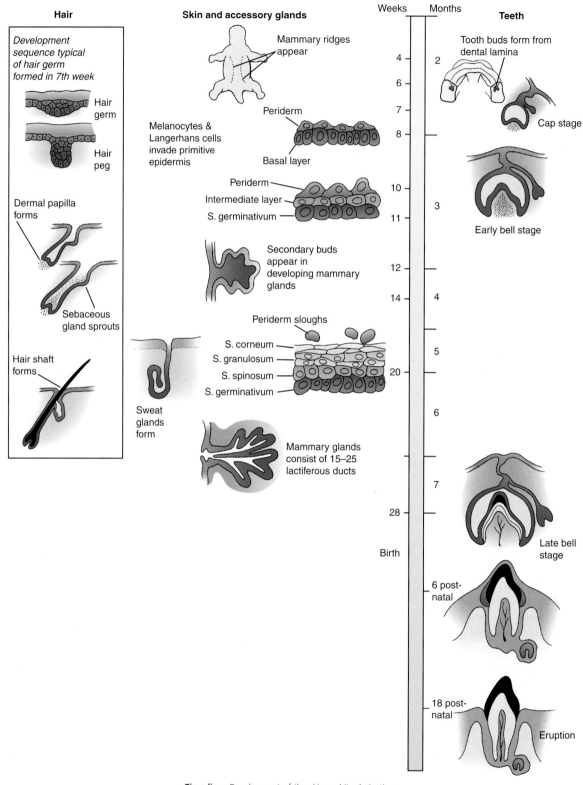

Time line. Development of the skin and its derivatives.

epithelial **enamel organ** formed from the bud. This stage of dental development is called the **cap stage** because the enamel organ sits on the papilla like a cap. By the 10th week, the dental lamina becomes a bell-shaped structure that completely covers the dental papilla. At the late **bell stage**, the cells of the enamel organ differentiate into enamel-producing **ameloblasts**, which begin to secrete organic matrix that mineralizes to form radially arranged prisms of enamel between themselves and the underlying papilla. The outermost cells of the papilla differentiate into **odontoblasts**, which secrete the dentin of the tooth. The inner cells of the dental papilla give rise to the tooth pulp. Nerves and blood vessels gain access to the pulp through the tips of the tooth roots.

| **Clinical Taster** | You are a pediatrician following a 3½-year-old girl with chronic constipation that started around the beginning of "potty training." You get a message from your answering service that the patient's mother |

called during the night from the emergency room. Apparently, they rushed the girl to the hospital in the late evening when they found that she had rectal prolapse (protrusion of the rectum out through the anus) after straining to stool.

You see the girl with her mother later that day for follow-up. The girl was seen by a surgeon in the emergency room who had reduced the prolapsed rectum without surgery and prescribed an enema and stool softeners. The surgeon had mentioned to the family that their pediatrician would talk to them about conditions like cystic fibrosis that can be associated with rectal prolapse, and would arrange to test for such conditions.

While examining the toddler's abdomen for impacted stool, you notice that she has pale, velvety skin and an unusual number of bruises and atrophic scars (widened paper-like scars) on her shins. The mother reminds you that the girl was born one month premature after her "water broke early" and that she was a "floppy" baby who starting walking late. Her mother states that the girl inherited her father's "double jointedness," and the girl proceeds to demonstrate just how flexible her joints are (Fig. 7-1). You also find her skin to be hyperextensible.

You tell the mother that testing for cystic fibrosis is certainly reasonable, but that you suspect the diagnosis of **Ehlers-Danlos syndrome (EDS)**, which is a hereditary connective tissue disorder. EDS is actually a group of disorders caused by mutations in several genes involved in the formation of the structural components of skin and joints. Classical EDS is caused by mutations in *COLLAGEN TYPE* I and V genes. You reassure the mother that her daughter's condition can be managed by restricting certain types of activities and by monitoring for more significant complications like dilation of the aortic root.

Origin of Epidermis and Dermis of Skin

Surface Ectoderm Forms Epidermis

The surface ectoderm covering of the embryo is initially a single-cell layer thick. After neurulation in the 4th week, the surface ectoderm proliferates to form a new outer layer of simple squamous epithelium called the **periderm** (Fig. 7-2A). The underlying layer of proliferating cells is now called the **basal layer** and is separated from the dermis by the basement membrane containing *Collagens*, *Laminin*, and *Fibronectin*. The cells of the periderm are gradually sloughed into the amniotic fluid. The periderm is normally shed completely by the 21st week, but in some fetuses it persists until birth, forming a "shell" or "cocoon" around the newborn infant that is removed by the physician or

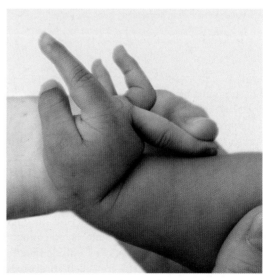

Figure 7-1. Demonstration of painless hyperflexibility of the right third metacarpal-phalangeal joint in a child.

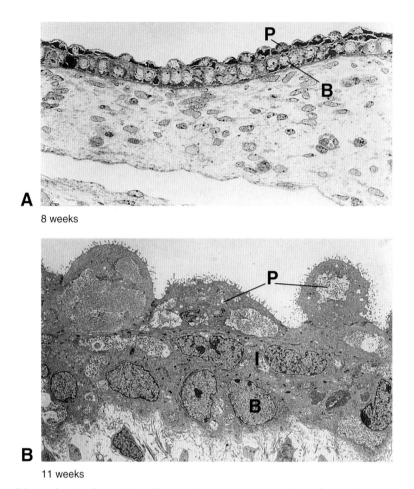

A
8 weeks

B
11 weeks

Figure 7-2. Differentiation of the ectoderm into the primitive epidermis. *A*, Between 8 and 9 weeks, the surface ectoderm has begun to proliferate to form a periderm layer (P). The proliferating layer is now called the basal layer (B). *B*, By week 11, the basal layer (B) produces an intermediate layer (I) while a complete but irregular outer layer of periderm (P) is still apparent.

shed spontaneously during the first weeks of life. These babies are called **collodion babies**.

In the 11th week, proliferation of the basal layer produces a new **intermediate layer** just deep to the periderm (Fig. 7-2*B*). This layer is the forerunner of the outer layers of the mature epidermis. The basal layer, now called the **germinative layer** or **stratum germinativum**, constitutes the layer of stem cells that will continue to replenish the epidermis throughout life. The cells of the intermediate layer contain the *Keratin* proteins characteristic of differentiated epidermis; therefore, these cells are called **keratinocytes**.

During the early part of the 5th month, at about the time that the periderm is shed, the intermediate layer is replaced by the three definitive layers of

keratinocytes: the inner **stratum spinosum** (or **spinous layer**), the middle **stratum granulosum** (or **granular layer**), and the outer **stratum corneum** (or **horny** or **cornified layer**) (Figs. 7-3, 7-4). This transformation, which involves **apoptosis (programmed cell death)**, begins at the cranial end of the fetus and proceeds caudally. The layers of the epidermis represent a maturational series: presumptive keratinocytes are constantly produced by the stratum germinativum, they differentiate as they pass outward to the stratum corneum, and, finally, they are sloughed from the surface of the skin.

The cells of the stratum germinativum are the only dividing cells of normal epidermis. These cells contain a dispersed network of primary *Keratin* filaments specific

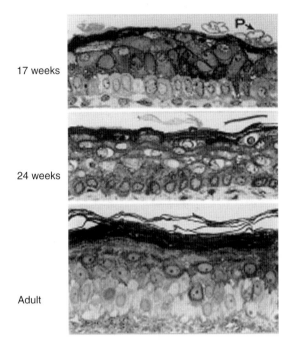

17 weeks

24 weeks

Adult

Figure 7-3. Differentiation of the mature epidermis. The periderm (P) is sloughed during the 4th month and normally is absent by week 21. The definitive epidermal layers, including the stratum spinosum, stratum granulosum, and stratum corneum, begin to develop during the 5th month.

IN THE RESEARCH LAB

MOLECULAR REGULATION OF SKIN DIFFERENTIATION

The "decision" of a cell in the stratum germinativum to remain in the pool of proliferating cells or to move into the stratum spinosum and begin differentiating is regulated by autocrine and paracrine factors. Cells in the stratum germinativum secrete *Interleukin 1* (a cytokine), which induces the expression of *Granulocyte macrophage colony stimulating factor* (*Gm-csf*) and *Fgf7* in the underlying dermis. *Gm-csf* and *Fgf7* signal back to the keratinocytes, promoting proliferation and differentiation.

The transcription factor *p63* is expressed in the stratum germinativum and regulates cell proliferation, the expression of cell-adhesion molecules, and differentiation. In the *p63* mouse mutant, ectodermal development is normal until E13.5, at which point the developing epidermis would normally start to stratify. Stratification does not occur in the *p63* null mouse and at birth the epidermis is almost entirely absent (Fig. 7-5). *Notch* signaling, which has the highest activity in the stratum germinativum, is needed for cell cycle exit (by inducing *p21* expression) and differentiation of the spinous layer, including the induction of expression of *Keratins Krt1* and *Krt10* and *Involucrin* (see Fig. 7-4). Therefore, loss of *Notch* function results in excess cell proliferation. *p63* upregulates the expression of the *Notch* ligands *Jagged 1* and *2* in the stratum germinativum.

Interferon regulatory factor 6 (*Ifr6*) and the kinase *Ikkα* (mutations in the related human kinase *IKKγ/NEMO* are

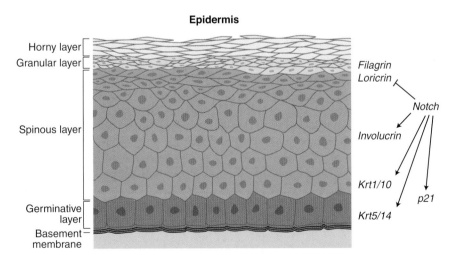

Figure 7-4. Differential expression of *Keratins* and envelope proteins during differentiation of the skin. The first stages of differentiation are induced by *Notch* signaling, whereas the last stages are inhibited by *Notch*.

discussed in the following "In the Clinic") are needed for the next phase of skin development, the formation of the granular and horny layers. In their absence, the germinativum and spinous layers are hyperproliferative, and do not differentiate further. In contrast to *Irf6* and *Ikkα*, *Notch* signaling represses formation of the granular layer by inhibiting the onset of *Filaggrin* and *Loricrin* expression (see Fig. 7-4).

IN THE CLINIC

INHERITED SKIN DISEASES

Inherited skin diseases can be caused by mutations in *Transglutaminases*, envelope proteins, desmosomes, *Keratins*, *Connexins*, and *Proteases*, as well as by abnormalities in lipid metabolism. In the adult, imbalances in this complex dynamic control system can also result in skin disorders. For example, excessive levels of *TRANSFORMING GROWTH FACTOR-α* can result in **psoriasis** and other hyperproliferative skin diseases.

The structural integrity of the epidermis is critical to its function and is achieved in part by the assembly of cell-type specific *Keratins* and desmosomal proteins into a network that provides tensile strength to the epithelium. Mutations in *Keratins* and desmosomal proteins lead to **skin fragility syndromes** that manifest as blistering or separation of the epidermis at the level at which the mutated gene plays a critical role in adhesion. To date more than 400 **KERATIN** (*KRT*) mutations have been reported. For example, dominant-negative mutations in genes encoding *KRT5* and *KRT14*, specifically expressed in the stratum germinativum, cause **epidermal bullosa simplex** (EBS), in which the germinativum is exceptionally fragile and leads to blistering. The most severe form, **Dowling-Meara EBS**, can be life threatening for neonates. In contrast, mutations in genes encoding *KRT1* or *KRT10* are associated with **bullous congenital ichthyosiform erythroderma** and cause blistering in the suprabasal layers and also reddening of the skin. However, because the stratum germinativum, which contains the stem cell population, is intact, with time the blistering resolves to form thickened ichthyotic skin (discussed in next paragraph) resulting from excessive proliferation of the germinativum. Mutations in genes encoding *DESMOPLAKIN*, a component of the desmosome cell adhesion complex, or the associated proteins, *DESMOGLEINS 1* and *4* and *PLAKOPHILIN 1*, also result in skin fragility defects (Fig. 7-6). Similarly, mutations in *Laminin β3*, a component of the basement membrane, cause blistering skin defects due to abnormal germinativum cell adherence in **junctional epidermolysis bullosa.**

A number of heritable disorders result in excessive keratinization of the skin, or **ichthyosis.** For example, infants suffering from **lamellar ichthyosis** have skin that cannot be shed properly and scales off in flakes, sometimes over the whole body. Due to the excess skin, these infants can be born as collodion babies (i.e., encased in a shiny thin film). **Lamellar ichthyosis** can be the result of mutations in *TRANSGLUTAMINASE 1*, the enzyme required for cornification; infants affected by the disorder also have permeability defects and require special care but are usually viable. **Harlequin fetuses**, in contrast, have rigid, deeply cracked skin and usually die shortly after birth. These babies have defects in the mechanisms that bundle keratin fibers and regulate formation of lamellar granules in the cells of the stratum granulosum. As a consequence, keratinocytes do not mature properly and cannot be sloughed from the surface of the stratum corneum.

Because different ectodermal areas express unique combinations of *Keratins*, mutations in a particular *keratin* can have regionalized effects. Mutations in *KRT3* and *KRT12*, the corneal-specific *Keratins*, result in **Meesmann epithelial corneal dystrophy**, which is characterized by cell fragility and the formation of cysts. On the other hand, mutations in *KRT4* and *KRT13* cause **white sponge naevus**, a syndrome that affects the oral keratinocytes and is characterized by the formation of patches of loose, white epithelium. *KRT9* is expressed specifically in the palms of the hands and soles of the feet, and mutation in *KRT9* thus results in **epidermolytic palmoplantar keratoderma**, the thickening of the skin in the hands and feet.

Defects in the skin can be **mosaic** within an area. This is demonstrated by skin defects that follow the **lines of Blaschko** (originally described in 1901 by the German dermatologist Alfred Blaschko), which can occur in several human syndromes, such as **hypohidrotic ectodermal dysplasia** (see below) and X-linked **incontinentia pigmenti.** The latter syndrome is caused by mutations in *IkBKG*, the product of which is called IKKγ/NEMO. In this syndrome, the mutant cells are eliminated by apoptosis induced by the cytokine *Tumor necrosis factor-α*. These defects occur as "M-" or "V"-shaped patterns on the abdomen and back, as proximally and distally oriented lines along the limbs, and as anteriorly and posteriorly curved lines along the face. These lines/patches of malformed skin reflect a common origin resulting from a defect in the development of a progenitor cell (e.g., following X-inactivation or somatic mutation). Basal cell carcinoma and common dermatologic disorders such as psoriasis and eczema can also occur in these patterns.

Control   *p63* ablated

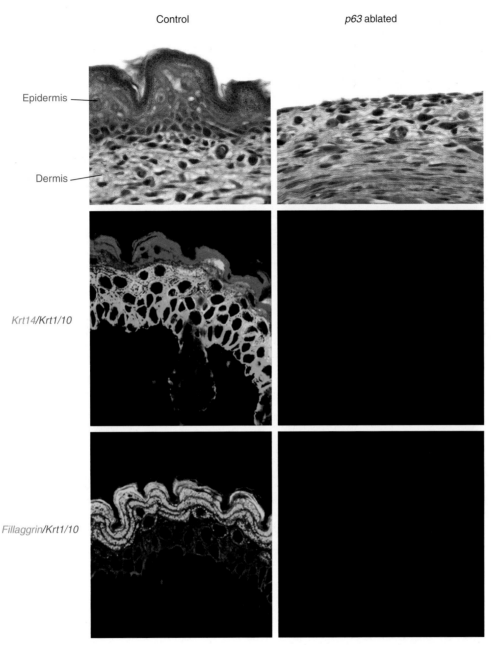

Epidermis

Dermis

Krt14/Krt1/10

Fillaggrin/Krt1/10

Figure 7-5. The absence of skin differentiation in mice following loss of the transcription factor *p63*.

to this layer, such as *K5* and *K14*, and are connected by cell-to-cell membrane junctions called **desmosomes.** Together with adherens junctions, desmosomes provide a tight, impervious structure resistant to water uptake or loss and infection (see Fig. 7-4). In addition, desmosomes help to distribute force evenly over the epidermis. Cells of the stratum germinativum are connected to the basement membrane by hemidesmosomes, which contain *Integrins*. This attachment is essential for cell survival and determines the orientation of cell divisions. As the cells in the stratum germinativum move into the overlying stratum spinosum (four to eight cells thick; see Fig. 7-4), the *K5* and K14 intermediate filaments are replaced by two secondary *Keratin* proteins, *K1* and *K10*. These are crosslinked by disulphide bonds to provide further strength.

199

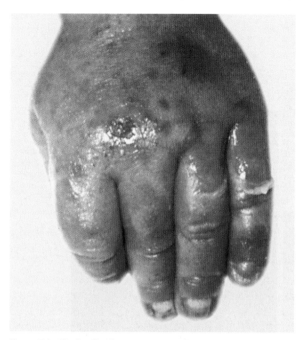

Figure 7-6. Skin fragility due to mutation in the *PLAKOPHILIN* gene.

Once the cells have moved into the stratum granulosum, they produce **envelope proteins** such as *Involucrin*, *Loricrin*, and *Envoplakin*, which line the inner surface of the plasma membrane, and the enzyme *Transglutaminase*, which crosslinks the envelope proteins. This layer also produces a protein called *Filaggrin*, which aggregates with the *Keratin* filaments to form tight bundles, helping to flatten the cell. Lipid-containing granules (**lamellar granules**) are

also produced that help seal the skin. Finally, in the process called **cornification**, lytic enzymes are released within the cell, metabolic activity ceases, and enucleation occurs, resulting in the loss of cell contents including the nucleus. Consequently, the keratinocytes that enter the stratum corneum are flattened, scalelike, and terminally differentiated keratinocytes, or **squames**.

In addition to keratinocytes, the epidermis contains a few types of less abundant cells, including melanocytes, Langerhans cells, and Merkel cells. As mentioned in Chapter 4, the pigment cells, or **melanocytes**, of the skin differentiate from neural crest cells that detach from the neural tube in the 6th week and migrate to the developing epidermis. Although morphologic and histochemical studies do not detect melanocytes in the human epidermis until the 10th to 11th weeks, studies using monoclonal antibodies directed against antigens characteristic of melanocyte precursors have identified these cells in the epidermis as early as the 6th to 7th weeks (Fig. 7-7A). Thus, it may take neural crest cells only a few days to a week to migrate to the epidermis. Melanocytes are also found in the dermis during fetal life, but the vast majority of these are probably in transit to the epidermis.

The density of melanocytes increases during fetal life, reaching a peak of about 2300 cells/mm^3 at the end of the 3rd month, after which melanocyte density drops to the final value of about 800 cells/mm^3. Melanocytes represent between 5% and 10% of the cells of the epidermis in the adult. In the 10th week, many melanocytes become associated with developing hair follicles (discussed later in the chapter), where they function to donate pigment to the hairs.

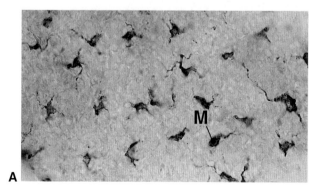

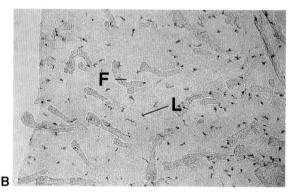

Figure 7-7. Specialized cells of the epidermis. *A*, Melanocytes (M) first appear in the embryonic epidermis during the 6th and 7th weeks. *B*, Langerhans cells (L) migrate into the epidermis from the bone marrow starting in the seventh week. F, hair follicle.

Melanocytes function as a sunscreen, protecting the deeper layers of the skin from solar radiation, which can cause not only sunburn but also, in the long run, cancer. Unfortunately, melanocytes themselves are relatively likely to produce tumors. Most of these remain benign, but sometimes they give rise to the highly malignant type of cancer called **melanoma**.

Langerhans cells are the macrophage immune cells of the skin, functioning both in contact sensitivity (allergic skin reactions) and in immune surveillance against invading microorganisms. They arise in the bone marrow and first appear in the epidermis by the 7th week (Fig. 7-7*B*). Langerhans cells continue to migrate into the epidermis throughout life.

Merkel cells are pressure-detecting mechanoreceptors that lie at the base of the epidermis and are associated with underlying nerve endings in the dermis. They contain keratin and form desmosomes with adjacent keratinocytes. They arise from neural crest cells and appear in the 4th to 6th months.

Mesoderm Forms Dermis, Except in the Head

The dermis, or **corium**—the layer of skin that underlies the epidermis and contains blood vessels, hair follicles, nerve endings, sensory receptors, and so forth—is a tissue with a triple embryonic origin. In the trunk, the majority of the dermis is derived from the somatic layer of the lateral plate mesoderm, but part of it is derived from the dermatomal divisions of the somites (discussed in Ch. 8). In contrast, in the head most of the dermis is derived from neural crest cells, and thus originates from ectoderm.

During the 3rd month, the outer layer of the developing dermis proliferates to form ridgelike **dermal papillae** that protrude into the overlying epidermis (Fig. 7-8). The intervening protrusions of the epidermis into the dermis are called **epidermal ridges**. This superficial region of the dermis is called the **papillary layer**, whereas the thick underlying layer of dense,

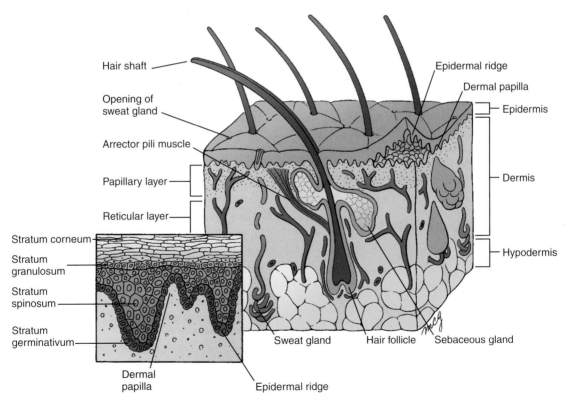

Figure 7-8. Definitive organization of the dermis and epidermis. The pattern of interdigitating dermal papillae and epidermal ridges first develops during the 3rd month. Sebaceous glands develop from the epidermal lining of the hair follicles, appearing about 1 month after a given hair bud is formed.

irregular connective tissue is called the **reticular layer**. The dermis is underlain by subcutaneous fatty connective tissue called the **hypodermis (subcorium)**. The dermis differentiates into its definitive form in the 2nd and 3rd trimesters, although it is thin at birth and thickens progressively through infancy and childhood.

The pattern of external ridges and grooves produced in the skin by the dermal papillae varies from one part of the body to another. The palmar and plantar surfaces of the hands and feet carry a familiar pattern of whorls and loops, the eyelids have a diamond-shaped pattern, and the ridges on the upper surface of the trunk resemble a cobweb. The first skin ridges to appear are the whorls on the palmar and plantar surfaces of the digits, which develop in the 11th and 12th weeks. The entire system of surface patterns is established early in the 5th month of fetal life. Thereafter, each patch of skin retains its characteristic pattern even if it is transplanted to a different part of the body.

Blood vessels form within the subcutaneous mesenchyme, deep to the developing dermis, in the 4th week. These branch to form a single layer of vessels in the dermis by the late 6th week and two parallel planes of vessels by the 8th week. Branches of these vessels follow nerves within the dermis and enter the papillary layer to become associated with the hair follicles. These branches may disappear and reappear during different stages of hair follicle differentiation.

It is estimated that the skin of the neonate contains 20 times more blood vessels than it needs to support its own metabolism. This excess is required for thermoregulation. Much of the definitive vasculature of the skin develops in the first few weeks after birth.

Development of Skin Derivatives

In many regions of the body, the skin gives rise to specialized structures that have a number of functions. The **sebaceous glands** produce sebum, an oily substance that protects the skin against friction and dehydration; the **hair** and **sweat glands** are involved in heat regulation; the **teeth** and **salivary glands** (discussed in Ch. 16) are essential for mastication; and the **lacrimal glands** produce tears. The **mammary gland** in females provides both nutrition and a source of immunity for the breastfeeding infant.

Development of all of these skin derivatives depends on **epithelial-mesenchymal interactions**. All are characterized by the development of an ectodermal placode, followed by condensation of cells in the underlying mesenchyme, and then invagination of the epithelium into the underlying dermis.

In addition, the development of skin derivatives requires many common pathways. Misexpression of the *Wnt* antagonist *Dkk1* arrests development at the placode stage of all the ectodermal derivatives analyzed (hair, tooth, and mammary gland). Loss of function of *Ectodysplasin* (*Eda*), its receptor (*Edar*), components of the signaling pathway (e.g., *Edaradd*), or *p63* in mice affects all the ectodermal derivatives (see the following "In the Clinic"). Misexpression of *Eda* using a *Keratin* promoter can also induce the formation of ectopic hair, nipples, and teeth. The *Hedgehog* and *Fgf* signaling pathways are also used during the development of the majority, if not all, of the ectodermal derivatives.

Recombination experiments between the dermis and ectoderm have shown that the dermis specifies the shape and pattern of the ectodermal derivative. Therefore, mammary dermis will induce ectopic mammary glands when recombined with ventral back ectoderm. Salivary gland mesenchyme will also induce the mammary gland epithelium to form many branches characteristic of salivary glands, rather than forming a duct, although the mammary epithelium retains its original differentiation characteristics. This role of the dermis in patterning is also illustrated in Chapter 16, which discusses how neural crest cells determine the pattern of feathers in birds, as well as the rate of feather growth (see Fig. 16-17C).

IN THE CLINIC

ANOMALIES OF SKIN DERIVATIVES

Mutations in the transmembrane protein, *ECTODYSPLASIN* (*EDA*), its receptor (*EDAR*), or components of this signaling pathway (*Edaradd*, *Ikkγ*/*Nemo*) result in **hypohidrotic ectodermal dysplasia (HED)**, which affects many, if not all, of the ectodermal derivatives (Fig. 7-9). *EDA* is a member of the *TNF* (*TUMOR NECROSIS FACTOR*) family of cytokines. In patients with hypohidrotic ectodermal dysplasia, hair is absent or thin; nails, sweat, and sebaceous glands are hypoplastic; skin is dry; and the teeth are absent, malformed, and/or small. Hypohidrotic ectodermal dysplasia can be life threatening, as it sometimes is in children with HED who are unable to sweat and are thus susceptible to

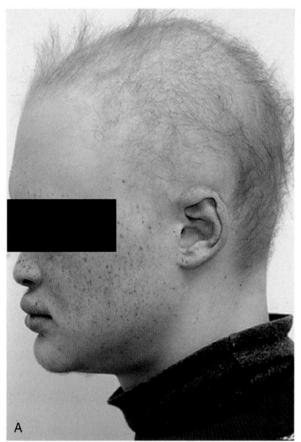

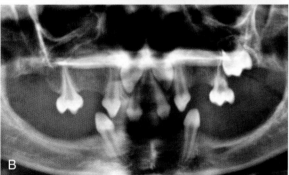

Figure 7-9. Sparse hair and dental abnormalities are characteristics of hypohidrotic ectodermal dysplasia. *A*, Patient from lateral view. *B*, X-ray of teeth.

febrile seizures and hyperthermia during hot weather. Four known mouse mutants mimic this syndrome: *tabby* (*Eda* mutation), *downless* (*Edar* mutation), *sleek* (*Edar* mutation), and *crinkle* (*Edaradd* mutation). In *tabby* mice, injection of *Eda* protein into a pregnant mother can prevent the majority of the defects in the mutant embryos.

Mutations in the transcription factor *TUMOR PROTEIN P73-LIKE* (*TP73L*; also known as *P63*) result in several syndromes that affect ectodermally derived structures. Examples include **ADULT** (a̲c̲ro-d̲ermato-u̲ngual-l̲acrimal-t̲ooth) syndrome, **ectrodactyly ectodermal dysplasia-cleft lip/palate**, or **a̲nkyloblepharon-e̲ctodermal dysplasia c̲lefting syndrome** (AEC, also called Hay-Wells syndrome). Ankyloblepharon is the fusion of the eyelids.

However, the different ectodermal derivatives can also be differentially affected in syndromes. Mutation in the homeobox gene *DLX3* causes **tricho-dento-osseous syndrome**, affecting the hair and teeth. Additionally, the skull bones of those affected by this syndrome have an abnormally high density. In **nail-tooth dysplasia**, which is the result of mutations in the homeobox gene *MSX1*, nail and teeth are dysplastic. On the other hand, in the rare syndrome **hypotrichosis-lymphedema-telangiectasia**, which results from a mutation in the transcription factor *SOX18*, hair is the only abnormal ectodermal derivative.

Development of Hair

Hair follicles first appear at the end of the 2nd month on the eyebrows, eyelids, upper lip, and chin. Hair follicles do not appear in other regions until the 4th month. Most, if not all, hair follicles are present by the 5th month, and it is believed that novel hair follicles do not form after birth. About 5 million hair follicles develop in both males and females. The differences between the two sexes in the distribution of various kinds of hairs are caused by the different concentrations of circulating sex steroid hormones.

The hair follicle first appears as a small concentration of ectodermal cells, called a **hair germ**, in the basal layer of the primitive, two-layered epidermis (Fig. 7-10*A*). Hair germs are thought to be induced by the underlying dermis. The hair germ recruits dermal cells to form a dermal condensate that promotes further differentiation of the hair germ. The hair germ proliferates to form a rodlike **hair peg** that pushes down into the dermis (Fig. 7-10*B-F*). Within the dermis, the tip of the hair peg expands, forming a **bulbous hair peg**, and the dermis cells just beneath the tip of the bulb proliferate to form a small hillock called the **dermal papilla**. About four weeks after the hair germ begins to grow, the dermal papilla invaginates into the expanded base of the hair bulb (see Fig. 7-10*E*, *F*). Except in the case of the eyebrows and eyelashes, the dermal root sheath of the follicle becomes associated with a bundle of smooth muscle cells called

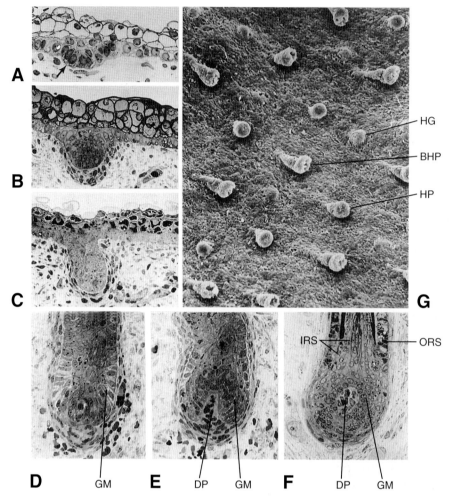

Figure 7-10. Development of the hair follicle. *A,* Hair germ at 80 days. *B,* Elongating hair germ later in the 1st trimester. *C,* Hair peg in the 2nd trimester. *D-F,* Development of the follicle base from the elongated hair peg stage to the bulbous hair peg stage. The dermal papilla (DP) invaginates into the base of the developing follicle, inducing the germinal matrix (GM). In *F,* the hair shaft can be seen growing up the center of the follicle, and the inner and outer epidermal root sheaths (IRS and ORS) are differentiating. *G,* Scanning electron micrograph of the undersurface of the developing epidermis, showing hair germs (HG), hair pegs (HP), and bulbous hair pegs (BHP) growing into the dermis (epidermis was removed from the dermis in the preparation to show the deep side of the epidermis).

the **arrector pili** muscle, which functions to erect the hair (making goose flesh) (see Fig. 7-8). The stem cells of the follicular epithelium that regenerate the follicle periodically during postnatal life are found near the site of the attachment of the arrector pili muscle in the **bulge** (Fig. 7-11; also discussed in Ch. 10). There are four phases of hair growth. These consist of a growth phase (**anagen**), regression phase (**catagen**), resting phase (**telogen**), and shedding phase (**exogen**).

The layer of proliferating ectoderm that overlies the dermal papilla in the base of the hair bulb becomes the **germinal matrix**. The germinal matrix is responsible for producing the hair shaft (see Fig. 7-10*D-F*): proliferation of the germinal matrix produces cells that undergo a specialized process of keratinization and are added to the base of the hair shaft. The growing hair shaft is thus pushed outward through the follicular canal. If the hair is to be colored, the maturing keratinocytes incorporate pigment

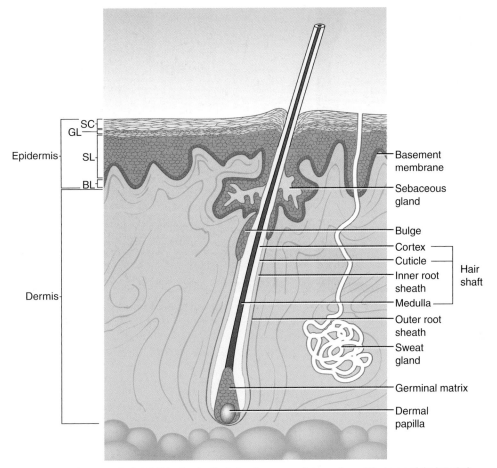

Figure 7-11. Structure of a hair follicle showing the bulge, the source of stem cells, and the layers of the hair shaft.

produced by the melanocytes of the hair bulb. The epidermal cells lining the follicular canal constitute the **inner** and **outer epidermal root sheaths** (see Fig. 7-10F).

The first generation of hairs formed is fine and unpigmented and are collectively called **lanugo**. These hairs first appear during the 12th week. They are mostly shed before birth and are replaced by coarser hairs during the perinatal period. Postnatally, there are two types of hair, the **vellus**—the nonpigmented hairs that do not project deep into the dermis—and the **terminal hairs**—pigmented hairs that penetrate into the fatty dermal tissues. At puberty, the rising levels of sex hormones cause the fine body hair to be replaced by coarser hairs on some parts of the body: the axilla and pubis of both sexes, the face, and (in some races) the chest and back of males.

IN THE RESEARCH LAB

REGULATION OF HAIR PATTERNING AND DIFFERENTIATION

Establishment of the hair placode requires *Eda/Edar* and *Wnt* signaling, and misexpression of *Eda* or *Wnt* components (e.g., *β-Catenin*, *Lef-1*) induces formation of ectopic placodes. Conversely blocking *Edar/Wnt* signaling prevents placode formation. *Eda* signaling is active in the ectoderm, whereas *Wnt* signaling is active first in the ectodermal placode and then in the underlying mesenchyme (Fig. 7-12). Spacing of hair follicles is controlled by an interplay of *Eda/Wnts*, with several other secreted factors, including *Fgfs*, *Follistatin*, and *Tgfβ2*, which all promote placode development. In contrast, *Bmp/Tgfβ1* signaling inhibits placode development. Patterning of the hair follicles may also be influenced by *Wnt* signaling via the **planar cell**

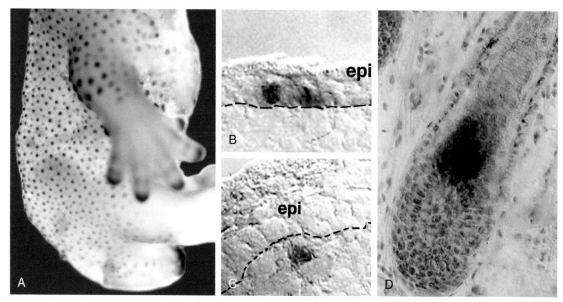

Figure 7-12. *Shh* and *Wnt* signaling pathways are active in the early development and morphogenesis of the hair follicle. **A**, *Ptc1* expression, indicative of active *Shh* signaling, in the hair placodes. **B–D**, Regions of *Wnt/β-Catenin* signaling: first in ectoderm **B**, subsequently in the mesenchyme in the forming germinal matrix **C**, and then in the differentiating hair shaft **D**.

polarity pathway (discussed in Ch. 5). In the *Frizzled 6* (a *Wnt* receptor) knockout mouse, the hairs and hair whorls are randomized and misoriented. This is analogous to the key role of *Frizzled* signaling in Drosophila during the specification of the orientation of bristles and the ommatidia of the eye. Once the placode has been established, the ectoderm invaginates to form the early hair follicle; this process is controlled by *Shh*, which is mitogenic (see Fig. 7-12). *Shh* also signals to the underlying dermal papillae. In *Shh* mouse mutants, hair development is arrested at the early peg stage.

An individual hair consists of the hair shaft and the outer (or external) and inner (or internal) root sheaths (see Figs. 7-10, 7-11). The hair shaft consists of three concentric layers: cuticle, cortex, and medulla (from outside to inside). The hair shaft and inner root sheath are keratinized. Studies of hair follicle development have shown that the progenitor cells or stem cells arise in the **bulge** (also discussed in Ch. 10 in relation to the origin of peripheral nervous system stem cells), which lies just below the sebaceous gland (see Fig. 7-11). Cells from the bulge migrate downwards into the matrix of the hair follicle and upwards towards the sebaceous gland. Fate mapping studies have shown that these progenitors can also contribute to the epidermis following wounding. In the matrix, the cells proliferate under the influence of *Shh* before undergoing terminal

differentiation. *Bmp* and *Wnt* signaling are also active in the hair shaft precursors and induce the formation of the hair shaft (see Fig. 7-12). Blocking *Bmp* signaling with the *Bmp* antagonist, *Noggin*, prevents hair shaft differentiation. Similarly, in *Lef1* mouse mutants, the few hairs that develop are not keratinized appropriately. Differentiation of the inner root sheath requires *Gata3* and *Notch* signaling, whereas the transcription factor *Sox9* is required for outer root sheath differentiation. *FoxN1*, a transcription factor mutated in the *nude* mouse and in a rare human syndrome, is required for keratinization. A consequence of this mutation is that hairs develop but they do not penetrate through the epidermis. Therefore, mouse *FoxN1* mutants are nude, that is, they lack hair. Humans with a mutation in this gene lack nails and all hair, including the eyelashes and eyebrows, and are subject to immune disorders.

IN THE CLINIC

HAIR ANOMALIES

Hair abnormalities can range from **hypertrichosis** (excess hair) to **atrichia** (congenital absence of hair) to structural/morphologic defects. In addition, hair abnormalities can arise from 1) hair cycle defects, the most common cause of hair abnormalities in humans; 2) immunologic defects in which the skin and hair proteins become targets of the immune system; and 3) sebaceous gland abnormalities. In women, at puberty vellus hairs can be transformed into terminal hairs, for example, on the upper lip and lower leg. This is known as **Hirsutism**.

Defective hair development can encompass all stages of hair differentiation. Like in the skin, mutations can occur in signaling pathways, *Proteases*, gap-junctions, and structural proteins such as desmosomes and *Keratins*. In **hypohidrotic ectodermal dysplasia** (discussed in the preceding "In the Clinic"), which affects the *EDA/EDAR* signaling pathway, the first stage of hair development (formation of the hair placode) does not occur. In contrast, mutations in structural proteins such *PLAKOPHILIN 1* and *DESMOPLAKIN 1* (both desmosomal proteins) and *KERATINS* affect differentiation and morphogenesis of the hair. For example, mutations in the hair *KERATINS KRTHB6* and *KRTHB1* result in **monilethrix**, in which the hair is "beaded" and fragile, and thus easily lost. Mutations in *DESMOPLAKIN 1* cause skin fragility and wooly hair.

Finally, as the hair goes through the phases of cyclic regeneration (i.e., anagen, catagen, telogen, and exogen; as discussed earlier in the chapter), a variety of stressors or illnesses (e.g., chemotherapy and pregnancy) can shift the hair cycle toward the telogen phase, resulting in excessive hair shedding—called **telogen effluvium**—several months later. Normally, during catagen, apoptosis of the matrix cells in the bulb and outer root sheath prevents further growth of the hair, but an epithelial strand between the bulge and the dermal papillae remains. This contact is necessary for the dermal papillae to induce new hair growth in the bulge where hair progenitor cells are located. If the epithelial cord is destroyed—for example as a consequence of mutations in the zinc-finger corepressor *HAIRLESS* or the *VITAMIN D RECEPTOR*—the dermal papillae are stranded within the dermis and the hair cannot regrow.

Tumors may also arise within epithelial structures. **Pilomatricoma**, a benign tumor of the hair follicle matrix cells, results from constitutive activation of β-*CATENIN*. **Gorlin syndrome (nevoid basal cell carcinoma syndrome; NBCCS)** is an autosomal dominant disorder occurring in about 1:50,000 to 1:100,000 individuals. These patients are afflicted with basal cell carcinomas that begin forming early in life. NBCCS patients also have increased susceptibility to other carcinomas such as meningiomas, fibromas, and rhabdomyosarcomas. Non-neoplastic disorders of epidermal derivatives also characterize NBCCS, including **odontogenic keratocysts** (arising from the dental lamina) and pathognomonic **dyskeratotic pitting** of the hands and feet. These tumors have the molecular and morphologic characteristics of undifferentiated hair follicles. NBCCS is the result of mutations in *PTCH*, the receptor that represses *HEDGEHOG* signaling. Hence, the syndrome results from increased *HEDGEHOG* signaling activity. Given the key role of the *HEDGEHOG* family during embryogenesis, developmental defects and postnatal growth defects are also present in this syndrome, including skeletal, facial, and dental anomalies, as well as neural tube closure defects.

Development of Sebaceous, Sweat, and Apocrine Glands

Several types of glands are produced by downgrowth of the epidermis. Three types of glands—the sebaceous glands, apocrine glands, and sweat glands—are widespread over the body. The milk-producing mammary glands represent a specialized type of epidermal gland.

The **sebaceous glands** produce the oily **sebum** that lubricates the skin and hair. Over most of the body, these glands form as diverticula of the hair follicle shafts, budding from the side of the root sheath about four weeks after the hair germ begins to elongate (see Fig. 7-8). In some areas of hairless skin—such as the glans penis of males and the labia minora of females—sebaceous glands develop as independent down growths of epidermis. The bud grows into the dermis tissue and branches to form a small system of ducts ending in expanded secretory acini (alveoli). The acini secrete by a **holocrine** mechanism; that is, entire secretory cells that are filled with vesicles of secretory products break down and are shed. The basal layer of the acinar epidermis consists of proliferating stem cells that constantly renew the supply of maturing secretory cells.

Mature sebaceous glands are present on the face by six months of development. Sebaceous glands are highly active in the fetus, and the sebum they produce combines with desquamating epidermal cells and remnants of the periderm to form a waterproof protective coating for the fetus called the **vernix caseosa**. After birth, the sebaceous glands become relatively inactive, but at puberty they again begin to secrete large quantities of sebum in response to the surge in circulating sex steroids.

The **apocrine glands** are highly coiled, unbranched glands that develop in association with hair follicles. They initially form over most of the body, but in the later months of fetal development they are lost except in certain areas, such as the axillae, mons pubis,

7

prepuce, scrotum, and labia minora. They begin to secrete at puberty, producing a complex mix of substances that are modified by bacterial activity into odorous compounds. These compounds may function mainly in social and sexual communication. The secretory cells lining the deep half of the gland secrete their products by an **apocrine** mechanism: small portions of cytoplasm-containing secretory vesicles pinch off and are released into the lumen of the gland.

The **sweat glands** first appear at about 20 weeks as buds of stratum germinativum that grow down into the underlying dermis to form unbranched, highly coiled glands (Fig. 7-13). The central cells degenerate to form the gland lumen, and the peripheral cells differentiate into an inner layer of secretory cells and an outer layer of **myoepithelial cells**, which are innervated by sympathetic fibers and contract to expel sweat from the gland (see Fig. 7-13). The secretory cells secrete fluid directly across the plasma membrane (**eccrine** secretion). Sweat glands form over the entire body surface except for a few areas such as the nipples. Large sweat glands develop as buds of the root sheath of hair follicles, superficial to the buds of sebaceous glands, in the axilla and areola.

As discussed earlier in the chapter, sweat glands fail to develop in the X-linked genetic disorder **hypohidrotic ectodermal dysplasia.** Infants with this disorder are vulnerable to potentially lethal **hyperpyrexia** (extremely high fever) or **hyperthermia** (overheating).

Development of Mammary Glands

In the 4th week, a pair of epidermal thickenings called the **mammary ridges** develop along either side of the body from the area of the future axilla to the future inguinal region and medial thigh (Fig. 7-14). In humans, these ridges normally disappear except at the site of the breasts. The remnant of the mammary ridge produces the **primary bud** of the mammary gland in the 5th week (see Fig. 7-14A, B). This bud grows down into the underlying dermis towards the presumptive fat pad that will induce the duct to branch. In the 10th week the primary bud begins to branch, and by the 12th week several **secondary buds** have formed (see Fig. 7-14C). These buds lengthen and branch throughout the remainder of gestation, and the resulting ducts canalize (see Fig. 7-14D, E).

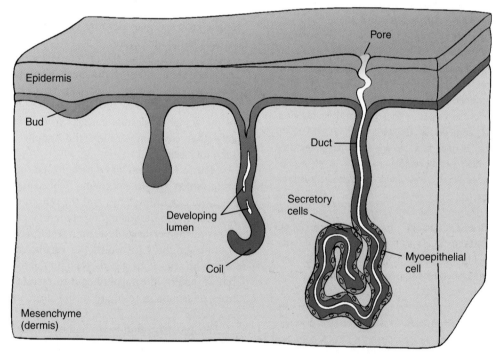

Figure 7-13. Development of sweat glands. Sweat glands first appear as elongated down growths of the epidermis at about 20 weeks. The outer cells of the down growth develop into a layer of smooth muscle, whereas the inner cells become the secretory cells of the gland.

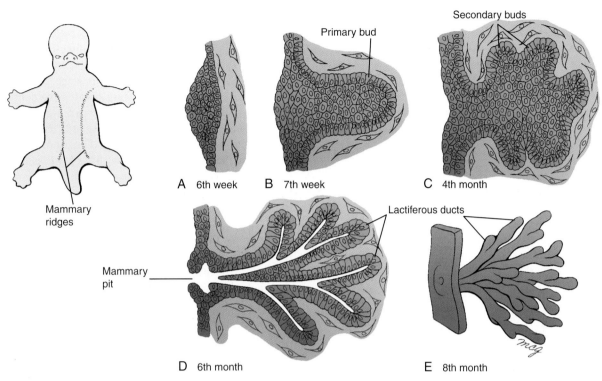

Figure 7-14. Development of the mammary glands. The mammary ridges first appear in the 4th week as thickened lines of epidermis that extend from the thorax to the medial thigh. *A, B,* In the region of the future mammary glands, the mammary ridge ectoderm then forms the primary mammary buds. *C, D,* Secondary buds form during the 3rd month and become canalized to form lactiferous ducts during the last 3 months of fetal life. *E,* Organization of lactiferous ducts around the developing nipple in the 8th month.

At birth, the mammary glands consist of 15 to 25 **lactiferous ducts**, which open onto a small superficial depression called the **mammary pit** (see Fig. 7-14*D, E*). Proliferation of the underlying mesoderm usually converts this pit to an everted nipple within a few weeks after birth, although occasionally the nipple remains depressed (**inverted nipple**). The skin surrounding the nipple also proliferates to form the areola.

Occasionally, one or more supernumerary nipples (**polythelia**) or supernumerary breasts (**polymastia**) form along the line of the mammary ridges. The most common location is just below the normal breast. Supernumerary nipples are about as common in males as in females. More rarely, an ectopic nipple forms off the line of the mammary ridge as a consequence of migration of mammary tissue. Supernumerary breasts are often discovered at puberty or during pregnancy, when they enlarge or even lactate in response to stimulatory hormones.

IN THE RESEARCH LAB

WNT SIGNALING AND DEVELOPMENT OF MAMMARY GLAND

As with the hair follicles, development of the mammary gland is controlled by *Wnt* signaling, and *Wnt6, 10a,* and *10b* are expressed in the early mammary ectoderm. Mutation of *Lef1*, a transcription factor involved in *Wnt/β-Catenin* signaling, or misexpression of the *Wnt* inhibitor *Dkk1*, results in the failure of the buds to develop appropriately. The T-box transcription factor *Tbx3* regulates the expression of *Wnt10b* and *Lef1*. Therefore, in *Tbx3* mouse mutants, the mammary glands also do not develop. Mutations of *Tbx3* in humans result in **ulnar-mammary syndrome**, characterized by the abnormal development of the limb, mammary gland, and other apocrine glands.

Other factors essential for mammary gland development include *Fgfs, Pthrp,* and *Ihh. Pthrp (Parathyroid hormone-related peptide)* is expressed in the ectoderm and signals to the underlying mesenchyme, which expresses the *Pthrp* receptor (r1). In *Pthrp* and *Pthrp receptor* (r1) mouse mutants, the mammary bud forms but the ductal tube and nipples do not develop. Misexpression of *Pthrp* can also induce nipple formation in the ventral ectoderm. In humans, loss-of-function mutations in *PTHRP RECEPTOR* (R1) cause **Blomstrand chondrodysplasia** (also discussed in Ch. 8). Patients with this syndrome have endochondral bone defects and absence of the breasts, and hence absence of the nipples.

Development of Nails

The nail anlagen first appear as epidermal thickenings at the tips of the digits (Fig. 7-15). These thickenings form at about 10 weeks on the fingers and at about 14 weeks on the toes. Almost immediately, the nail anlagen migrate proximally on the dorsal surface of the digits. The nail anlage forms a shallow depression called the **nail field**, which is surrounded laterally and proximally by ectodermal **nail folds** (see Fig. 7-15A, B). The stratum germinativum of the proximal nail fold proliferates to become the **formative zone** (also called the **formative root** or **matrix**), that produces the horny **nail plate** (see Fig. 7-15C). Like a hair, the nail plate is made of compressed keratinocytes. A thin layer of epidermis called the **eponychium** initially covers the nail plate, but this layer normally degenerates, except at the nail base. Fate mapping studies of the ventral ectoderm have shown that the boundaries of dorsal versus ventral ectoderm derivatives lie at the distal tip of **hyponychium** (the layer beneath the free edge of the nail) (Fig. 7-15D, E). The growing nails reach the tips of the fingers by the 8th month and the tips of the toes by birth. The degree of nail growth can be used as an indicator of prematurity.

Development of Teeth

In the 6th week, a U-shaped ridge of epidermis called the **dental lamina** appears on the upper and lower jaws (Figs. 7-16A, 7-17A, E). In the 7th week, ten centers of epidermal cell proliferation develop at intervals on each dental lamina and grow down into the underlying mesenchyme. A condensation of mesenchyme appears under and around each of these 20 ingrowths. The composite structure consisting of the dental lamina ingrowth and the underlying mesenchymal condensation is called a **tooth bud** (see Figs. 7-16A, 7-17B, F).

During the 8th week, instructive influences from the epidermis cause the mesenchymal condensation to invade the base of the dental lamina ingrowth, forming a hillock-shaped mesenchymal *dental papilla* (Fig. 7-17C, G; see Fig. 7-16A). This stage of tooth development is called the **cap stage** because the dental lamina invests the top of the papilla like a cap. The mesenchyme surrounding the papilla and its dental lamina cap condenses to form an enclosure called the **dental sac** (see Fig. 7-16A). By 14 weeks, the dental papilla has deeply invaginated the dental lamina and constitutes the core of the developing tooth. This is called the **bell stage** of tooth development, because the dental lamina looks like a bell resting over the dental papilla (Fig. 7-17D, H; see Fig. 7-16B).

During the bell stage, the outermost cells of the dental papilla become organized into a layer just adjacent to the inner enamel epithelium. These cells differentiate into the **odontoblasts**, which will produce the **dentin** of the teeth (see Fig. 7-16B). At this stage, the dental lamina differentiates to form the **enamel organ**, which will produce the **enamel layer** of the tooth. First, the dental lamina becomes a three-layered structure, consisting of an **inner enamel epithelium** overlying the dental papilla; a central layer, the **enamel (stellate) reticulum** composed of star-shaped cells dispersed in an extracellular layer; and an **outer enamel epithelium**.

In the 7th month, the odontoblasts begin to secrete the nonmineralized matrix of the dentin, called **predentin**, which later progressively calcifies to form **dentin**. Production of predentin is induced by signals from the inner enamel epithelium and begins at the apex of the tooth and moves downward (see Fig. 7-16B). As the odontoblasts migrate downwards, they leave long cell processes (**odontoblastic processes**) that extend through the thickness of the dentin behind them. The inner mesenchyme of the dental papilla becomes the tooth pulp. As soon as dentin is formed, the odontoblasts in turn induce cells of the inner epithelium to differentiate into enamel-producing **ameloblasts**, which begin to secrete rod-shaped enamel prisms between themselves and the underlying dentin (Fig. 7-16B, C).

The 20 tooth buds give rise directly to the **primary (deciduous** or **milk) teeth**, consisting in each half-jaw of two incisors, one canine, and two premolars. However, early in the cap stage the dental lamina superficial to each tooth bud produces a small diverticulum that migrates to the base of the primary tooth

Text continued on page 214.

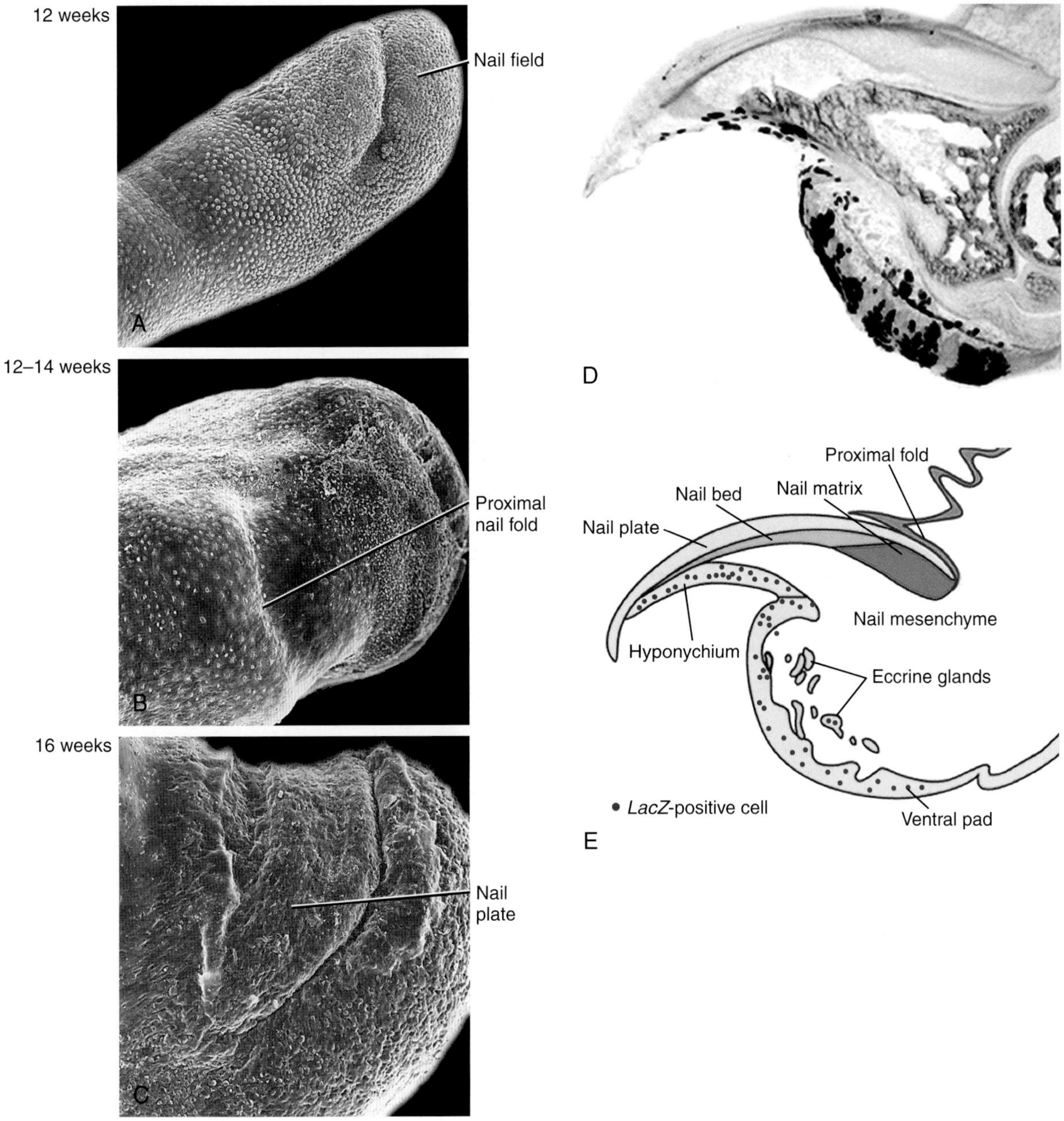

Figure 7-15. Development of the nails. *A-C,* Scanning electron micrographs showing development between 12 and 16 weeks. *A,* Formation of the nail field. *B,* The margin of the proximal nail fold is clearly defined by 12 to 14 weeks. *C,* The nail plate is apparent by 16 weeks. *D, E,* The boundary between the dorsal and ventral ectodermal derivatives is shown in the light micrograph by the presence of *LacZ*-expressing cells (blue) along the ventral surface. The drawing provides an explanation of the morphology seen in the light micrograph.

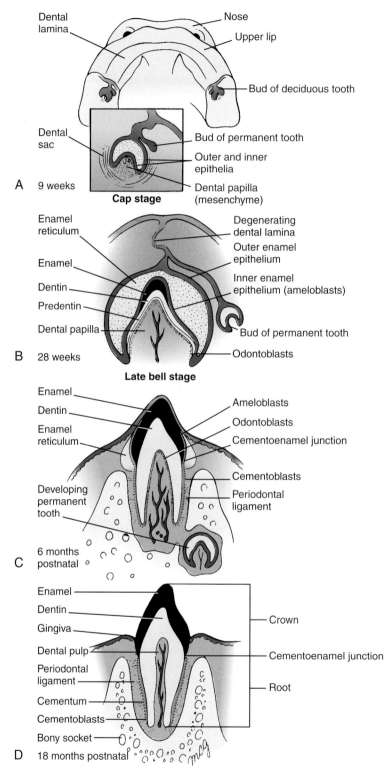

A 9 weeks
Cap stage

B 28 weeks
Late bell stage

C 6 months postnatal

D 18 months postnatal

Figure 7-16. *A-D,* Development and eruption of the primary dentition. Notice that the ectodermal dental lamina gives rise to the enamel organ, which secretes the enamel of the tooth, whereas the neural crest cells that initially form the dental papilla differentiate into the odontoblasts, which secrete dentin.

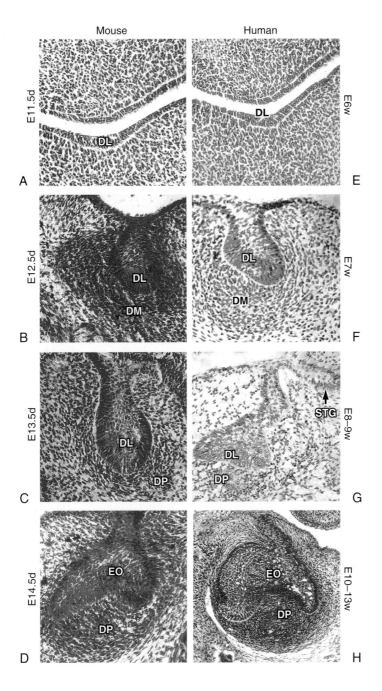

Figure 7-17. Early stages in molar tooth development. *A-D*, Development in the mouse embryo from day 11.5 through 14.5. *E-H*, Development in the human embryo from week 6 through 10 to 13. In both mice and humans, development of the tooth begins with formation of the dental lamina (DL; panels *A*, *E*); its expansion to form the tooth bud, which consists of the thickened and folded dental lamina and underlying dental mesenchyme (DM; panels *B*, *F*); invagination of the dental lamina by the growth of the condensed dental mesenchyme called the dental papilla (DP) at the cap stage (*C*, *G*), with formation of the secondary tooth germ (STG); and development of the enamel organ (EO; panels *D*, *H*) at the bell stage.

bud and becomes the bud of the **secondary (permanent)** tooth that will replace it (see Fig. 7-16A-C). These secondary teeth develop to the bell stage and arrest until about 6 years of age. Then they start to develop secondarily, destroying the root of the primary tooth in the process. The buds of the permanent molars, which do not have a deciduous precursor, arise during postnatal life from a pencil-like extension of the dental lamina that burrows back into the posterior jaw from the hindmost primary tooth buds. The full human dentition consists of 32 teeth, including three molars, but the third molars (wisdom teeth) often fail to develop or to erupt.

The roots of the teeth begin to form in late fetal and early postnatal life. At the junction of the inner and outer enamel epithelia, **the cervical loop**, the cells proliferate and elongate to form the **epithelial root sheath** (Fig. 7-16D). The mesenchyme just internal to the epithelial sheath differentiates into odontoblasts, which produce dentin. Each root contains a narrow canal of dental pulp by which nerves and blood vessels enter the tooth (see Fig. 7-16D).

The tooth roots are enclosed in extensions of the mesenchymal dental sac. The inner cells of the dental sac differentiate into **cementoblasts**, which secrete a layer of **cementum** to cover the dentin of the root. At the neck of the tooth root, the cementum meets the enamel at a **cementoenamel junction** (see Fig. 7-16C, D). The outermost cells of the dental sac participate in bone formation as the jaws ossify and also form the **periodontal ligament** that holds the tooth to its bony socket, or **alveolus**.

The primary teeth start to erupt at about 6 months after birth. Mandibular teeth usually erupt earlier than the corresponding maxillary teeth. The primary dentition is usually fully erupted by 2 years. Between approximately age 6 and 8 years, the primary teeth begin to be shed and are replaced by the permanent teeth.

IN THE RESEARCH LAB

TOOTH INDUCTION

Experiments in which dental laminae and mesenchymal components have been cultured with and without each other have shown that tooth development requires both components. Initially, the instructive signal is present in the epithelium, and if early odontogenic epithelium is recombined with nonodontogenic mesenchyme, teeth will develop. Crucially, the nonodontogenic mesenchyme must be derived from neural crest cells, as teeth will not form when odontogenic epithelium is recombined with trunk-derived mesenchyme. Later, during tooth development, the ectomesenchyme becomes instructive, that is, it can specify tooth development in nonodontogenic or naïve epithelium. This "transfer" of inducing ability correlates with a switch in *Bmp4* expression from the epithelium to the underlying mesenchyme.

Odontogenic development starts with the specification of the odontogenic field. This is achieved by antagonistic interactions between *Fgf8* and *Bmp4* signaling in the oral epithelium. Subsequent development requires multiple factors including *Shh*, *Bmps*, *Fgfs*, and *Wnts*; loss of these signals results in the arrest of tooth development before the bud stage. *Shh*, which is expressed in the odontogenic epithelium, is mitogenic, as it is in hair follicles. Enamel knots—transient, nonproliferative structures in the enamel organ that express a number of signaling molecules (*Shh*; *Bmp2, 4, 7*; *Fgf4, 9*)—are thought to act as signaling centers, promoting proliferation and folding of the adjacent epithelium. Thus, they specify the number of cusps that a tooth will form. The primary enamel knot forms at the center of the inner enamel epithelium. In molar teeth, secondary enamel knots develop. Aberrant enamel knot formation/morphogenesis, for example following loss of *Eda* signaling or loss of the *Bmp* antagonist *Ectodin*, is associated with changes in cusp number/morphology.

Patterning of different types of teeth is thought to occur by the differential expression of homeobox genes in the cranial mesenchyme: for example, the homeobox gene *Barx1* has been proposed to specify molars, whereas *Msx1/2* expression has been proposed to specify incisors. Definitive evidence for this proposal is lacking, although the transformation of skeletal structures following loss of both *Dlx5/6* in the developing face (discussed in Ch. 16) makes this proposal likely.

IN THE CLINIC

TOOTH ANOMALIES

Malformations in teeth can arise from patterning defects or from abnormalities in differentiation. For example, the presence of a single maxillary incisor at the mild end of the holoprosencephaly spectrum (discussed in Ch. 16) is due to failure to specify (i.e., pattern) the embryonic midline. In contrast, defective development of enamel or dentin, such as occurs in **amelogenesis imperfecta** (*DLX3* mutations) and **dentinogenesis imperfecta** (*DENTIN SIALOPHOSPHOPROTEIN* mutations), involves faulty differentiation. Enamel defects can also be caused by **vitamin A deficiency**, or the enamel may be discolored following exposure to antibiotics such as **tetracyclines**.

Alternatively, there may be too few teeth (**hypodontia**; or **oligodontia**, when more than six teeth are absent) or excess or supernumerary teeth (**hyperdontia**). Hypodontia typically affects the secondary dentition and can be the result of mutations in the *WNT* signaling component *AXIN2* or in the transcription factors *PAX9*, *PITX2*, or *MSX1*. Hyperdontia resulting from *RUNX2* mutations (associated with **cleidocranial dysplasia**) can include the generation of a third set of teeth. In these patients the dental lamina is hyperproliferative. Loss or gain of teeth can also be a secondary consequence of facial clefting.

Suggested Readings

Alonso L, Fuchs E. 2003. Stem cells of the skin epithelium. Proc Natl Acad Sci U S A 100(Supp. 1):11830-11835.

Alonso L, Fuchs E. 2003. Stem cells in the skin: waste not, Wnt not. Genes Dev 17:1189-1200.

Athar M, Tang X, Lee JL, Kopelovich L, Kim AL. 2006. Hedgehog signaling in skin development and cancer. Exp Dermatol 15:667-677.

Botchkarev VA, Sharov AA. 2004. BMP signaling in the control of skin development and hair follicle growth. Differentiation 72:512-526.

Brunner HG, Hamel BC, Bokhoven Hv H. 2002. P63 gene mutations and human developmental syndromes. Am J Med Genet 112:284-290.

Callahan CA, Oro AE. 2001. Monstrous attempts at adnexogenesis: regulating hair follicle progenitors through Sonic hedgehog signaling. Curr Opin Genet Dev 11:541-546.

Candi E, Schmidt R, Melino G. 2005. The cornified envelope: a model of cell death in the skin. Nat Rev Mol Cell Biol 6:328-340.

Cobourne MT, Miletich I, Sharpe PT. 2004. Restriction of sonic hedgehog signalling during early tooth development. Development 131:2875-2885.

Courtois G. 2005. The NF-kappaB signaling pathway in human genetic diseases. Cell Mol Life Sci 62:1682-1691.

Fuchs E, Merrill BJ, Jamora C, DasGupta R. 2001. At the roots of a never-ending cycle. Dev Cell 1:13-25.

Fuchs E, Raghavan S. 2002. Getting under the skin of epidermal morphogenesis. Nat Rev Genet 3:199-209.

Hennighausen L, Robinson GW. 2001. Signaling pathways in mammary gland development. Dev Cell 1:467-475.

Hennighausen L, Robinson GW. 2005. Information networks in the mammary gland. Nat Rev Mol Cell Biol 6:715-725.

Huysseune A, Thesleff I. 2004. Continuous tooth replacement: the possible involvement of epithelial stem cells. Bioessays 26:665-671.

Irvine AD, Christiano AM. 2001. Hair on a gene string: recent advances in understanding the molecular genetics of hair loss. Clin Exp Dermatol 26:59-71.

Itin PH, Fistarol SK. 2004. Ectodermal dysplasias. Am J Med Genet C Semin Med Genet 131C:45-51.

Jernvall J, Thesleff I. 2000. Reiterative signaling and patterning during mammalian tooth morphogenesis. Mech Dev 92:19-29.

Kalinin AE, Kajava AV, Steinert PM. 2002. Epithelial barrier function: assembly and structural features of the cornified cell envelope. Bioessays 24:789-800.

Lane EB, McLean WH. 2004. Keratins and skin disorders. J Pathol 204:355-366.

Mack JA, Anand S, Maytin EV. 2005. Proliferation and cornification during development of the mammalian epidermis. Birth Defects Res C Embryo Today 75:314-329.

McLean WH. 2003. Genetic disorders of palm skin and nail. J Anat 202:133-141.

Mecklenburg L, Tychsen B, Paus R. 2005. Learning from nudity: lessons from the nude phenotype. Exp Dermatol 14:797-810.

Mikkola ML, Millar SE. 2006. The mammary bud as a skin appendage: unique and shared aspects of development. J Mammary Gland Biol Neoplasia 11:187-203.

Mikkola ML, Thesleff I. 2003. Ectodysplasin signaling in development. Cytokine Growth Factor Rev 14:211-224.

Miletich I, Sharpe PT. 2004. Neural crest contribution to mammalian tooth formation. Birth Defects Res C Embryo Today 72:200-212.

Millar SE. 2002. Molecular mechanisms regulating hair follicle development. J Invest Dermatol 118:216-225.

Morasso MI, Radoja N. 2005. Dlx genes, p63, and ectodermal dysplasias. Birth Defects Res C Embryo Today 75:163-171.

Niemann C, Watt FM. 2002. Designer skin: lineage commitment in postnatal epidermis. Trends Cell Biol 12:185-192.

O'Shaughnessy RF, Christiano AM. 2004. Inherited disorders of the skin in human and mouse: from development to differentiation. Int J Dev Biol 48:171-179.

Ohazama A, Sharpe PT. 2004. TNF signalling in tooth development. Curr Opin Genet Dev 14:513-519.

Owens DW, Lane EB. 2003. The quest for the function of simple epithelial keratins. Bioessays 25:748-758.

Pispa J, Thesleff I. 2003. Mechanisms of ectodermal organogenesis. Dev Biol 262:195-205.

Porter RM. 2003. Mouse models for human hair loss disorders. J Anat 202:125-131.

Robinson GW. 2004. Identification of signaling pathways in early mammary gland development by mouse genetics. Breast Cancer Res 6:105-108.

Rogers GE. 2004. Hair follicle differentiation and regulation. Int J Dev Biol 48:163-170.

Schmidt-Ullrich R, Paus R. 2005. Molecular principles of hair follicle induction and morphogenesis. Bioessays 27:247-261.

Thesleff I. 2003. Epithelial-mesenchymal signalling regulating tooth morphogenesis. J Cell Sci 116:1647-1648.

Thesleff I, Keranen S, Jernvall J. 2001. Enamel knots as signaling centers linking tooth morphogenesis and odontoblast differentiation. Adv Dent Res 15:14-18.

Tiede S, Paus R. 2006. Lhx2-decisive role in epithelial stem cell maintenance, or just the "tip of the iceberg"? Bioessays 28:1157-1160.

Tucker A, Sharpe P. 2004. The cutting-edge of mammalian development; how the embryo makes teeth. Nat Rev Genet 5:499-508.

van Bokhoven H, McKeon F. 2002. Mutations in the p53 homolog p63: allele-specific developmental syndromes in humans. Trends Mol Med 8:133-139.

7

van Steensel MA, van Geel M, Steijlen PM. 2004. Molecular genetics of hereditary hair and nail disease. Am J Med Genet C Semin Med Genet 131C:52-60.

Veltmaat JM, Mailleux AA, Thiery JP, Bellusci S. 2003. Mouse embryonic mammogenesis as a model for the molecular regulation of pattern formation. Differentiation 71:1-17.

Villavicencio EH, Walterhouse DO, Iannaccone PM. 2000. The sonic hedgehog-patched-gli pathway in human development and disease. Am J Hum Genet 67:1047-1054.

Vorbach C, Capecchi MR, Penninger JM. 2006. Evolution of the mammary gland from the innate immune system? Bioessays 28:606-616.

Watt FM, Lo Celso C, Silva-Vargas V. 2006. Epidermal stem cells: an update. Curr Opin Genet Dev 16:518-524.

Widelitz RB, Baker RE, Plikus M, et al. 2006. Distinct mechanisms underlie pattern formation in the skin and skin appendages. Birth Defects Res C Embryo Today 78:280-291.

Wilson A, Radtke F. 2006. Multiple functions of Notch signaling in self-renewing organs and cancer. FEBS Lett 580:2860-2868.

Yin T, Green KJ. 2004. Regulation of desmosome assembly and adhesion. Semin Cell Dev Biol 15:665-677.

Zhang YD, Chen Z, Song YQ, et al. 2005. Making a tooth: growth factors, transcription factors, and stem cells. Cell Res 15:301-316.

Development of the Musculoskeletal System

8

Summary Development of bone and muscle occurs within mesenchymal regions of the embryo after the tube-within-a-tube body plan is established during the 4th week of gestation. Bone formation occurs in two ways. During **endochondral ossification**, a cartilage model first forms and is eventually replaced with bone. This type of ossification underlies formation of the axial (vertebral column and ribs) and appendicular (limb) skeletons, with the exception of part of the clavicles. During **intramembranous ossification**, bone forms directly from mesenchymal cells without the prior formation of cartilage. This type of ossification underlies formation of the majority of bones of the face and skull.

Three types of cells act in endochondral bone development: **chondrocytes, osteoblasts**, and **osteoclasts**. The former two function in secreting cartilage and bone matrix, respectively, whereas the latter is involved in bone resorption. Only the latter two cell types act in membranous ossification.

Three types of muscles form in the embryo: skeletal, smooth, and cardiac. Skeletal, or voluntary, muscle—the focus of this chapter—develops in association with bone as part of the musculoskeletal system. Smooth muscle develops in association with formation of the walls of the viscera, blood vessels, and glands. Cardiac muscle develops only in the heart. Development of smooth and cardiac muscle is discussed in relation to development of the gut tube and urogenital system (discussed in Chs. 14 and 15) and to the heart (discussed in Ch. 12).

Muscle development occurs in the embryo through the formation of **myoblasts**, which undergo extensive proliferation to form terminally differentiated, postmitotic **myocytes**. Myocytes express *Actin, Myosin*, and other contractile proteins and fuse to form contractile **myofibrils**. Striated muscle development involves both prenatal and postnatal events: **primary myogenesis** (occurs during the stage of the embryo) and **secondary myogenesis** (occurs during the stage of the fetus) lay down the muscular system, and **satellite cells** act in muscle growth postnatally and in response to exercise or muscle damage.

The muscles and bones of the trunk derive from the **somites**. Each somite forms two distinct zones: a **sclerotome** and a **dermomyotome**. The former gives rise to the bones of the axial skeleton. The latter gives rise to the **dermatome**—which forms the dermis of the back skin of the trunk and neck (with the remainder of the dermis of these regions forming from **lateral plate mesoderm**)—and the **myotome**—which forms the muscles of the trunk. The myotome also gives rise to the musculature of the limbs (discussed in Ch. 18) and tongue (discussed in Ch. 16). The dermis and bones of the limbs form from **lateral plate mesoderm** (discussed in Ch. 18). As discussed in Chapter 16, the bones of the head and neck arise from **neural crest cells**, as does most of the dermis of the head, whereas the facial, masticatory, and laryngeal muscles arise from unsegmented paraxial (head) mesoderm.

Shortly after formation of the somitic myotome, the myotome splits into a dorsal **epimere** and ventral **hypomere**. The epimere forms the deep **epaxial muscles** of the back, which are innervated by the dorsal ramus of the spinal nerve. In contrast, the hypomere forms the **hypaxial muscles** of the lateral and ventral body wall in the thorax and abdomen, which are innervated by the ventral ramus of the spinal nerve. The innervation of these muscles is discussed further in Chapter 10.

Formation of the vertebral column involves the important process of **resegmentation** of the sclerotomes of the somites. During resegmentation, the sclerotome of each somite subdivides into cranial and caudal segments, each of which fuses, respectively, with the adjacent caudal or cranial segment. Resegmentation allows motor axons and dorsal root ganglia to lie between vertebrae, rather than running through them.

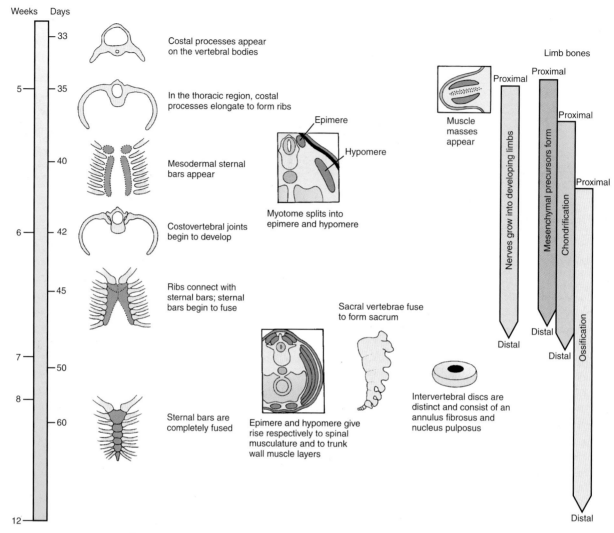

Weeks Days

33 — Costal processes appear on the vertebral bodies

5 — 35 — In the thoracic region, costal processes elongate to form ribs

Epimere

Hypomere

40 — Mesodermal sternal bars appear

Myotome splits into epimere and hypomere

6 — 42 — Costovertebral joints begin to develop

45 — Ribs connect with sternal bars; sternal bars begin to fuse

Sacral vertebrae fuse to form sacrum

7 — 50 —

8 — 60 — Sternal bars are completely fused

Epimere and hypomere give rise respectively to spinal musculature and to trunk wall muscle layers

Intervertebral discs are distinct and consist of an annulus fibrosus and nucleus pulposus

12 —

Muscle masses appear

Limb bones

Proximal

Proximal

Proximal

Nerves grow into developing limbs

Mesenchymal precursors form

Chondrification

Ossification

Distal

Distal

Distal

Proximal

Proximal

Distal

Time line. Formation of the musculoskeletal system.

A newlywed couple, both divorcees with previous children, decides to have a child together. The woman becomes pregnant within a few months of trying and, due to her "advanced maternal age" of 38, her obstetrician recommends first trimester screening. This testing indicates an elevated chance (1 in 25) of trisomy 18. Amniocentesis shows a normal karyotype of 46,XX, and a follow-up ultrasound at 20 weeks shows that the length of the long bones is below normal. Otherwise, the pregnancy progresses normally.

The couple delivers a healthy girl at 39 weeks gestational age without complications. Over the next few months the family becomes increasingly concerned that their daughter seems to have short arms and legs and bears little resemblance to either parent. The girl is referred to the genetics clinic and is noted to have **rhizomelia** (shortening of the proximal limbs), short fingers, large head, and a flat nasal bridge (Fig. 8-1). X-rays confirm the diagnosis of **achondroplasia**. The parents are told that their daughter's adult height will be around 4 feet. They are reassured somewhat when they learn that she should have normal intelligence and a normal life expectancy.

Achondroplasia, which is Greek meaning "without cartilage formation," is the most common and most recognizable form of dwarfism. It is caused by mutations in the *Fibroblast growth factor receptor 3 (FGFR3)*. In contrast to aneuploidy syndromes, like trisomy 18, achondroplasia is associated with advanced *paternal* age, with 80% of cases resulting from new mutations in the *FGFR3* gene.

Tissue Origins and Differentiation of Musculoskeletal System

Overview of Bone Development

There are two types of bones in the body: those that develop via **endochondral ossification** and those that develop via **intramembranous ossification**. During endochondral bone development, a cartilaginous template forms preceding ossification. This pathway of differentiation is used by all the **axial** (vertebral column and ribs) and **appendicular** (limb) **bones** of the body, with the exception of part of the clavicle. The cranial base, sensory capsules, and pharyngeal arch cartilages also form via endochondral ossification (discussed in Ch. 16). Alternatively, bones may develop by intramembranous ossification directly from the mesenchyme. These bones typify the majority of bones of the face and skull and are called **dermal** or **membrane bones**.

Endochondral bones are formed by three cell types: **chondrocytes** (cartilage cells), **osteoblasts** (bone-forming cells), and **osteoclasts** (bone-resorbing cells). Chondrocytes have three tissue origins: the **paraxial mesoderm** forms the axial skeleton, including the occipital portion of the cranial base; the **lateral plate mesoderm** forms the appendicular skeleton and sternum; and **neural crest cells** (i.e., *ectodermal* cells) give rise to the cartilaginous elements in the face and neck.

The origin of osteoblasts and osteoclasts is less diverse: osteoblasts arise from **mesenchymal stem cells** and osteoclasts arise from the **hematopoietic** system.

Dermal bones develop from **neural crest cells** (facial bones and the frontal bone of the skull) or unsegmented **paraxial (head) mesoderm** (e.g., parietal bone of the skull). In dermal bones, the osteoblasts directly differentiate within the mesenchyme.

Overview of Muscle Development

The striated muscles of the trunk and limb are derived from the segmented **paraxial mesoderm**, that is, the **somites**. The tongue musculature also arises from the **somites** (the so-called occipital somites; discussed in Ch. 16), whereas all other craniofacial muscles arise from the unsegmented **paraxial mesoderm** and **prechordal plate mesoderm** (i.e., head mesoderm). The tongue and limb myoblast precursors undergo extensive migration to reach their final destination. Initially the myogenic cells, the **myoblasts**, proliferate but then they exit the cell cycle and terminally differentiate to form **myocytes**. The myocytes express contractile proteins such as *Actin* and *Myosin* and fuse to form a **myofiber**, which is a multinucleated **syncytium** (i.e., a mass of cells each containing multiple nuclei) containing the contractile **myofibrils**. The tongue and extraocular muscles express unique *Myosin* heavy chains needed for the function of mastication and eye movement, respectively.

Striated muscle development occurs in three waves. First, there is **primary myogenesis**, which occurs in

8

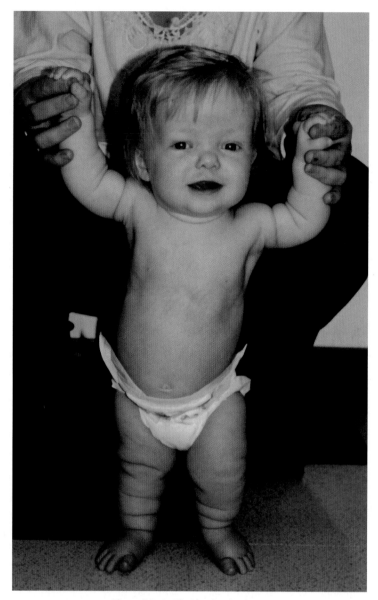

Figure 8-1. A girl with achondroplasia.

the embryo. This is followed by **secondary myogenesis**, which occurs in the fetus and gives rise to the bulk of fetal muscle. Finally, postnatal muscle growth involves **satellite cells**, small quiescent cells underlying the basal lamina of the muscle fiber. In response to exercise or muscle damage, satellite cells form myocytes, which permit further muscle growth. The satellite cells in the trunk and limb also arise from the **somites**.

The smooth muscle of the gut and cardiac muscle forms from **splanchnic mesoderm**, whereas the smooth muscle contributing to blood vessels and hair follicles arises locally within the mesoderm. Smooth muscle can also form from neural crest cells. For example, the iris and ciliary muscles are derived from cranial neural crest cells, as is the smooth muscle of the dermis of the head and neck.

IN THE RESEARCH LAB

COMMITMENT TO MUSCULOSKELETAL LINEAGE

Commitment to the chondrogenic, osteoblastic, and myogenic lineages is determined by distinct transcription factors. Commitment to the chondrogenic lineage requires the transcription factor **Sox9**, which regulates **Collagen type II** expression, a key constituent of the early cartilaginous matrix. Commitment to the osteoblastic lineage requires **Runx2** (*Runt-related transcription factor 2*, also known as *Cbfa1* or *Core binding factor 1*), a transcription factor. Misexpression of *Runx2* in primary fibroblasts can induce the expression of bone markers such as *Osteocalcin*, *Bone sialoprotein*, and *Collagen Type I*. Gene inactivation of the transcription factor *Sox9* in mice affects the early development of all cartilaginous bones. In contrast, loss of function of *Runx2* in mice results in ossification defects resulting from the lack of osteoblasts; however, the cartilaginous templates of the endochondral bone still form (Fig. 8-2). *Osterix*, a zinc finger transcription factor that is downstream of *Cbfa1*, is also essential for osteoblast development; in the absence of *Osterix*, osteoblasts also do not differentiate.

Mutations in *SOX9* and *RUNX2* also occur in humans. Mutations in *SOX9* result in **campomelic dysplasia**, typified by the bowing of the long bones and defects in all endochondral bones. Campomelic dysplasia is also associated with XY sex reversal in males (discussed in Ch. 15). Mutations in *RUNX2* cause **cleidocranial dysplasia**, characterized by clavicular hypoplasia (that allows the juxtaposition of the shoulders), large open sutures in the skull, a wide pubic symphysis, and dental abnormalities such as delayed erupting or supernumerary teeth.

Striated muscle development is characterized by the commitment to the myogenic lineage by the expression of the **myogenic (or muscle) regulatory factors** (MRFs), the basic-helix-loop-helix transcription factors **Myf5** and **MyoD**. This is followed by expression of two other MRFs, **Myogenin** and **Mrf4**, and, finally, terminal differentiation to form **myocytes**, characterized by the expression of contractile proteins such as the **Myosin heavy chains** (*MyHC*). When either *Myf5* or *MyoD* are individually inactivated in mice, there are no muscle defects, but loss of both *Myf5* and *MyoD* results in a complete absence of muscle development. **Satellite cells** depend for survival on the paired-box transcription factor **Pax7**; in its absence, satellite cells initially develop but they fail to survive.

8

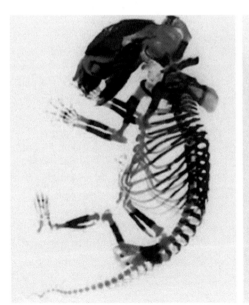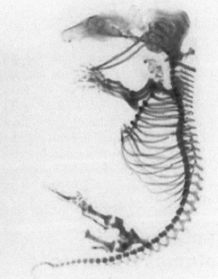

Figure 8-2. The role of *Runx2* in bone development. Wild-type mouse embryo (left) and a *Runx2* null embryo (right) have been stained with alcian blue and alizarin red to show cartilage (blue) and bone (red) differentiation. In the absence of *Cbfa1*, the osteoblasts (the bone-forming cells) do not develop.

Somites Differentiate into Sclerotome, Myotome, and Dermatome

As discussed in Chapter 4, the **somites** are transient segmented structures derived from **paraxial mesoderm**. They contain the progenitors of the axial skeleton, trunk musculature and associated tendons, trunk dermis, endothelial cells, and meninges of the spinal cord. Somites are initially epithelial balls with a central cavity that contains a population of loose **core cells**, the **somitocoele** cells (Fig. 8-3A, B). Shortly after forming, each somite separates into subdivisions that give rise to specific mesodermal components. The ventromedial part of the somite undergoes an **epithelial-to-mesenchymal transformation**, and these cells, together with the core cells, form the **sclerotome;** after formation of the sclerotome, the remainder of the somite consists of a dorsal epithelial layer called the **dermomyotome** (Fig. 8-3C; see Fig. 8-3A). The sclerotome will develop into the **vertebrae** and **ribs**. As shown in Figures 8-3A and 8-4, cells in the ventral portion of the sclerotome migrate to surround the **notochord** and form the rudiment of the **vertebral body**; those in the dorsal portion of the sclerotome surround the neural tube and form the rudiment of the **vertebral arch** and **vertebral spine**; and more laterally located sclerotome forms the **vertebral transverse process** and **ribs**.

The dermomyotome initially retains its epithelial structure (see Fig. 8-3C) and contains the presumptive myogenic and dermal cells. The dermomyotome gives rise to the myotome, containing committed muscle cells (see Fig. 8-3A). The compartmentalized structure of the somite also controls pathways of neural crest cell and motor axon migration and, hence, is responsible for the segmentation of the peripheral nervous system (discussed in Ch. 10). The factors involved in specification and patterning of the sclerotome and myotome are discussed in Chapter 4 (also see Fig. 4-25).

Resegmentation of Sclerotomes

There is a cranial-caudal difference in the sclerotome marked by differences in both gene expression and cell density. The caudal portion of each sclerotome is cell dense, with higher cell proliferation, whereas the cranial portion is less cell dense. These differences result in segmentation of the neural crest cells and motor axons, which can only migrate towards the cranial portion of the sclerotome, as the caudal portion of the sclerotome is inhibitory for migration (Fig. 8-5C). The division between the cranial and caudal portions of each sclerotome is characterized by a line of transversely arranged cells known as the **intrasegmental boundary**, or **von Ebner's fissure (Fig. 8-6)**. In later development, the sclerotomes split along this fissure, and the caudal segment of each sclerotome fuses with the cranial segment of the sclerotome caudal to it, with each of the two segments of the sclerotome contributing to a vertebra. This process is called **resegmentation of the sclerotomes**. Resegmentation thus produces vertebrae that lie **intersegmentally**.

IN THE RESEARCH LAB

SUBDIVISION OF SCLEROTOME

The cranial and caudal halves of each sclerotome are marked by the expression of different genes, which establish in the two halves different cell-adhesive properties. For example, the cranial half of each sclerotome expresses *EphA4* and *EphB3* (*Ephrin* receptors) and *Tbx18* (a T-box transcription factor), whereas the caudal half of each sclerotome expresses *EphB1* and *EphB4* (two other Ephrin receptors), *Ephrin-B1* (an *Ephrin* ligand), (*Delta 1* (a ligand for the *Notch* signaling pathway), and *Uncx4.1* (a homeobox-containing transcription factor) (the expression patterns of *EphB3* and *Ephrin-B1* are illustrated in Fig. 8-5). Importantly, this division of the sclerotome into cranial and caudal halves determines the migration pathway of neural crest cells and motor axons, thereby establishing the segmentation of the peripheral nervous system. Of particular relevance are the *EphB3* receptor and its ligand, *Ephrin-B1*, which together control cell mixing and segregation. As just stated, *EphB3* is expressed in the cranial half of the sclerotome and in migrating neural crest cells, whereas *Ephrin-B1* is expressed in the caudal half of the sclerotome. *EphB3*-expressing cells cannot mix with, and actually avoid, cells expressing the ligand *Ephrin-B1* (i.e., cells in the caudal half of the sclerotome). This is illustrated by plating cells on alternative strips of *Ephrin-B1* and non–*Ephrin-B1*-expressing cells: neural crest cells migrate in stripes, avoiding *Ephrin-B1*.

The fate of cells developing in different regions of the sclerotome during formation of the vertebrae are controlled by distinct genes. For example, mutation of *Uncx4.1* in mice results in loss of the pedicles and transverse processes of

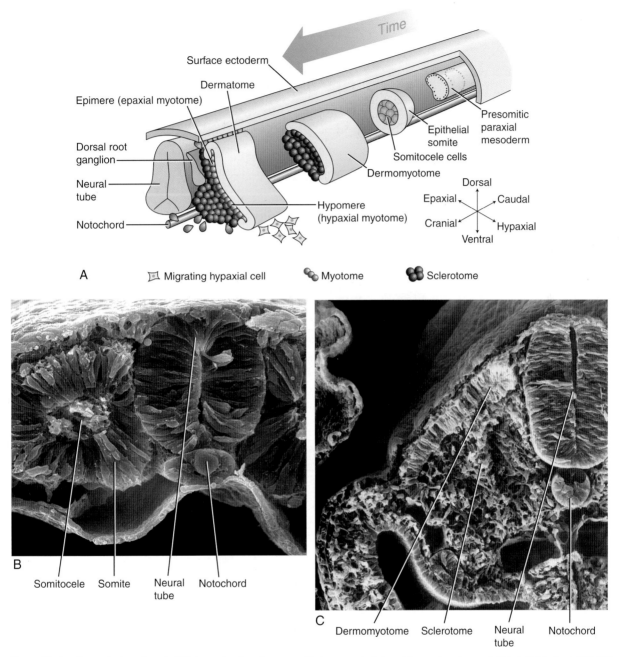

Figure 8-3. Development of somites. *A*, With increasing time the presomitic (unsegmented) paraxial mesoderm becomes segmented to form epithelial somites. These form two initial subdivisions: sclerotome and dermomyotome, and later the dermomyotome forms the dermatome and myotome. *B, C*, Scanning electron micrographs showing somites in cross-section before and after formation of the sclerotome and dermomyotome.

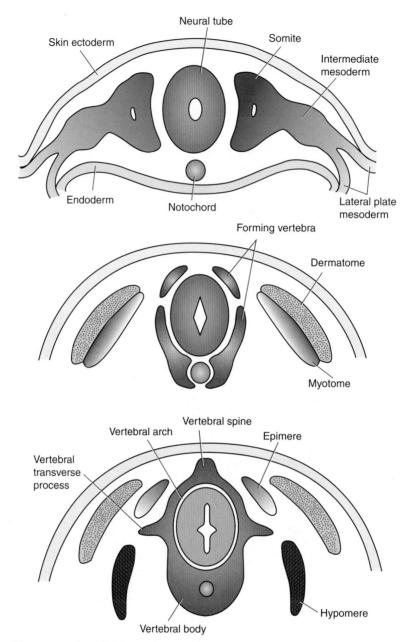

Figure 8-4. Contributions of the somites to the axial skeleton and associated structures. Subdivision of the somite involves the formation of sclerotome cells, which quickly surround the notochord, to form the rudiment of the vertebral body; and the neural tube, to form the rudiment of the vertebral arch, vertebral spine, transverse process, and ribs (not shown). With formation of the sclerotome, the dorsal part of the somite forms the dermomyotome, which quickly gives rise to the dermatome and myotome. The former forms the dermis and the latter splits into an epimere and a hypomere, which form the epaxial and hypaxial muscles, respectively.

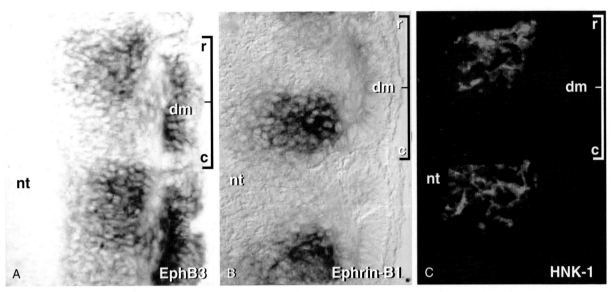

Figure 8-5. The complementary expression of *EphB3* receptor, *A*, and its ligand, *Ephrin B1*, *B*, in the cranial (r) and caudal (c) segments of the sclerotome. *C*, Neural crest cells, marked by the antibody HNK-1, migrate only through the cranial (r) half of each sclerotome and are excluded from its caudal (c) half. Brackets in *A* and *B* indicate the cranial-caudal extent of the somite; dm, dermatome (*A*); nt (*A-C*), neural tube side of each illustration.

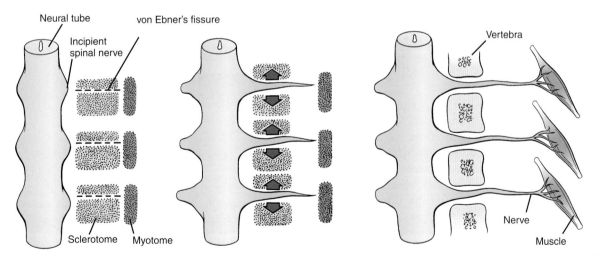

Figure 8-6. Resegmentation of the sclerotomes to form the vertebrae. Each sclerotome splits into cranial and caudal segments. As the segmental spinal nerves grow towards the cranial portion of the somite to innervate the myotomes, the cranial segment of each sclerotome recombines with the caudal segment of the next cranial sclerotome to form a vertebral rudiment.

the vertebrae, as well as the proximal portion of the ribs, whereas loss of *Tbx18* function results in the expansion of these regions. *Pax1* mutations affect the vertebral bodies and intervertebral disc, but the vertebral spine and neural arch are unaffected. These latter regions of the vertebrae are controlled by the homeobox genes *Msx1* and *2*. In contrast to the regulation of *Pax1* by *Shh* (as discussed in Ch. 4), *Msx1 and 2* expression is regulated by *Bmp4*, which is expressed by the ectoderm and roof plate of the neural tube. Development of the ribs depends on *Fgf* signals from the myotome. Therefore, in the *splotch* (*Pax3*) mouse mutant in which the dermomyotome and myotome do not develop appropriately, there are secondary consequences on development of the distal portions of the ribs, which are malformed.

Figure 8-6 illustrates the process of resegmentation of the sclerotomes.

The sclerotomes of the most cranial four somites, the so-called occipital somites, fuse to form the occipital bone of the skull base. The more caudal somites in the series are the cervical somites. Eight cervical somites develop in the embryo, but these somites form only *seven* cervical sclerotomes. This is explained by the fact that the sclerotome of the 1st cervical somite is "lost" as it fuses with the caudal half of the 4th occipital sclerotome and, therefore, contributes to the base of the skull (Fig. 8-7). The caudal half of the 1st cervical sclerotome then fuses with the cranial half of the 2nd cervical sclerotome to form the 1st cervical vertebra (the atlas), and so on down the spine. The 8th cervical sclerotome thus contributes its cranial half to the 7th cervical vertebra and its caudal half to the 1st thoracic vertebra.

As a result of sclerotomal resegmentation, the intersegmental arteries, which initially passed through the sclerotomes, now pass over the vertebral body. Also, the segmental spinal nerves, which were initially growing towards the cranial portion of the sclerotome, now exit between the vertebrae. However, it is important to remember that even though there are seven cervical vertebrae, there are *eight* cervical spinal nerves. The 1st spinal nerve exits between the base of the skull and the 1st cervical vertebra (in alignment with the 1st cervical somite), and thus the 8th spinal nerve exits above the 1st thoracic vertebra (in alignment with the 8th cervical somite). From this point onward, each spinal nerve exits just below the vertebra of the same number (see Fig. 8-7). Finally, each sclerotome is associated with an overlying myotome,

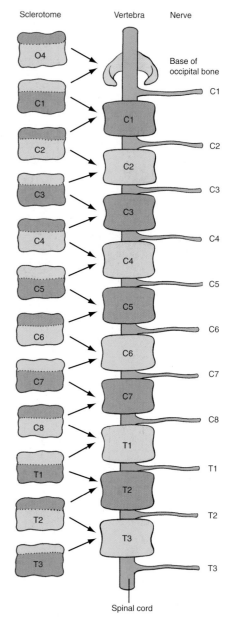

Figure 8-7. The mechanism by which the cervical region develops eight cervical nerves but only seven cervical vertebrae. The ventral roots of spinal nerves grow out from the spinal cord toward the sclerotome. With resegmentation of the sclerotomes, the cranial half of the first sclerotome fuses with the occipital bone of the skull. As a result, the nerve projecting to cervical somite one is now located rostral to the first cervical vertebrae. In the thoracic, lumbar, and sacral regions, the number of spinal nerves matches the number of vertebrae.

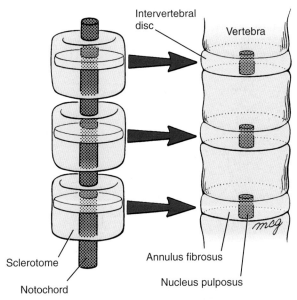

Intervertebral disc

Vertebra

Sclerotome

Notochord

Annulus fibrosus

Nucleus pulposus

Figure 8-8. Contribution of the sclerotome and notochord to the intervertebral disc. When the sclerotome splits, cells remaining in the plane of division coalesce to form the annulus fibrosus of the disc, and the notochordal cells enclosed by this structure differentiate to form the nucleus pulposus of the disc. The regions of the notochord enclosed by the developing vertebral bodies degenerate and disappear.

which contains the developing muscle plate. Therefore, following resegmentation, the myotome that was initially associated with one sclerotome becomes attached to two adjacent vertebrae and crosses the intervertebral space.

At the intrasegmental boundary the fibrous intervertebral discs develop (Fig. 8-8). The original core of each disc is composed of cells of notochordal origin (see Fig. 8-4) that will die, leaving a gelatinous core, the **nucleus pulposus**, whereas the surrounding **annulus fibrosus** develops from sclerotomal cells that are left in the region of the resegmentating sclerotome as its cranial and caudal halves split apart.

Small lateral mesenchymal condensations called **costal processes** develop in association with the vertebral arches of all the developing neck and trunk vertebrae (Fig. 8-9A). Concomitantly, transverse processes grow laterally along the dorsal side of each costal process. In the cervical vertebrae, the costal and transverse processes give rise to the lateral and medial boundaries of the **foramina transversaria** (or **transverse foramen**) that transmit the vertebral arteries. In the lumbar region, the costal processes do not project distally and contribute to the transverse

processes. The costal processes of the first two or three sacral vertebrae contribute to the development of the lateral sacral mass, or **ala**, of the **sacrum**.

However, in the thoracic region, the distal tips of the costal processes lengthen to form **ribs**. The ribs begin to form and lengthen on day 35. The first seven ribs connect ventrally to the sternum via **costal cartilages** by day 45 and are called the **true ribs**. The five lower ribs do not articulate directly with the sternum and are called the **false ribs**. The ribs develop as cartilaginous precursors that later ossify by endochondral ossification. Primary ossification centers (i.e., regions where ossification first begins) form near the angle of each rib in the 6th week, and further ossification occurs in a distal direction. Secondary ossification centers (regions where ossification begins secondarily to those constituting the primary ossification centers) develop in the tubercles and heads of the ribs during adolescence.

The sternum develops from a pair of longitudinal mesenchymal condensations, the **sternal bars**, which form in the ventrolateral body wall (Fig. 8-9B). As the most cranial ribs make contact with them in the 7th week, the sternal bars meet along the midline and begin to fuse. Fusion commences at the cranial end of the sternal bars and progresses caudally, finishing with the formation of the xiphoid process in the 9th week. Like the ribs, the sternal bones ossify from cartilaginous precursors. The sternal bars ossify in craniocaudal succession from the 5th month until shortly after birth, producing the definitive bones of the **sternum**: the **manubrium, body of the sternum**, and **xiphoid process**.

IN THE RESEARCH LAB

SPECIFICATION OF VERTEBRAE IDENTITY

Although somites throughout the trunk are morphologically indistinguishable from one another, they become specified to form structures characteristic of particular body levels. Moreover, the characteristic development of specific vertebrae seems to be related to the intrinsic properties of their particular somitic precursor. Somites transplanted to another region will form structures typical of the region of their origin. For example, thoracic somites transplanted to the lumbar region form typical thoracic vertebrae and ribs at the ectopic lumbar site. Based on experiments such as these, it has been suggested that somites acquire their regional specificity in the paraxial mesoderm prior to its segmentation into somites.

8

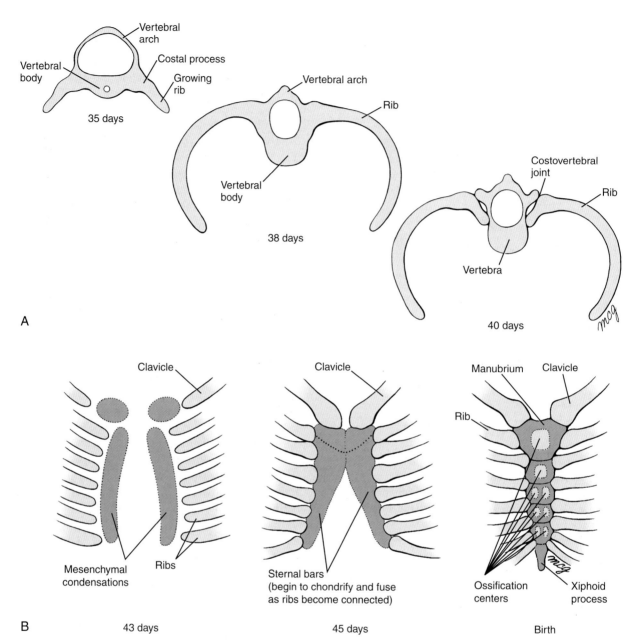

Figure 8-9. Development of the ribs and sternum. *A,* The costal processes of the vertebrae in the thoracic region begin to elongate in the 5th week to form the ribs. Late in the 6th week, the costovertebral joints form and separate the ribs from the vertebrae. *B,* Paired mesenchymal condensations called *sternal bars* form within the ventral body wall at the end of the 6th week. These bars quickly fuse together at their cranial ends, while their lateral edges connect with the distal ends of the growing ribs. The sternal bars then fuse across the midline in a cranial-to-caudal direction. Ossification centers appear within the sternum as early as 60 days, but the xiphoid process does not ossify until birth.

Specific numbers of presumptive cervical, thoracic, lumbar, sacral, and coccygeal somites are formed in human embryos, which results in a relatively invariant number of each type of vertebrae (7, 12, 5, 5, and 4, respectively). However, significant variation in the numbers of somites and vertebrae occur among different vertebrate organisms. For example, the number of cervical vertebrae in amphibians is only 3 or 4, whereas the number of cervical vertebrae in geese is 17. Mice and even giraffes possess the same number of cervical vertebrae as do humans (7), but mice have 13 (not 12) thoracic vertebrae, 6 (not 5) lumbar vertebrae, and 4 (not 5) sacral vertebrae. Snakes have hundreds of vertebrae. What factors specify regional differences in the vertebrae? And how is the number of vertebrae in any given region determined?

Interestingly, the most cranial expression of the vertebrate *Hox* genes, as shown by in situ hybridization or use of the *LacZ* reporter gene, typically occurs at approximate boundaries between somites (Fig. 8-10). This arrangement results in unique combinations of *Hox* gene expression at virtually every segment of the trunk, an organization consistent with a model of *Homc* arthropod segment specification formulated by Edward Lewis that states that homeotic genes may specify segment diversity through a **combinatorial code**.

Loss-of-function and gain-of-function mutations of *Hox* genes normally expressed in the trunk result in intriguing alterations of the identity of skeletal segments in the mouse. For example, a null mutation in mice of *Hoxc8* leads to transformation of the first lumbar vertebra into a 14th thoracic vertebra, complete with ribs (see Fig. 8-10 and note that the caudal expression domain of *Hoxc8* extends to the first lumbar vertebra). Moreover, the eighth rib, not the seventh rib, is now the most caudal rib directly attached to the sternum, which also develops an additional ossification center or sternebra. Loss of multiple *Hox8* paralogs has similar effects, but in addition, the first sacral vertebra is transformed into one with a lumbar identity, which also is associated with a shift in the position of the hindlimb. The cranial expression domain of *Hox10* genes falls at the thoracic/lumbar transition during early somitogenesis (see Fig. 8-10). Loss of all the *Hox10* paralogs results in the loss of vertebrae with lumbar characteristics—these develop as thoracic vertebrae, complete with ribs (Fig. 8-11A). Thus, null mutations of either *Hox8* or *10* genes **"cranialize"** somitic segments of the trunk.

Conversely, gain of *Hox* gene expression **"caudalizes"** the vertebrae. Therefore, if *Hoxa10* is misexpressed throughout the presomitic (unsegmented paraxial) mesoderm, thoracic vertebrae are respecified to form vertebrae with lumbar characteristics, that is, they lack ribs (Fig. 8-11B). This effect is opposite to the effect that occurs with the loss of *Hox10* paralog group described above. Importantly, misexpression of *Hoxa10* in the presomitic mesoderm or later in the somites has different effects. Only when *Hoxa10* is misexpressed in the presomitic mesoderm are the vertebrae transformed. In contrast, misexpression later, after somitogenesis has occurs, results only in relatively minor rib abnormalities.

Hox gene expression is regulated by the segmentation clock in the presomitic mesoderm (discussed in Ch. 4). This clock is controlled by *Notch, Fgf, Wnt*, and retinoid signaling, which are integrated to determine the epithelization and identity via the *Hox* code of the somite. Therefore, changes in the segmentation clock will result in a transformation of vertebrae (see the following "In the Clinic" section). **Retinoic acid** in the presomitic mesoderm regulates *Hox* gene expression, in part by the induction of another homeobox gene, *Caudal*. Genetic loss of function of two or more members of the family of **Retinoic acid receptors** results in the **cranialization** of vertebral segments (Fig. 8-12). This effect is similar to that observed in the homeotic null mutations of *Hox8* and *10* genes described above. Conversely, the ectopic application of excess retinoic acid results in the **caudalization** of vertebral segments, similar to that occurring in the *Hoxa10* "homeotic" gain-of-function mutant (see Fig. 8-12).

The mechanism by which segmental identity is achieved in vertebrates is undoubtedly far more complex than implied by this brief discussion. For example, in contrast to the loss-of-function *Hox* mutations discussed above, a loss-of-function mutation of *Hoxa6* has been shown to caudalize the 7th cervical vertebra as indicated by its development of a rib. Some other *Hox* gene knockouts simultaneously cranialize one region of the spine and caudalize another region. Thus, although retinoic acid and *Hox* genes seem to play a role in cranial-caudal specification of the vertebrae, they may only establish the general pattern of regional specification. Other factors, including the ability of some members of the *Hox* family to antagonize the function of other *Hox* genes, may fine-tune the regulation of specific segmental differentiation.

8

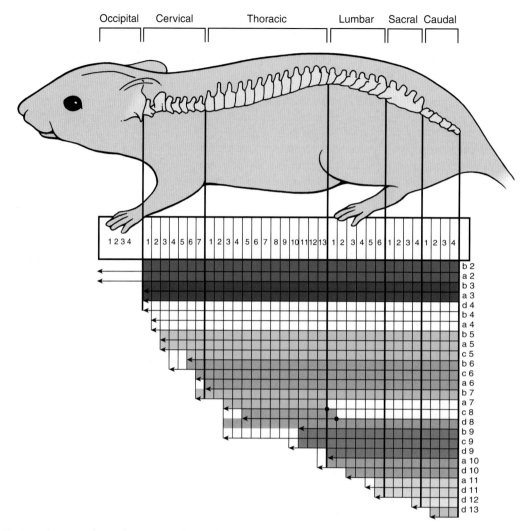

Figure 8-10. *Hox* code patterns the vertebrae. Diagram showing the expression boundaries of *Hox* gene expression along the cranial-caudal axis of the body. *Hox* genes are expressed in nested patterns along the cranial-caudal axis with each vertebrae, or small groups of vertebrae, having a distinct combinatorial *Hox* code. The boundaries of some *Hox* genes correlate with changes in vertebrae identity and the formation of appendages (i.e., the forelimbs always form at the cervical to thoracic boundary, whereas the hindlimbs always form at the lumbar to sacral boundary). This correlation between *Hox* gene expression and vertebrae identity is conserved across species. The expression domains of most, but not all, known *Hox* genes are illustrated.

IN THE CLINIC

VERTEBRAL DEFECTS

A number of spinal defects are caused by abnormal induction of the sclerotomes. **Spina bifida occulta** or **cleft vertebrae**, where the neural tube itself is morphologically unaffected (i.e., it is closed), is caused by abnormal induction of the vertebral arch rudiments by the neural tube/ectoderm. Defective induction and morphogenesis of vertebral bodies on one side of the body may result in a severe congenital **scoliosis** (lateral bending of the spinal column), which may require surgical correction. Cleft vertebrae may also be a secondary consequence of failure of neural tube closure, as in **spina bifida aperta**. Spina bifida is further discussed in Chapter 4.

In addition, rib defects may accompany defects in the specification of vertebrae or of their correct number. Such defects occur in a heterogeneous group of conditions including **spondylocostal dysostosis** (also called **Jarcho-Levin syndrome**), **VATER/VACTERL** (vertebral-anal-cardiac-tracheo-esophageal-renal-limb), and **Alagille syndrome**, as well as

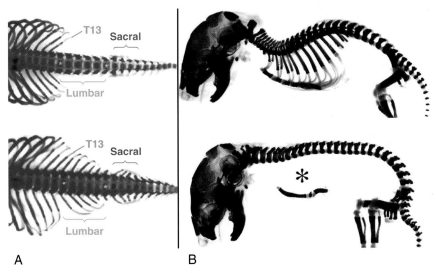

Figure 8-11. Homeotic transformations. *A,* Loss of the *Hox10* paralogs converts lumbar and sacral vertebrae into thoracic vertebrae complete with ribs. *B,* Gain of *Hoxa10* function in the presomitic mesoderm converts thoracic vertebrae into lumbar vertebrae lacking ribs. The sternum forms in the area superficial to (below) the asterisk.

in **Klippel-Feil anomaly** (these conditions are also discussed in Chs. 3, 5, and 12 to 14). Typically, spondylocostal dysostosis is characterized by vertebral defects such as hemivertebrae, rib fusions, and kyphoscoliosis (spine curvature in both lateral and anterior-posterior planes). Because the vertebral column is short, the arms appear to be relatively long. Mutations in *Delta-3,* a ligand for the *Notch* signaling pathway, have been linked to spondylocostal dysostosis. Similarly, mutations in *Lunatic fringe*—an intracellular factor that modulates *Notch receptors,* thereby altering their affinity for their ligands—and mutations in *Mesp2*—a basic helix-loop-helix transcription factor—can cause spondylocostal dysostosis (Fig. 8-13*A*). **Klippel-Feil anomaly** (Fig. 8-13*B*) affects the cervical and thoracic vertebrae such that the neck is shorter with restricted movement (cervical vertebrae are sometimes fused). In **Alagille syndrome** (resulting from mutations in *JAGGED1,* a *Notch* ligand) butterfly vertebrae are a feature in approximately 60% of cases (Fig. 8-13*C*). All the above-mentioned genes are linked to the *Notch* signaling pathway and are necessary for functioning of the segmentation clock (discussed in Ch. 4), which regulates *Hox* gene expression in the presomitic mesoderm.

Myotomes and Dermatomes Develop at Segmental Levels

As mentioned above, as the sclerotome forms, the dorsal part of the somite remains epithelial and is called the **dermomyotome**. This structure quickly separates into two structures: a **dermatome** and a **myotome** (Fig. 8-14; also see Fig. 8-3 and 8-4). The dermatomes contribute to the dermis (including fat and connective tissue) of the neck and the back. However, as discussed in Chapter 7, most of the dermis is derived from somatopleuric lateral plate mesoderm (also, as discussed in Ch. 16, the dermis of the head is derived from neural crest cells).

The myotomes differentiate into myogenic (muscle-producing) cells (see Fig. 8-14). Each myotome splits into two structures: a dorsal **epimere** and a ventral **hypomere** (see Fig. 8-3 and 8-4). The epimeres give rise to the deep **epaxial muscles** of the back, including the **erector spinae** and **transversospinalis** groups. These are innervated by the **dorsal ramus of the spinal nerve**. The hypomeres form the **hypaxial muscles** of the lateral and ventral body wall in the thorax and abdomen. These are innervated by the **ventral ramus of the**

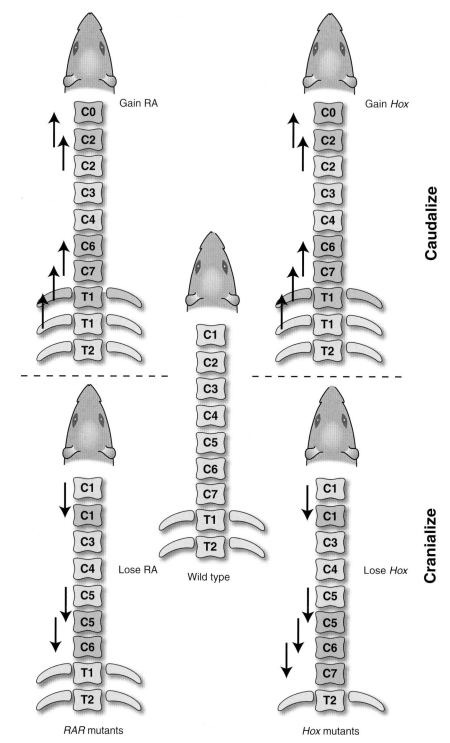

Figure 8-12. Homeotic transformations following gain and loss of either *Hox* gene function (right) or retinoid acid signaling (left).

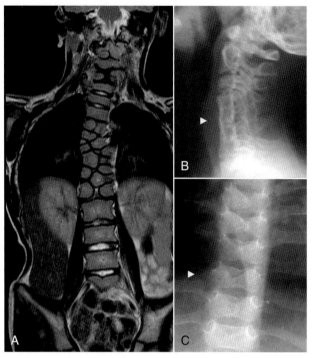

Figure 8-13. Different types of vertebral defects. *A*, Patient with an *MESP2* mutation showing severe vertebral segmentation defects. *B*, Klippel-Feil anomaly showing fused cervical vertebral bodies (arrowhead). *C*, Alagille syndrome showing "butterfly" vertebrae (arrowhead marks one vertebra; note the deep midline cleft in each vertebra).

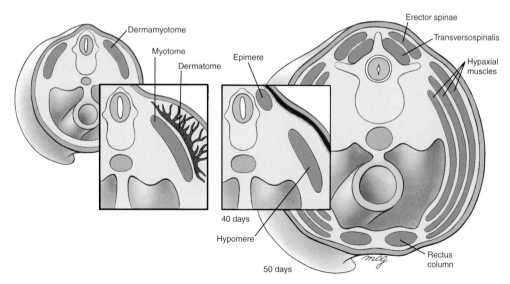

Figure 8-14. Fate of the dermomyotome. Each dermomyotome splits into a dermatome and a subjacent myotome. Dermatome cells migrate to the surface ectoderm of the corresponding segmental region. There, with cells from the lateral plate mesoderm, they form the dermis. Each myotome splits first into a dorsal epimere and ventral hypomere. The epimere forms the deep muscles of the back. In the thoracic region, the hypomere splits into three layers of the anterolateral muscles; in the abdominal region, a fourth ventral segment also differentiates and forms the rectus abdominis muscle.

spinal nerve. The hypaxial muscles include three layers of **intercostal muscles** in the thorax (**external** and **inner intercostals**, and **innermost intercostals**), the homologous three layers of the abdominal musculature (the **external oblique, internal oblique**, and **transversus abdominis**), and the **rectus abdominis** muscles that flank the ventral midline. The rectus column is usually limited to the abdominal region, but occasionally it develops on either side of the sternum as a **sternalis muscle**. In the cervical region, hypaxial myoblasts form the strap muscles of the neck, including the **scalene** and **infrahyoid** muscles. In the lumbar region, the hypomeres form the **quadratus lumborum** muscles. At limb-forming levels, somitic hypaxial myoblasts also invade the developing limb buds and give rise to the **limb musculature**. In the occipital region, somitic (i.e., occipital; discussed in Ch. 16) hypaxial myoblasts migrate along the hypoglossal cord to form the **intrinsic** and **extrinsic tongue musculature**. In addition to the musculature, the tendons in the body wall also arise from the somite in close association with the myotome.

IN THE RESEARCH LAB

MYOGENIC COMMITMENT IN SOMITE

Wnt signaling is necessary for both hypaxial and epaxial muscle development *and two pathways have been implicated*. Wnt signaling via the classical canonical pathway induces epaxial muscle formation, whereas *both epaxial and* hypaxial muscle differentiation *require* a novel PKA/Creb (protein Kinase A/cAMP response element binding protein) Wnt signalling pathway. In the epaxial myotome, *Wnt* signaling induces the expression of the *Bmp* antagonist *Noggin* in the dorsal medial lip (Fig. 8-15*A*). *Noggin* blocks the repressive action of *Bmps* (produced by both the dorsal neural tube and lateral plate mesoderm), resulting in the onset of *Myf5* expression. Myogenic commitment is followed by the migration of the cells into the myotome from all the edges of the dermomyotome (Fig 8-15). The cells in the myotome switch on the expression of *MyoD*, become postmitotic, and differentiate. Bipotential cells in the central dermomyotome give rise to the second wave of myogenic progenitors (Fig 8-15*B*). The cells divide perpendicularly to the dermotome: those that enter the myotome are the progenitors of the secondary myogenesis in the axial muscle. These cells are characterized by *Frek* (a *Fibroblast growth factor receptor*), *Pax3*, and *Pax7* expression. They are mitotically active and are not yet committed to the myogenic pathway. The other cells arising from these divisions do not express these genes and form the dermis.

Myostatin (also known as *Gdf8, Growth differentiation factor8*), a member of the *Tgfβ* family, is a negative regulator of muscle differentiation. Naturally occurring mutations in **Myostatin** occur in large doubled-muscled cattle, such as the Belgian Blue and Piedmontese, as a result of muscle hypertrophy and hyperplasia. *MYOSTATIN* mutations have been reported in humans and are linked to increased muscle strength.

A novel compartment has been identified at the rostral and caudal ends of the somite: the **syndetome**. The syndetome is characterized by *Scleraxis* expression and contains the **tendon** progenitors. Syndetome development is regulated by *Fgf8* signaling from the myotome.

Long Bone and Joint Development

With the exception of part of the clavicle, the bones of the limbs and girdles (constituting the **appendicular skeleton**) form by **endochondral ossification**. Part of the clavicle, in contrast, is a **membrane bone**.

Most of the endochondral bones of the limb are long bones. Their development begins as mesenchymal cells condense (long bone development is summarized in Fig. 8-16*A*). In response to growth factors, **chondrocytes** differentiate within this mesenchyme and begin to secrete molecules characteristic of the extracellular matrix of cartilage, such as *Collagen type II* and *Proteoglycans*.

Distinct layers of chondrocytes form (Fig. 8-16*B*). At the end, or **epiphyses**, of the elements are the resting chondrocytes, the progenitor cells for cartilage growth. Towards the center, or **diaphysis**, of the long bone, there is a proliferating layer of chondrocytes, then a **prehypertrophic** zone in which the chondrocytes have enlarged. Finally, at the center are enlarged terminally differentiated, or **hypertrophic**, chondrocytes that are surrounded by calcified matrix. Hypertrophic chondrocytes express *Collagen type X*.

Following terminal differentiation (i.e., hypertrophy) the process of **ossification** commences in the **primary ossification center** at the center of the long bone (see Fig. 8-16*A*). Ossification begins when the developing bone is invaded by multiple blood vessels that branch from the limb vasculature (discussed in Ch. 13). One of these vessels eventually becomes dominant and gives rise to the **nutrient artery** that

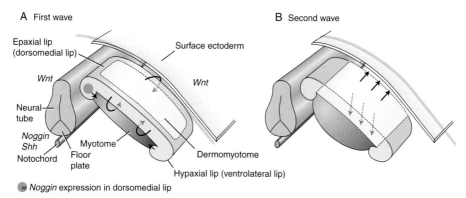

A First wave

Epaxial lip
(dorsomedial lip)

Surface ectoderm

Wnt

Wnt

Neural tube

*Noggin
Shh*
Notochord

Myotome

Floor plate

Dermomyotome

Hypaxial lip (ventrolateral lip)

B Second wave

● = *Noggin* expression in dorsomedial lip

Figure 8-15. Development of the myotome. *A*, Myogenic cells in the myotome first form from the edges of the dermomyotome (i.e., the epaxial and hypaxial lips, and cranial and caudal borders) in response to *Wnt* signaling. Arrows indicate the directions of cell movements from the dermomyotome into the myotome in the first wave of cell migration. *B*, Myogenic cells then arise from the central region of the dermomyotome, which also gives rise to cells in the dermis. Arrows indicate cell movements from the dermomyotome into the myotome (curved arrows) in the first wave of cell migration (*A*), and from the dermomyotome into the myotome (dashed arrows) and from the dermomyotome into the dermis (solid arrows) in the second wave of cell migration (*B*).

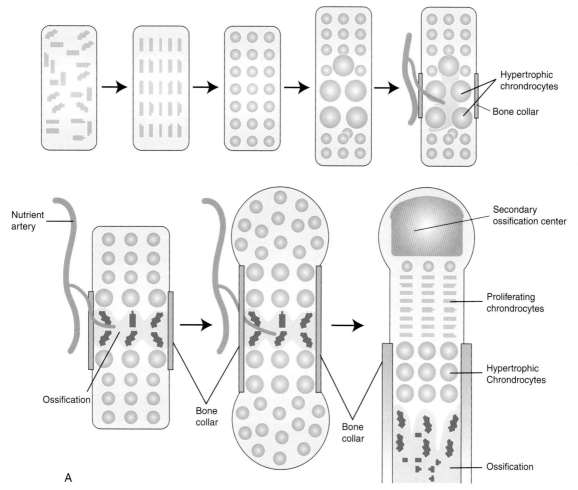

Hypertrophic chondrocytes

Bone collar

Nutrient artery

Secondary ossification center

Proliferating chondrocytes

Hypertrophic Chondrocytes

Ossification

Bone collar

Bone collar

Ossification

A

Figure 8-16. Long bone development. *A*, Summary of long bone development.

Continued

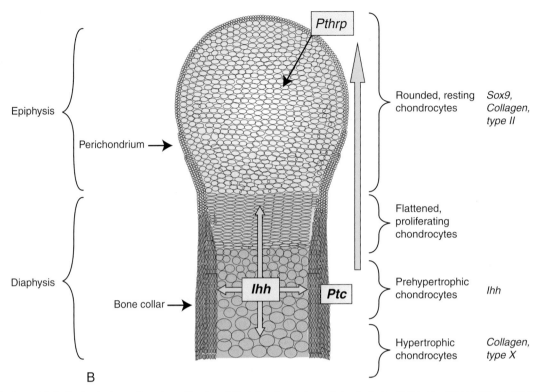

B

Figure 8-16, cont'd. *B,* The developing cartilage element has four distinct chondrocyte layers. *Indian hedgehog (Ihh)* is one of the crucial genes that regulates the differentiation of the chondrocytes; it signals through the *Patched (Ptc)* receptor.

nourishes the bone. The establishment of the vasculature brings in the preosteoblastic cells that differentiate into osteoblasts and replace the hypertrophic chondrocytes. The osteoblasts lay down *Collagen type I* and mineralized matrix. Ossification spreads from the primary ossification center toward the epiphyses of the anlage to form a loose **trabecular network** of bone.

In addition to osteoblasts, the blood vessels bring in cells called **osteoclasts**, which break down previously formed bone. These are important for remodeling of the growing bone. Bone is continually remodeled throughout development and adult life.

The region surrounding the diaphysis ossifies to form a **primary bone collar** around the circumference of the bone. This primary bone collar thickens as osteoblasts differentiate in progressively more peripheral layers of the perichondrium to form **cortical bone**.

At birth, the **diaphyses**—or shafts of the limb bones (consisting of a bone collar and trabecular core)—are completely ossified, whereas the ends of the bones, called the **epiphyses**, are still cartilaginous. After

birth **secondary ossification centers** develop in the epiphyses, which gradually ossify. However, a layer of cartilage called the **epiphyseal cartilage plate** (**growth plate** or **physis**) persists between the epiphysis and the growing end of the diaphysis (**metaphysis**). In the epiphyseal cartilage plate, distinct zones of chondrocytes are present, and because growth is predominantly along the long axis of the bones, the chondrocytes are arranged in columns. Continued proliferation of the chondrocytes followed by differentiation and replacement by bone in this growth plate allows the diaphysis to lengthen. Finally, when the growth of the body is complete at about 20 years of age, the epiphyseal growth plate completely ossifies.

The process of ossification is similar in other endochondral bones, although some cartilage elements such as the cartilages of the larynx, intervertebral discs, and pinna do not ossify. The chondrocostal cartilages also remain unossified until about 50 years old.

Figure 8-17 illustrates the process by which the **diarthrodial (synovial) joints** connecting the limb bones develop. First, the mesenchyme of the interzones

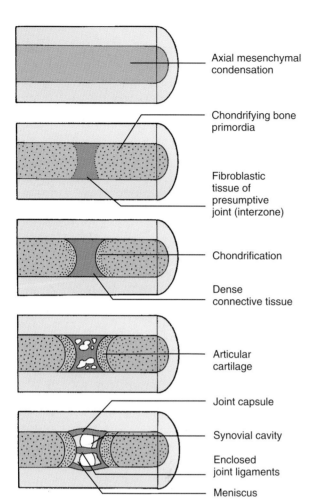

Axial mesenchymal condensation

Chondrifying bone primordia

Fibroblastic tissue of presumptive joint (interzone)

Chondrification

Dense connective tissue

Articular cartilage

Joint capsule

Synovial cavity

Enclosed joint ligaments

Meniscus

Figure 8-17. Formation of joints. Cartilage, ligaments, and capsular elements of the joints develop from the interzone regions of the axial mesenchymal condensations that form the long bones of the limbs.

between the chondrifying bone primordia differentiates into **fibroblastic tissue** (undifferentiated connective tissue). This tissue then further differentiates into three regions: a cartilage layer at either end of the future joint (the **articular cartilage**), in contact with the adjacent bone primordia, and a central region of dense connective tissue. The connective tissue of this central region gives rise to the internal elements of the joint. Proximally and distally, it condenses to form the **synovial tissue** that will line the future joint cavity. Its central zone gives rise to the **menisci** and **enclosed joint ligaments**, such as the cruciate ligaments of the knee. Vacuoles form within connective tissue and coalesce (that is, the central region of the dense connective tissue cavitates) to form the **synovial cavity**.

The **joint capsule** arises from the mesenchymal sheath surrounding the entire interzone.

Synchondroidal or **fibrous joints** such as those connecting the bones of the pelvis, also develop from interzones. However, as also discussed in Chapter 18, the interzone mesenchyme simply differentiates into a single layer of fibrocartilage.

IN THE RESEARCH LAB

MOLECULAR REGULATION OF BONE AND JOINT DEVELOPMENT

The first step of chondrogenesis requires *Bmp* and *Fgf* induction of *Sox9* expression, which in turn regulates *Collagen type II* expression. In the absence of *Sox9*, the cartilaginous condensations do not form. *Sox5* and *Sox6* are coexpressed with *Sox9* in the nonhypertrophic chondrocytes and are also required for chondrogenesis. In *Sox5, 6* double mouse mutants, the early cartilage condensation forms, but the cells do not differentiate.

Once the chondrocyte layers and the perichondrium—the fibroblastic layer surrounding the cartilaginous element—have formed, development of the skeleton involves an interplay between the perichondrium and the chondrocytes (see Fig. 8-16B). *Indian hedgehog* (*Ihh*), expressed by the prehypertrophic chondrocytes, signals to the periarticular perichondrium to induce *Parathyroid hormone–related protein* (*Pthrp*) expression. *Pthrp* expression in turn signals to the proliferating and prehypertrophic chondrocytes, which express the *Pthrp receptor*. This signaling loop prevents hypertrophy. *Sox9* expression in the resting and proliferating chondrocytes also delays hypertrophy, whereas *Runx2* is needed for hypertrophy in some cartilage elements.

Activating *PTHRP RECEPTOR 1* mutations in humans cause **Jansen-type metaphyseal chondrodysplasia**, characterized by short limbs and dwarfism, whereas inactivating *PTHRP RECEPTOR 1* mutations result in **Blomstrand chondrodysplasia**, marked by accelerated bone formation and premature death.

Independent of *Pthrp*, *Ihh* regulates chondrocyte proliferation and promotes hypertrophy. *Ihh* also induces the development of the bone collar around the diaphysis of the cartilage element. Vascularization is induced by *Vascular endothelial growth factor* (*Vegf*) expressed by hypertrophic chondrocytes. *Runx2* expression in the hypertrophic chondrocytes regulates *Vegf* expression.

Members of the *Wnt* signaling family also control chondrogenesis. Different members can promote condensation (*Wnt5a*), or delay (*Wnt5b*) or promote (*β-Catenin* signaling)

8

hypertrophy. Importantly, *Wnt* signaling (specifically, *Wnt9a*—previously called *Wnt14*—and *Wnt4*) via the *β-Catenin* pathway regulates joint development by preventing chondrogenic differentiation in the joint interzone.

Gdf5 (*Growth and differentiation factor 5*), which is downstream of *Wnt9a*, is also expressed in the joint interzone (Fig. 8-18). In mice and in humans, *Gdf5* is necessary for the development of some of the appendicular joints, but its precise role in this process is unknown because over expression of *Gdf5*, unlike *Wnt9a*, does not induce/maintain joint formation. *Gdf6* (*Growth and differentiation factor 6*) is also expressed in developing joints, and the *Gdf5/6* double mouse mutant lacks both appendicular and axial joints.

Following specification of the joint, its cavitation to form the joint (synovial) cavity is achieved by the secretion of *Hyaluronan* (also called *Hyaluronic acid* or *Hyaluronate*, a glycosaminoglycan that readily absorbs water, thereby creating tissue spaces). Movement promotes *Hyaluronan* synthesis; if movement is prevented during development (e.g., by neuromuscular paralysis), the joints either do not cavitate or, if they have started to cavitate, they fuse and the joint becomes fixed.

Osteoblast development is controlled by the transcription factors, *Runx2* and *Osterix* and requires canonical *Wnt* signaling (see following "In the Clinic" for additional discussion). *Runx2* induces the differentiation of the early pre-osteoblast, preventing a mesenchymal cell forming other cell-types, whereas *β-Catenin* signaling and *Osterix* are required for further differentiation into osteoblasts. Terminal differentiation of osteoblasts (i.e., the formation of osteocytes) requires the transcription factor *Atf4*.

Osteoclast development depends on osteoblasts. First, osteoblasts express *Macrophage colony stimulating factor*, which promotes the proliferation and survival of osteoclast precursors and also upregulates the expression of a receptor called *Rank* (*Receptor activator of nuclear factor kappa B*). Osteoblasts also express the ligand *Rankl*, which binds to the *Rank* receptor on osteoclasts and osteoclast precursors. This interaction promotes differentiation of the osteoclasts and activates mature osteoclasts. Emphasizing this importance, gene inactivation of either *Rank* or *Rankl* results in a complete absence of osteoclasts. The interplay between osteoblasts and osteoclasts is also negatively controlled by the production of *Osteoprotegerin*, a *Rankl* decoy receptor (a receptor directly secreted into the extracellular space), secreted by the osteoblasts. In this case, *Osteoprotegerin* binds to *Rankl*, preventing its binding to *Rank* on the osteoclast progenitor.

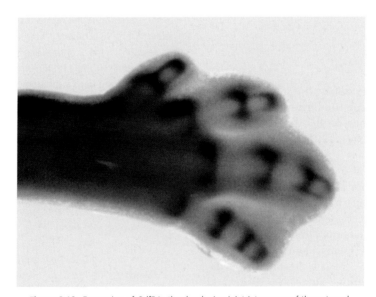

Figure 8-18. Expression of *Gdf5* in the developing joint interzones of the autopod.

IN THE CLINIC

DEFECTS IN SKELETAL DEVELOPMENT

Defects in skeletal development may be the result of defects in growth factor signaling (*Fgf* and *Gdf5*), transcription factors (e.g., *Sox9* and *Cbfa1*), and matrix components (*Collagens types I, II,* and *X*). These can include syndromes where all endochondral bones are affected, as in **achondroplasia**. Alternatively, these can include conditions in which a subset of skeletal structures is affected, as in **Grebe type chondrodysplasia** (Fig. 8-19), which specifically affects the appendicular skeleton, or as in spondylocostal dysplasia syndromes, discussed earlier in this chapter. Similarly, membranous bones can be specifically affected, as in **craniosynostosis** (discussed in the first "In the Clinic" of Ch. 16). Defects in skeletal development may be linked to changes in patterning, as in some spondylocostal abnormalities (other examples are discussed in Ch. 18), or they may reflect intrinsic changes in skeletal tissues. The different skeletal syndromes are summarized in Figure 8-20.

Achondroplasia, an autosomal dominant syndrome, is the most common form of dwarfism. It is characterized by shortening of the long bones, a small midface resulting from defects in the cranial base (the latter is derived from endochondral bones as discussed in Ch. 16), and curvature of the spine. Achondroplasia is the result of a mutation of the *Fibroblast growth factor receptor 3* (*FGFR3*). Mutations in *FGFR3* can also cause the more severe, neonatally lethal syndromes such as **thanatophoric dysplasia type I** and **II**, and other skeletal syndromes. Although mutations in *FGF* can be associated with craniosynostosis (e.g., in **Muenke syndrome**), in general *FGFR1* and *2* mutations are linked with craniosynostosis (i.e., abnormal growth of the sutures as discussed in Ch. 16). *FGFR3* mutations, on the other hand, are associated with defects in endochondral growth. However, in all cases, the *FGFR* mutations result in constitutive activation of the *FGF* signaling pathway. Animal models with *Fgfr3* mutations have been used to show that the abnormal skeletal growth is due to decreased chondrocyte proliferation.

8

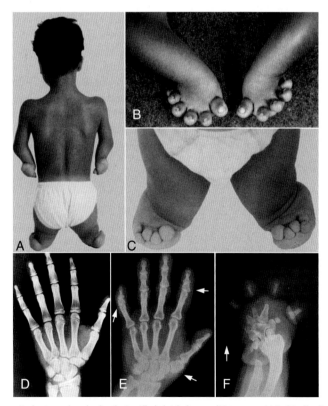

Figure 8-19. Mutations in *GDF5* cause Grebe-type chondrodysplasia. All skeletal abnormalities are restricted to the limb. *A,* Ten-year-old boy with a *GDF5* mutation showing severe lower limb and upper limb anomalies. *B, C,* Enlarged views of the upper and lower limbs, respectively. *D,* Normal hand of a 10-year-old child. *E,* Child with a heterozygous mutation showing shortened phalangeal elements (marked with arrows). *F,* Child with a homozygous mutation showing severe carpal and phalangeal anomalies, as well as distal anomalies of the radius and ulna.

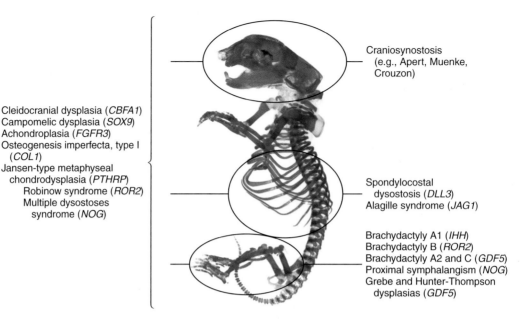

Craniosynostosis
(e.g., Apert, Muenke, Crouzon)

Cleidocranial dysplasia (*CBFA1*)
Campomelic dysplasia (*SOX9*)
Achondroplasia (*FGFR3*)
Osteogenesis imperfecta, type I
(*COL1*)
Jansen-type metaphyseal
chondrodysplasia (*PTHRP*)
Robinow syndrome (*ROR2*)
Multiple dysostoses
syndrome (*NOG*)

Spondylocostal
dysostosis (*DLL3*)
Alagille syndrome (*JAG1*)

Brachydactyly A1 (*IHH*)
Brachydactyly B (*ROR2*)
Brachydactyly A2 and C (*GDF5*)
Proximal symphalangism (*NOG*)
Grebe and Hunter-Thompson
dysplasias (*GDF5*)

Figure 8-20. Summary diagram showing that different gene mutations in humans affect different regions of the skeleton (mouse skeleton shown).

In contrast, some syndromes affect discrete groups of bones. This is typified by **Grebe** and **Hunter-Thompson type chondrodysplasias** and **brachydactyly types C** and **A2** (see Figs. 8-19, 8-20). These are all characterized by shortening of the appendicular skeleton (*brachydactyly* means short fingers), and they all can result from mutations in *GDF5*. *GDF5* promotes chondrogenesis by increasing the size of the initial chondrocyte condensations and increasing chondrocyte proliferation. Grebe and Hunter-Thompson syndromes can affect all limb skeletal elements, with increasing severity in a proximal-to-distal direction; in the brachydactyly syndromes only the phalanges are affected (shortened). Both the Grebe and Hunter-Thompson syndromes are autosomal recessive, but Grebe-type chondrodysplasia is more severe than the Hunter-Thompson–type. This is attributed to the different mutations in the *GDF5* gene (so-called **genotype-phenotype correlations**). The Hunter-Thompson-type chondrodysplasia is predicted to be loss of function, whereas in Grebe-type chondrodysplasia, the mutated *GDF5* protein is able to form dimers with other *BMP* members, which cannot be secreted. Therefore, Grebe syndrome is the result of loss of *GDF5* function, as in Hunter-Thompson syndrome, together with a dominant negative effect on other members of the *BMP* family. The brachydactyly phenotypes are milder: in these syndromes, only one copy of *GDF5* is mutated/nonfunctional.

GDF5 mutations are also found in autosomal dominant **proximal symphalangism**, the fusion of the inter-phalangeal, wrist, and ankle joints. Analysis of one of these *GDF5* mutations has shown that it is a gain-of-function mutation, with the mutant protein showing increased binding to the *BMPR1A* receptor. Mutations in *NOGGIN*, a *BMP* antagonist, also result in proximal symphalangism and **multiple synostoses syndrome type 1**, which is characterized by the fusion of the limb joints and craniofacial anomalies that are typified by conductive hearing loss and a broad nose. This syndrome can also involve synostoses of the vertebrae. Likewise, the *Noggin* mutant mouse has multiple fusions of the bones in both the appendicular and axial skeletons.

The study of these human skeletal mutations has taught us that increased *BMP/GDF5* activity causes joint fusions, and blocking *BMP* activity is necessary both for normal joint development in the embryo and maintenance of the joint cavity postnatally. In addition, loss of *BMP/GDF5* signaling results in defective growth of the skeleton. Moreover, the mouse mutants *short ear* and *brachypod*, which have mutations in *Bmp5* and *Gdf5*, respectively, exhibit distinct defects: *Short ear* mutant mice have defects in the external ear, sternum, and ribs; whereas *brachypod* mutant mice have defects restricted to the appendicular skeleton. Collectively, these findings have led to the idea that a mosaic pattern of *Bmp* signaling determines the patterning and development of individual skeletal elements.

Other genes are also essential for osteoblast and osteoclast development and function. A decrease in the number of functional osteoblasts, and/or an increase in the number of osteoclasts, results in **osteoporosis**, the loss of bone mass, associated with increased skeletal fragility and bone fracture. The converse situation results in an excess bone mass, or **osteopetrosis**. Mutations in the *LIPOPROTEIN RECEPTOR PROTEIN*, *LRP5*, a *WNT* coreceptor, result in either an increase in bone mass or a decrease (**osteoporosis pseudoglioma syndrome**) in bone mass, both of which are attributed to changes in osteoblast development. *LRP5* controls osteoblast proliferation, differentiation, and survival, and the *LRP5* mutations that result in a decrease in bone mass are due to loss of *LRP5* function. Other mutations that cause osteoporosis occur in the *RANKL DECOY RECEPTOR* gene *OSTEOPROTEGERIN* (discussed earlier in the chapter). Loss of this decoy receptor increases the *RANK/RANKL* interaction between osteoclast progenitors and osteoblasts, enhancing osteoclast differentiation.

The mutations in *LRP5* that result in a gain of bone mass affect the ability of the *WNT* antagonist *DICKKOPF 1* to bind to the *LRP5* receptor and block *WNT* signaling. Hence, these mutations result in increased *WNT* signaling via the *β-CATENIN* pathway. Other mutations that result in osteopetrosis include those that affect different aspects of osteoclast function. Mutations in the vacuolar proton pump, as in **infantile malignant osteopetrosis**, prevent the establishment of the acidic environment necessary to dissolve the mineral matrix. *CATHEPSIN K* is a secreted osteoclast enzyme that works at low pH to degrade exposed organic residues. Mutations in *CATHEPSIN K* result in **pycnodysostosis**, another condition with enhanced bone mass.

In addition to mutations in genes expressed in skeletal tissues, defects in tissues outside the skeleton may affect its development. Postnatal growth is regulated hormonally, and defects in the pituitary gland, as in **acromegaly**—a condition in which growth hormone production is increased—increases the size of the hands, feet, and face.

Development of Limb Muscles

Both axial muscles of the trunk and muscles of limb develop similarly, with both groups of muscles arising from somitic myotomes and migrating ventrally —along the dorsolateral body wall into the ventral body wall in the case of axial muscles, and ventrally into the limb buds in the case of limb muscles.

Both groups of muscles are innervated by spinal nerves bordering their level of origin (by dorsal and ventral rami in the case of axial muscles, and by ventral rami only in the case of limb muscles). As discussed in Chapters 10 and 11, the muscle of the diaphragm also arises from somitic myotomes (specifically cervical myotomes 3, 4, and 5). Thus, as the diaphragm descends to form a partition separating the pleural and abdominal cavities, it carries its innervation—the **phrenic nerves**—with it, explaining why a thoracic/abdominal structure is innervated by nerves originating from the cervical region.

In human embryos, migration of the myogenic precursors into the limb buds starts during the 5th week of development. The invading myoblasts form two large condensations in the dorsal and ventral limb bud (Fig. 8-21). The dorsal muscle mass gives rise in general to the **extensors** and **supinators** of the upper limb and to the **extensors** and **abductors** of the lower

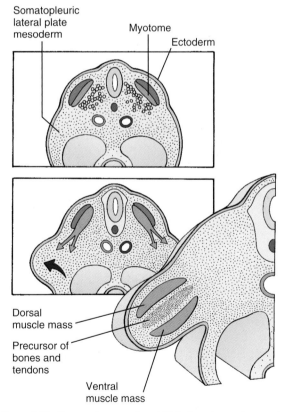

Figure 8-21. The muscle progenitors initially form two major muscle masses as the limb bud forms (arrow). The ventral muscle mass gives rise mainly to the flexors, pronators, and adductors, where as the dorsal muscle mass gives rise mainly to extensors, supinators, and abductors.

Table 8-1 Muscles Derived from the Ventral and Dorsal Muscle Masses of the Limb Buds

Ventral Muscle Mass	Dorsal Muscle Mass
Upper Limb	**Upper Limb**
Anterior compartment of arm and forearm	Posterior compartment muscles of arm and forearm
All muscles on palmar surface of hand	Deltoid
Lower Limb	Lateral compartment muscles of forearm and hand
Medial compartment muscles of thigh	Latissimus dorsi
Posterior compartment muscles of thigh except for short head of biceps femoris	Rhomboids
Posterior compartment muscles of leg	Levator scapulae
All muscles on plantar surface of foot	Serratus anterior
Obturator internus	Teres major and minor
Gemellus superior and inferior	Subscapularis
Quadratus femoris	Supraspinatus
	Infraspinatus
	Lower Limb
	Anterior compartment muscles of thigh and leg
	Tensor fascia latae
	Short head of biceps femoris
	Lateral compartment muscles of leg
	Muscles of the dorsum of foot
	Gluteus maximus, medius, and minimus
	Piriformis
	Iliacus
	Psoas

limb, whereas the ventral muscle mass gives rise to the **flexors** and **pronators** of the upper limb and to the **flexors** and **adductors** of the lower limb (Table 8-1). Experimental studies in animal models have shown that as these progenitor cells migrate toward the limb bud, they are bipotential and can form myocytes and/or endothelial cells (see following "In the Research Lab"). In contrast to limb muscles, which arise from the somitic myotomes, the limb tendons arise from the lateral plate mesoderm.

IN THE RESEARCH LAB

MIGRATION OF MUSCLE PROGENITORS

Classical quail-chick recombination experiments (discussed in Ch. 5) showed that the limb myogenic cells arise from the somites. Therefore, if a quail somite is transplanted into a chick host, the limb muscles will be of quail origin (Fig. 8-22). Importantly, experiments such as these have shown that

the limb muscles are patterned by the surrounding connective tissues, as in other regions of the body.

As discussed earlier in this chapter, the myogenic cells that give rise to the limb, tongue, and diaphragm muscles delaminate from the myotome to migrate into their respective final environments. Delamination and migration of muscle progenitors requires several factors. In the limb bud (Fig. 8-23) these include *Pax3* (a paired-box transcription factor), *c-Met* (a proto-oncogene; that is, a normal gene that when mutated can become an oncogene, resulting in the development of cancer), *Hgf* (*Hepatocyte growth factor*)/*scatter factor*, and *Lbx1* (homolog of the Drosophila *Lady bird late* gene, a homeobox transcription factor). In response to *Hgf* signaling in the early limb bud, *c-Met*–expressing cells in the somitic myotome delaminate and start to migrate. *Pax3* regulates the expression of *c-Met*—the *Hgf receptor* that is necessary for migration. Therefore, in the **splotch** mouse (*Pax3* mutant), the limb (and also the diaphragm) muscles are absent. The transcription factor *Lbx1* is also required. In *Lbx1* mutants

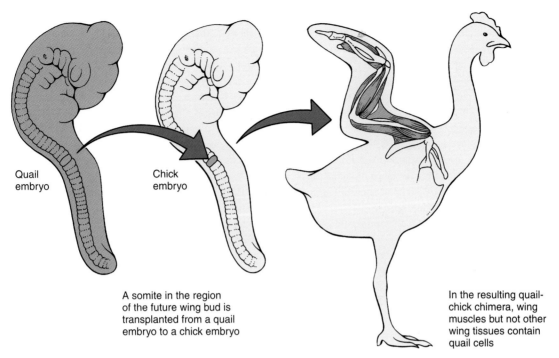

Quail
embryo

Chick
embryo

A somite in the region
of the future wing bud is
transplanted from a quail
embryo to a chick embryo

In the resulting quail-
chick chimera, wing
muscles but not other
wing tissues contain
quail cells

Figure 8-22. Summary diagram showing cell-tracing experiment using quail-chick transplantation chimeras. This experiment demonstrated that the musculature of the limbs forms from somitic mesoderm, whereas the limb bones form from lateral plate mesoderm. Quail somites, transplanted to the axial level at which limb bud development occurs, give rise to limb myocytes.

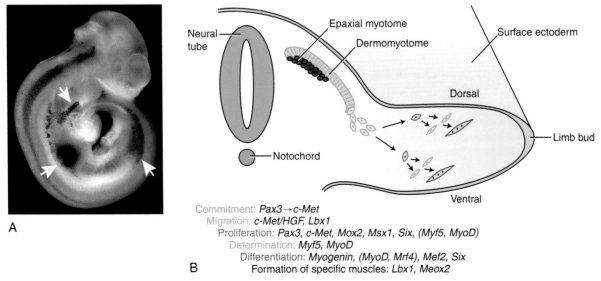

A

B

Commitment: *Pax3→c-Met*
Migration: *c-Met/HGF, Lbx1*
Proliferation: *Pax3, c-Met, Mox2, Msx1, Six, (Myf5, MyoD)*
Determination: *Myf5, MyoD*
Differentiation: *Myogenin, (MyoD, Mrf4), Mef2, Six*
Formation of specific muscles: *Lbx1, Meox2*

Figure 8-23. Regulation of limb myogenesis. *A,* Expression of *Lbx1,* a gene necessary for migration in the migratory limb and tongue muscle precursors (arrows). *B,* Summary diagram showing the molecular regulators of limb myogenesis.

myogenic precursors delaminate but do not migrate appropriately; consequently, hindlimb muscles are totally absent but flexor muscles (ventral muscle mass) form in the forelimb. Once within the limb bud, the premyogenic cells proliferate (requires several genes as listed in Fig. 8-23) and become committed to the myogenic pathway. This commitment requires *Pax3*, which regulates the expression of *Myf5* (discussed earlier in this chapter). *Meox2* (a homeobox gene; also called Mox2) is needed for the development of the appropriate number of myogenic cells in the limb, which in turn leads to the formation of the full range of normal limb muscles; in the absence of *Meox2* function, some of the limb muscles do not form or are abnormally patterned.

Recent fate mapping studies have shown the surprising result that the ventral muscle mass of the hindlimb also gives rise to the perineal muscles (i.e., the muscles located in the perineal region; development of this area is discussed in Ch. 15). These muscles include the external anal sphincter, superficial transverse perineal muscle, ischiocavernosus muscle, bulbospongiosus muscle, deep transverse perineal muscle, and sphincter urethrae muscle. During their formation, the prospective perineal muscles move caudally from the hindlimbs to the forming perineal region.

MUSCLE CELL AND FIBER TYPE COMMITMENT

Cell lineage studies in which an individual premigratory hypaxial cell is labeled with a unique molecular tag have shown that as the cells leave the somite they are not yet committed to either an endothelial or myogenic cell fate (as discussed in Ch. 13, paraxial mesoderm also contributes to the endothelium of intraembryonic blood vessels). Thus, endothelial and myogenic differentiation occurs as a result of local environmental cues within the limb bud. Similarly, early myogenic cells are not yet committed to become either **slow** or **fast** myocytes. The distribution of slow and fast myotubes determines how a muscle functions. Simplistically, slow myocytes are characterized by the expression of slow *Myosin heavy chain* (*MyHC*); slow myocytes contract slowly and have oxidative metabolism (i.e., aerobic metabolism). Consequently, these fibers do not fatigue quickly and are involved in the maintenance of posture. In contrast, "fast" fibers tend to express fast *MyHCs*, contract rapidly with high force, and have glycolytic metabolism (i.e., anaerobic metabolism). "Fast" fibers are needed for movement. As in cell fate determination, local environmental cues also control slow and fast fiber differentiation within the limb bud.

REGIONAL DIFFERENCES IN DEVELOPMENT OF MUSCLES

The development of axial and limb muscles has been emphasized in this chapter on musculoskeletal development.

However, it is important to point out that differences exist between what has been described here for the development of axial and limb muscles and for the development of the craniofacial muscles (discussed in Ch. 16). For example, as discussed earlier in this "In the Research Lab," although *Pax3* mutations affect the development of the trunk and limb muscles, the craniofacial musculature is unaffected. Conversely, inactivation of *Capsulin* and *MyoR*, two transcription factors related to the myogenic regulatory factors (discussed earlier in the chapter), results in the loss of a subset of jaw muscles, leaving the majority of axial muscles unaffected. Reflecting the different molecular networks, regulation of *Myf5* is controlled by distinct enhancers in the head and trunk. Also, whereas *Wnt* signaling is necessary for myogenic commitment in the trunk and limb, *Wnt* signaling is inhibitory for myogenesis in the head.

IN THE CLINIC

MUSCULAR DYSTROPHY

Muscular abnormalities include the devastating muscular dystrophies where functional muscle mass is either not maintained or the satellite cells, the progenitors for postnatal growth and muscle repair, are defective. The X-linked **Duchenne muscular dystrophy**, with the milder condition, **Becker type muscular dystrophy**, are both due to mutations in *DYSTROPHIN*, a large protein (encoded by the largest gene in the human genome) that links intracellular cytoskeletal proteins with the sarcolemma, the plasma membrane of the muscle fiber. Duchenne muscular dystrophy occurs in 1 in 3500 male infants and affects most of the muscles of the body. Other dystrophies may affect a subset of muscles, such as **oculopharyngeal muscular dystrophy** (due to mutations in *PABPN1*, *POLYADENYLATE-BINDING PROTEIN, NUCLEAR 1*), which affects the neck, face, and proximal limb muscles. Muscular defects can also include the absence of specific muscles; for example, in the sporadic **Poland anomaly**, in which the pectoralis major muscle is absent on one side of the body, or in **prune-belly syndrome**, in which the abdominal wall muscles fail to develop. Finally, muscle weakness may have an extrinsic component resulting from defects in motor nerve innervation. This is typified by **Duane anomaly**, characterized by lateral gaze palsy (abnormal eye movements). In Duane anomaly, there are abnormalities in cranial nerve VI (abducens nerve), which innervates the lateral rectus, the extraocular eye muscle that moves the globe laterally.

Suggested Readings

Arber S, Burden SJ, Harris AJ. 2002. Patterning of skeletal muscle. Curr Opin Neurobiol 12:100-103.

Archer CW, Dowthwaite GP, Francis-West P. 2003. Development of synovial joints. Birth Defects Res C Embryo Today 69:144-155.

Bailey P, Holowacz T, Lassar AB. 2001. The origin of skeletal muscle stem cells in the embryo and the adult. Curr Opin Cell Biol 13:679-689.

Bodine PV, Komm BS. 2006. Wnt signaling and osteoblastogenesis. Rev Endocr Metab Disord 7:123-139.

Boyle WJ, Simonet WS, Lacey DL. 2003. Osteoclast differentiation and activation. Nature 423:337-342.

Brent AE, Tabin CJ. 2002. Developmental regulation of somite derivatives: muscle, cartilage and tendon. Curr Opin Genet Dev 12:548-557.

Bruzzaniti A, Baron R. 2006. Molecular regulation of osteoclast activity. Rev Endocr Metab Disord 7:33-39.

Buckingham M. 2006. Myogenic progenitor cells and skeletal myogenesis in vertebrates. Curr Opin Genet Dev 16:525-532.

Buckingham M, Bajard L, Daubas P, et al. 2006. Myogenic progenitor cells in the mouse embryo are marked by the expression of Pax3/7 genes that regulate their survival and myogenic potential. Anat Embryol (Berl) 211(Suppl 1):51-56.

Carapuco M, Novoa A, Bobola N, Mallo M. 2005. Hox genes specify vertebral types in the presomitic mesoderm. Genes Dev 19:2116-2121.

Christ B, Huang R, Scaal M. 2004. Formation and differentiation of the avian sclerotome. Anat Embryol (Berl) 208:333-350.

Christ B, Huang R, Wilting J. 2000. The development of the avian vertebral column. Anat Embryol (Berl) 202:179-194.

Davies KE, Nowak KJ. 2006. Molecular mechanisms of muscular dystrophies: old and new players. Nat Rev Mol Cell Biol 7:762-773.

de Crombrugghe B, Lefebvre V, Nakashima K. 2001. Regulatory mechanisms in the pathways of cartilage and bone formation. Curr Opin Cell Biol 13:721-727.

Durbeej M, Campbell KP. 2002. Muscular dystrophies involving the dystrophin-glycoprotein complex: an overview of current mouse models. Curr Opin Genet Dev 12:349-361.

Evans DJ, Valasek P, Schmidt C, Patel K. 2006. Skeletal muscle translocation in vertebrates. Anat Embryol (Berl) 211(Suppl 1):43-50.

Frugier T, Nicole S, Cifuentes-Diaz C, Melki J. 2002. The molecular bases of spinal muscular atrophy. Curr Opin Genet Dev 12:294-298.

Glass DA 2nd, Karsenty G. 2006. Molecular bases of the regulation of bone remodeling by the canonical Wnt signaling pathway. Curr Top Dev Biol 73:43-84.

Gridley T. 2003. Notch signaling and inherited disease syndromes. Hum Mol Genet 12(Spec No 1):R9-R13.

Gridley T. 2006. The long and short of it: somite formation in mice. Dev Dyn 235:2330-2336.

Hall BK, Miyake T. 2000. All for one and one for all: condensations and the initiation of skeletal development. Bioessays 22:138-147.

Horowitz MC, Lorenzo JA. 2004. The origins of osteoclasts. Curr Opin Rheumatol 16:464-468.

Joulia-Ekaza D, Cabello G. 2006. Myostatin regulation of muscle development: molecular basis, natural mutations, physiopathological aspects. Exp Cell Res 312:2401-2414.

Kalcheim C, Ben-Yair R. 2005. Cell rearrangements during development of the somite and its derivatives. Curr Opin Genet Dev 15:371-380.

Karsenty G. 2001. Minireview: transcriptional control of osteoblast differentiation. Endocrinology 142:2731-2733.

Karsenty G, Wagner EF. 2002. Reaching a genetic and molecular understanding of skeletal development. Dev Cell 2:389-406.

Krishnan V, Bryant HU, Macdougald OA. 2006. Regulation of bone mass by Wnt signaling. J Clin Invest 116:1202-1209.

Kronenberg HM. 2003. Developmental regulation of the growth plate. Nature 423:332-336.

Lai LP, Mitchell J. 2005. Indian hedgehog: its roles and regulation in endochondral bone development. J Cell Biochem 96:1163-1173.

Lohnes D. 2003. The Cdx1 homeodomain protein: an integrator of posterior signaling in the mouse. Bioessays 25:971-980.

Matsuoka T, Ahlberg PE, Kessaris N, et al. 2005. Neural crest origins of the neck and shoulder. Nature 436:347-355.

McKinsey TA, Zhang CL, Olson EN. 2001. Control of muscle development by dueling HATs and HDACs. Curr Opin Genet Dev 11:497-504.

McKinsey TA, Zhang CL, Olson EN. 2002. Signaling chromatin to make muscle. Curr Opin Cell Biol 14:763-772.

McLean W, Olsen BR. 2001. Mouse models of abnormal skeletal development and homeostasis. Trends Genet 17:S38-S43.

Monsoro-Burq AH. 2005. Sclerotome development and morphogenesis: when experimental embryology meets genetics. Int J Dev Biol 49:301-308.

Mundlos S. 1999. Cleidocranial dysplasia: clinical and molecular genetics. J Med Genet 36:177-182.

Mundy GR, Elefteriou F. 2006. Boning up on ephrin signaling. Cell 126:441-443.

Nakashima K, de Crombrugghe B. 2003. Transcriptional mechanisms in osteoblast differentiation and bone formation. Trends Genet 19:458-466.

Noden DM, Francis-West P. 2006. The differentiation and morphogenesis of craniofacial muscles. Dev Dyn 235:1194-1218.

Olsen BR, Reginato AM, Wang W. 2000. Bone development. Annu Rev Cell Dev Biol 16:191-220.

Pacifici M, Koyama E, Iwamoto M. 2005. Mechanisms of synovial joint and articular cartilage formation: recent advances, but many lingering mysteries. Birth Defects Res C Embryo Today 75:237-248.

Parker MH, Seale P, Rudnicki MA. 2003. Looking back to the embryo: defining transcriptional networks in adult myogenesis. Nat Rev Genet 4:497-507.

Pourquie O, Kusumi K. 2001. When body segmentation goes wrong. Clin Genet 60:409-416.

Pownall ME, Gustafsson MK, Emerson CP, Jr. 2002. Myogenic regulatory factors and the specification of muscle progenitors in vertebrate embryos. Annu Rev Cell Dev Biol 18:747-783.

Ralston SH, de Crombrugghe B. 2006. Genetic regulation of bone mass and susceptibility to osteoporosis. Genes Dev 20:2492-2506.

Reddy SV. 2004. Regulatory mechanisms operative in osteoclasts. Crit Rev Eukaryot Gene Expr 14:255-270.

Sparrow DB, Chapman G, Turnpenny PD, Dunwoodie SL. 2007. Disruption of the somitic molecular clock causes abnormal vertebral segmentation. Birth Defects Res C Embryo Today 81:93-110.

Scaal M, Christ B. 2004. Formation and differentiation of the avian dermomyotome. Anat Embryol (Berl) 208:411-424.

8

Teitelbaum SL, Ross FP. 2003. Genetic regulation of osteoclast development and function. Nat Rev Genet 4:638-649.

Turnpenny PD, Alman B, Cornier AS, et al. 2007. Abnormal vertebral segmentation and the notch signaling pathway in man. Dev Dyn 236:1456-1474.

van Deutekom JC, van Ommen GJ. 2003. Advances in Duchenne muscular dystrophy gene therapy. Nat Rev Genet 4:774-783.

Vasyutina E, Birchmeier C. 2006. The development of migrating muscle precursor cells. Anat Embryol (Berl) 211 (Suppl 1):37-41.

Wada T, Nakashima T, Hiroshi N, Penninger JM. 2006. RANKL-RANK signaling in osteoclastogenesis and bone disease. Trends Mol Med 12:17-25.

Wellik DM, Capecchi MR. 2003. Hox10 and Hox11 genes are required to globally pattern the mammalian skeleton. Science 301:363-367.

Yang X, Karsenty G. 2002. Transcription factors in bone: developmental and pathological aspects. Trends Mol Med 8:340-345.

Yoon BS, Lyons KM. 2004. Multiple functions of BMPs in chondrogenesis. J Cell Biochem 93:93-103.

Yusuf F, Brand-Saberi B. 2006. The eventful somite: patterning, fate determination and cell division in the somite. Anat Embryol (Berl) 211(Suppl 1):21-30.

Zelzer E, Olsen BR. 2003. The genetic basis for skeletal diseases. Nature 423:343-348.

Zhao C, Irie N, Takada Y, et al. 2006. Bidirectional ephrinB2-EphB4 signaling controls bone homeostasis. Cell Metab 4:111-121.

Development of the Central Nervous System

9

Summary Even before neurulation begins, the primordia of the three **primary brain vesicles**—the **prosencephalon, mesencephalon**, and **rhombencephalon**—are visible as broadenings in the neural plate. During the 5th week, the prosencephalon subdivides into the **telencephalon** and **diencephalon**, and the rhombencephalon subdivides into the **metencephalon** and **myelencephalon**. Thus, along with the mesencephalon, there are five **secondary brain vesicles**. During this period the hindbrain is divided into small repetitive segments called **rhombomeres**. The extension of the neural tube caudal to the rhombomeres constitutes the **spinal cord**.

The primordial brain portion of the neural tube undergoes flexion at three points. At two of these, the **mesencephalic (cranial) flexure** and **cervical flexure**, the bends are ventrally directed. At the **pontine flexure**, the bend is dorsally directed.

Cytodifferentiation of the neural tube begins in the rhombencephalon at the end of the 4th week. During this process, the neural tube neuroepithelium proliferates to produce the neurons, glia, and ependymal cells of the central nervous system. The young neurons, born in the **ventricular zone** that surrounds the central lumen, migrate peripherally to establish the **mantle zone**, the precursor of the gray matter, wherein lie the majority of mature neurons. Axons extending from mantle layer neurons establish the **marginal zone** (the future white matter) peripheral to the mantle zone. In areas of the brain that develop a cortex, including the cerebellum and cerebral hemispheres, the pattern of generation and migration of neurons is more complex.

The mantle zone of the spinal cord and brain stem is organized into a pair of **ventral (basal) plates** and a pair of **dorsal (alar) plates**. Laterally, the two plates abut at a groove called the **sulcus limitans;** dorsally and ventrally, they are connected by non-neurogenic structures called, respectively, the **roof plate** and **floor plate. Association neurons** form in the dorsal plates, and one or two cell columns (depending on the level) form in the ventral plates: the **somatic motor column** and the **visceral motor column**.

The nuclei of the 3rd to 12th cranial nerves are located in the brain stem (mesencephalon, metencephalon, and myelencephalon). Some of these cranial nerves are motor, some are sensory, and some are mixed, arising from more than one nucleus. The cranial nerve motor nuclei develop from the brain stem basal plates, and the associational sensory nuclei develop from the brain stem alar plates. The brain stem cranial nerve nuclei are organized into seven longitudinal columns, which correspond closely to the types of function they subserve. From ventromedial to dorsolateral, the three basal columns contain **somatic efferent, branchial (or special visceral) efferent,** and **(general) visceral efferent motoneurons**, and the four alar columns contain **general visceral afferent, special visceral afferent** (subserving the special sense of taste), **general somatic afferent**, and **special somatic afferent** (subserving the special senses of hearing and balance) **associational neurons**.

The myelencephalon gives rise to the **medulla oblongata**, the portion of the brain most similar in organization to the spinal cord. The metencephalon gives rise to the **pons**, a bulbous expansion that consists mainly of the massive white matter tracts serving the cerebellum, and to the **cerebellum**. A specialized process of neurogenesis in the cerebellum gives rise to the gray matter of the **cerebellar cortex**, as well as to the **deep cerebellar nuclei**. The cerebellum controls posture, balance, and the smooth execution of movements by coordinating sensory input with motor functions.

The mesencephalon contains nuclei of two cranial nerves as well as various other structures. In particular, the alar plates give rise to the **superior** and **inferior colliculi**, which are visible as round protuberances on the dorsal surface of the midbrain. The superior colliculi control ocular reflexes; the inferior colliculi serve as relays in the auditory pathway.

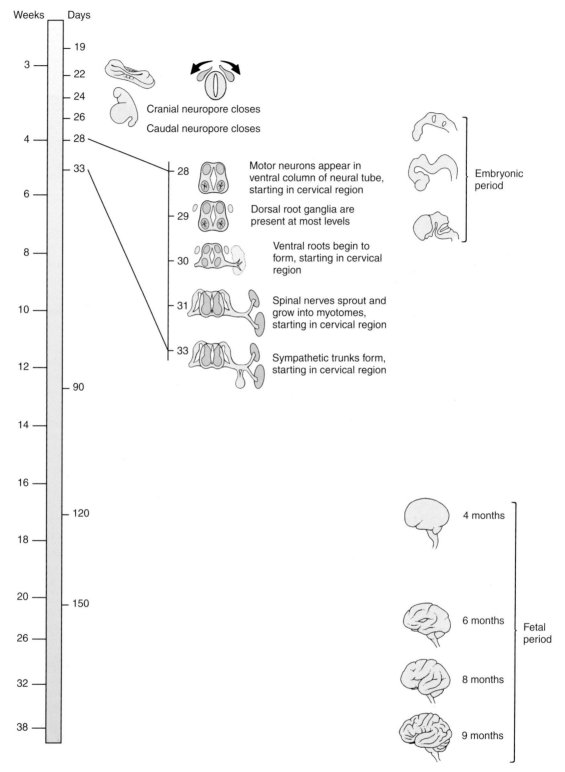

Weeks | Days

3 — 19
— 22
— 24
— 26
4 — 28

Cranial neuropore closes

Caudal neuropore closes

33

28 — Motor neurons appear in ventral column of neural tube, starting in cervical region

29 — Dorsal root ganglia are present at most levels

30 — Ventral roots begin to form, starting in cervical region

31 — Spinal nerves sprout and grow into myotomes, starting in cervical region

33 — Sympathetic trunks form, starting in cervical region

Embryonic period

6

8

10

12 — 90

14

16

18 — 120

20 — 150

26

32

38

4 months

6 months

8 months

9 months

Fetal period

Time line. Development of the brain and spinal cord.

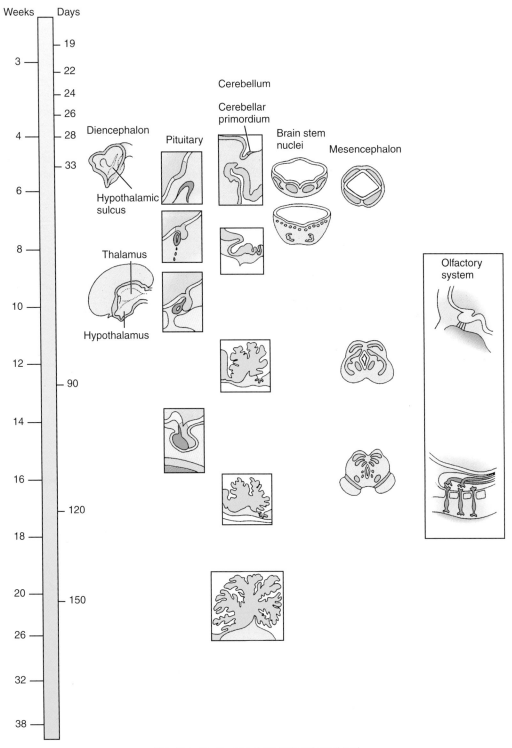

Time line. Development of the brain and spinal cord.

9

The forebrain has no basal plate. The alar plate of the diencephalon is divided into a dorsal portion and a ventral portion by a deep groove called the **hypothalamic sulcus**. The **hypothalamic swelling** ventral to this groove differentiates into the nuclei collectively known as the **hypothalamus**, the most prominent function of which is to control visceral activities such as heart rate and pituitary secretion. Dorsal to the hypothalamic sulcus, the large **thalamic swelling** gives rise to the **thalamus**, by far the largest diencephalic structure, which serves as a relay center, processing information from subcortical structures before passing it to the cerebral cortex. Finally, a dorsal swelling, the **epithalamus**, gives rise to a few smaller structures, including the pineal gland.

A ventral outpouching of the diencephalic midline, called the **infundibulum**, differentiates to form the **posterior pituitary**. A matching diverticulum of the stomodeal roof, called **Rathke's pouch**, grows to meet the infundibulum and becomes the **anterior pituitary**. Cranial diencephalic outpouchings also form the eyes, as discussed in Chapter 17.

The telencephalon is subdivided into a dorsal **pallium** and ventral **subpallium**. The latter forms the large neuronal nuclei of the **basal ganglia (corpus striatum, globus pallidus)** that are crucial to executing commands from the **cerebral hemispheres**. These cortical structures arise as lateral outpouchings of the pallium and grow rapidly to cover the diencephalon and mesencephalon. The hemispheres are joined by the cranial **lamina terminalis** (representing the zone of closure of the cranial neuropore) and by axon tracts called **commissures**, particularly the massive **corpus callosum**. The **olfactory bulbs** and **olfactory tracts** arise from the cranial telencephalon and receive input from the primary olfactory neurosensory cells, which differentiate from the nasal placodes and line the roof of the nasal cavity.

The expanded **primitive ventricles** formed by the neural canal in the secondary brain vesicles give rise to the ventricular system of the brain. The cerebrospinal fluid that fills the ventricle system is produced mainly by secretory **choroid plexuses** in the lateral, third, and fourth ventricles, which are formed by the ependyma and overlying vascular pia. The third ventricle also contains specialized ependymal secretory structures called **circumventricular organs.**

Clinical Taster

A mother brings her 4-year-old son to you for a second opinion regarding his bedwetting. She tells you that the problem has been getting worse, but their previous doctor continued to dismiss it as normal behavior. She states her concern that her son now has trouble staying dry even during the day, when he previously was able to stay dry both day and night. She worries that her son does not seem to sense when his bladder is full.

Your history reveals that the boy was born prematurely, resulting in several other ongoing medical issues, including eye and lung problems. During his stay in the neonatal intensive care unit (NICU), he had an ultrasound that revealed a minor bleed in his brain. The mother was told that this was very common and that they would have to "wait and see" if this was going to affect his development. More recently, she was told by her pediatrician that her son might be showing mild manifestations of cerebral palsy (CP), based on his poor coordination and his tendency to "toe walk," and that these signs of CP could be related to the bleeding he had in his brain. Obviously, she is confused and concerned, so she asks you if CP tends to get worse over time. She states that her son's stumbling and inability to walk long distances seem to be getting worse, along with his poor bladder control.

On examination you are alarmed to find decreased muscle mass and absent deep tendon reflexes in both lower extremities. The boy also has exaggerated arches in both feet, which could explain his abnormal gait, and you identify an unusual dimple at the base of his spine that is slightly off center. You order an MRI (magnetic resonance imaging) of the spinal cord, and the diagnosis of terminal **syringomyelia** (a fluid-filled cyst of the spinal cord) with a **tethered cord** (an abnormal attachment of the spinal cord to the sacrum) is made.

A variety of occult congenital anomalies of the spinal cord, including **tethered cord syndrome** (TCS), can lead to progressive neurologic dysfunction. Signs and symptoms include bladder and bowel dysfunction, motor or sensory abnormalities in the legs, loss of muscle mass, and bony deformities of the feet. The pathogenesis of the neurologic impairment in TCS is unknown, but it has been hypothesized that traction on the spinal cord, created by its tethering to the adjacent elongating tissues as they grow, results in decreased blood flow and spinal cord ischemia. With early diagnosis, untethering surgery can sometimes prevent, or even reverse, these sequelae.

Structural Divisions of Nervous System

The nervous system of vertebrates consists of two major *structural* divisions: a **central nervous system (CNS)** and a **peripheral nervous system (PNS)**. The CNS consists of the brain and spinal cord. The development of the CNS is discussed in this chapter. The PNS consists of all components of the nervous system outside of the CNS. Thus, the PNS consists of cranial nerves and ganglia, spinal nerves and ganglia, autonomic nerves and ganglia, and the enteric nervous system. The development of the PNS is discussed in Chapter 10.

Functional Divisions of Nervous System

The nervous system of vertebrates consists of two major *functional* divisions: a **somatic nervous system** and a **visceral nervous system**. The somatic nervous system innervates the skin and most skeletal muscles (i.e., it provides both sensory and motor components). Similarly, the visceral nervous system innervates the viscera (organs of the body), and smooth muscle and glands in the more peripheral part of the body. The visceral nervous system is also called the **autonomic nervous system**. It consists of two components: the **sympathetic division** and the **parasympathetic division**. The somatic and visceral nervous systems are discussed in both this chapter (CNS components) and in Chapter 10 (PNS components).

Both divisions of the autonomic nervous system consist of two-neuron pathways. Because the peripheral autonomic neurons reside in ganglia, the axons of the central sympathetic neurons are called **preganglionic fibers**, and the axons of the peripheral sympathetic neurons are called **postganglionic fibers**. This terminology is used for both sympathetic pathways and parasympathetic (discussed later in the chapter) pathways. Sometimes preganglionic fibers are also called *presynaptic fibers*, and postganglionic fibers, *postsynaptic fibers*. They are so called because the axons of the preganglionic fibers *synapse* on the cell bodies of postganglionic neurons in the autonomic ganglia.

Primary Brain Vesicles Subdivide to Form Secondary Brain Vesicles

Chapters 3 and 4 describe how during neurulation the rudiment of the central nervous system arises as a neural plate from the ectoderm of the embryonic disc and folds to form the neural tube. The presumptive brain is visible as the broad cranial portion of the neural plate (see Fig. 3-20). Even on day 19, before bending of the neural plate begins, the three major divisions of the brain—the **prosencephalon (forebrain)**, **mesencephalon (midbrain)**, and **rhombencephalon (hindbrain)**—are demarcated by indentations in the neural plate. The future eyes appear as outpouchings from the forebrain neural folds by day 22 (discussed in Ch. 17). Bending of the neural plate begins on day 22, and the cranial neuropore closes on day 24. The three brain divisions are then marked by expansions of the neural tube called **primary brain vesicles** (Fig. 9-1A, B).

By day 21, an additional series of narrow swellings called **neuromeres** becomes apparent in the future brain (Fig. 9-1C; see Fig. 9-1A, B). These are prominent in the hindbrain, where seven or eight **rhombomeres** (depending on the species) partition the neural tube into approximately equal-sized segments. The rhombomeres are transient structures and become indistinguishable by the early 6th week.

During the 5th week, the mesencephalon enlarges and the prosencephalon and rhombencephalon each subdivide into two portions, thus converting the three primary brain vesicles into five **secondary brain vesicles** (Fig. 9-1D; see Fig. 9-1C). The prosencephalon divides into a cranial **telencephalon** ("endbrain") and a caudal **diencephalon** ("between-brain"). The diencephalon, like the rhombencephalon, becomes subdivided into a series of three or four **prosomeres**. The rhombencephalon divides into a cranial **metencephalon** ("behind-brain," consisting of rhombomeres 1 and 2) and a caudal **myelencephalon** ("medulla-brain," consisting of the remaining rhombomeres). Within each of the brain vesicles, the neural canal is expanded into a cavity called a **primitive ventricle**. These primitive ventricles will become the definitive ventricles of the mature brain (see Fig. 9-23). The rhombencephalon cavity becomes the **fourth ventricle**, the mesencephalon cavity becomes the **cerebral**

9

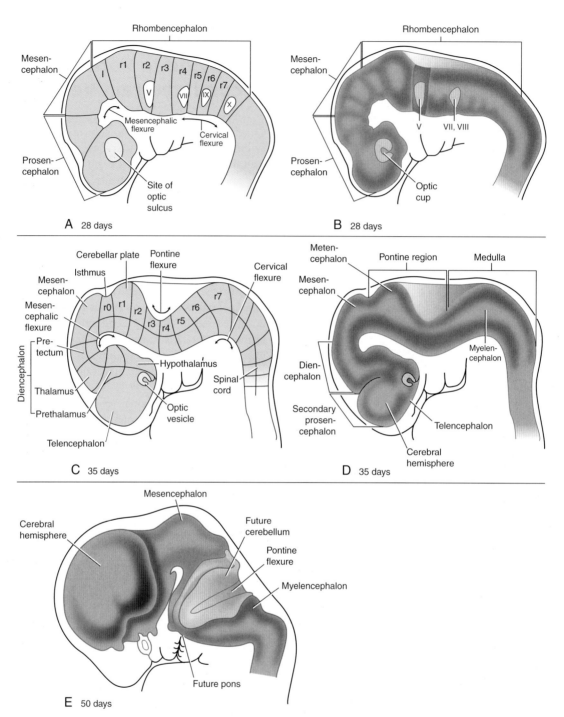

Figure 9-1. Early development of the brain. *A, B,* By day 28, the future brain consists of three primary brain vesicles (the prosencephalon, mesencephalon, and rhombencephalon). The locations of the mesencephalic and cervical flexures are indicated, as are the positions of the isthmus (I), rhombomeres (r1-r7), and some cranial nerve ganglia (roman numerals). *C-E,* Further subdivision of the brain vesicles creates five secondary vesicles: the enlarged mesencephalon, the metencephalon, and myelencephalon (that arise from the rhombencephalon) and the diencephalon and telencephalon (that arise from the prosencephalon). The cerebral hemispheres appear and expand rapidly. The pontine flexure folds the metencephalon back against the myelencephalon.

aqueduct (of Sylvius), the diencephalon cavity becomes the **third ventricle**, and the telencephalon cavity becomes the paired **lateral ventricles** of the cerebral hemispheres. After the closure of the caudal neuropore, the developing brain ventricles and the central canal of the more caudal **spinal cord** are filled with **cerebrospinal fluid**, a specialized dialysate of blood plasma.

IN THE RESEARCH LAB

One of the major challenges facing the embryo is how to generate a very large number of different neuronal cell types and at the same time ensure that each of them forms at its correct position in the neural tube. Distinguished and defined by the specificity of their connections with other neurons, the neuronal cell types of the CNS number in the many hundreds, or even thousands, and the embryo has to get the right cells in the right places for the system then to wire up appropriately and function correctly. The highly elaborate patterning of cell specification and the subsequent formation of precise connections between remote cells during development sets the CNS far apart from other organ systems; how these processes are controlled is thus an important question for researchers.

POSITIONAL INFORMATION PATTERNS NEURAL PLATE AND TUBE

In addressing the issue of **cell patterning**, it is helpful to think in terms of a Cartesian system of **positional information**, in which naive cells may sense their position on orthogonal gradients of **morphogens** acting along the cranial-caudal (CrCd) and medial-lateral (ML) axes of the neural plate. Cells would acquire a unique "grid reference" by measuring the ambient concentration of morphogen on each of the intersecting axes and would then interpret this, their **positional value**, by selecting an appropriate fate from the range made available in the genome. This concept is undoubtedly simplistic but not wholly unrealistic.

The events of pattern formation can be summarized as first, the polarization of the entire CrCd axis of the CNS primordium and next, the setting up of discrete morphogen sources at particular positions along the axis that act as local **signaling centers**, informing neighboring cells about their position and fate (Fig. 9-2A, B). Similar events occur on the ML axis of the neural plate (later the dorsal-ventral, DV, axis of the neural tube) except that, being considerably shorter than the CrCd axis, morphogen sources established at the dorsal and ventral poles are sufficient to pattern the entire axis (Fig. 9-2C).

At gastrulation, when a region of the dorsal ectoderm is set aside to be the **neural plate** (Ch. 3), the CrCd axis is polarized by a gradient of **Wnt** molecules diffusing from the caudal pole of the neural plate and by counteracting Wnt inhibitors at the cranial pole. In the absence of Wnt signaling, the default neural fate of cranial is realized. Higher Wnt levels effectively confer successively more caudal neural fates. Gradients of **retinoid** signaling, also high at the caudal end of the embryo, operate in addition to Wnts to polarize the CrCd axis. The initially coarse regional subdivision of the CrCd axis is manifest by the expression of **transcriptional control genes** in distinct domains that dictate the direction of their subsequent development. For example, Otx2 is expressed only in the cranial neural plate (forebrain and midbrain), whereas Hox genes are expressed in nested subdomains of the caudal neural plate (hindbrain and spinal cord). Another transcriptional control gene, Gbx2, is expressed between the Otx2 and Hox expression domains.

Gbx2 and Otx2 proteins mutually repress each other's expression, so their domains abut at a sharp line—this will become the midbrain/hindbrain boundary (see Fig. 9-2A). At this interface between gene expression domains (an area known as the **isthmus**), a band of cells differentiates that secrete **Fibroblast growth factor 8** (Fgf8), which signals the formation of optic tectum in the Otx2 expression domain and cerebellum in the Gbx2 domain. Fgf8 is also released from a signaling center at the cranial pole of the axis (called the **anterior neural ridge**; ANR), inducing the local expression of transcription factors such as Bf1 (also known as FoxG1) that establish the telencephalon as a distinct region of the forebrain (see Fig. 9-2A). Similarly, a further signaling center develops in the middle of the diencephalon (at the **zona limitans intrathalamica**, ZLI) that releases another morphogen, **Sonic hedgehog** (Shh), which signals the formation of prethalamus cranially and thalamus caudally (see Fig. 9-2A).

As the initially flat neural plate neurulates to form the neural tube, distinct signaling centers form at both ventral and dorsal midlines, along almost the entire length of the CrCd axis (also discussed in Ch. 4). The ventral pole cells, constituting the **floor plate of the neural tube**, secrete Shh, whereas the dorsal cells, constituting the **roof plate of the neural tube**, secrete **Bone morphogenetic proteins** (Bmps). In the context of midbrain, hindbrain, and spinal cord, Shh signaling from the floor plate induces the formation of a variety of neuronal cell types according to the concentration of Shh—at high levels, close to the floor plate, motoneurons are induced, whereas a diversity of interneurons is induced at successively lower Shh levels

9

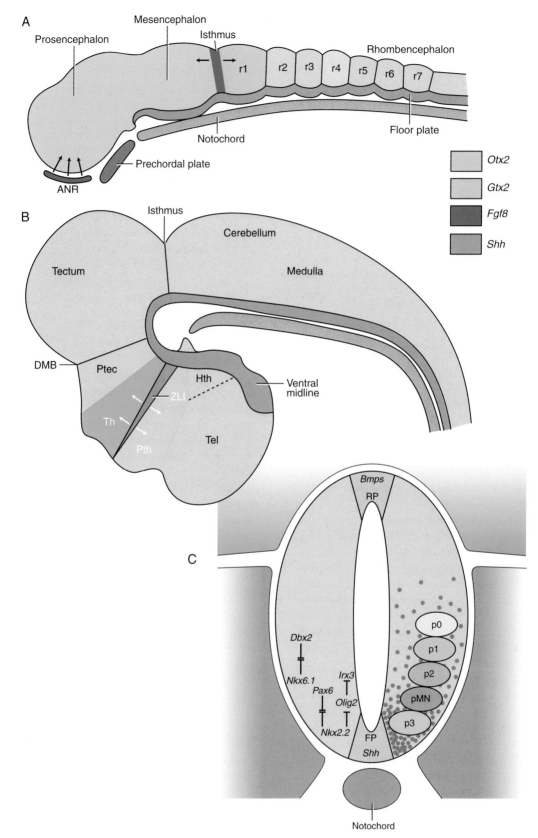

Figure 9–2. For legend, see next page.

Figure 9-2. The early embryonic neural axis is subdivided and partitioned by the actions of local signaling centers in both the cranial-caudal (*A*, *B*) and dorsal-ventral (*C*) axes. In the earlier embryo (*A*), signaling boundaries develop between rhombomeres (r1-r7) and at the midbrain-hindbrain boundary (isthmus). The latter expresses the signaling molecule *Fgf8*, which triggers development of the optic tectum in the caudal midbrain and cerebellum in r1. At the cranial tip of the neural plate, a row of cells that earlier expressed *Wnt* inhibitors develops into the anterior neural ridge (ANR); the *Fgfs* released by ANR cells are involved in specifying development of the telencephalon (Tel). Later in development (*B*) another major signaling center (the zona limitans intrathalamica, ZLI) develops in the mid-diencephalon and regulates the development of thalamus (Th) and prethalamus (Pth). DMB: diencephalic/mesencephalic boundary; Hth: hypothalamus; Ptec: pretectum. *C*, Cross section through the dorsal-ventral (DV) axis of the neural tube. Ventral midline cells (floor plate, FP) express the morphogen *Sonic hedgehog* (*Shh*), which diffuses through the ventral regions forming a concentration gradient. Different transcription factors are induced at different *Shh* concentrations, such that their expression domains subdivide the DV axis. Some of these factors (shown on left of figure) mutually repress each other's expression, effectively sharpening the interfaces between their domains. The transcription factors expressed in each domain direct the expression of downstream genes that regulate progenitor cell identity. Shown on the right side are the progenitors for motoneurons (pMN) and for four different types of interneuron (p0-p3). *Bmps* are expressed in the roof plate (RP) and induce dorsal interneurons.

impinging on precursor cells at successively more dorsal positions in the basal plate (see Fig. 9-2*C*). The *Bmp* gradient from the roof plate counteracts the *Shh* gradient and is responsible for the elaboration of a range of alar plate cell types (see Fig. 9-2*C*).

How CrCd and DV signals interact to confer position in two dimensions is not fully understood. However, it is clear that the signals from the dorsal and ventral poles are essentially uniform along the length of the CrCd axis, yet they induce different cell types at different CrCd positions. For example, *Shh* from the midbrain floor plate induces the formation of oculomotor neurons at one CrCd position and dopaminergic neurons of the substantia nigra at another CrCd position. One explanation is that the uniform ventral signal in this case acts on a preexisting bias, or **competence**, of the receiving cells that is conferred during patterning of the CrCd axis.

Having achieved a correct spatial pattern of differentiation, with individual neuronal subtypes either in their correct positions or specified to migrate into new settling positions, the next major event in brain development is the outgrowth of axons to form connections with other neurons—the substrate of forming neural networks. A well-studied example is the visual system, where the sequential processes of cell patterning, axon outgrowth, and the formation of appropriate connection are all accessible. The development of the visual system will be considered later in this chapter.

Formation of Brain Flexures

Between the 4th and 8th weeks, the brain tube folds sharply at three locations (Fig. 9-1*E*; see Fig. 9-1*C*, *D*). The first of these folds to develop is the **mesencephalic** flexure (**cranial** or **cephalic flexure**), centered at the midbrain region. The second fold is the **cervical flexure**, located near the juncture between the myelencephalon and the spinal cord. Both of these flexures involve a ventral folding of the brain tube. The third fold, a reverse, dorsally directed flexion called the **pontine flexure**, begins at the location of the developing pons. By the 8th week, the deepening of the pontine flexure has folded the metencephalon (including the developing cerebellum) back onto the myelencephalon.

Cytodifferentiation of Neural Tube

Cytodifferentiation of the neural tube commences in the rhombencephalic region just after the occipitocervical neural folds fuse and proceeds cranially and caudally as the tube zips up. The precursors of most of the cell types of the future central nervous system—neurons, some types of glial cells, and ependymal cells that line the central canal of the spinal cord and the ventricles of the brain—are produced by proliferation in the layer of neuroepithelial cells that immediately surrounds the neural canal (Fig. 9-3). This layer of proliferating cells is called the **ventricular layer** of the differentiating neural tube. The first wave of cells produced in the ventricular layer consists of postmitotic **young neurons**, which migrate peripherally to establish a second layer containing cell bodies, the **mantle layer**, external to the ventricular layer. This **neuron**-containing layer develops into the

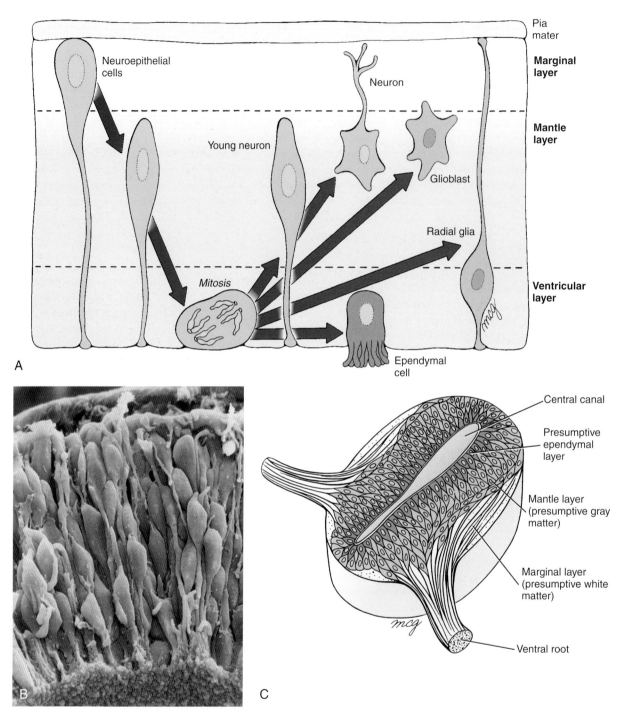

Figure 9-3. Cytodifferentiation of the neural tube. *A, B,* Neuroepithelial cells are elongated and span the entire thickness of the wall of the early neural tube prior to their rounding up at the luminal side for mitosis. Waves of mitosis and differentiation form postmitotic young neurons, which migrate away from the luminal side to form definitive neurons and glioblasts, some of which form radial glia (or Bergmann glia in the cerebellum). Such a wave is illustrated in *A,* which shows progression in time from left to right. *A, C,* As neurons form, the neural tube becomes stratified into a ventricular layer (adjacent to the neural canal), mantle layer (containing neuronal cell bodies), and marginal layer (containing nerve fibers).

gray matter of the central nervous system. The neuronal processes (axons) that sprout from the mantle layer neurons grow peripherally to establish a third layer, the **marginal layer**, which contains no neuronal cell bodies and becomes the **white matter** of the central nervous system. The white matter is so called because of the whitish color imparted by the fatty myelin sheaths that wrap around many of axons. In the CNS, these sheaths are formed by oligodendrocytes (discussed in the next section; in the PNS, myelin sheaths are formed by neural crest cell–derived Schwann cells; Schwann cells are discussed in Ch. 10). The marginal layer contains axons entering and leaving the CNS, as well as the axon tracts coursing to higher or lower levels in the CNS.

After production of neurons is waning in the ventricular layer, this layer begins to produce a new cell type, the **glioblast** (see Fig. 9-3A). These cells differentiate into the **glia** of the CNS-the **astrocytes** and **oligodendrocytes**. Glia provide metabolic and structural support to the neurons of the central nervous system. The last cells produced by the ventricular layer are the **ependymal cells;** these line the brain ventricles and central canal of the spinal cord (see Fig. 9-3A, C). Elaborations of the ependyma are responsible for producing **cerebrospinal fluid (CSF)**, which fills the brain ventricles, central canal of the spinal cord, and subarachnoid space that surrounds the CNS. The CSF is under pressure and thus provides a fluid jacket that protects and supports the brain.

Differentiation of Spinal Cord

The differentiation of the spinal cord is relatively simple compared to that of the brain, so we will begin our discussion with the spinal cord. Starting at the end of the 4th week, the neurons in the mantle layer of the spinal cord become organized into four plates that run the length of the cord: a pair of **dorsal** or **alar plates (columns)** and a pair of **ventral** or **basal plates (columns)** (Fig. 9-4). Laterally, the two plates abut at a groove called the **sulcus limitans;** dorsally and ventrally they are connected by non-neurogenic structures called, respectively, the **roof plate** and the **floor plate**. The cells of the ventral columns become the **somatic motoneurons** of the spinal cord and

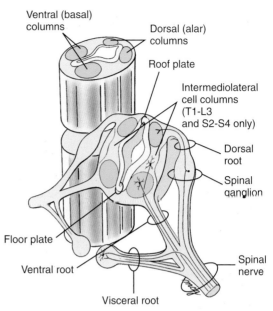

Figure 9-4. Neurons within the mantle layer of the neural tube become organized into two ventral motor (basal) columns and two dorsal sensory (alar) columns throughout most of the length of the spinal cord and hindbrain. Intermediolateral cell columns also form at spinal levels T1-L3 and S2-S4.

9

innervate somatic motor structures such as the voluntary (striated) muscles of the body wall and extremities. The cells of the dorsal columns develop into **association neurons**. These neurons synapse with *afferent* (incoming) fibers from the sensory neurons of the dorsal root ganglia (discussed in Ch. 10). In addition, the axon of an association neuron may synapse with motoneurons on the same (ipsilateral) or opposite (contralateral) side of the cord, forming a reflex arc—or it may ascend to the brain. The outgoing (*efferent*) motor neuron fibers exit via the ventral roots.

In most regions of the cord—at all 12 thoracic levels, at lumbar levels L1 and L2, and at sacral levels S2 to S4—the neurons in more dorsal regions of the ventral columns segregate to form **intermediolateral cell columns**. The thoracic and lumbar intermediolateral cell columns contain the **visceral motoneurons** that constitute the central **autonomic motoneurons of the sympathetic division**, whereas the intermediolateral cell columns in the sacral region contain the **visceral motoneurons** that constitute the central **autonomic motoneurons of the parasympathetic division**. The structure and function of these systems are discussed in the Chapter 10 (where the peripheral components are described). In general, at any given level of the brain or spinal cord, the motoneurons form before the sensory elements.

Overview of Spinal Nerves

Spinal nerves consist of (1) a dorsal root, containing neurons whose cell bodies reside in the dorsal root ganglion; (2) a ventral root, containing neurons whose cell bodies reside in the ventral spinal cord grey matter (ventral columns); and (3) at levels in which intermediolateral cell columns are present, a visceral root, containing neurons whose cell bodies reside within the intermediolateral cell column (see Fig. 9-4). The region where these roots join and extend peripherally constitutes the spinal nerve. Spinal nerves are discussed in more detail in Chapter 10.

Differentiation of Brain

For purposes of description, the brain can be divided into two parts: the **brain stem**, which represents the cranial continuation of the spinal cord and is similar to it in organization, and the **higher centers**, which are extremely specialized and retain little trace of a spinal cord–like organization. The brain stem consists of the myelencephalon, the metencephalon derivative called the **pons**, and the mesencephalon. The higher centers consist of the cerebellum (derived from the metencephalon) and the forebrain.

Brain Stem

The fundamental pattern of alar columns, basal columns, dorsal sensory roots, and ventral motor roots described earlier in the chapter for the spinal cord also occurs, albeit more elaborately, in the brain stem. This pattern is altered during development as some groups of neurons migrate away from their site of origin to establish a nucleus elsewhere. Also, as in the spinal cord, the brain stem is organized into a ventricular zone (containing proliferating neuroepithelial cells that generate young neurons and glioblasts), mantle zone, and marginal zone.

Overview of cranial nerves
All of the 12 cranial nerves except the first (olfactory) and second (optic) have nuclei located in the brain stem. These nuclei are among the earliest structures to develop in the brain and hence are discussed here; cranial nerves are discussed in more detail in Chapter 10. The basal plates of the rhombencephalon form the earliest neurons in the CNS. By day 28, all brain stem cranial nerve motor nuclei are distinguishable. As in the spinal cord, the alar plates of the brain stem form somewhat later than the basal plates, appearing in the middle of the 5th week. The cranial nerve associational nuclei are all distinguishable by the end of the 5th week.

Although cranial nerves show homologies to spinal nerves, they are much less uniform in composition. Three cranial nerves are exclusively sensory (I, II, and VIII); four are exclusively motor (IV, VI, XI, and XII); one is mixed sensory and motor (i.e., mixed; V); one is motor and parasympathetic (III); and three include sensory, motor, and parasympathetic fibers (VII, IX, and X). Nevertheless, the motor and sensory axons of the cranial nerves bear the same basic relation to the cell columns of the brain that the ventral and dorsal roots bear to the cell columns of the spinal cord. Table 9-1 summarizes the relations of the cranial nerves to the subdivisions of the brain.

Organization of columns
In the same way that the basal plates of the spinal cord are organized into somatic motor and autonomic (visceral) motor columns (discussed earlier in the chapter), the basal and alar cranial nerve nuclei of the brain stem are organized into seven columns that subserve particular functions. Although seven columns form, some textbooks described only *six* functions, three motor and three sensory. The columns are as follows (Fig. 9-5; numbers listed below correspond to the numbers shown in Figs. 9-5 and 9-6):

Motor Functions (Basal Columns)
1. *Somatic efferent* neurons in the brain innervate the extrinsic ocular muscles and the muscles of the tongue (III, IV, VI, and XII).

2. *Branchial efferent* (alternatively called *special visceral efferent*) neurons serve the striated muscles derived from the pharyngeal arches and ensheathed by connective tissue derived from cranial neural crest cells (V, VII, IX, X). The motor nucleus of the accessory nerve (XI) is branchial efferent because it forms part of this column; even though the trapezius and sternocleidomastoid muscles that it innervates are not

Table 9-1 Location of the Cranial Nerve Nuclei.

Brain Region	Associated Cranial Nerves
Telencephalon	Olfactory (I)
Diencephalon	Optic (II)
Mesencephalon	Oculomotor (III)
Metencephalon	Trochlear (IV) (arises in the metencephalon but is later displaced into the mesencephalon) Trigeminal (V) (trigeminal sensory nuclei arise in the metencephalon and myelencephalon but are later displaced partly into the mesencephalon; the trigeminal motor nucleus arises in the metencephalon and remains there) Abducens (VI) Facial (VII) Vestibulocochlear (VIII)
Myelencephalon	Glossopharyngeal (IX) Vagus (X) Accessory (XI) Hypoglossal (XII)

obviously derived from pharyngeal arch mesoderm, their connective tissue derives from cranial neural crest cells.

3. *Visceral efferent* (alternatively called *general visceral efferent*) neurons serve the parasympathetic pathways innervating the sphincter pupillae and ciliary muscles of the eyes (III) and (via the glossopharyngeal, IX, and vagus nerve, X) the smooth muscle and glands of the thoracic, abdominal, and pelvic viscera, including the heart, airways, and salivary glands.

Sensory Functions (Alar Columns)
4. *Visceral afferent* (alternatively called *general visceral afferent*) association neurons receive impulses via the vagus nerve from sensory receptors in the walls of the thoracic, abdominal, and

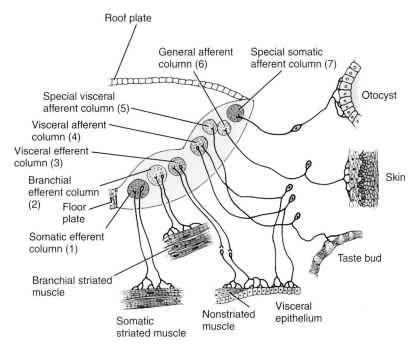

Figure 9-5. Organization of the brain stem cranial nerve nuclei. The basal columns give rise to motor (efferent) cranial nerve nuclei and the alar columns to associational (afferent) cranial nerve nuclei. These nuclei can be grouped into seven discontinuous columns (numbers in parentheses correspond to the numbering describing these columns in the text), each subserving a specific type of function.

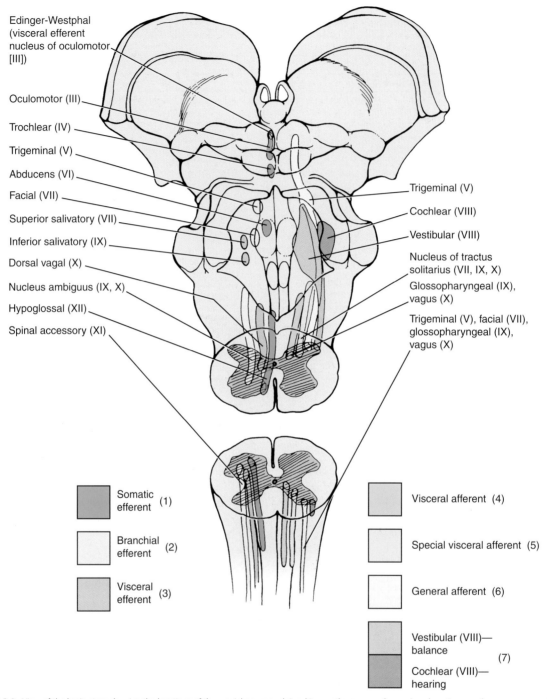

Figure 9-6. View of the brain stem showing the locations of the cranial nerve nuclei making up the seven columns (numbers in parentheses correspond to the numbers describing these columns in the text). The efferent nuclei are shown on the left and the afferent nuclei on the right.

pelvic viscera (referred to as interoceptive sensory receptors).

5. *Special afferent* association neurons subserve the special senses. This function is sometimes subdivided into two functions—*special visceral afferent* (taste; VII, IX) and *special somatic afferent* (hearing and balance; VIII)—to match the two columns of special afferent nuclei that develop in the brain stem.

6. *General afferent* (alternatively called *general somatic afferent*) association neurons in the brain subserve "general sensation" (e.g., touch, temperature, pain) over the head and neck, as well as for the mucosa of the oral and nasal cavities and the pharynx (V, VII, IX).

The number of columns present at different levels of the brain stem varies, with all columns being present in the rhombencephalon and only two columns being present in the mesencephalon (see Fig. 9-6). The distribution of the columns in the brain stem is as follows (columns are numbered as described immediately above and as labeled in Figs. 9-5 and 9-6):

1. The *somatic efferent* column consists of the nucleus of the hypoglossal nerve (XII) in the caudalmost rhombencephalon, that of nerve VI more cranially in the rhombencephalon, that of nerve IV in the most cranial rhombencephalon (later displaced into the caudal midbrain), and that of nerve III in the mesencephalon.

2. The *branchial efferent* column contains three nuclei serving nerves V, VII, and IX through XI and is confined to the rhombencephalon. The branchial efferent nuclei serving nerves V and VII are located cranially in the rhombencephalon; caudally, the elongated nucleus ambiguus supplies branchial efferent fibers for nerves IX, X, and XI.

3. The *visceral efferent* column includes two nuclei located in the rhombencephalon. The salivatory nuclei provide preganglionic parasympathetic innervation to the salivary and lacrimal glands via nerves VII and IX. Just caudal to this nucleus is the dorsal nucleus of the vagus, which contains preganglionic parasympathetic neurons innervating the viscera. The Edinger-Westphal nucleus (III) is located in the mesencephalon.

4. The general *visceral afferent* column consists of the nucleus that receives interoceptive

information via the glossopharyngeal (IX) and vagus nerve (X).

5. The first *special afferent* column (sometimes called the *special visceral afferent* column) consists of the nucleus of the tractus solitarius, which receives taste impulses via the facial (VII), glossopharyngeal (IX), and vagus (X) nerves.

6. The *general afferent* column consists of the neurons that receive impulses of general sensation from areas of the face served by the trigeminal (V) and facial (VII) nerves and from the oral, nasal, external auditory, and pharyngeal and laryngeal cavities (V, VII, IX, and X).

7. The second *special afferent* column (sometimes called the *special somatic afferent column*) consists of the cochlear and vestibular nuclei, which subserve the special senses of balance and hearing (VIII).

Not all nuclei that develop within the basal and alar columns remain where they form. For example, the branchial efferent nucleus of the facial nerve travels first caudally and then laterally, circumnavigating the abducens nucleus, to form the internal genu of the facial nerve. The nucleus ambiguus also migrates, as do some of the noncranial nerve nuclei of the rhombencephalon, such as the olivary and pontine nuclei, which arise from the rhombic lip but migrate to a ventral position (Fig. 9-7). Many CNS neurons "reel out" their axons behind them as they migrate; thus, the migratory path of a nucleus often can be reconstructed by tracing its axons.

Rhombencephalon

In contrast to the spinal cord, where the roof and floor plates are narrow and lie at the bottom of deep grooves (see Fig. 9-4), in the rhombencephalon, the walls of the neural tube splay open dorsally so that the roof plate is stretched and widened and the two sides of the hindbrain become disposed at an obtuse angle to one another (see Fig. 9-7). The rhombencephalic neural canal (future fourth ventricle) is rhombus (diamond) shaped in dorsal view, with the widest point located at the pontine flexure. The dorsal margin of the alar plate, adjoining the massively expanded roof plate, is called the **rhombic lip**. Its metencephalic portion contributes to the granule cells of the cerebellum (discussed below).

The thin rhombencephalic roof plate consists mainly of a layer of ependyma and is covered by a

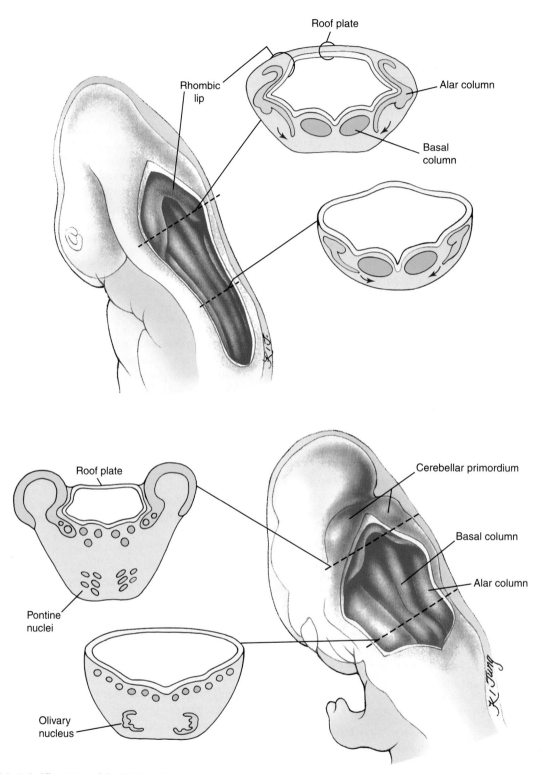

Figure 9-7. Early differentiation of the rhombencephalon. The roof plate in the rhombencephalic region forms a wide, transparent membrane over the fourth ventricle. The basal and alar columns give rise to the motor and associational nuclei, respectively, of most of the cranial nerves, as well as to other structures. Extensions of the alar columns also migrate ventrally to form pontine and olivary nuclei.

well-vascularized layer of pia mater called the **tela choroidea**. On either side of the midline, the pia and ependyma form a zone of minute, finger-like structures projecting into the fourth ventricle. This zone, called a **choroid plexus**, is specialized to secrete cerebrospinal fluid. Similar choroid plexuses develop in the ventricles of the forebrain (discussed later in the chapter). Cerebrospinal fluid circulates constantly through the central canal of the spinal cord and the ventricles of the brain and also through the subarachnoid space surrounding the CNS, from which it is reabsorbed into the blood. The fluid gains access to the subarachnoid space via three holes that open in the roof plate of the fourth ventricle: a single **median aperture (foramen of Magendie)** and two **lateral apertures (foramina of Luschka).**

Formation of medulla oblongata, pons, and cerebellum

The myelencephalon (consisting of rhombomeres 3 to 8) differentiates to form the **medulla oblongata**, which is the portion of the brain most similar to the spinal cord. In addition to housing many cranial nerve nuclei, the medulla serves as a relay center between the spinal cord and the higher brain centers and also contains centers and nerve networks that regulate respiration, heartbeat, reflex movements, and a number of other functions.

The metencephalon (rhombomeres 1 and 2) gives rise to two structures: the **pons**, which functions mainly to relay signals that link both the spinal cord and the cerebral cortex with the cerebellum; and the **cerebellum**, which is a center for balance and postural control. (Although the cerebellum is part of the higher centers, rather than part of the brain stem, it is discussed here because it is derived from the rhombencephalon.) The pons (Latin, for "bridge") contains massive axon tracts (Fig. 9-8) that arise mainly from the marginal layer of the basal columns of the metencephalon. In addition, ventrally located **pontine nuclei** relay input from the cerebrum to the cerebellum (see Fig. 9-7).

The cerebellum is derived from both the alar plates of the metencephalon and the adjacent rhombic lips; the latter give rise to **cerebellar granule cells** and the deep cerebellar nuclei (discussed below). The rudiment of the cerebellum is first recognizable as a pair of thickened **cerebellar plates** or **cerebellar primordia** (Fig. 9-9; see also Fig. 9-7). By the 2nd month, the cranial portions of the growing cerebellar plates meet across the midline, forming a single primordium that covers the fourth ventricle. This primordium initially bulges only into the fourth ventricle and does not protrude dorsally. However, by the middle of the 3rd month, the growing cerebellum begins to bulge dorsally, forming a dumbbell-shaped swelling at the cranial end of the rhombencephalon.

At this stage, the developing cerebellum is separated into cranial and caudal portions by a transverse groove called the **posterolateral fissure** (see Fig. 9-9D). The caudal portion, consisting of a pair of **flocculonodular lobes**, represents the most primitive part of the cerebellum. The larger cranial portion consists of a narrow median swelling called the **vermis** connecting a pair of broad **cerebellar hemispheres**. This cranial portion grows much faster than the flocculonodular lobes and becomes the dominant component of the mature cerebellum.

The cerebellar vermis and hemispheres undergo an intricate process of transverse folding as they develop. The major **primary fissure** deepens by the end of the 3rd month and divides the vermis and hemispheres into a cranial **anterior lobe** and a caudal **middle lobe** (see Fig. 9-9C, D). These lobes are further divided into a number of **lobules** by the development of additional transverse fissures (starting with the **secondary** and **prepyramidal fissures**), and the surface of the lobules is thrown into closely packed, leaflike transverse gyri called **folia**. These processes of fissure formation and foliation continue throughout embryonic, fetal, and postnatal life, and they vastly increase the surface area of the cerebellar cortex (see Fig. 9-9E, F).

The cerebellum has two types of gray matter: a group of internal **deep cerebellar nuclei** and an external **cerebellar cortex**. Four deep nuclei form on each side: the **dentate, globose, emboliform**, and **fastigial nuclei**. All input to the cerebellar cortex is relayed through these nuclei. The cerebellar cortex has an extremely regular cytoarchitecture that is similar over the entire cerebellum. The cell types of the cortex are arranged in layers.

The deep nuclei and cortex of the cerebellum are produced by a complex process of neurogenesis and neuronal migration (Fig. 9-10). As elsewhere in the neural tube, the neuroepithelium of the metencephalon undergoes an initial proliferation to produce ventricular, mantle, and marginal layers (see Fig. 9-10A). However, in the 3rd month, a second layer of proliferating cells forms over the marginal zone. It is derived from the most cranial rhombic lips. This new outer layer of proliferation and neurogenesis is called the **external germinal layer** (or, sometimes, the **external granular layer**; see Fig. 9-10B).

9

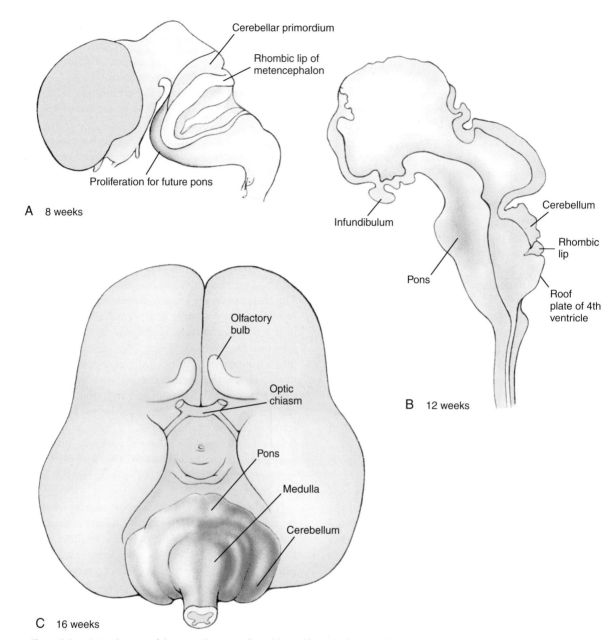

Figure 9-8. *A-C,* Development of the pons. The pons is formed by proliferation of cell and fiber tracts on the ventral side of the metencephalon.

Starting in the 4th month, the germinal layers undergo highly regulated cell divisions that produce the various populations of cerebellar neurons (see Fig. 9-10C). The *ventricular* layer produces four types of neurons that migrate to the cortex: the **Purkinje cells, Golgi cells, basket cells,** and **stellate cells,** as well as their associated glia (astrocytes—including Bergmann glia, which are discussed below—and oligodendrocytes). The remaining cells of the cerebellar cortex, the **granule cells,** arise from the *external germinal* layer. The external germinal layer also gives rise to the **primitive nuclear neurons,** which migrate to form the **deep cerebellar nuclei** (see Fig. 9-10D).

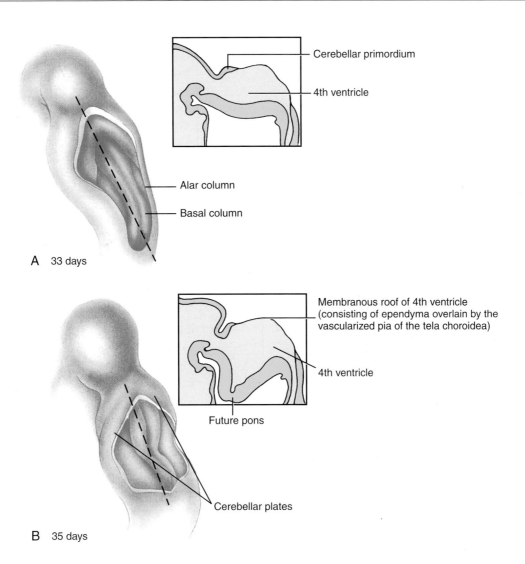

Cerebellar primordium

4th ventricle

Alar column

Basal column

A 33 days

Membranous roof of 4th ventricle (consisting of ependyma overlain by the vascularized pia of the tela choroidea)

4th ventricle

Future pons

Cerebellar plates

B 35 days

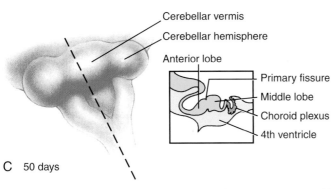

Cerebellar vermis

Cerebellar hemisphere

Anterior lobe

Primary fissure

Middle lobe

Choroid plexus

4th ventricle

C 50 days

Figure 9-9. Development of the cerebellum and the choroid plexus of the fourth ventricle. *A, B,* Proliferation of cells in the metencephalic alar plates and adjacent rhombic lips forms the cerebellar plates. *C,* Further growth creates two lateral cerebellar hemispheres and a central vermis. The primary fissure forms and divides the cerebellum into anterior and middle lobes. A choroid plexus develops in the roof plate of the fourth ventricle.

Continued

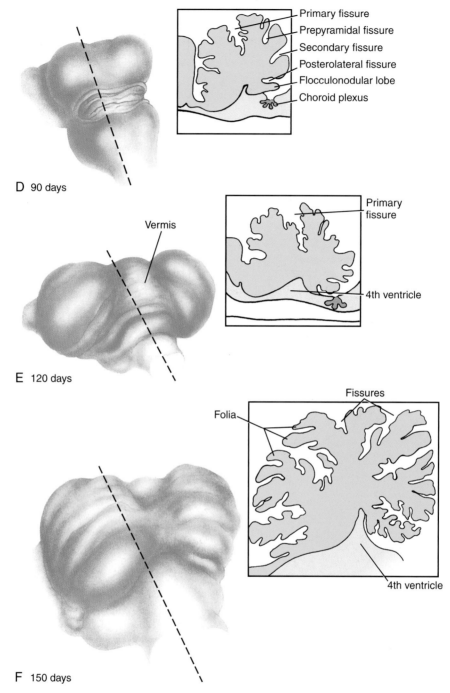

D 90 days

Primary fissure
Prepyramidal fissure
Secondary fissure
Posterolateral fissure
Flocculonodular lobe
Choroid plexus

Vermis

Primary fissure

4th ventricle

E 120 days

Fissures
Folia

4th ventricle

F 150 days

Figure 9-9. **Cont'd,** *D-F,* Continued fissuration subdivides the expanding cerebellum into further lobes and then, starting in the 3rd month, into lobules and folia. This process greatly increases the area of the cerebellar cortex.

As each newly born Purkinje cell migrates from the ventricular layer toward the cortex, it reels out an axon that maintains synaptic contact with neurons in the developing cerebellar nuclei. These axons will constitute the only efferents of the mature cerebellar cortex. The Purkinje cells form a distinct **Purkinje cell layer** just underlying the external germinal layer, which is initially multilayered but becomes a single layer when foliation is complete. Basket and stellate cells also migrate radially from the ventricular layer, closely associated with the Purkinje cells, and form the **molecular layer** of the definitive cortex. Once the granule cells begin to differentiate, they migrate (in a direction that is opposite of that of the Purkinje, basket, and stellate cells) from the external germinal layer through the developing molecular layer toward the ventricular layer. Here they form the **internal germinal layer** or **internal granular layer** of the developing cortex (see Fig. 9-10B), simply called the **granular layer** of the definitive cortex (see Fig. 9-10D). Granule cells migrate along the elongated fibers of glial cells called **Bergmann (radial) glia**. The bifurcated axons of granule cells course transversely in the outermost, molecular layer of the cortex, passing through and synapsing with the fanlike array of Purkinje cell dendrites (see Fig. 9-10D).

IN THE CLINIC

CELLULAR AND MOLECULAR BASIS OF CEREBELLAR MALFORMATIONS AND DYSFUNCTION

A variety of malformations occur in the development of the human cerebellum, including **hypoplasias** (under-**dysplasias** (abnormal tissue development), and **heterotopias** (misplaced cells). More subtle developmental defects

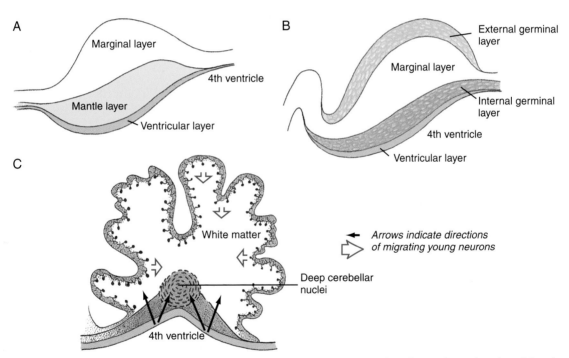

Figure 9-10. Cytodifferentiation of the cerebellum. *A*, During the 2nd month, typical ventricular, mantle, and marginal zones have formed throughout the metencephalon region, the dorsal part of which (alar plates and associated rhombic lips) forms the cerebellum. *B*, During the 3rd month, two additional layers have formed: an external germinal layer (derived from the metencephalic rhombic lips) and an internal germinal layer (composed of granule cells born in the external germinal layer that subsequently migrate toward the ventricle to form this layer). Neurons residing earlier in the mantle zone (and born in the ventricular zone; namely, stellate, basket, Golgi, and Purkinje cells) have dispersed into the marginal zone, where they will subsequently arrange into a distinct pattern. *C*, Neurons (granule cells) produced by the external germinal layer continue to migrate inward (open arrows), while neurons produced by the ventricular zone continue to migrate outward (closed arrows); some of these latter neurons form the deep cerebellar nuclei.

Continued

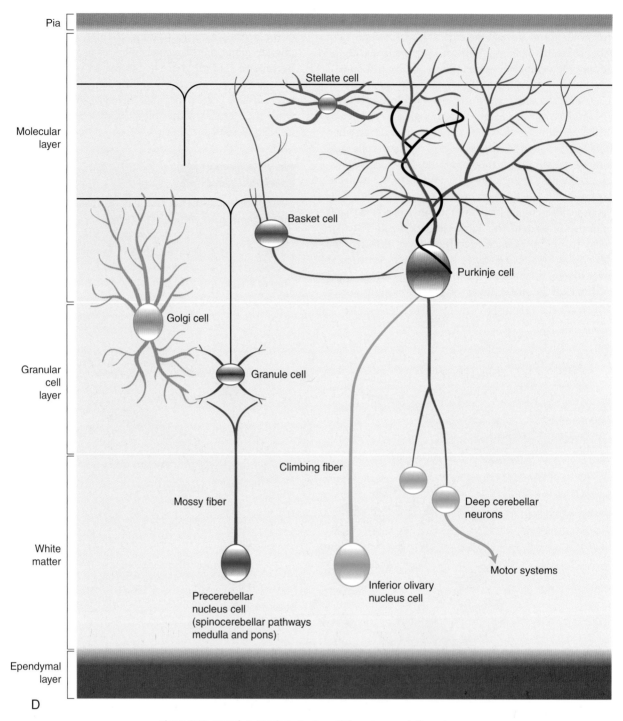

Pia

Molecular layer

Stellate cell

Basket cell

Purkinje cell

Golgi cell

Granule cell

Granular cell layer

White matter

Climbing fiber

Mossy fiber

Deep cerebellar neurons

Motor systems

Inferior olivary nucleus cell

Precerebellar nucleus cell (spinocerebellar pathways medulla and pons)

Ependymal layer

D

Figure 9-10. Cont'd, *D*, Histologic structure of the mature cerebellar cortex.

in the organization of the cerebellar cortical circuits might underlie a plethora of other disorders. **Schizophrenia**, for instance, which affects up to 1% of adult humans, might be related to early defects in neuronal migration, the expression of neurotransmitter receptors, or myelination, not only in the forebrain (the area usually thought to be affected in most mental illnesses) but, surprisingly, also in the cerebellar cortex. Another subset of cerebellar abnormalities result from degeneration. Cerebellar disorders often result in **ataxias** (disruptions of coordination).

Cerebellar ataxias can result from either environmental toxins or genetic anomalies. Mercury, an environmental toxin, may cause focal damage to the granular layer of the cerebellum and ataxia in humans following exposure. Genetic causes of ataxia include both chromosomal anomalies and single-gene mutations. Trisomy 13 results in gross brain abnormalities affecting the cerebellum and cerebrum. In the cerebellum, the vermis is hypoplastic and neurons are heterotopically located in the white matter. Cerebellar dysplasia, usually of the vermis, is also characteristic of trisomy 18, and Down syndrome (trisomy 21) may involve abnormalities of the Purkinje and granule cell layers. A variety of chromosome deletion syndromes, including 5p− (**cri du chat**), 13q−, and 4p−, also may cause cerebellar anomalies.

A large number of cerebellar ataxias are inherited, with autosomal recessive, autosomal dominant, X-linked, and mitochondrial inheritance all having been observed. There are several autosomal recessive cerebellar ataxias, one of the most common being **Friedreich ataxia**, which affects the dorsal root ganglia, spinal cord, and cerebellum. It is a progressive disorder with onset in childhood characterized by clumsy gait, ataxia of the upper limbs, and dysarthria (disturbed speech articulation). Other autosomal recessive cerebellar ataxia syndromes include **ataxia-telangiectasia, Marinesco-Sjogren syndrome, Gillespie syndrome, Joubert syndrome,** and the growing class of disorders termed **congenital disorders of glycosylation**. The latter three disorders often present with gross cerebellar malformations that can be diagnosed after birth with CT (computed tomography) or MRI (magnetic resonance imaging).

More than thirty autosomal dominant **spinocerebellar ataxia syndromes** (SCA) have been mapped, and the gene has been identified in about half of these. Many of these conditions are caused by unstable CAG **trinucleotide repeat** tracts within the coding region of the genes. CAG codes for the amino acid glutamine, and these **polyglutamine disorders** occur when the tract of glutamine residues reaches a disease-causing threshold. Expanded CAG trinucleotide repeats are

unstable and can increase in size as they are passed from one generation to the next, with earlier onset and more severe disease. This worsening of the disease in successive generations is called **genetic anticipation**.

The mutations that cause some of the recessive heritable cerebellar ataxias are known to affect the metabolism of mucopolys accharides, lipids, and amino acids. In the cerebellum, these mutations cause effects such as a deficiency of Purkinje cells (mucopolysaccharidosis III), abnormal accumulation of lipid (juvenile ganglioidosis), and reduced myelin formation (phenylketonuria). The disorder called **olivopontocerebellar atrophy** seems in some cases to be caused by a deficiency in the excitatory neurotransmitter glutamate, resulting in turn from a deficiency in the enzyme glutamate dehydrogenase.

IN THE RESEARCH LAB

MOUSE MUTANTS WITH CEREBELLAR ATAXIAS

A more detailed understanding of the cellular and molecular mechanisms that cause various cerebellar anomalies has been gained by research on a series of mouse mutants that display a broad array of cerebellar ataxias. The strange gaits of many of these mouse mutants can be correlated with defects in cerebellar cytoarchitecture. For example, the high-stepping, broad-based gait of the *stumbler* mutant is apparently caused by defects in Purkinje cells. The *meander tail* mutant also has Purkinje cell deficits, but only in the anterior lobe of the cerebellum. The *vibrator* mouse displays a rapid postural tremor caused by progressive degeneration of cerebellar neurons. This phenotype has been linked to mutations in the gene encoding *phosphatidylinositol transfer protein alpha*. *Tottering* and *leaner* mice exhibit symptoms of ataxia and epilepsy, which are likely due to mutations in the *calcium channel alpha(1A) subunit* gene. In humans, mutations in this gene have been linked to familial hemiplegic migraine, episodic ataxia type 2, and chronic spinocerebellar ataxia type 6.

Normally, the granule cells that arise in the external germinal layer of the developing cerebellum produce bipolar processes and then migrate inward along Bergmann glia (astrocyte) fibers to populate the internal granule cell layer, reeling out an axon behind them as they travel. In the homozygous recessive *weaver* mutant, the granule cells fail to produce processes, fail to migrate, and then die prematurely.

Weaver mice harbor a missense mutation in the gene coding for the *G protein–coupled inward-rectifying potassium channel (Girk2)*. How this defect leads to granule cell death remains unclear. However, a series of experiments, using wild-type and *weaver* astrocytes and granule cells mixed in vitro, showed that wild-type granule cells interact normally with *weaver* astrocytes, but *weaver* granule cells do not interact with wild-type astrocytes and do not migrate along astrocyte processes. Thus, the *weaver* mutation has a direct effect on granule cells but not on astrocytes.

Granule cells also interact with Purkinje cells as well as astrocytes, and this interaction is required for granule cell survival. In the normal cerebellum, the relative number of granule cells is matched to the number of Purkinje cells. This matching is accomplished by a process of **histogenetic cell death**, by which the great overabundance of granule cells initially produced by the external germinal layer is reduced to the correct number. Various experiments have indicated that this process is automatically controlled by the number of Purkinje cells: apparently, granule cells die unless they make contact with the dendritic arbor of a Purkinje cell. *Sonic hedgehog* is expressed by Purkinje cells and is required for granule cell proliferation, and likely, survival.

The role of Purkinje cells in granule cell survival was examined in two ways. In one experiment, *staggerer*–wild-type chimeras were made by aggregating eight-cell *staggerer* mutant mouse embryos with wild-type embryos and then reinserting them into the uterus of a pseudopregnant mother (**aggregation chimeras** are an alternative to injection chimeras, described in Ch. 5, for making mouse chimeras). The death of Purkinje cells in the *staggerer* mouse embryos beginning in late gestation (*staggerer* mice harbor a mutation in *RAR-related orphan receptor alpha*, but the cause of Purkinje cell death is unknown) resulted in the birth of animals with widely different numbers of normal and wild-type Purkinje cells. Examination revealed a linear relationship between the number of granule cells and the number of wild-type Purkinje cells, confirming the hypothesis that granule cell survival depends on the presence of appropriate Purkinje cell targets. In another experiment, transgenic technology was used to kill Purkinje cells. It was found that overlying granule cells stopped their proliferation, and the internal granule layer of the cerebellar cortex (normally formed by migrating granule cells; discussed above) failed to form.

Mesencephalon

Much of the mesencephalon is composed of white matter, principally the massive tracts that connect the forebrain with the hindbrain and spinal cord.

The midbrain also contains a number of important neuronal centers, including four cranial nerve nuclei.

As mentioned earlier in the chapter, the motor nuclei of the oculomotor (III) and trochlear (IV) nerves are located in the mesencephalon, as is a portion of the sensory nucleus of the trigeminal nerve (V) called the **mesencephalic trigeminal nucleus** (Fig. 9-11). However, of these nuclei, only those serving the oculomotor nerve and the trigeminal nerve arise from mesencephalic neuroepithelial cells; the trochlear nuclei originate in the metencephalon and are secondarily displaced into the mesencephalon. The two nuclei of the oculomotor nerve are the somatic motor **oculomotor nucleus**, which controls the movements of all but the superior oblique and lateral rectus extrinsic ocular muscles, and the general visceral efferent **Edinger-Westphal nucleus**, which supplies parasympathetic pathways to the pupillary constrictor and the ciliary muscles of the globe.

The **superior** and **inferior colliculi** are visible as four prominent swellings on the dorsal surface of the midbrain (see Fig. 9-11*C*). The superior colliculi receive axons from the retinae and mediate ocular reflexes. In contrast, the inferior colliculi form part of the perceptual pathway by which information from the cochlea is relayed to the auditory areas of the cerebral hemispheres. The colliculi are formed by mesencephalic alar plate cells that proliferate and migrate medially. The dorsal thickening produced by these cells is subsequently divided by a midline groove into a pair of lateral **corpora bigemina** (see Fig. 9-11*B*), which are later subdivided into inferior and superior colliculi by a transverse groove. The synapses of axons from retinal ganglion cells form precise spatial maps in the superior colliculi of the corresponding sensory fields of the retina.

During development, the primitive ventricle of the mesencephalon becomes the narrow **cerebral aqueduct** (see Fig. 9-11*C*). The cerebrospinal fluid produced by the choroid plexuses of the forebrain normally flows through the cerebral aqueduct to reach the fourth ventricle. However, various conditions can cause the aqueduct to become blocked during fetal life. Obstruction of the flow of cerebrospinal fluid through the aqueduct results in the congenital condition called **hydrocephalus**, in which the third and lateral ventricles are swollen with fluid, the cerebral cortex is abnormally thin, and the sutures of the skull are forced apart allowing the calvarial bones to increase in size (Fig. 9-12).

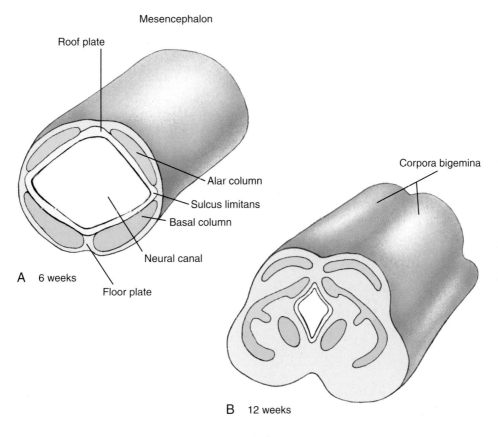

Mesencephalon

Roof plate

Alar column

Sulcus limitans

Basal column

Neural canal

A   6 weeks

Floor plate

Corpora bigemina

B   12 weeks

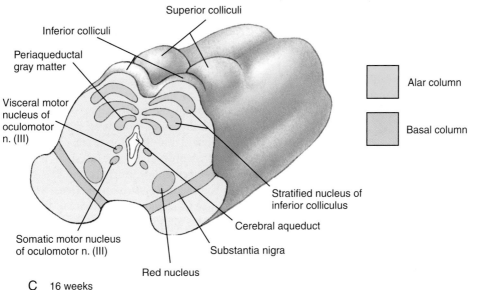

Superior colliculi

Inferior colliculi

Periaqueductal
gray matter

Visceral motor
nucleus of
oculomotor
n. (III)

Alar column

Basal column

Stratified nucleus of
inferior colliculus

Cerebral aqueduct

Somatic motor nucleus
of oculomotor n. (III)

Substantia nigra

Red nucleus

C   16 weeks

Figure 9-11. Development of the mesencephalon. *A, B,* A shallow longitudinal groove develops on the dorsal surface of the mesencephalon between weeks 6 and 12, creating the corpora bigemina. *C,* Over the next month, a transverse groove subdivides these swellings to produce the superior and inferior colliculi. The mesencephalic alar columns form the stratified nuclear layers of the colliculi, the periaqueductal gray matter, and the substantia nigra. The mesencephalic basal columns form the red nuclei and nuclei of the oculomotor nerve.

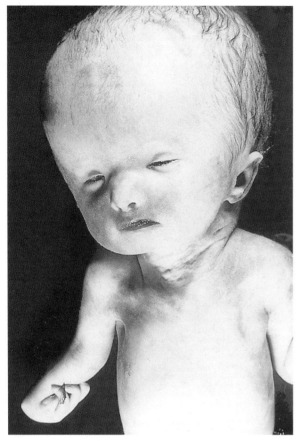

Figure 9-12. Hydrocephalus. Obstruction of the cerebral aqueduct causes the developing forebrain ventricles to become swollen with cerebrospinal fluid. Infants born with this condition may be retarded. However, incipient hydrocephalus can now be detected in utero using ultrasonography and can be corrected by inserting a pressure valve that allows the excess cerebrospinal fluid to vent into the amniotic cavity.

Higher Centers

As discussed above, the higher centers consist of the cerebellum (derived from the metencephalon) and the forebrain. The development of the cerebellum was discussed in the preceding section as part of the discussion of development of the rhombencephalon; hence, this section discusses only the development of the forebrain and its derivatives.

Forebrain

The prosencephalon consists of two secondary brain vesicles, the diencephalon and the telencephalon. The walls of the diencephalon differentiate to form a number of neuronal centers and tracts that are described later. In addition, the roof plate, floor plate, and ependyma of the diencephalon give rise to several specialized structures through mechanisms that are relatively unique. These structures include the **choroid plexus** and **circumventricular organs, posterior lobe of the pituitary gland (neurohypophysis),** and **optic vesicles.** The origin of the optic cups from the diencephalic neural folds is described in Chapter 17.

The thin dorsal telencephalon (**pallium**) gives rise to the **cerebral hemispheres** and to the commissures and other structures that join them. It also forms the **olfactory bulbs** and **olfactory tracts,** which along with the olfactory centers and tracts of the cerebral hemispheres constitute the **rhinencephalon** ("nose-brain"). The thicker ventral part of the telencephalon, the **subpallium,** budges into the neural canal to form the ganglion eminences that later make up the **basal ganglia.**

Diencephalon. As mentioned earlier in the chapter, the walls of the diencephalon are formed by alar plates; basal plates are lacking. The alar plates form three subdivisions that have been described as neuromeres (called **prosomeres**), similar to the rhombomeres of the hindbrain: a rostral neuromere that forms the **prethalamus** and **hypothalamus,** a middle neuromere that forms the **thalamus** and **epithalamus,** and a caudal neuromere that forms the **pretectum** (Fig. 9-13; see Fig. 9-2B). The thalamus and hypothalamus differentiate to form complexes of nuclei that serve a diverse range of functions. The thalamus acts mainly as the relay center for the cerebral cortex: it receives all the information projecting to the cortex from subcortical structures, processes it as necessary, and relays it to the appropriate cortical area(s). Within the thalamus, the sense of sight is handled by the **lateral geniculate nucleus** and the sense of hearing by the **medial geniculate nucleus.** The hypothalamus regulates the endocrine activity of the pituitary as well as many autonomic responses. It participates in the limbic system, which controls emotion and coordinates emotional state with the appropriate visceral responses. The hypothalamus also controls the level of arousal of the brain (sleep and waking). The small epithalamus gives rise to a few more minor structures described later in the chapter.

At the end of the 5th week, the thalamus and hypothalamus are visible as swellings on the inner surface of the diencephalic neural canal, separated by a deep groove called the **hypothalamic sulcus** (see Fig. 9-13A).

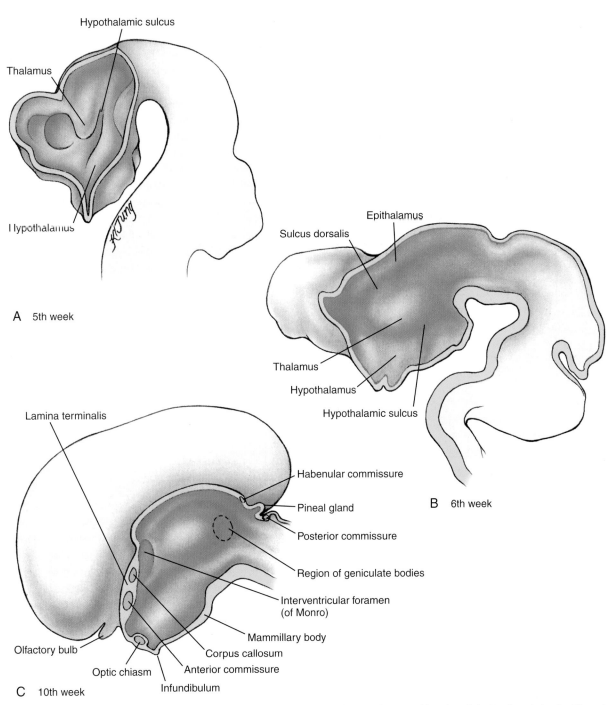

Figure 9-13. Development of the diencephalon. *A*, The thalamus and hypothalamus become demarcated by a hypothalamic sulcus during the 5th week. *B*, By the end of the 6th week, the thalamus is clearly differentiated from the more dorsal epithalamus by a shallow groove called the *sulcus dorsalis*. *C*, By 10 weeks, additional specializations of the diencephalon are apparent, including the mamillary body, the pineal gland, and the posterior lobe of the pituitary. The optic sulci, the posterior and habenular commissures, and the geniculate bodies are also specializations of the diencephalon.

The thalamus grows disproportionately after the 7th week and becomes the largest element of the diencephalon. The two thalami usually meet and fuse across the third ventricle at one or more points called **interthalamic adhesions** (Fig. 9-14*C*).

By the end of the 6th week, a shallow groove called the **sulcus dorsalis** separates the thalamus from the epithalamic swelling, which forms in the dorsal rim of the diencephalic wall and the adjoining roof plate (see Fig. 9-13*B, C*). The epithalamic roof plate evaginates to form a midline diverticulum that differentiates into the endocrine **pineal gland**. The epithalamus also forms a neural structure called the **trigonium habenulae** (including the **nucleus habenulae**) and two small commissures, the **posterior** and **habenular commissures**. The growth of the thalamus eventually obliterates the sulcus dorsalis and displaces the epithalamic structures dorsally.

Retinal fibers from the optic cups project to the lateral geniculate nuclei. As described in Chapter 17, the axons from the retinal ganglion cells grow back through the optic nerves to the diencephalon. Just before they enter the brain, axons growing from both eyes meet to form the **optic chiasm** (Fig. 9-14*A*; see Fig. 9-13*C*), a joint midline structure in which the axons from the inner (nasal) side of each eye cross over to the other side of the brain (decussate), whereas those of the outer (temporal) side of each eye remains on the same side; axons relaying information from the left half of the visual field of both eyes project to the right side of the brain and vice versa. The resulting bundles of ipsilateral and contralateral fibers then project back to the lateral geniculate nucleus, where they synapse to form a map of the visual field. Not all retinal fibers project to the lateral geniculate nuclei; as mentioned earlier in the chapter, some of them terminate in the superior colliculus, where they mediate ocular reflex control.

Cranial to the epithalamus, the diencephalic roof plate remains epithelial. This portion of the roof plate differentiates along with the overlying pia to form the paired **choroid plexuses** of the third ventricle (see Fig. 9-14*C*). Elsewhere in the third ventricle, the ependyma forms a number of unique secretory structures that add specific metabolites and neuropeptides to the cerebrospinal fluid. These structures, collectively known as the **circumventricular organs**, include the **subfornical organ**, the **organum vasculosum of the lamina terminalis**, and the **subcommissural organ**.

IN THE RESEARCH LAB

DEVELOPMENT OF VISUAL SYSTEM: EXAMPLE OF HOW NERVOUS SYSTEM WIRES ITSELF

The projection neurons of the retinae (**retinal ganglion cells**) produce axons that grow across the retinae and thence through the optic nerves and tracts to synapse in the **lateral geniculate nucleus** (or body; LGN) of the thalamus and superior colliculi (SC) of the dorsal midbrain (tectum). Lateral geniculate axons then relay visual information to the visual cortex (Fig. 9-15). Development of this system, which is characterized by highly precise, point-to-point mapping of retinal cells to the higher brain centers, raises a number of key questions about **axonal guidance** and the formation of **topographic neural connections**.

It will become apparent below that among the molecules used to guide axons to their targets are some of the same molecules that the embryo uses earlier as morphogens to pattern cell differentiation—an example of how a relatively small set of signaling molecules is used repeatedly for different tasks at different times and in different developmental contexts. However, before considering neuronal connectivity in the visual system, we must first examine how cell pattern is formed in the retinae and how this translates into the transcriptional control of molecules involved in the navigation of retinal axons.

Cell Pattern in Neural Retinae

As discussed in Chapter 17, each retina consists of two components, the **neural retina**, which receives visual information and transmits it to the brain via the retinal ganglion cells, and the pigment epithelium, which lies behind the neural retina. The neural retina itself consists of several cell layers in all, but here we will consider only that which lines its inner surface: the layer of retinal ganglion cells (RGC) that project in point-to-point fashion to the visual centers, creating a map of visual space in the brain. To ensure this precisely patterned connectivity, individual neurons in the RGC layer must be endowed with positional identity. Just as for the CNS axis as a whole, this is achieved by patterning along each of its planar axes, CrCd (cranial-caudal; alternatively referred to as nasal-temporal, to denote its orientation in the skull) and DV (dorsal-ventral). Both axes of the neural retina are specified before neurogenesis, even before the retina emerges as a distinct layer of the optic vesicle.

An early step in the subdivision of the optic vesicles involves the expression of two forkhead genes, *Bf1* and *Bf2*, in complementary fashion along the CrCd axis, *Bf1* being highly expressed at the cranial (nasal) pole of the retina and *Bf2* at the caudal (temporal) pole. The cranial domain is then

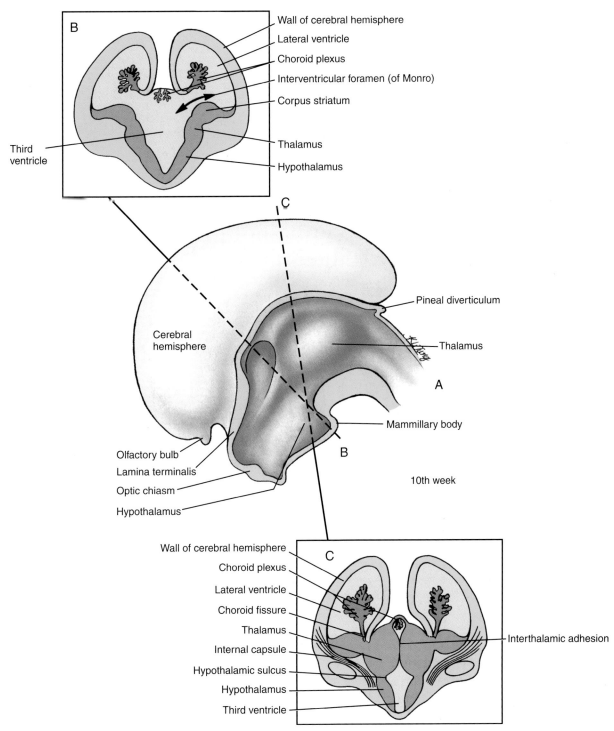

Figure 9-14. *A-C,* Development of the cerebral hemispheres and lateral ventricles, as seen in sagittal view (*A*) and in sections *B, C* at the level indicated in *A.* The lateral ventricle in each hemisphere communicates with the third ventricle through an interventricular foramen (of Monro). The choroid fissure running the length of each lateral ventricle contains a choroid plexus, which produces cerebrospinal fluid. The fibers growing to and from the cerebral cortex form the massive fiber bundle called the *internal capsule.* The thalami function mainly as relay centers that process information destined for the cerebral hemispheres. The growing thalami meet across the third ventricle, forming the interthalamic adhesion.

Secondary visual neuron on temporal side of retina–*projects to ipsilateral side of brain*

Secondary visual neuron on nasal side of retina–*projects to contralateral side of brain*

Pathway of temporal secondary neurons

Pathway of nasal secondary neurons (decussating at the chiasm)

Pathway of tertiary neurons

Lateral geniculate body

Pathway of tertiary neurons

Primary visual cortex

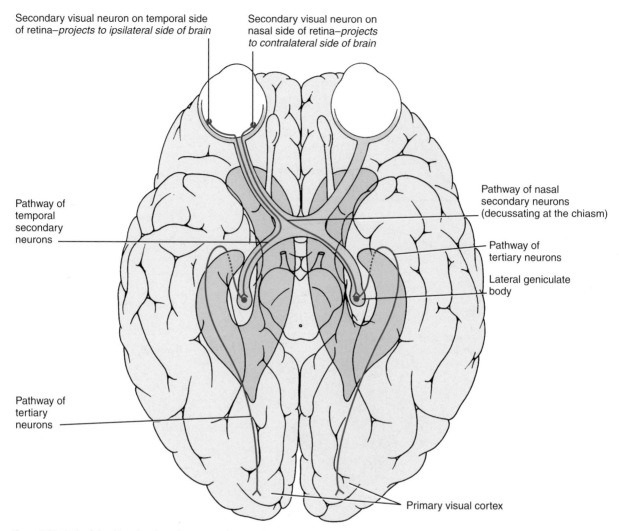

Figure 9-15. Path of visual impulses from the retinae. The secondary neurons of the visual pathway undergo partial decussation across the optic chiasm so that each visual cortex receives the information from the contralateral visual field. As shown, the axons from the nasal half of each retina cross over in the chiasm to enter the contralateral visual tract, whereas axons from the temporal half of each retina enter the ipsilateral visual tract. These secondary axons synapse in the lateral geniculate bodies with the tertiary neurons of the visual pathway, which project to the primary visual cortex in the occipital lobe. The synapses in the lateral geniculate bodies and the visual cortex are arranged so as to form a spatial map of the visual field. Dark blue marks the position of the lateral ventricles

further subdivided by the expression of two homeobox genes, *Soho* (for *Sense organ homeobox*) and *Gh6* (*Gallus homeobox 6*). Each of these transcriptional control genes plays a part in patterning the CrCd axis, as both knockout and overexpression studies result in altered positional identity of RGCs, revealed by their aberrant projections. However, it remains unclear how the patterned expression of these genes is directed by upstream signals.

The DV axis is patterned slightly later than the CrCd axis, at the optic cup stage. Here, it seems that the governing

mechanism involves a gradient of *Bmp4* (*Bone morphogenetic protein 4*) diffusing from the dorsal pole and a complementary gradient of a *Bmp* antagonist (*Ventroptin*) diffusing from the ventral pole. High levels of *Bmp* signaling induce the expression of a transcriptional control gene, *Tbx5*, in the dorsal retina, whereas high levels of *Ventroptin* associate with expression of the homeobox gene *Vax2* and the paired box gene *Pax2* in the ventral retina. Ectopic misexpression of *Tbx5* dorsalizes the retina. Conversely, misexpression of *Vax2* results in ventralization, including the downregulation of the dorsal factors *Bmp4* and *Tbx5*, and the misprojection of dorsal RGC axons. How the retinal polarity conferred by these transcription factors translates into the graded expression of axon guidance receptor molecules is considered next.

Spatial Targeting of Retinal Axons

As discussed further in Chapter 10, a specialized structure at the tip of the axon called the **growth cone** is responsible for neuronal pathfinding (Fig. 9-16; see Fig. 10–2). The first task for the retinal ganglion cell growth cones, after they enter the axon layer that lines the inner surface of the retina, is to grow to the **optic disc** and then turn sharply to funnel into the **optic nerve** (Fig. 9-17). Outgrowth of retinal ganglion cell axons and guidance of their growth cones to the optic disc seems to require interaction with radial glia endfeet (specializations of the luminal side of radial glia) within the inner layer of the neural retina and associated cell adhesion and extracellular matrix molecules. Indeed, many such substratum-associated or diffusible factors seem to play a role in the guidance of RGC growth cones, either within the retina or in the optic nerve. These include *Laminin, L1, Axonin-1, Ncam, Netrins, Slits, Semaphorins, Ephrins, Hedgehogs,* and *sFrps*. Some of these molecules act as attractants, whereas others act as repellants, serving to restrict axons to a localized pathway by surround repulsion. In addition, the survival of RGCs within the retina may be supported by **trophic factors**, including a factor produced by pigment epithelial cells. Other trophic factors that support survival of RGCs include *Bdnf* and *Neurotrophin 4/5*.

Directional growth by RGC growth cones towards the centrally located optic disc is particularly influenced by attractive interactions involving the **Laminin** and **Netrin** signaling pathways, but is also regulated by their repulsion from the periphery of the neural retina. A zinc-finger gene, **Zic3**, which is expressed strongly in the peripheral retina with a decreasing gradient towards the optic disc, seems to regulate the expression of (so far unidentified) axon repellant factors. When the growth cone reaches the optic disc, its morphology changes from a simple tapered cone to a complex, actively pleomorphic structure that puts out numerous cell processes called **filopodia** (see Fig. 9-16). The filopodia, especially, have been implicated in the sensing and transducing of environmental signals that guide the growth cone to its target. The increased morphologic complexity of the growth cone at such **choice points** reflects its response to the environmental signals that determine its behavior. The retinal axon growth cones change back to a simple, tapered shape once they have plunged into the optic nerve, but they become complex again when they reach the **optic chiasm**, where they must decide whether to cross into the other side of the brain.

Half of the Retinal Ganglion Axons Cross Midline

In the majority of submammalian vertebrates, whose left and right visual fields are separate, all retinal axons cross at the optic chiasm and innervate the contralateral side of the brain. In humans, half the axons from each retina (those of the medial or nasal half) cross over to the other side and form the contralateral optic tract, whereas axons from the

9

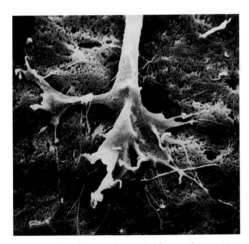

Figure 9-16. Scanning electron micrograph of a growth cone. Note numerous filopodia and lamellipodia.

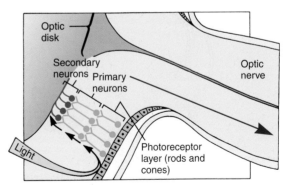

Figure 9-17. Organization of neurons in the retina and optic nerve. Photoreceptor cells, the rods and cones, form the deepest layer of the neural retina (the layer furthest from the vitreous humor). The information from the rods and cones is gathered by a layer of short primary visual neurons, which synapse in the retina with the secondary visual neurons. The axons of these secondary neurons traverse the surface of the retina and then travel via the optic nerve to the brain.

lateral (or temporal) half turn into the ipsilateral optic tract, where they join axons that have already crossed over from the contralateral nasal retina (Fig. 9-18; also see Fig. 9-15). The decision for an RGC axon to remain ipsilateral rather than to cross **(decussate)** at the chiasm exists only for animals with **binocular** vision, where the visual fields of left and right eyes overlap and information from the visual field is relayed from both eyes to one side of the brain. How in the case of binocularity do some retinal axons know to cross at the optic chiasm whereas others know not to cross?

The mouse optic chiasm has featured prominently as a model for addressing this question, being particularly amenable to genetic manipulation, despite the fact that in mice only a small part of the visual field is shared by both eyes and a correspondingly small region of the retina (the **ventrotemporal crescent**) projects ipsilaterally (Fig. 9-19). Recent studies have revealed the matched expression of an axon-repellant molecule (*Ephrin-B2*) by midline glial cells at the chiasm, and a receptor (*EphB1*) for this ligand exclusively

on RGC of the ventrotemporal retina. **Ephrins** are a large family of ligands that may cause collapse of the growth cone with loss or slowing of its locomotor activity when sensed by a neuron that expresses a *Receptor tyrosine kinase* of the **Eph** family (*Ephrins* are discussed in more detail in Ch. 5). Significantly, when the function of *Ephrin-B2* is blocked, all axons project contralaterally, recapitulating the primitive "default" condition for the monocular visual pathway. Normally, *Ephrin-B2* function causes those growth cones that are sensitive to it to be repelled from the midline and join the pathway provided by axons crossing from the other side. Interestingly, the metamorphosis of frogs is accompanied by the acquisition of an ipsilateral visual projection: as the side-facing eyes of a tadpole rotate up towards the top of the head, so the originally separate visual fields overlap to some extent and retinal axons begin to project to the ipsilateral tectum. This correlates with the onset of *Ephrin-B2* expression in the chiasm and of *EphB1* in the ventrotemporal retina—again consistent with a pivotal

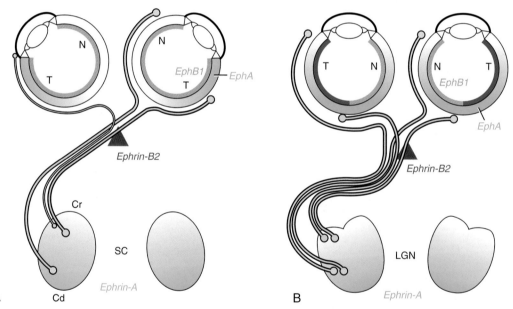

Figure 9-18. Visual mapping in mouse and human. In the mouse (*A*), the large majority of retinal ganglion cells (RGC) project to the mesencephalic superior colliculus (SC) and a minority project to the diencephalic lateral geniculate nucleus (not shown). The visual field is only partly binocular, so that only a small contingent of axons from the temporal hemiretina (T) project to the ipsilateral SC, whereas all the others project contralaterally. The ipsilateral RGC express *EphB1* receptors, which regulate their exclusion from the midline chiasm cells that express *Ephrin-B2*. *EphA* receptors are expressed in a decreasing temporal-to-nasal gradient, complementary to the gradient of *Ephrin-A* ligands in the SC. Axons from the temporal hemiretina (T) are excluded from caudal (cd) SC by repulsive interactions between the *EphA*s and *Ephrin-A*s and thus project to the cranial SC (cr). Nasal RGC (N) project to the caudal SC (P). In humans (*B*), the large majority of RGC project to the LGN and only a minority project to the SC (not shown). The visual field is binocular, so that the entire temporal hemiretina projects ipsilaterally, and the entire nasal hemiretina projects contralaterally. Ipsilateral and contralaterally projecting RGC from both eyes that see the same point in space terminate at the same craniocaudal position in the LGN but in adjacent eye-specific layers.

role for *Eph/Ephrin* signaling in effecting the ipsilateral routing of axons. Regulating the noncrossing phenotype of ventrotemporal RGC, and likely upstream of *EphB1* expression, is a zinc-finger transcription factor, *Zic2*, which is expressed exclusively in these cells. In genetic loss-of-function experiments in mice, the ventrotemporal RGC project contralaterally.

The deflection of temporal axons back into the ipsilateral optic tract also depends on the presence of the axons from the opposite eye that have already crossed over in the chiasm and constructed a **pre-formed pathway** on which ipsilateral axons can adhere. If the opposite eye is removed in a mouse embryo, so that the crossing axons never develop, the ipsilaterally targeting axons of the remaining eye pause for a long period at the chiasm and may never project further. Normal formation of the ipsilateral tract seems to depend on adhesive interactions with the already crossed axons, for which a candidate is the immunoglobulin family cell adhesion molecule *L1*. In mice lacking this protein, the ipsilateral projection is severely diminished.

Another factor influencing the choice of axonal pathway at the chiasm is the presence of *Melanin*, which is normally expressed by chiasm cells. In ocular albinos of numerous species, many axons go to the wrong side of the brain, resulting in targeting anomalies that degrade visual acuity and may alter the visible morphology of the lateral geniculate nuclei.

Retinal Ganglion Cell (RGC) Axons Form a Precise Map of Visual Space when They Synapse in Tectum and Lateral Geniculate Nucleus

Each retinal axon courses to the correct region in the **lateral geniculate nucleus** (LGN) and synapses with the correct target neurons, thus reproducing in the LGN the spatial information from the retina, point-to-point. A similar feat is accomplished by the axons of the LGN, which grow back to the occipital lobe of the cerebrum, where they map onto the **primary visual (striate) cortex**. Axons from right and left eyes synapse in distinct, eye-specific layers of the LGN. By means of these neural maps, passed on between

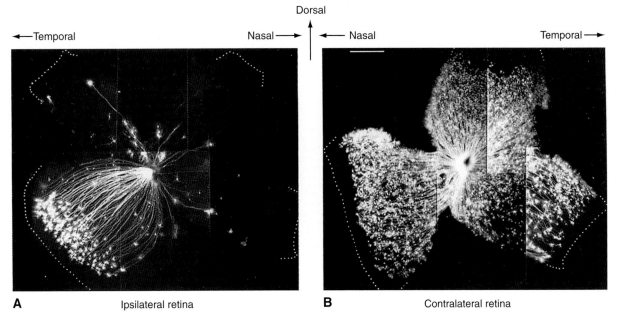

Dorsal

←—Temporal   Nasal —→ | ←— Nasal   Temporal —→

A   Ipsilateral retina   **B**   Contralateral retina

Figure 9-19. A "tract-tracing" technique used to show the projection of secondary retinal neurons to a particular locus in the optic tract. The use of dyes to analyze the arrangement of the axons projected by distant neurons is a time-honored neurobiologic technique. In this example, a crystal of the carbocyanine dye Dil was inserted into the optic tract of a 16.5-day mouse embryo at a site caudal to the optic chiasm. After the dye had time to diffuse along the axons, the ipsilateral, *A,* and contralateral, *B,* retinae were mounted flat on a microscope slide and examined with a fluorescence microscope to determine which of the axons were back-filled with dye. The back-filled axons can be assumed to represent the axon population that projects to the site of the crystal in the optic tract. In the ipsilateral retina, *A,* secondary neurons located mainly in the ventrotemporal crescent project to the site of the crystal, whereas in the contralateral retina, *B,* neurons from all areas project to this site. This pattern is characteristic of the adult retina. Fibers from the ipsilateral and contralateral retinae are intermingled in the optic tract at the site of the crystal.

successive stages in the neural pathway, a representation of the visual world is transmitted to the cortex, which integrates the right and left visual fields and forms an image that is congruent between the two eyes (see Fig. 9-18).

Precise visual maps are also reproduced by the targeting of specific populations of RGC axons to the **superior colliculi** (SC)—the homolog of the submammalian tectum. In humans and other primates, where vision is a dominant sense, only a small minority of RGC axons project to the SC, whereas the large majority of RGC axons project to the LGN. In rodents, which lack high visual acuity, the situation is reversed—with the large majority of RGC axons projecting to the SC. The SC, along with other regions of the tectum including the inferior colliculi, integrates visual, auditory, and somatosensory information and coordinates reflex responses to movement, sound, and somatic sensation.

The question of how visual mapping is achieved is of interest not only in itself but also because spatial maps are a common and characteristic feature of the CNS, especially the sensory systems. A number of studies have begun to shed light on the intricate puzzle of how maps are formed, most of which have involved experimenting with the retinotectal/retinocollicular projection of zebrafish, Xenopus, chick, and mouse embryos. The visual map is created in two steps. First, a number of **activity-independent cues** guide the growing retinal axons to the approximately correct point (**termination zone**) in the tectum/SC, where they arborize extensively and synapse to form a rough map. Second, these initial, somewhat unfocussed synapses are then sharpened by **activity-dependent** pruning of axonal arbors, by secondary axonal reconnection, and by cell death of inappropriately targeted cells to form a highly tuned point-to-point map.

The synapses of RGC axons in the optic tectum re-produce the spatial order of the retina on two orthogonal axes, such that the temporonasal (TN) axis of the retina maps to the cranial-caudal (CrCd) axis of the tectum, and the dorsoventral (DV) axis of the retina maps to the mediallateral (LM) axis of the tectum (see Fig. 9-18). The relationship is such that the axes of retina and tectum are in inverse orientation: that is, nasal retina (originally *cranial* on the neuraxis) maps to *caudal* tectum and *ventral* retina maps to medial (originally *dorsal*) tectum. This inversion effectively corrects the inversion of the visual field produced by the lens.

Having traversed the surface of the diencephalon to reach the dorsal midbrain, retinal axon growth cones enter the tectum at its cranial border and grow towards its caudal border; that is, they grow near parallel to the midline (Fig. 9-20). In chick and mouse embryos, axons may overshoot their termination zone by a considerable distance, and appropriate retinotopic connectivity occurs through the interstitial branching of collaterals from the main axon shaft. Interstitials bud off at roughly the correct position on the CrCd axis, which may be some distance back from the growth cone, and then grow at right angles to the axon shaft to reach their correct termination zone on the ML axis. In fish and frog, by contrast, the correct termination zone is reached directly by the primary growth cone. In these species, which grow continuously throughout life, the retinotectal projection changes constantly to incorporate the radial increments of retinal growth into a tectal map with two orthogonal dimensions.

However, in all species once an axon or collateral reaches the CrCd and ML position that maps to the position of the parent neuron in the retina, it invades the tectum and arborizes extensively in the retinorecipient layers. This point-to-zone mapping is thought to be controlled, at least in part, by complementary gradients of *Ephrins* expressed in the tectum and of *Eph* receptors expressed in the retina. For example, *Ephrin-A2* and *Ephrin-A5* are expressed in increasing cranial to caudal gradients, whereas their *EphA* receptor is expressed in an increasing nasal to temporal gradient. The *Ephrin-As* are powerful repellants of growth cones and inhibitors of interstitial branching. Because the level of *EphA* receptor on a cell determines the degree to which its axon (or branching capacity) is inhibited by *Ephrin-As*, temporal axons are subject to more intense repulsion than nasal axons, and are thereby confined to the anterior tectum. Countergradients of receptor and ligand may sharpen the ability of axons across the nasal-temporal axis to find their correct termination zone in the tectum according to particular thresholds of inhibition.

A similar mechanism involving complementary gradients of *Ephrin-B* ligands and *EphB* receptors operates in mapping the DV axis of the retina onto the LM axis of the tectum. Here, however, the evidence from both frogs and mice points to an attractant interaction rather than a repellant one, with high *EphB* expressing ventral RGC projecting to high *Ephrin-B* expressing medial tectum.

More than 40 years ago, work on the visual system of frogs led Sperry to propose a **chemoaffinity hypothesis** for topographic mapping, which held that each position in the optic tectum has a unique address dictated by the gradient distribution of molecular labels along orthogonal axes, matched by an equivalent distribution of labels in the retina. This hypothesis, long neglected in favor of more mechanical mechanisms for axon guidance, has been substantially vindicated by the discovery of *Eph/Ephrin* gradients and their central role in retinotectal mapping.

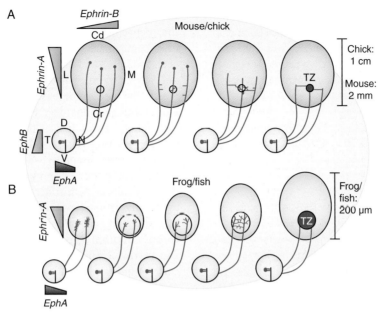

Figure 9-20. Development of visual projections in amniotes (chick, mouse) *A*, and in anamniotes (frog, fish) *B*. In all species, the temporonasal axis of the retina (TN) maps to the cranial-caudal axis of the tectum/superior colliculus (CrCd) and the dorsal-ventral axis of the retina (DV) maps to the medial-lateral axis (ML) of the tectum/superior colliculus. The termination zones (TZ) of retinal ganglion cells (RGC) are established according to position on orthogonal gradients of *Ephrin-As* (CrCd axis) and *Ephrin-Bs* (LM axis). In amniotes, the termination zones are set up by collaterals that bud interstitially from the main axon shaft, which itself may extend well beyond the TZ. In anamniotes, the TZs are set up directly by the growth cones of RGC. In both cases, there is extensive arborization in the TZ before final point-to-point mapping is achieved by secondary refinement of activity-dependent pruning.

We saw above how certain transcription factors may confer polarity on the neural retina and positional identity on the RGC. However, in only a few examples is it yet seen that these factors regulate the *Eph/Ephrin* system, which is the essential readout of retinal position information. For example, overexpression of either *Soho* and *Gh6* on the CrCd axis can repress expression of *EphAs*, leading to pathway errors and mapping defects. On the DV axis, ectopic expression of *Vax* induces *EphB* in the dorsal retina, whereas knocking out *Vax2* leads to the loss of *EphB* expression, dorsalization of the ventral retina, and the shift of ventrotemporal axon terminations from medial to lateral regions of the superior colliculus. The search for genes involved in upstream regulatory control of the tectal gradients has revealed few candidates: the most prominent of these is the homeobox gene **Engrailed**, which regulates the expression of *Ephrin-A* ligands in the caudal midbrain and has a similarly graded expression pattern.

Binocular Visual System of Humans Also Involves Ephs and Ephrins in Guidance and Mapping

Retinal mapping in humans and other primates with fully binocular vision is characterized by the congruent mapping of hemiretinas from both eyes onto the same target—the LGN on one side of the thalamus. Just as in rodents, where *EphB1* expression in the ventrotemporal retina regulates ipsilateral passage at the chiasm, so in humans this receptor is expressed in the entire temporal hemiretina and its repellant ligand, *Ephrin-B2*, is expressed at the optic chiasm (see Fig. 9-18). Similarly, the *Ephrin-A* gradients that segregate temporal and nasal axons in the tectum of birds and the mouse SC are also formed in the human LGN, in complementary fashion to *EphA* gradients in the retina.

Fine-Tuning the Visual Map Depends on Neuronal Activity

Several studies indicate that feedback in the form of neural impulses from the retina is important in refining the coarse-grained visual map formed by the **activity-independent** axon guidance mechanisms. Fine-tuning the visual map depends as much on the retraction from inappropriate targets as it does on growth to appropriate targets. Indeed, when correlated electrical activity is inhibited within the visual system by sodium channel blockers such as tetrodotoxin (TTX), axons are not retracted from inappropriate targets and large, more diffuse termination zones persist. Moreover, it has been demonstrated in cultured neurons that neurite retraction depends on the density of voltage-activated calcium channels following stimulation. It has been demonstrated in several vertebrate systems that the final pattern of point-to-point synaptic connections depends on matching the frequency and duration of impulse activity—cells that fire together wire together. Matching coactive retinal inputs to the tectum/SC requires the activity of the *N-methyl-D-aspartate* (*NMDA*) *receptor*: blocking excitatory transmission with *NMDA receptor* inhibitors such as 2-amino-5-phosphonovalerate (APV) disorganizes the retinotopic map.

It is also becoming clear that the visual system is extensively modified by the **death of neurons** even as it is being formed. As in other areas of the nervous system, far more neurons are initially produced than survive in the mature system. For example, it is estimated that three to four million ganglion cells arise in the human retina, but only just over a million survive in the adult. Many of the original synaptic connections made by these cells are eliminated by a pruning process that participates in tuning the visual maps in the LGN and superior colliculus.

During the 3rd week, a diverticulum called the **in-fundibulum** develops in the floor of the third ventricle and grows ventrally toward the stomodeum (Fig. 9-21; see also Fig. 9-13C). Simultaneously, an ectodermal placode appears in the roof of the stomodeum (an ectodermal lined space near the future mouth opening, between the maxillary and mandibular processes; discussed in Ch. 16) and invaginates to form a diverticulum called **Rathke's pouch**, which grows dorsally toward the infundibulum. Rathke's pouch eventually loses its connection with the stomodeum and forms a discrete sac that is apposed to the cranial surface of the infundibulum. This sac differentiates to form the **adenohypophysis** of the pituitary. The cells of its anterior surface give rise to the **anterior lobe** proper of the pituitary, and a small group of cells on the posterior surface of the pouch form the functionally distinct **pars intermedia**. Meanwhile, the distal portion of the infundibulum differentiates to form the **posterior pituitary (neurohypophysis)**. The lumen of the infundibulum is obliterated by this process, but a small proximal pit, the **infundibular recess**, persists in the floor of the third ventricle.

Telencephalon. The cerebral hemispheres first appear on day 32 as a pair of bubble-like outgrowths of the telencephalon. By 16 weeks, the rapidly growing hemispheres are oval and have expanded back to cover the diencephalon. The thin roof and lateral walls of each hemisphere represent the future **cerebral cortex** (Fig. 9-22A). The floor is thicker and contains neuronal aggregations called the **ganglionic eminences**, which give rise to the **basal ganglia** (**corpus striatum** and **globus pallidus**) (see Fig. 9-14B). As the growing hemispheres press against the walls of the diencephalon, the meningeal layers that originally separate the two structures disappear, so that the neural tissue of the thalami becomes continuous with that of the floor of the cerebral hemispheres. This former border is eventually crossed by a massive axon bundle called the **internal capsule**, which passes through the corpus striatum (giving it its striated appearance) and carries axons from the thalamus to the cerebral cortex (and vice versa) as well as from the cerebral cortex to lower regions of the brain and spinal cord (see Fig. 9-14C).

The cerebral hemispheres are initially smooth surfaced. However, like the cerebellar cortex, the cerebral cortex folds into an increasingly complex pattern of gyri (ridges) and sulci (grooves) as the hemispheres grow. This process begins in the 4th month with the formation of a small indentation called the **lateral cerebral fossa** in the lateral wall of each hemisphere (Fig. 9-22B; see Fig. 9-22A). The caudal end of each lengthening hemisphere curves ventrally and then grows forward across this fossa, creating the **temporal lobe** of the cerebral hemisphere and converting the fossa into a deep cleft called the **lateral cerebral sulcus**. The portion of the cerebral cortex that originally forms the medial floor of the fossa is covered by the temporal lobe and is called the **insula**.

By the 6th month, several other cerebral sulci have formed. These include the **central sulcus**, which separates the frontal and parietal lobes, and the **occipital sulcus**, which demarcates the occipital lobe. The detailed pattern of gyri that ultimately forms on the cerebral hemispheres varies somewhat from individual to individual. The gyri and sulci effectively increase the surface area of the brain such that when fully grown, it is the size of a pillowcase.

Each cerebral hemisphere contains a diverticulum of the telencephalic primitive ventricle called the **lateral ventricle**. The lateral ventricle initially occupies most of the volume of the hemisphere but is progressively constricted by the thickening of the cortex. However, along the line between the floor and the medial wall of the hemisphere, the cerebral wall does not thicken but instead remains

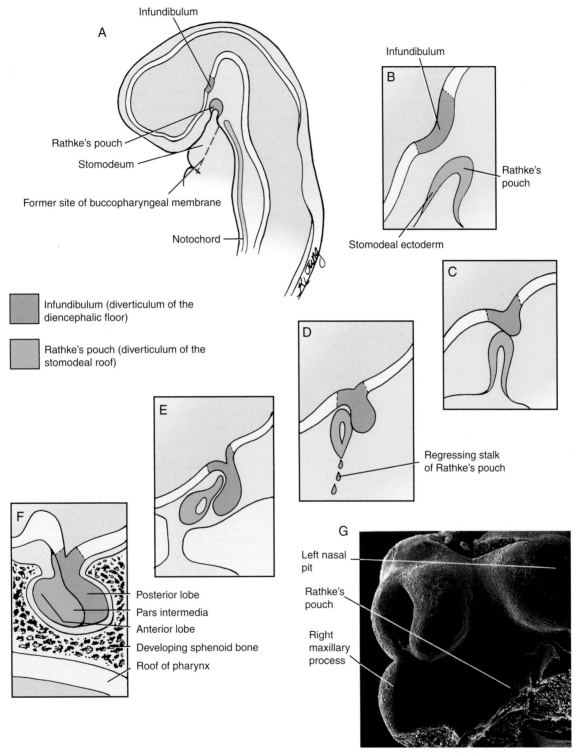

9

Figure 9-21. *A-F*, Development of the pituitary. The pituitary gland is a compound structure. The posterior lobe forms from a diverticulum of the diencephalic floor called the *infundibulum*, whereas the anterior lobe and pars intermedia form from an evagination of the ectodermal roof of the stomodeum called *Rathke's pouch*. Rathke's pouch detaches from the stomodeum and becomes associated with the developing posterior pituitary. *G*, Scanning electron micrograph of the roof of the embryonic oral cavity, showing the opening to Rathke's pouch.

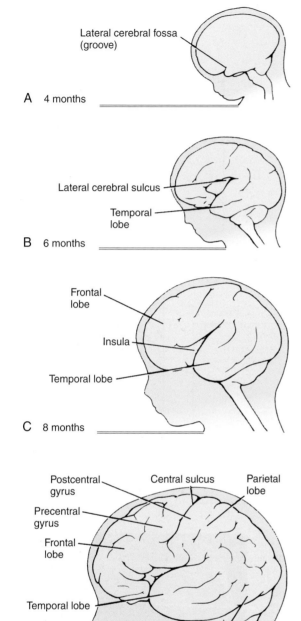

A 4 months — Lateral cerebral fossa (groove)

B 6 months — Lateral cerebral sulcus, Temporal lobe

C 8 months — Frontal lobe, Insula, Temporal lobe

D 9 months — Postcentral gyrus, Central sulcus, Parietal lobe, Precentral gyrus, Frontal lobe, Temporal lobe, Occipital lobe

Figure 9-22. Growth and folding of the cerebral hemispheres during fetal life. Growth of the cerebral hemispheres is continuous throughout embryonic and fetal development and continues after birth. *A, B,* In the 4th month, the formation of the narrow lateral cerebral fossa delineates the temporal lobe of the cerebral hemisphere. By the 6th month, additional clefts delineate the frontal, parietal, and occipital lobes. *C, D,* Additional sulci and gyri form throughout the remainder of fetal life.

thin and epithelial. This zone forms a longitudinal groove in the ventricle; the groove is called the **choroid fissure** (see Fig. 9-14C). A choroid plexus develops along the choroid fissure. As shown in Figure 9-23, the lateral ventricle extends the whole length of each hemisphere, reaching anteriorly into the frontal lobe and, at its posterior end, curving around to occupy the temporal lobe. The opening between each lateral ventricle and the third ventricle persists as the **interventricular foramen (foramen of Monro)**.

The neuroepithelium of the cerebral hemispheres is initially much like that of other parts of the neural tube. However, studies on cerebral histogenesis have shown that the process of proliferation, migration, and differentiation by which the mature cortex is produced is unique. The cerebral cortex is made up of several cell layers (or laminae) that vary in number from three in the phylogenetically oldest parts to six in the dominant **neocortex**. In other regions of the CNS the white matter (axons) forms outside the grey matter (neuronal cell bodies); this situation is reversed in the cerebral cortex. Here, axons enter and leave through an intermediate zone that lies deep to the grey matter and thus forms the outer surface of the brain. The details of how this inside-out arrangement of grey and white matter develops are complex and still poorly understood. To summarize, the proliferating cells of the ventricular layer undergo a series of regulated divisions to produce waves of neurons that migrate peripherally and establish the neuronal layers of the cortex. Axons extend from these cells on the inner or deep surface of the neuronal layers, between them and the ventricular zone. Furthermore, the cortical layers are laid down in a sequence from *deep* to *superficial*: that is, the neurons of each wave migrate through the preceding layers to establish a more superficial layer. As the production of neurons tapers off, the ventricular layer gives rise to the various kinds of glia and then to the ependyma.

Let us now examine the process in more detail (Fig. 9-24A). The first neurons produced from the ventricular zone form a superficial layer, the **preplate**, which immediately underlies the developing pia. Axons extend from these neurons on the *inner* side of the preplate, establishing an **intermediate zone**. The next neurons to be born migrate into the middle of the preplate and split it into a superficial **marginal zone** (future lamina I) and deep **subplate**, forming a middle layer called the **cortical plate**. Young neurons migrate on the surfaces of a preformed array of **radial glial cells**, whose processes span the full thickness of the cortex. Axons from neurons in the

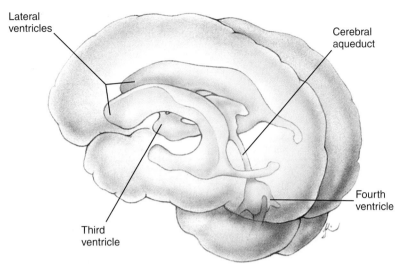

Lateral
ventricles

Cerebral
aqueduct

Fourth
ventricle

Third
ventricle

Figure 9-23. The cerebral ventricles. The expansions of the neural canal in the primary and secondary brain vesicles and cerebral hemispheres give rise to the cerebral ventricles. The ventricle system consists of the lateral ventricles in the cerebral hemispheres, the third ventricle in the diencephalon, the narrow cerebral aqueduct (of Sylvius) in the mesencephalon, and the fourth ventricle in the rhombencephalon.

cortical plate and subplate join those already in the intermediate zone, which will later become the **white matter** of the cortex. The early neurons of the cortical plate form the deep layers (laminae VI and V) of the finished cortex, whereas later-born cells migrate radially from the ventricular zone across the intermediate zone and subplate, through the earlier layers VI and V of the cortical plate. In the process they establish, in sequence, the more superficial laminae IV, III, and (finally) II. As neurogenesis proceeds, new neurons are increasingly formed in an accessory germinative zone lying deep to the ventricular zone, called the **subventricular zone.**

The above describes the generation of the principal excitatory neurons of the neocortex—the **pyramidal cells**—the large neurons that project to subcortical targets and to the contralateral hemisphere. More numerous but smaller than the pyramidal neurons are the inhibitory interneurons—the **granule cells**. The majority of the latter do not arise from either the ventricular zone or the subventricular zone of the cortical area in which settle; rather, they originate in the ganglionic eminences of the ventral telencephalon and migrate dorsally into the cortex via a tangential route (Fig. 9-24*B*).

Whereas laminae II to VI are the principal constituents of the grey matter in the adult neocortex, the first-born neurons that contribute to lamina I and the subplate disappear later in development; however,

their transient existence is crucial to normal cortical histogenesis. Lamina I, the marginal zone, contains transient neurons called **Cajal-Retzius cells**, the majority of which originate in a dorsal midline structure of the telencephalon (the cortical hem) and migrate tangentially into lamina I. Through their secretion of the large glycoprotein *Reelin*, Cajal-Retzius cells are believed to orchestrate the inside-to-outside migration of neurons into the cortical plate. In the absence of *Reelin*, or of other proteins in the *Reelin* signaling pathway, successive waves of young neurons pile up on the inside of their predecessors rather than passing through to form a more superficial layer. The neurons of the subplate, which are the first of the cerebral cortex to extend axons, are thought to be crucial in guiding the ordered ingrowth of thalamic axons towards their appropriate presumptive cortical area.

IN THE CLINIC

CONGENITAL MALFORMATIONS OF CEREBRAL CORTEX

Like the human cerebellum, the human cerebrum is subject to a variety of developmental disorders that result from abnormal cell migration, differentiation, survival, or proliferation. The most severe of these abnormalities are obvious in early development, but some do not manifest

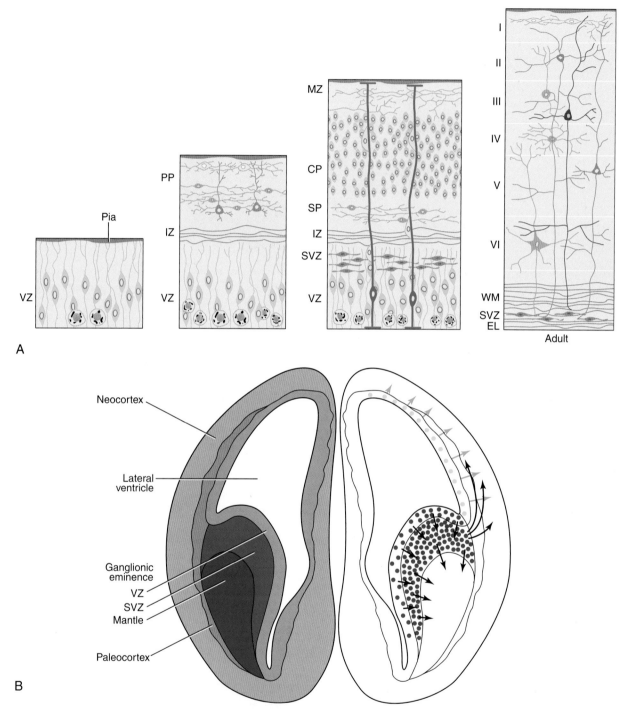

Figure 9-24. *A,* Cytodifferentiation and lamination of the neocortex. The diagram shows a series of four stages in section. The green cells in the marginal zone (MZ) are the Cajal-Retzius cells. CP, cortical plate; EL, ependymal layer; IZ, intermediate zone; PP, preplate; SP, subplate; WM, white matter; I-VI, numbered layers of neocortex. *B,* Migration of interneurons (nonpyramidal cells) from their origin in the ventricular and subventricular zones (VZ, SVZ) of the ganglionic eminences via tangential pathways (arrows on right side) to the neocortex. A small minority of cortical interneurons arise from the cortical germinative zones (yellow). The germinative zones of the ganglionic eminences also produce the neurons of the corpus striatum and globus pallidus (basal ganglia).

themselves until later in life. Diagnosis can be made from gross specimens or by magnetic resonance imaging (MRI), computed tomography (CT), or ultrasonography.

Classical lissencephaly (incidence of at least 1 in 100,000 live births) is a condition that results from incomplete neuronal migration to the cerebral cortex during the 3rd and 4th months of gestation. Brains from patients with lissencephaly have a smoothened cerebral surface due to a combination of **pachygyria** (broad, thick gyri), **agyria** (lack of gyri), and widespread neuronal **heterotopia** (cells in aberrant positions compared with those of normal brain). Enlarged ventricles and malformation of the corpus callosum are also common. As newborns, these patients often appear normal but sometimes have apnea, poor feeding, or abnormal muscle tone. Patients typically later develop seizures, profound mental retardation, and mild spastic quadriplegia.

Subcortical band heterotopia (SBH) is also believed to result from aberrant migration of differentiating neuro-epithelial cells. These patients have bilateral circumferential and symmetric ribbons of gray matter located just beneath the cortex and separated from it by a thin band of white matter, which led to the term *double cortex syndrome*. Seizures, mild mental retardation, and some behavioral abnormalities are often present in infancy. However, intelligence can be normal and seizures may begin later in life. A related syndrome, **X-linked lissencephaly** and **SBH**, also occurs in which homozygous males have lissencephaly and heterozygous females have SBH.

Recent studies have identified two genes that are linked to lissencephaly and SBH. One, *LIS1*, maps to chromosome 17p13 and encodes a protein that functions as a regulatory subunit of PLATELET-ACTIVATING FACTOR ACETYLHYDRO-LASE, which degrades PLATELET ACTIVATING FACTOR and is also involved in microtubule dynamics. In regards to its latter role, PLATELET-ACTIVATING FACTOR ACETYLHYDROLASE controls the distribution and function of the microtubule motor DYNEIN, thereby controlling the movement of the nucleus during neuronal migration. Studies of mice with targeted *Lis-1* mutations suggest that this protein is necessary for normal pyramidal cell migration and neurite outgrowth. Another gene, called *DOUBLECORTIN*, is located on the X chromosome and is mutated in patients with X-linked lissencephaly and SBH. The protein product of *DOUBLECORTIN* is highly expressed in fetal neurons and their precursors during cortical development. Like PLATELET-ACTIVATING FACTOR ACETYLHYDROLASE, the DOUBLE-CORTIN protein is associated with microtubules, suggesting that it is also involved in cell migration through interactions with the cytoskeleton.

As described in Chapter 16, the nasal placodes form at the end of the 4th week. Very early, some cells in the nasal placode differentiate to form the **primary neurosensory cells** of the future olfactory epithelium. At the end of the 5th week, these cells sprout axons that cross the short distance to penetrate the most cranial end of the telencephalon (Fig. 9-25A). The subsequent ossification of the ethmoid bone around these axons creates the perforated cribriform plates.

In the 6th week, as the nasal pits differentiate to form the epithelium of the nasal passages, the area at the tip of each cerebral hemisphere (where the axons of the primary neurosensory cells synapse) begins to form an outgrowth called the **olfactory bulb** (Fig. 9-25B-D). The cells in the olfactory bulb that synapse with the axons of the primary sensory neurons differentiate to become the secondary sensory neurons (mitral cells) of the olfactory pathways. The axons of these cells synapse in the olfactory centers of the cerebral hemispheres. As the changing proportions of the face and brain lengthen the distance between the olfactory bulbs and their point of origin on the hemispheres, the axons of the secondary olfactory neurons lengthen to form stalk-like CNS **olfactory tracts**. Traditionally, the olfactory tract and bulb together are referred to as the **olfactory nerve.**

9

IN THE CLINIC

KALLMANN SYNDROME

Kallmann syndrome is characterized by **anosmia** (loss of sense of smell) or **hyposmia** (diminished sense of spell) and **hypogonadism** (small gonads). It affects between 1 in 10,000 and 1 in 60,000 people, and occurs five times more frequently in males than in females. Anosmia or hyposmia results because the olfactory bulbs and olfactory nerves fail to develop properly. Hypogonadism results because the hypothalamus fails to produce sufficient *GnRH* (*Gonadotropin-releasing hormone*), a hormone required for normal development of the gonads (discussed in Ch. 15).

The failure of the hypothalamus to produce sufficient *GnRH* is secondary to a neuronal migration defect. *GnRH* neurons originate in the olfactory placodes and migrate to the developing hypothalamus via the olfactory bulbs. The gene responsible for the X-linked form of Kallmann syndrome, *KAL1*, has been identified. It encodes an extracellular matrix glycoprotein protein called ANOSMIN-1. Kallmann also results from mutations in other genes including *FGFR1*, *PROKINETICIN2*, and its receptor (a cysteine-rich protein secreted by the suprachiasmatic nucleus

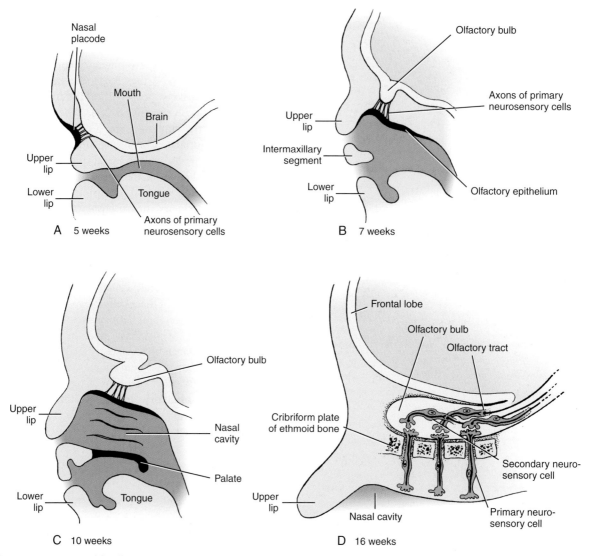

Figure 9-25. Formation of the olfactory tract as seen in sagittal views. *A*, During the 5th week, cells of the nasal placode differentiate into the primary neurosensory cells of the olfactory tract and produce axons that grow into the presumptive olfactory bulb of the adjacent telencephalon. There they synapse there with secondary neurons. *B-D*, As development continues, the elongating axons of the secondary olfactory neurons in the olfactory bulb produce the olfactory tract.

and involved in the circadian clock). The syndrome can be inherited as an autosomal dominant or autosomal recessive trait, or as a digenic trait. With identification of the genes involved, Kallmann syndrome can be diagnosed during in vitro fertilization and preimplantation genetic diagnosis (discussed in Ch. 1).

The commissures that connect the right and left cerebral hemispheres form from a thickening at the cranial end of the telencephalon, which represents the zone of final neuropore closure. This area can be divided into a dorsal **commissural plate** and a ventral **lamina terminalis**.

The first axon tract to develop in the commissural plate is the **anterior commissure**, which forms during the 7th week and interconnects the olfactory bulbs and olfactory centers of the two hemispheres (Fig. 9-26). During the 9th week, the **hippocampal**, or **fornix commissure**, forms between the right and left hippocampi (a phylogenetically old portion of the cerebral hemisphere that is located adjacent to the choroid fissure). A few days later, the massive, arched **corpus**

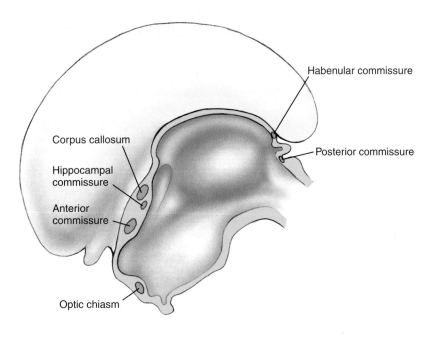

A   10 weeks

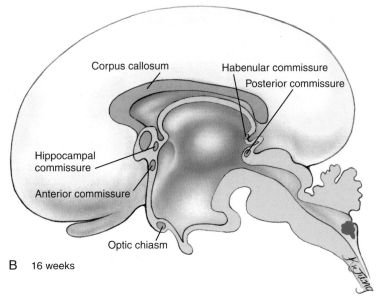

B   16 weeks

Figure 9-26. Formation of the commissures at 10, *A*, and 16, *B*, weeks. The telencephalon gives rise to commissural tracts that integrate the activities of the left and right cerebral hemispheres. These include the anterior and hippocampal commissures and the corpus callosum. The small posterior and habenular commissures arise from the epithalamus.

callosum begins to form, linking together the right and left neocortices along their entire length. The most anterior part of the corpus callosum appears first, and its posterior extension (the **splenium**) forms later in fetal life.

Growth of Brain

Although growth of the brain is rapid during fetal life (see Fig. 9-22), the brain at birth is only about 25% of its adult volume. Some of the postnatal growth of the brain is the result of increases in the size of neuronal cell bodies and the proliferation of neuronal processes. However, most of this growth results from the myelination of nerve fibers. The brain reaches its final size at around 7 years of age.

The manner in which the 10 billion to 1 trillion neurons of the human brain become organized and interconnected is a problem of daunting complexity. As discussed in this chapter, not only do the neurons themselves proliferate, migrate, and differentiate according to a precise pattern, but also their cell processes display phenomenal pathfinding abilities.

IN THE CLINIC

BRAIN SIZE

Microcephaly, typically defined as small head, results from the formation of a small brain (Fig. 9-27). Recently genes have been identified that play roles in dramatically regulating brain growth. One gene, *ASPM* (*ABNORMAL SPINDLE-LIKE*

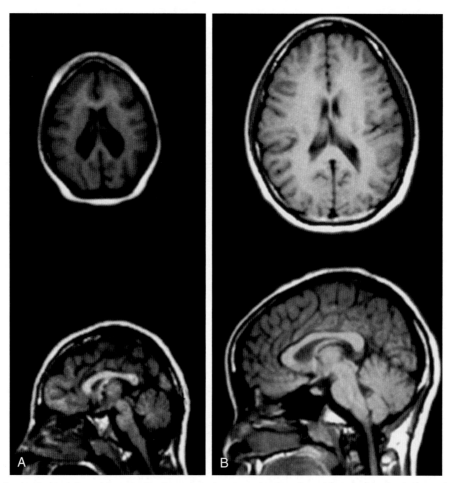

Figure 9-27. MRIs showing the head of an adolescent with microcephaly, *A*, compared to that of an adolescent with a head of normal size, *B*. The top row shows images taken in the coronal plane; the bottom row shows images taken in the sagittal plane.

MICROCEPHALY ASSOCIATED), a homolog of the *Drosophila Abnormal spindle* gene, is mutated in the most common form of autosomal recessive primary microcephaly in humans. *ASPM* plays an essential role in embryonic neuroblasts in normal mitotic spindle function, and it is expressed in proliferating regions of the cerebral cortex during neurogenesis.

Brains that are lissencephalic are also microcephalic. One link between these two brain defects involves two genes, *LIS1* (as discussed earlier in the chapter, results in lissencephaly when mutated) and a second gene called *NDE1*. *NDE1*, formerly known as *mNUDE* and homologous to the *Nude* gene of the filamentous fungi *A. nidulans*, has been shown to directly interact with *LIS1*. In *A. nidulans*, *Nude* localizes to the microtubule organizing center and regulates microtubule organization. Genetic ablation of *Nde1* function in mice results in microcephaly, with the most striking reduction in brain size occurring in the cerebral cortex. It is unknown whether *NDE1* is mutated in patients with microcephaly.

Another gene that regulates brain size is *β-Catenin*. When over expressed in mice, the brain grows to almost twice its normal size. In addition, foliation of the brain is increased, such that the cerebral cortex of the mouse more closely resembles that of the human.

Suggested Readings

Anderson S. 2004. Tlx genes make an exciting choice. Nat Neurosci 7:421-422.

Anderson SA, Marin O, Horn C, Jennings K, Rubenstein JL. 2001. Distinct cortical migrations from the medial and lateral ganglionic eminences. Development 128:353-363.

Appel B, Eisen JS. 2003. Retinoids run rampant: multiple roles during spinal cord and motor neuron development. Neuron 40:461-464.

Araujo SJ, Tear G. 2003. Axon guidance mechanisms and molecules: lessons from invertebrates. Nat Rev Neurosci 4:910-922.

Arevalo JC, Chao MV. 2005. Axonal growth: where neurotrophins meet Wnts. Curr Opin Cell Biol 17:112-115.

Assadi AH, Zhang G, Beffert U, et al. 2003. Interaction of reelin signaling and Lis1 in brain development. Nat Genet 35:270-276.

Barbieri AM, Broccoli V, Bovolenta P, et al. 2002. Vax2 inactivation in mouse determines alteration of the eye dorsal-ventral axis, misrouting of the optic fibres and eye coloboma. Development 129:805-813.

Bardin AJ, Le Borgne R, Schweisguth F. 2004. Asymmetric localization and function of cell-fate determinants: a fly's view. Curr Opin Neurobiol 14:6-14.

Barres BA, Barde Y. 2000. Neuronal and glial cell biology. Curr Opin Neurobiol 10:642-648.

Baumer N, Marquardt T, Stoykova A, et al. 2002. Pax6 is required for establishing naso-temporal and dorsal characteristics of the optic vesicle. Development 129:4535-4545.

Bertrand N, Castro DS, Guillemot F. 2002. Proneural genes and the specification of neural cell types. Nat Rev Neurosci 3:517-530.

Bertrand N, Dahmane N. 2006. Sonic hedgehog signaling in forebrain development and its interactions with pathways that modify its effects. Trends Cell Biol 16:597-605.

Bibel M, Barde YA. 2000. Neurotrophins: key regulators of cell fate and cell shape in the vertebrate nervous system. Genes Dev 14:2919-2937.

Bond J, Roberts E, Mochida GH, et al. 2002. ASPM is a major determinant of cerebral cortical size. Nat Genet 32:316-320.

Briscoe J, Ericson J. 2001. Specification of neuronal fates in the ventral neural tube. Curr Opin Neurobiol 11:43-49.

Brown A, Yates PA, Burrola P, et al. 2000. Topographic mapping from the retina to the midbrain is controlled by relative but not absolute levels of EphA receptor signaling. Cell 102:77-88.

Brunet I, Weinl C, Piper M, et al. 2005. The transcription factor Engrailed-2 guides retinal axons. Nature 438:94-98.

Burgess R, Lunyak V, Rosenfeld M. 2002. Signaling and transcriptional control of pituitary development. Curr Opin Genet Dev 12:534-539.

Campbell K. 2003. Dorsal-ventral patterning in the mammalian telencephalon. Curr Opin Neurobiol 13:50-56.

Carmeliet P, Tessier-Lavigne M. 2005. Common mechanisms of nerve and blood vessel wiring. Nature 436:193-200.

Caspary T, Anderson KV. 2003. Patterning cell types in the dorsal spinal cord: what the mouse mutants say. Nat Rev Neurosci 4:289-297.

Chao MV. 2003. Neurotrophins and their receptors: a convergence point for many signalling pathways. Nat Rev Neurosci 4:299-309.

Charron F, Tessier-Lavigne M. 2005. Novel brain wiring functions for classical morphogens: a role as graded positional cues in axon guidance. Development 132:2251-2262.

Chenn A, Walsh CA. 2002. Regulation of cerebral cortical size by control of cell cycle exit in neural precursors. Science 297:365-369.

Chien C-B. 2005. Guidance of Axons and Dendrites. In: Rao MS, Jacobson M, editors. Developmental Neurobiology. New York: Kluwer Academic/Plenum Pubs. pp 241-268.

Colognato H, ffrench-Constant C. 2004. Mechanisms of glial development. Curr Opin Neurobiol 14:37-44.

Conti L, Cattaneo E. 2005. Controlling neural stem cell division within the adult subventricular zone: an APPealing job. Trends Neurosci 28:57-59.

Cooke JE, Moens CB. 2002. Boundary formation in the hindbrain: Eph only it were simple. Trends Neurosci 25:260-267.

Corfas G, Roy K, Buxbaum JD. 2004. Neuregulin 1-erbB signaling and the molecular/cellular basis of schizophrenia. Nat Neurosci 7:575-580.

Dasen JS, Rosenfeld MG. 2001. Signaling and transcriptional mechanisms in pituitary development. Annu Rev Neurosci 24:327-355.

Debski EA, Cline HT. 2002. Activity-dependent mapping in the retinotectal projection. Curr Opin Neurobiol 12:93-99.

Dickson BJ. 2005. Wnts send axons up and down the spinal cord. Nat Neurosci 8:1130-1132.

Dickson BJ, Keleman K. 2002. Netrins. Curr Biol 12:R154-R155.

9

Diez del Corral R, Storey KG. 2004. Opposing FGF and retinoid pathways: a signalling switch that controls differentiation and patterning onset in the extending vertebrate body axis. Bioessays 26:857-869.

Dityatev A, Schachner M. 2003. Extracellular matrix molecules and synaptic plasticity. Nat Rev Neurosci 4:456-468.

Drescher U. 2005. A no-Wnt situation: SFRPs as axon guidance molecules. Nat Neurosci 8:1281-1282.

Feldheim DA, Kim YI, Bergemann AD, et al. 2000. Genetic analysis of ephrin-A2 and ephrin-A5 shows their requirement in multiple aspects of retinocollicular mapping. Neuron 25:563-574.

Feng Y, Walsh CA. 2004. Mitotic spindle regulation by Nde1 controls cerebral cortical size. Neuron 44:279-293.

Ferguson KL, Slack RS. 2003. Growth factors: can they promote neurogenesis? Trends Neurosci 26:283-285.

Fishell G, Kriegstein AR. 2003. Neurons from radial glia: the consequences of asymmetric inheritance. Curr Opin Neurobiol 13:34-41.

Garner CC, Nash J, Huganir RL. 2000. PDZ domains in synapse assembly and signalling. Trends Cell Biol 10:274-280.

Gavalas A. 2002. ArRAnging the hindbrain. Trends Neurosci 25:61-64.

Gavalas A, Krumlauf R. 2000. Retinoid signalling and hindbrain patterning. Curr Opin Genet Dev 10:380-386.

Ghysen A, Dambly-Chaudiere C. 2000. A genetic programme for neuronal connectivity. Trends Genet 16:221-226.

Gilthorpe JD, Papantoniou EK, Chedotal A, et al. 2002. The migration of cerebellar rhombic lip derivatives. Development 129:4719-4728.

Gleeson JG, Walsh CA. 2000. Neuronal migration disorders: from genetic diseases to developmental mechanisms. Trends Neurosci 23:352-359.

Goldberg JL. 2003. How does an axon grow? Genes Dev 17:941-958.

Goldman S. 2003. Glia as neural progenitor cells. Trends Neurosci 26:590-596.

Gomez-Skarmeta JL, Campuzano S, Modolell J. 2003. Half a century of neural prepatterning: the story of a few bristles and many genes. Nat Rev Neurosci 4:587-598.

Graw J. 2003. The genetic and molecular basis of congenital eye defects. Nat Rev Genet 4:876-888.

Grunwald IC, Klein R. 2002. Axon guidance: receptor complexes and signaling mechanisms. Curr Opin Neurobiol 12:250-259.

Guan KL, Rao Y. 2003. Signalling mechanisms mediating neuronal responses to guidance cues. Nat Rev Neurosci 4:941-956.

Guthrie S. 2001. Axon guidance: Robos make the rules. Curr Biol 11:R300-R303.

Hagg T. 2005. Molecular regulation of adult CNS neurogenesis: an integrated view. Trends Neurosci 28:589-595.

Hansen MJ, Dallal GE, Flanagan JG. 2004. Retinal axon response to ephrin-as shows a graded, concentration-dependent transition from growth promotion to inhibition. Neuron 42:717-730.

Hebert JM. 2005. Unraveling the molecular pathways that regulate early telencephalon development. Curr Top Dev Biol 69:17-37.

Herrera E, Brown L, Aruga J, et al. 2003. Zic2 patterns binocular vision by specifying the uncrossed retinal projection. Cell 114:545-557.

Hindges R, McLaughlin T, Genoud N, et al. 2002. EphB forward signaling controls directional branch extension and arborization required for dorsal-ventral retinotopic mapping. Neuron 35:475-487.

Huang EJ, Reichardt LF. 2001. Neurotrophins: roles in neuronal development and function. Annu Rev Neurosci 24:677-736.

Huang EJ, Reichardt LF. 2003. Trk receptors: roles in neuronal signal transduction. Annu Rev Biochem 72:609-642.

Huberman AD, Murray KD, Warland DK, et al. 2005. Ephrin-As mediate targeting of eye-specific projections to the lateral geniculate nucleus. Nat Neurosci 8:1013-1021.

Hutson LD, Chien CB. 2002. Wiring the zebrafish: axon guidance and synaptogenesis. Curr Opin Neurobiol 12:87-92.

Hutson LD, Chien CB. 2002. Pathfinding and error correction by retinal axons: the role of astray/robo2. Neuron 33:205-217.

Jacob J, Hacker A, Guthrie S. 2001. Mechanisms and molecules in motor neuron specification and axon pathfinding. Bioessays 23:582-595.

Jenny M, Uhl C, Roche C, et al. 2002. Neurogenin3 is differentially required for endocrine cell fate specification in the intestinal and gastric epithelium. Embo J 21:6338-6347.

Jin Y. 2002. Synaptogenesis: insights from worm and fly. Curr Opin Neurobiol 12:71-79.

Joyner AL. 2002. Establishment of anterior-posterior and dorsal-ventral pattern in the early central nervous system. In: Rossant J, Tam P, editors. Mouse Development. Patterning, Morphogenesis, and Organogenesis. New York: Academic Press. pp 107-126.

Joyner AL, Liu A, Millet S. 2000. Otx2, Gbx2 and Fgf8 interact to position and maintain a mid-hindbrain organizer. Curr Opin Cell Biol 12:736-741.

Jurata LW, Thomas JB, Pfaff SL. 2000. Transcriptional mechanisms in the development of motor control. Curr Opin Neurobiol 10:72-79.

Katz LC, Crowley JC. 2002. Development of cortical circuits: lessons from ocular dominance columns. Nat Rev Neurosci 3:34-42.

Kerjan G, Dolan J, Haumaitre C, et al. 2005. The transmembrane semaphorin Sema6A controls cerebellar granule cell migration. Nat Neurosci 8:1516-1524.

Kiecker C, Lumsden A. 2004. Hedgehog signaling from the ZLI regulates diencephalic regional identity. Nat Neurosci 7:1242-1249.

Kiecker C, Lumsden A. 2005. Compartments and their boundaries in vertebrate brain development. Nat Rev Neurosci 6:553-564.

Kiefer JC, Jarman A, Johnson J. 2005. Pro-neural factors and neurogenesis. Dev Dyn 234:808-813.

Kitamura K, Yanazawa M, Sugiyama N, et al. 2002. Mutation of ARX causes abnormal development of forebrain and testes in mice and X-linked lissencephaly with abnormal genitalia in humans. Nat Genet 32:359-369.

Klein R. 2004. Eph/ephrin signaling in morphogenesis, neural development and plasticity. Curr Opin Cell Biol 16:580-589.

Knoblich JA. 2001. Asymmetric cell division during animal development. Nat Rev Mol Cell Biol 2:11-20.

Kokaia Z, Lindvall O. 2003. Neurogenesis after ischaemic brain insults. Curr Opin Neurobiol 13:127-132.

Korzh V, Strahle U. 2002. Proneural, prosensory, antiglial: the many faces of neurogenins. Trends Neurosci 25:603-605.

Koshiba-Takeuchi K, Takeuchi JK, et al. 2000. Tbx5 and the retinotectum projection. Science 287:134-137.

Kriegstein AR, Noctor SC. 2004. Patterns of neuronal migration in the embryonic cortex. Trends Neurosci 27:392-399.

Kruger RP, Aurandt J, Guan KL. 2005. Semaphorins command cells to move. Nat Rev Mol Cell Biol 6:789-800.

Kuan CY, Roth KA, Flavell RA, Rakic P. 2000. Mechanisms of programmed cell death in the developing brain. Trends Neurosci 23:291-297.

Lambot MA, Depasse F, Noel JC, Vanderhaeghen P. 2005. Mapping labels in the human developing visual system and the evolution of binocular vision. J Neurosci 25:7232-7237.

Le Douarin NM, Halpern ME. 2000. Discussion point. Origin and specification of the neural tube floor plate: insights from the chick and zebrafish. Curr Opin Neurobiol 10:23-30.

Lee KJ, Dietrich P, Jessell TM. 2000. Genetic ablation reveals that the roof plate is essential for dorsal interneuron specification. Nature 403:734-740.

Levine JM, Reynolds R, Fawcett JW. 2001. The oligodendrocyte precursor cell in health and disease. Trends Neurosci 24:39-47.

Lin H. 2002. The stem-cell niche theory: lessons from flies. Nat Rev Genet 3:931-940.

Lindvall O, Kokaia Z, Martinez-Serrano A. 2004. Stem cell therapy for human neurodegenerative disorders-how to make it work. Nat Med 10(Suppl):S42-S50.

Liu A, Niswander LA. 2005. Signalling in development: Bone morphogenetic protein signalling and vertebrate nervous system development. Nat Rev Neurosci 6:945-954.

Liu BP, Strittmatter SM. 2001. Semaphorin-mediated axonal guidance via Rho-related G proteins. Curr Opin Cell Biol 13:619-626.

Liu Y, Rao M. 2003. Oligodendrocytes, GRPs and MNOPs. Trends Neurosci 26:410-412.

Lumsden A. 2004. Segmentation and compartition in the early avian hindbrain. Mech Dev 121:1081-1088.

Lupo G, Harris WA, Lewis KE. 2006. Mechanisms of ventral patterning in the vertebrate nervous system. Nat Rev Neurosci 7:103-114.

Lupo G, Liu Y, Qiu R, et al. 2005. Dorsoventral patterning of the Xenopus eye: a collaboration of Retinoid, Hedgehog and FGF receptor signaling. Development 132:1737-1748.

Machold R, Fishell G. 2002. Hedgehog patterns midbrain ARChitecture. Trends Neurosci 25:10-11.

Mann F, Miranda E, Weinl C. 2003. B-type Eph receptors and ephrins induce growth cone collapse through distinct intracellular pathways. J Neurobiol 57:323-336.

Mann F, Ray S, Harris W, Holt C, et al. 2002. Topographic mapping in dorsoventral axis of the Xenopus retinotectal system depends on signaling through ephrin-B ligands. Neuron 35:461-473.

Maricich SM, Gilmore EC, Herrup K. 2001. The role of tangential migration in the establishment of mammalian cortex. Neuron 31:175-178.

Marillat V, Sabatier C, Failli V, et al. 2004. The slit receptor Rig-1/Robo3 controls midline crossing by hindbrain precerebellar neurons and axons. Neuron 43:69-79.

Marti E, Bovolenta P. 2002. Sonic hedgehog in CNS development: one signal, multiple outputs. Trends Neurosci 25:89-96.

McCaffery P, Drager UC. 2000. Regulation of retinoic acid signaling in the embryonic nervous system: a master differentiation factor. Cytokine Growth Factor Rev 11:233-249.

McGee AW, Strittmatter SM. 2003. The Nogo-66 receptor: focusing myelin inhibition of axon regeneration. Trends Neurosci 26:193-198.

McKay B, Sandhu HS. 2002. Use of recombinant human bone morphogenetic protein-2 in spinal fusion applications. Spine 27:S66-S85.

McLaughlin T, Hindges R, O'Leary DD. 2003. Regulation of axial patterning of the retina and its topographic mapping in the brain. Curr Opin Neurobiol 13:57-69.

McMahon AP. 2000. Neural patterning: the role of Nkx genes in the ventral spinal cord. Genes Dev 14:2261-2264.

Moens CB, Prince VE. 2002. Constructing the hindbrain: insights from the zebrafish. Dev Dyn 224:1-17.

Mori T, Buffo A, Gotz M. 2005. The novel roles of glial cells revisited: the contribution of radial glia and astrocytes to neurogenesis. Curr Top Dev Biol 69:67-99.

Mui SH, Hindges R, O'Leary DD, et al. 2002. The homeodomain protein Vax2 patterns the dorsoventral and nasotemporal axes of the eye. Development 129:797-804.

Murase S, Horwitz AF. 2004. Directions in cell migration along the rostral migratory stream: the pathway for migration in the brain. Curr Top Dev Biol 61:135-152.

Nakagawa S, Brennan C, Johnson KG, et al. 2000. Ephrin-B regulates the Ipsilateral routing of retinal axons at the optic chiasm. Neuron 25:599-610.

Nakamura H, Watanabe Y. 2005. Isthmus organizer and regionalization of the mesencephalon and metencephalon. Int J Dev Biol 49:231-235.

Nguyen L, Rigo JM, Rocher V, et al. 2001. Neurotransmitters as early signals for central nervous system development. Cell Tissue Res 305:187-202.

Ohnuma S, Philpott A, Harris WA. 2001. Cell cycle and cell fate in the nervous system. Curr Opin Neurobiol 11:66-73.

O'Leary DD, Nakagawa Y. 2002. Patterning centers, regulatory genes and extrinsic mechanisms controlling arealization of the neocortex. Curr Opin Neurobiol 12:14-25.

Olson EC, Walsh CA. 2002. Smooth, rough and upside-down neocortical development. Curr Opin Genet Dev 12:320-327.

Packard M, Mathew D, Budnik V. 2003. Wnts and TGF beta in synaptogenesis: old friends signalling at new places. Nat Rev Neurosci 4:113-120.

Parnavelas JG. 2000. The origin and migration of cortical neurones: new vistas. Trends Neurosci 23:126-131.

Parnavelas JG, Alifragis P, Nadarajah B. 2002. The origin and migration of cortical neurons. Prog Brain Res 136:73-80.

Parras CM, Schuurmans C, Scardigli R, et al. 2002. Divergent functions of the proneural genes Mash1 and Ngn2 in the specification of neuronal subtype identity. Genes Dev 16:324-338.

Patten I, Placzek M. 2002. Opponent activities of Shh and BMP signaling during floor plate induction in vivo. Curr Biol 12:47-52.

Perrone-Capano C, Di Porzio U. 2000. Genetic and epigenetic control of midbrain dopaminergic neuron development. Int J Dev Biol 44:679-687.

Peters MA. 2002. Patterning the neural retina. Curr Opin Neurobiol 12:43-48.

Pevny L, Placzek M. 2005. SOX genes and neural progenitor identity. Curr Opin Neurobiol 15:7-13.

Pevny L, Rao MS. 2003. The stem-cell menagerie. Trends Neurosci 26:351-359.

Pfeiffenberger C, Cutforth T, Woods G, et al. 2005. Ephrin-As and neural activity are required for eye-specific patterning during retinogeniculate mapping. Nat Neurosci 8:1022-1027.

Piper M, Little M. 2003. Movement through Slits: cellular migration via the Slit family. Bioessays 25:32-38.

Placzek M, Briscoe J. 2005. The floor plate: multiple cells, multiple signals. Nat Rev Neurosci 6:230-240.

Placzek M, Dodd J, Jessell TM. 2000. Discussion point. The case for floor plate induction by the notochord. Curr Opin Neurobiol 10:15-22.

Price SR, Briscoe J. 2004. The generation and diversification of spinal motor neurons: signals and responses. Mech Dev 121: 1103-1115.

Ragsdale CW, Grove EA. 2001. Patterning the mammalian cerebral cortex. Curr Opin Neurobiol 11:50-58.

Rakic P. 2002. Neurogenesis in adult primate neocortex: an evaluation of the evidence. Nat Rev Neurosci 3:65-71.

Rallu M, Corbin JG, Fishell G. 2002. Parsing the prosencephalon. Nat Rev Neurosci 3:943-951.

Ramos C, Robert B. 2005. msh/Msx gene family in neural development. Trends Genet 21:624-632.

Rao Y, Wong K, Ward M, Jurgensen C, Wu JY. 2002. Neuronal migration and molecular conservation with leukocyte chemotaxis. Genes Dev 16:2973-2984.

Redies C, Puelles L. 2001. Modularity in vertebrate brain development and evolution. Bioessays 23:1100-1111.

Reiner O. 2000. LIS1. let's interact sometimes . . . (part 1). Neuron 28:633-636.

Rhinn M, Brand M. 2001. The midbrain—hindbrain boundary organizer. Curr Opin Neurobiol 11:34-42.

Rhinn M, Picker A, Brand M. 2006. Global and local mechanisms of forebrain and midbrain patterning. Curr Opin Neurobiol 16:5-12.

Roegiers F, Jan YN. 2004. Asymmetric cell division. Curr Opin Cell Biol 16:195-205.

Ross SE, Greenberg ME, Stiles CD. 2003. Basic helix-loop-helix factors in cortical development. Neuron 39:13-25.

Rowitch DH. 2004. Glial specification in the vertebrate neural tube. Nat Rev Neurosci 5:409-419.

Rowitch DH, Lu QR, Kessaris N, Richardson WD. 2002. An 'oligarchy' rules neural development. Trends Neurosci 25:417-422.

Ruizi Altaba A, Nguyen V, Palma V. 2003. The emergent design of the neural tube: prepattern, SHH morphogen and GLI code. Curr Opin Genet Dev 13:513-521.

Ruizi Altaba A, Palma V, Dahmane N. 2002. Hedgehog-Gli signalling and the growth of the brain. Nat Rev Neurosci 3:24-33.

Sakuta H, Suzuki R, Takahashi H, et al. 2001. Ventroptin: a BMP-4 antagonist expressed in a double-gradient pattern in the retina. Science 293:111-115.

Salinas PC. 2003. The morphogen sonic hedgehog collaborates with netrin-1 to guide axons in the spinal cord. Trends Neurosci 26:641-643.

Schulte D, Cepko CL. 2000. Two homeobox genes define the domain of EphA3 expression in the developing chick retina. Development 127:5033-5045.

Schuurmans C, Guillemot F. 2002. Molecular mechanisms underlying cell fate specification in the developing telencephalon. Curr Opin Neurobiol 12:26-34.

Schwab ME. 2004. Nogo and axon regeneration. Curr Opin Neurobiol 14:118-124.

Scully KM, Rosenfeld MG. 2002. Pituitary development: regulatory codes in mammalian organogenesis. Science 295:2231-2235.

Shaham S. 2005. Glia-neuron interactions in nervous system function and development. Curr Top Dev Biol 69:39-66.

Shewan D, Dwivedy A, Anderson R, Holt CE. 2002. Age-related changes underlie switch in netrin-1 responsiveness as growth cones advance along visual pathway. Nat Neurosci 5:955-962.

Sisodiya SM. 2004. Malformations of cortical development: burdens and insights from important causes of human epilepsy. Lancet Neurol 3:29-38.

Song H, Poo M. 2001. The cell biology of neuronal navigation. Nat Cell Biol 3:E81-E88.

Stoker AW. 2001. Receptor tyrosine phosphatases in axon growth and guidance. Curr Opin Neurobiol 11:95-102.

Strahle U, Lam CS, Ertzer R, Rastegar S. 2004. Vertebrate floor-plate specification: variations on common themes. Trends Genet 20:155-162.

Takahashi H, Liu FC. 2006. Genetic Patterning of the mammalian telencephalon by morphogenetic molecules and transcription factors. Birth Defects Res C Embryo Today 78:256-266.

ten Donkelaar HJ, Lammens M, Wesseling P, Thijssen HO, Renier WO. 2003. Development and developmental disorders of the human cerebellum. J Neurol 250:1025-1036.

Tissir F, Goffinet AM. 2003. Reelin and brain development. Nat Rev Neurosci 4:496-505.

Torborg CL, Hansen KA, Feller MB. 2005. High frequency, synchronized bursting drives eye-specific segregation of retinogeniculate projections. Nat Neurosci 8:72-78.

Toyo-oka K, Shionoya A, Gamebllo MJ, et al. 2003. 14-3-3epsilon is important for neuronal migration by binding to NUDEL: a molecular explanation for Miller-Dieker syndrome. Nat Genet 34:274-285.

Vallee RB, Tai C, Faulkner NE. 2001. LIS1: cellular function of a disease-causing gene. Trends Cell Biol 11:155-160.

van Horck FP, Weinl C, Holt CE. 2004. Retinal axon guidance: novel mechanisms for steering. Curr Opin Neurobiol 14:61-66.

Voorn P, Vanderschuren LJ, Groenewegen HJ, et al. 2004. Putting a spin on the dorsal-ventral divide of the striatum. Trends Neurosci 27:468-474.

Walsh CA, Goffinet AM. 2000. Potential mechanisms of mutations that affect neuronal migration in man and mouse. Curr Opin Genet Dev 10:270-274.

Watanabe Y, Nakamura H. 2000. Control of chick tectum territory along dorsoventral axis by Sonic hedgehog. Development 127:1131-1140.

Wegner M, Stolt CC. 2005. From stem cells to neurons and glia: a Soxist's view of neural development. Trends Neurosci 28:583-588.

Weinstein BM. 2005. Vessels and nerves: marching to the same tune. Cell 120:299-302.

Wilkinson DG. 2001. Multiple roles of EPH receptors and ephrins in neural development. Nat Rev Neurosci 2:155-164.

Williams SE, Mann F, Erskine L, et al. 2003. Ephrin-B2 and EphB1 mediate retinal axon divergence at the optic chiasm. Neuron 39:919-935.

Williams SE, Mason CA, Herrera E. 2004. The optic chiasm as a midline choice point. Curr Opin Neurobiol 14:51-60.

Wilson L, Maden M. 2005. The mechanisms of dorsoventral patterning in the vertebrate neural tube. Dev Biol 282:1-13.

Wilson SW, Houart C. 2004. Early steps in the development of the forebrain. Dev Cell 6:167-181.

Wingate RJ. 2001. The rhombic lip and early cerebellar development. Curr Opin Neurobiol 11:82-88.

Wodarz A. 2005. Molecular control of cell polarity and asymmetric cell division in Drosophila neuroblasts. Curr Opin Cell Biol 17:475-481.

Wong K, Park HT, Wu JY, Rao Y. 2002. Slit proteins: molecular guidance cues for cells ranging from neurons to leukocytes. Curr Opin Genet Dev 12:583-591.

Woods CG. 2004. Human microcephaly. Curr Opin Neurobiol 14:112-117.

Wurst W, Bally-Cuif L. 2001. Neural plate patterning: upstream and downstream of the isthmic organizer. Nat Rev Neurosci 2:99-108.

Wynshaw-Boris A, Gambello MJ. 2001. LIS1 and dynein motor function in neuronal migration and development. Genes Dev 15:639-651.

Yamada K, Watanabe M. 2002. Cytodifferentiation of Bergmann glia and its relationship with Purkinje cells. Anat Sci Int 77:94-108.

Yates PA, Roskies AL, McLaughlin T, O'Leary DD. 2001. Topographic-specific axon branching controlled by ephrin-As is the critical event in retinotectal map development. J Neurosci 21:8548-8563.

Yoon K, Gaiano N. 2005. Notch signaling in the mammalian central nervous system: insights from mouse mutants. Nat Neurosci 8:709-715.

Yoshikawa S, Thomas JB. 2004. Secreted cell signaling molecules in axon guidance. Curr Opin Neurobiol 14:45-50.

Zervas M, Blaess S, Joyner AL. 2005. Classical embryological studies and modern genetic analysis of midbrain and cerebellum development. Curr Top Dev Biol 69:101-138.

Zhang J, Jin Z, Bao ZZ. 2004. Disruption of gradient expression of Zic3 resulted in abnormal intra-retinal axon projection. Development 131:1553-1562.

Zhong J, Deng J, Phan J, et al. 2005. Insulin-like growth factor-I protects granule neurons from apoptosis and improves ataxia in weaver mice. J Neurosci Res 80:481-490.

Zhu X, Lin CR, Prefontaine GG, et al. 2005. Genetic control of pituitary development and hypopituitarism. Curr Opin Genet Dev 15:332-340.

Zou Y. 2004. Wnt signaling in axon guidance. Trends Neurosci 27:528-532.

9

Development of the Peripheral Nervous System

10

Summary The nervous system consists of complex networks of neurons that carry information from the sensory receptors in the body to the central nervous system (CNS); integrate, process, and store it; and return motor impulses to various effector organs in the body. The development of the CNS is discussed in Chapter 9; this chapter discusses the development of the peripheral nervous system (PNS).

The PNS and its central pathways are traditionally divided into two systems. The **somatic nervous system** is responsible for carrying conscious sensations and for innervating the voluntary (striated) muscles of the body. The **autonomic nervous system** is strictly motor and controls most of the involuntary, visceral activities of the body. The autonomic system itself consists of two divisions: the **parasympathetic division**, which, in general, promotes the anabolic visceral activities characteristic of periods of peace and relaxation, and the **sympathetic division**, which controls the involuntary activities that occur under stressful "fight or flight" conditions. Each of these systems are composed of two-neuron pathways consisting of preganglionic and postganglionic neurons. As discussed in Chapters 4 and 14, the gut contains its own nervous system called the **enteric nervous system**.

Neurons originate from three embryonic tissues: the **neuroepithelium** lining the neural canal, **neural crest cells**, and specialized regions of ectoderm in the head and neck called **ectodermal placodes**. Neurons of the CNS arise from the neuroepithelium (discussed in Ch. 9), whereas those of the PNS arise from neural crest cells and ectodermal placodes.

Trunk ganglia are formed by migrating neural crest cells. These ganglia include: 1) sensory **dorsal root ganglia** that condense next to the spinal cord in register with each pair of somites and consist of sensory neurons that relay information from receptors in the body to the CNS and their supporting **satellite cells**; 2) **sympathetic chain ganglia** that also flank the spinal cord (but more ventrally) and the **prevertebral (or preaortic) ganglia** that form next to branches of the abdominal aorta and contain the peripheral (postganglionic) neurons of the two-neuron sympathetic pathways; and 3) the **parasympathetic ganglia** embedded in the walls of the visceral organs and containing the peripheral (postganglionic) neurons of the two-neuron parasympathetic division. The parasympathetic ganglia that reside within the gut are termed **enteric ganglia**.

As neural crest cells of the trunk coalesce to form spinal ganglia, somatic motor axons begin to grow out from the basal columns of the spinal cord, forming a pair of **ventral roots** at the level of each somite. These somatic motor fibers are later joined by autonomic motor fibers arising in the intermediolateral cell columns. The somatic motor fibers grow into the myotomes and thus come to innervate the voluntary muscles. The autonomic (preganglionic) fibers, in contrast, terminate in the autonomic ganglia (sympathetic and parasympathetic), where they synapse with cell bodies of the peripheral (postganglionic) autonomic neurons that innervate the appropriate target organs.

The central (preganglionic) neurons of the sympathetic division develop in the intermediolateral cell columns of the **thoracolumbar** spinal cord (T1 through L2 or L3). The thinly myelinated axons of these cells leave the spinal cord in the ventral root but immediately branch off to form a **white ramus**, which enters the corresponding chain ganglion. Some of these fibers synapse with peripheral (postganglionic) sympathetic neurons in the chain ganglion; others pass onward to synapse in another chain ganglion or in one of the prevertebral ganglia. The unmyelinated axons of the peripheral (postganglionic) sympathetic chain ganglion neurons re-enter the spinal nerve via a branch called the **gray ramus**.

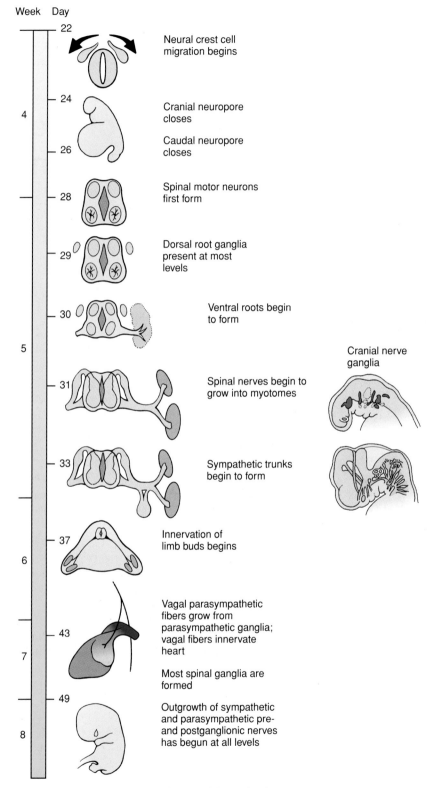

Week　Day

22 — Neural crest cell migration begins

4

24 — Cranial neuropore closes

26 — Caudal neuropore closes

28 — Spinal motor neurons first form

29 — Dorsal root ganglia present at most levels

30 — Ventral roots begin to form

5

Cranial nerve ganglia

31 — Spinal nerves begin to grow into myotomes

33 — Sympathetic trunks begin to form

37 — Innervation of limb buds begins

6

43 — Vagal parasympathetic fibers grow from parasympathetic ganglia; vagal fibers innervate heart

7

Most spinal ganglia are formed

49 — Outgrowth of sympathetic and parasympathetic pre- and postganglionic nerves has begun at all levels

8

Time line. Development of the peripheral nervous system.

The ganglia of the head consist of two types: the **cranial nerve ganglia**, the neurons of which arise from either neural crest cells or ectodermal placodes, depending on the particular ganglion (glial cells arise exclusively from neural crest cells in all ganglia); and the **cranial parasympathetic ganglia**, which arise from neural crest cells.

The central (preganglionic) neurons of the parasympathetic pathways are located in the brain stem and in the spinal cord at levels S2 through S4. The parasympathetic division is thus called a **craniosacral system.** Parasympathetic fibers from the hindbrain reach the parasympathetic ganglia of the neck and trunk viscera via the **vagus nerve,** whereas the sacral parasympathetic fibers innervate hindgut and pelvic visceral ganglia via the **pelvic splanchnic nerves.**

Clinical Taster

A toddler is brought to the emergency department after biting off the right anterolateral part of his tongue. While an oral surgeon is suturing the tongue, the staff notices other suspicious injuries. These include lacerations of the gums with missing teeth (Fig. 10-1A), a burn on the left index finger (Fig. 10-1B), and multiple other small cuts and bruises. An X-ray of the face, done to investigate the broken teeth, reveals an occult fracture of the parietal bone. An inquiry is begun by child protective services (CPS).

The parents claim that the injuries are all "self-inflicted," and describe the boy as having "no pain." They explain that the broken teeth are a result of biting on toys and that the burned finger occurred when the child touched a hot grill. He does not cry with any of these significant injuries, including the bitten tongue, and they express their surprise when the skull fracture is discovered. His medical records show that he has been admitted to the hospital several times with high fever and presumed sepsis (severe infection) that was treated with antibiotics. The family has noticed that he becomes flushed and lethargic in the heat, and they have never seen him sweat. The boy cries little with the procedure to repair his tongue and is indifferent to the needle sticks needed to obtain lab tests. The CPS investigation uncovers no evidence of abuse. The family has two older children who are healthy and well cared for.

Neurology is consulted and they obtain a skin biopsy that shows a paucity of small nerve fibers in the skin and an absence of innervation of the sweat glands. Based on the clinical history and on these histologic findings, the diagnosis of **congenital insensitivity to pain with anhidrosis** (CIPA; anhidrosis means lack of sweating) is made. Confirmatory sequencing of the *NTKR1* gene uncovers two deleterious mutations, each carried by one parent. *NTKR1* is a receptor for *NERVE GROWTH FACTOR* and is required for the development of nociceptive (pain) sensory innervation of the skin, and for autonomic innervation of the eccrine sweat glands.

10

Structural Divisions of Nervous System

As discussed in Chapter 9, the nervous system of vertebrates consists of two major *structural* divisions: a **central nervous system (CNS)** and a **peripheral nervous system (PNS).** The CNS consists of the brain and spinal cord. The development of the CNS is discussed in Chapter 9. The PNS consists of all components of the nervous system outside of the CNS. Thus, the PNS consists of cranial nerves and ganglia, spinal nerves and ganglia, autonomic nerves and ganglia, and the enteric nervous system. The development of the PNS is discussed in this chapter.

Functional Divisions of Nervous System

As discussed in Chapter 9, the nervous system of vertebrates consists of two major *functional* divisions: a **somatic nervous system** and a **visceral nervous system.** The somatic nervous system innervates the skin and most skeletal muscles (i.e., it provides both sensory and motor components). Similarly, the visceral nervous system innervates the viscera (organs of the body) and smooth muscle and glands in the more peripheral part of the body. The visceral nervous system is also called the **autonomic nervous system.** It consists of two components: the **sympathetic division** and the **parasympathetic division.** The somatic

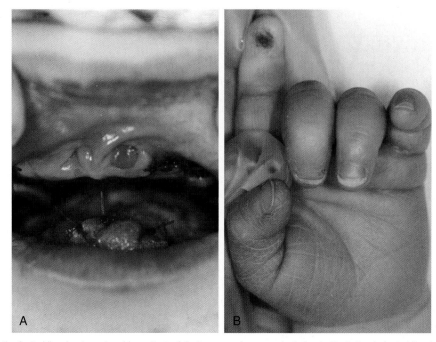

Figure 10-1. *A*, Mouth of a toddler showing sutured lacerations of the tongue and gums and missing teeth. *B*, Hand of a toddler showing burn on the left index finger.

and visceral nervous systems are discussed both in Chapter 9 (CNS components) and in this chapter (PNS components).

Both divisions of the autonomic nervous system consist of two-neuron pathways. Because the peripheral autonomic neurons reside in ganglia, the axons of the central sympathetic neurons are called **preganglionic fibers** and the axons of the peripheral sympathetic neurons are called **postganglionic fibers**. This terminology is used for both sympathetic pathways and parasympathetic (discussed later in the chapter) pathways. Sometimes preganglionic fibers are also called *presynaptic fibers*, and postganglionic fibers, *postsynaptic fibers*, because the axons of the preganglionic fibers *synapse* on the cell bodies of postganglionic neurons in the autonomic ganglia.

Origin of PNS

Chapters 3 and 4 describe how during neurulation the rudiment of the central nervous system arises as a neural plate from the ectoderm of the embryonic disc and folds to form the neural tube (the rudiment of the brain and spinal cord). The PNS arises from the neural tube and two groups of cells outside of the neural tube: neural crest cells and ectodermal placodes. The PNS develops as an integrated system, essentially in cranial-to-caudal sequence. However, for the sake of simplicity, the development of the trunk (associated with the spinal cord) and cranial (associated with the brain) portions of the PNS will be discussed separately. The sympathetic division of the autonomic nervous system arises in association with the trunk (thoracolumbar levels of the spinal cord), whereas the parasympathetic division of the autonomic nervous system arises in association with the brain and caudal spinal cord (craniosacral levels of the CNS).

IN THE RESEARCH LAB

SPECIFICATION AND PLASTICITY OF PRECURSOR CELLS OF PNS

As just mentioned, the PNS arises from both neural crest cells and ectodermal placodes. How are these structures determined in the early embryo and to what extent are they able to change their fate? Induction of neural crest cells is discussed in Chapter 4. Consequently, in this section, induction of ectodermal placodes is discussed, followed by consideration of the plasticity of neural crest cells and ectodermal placodes.

Induction of Ectodermal Placodes

As discussed later in the chapter, **ectodermal placodes** (so-called **neurogenic placodes**) contribute to some of the ganglia of the cranial nerves. These ganglia are derived from **epiphayngeal placodes**, associated with pharyngeal arches 1 to 4, **retinal disc placodes**, **nasal placodes**, and **otic (acousticovestibular) placodes**. How do these placodes arise?

Prospective cranial neural crest cells and ectodermal placodal cells arise together from a horseshoe-shaped band of ectoderm (with the two limbs of the horseshoe pointing caudally) partially encircling the cranial borders of the early neural plate (see Fig. 3-10D). This positioning apparently involves the expression of genes such as the transcription factor, *Dlx5*. Signals from surrounding tissues act on this band to specify cranial neural crest cells or ectodermal placodal cells.

The neurogenic placodes as well as the non-neurogenic **lens placodes** (discussed in Ch. 17) are induced, at least in part, by the underlying head mesoderm. Signals from the mesoderm suppress both *Bmp* and *Wnt* signaling in the preplacodal ectoderm. In addition, the mesoderm secretes *Fgf*, which in the presence of attenuated *Bmp* and *Wnt* signaling, results in preplacodal specification. Additional factors secreted by surrounding tissues act on the preplacodal ectoderm to specify specific types of placodes. For most ectodermal placodes, the specific tissue interactions involved and the identity of the secreted signals remain unknown. The best-studied examples of such tissue interactions and secreted signals involve the non-neurogenic lens placode and the neurogenic retinal disc placode and otic placode. These are discussed in Chapter 17.

Plasticity of Neural Crest Cells and Ectodermal Placodes

Heterotopic transplantation studies have revealed that both neural crest cells and ectodermal placodes are highly plastic at the time of their formation. In these studies, small groups of prospective neural crest cells or small patches of preplacodal ectoderm are transplanted from their normal site of origin to an ectopic site. Typically, quail tissues are transplanted heterotopically to chick embryos, so that donor and host tissues can be specifically traced during subsequent development (discussed in Ch. 5; see Fig. 5-8). Preplacodal cells are generally transplanted from one prospective placode to another (e.g., lens to otic or vice versa), where they readily adapt to their new environment and change their fate, that is, they exhibit plasticity. Neural crest cells are generally transplanted from one craniocaudal level to another, including the placement of trunk neural crest cells in the head and vice versa. As discussed in Chapter 4, neural crest cells give rise to a large number of cell types, including cartilage, bone, melanocytes, endocrine tissues, PNS neurons, and glial cells. Only head (cranial) neural crest cells are capable of forming bone and cartilage in transplantation studies, although isolated trunk neural crest cells subjected to various signaling molecules in vitro are capable of forming cartilage in some cases. Thus, neural crest cells at the time of their migration also display considerable plasticity.

Despite having early plasticity at the time of their formation, generally by about late neurulation stages, the fates of both neural crest cells and placodal cells as *populations* become fixed. Hence, heterotopic transplantation typically results at these stages in the formation of ectopic structures commensurate with the *origin—not the new position—*of the transplanted tissue.

NEURAL CREST CELLS AND THEIR DERIVATIVES AS STEM CELLS

As just discussed, neural crest cells give rise to a large number of different cell types and, consequently, they act like typical stem cells (*embryonic stem cells* are discussed in Ch. 5). This stem cell nature occurs not only within migrating neural crest cells but also continues in their progeny (i.e., in tissues and organs formed by neural crest cells) as *individual* cells. For example, pluripotent neural crest cells (i.e., stem cells) have been identified in the embryonic chick dorsal root ganglion, sympathetic ganglion, and cardiac outflow tract. Neural crest cell stem cells are present also in the mammalian embryonic sciatic nerve, and in the embryonic and adult gut. However, the developmental potentials of these cells are more restricted than for migrating neural crest cells, and they vary according to the location of the cells.

Surprisingly, pluripotent neural crest cells that can give rise to all cranial neural crest cell derivatives have been isolated from the bulge of adult mammalian hair follicles. The follicular bulge is an epidermal structure of the hair follicle that serves as a niche for keratinocyte stem cells, which form new epidermis, sebaceous gland, and hair (discussed in Ch. 7). Thus, the bulge contains a mixed population of stem cells consisting of both keratinocyte stem cells and neural crest cell stem cells. Highly motile neural crest cell–derived stem cells (**epidermal neural crest cell stem cells**) emigrate from bulge explants dissected from adult hair follicles (Fig. 10-2). Remarkably, more than 88% of these migrating cells are pluripotent stem cells that can generate all cranial neural crest derivatives.

Because of their existence in humans, their accessibility, and high degree of physiologic plasticity, neural crest cell stem cells in the periphery of the adult organism are promising candidates for cell replacement therapy.

10

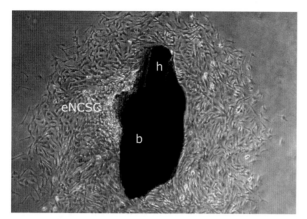

Figure 10-2. Bulge explant four days after onset of epidermal neural crest cell stem cell (eNCSC) emigration. The bulge (b), which was dissected from an adult mouse whisker follicle, releases numerous highly motile eNCSC, which divide rapidly in culture. The hair (h) is visible within the bulge.

IN THE CLINIC

NEUROFIBROMATOSIS TYPE 1 (NF-1)

Neurofibromatosis-type1 is a prevalent familial tumor disposition that affects 1 in 3500 individuals worldwide. It is a progressive disease with multiple deficits, including benign and malignant tumors of the peripheral and central nervous systems. The gene mutated in neurofibromatosis-type 1, *NEUROFIBROMIN* (*NF1*), is a **tumor suppressor gene** that inactivates the **proto-oncogene** *RAS*. Patients with NF1 are heterozygous for the inactivating mutations of the *NF-1* gene. Thus, *RAS* function is upregulated in NF-1 patients. One hallmark in NF-1 is the presence of numerous benign cutaneous tumors, called **neurofibromas.** These tumors contain multiple cell types, including Schwann cells, neurons, fibroblasts, and mast cells. As discussed in Chapter 4, the first two of these cell types are derived from neural crest cells. There is evidence that the second wild-type allele is lost in NF-1 patients through subsequent somatic deletion (the so-called **two-hit hypothesis**), which leads to certain types of tumors (e.g., malignant peripheral nerve sheath tumor). However, because of the infrequency of somatic deletion and frequency of neurofibromas developing in NF patients, second mutations are likely not required for neurofibroma formation.

Both paracrine and/or cell-autonomous events are known to trigger neurofibroma formation. For example, the onset of puberty and pregnancy are often associated with a major increase in the number and size of neurofibromas. Both circumstances involve hormonal changes and an increase in subcutaneous adipose tissue deposits. Therefore, potentially hormonal and/or paracrine mechanisms may be responsible for tumorigenesis in some NF-1 patients. In this regard, there is an interesting convergence of two observations: first, hair follicles from normal-looking skin of NF-1 patients are often surrounded by numerous S100-positive neural crest cell–derived Schwann cells, or Schwann cell progenitors; and second, as discussed in the preceding section, hair follicles contain neural crest cell stem cells. Therefore, it is conceivable that mitogens produced by adipocytes and/or female hormones promote proliferation of neural crest stem cells in hair follicles of NF-1 patients, leading to neurofibroma formation.

IN THE RESEARCH LAB

NEUROGENESIS IN PNS

The process of neurogenesis occurs similarly in the CNS and PNS and involves a series of steps in which multipotential precursor cells (i.e., stem cells) become progressively restricted in their fate over time. During this process, cells generally transform from multipotent precursors (e.g., capable of forming all types of neurons and glia) to restricted neuronal (or glial) precursors (e.g., capable of forming only neurons or only glial, but not both) to differentiated cell types (i.e., a specific type of neuron). Within the CNS, these precursors arise from the neural plate; within the PNS, they arise from neural crest cells and ectodermal placodes. Initially cells in these rudiments rapidly divide to expand the number of cells in the population. However, over time the division of these cells becomes asymmetric such that one daughter cell derived from a particular mitotic division remains mitotically active and undifferentiated, whereas the other daughter cell becomes postmitotic, migrates away from its site of generation, and begins to differentiate.

Several genes play essential roles in regulating neurogenesis. These include both positive regulators and negative regulators. Examples of the former include the basic helix-loop-helix (bHLH) transcription factors known as the **proneural genes**. In vertebrates, these include genes such as *Mash* (the mammalian ortholog of Drosophila *Achaete-Scute* genes). Other vertebrate proneural genes include *Math*, *NeuroD*, and the *Neurogenins* (the latter three are vertebrate—mammalian in the case of *Math*—orthologs of Drosophila *Atonal* genes). Expression of these proneural genes is both sufficient and necessary for the formation of neurons. Examples of the negative regulators of neurogenesis include members of the *Notch* signaling pathway (discussed in Ch. 5). Through a process called **lateral inhibition**, which involves *Notch* signaling, a neuronal precursor cell inhibits its neighbors from differentiating as neurons (e.g., by secreting a *Notch* ligand such as *Delta*, which binds to the neighbor's *Notch* receptors). Lateral inhibition thus regulates the number of neurons born in any one region of the developing nervous system and allows for the generation of supporting glial cells. Nevertheless, many more neurons are actually born than required. Hence, through a subsequent process of **programmed cell death**, the number of definitive neurons is reduced to the characteristic number for each area of the CNS and PNS.

Development of Trunk PNS

The trunk PNS consists of spinal nerves and ganglia, autonomic nerves and ganglia, and the enteric nervous system. Sympathetic nerves course through spinal nerves at the thoracolumbar level to reach their ganglia. In addition, parasympathetic nerves course through sacral spinal nerves to reach their ganglia. Thus, the development of spinal nerves (and ganglia) and associated autonomic nerves (sympathetic at thoracolumbar levels and parasympathetic at sacral levels) is considered together. The development of the enteric nervous system is discussed in Chapter 4, and in Chapter 14 in the context of the development of the gut wall.

Development of Spinal Nerves and Ganglia

Ventral Column Motor Axons Are First to Sprout from Spinal Cord

The first axons to emerge from the spinal cord are produced by somatic motoneurons in the ventral gray columns. These fibers appear in the cervical region on about day 30 (Fig. 10-3) and (like so many other embryonic processes) proceed in a craniocaudal wave down the spinal cord.

The ventral motor axons initially leave the spinal cord as a continuous broad band. However, as they grow toward the sclerotomes, they rapidly condense to form discrete segmental nerves. Although these axons will eventually synapse with muscles derived from the developing myotomes, their initial guidance depends only on the sclerotomes and not on myotomal or dermatomal elements of the somite. As discussed in Chapter 8, neural crest cells migrate within the cranial half of each sclerotome; ventral column axons migrate within the cranial half of each sclerotome as

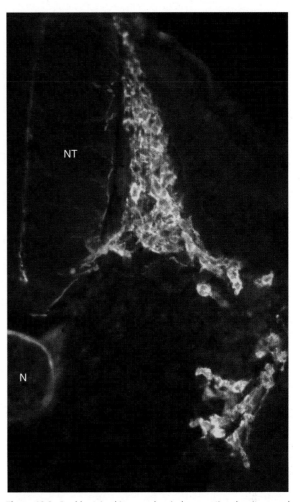

Figure 10-3. Double-stained immunochemical preparation showing neural crest cells (in a chick embryo stained with HNK-1 antibody; yellow) and ventral motoneuron fibers (labeled with E/C8, an antibody against neurofilament-binding protein; red). Neural crest cells are migrating through the cranial half of the sclerotome. NT, neural tube; N, notochord.

well (see Fig. 10-3). As a result, these growing axons pass close to the developing dorsal root ganglion at each level.

The pioneer axons that initially sprout from the spinal cord are soon joined by additional ventral column motor axons, and the growing bundle is now called a **ventral root** (Fig. 10-4). At spinal levels T1 through L2 or L3, the ventral root is later joined by axons from the sympathetic motoneurons developing in the intermediolateral cell columns at these levels (see Fig. 10-4 and later discussions in this chapter).

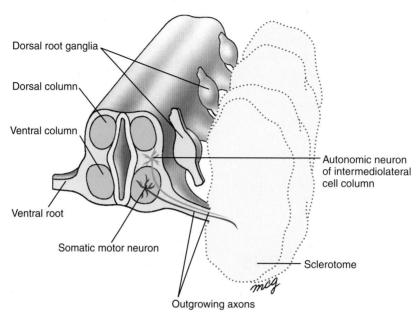

Figure 10-4. Outgrowth of the ventral roots and formation of the dorsal root ganglia. Axons growing from ventral column motoneurons at each segmental level of the spinal cord are guided by the sclerotome to form a ventral root. Dorsal root ganglia form in the same plane.

Somatic and Autonomic Motor Fibers Combine with Sensory Fibers to Form Spinal Nerves

As axons of the ventral motoneurons approach the corresponding dorsal root ganglion, the neurons in the dorsal root ganglion begin to extend axons bidirectionally. Each of these bipolar neurons, whose cell bodies reside within the dorsal root ganglion, has a branch that grows medially toward the dorsal column of the spinal cord and a branch that joins the ventral root and grows toward the periphery to innervate the target organ (Fig. 10-5). The bundle of axons that connect the dorsal root ganglion to the spinal cord is called the **dorsal root**. The central processes of dorsal root ganglion cells penetrate the dorsal columns of the spinal cord (Fig. 10-6), where they synapse with developing **association neurons.** These association neurons in turn sprout axons that either synapse with autonomic motoneurons in the intermediolateral cell columns or with somatic motoneurons in the ventral columns, or else they ascend to higher levels in the spinal cord in the form of **tracts.** The axons of some association neurons synapse with motoneurons on the same, or **ipsilateral**, side of the spinal cord, whereas others cross over to synapse with motoneurons on the opposite, or **contralateral**, side of the cord.

The mixed motor and sensory trunk formed at each level by the confluence of the peripheral processes of the dorsal root ganglion cells and the ventral roots is called a **spinal nerve** (see Fig. 10-5). The sympathetic fibers (preganglionic) that exit via the ventral roots at levels T1 through L2 or L3 soon branch from the spinal nerve and grow ventrally to enter the corresponding **sympathetic chain ganglion** (Fig. 10-7; also see Figs. 4-17, 4-20). This branch is called a **white ramus.** Some of the sympathetic fibers carried in the white ramus synapse directly with a neuron in the chain ganglion. This neuron becomes the second (peripheral or postganglionic or postsynaptic) neuron in a two-neuron sympathetic pathway and sprouts an axon that grows to innervate the appropriate peripheral target organ.

Not all preganglionic sympathetic fibers that enter a chain ganglion via the white ramus synapse there. The remainder project cranially or caudally and synapse in a more cranial or caudal chain ganglion or in one of the prevertebral (or preaortic) ganglia (see Fig. 4-17). These fibers, plus the chain ganglia themselves, constitute the **sympathetic trunk.** They are discussed later in the chapter.

The postganglionic fibers that originate in each chain ganglion form a small branch—the **gray ramus**—that grows dorsally to rejoin the spinal nerve,

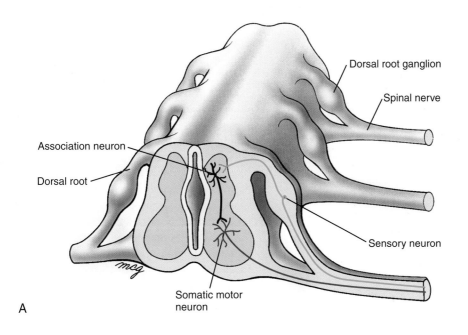

A

The dorsal root joins
the spinal cord out of
the plane of this section

B

Figure 10-5. *A,* Once the ventral roots are formed, sensory neurons within each dorsal root ganglion sprout processes that grow into the neural tube to synapse with association neurons in the dorsal column. Other processes grow outward from the dorsal root ganglion to join the ventral root, forming a typical spinal nerve. The dorsal root connects the dorsal root ganglion to the spinal cord. The axon of the association neuron in this illustration synapses with a motor neuron on the same side of the spinal cord at the same segmental level (axons may also display other patterns of connection; discussed in text). *B,* Double-stained immunochemical preparation showing neuronal cell bodies (green) and neurofilaments within nerve cell processes (red).

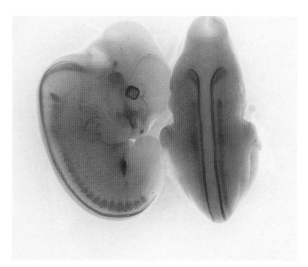

Figure 10-6. Dorsal and lateral views of transgenic mice that express the bacterial *lacZ* gene in tissues that also produce *Peripherin* (a neurofilament protein characteristic of PNS, but not CNS, neurons). The enzyme encoded by *lacZ* causes the cells producing it to turn blue when appropriately incubated. The blue stain is localized in small neurons of the neural crest cell–derived dorsal root ganglia and in the axons of these cells that penetrate the spinal cord in a region overlying the dorsal gray columns of the spinal cord (parasagittal stripes).

and then grows toward the periphery (see Fig. 10-7). Distal to the gray ramus, the spinal nerve thus carries sensory fibers, somatic motor fibers, and postganglionic sympathetic fibers.

Axons in Spinal Nerves Grow to Specific Sites

Motor and sensory axons in spinal nerves grow to specific targets in the body wall and extremities. Shortly after leaving the spinal column, each axon first chooses one of two routes, growing either dorsally toward the **epimere** or ventrally toward the **hypomere**. Thus, the spinal nerve splits into two **rami**. The axons that direct their path toward the epimere form the **dorsal ramus**, and the fibers that grow toward the hypomere form the **ventral ramus** (see Fig. 10-7). The presence of the epimere is required for the formation of the dorsal ramus. If a single epimere is removed from an experimental animal, the dorsal ramus of the corresponding spinal nerve will grow to innervate an adjacent epimere. However, if several successive epimeres are ablated, the corresponding dorsal rami do not form.

The axons of somatic motor fibers in the dorsal and ventral rami seek out specific muscles or bundles of muscle fibers and form synapses with the muscle fibers, whereas the postganglionic sympathetic motor fibers innervate the smooth muscle of blood vessels and sweat glands and erector pili muscles in the skin. The specific signals that guide motor fibers to their targets are not known. Inhibitory signaling from *Ephrins* in ventral muscles is thought to direct motor axons into dorsal nerve branches (also see the discussion of axonal guidance in the following "In the Research Lab"). Moreover, it has been suggested that sympathetic fibers use the developing vascular system as a guide. Conversely, recently it has been suggested that peripheral nerves provide a template that determines the organotypic pattern of blood vessel branching and arterial differentiation in the skin, via local secretion of *Vascular endothelial growth factor* (*Vegf*).

Sensory axons grow somewhat later than motor axons. For most of their length they follow the pathways established by the somatic and sympathetic motor fibers, but eventually they branch from the combined nerves and ultimately become associated with sensory end organs such as muscle spindles, temperature and touch receptors in the dermis of the skin, and pressure sensors and chemoreceptors in the developing vasculature. In many cases, the sensory neurons are responsible for inducing and maintaining the specialized sensory receptors.

IN THE CLINIC

HEREDITARY PERIPHERAL NEUROPATHIES

Motoneurons, whose cell bodies lie in the anterior horns of the spinal cord, may extend their axons for up to a meter in the PNS. Sensory neurons, whose cell bodies lie in the dorsal root ganglia, extend their central processes segmentally into the spinal cord, and their peripheral processes fasciculate with the axons of motoneurons to form mixed nerves. Axons in the PNS are myelinated by **Schwann cells**. Thus, the Schwann cell performs the role in the PNS subserved by astrocytes and oligodendrocyte in the CNS (discussed in Ch. 9). The signal for myelination comes from the axon, and myelination occurs in axons larger than 1 to 2 μm in diameter. Each segment of a myelinated axon is the territory of a single Schwann cell, the length of the segments correlating with the diameter of the axon. For unmyelinated fibers, single Schwann cells usually surround multiple axons. The myelin sheath is composed of compacted layers of the Schwann cell membrane. It is predominantly lipid, but contains several proteins that have

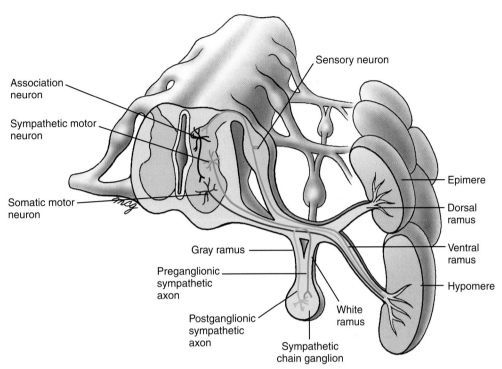

Figure 10-7. Organization of spinal nerves and associated chain ganglia at levels T1-L2 and S2-S4. In this example, the preganglionic fiber growing from the intermediolateral cell column exits the spinal nerve through a white ramus and synapses with a neuron in the chain ganglion at the same level. The postganglionic fiber then exits through the gray ramus and rejoins the same spinal nerve. Each spinal nerve splits into a dorsal primary ramus and a ventral primary ramus, which innervate the segmental epimere and hypomere, respectively. Both rami contain motor, sensory, and autonomic fibers.

key roles in maintaining the structure and compaction of the myelin and adhesion of the sheath to the axon. Several of these proteins and lipids may be important immunogens in disease.

Peripheral nerves are generally mixed nerves composed of sensory, motor, sympathetic, and parasympathetic fibers. The nerves are divided into fascicles surrounded by the **perineurium**, a connective tissue sheath, and are bound together by the **epineurium**, a similar connective tissue sheath. Individual nerve fibers are surrounded by a third sheath, the **endoneurium**. This sheath contains collagen, fibroblasts, mast cells, and resident macrophages. Endoneurial arterioles are supplied by a plexus of epineurial blood vessels with multiple systemic feeders. Circulating macromolecules are excluded from the endoneurium by the **blood-nerve barrier**, which is analogous to the blood-brain barrier and is formed by the endothelial cells and their tight junctions.

The long length of PNS axons, their dependence on axonal transport for renewal of structural membrane and

cytoskeletal components, and other factors make them especially vulnerable to damage. Major pathologies of the nerve involve axonal degeneration and demyelination. Damage to Schwann cells or myelin can result in segmental demyelination. In this process, the myelin sheath is stripped from a complete segment up to 1 mm in length. Macrophages remove myelin debris, and Schwann cells divide after segmental demyelination. Remyelination can begin quickly, within a few days, producing shorter segments of myelin, usually about 300 μm long.

Certain demyelinating diseases are hereditary. Specific diagnosis is now possible by genetic analysis of appropriate phenotypes, obviating the need for nerve biopsy in many cases. Diagnosis guides neurologic assessment and counseling of at-risk family members.

Charcot-Marie-Tooth Hereditary Neuropathy

Charcot-Marie-Tooth (CMT) hereditary neuropathy, also called *hereditary motor-sensory neuropathy (HMSN)*, is a group of chronic demyelinating polyneuro-pathies (i.e.,motor and sensory) that present in the first and second decades with slowly progressive distal weakness, wasting, and sensory loss, which is worse in the legs. High arches (pes cavus), hammer toes, ankle instability, and eventually deformity are common. Nerve hypertrophy may be seen. Slowed nerve conduction velocities, usually to 20 to 30 m/sec (normal ≥40 m/sec), without conduction block are typical. Biopsies show loss of myelinated fibers, signs of demyelination and remyelination, and onion bulbs (concentric laminar structures formed by Schwann cells). Ankle braces, special shoes, and corrective foot and ankle surgery are often helpful. Most patients remain ambulatory. Four separate types are currently recognized: types **CMT1, -2, -4,** and **-X.**

CMT1 is an autosomal dominant disease occurring in 50% of the CMT patients. It results from mutations in six different genes encoding **myelin** or myelin-related proteins, with most (70% to 80%) occurring in the *PMP22* (*PERIPHERAL MYELIN PROTEIN 22*) gene and 5% to 10% occurring in the *MPZ* (*MYELIN PROTEIN ZERO*) gene. Demyelination affects both motor and sensory nerves and results in muscle atrophy and sensory deficits.

CMT2 is predominantly an autosomal dominant disease causing chronic motor-sensory polyneuropathy of **axons,** without demyelination. It occurs in 20% to 40% of CMT patients. Electrophysiologic studies show signs of chronic distal muscle denervation and minor slowing of nerve conduction velocities. CMT1 and CMT2 patients present similarly with high arches and hammer toes, and a distal predominance of wasting, weakness, and sensory loss. CMT2 is genetically heterogeneous with mutations occurring in nine different genes, with roughly equal frequency. Some of these genes are known to be involved in axonal functioning, such as the *KINESIN* family member *KIF1B.*

CMT4 is a rare autosomal recessive disease that can cause abnormalities of **myelin** and/or **axons.** Patients present with typical CMT symptoms including muscle weakness and sensory loss. CMT4 results from mutations in seven different genes, with roughly equal frequency.

CMTX is an X-linked condition affecting 10% to 20% of CMT patients. Axonopathy and demyelination occur more severely in male subjects, who clinically resemble patients with CMT1 and CMT2. About half the female carriers are mildly affected. There is slowing of nerve conduction velocities to 30 to 40 m/sec. Pathologic changes suggest an **axon** defect, but the abnormal protein CONNEXIN-32 is a gap junction protein found in compacted **myelin.**

In addition to the four types of CMT, other CMT-like hereditary peripheral neuropathies exist such as **Refsum disease.** This disease is distinguished from CMT by the presence of additional symptoms including anosmia, deafness, retinitis, ichthyosis, and ataxia. It is caused by the accumulation of **phytanic acid** (a substance commonly present in foods) resulting from mutations in the gene encoding the enzyme PHYTANOYL-CoA HYDROXYLASE.

Pattern of Somatic Motor and Sensory Innervation Is Segmental

Motor and sensory nerves innervate the body wall and limbs in a pattern that is based on the segmental organization established by the somites. For example, the intercostal muscles between a given pair of ribs are innervated by the spinal nerve that grows out at that level. The sensory innervation of the skin is also basically segmental: each dermatome is innervated by the spinal nerve growing out at the same level. However, the sensory component of each spinal nerve also spreads to some extent into the adjacent dermatomes, so there is some overlap in dermatomal innervation (Fig. 10-8).

Pattern of Sympathetic Innervation Is Not Entirely Segmental

Sympathetic fibers traveling in the spinal nerves share the segmental distribution of the somatic motor and sensory fibers. Therefore, the segments of the body wall and extremities developing at levels T1 through L2 or L3 are innervated by postganglionic fibers originating from chain ganglia at the corresponding levels of the spinal cord. However, another pattern is required to provide sympathetic innervation to the remaining levels of the body wall and extremities, which correspond to cord levels lacking central sympathetic neurons. Chain ganglia develop in the cervical, lower lumbar, sacral, and coccygeal regions in addition to the thoracic and upper lumbar regions. How do these ganglia receive central sympathetic innervation? The answer (as hinted earlier) is that some of the preganglionic sympathetic fibers that enter chain ganglia at levels T1 through L2 or L3 travel cranially or caudally to another chain ganglion before synapsing. Some of these ascending or descending fibers supply the chain ganglia outside of T1 through L2 or L3 (Fig. 10-9).

The postganglionic fibers from each chain ganglion enter the corresponding spinal nerve via a gray ramus. As a result, the spinal nerves at levels T1 through L2 or L3 have both white and gray rami,

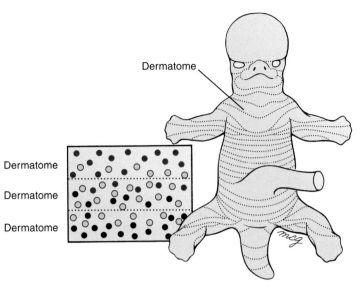

Figure 10-8. Dermatomal distribution of sensory innervation. Sensory fibers of each spinal nerve innervate receptors mainly in the corresponding body segment or dermatome. However, the innervation of adjacent dermatomes shows some overlap, so that ablation of a dorsal root does not entirely obliterate sensation in the corresponding dermatome.

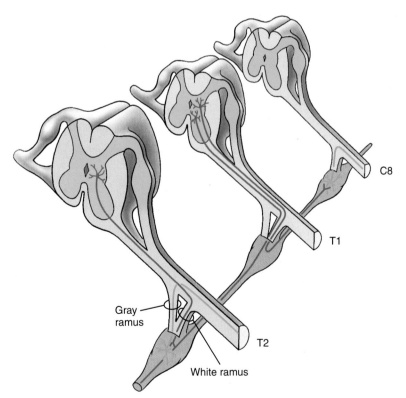

Figure 10-9. Preganglionic fibers growing from the intermediolateral cell column may synapse with a neuron in a chain ganglion at their own level, a lower level, or a higher level. This mechanism provides sympathetic innervation to spinal levels other than T1-L2, which lack a white ramus (i.e., C1-C8, L3 and L5, S1-S5, and the first coccygeal nerve).

whereas all other spinal nerves have just a gray ramus. Thus, the motor fibers linking chain ganglia to one another are exclusively preganglionic sympathetic fibers.

Sympathetic Innervation of Organs of Thorax and Head

The sympathetic supply to the heart originates at cord levels T1 through T4 (Fig. 10-10). Some of the fibers from T1 travel up the sympathetic trunk to synapse in the three cervical chain ganglia—the **inferior cervical ganglion** (which is sometimes fused with the chain ganglion at T1 to form the **stellate ganglion**), the **middle cervical ganglion**, and the **superior cervical ganglion**. Postganglionic fibers from these ganglia join postganglionic fibers emanating directly from nerves T1 through T4 to form the cardiac nerves, which innervate the heart muscle.

Postganglionic sympathetic fibers exiting directly from chain ganglia associated with levels T1 through T4, or from cervical ganglia innervated by preganglionic fibers originating at cord levels T1 to T4, also innervate the trachea and lungs.

Some postganglionic fibers arising from the superior cervical ganglion project to the various structures in the head that receive sympathetic innervation. These structures include the lacrimal glands, the dilator pupillae muscles of the iris, and the nasal and oral mucosa.

Sympathetic Innervation of Abdomen

The preganglionic sympathetic fibers destined to supply the gut arise from cord levels T5 through L2 or L3 and enter the corresponding chain ganglia. However, instead of synapsing there, they immediately leave the sympathetic trunk via the **splanchnic nerves**, which emerge directly from the chain ganglia (see Fig. 10-10). The splanchnic nerves innervate the various prevertebral (or preaortic) ganglia, which in turn send postganglionic fibers to the visceral end organs. The pattern of distribution is as follows:

Fibers from levels T5 through T9 come together to form the **greater splanchnic nerves** serving the **celiac ganglia**.

Fibers from T10 and T11 form the **lesser splanchnic nerves** serving the **aorticorenal ganglia**.

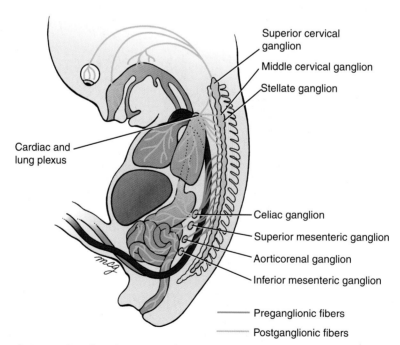

Figure 10-10. Some postganglionic sympathetic fibers do not join with spinal nerves. Postganglionic fibers emanating from cervical and thoracic chain ganglia follow blood vessels to structures in the head and pharynx and to the heart and lungs. The splanchnic nerves are preganglionic fibers that pass directly out of the chain ganglia at levels T5 to L2 to innervate neurons within the celiac, superior, mesenteric, aorticorenal, and inferior mesenteric ganglia. Postganglionic fibers from these ganglia grow out along blood vessels to innervate their visceral end organs.

Fibers from T12 alone form the least splanchnic nerves serving the superior mesenteric ganglia.

Fibers from L1 and L2 or L3 form the **lumbar splanchnic nerves** serving the **inferior mesenteric ganglia**.

The prevertebral (or preaortic) ganglia develop next to major branches of the descending aorta (i.e., the celiac, superior mesenteric, and inferior mesenteric arteries; discussed in Ch. 13, and in relation to the regions of the gut in Ch. 14). The postganglionic sympathetic axons from the prevertebral ganglia grow out along these arteries and thus come to innervate the same tissues that the arteries supply with blood (see Fig. 10-10). Thus, the postganglionic fibers from the celiac ganglia innervate the distal foregut region vascularized by the celiac artery—that is, the portion of the foregut from the abdominal esophagus through the duodenum to the entrance of the bile duct. Similarly, fibers from the superior mesenteric ganglia innervate the **midgut** (the remainder of the duodenum, the jejunum, and the ileum) plus the ascending colon and about two thirds of the transverse colon. The aorticorenal ganglia innervate the kidney and suprarenal gland, and the inferior mesenteric ganglia innervate the **hindgut**, including the distal one third of the transverse colon, the descending and sigmoid colons, and the upper two thirds of the anorectal canal.

Parasympathetic Innervation of Lower Abdomen, Pelvis, and Perineum

Parasympathetic preganglionic fibers arising in the sacral spinal cord emerge from the ventral rami of the cord and join together to form the **pelvic splanchnic nerves**. These nerves ramify throughout the pelvis and lower abdomen, innervating ganglia embedded in the walls of the descending and sigmoid colons, rectum, ureter, prostate, bladder, urethra, and phallus. The postganglionic fibers from these ganglia innervate smooth muscle or glands in the target organs (Fig. 10-11).

IN THE RESEARCH LAB

REGULATING AXONAL GUIDANCE IN PNS

The sensory neurons and motoneurons of the brain and spinal cord become interconnected in functional patterns, and axons grow out of the CNS and peripheral ganglia to innervate appropriate **target (end) organs** in the body. Peripheral axons travel to their target structures as they do

10

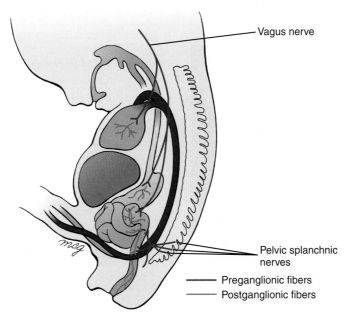

Vagus nerve

Pelvic splanchnic nerves

— Preganglionic fibers
-- Postganglionic fibers

Figure 10-11. The vagus nerve and pelvic splanchnic nerves provide preganglionic parasympathetic innervation to ganglia embedded in the walls of visceral organs. The preganglionic fibers originating at cord levels S2 through S4 issue from the cord at those levels and then branch off to form pelvic splanchnic nerves. The latter innervate the parasympathetic ganglia of the target viscera. The postganglionic parasympathetic fibers are relatively short.

within the CNS (discussed in Ch. 9)—that is, through the active locomotion of an apical structure called the **growth cone** (Fig. 10-12; see also Fig. 9-16). The growth cone guides the axon along the correct trajectory to its target by detecting and integrating various molecular guidance cues in and around the axon pathways. This activity of the growth cone is called **pathfinding.** Once the growth cone reaches its target, it halts and forms a synapse. Somatic motor and sensory fibers synapse directly with their target organs. In contrast, the axons of central autonomic neurons terminate in peripheral autonomic ganglia, where they synapse with the peripheral neuron of the two-neuron autonomic pathway.

The process of axon pathfinding is orchestrated by a complex interplay between highly conserved families of attractive and repulsive guidance molecules, among which the **Netrins, Slits, Semaphorins**, and **Ephrins** are the best understood. *Netrins* can guide axons from distances of up to a few millimeters, but in other cases they act only short-range. *Netrins* signal through the transmembrane proteins *Unc5* and *Unc40*. The latter belongs to the *Dcc* (*Deleted in colorectal carcinoma*) family of genes. *Slits* are large secreted proteins that can act as repellants and that signal through the *Roundabout* (*Robo*) family of receptors. Because *Slit1* and *Slit2* are expressed in cells that border the optic chiasm, the idea emerged that *Slits* may form a repulsive border and thus a corridor to guide retinal axons through the chiasm (discussed in Ch. 9). *Semaphorins* are a large family of cell surface and secreted guidance molecules (more than 30 have been identified to date), defined by the presence of a conserved "Sema" domain. They signal through the **Neuropilin** family of receptors, which in turn bind to a second family of receptors called the **Plexins**. *Semaphorin* is thought to act as a short-range inhibitory cue that deflects growth cones away from inappropriate regions or guides them through repulsive corridors. Conversely, for certain axons *Semaphorins* may act as attractants. *Ephrins* form a family of membrane-bound ligands for the *Eph* family of receptors that mainly act as repellants. *Ephrin-A* ligands in the superior colliculi and *EphA* receptors in the retinae, respectively, form complementary gradients, thus directing topographically correct connections (discussed in Ch. 9). Both "forward" signaling from ligand to receptor and "reverse" signaling from *Eph* receptors to their membrane-bound ligands occur. The ability to mediate either attraction or repulsion is a common theme among guidance molecules.

A few years ago, the prevailing view was that neuronal activity plays a role only during the terminal stages of target selection. This notion has now been challenged by evidence of **early episodes of spontaneous rhythmic electrical activity** in the embryonic spinal cord that depend on *GABA*-mediated excitatory currents (i.e., currents resulting from the release of the neurotransmitter *Gamma-aminobutyric acid*) and appear to be required for motor axons to navigate correctly to their peripheral targets. Inhibiting this early bursting activity with picrotoxin perturbs axonal guidance and causes a marked reduction in the expression of polysialylated *Neural cell adhesion molecule* (*Psa-Ncam*) and *EphA4*. These intriguing results suggest that early neuronal activity contributes to axonal pathfinding by regulating *Psa-Ncam* and guidance molecule expression on motor axons.

A recent new hypothesis on axonal pathfinding suggests a role for morphogens, including the **Hedgehog, Wnt**, and **Bone morphogenetic protein** (**Bmp**) families of proteins. Evidence comes from *Netrin*-deficient ventral spinal cord explants that were challenged with a local source of *Sonic hedgehog* (*Shh*). *Shh* attracted the growth cone. This event could be prevented by blocking the *Hedgehog* transducer *Smoothened*. Conversely, *Bmp* repulses commissural fibers in the dorsal spinal cord. Mice that lack the *Wnt* receptor *Frizzled3* show aberrant commissural neuron trajectories. These morphogens have an attractive feature that is desirable for guidance cues: they form gradients within the spinal cord. *Bmp*, which initially has a dorsalizing role, forms a dorsoventral gradient; *Shh*, having a ventralizing activity, forms a ventrodorsal gradient; and *Wnt4* forms a rostrocaudal gradient in the floor plate. Although these are exciting data, many questions remain. It is not known, for

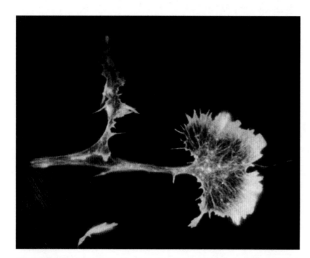

Figure 10-12. Axonal growth cone. The nerve cell body is at the left. The actin filaments in the fan-shaped growth cone are stained with rhodamine-labeled phalloidin. Rhodamine is a fluorescent molecule, and phalloidin (the toxin in the poisonous green fungus *Amanita phalloides*) binds strongly to actin filaments.

instance, how these molecules signal to the cytoskeleton to direct axon growth, rather than to the nucleus to determine cell fate.

It is thought that both guidance molecules and electrical neuronal activity converge in changing **calcium homeostasis** within the growth cone to regulate growth cone turning. Hotspots of intracellular free calcium occur closest to the source of the guidance factor. The amplitude of the calcium signal seems to decide the role of the guidance factor. For example, treatments that reduce calcium signals convert *Netrin-1*–induced growth cone steering from attraction to repulsion. Thus it is thought that a gradient of intracellular free calcium across the growth cone can mediate steering responses, with higher-amplitude calcium signals mediating attraction and lower-amplitude calcium signals mediating repulsion. Calcium signaling in turn is thought to affect the cytoskeleton in the growth cone by stabilizing the dynamically extending and retracting microtubules, which grow preferentially along the filopodial actin filaments. Subsequently, asymmetric extension of stabilized microtubule bundles within filopodia initiates growth cone turning towards the new direction.

Although many of the mechanisms discussed in this section have been elucidated in the CNS, many are likely to be conserved in the PNS. Overall, currently available information points to a complex system of diverse long-range and short-range cues, in which relative rather than absolute concentrations convey positional information.

Not all axons need to navigate pathways independently. It is likely that the first (the "pioneer") growth cones to traverse a route establish a pathway that is used by later growing axons. This mechanism would account for the formation of nerves, in which many axons travel together. The phenomenon of axonal pathfinding is a very active area of research, with obvious implications for the process of nerve regeneration after injury in children or adults.

Development of Cranial PNS

The cranial PNS consists of both cranial nerves and ganglia as well as autonomic (parasympathetic) nerves and ganglia. Parasympathetic nerves course through cranial nerves in the head, and sacral spinal nerves in the caudal trunk, to reach their ganglia. Those arising with sacral spinal nerves are discussed earlier in the chapter. The development of cranial nerves (and ganglia) and cranial parasympathetic nerves are considered together.

Development of Cranial Nerves, and Sensory and Parasympathetic Ganglia

The peripheral neurons of the cranial nerve sensory and parasympathetic pathways are housed in ganglia that lie outside the CNS. The cranial parasympathetic division consists of two-neuron pathways: the central neuron of each pathway resides in a peripheral nucleus, whereas the peripheral neuron resides in a ganglion located in the head or neck. The cranial sensory (afferent) and parasympathetic (visceral efferent) ganglia (Table 10-1; Fig. 10-13) appear during the end of the 4th week and beginning of the 5th week. The cranial nerve sensory ganglia contain the cell bodies of sensory neurons for the corresponding cranial nerves. The cranial nerve parasympathetic ganglia can be divided into two groups: the ganglia associated with the vagus nerve, which are located in the walls of the visceral organs (e.g., gut, heart, lungs, pelvic organs), and the parasympathetic ganglia of cranial nerves III, VII, and IX, which innervate structures in the head. The head receives sympathetic innervation via nerves from the cervical chain ganglia.

Origin of Cranial Nerve Sensory Ganglia

Experiments involving quail-chick transplantation chimeras (discussed in Ch. 5) have shown that neurons in the cranial nerve sensory ganglia have a dual origin (see Fig. 10-13; also see Fig. 4-19). Some are formed from neural crest cells in the same way as the neurons in the dorsal root ganglia of the spinal nerves, other neurons are derived from **ectodermal placodes**. Three of these placodes—the nasal placodes, retinal disc placodes (the thickened inner layer of the optic vesicles, also called the neural retinae), and otic placodes—are discussed in Chapters 16 and 17. In addition, a series of four **epipharyngeal** (also called **epibranchial**) **placodes** develop as ectodermal thickenings just dorsal to the four pharyngeal clefts, and a more diffuse **trigeminal placode** develops in the area between the epipharyngeal placodes and the lens placode. Epipharyngeal placodes give rise to neuronal precursors beginning roughly at the end of the 4th week of gestation. In contrast to neurons in the cranial nerve sensory ganglia, which can arise either from neural crest cells or ectodermal placodes, all glia in these ganglia are derived from neural crest cells.

The nasal placodes give rise to the primary neurosensory cells of the olfactory epithelium, and the axons of these cells form the olfactory nerve (I), which penetrates the olfactory bulb of the telencephalon. With some

10

Table 10-1 Origins of the Neurons in the Cranial Nerve Ganglia.

Cranial Nerve	Ganglion and Type	Origin of Neurons
Olfactory (I)	Olfactory epithelium (primary neurons of the olfactory pathway) (special afferent)	Nasal placode
Oculomotor (III)	Ciliary ganglion (visceral efferent)	Neural crest cells of the caudal diencephalon and cranial mesencephalon
Trigeminal (V)	Trigeminal ganglion (general afferent)	Neural crest cells of the caudal diencephalon and cranial mesencephalon; trigeminal placode
Facial (VII)	Superior ganglion of nerve VII (general and special afferent) Inferior (geniculate) ganglion of nerve VII (general and special afferent) Sphenopalatine ganglion (visceral efferent) Submandibular ganglion (visceral efferent)	Rhombencephalic neural crest cells; 1st epipharyngeal placode 1st epipharyngeal placode Rhombencephalic neural crest cells Rhombencephalic neural crest cells
Vestibulocochlear (VIII)	Acoustic (cochlear) ganglion (special afferent) Vestibular ganglion (special afferent)	Otic placode Otic placode plus contribution from neural crest cells
Glossopharyngeal (IX)	Superior ganglion (general and special afferent) Inferior (petrosal) ganglion (general and special afferent) Otic ganglion (visceral efferent)	Rhombencephalic neural crest cells 2nd epipharyngeal placodes Rhombencephalic neural crest cells
Vagus (X)	Superior ganglion (general afferent) Inferior (nodose) ganglion (general and special afferent) Vagal parasympathetic (enteric) ganglia (visceral efferent)	Rhombencephalic neural crest cells 3rd and 4th epipharyngeal placodes Rhombencephalic neural crest cells

exceptions, the remaining cranial nerve sensory ganglia show a regular stratification with respect to their origin: the ganglia (or portions of ganglia) that lie closer to the brain (i.e., the so-called proximal ganglia) are derived from neural crest cells, whereas the neurons of ganglia (or portions thereof) lying farther from the brain (i.e., the so-called distal ganglia) are formed by placode-derived cells. However, the supporting cells of all cranial nerve sensory ganglia are derived from neural crest cells.

The **trigeminal (semilunar) ganglion** of cranial nerve V has a mixed origin: the proximal portion arises mainly from diencephalic and mesencephalic neural crest cells, whereas most neurons in the distal portion arise from the diffuse trigeminal placode. The sensory ganglia associated with the second, third, fourth, and sixth pharyngeal arches are derived from the corresponding epipharyngeal placodes and from neural crest cells. Each of these nerves has both a proximal and a distal sensory ganglion. In general, the proximal-distal rule discussed in the preceding paragraph holds for these ganglia. The combined **superior ganglion** of nerves IX and X is formed by rhombencephalic neural crest cells, whereas the neurons of the **inferior (petrosal) ganglion** of nerve IX are derived from the second epipharyngeal placode, and those of the **inferior (nodose) ganglion** of nerve X are derived from the third and fourth epipharyngeal placodes. The **superior combined ganglion** of nerves VII and VIII is derived from both the first epipharyngeal placode and

the rhombencephalic neural crest cells, but the neurons of the **inferior (geniculate) ganglion** of nerve VII are derived exclusively from the first epipharyngeal placode. As mentioned in Chapter 17, the distal ganglia of cranial nerve VIII—the **vestibular ganglion** and the **cochlear ganglion**—differentiate from the otic placode.

Origin of Cranial Nerve Parasympathetic Ganglia

The origin of the neural crest cells giving rise to the various cranial nerve parasympathetic ganglia has been determined in experiments using quail-chick transplantation chimeras (discussed in Ch. 5). The neurons and glia in each ganglion (and thus the entire ganglion) arise from neural crest cells located at roughly the same level as the corresponding brain stem nucleus (compare Fig. 10-13 and 9-6; also see Fig. 4-19). Specifically, the **ciliary ganglion** of the oculomotor nerve (III) is formed by neural crest cells arising in the caudal part of the diencephalon and the cranial part of the mesencephalon; the **sphenopalatine** and **submandibular ganglia** of the facial nerve (VII) are formed by neural crest cells that migrate from the cranial rhombencephalon; and the **otic ganglion** of the glossopharyngeal nerve (IX) as well as the enteric ganglia served by the vagus nerve are derived from neural crest cells originating in the caudal portion of the rhombencephalon.

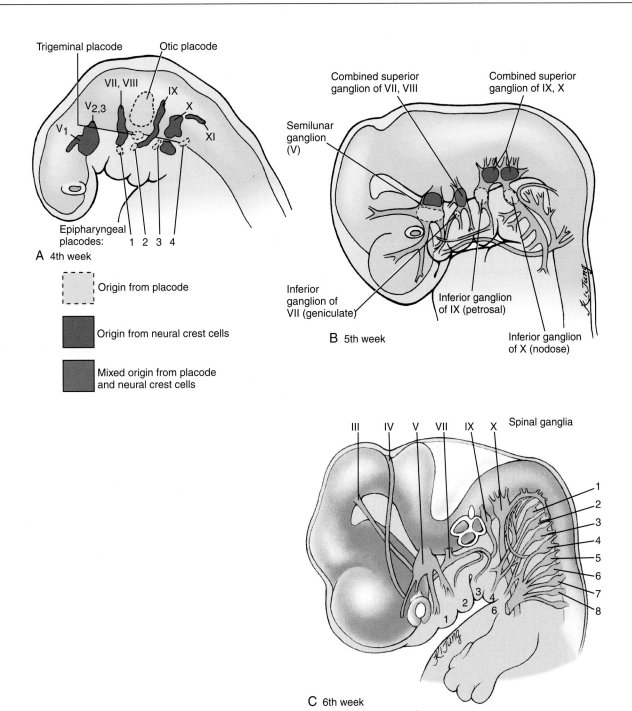

Figure 10-13. Development of the cranial nerves and their ganglia. *A, B,* Origin of cranial nerve ganglia from neural crest cells and ectodermal placodes. Cranial nerve parasympathetic ganglia arise solely from neural crest cells, whereas neurons in the cranial nerve sensory ganglia arise from either neural crest cells or placode cells. Glia in all cranial nerve ganglia are derived from neural crest cells. *C,* The definitive arrangement of cranial nerves is apparent by the 6th week.

Differences in Preganglionic and Postganglionic Fiber Length between Parasympathetic and Sympathetic Divisions of Autonomic Nervous System

Parasympathetic ganglia form close to the organs they are destined to innervate. This is in contrast to the sympathetic ganglia, which form relatively far from the organs they are destined to innervate. Thus, in general, preganglionic fibers of the parasympathetic division are relatively long and their postganglionic fibers are relatively short, whereas in the sympathetic division the situation is reversed.

The central (preganglionic or presynaptic) neurons of the two-cell parasympathetic pathways reside either in one of four motor nuclei in the brain (associated with cranial nerves III, VII, IX, and X) or in the intermediolateral cell columns of the sacral cord at levels S2 through S4. The cranial nuclei supply the head and the viscera superior to the hindgut, whereas the sacral neurons supply the viscera inferior to this point (see Fig. 10-11).

The preganglionic parasympathetic fibers associated with cranial nerves III, VII, and IX travel to parasympathetic ganglia located near the structures to be innervated, where they synapse with the second (postganglionic or postsynaptic) neuron of the pathway. Organs receiving parasympathetic innervation in this way include the dilator pupillae muscles of the eye, the lacrimal and salivary glands, and glands of the oral and nasal mucosa (discussed in Ch. 16). In contrast, the preganglionic parasympathetic fibers associated with cranial nerve X join with somatic motor and sensory fibers to form the **vagus nerve**. Some branches of the vagus nerve serve structures in the head and neck, but other parasympathetic and sensory fibers within the nerve continue into the thorax and abdomen, where the parasympathetic fibers synapse with postganglionic neurons in numerous small parasympathetic ganglia embedded in the walls of target organs such as the heart, liver, suprarenal cortex, kidney, gonads, and gut. The preganglionic vagal fibers, therefore, are very long, whereas the postganglionic fibers that penetrate the target organs are very short (see Fig. 10-11).

Suggested Readings

Araujo SJ, Tear G. 2003. Axon guidance mechanisms and molecules: lessons from invertebrates. Nat Rev Neurosci 4:910-922.

Arevalo JC, Chao MV. 2005. Axonal growth: where neurotrophins meet Wnts. Curr Opin Cell Biol 17:112-115.

Auer-Grumbach M. 2004. Hereditary sensory neuropathies. Drugs Today (Barc) 40:385-394.

Baker C. 2005. Neural crest and cranial ectodermal placodes. In: Rao MS, Jacobson M, editors. Developmental Neurobiology. New York: Kluwer Academic/Plenum Pubs. pp 67-127.

Baker CV, Bronner-Fraser M. 2000. Establishing neuronal identity in vertebrate neurogenic placodes. Development 127:3045-3056.

Baker CV, Bronner-Fraser M. 2001. Vertebrate cranial placodes I. Embryonic induction. Dev Biol 232:1-61.

Baker CV, Stark MR, Bronner-Fraser M. 2002. Pax3-expressing trigeminal placode cells can localize to trunk neural crest sites but are committed to a cutaneous sensory neuron fate. Dev Biol 249:219-236.

Basch ML, Garcia-Castro MI, Bronner-Fraser M. 2004. Molecular mechanisms of neural crest induction. Birth Defects Res C Embryo Today 72:109-123.

Begbie J, Ballivet M, Graham A. 2002. Early steps in the production of sensory neurons by the neurogenic placodes. Mol Cell Neurosci 21:502-511.

Begbie J, Graham A. 2001. Integration between the epibranchial placodes and the hindbrain. Science 294:595-598.

Begbie J, Graham A. 2001. The ectodermal placodes: a dysfunctional family. Philos Trans R Soc Lond B Biol Sci 356:1655-1660.

Bhattacharyya S, Bailey AP, Bronner-Fraser M, Streit A. 2004. Segregation of lens and olfactory precursors from a common territory: cell sorting and reciprocity of Dlx5 and Pax6 expression. Dev Biol 271:403-414.

Bixby S, Kruger GM, Mosher JT, Joseph NM, Morrison SJ. 2002. Cell-intrinsic differences between stem cells from different regions of the peripheral nervous system regulate the generation of neural diversity. Neuron 35:643-656.

Carmeliet P. 2003. Blood vessels and nerves: common signals, pathways and diseases. Nat Rev Genet 4:710-720.

Carmeliet P, Tessier-Lavigne M. 2005. Common mechanisms of nerve and blood vessel wiring. Nature 436:193-200.

Chai Y, Jiang X, Ito Y, et al. 2000. Fate of the mammalian cranial neural crest during tooth and mandibular morphogenesis. Development 127:1671-1679.

Charron F, Tessier-Lavigne M. 2005. Novel brain wiring functions for classical morphogens: a role as graded positional cues in axon guidance. Development 132:2251-2262.

Chien C-B. 2005. Guidance of Axons and Dendrites. In: Rao MS, Jacobson M, editors. Developmental Neurobiology. New York: Kluwer Academic/Plenum Pubs. pp 241-268.

Chilton JK. 2006. Molecular mechanisms of axon guidance. Dev Biol 292:13-24.

Cichowski K, Jacks T. 2001. NF1 tumor suppressor gene function: narrowing the GAP. Cell 104:593-604.

Cordes SP. 2001. Molecular genetics of cranial nerve development in mouse. Nat Rev Neurosci 2:611-623.

De Bellard ME, Rao Y, Bronner-Fraser M. 2003. Dual function of Slit2 in repulsion and enhanced migration of trunk, but not vagal, neural crest cells. J Cell Biol 162:269-279.

Dickson BJ, Keleman K. 2002. Netrins. Curr Biol 12:R154-R155.

Eberhart J, Barr J, O'Connell S, et al. 2004. Ephrin-A5 exerts positive or inhibitory effects on distinct subsets of EphA4-positive motor neurons. J Neurosci 24:1070-1078.

Eberhart J, Swartz ME, Koblar SA, et al. 2002. EphA4 constitutes a population-specific guidance cue for motor neurons. Dev Biol 247:89-101.

Erickson CA. 2003. Patterning of the neural crest. In: Tickle C, editor. Patterning in Vertebrate Development. Oxford: Oxford University Press. pp. 166-197.

Farlie PG, McKeown SJ, Newgreen DF. 2004. The neural crest: basic biology and clinical relationships in the craniofacial and enteric nervous systems. Birth Defects Res C Embryo Today 72:173-189.

Francis-West PH, Ladher RK, Schoenwolf GC. 2002. Development of the sensory organs. Sci Prog 85:151-173.

Gammill LS, Bronner-Fraser M. 2002. Genomic analysis of neural crest induction. Development 129:5731-5741.

Gammill LS, Bronner-Fraser M. 2003. Neural crest specification: migrating into genomics. Nat Rev Neurosci 4:795-805.

Gershon MD. 2003. Serotonin and its implication for the management of irritable bowel syndrome. Rev Gastroenterol Disord 3 (Suppl 2):S25-S34.

Gershon MD. 2004. Review article: serotonin receptors and transporters — roles in normal and abnormal gastrointestinal motility. Aliment Pharmacol Ther 20 (Suppl 7):3-14.

Ghysen A, Dambly-Chaudiere C. 2000. A genetic programme for neuronal connectivity. Trends Genet 16:221-226.

Goldberg JL. 2003. How does an axon grow? Genes Dev 17:941-958.

Goulding M. 2004. How early is firing required for wiring? Neuron 43:601-603.

Graham A, Begbie J. 2000. Neurogenic placodes: a common front. Trends Neurosci 23:313-316.

Graham A, Begbie J, McGonnell I. 2004. Significance of the cranial neural crest. Dev Dyn 229:5-13.

Grunwald IC, Klein R. 2002. Axon guidance: receptor complexes and signaling mechanisms. Curr Opin Neurobiol 12:250-259.

Guan KL, Rao Y. 2003. Signalling mechanisms mediating neuronal responses to guidance cues. Nat Rev Neurosci 4:941-956.

Guthrie S. 2001. Axon guidance: Robos make the rules. Curr Biol 11:R300-R303.

Hanson MG, Landmesser LT. 2004. Normal patterns of spontaneous activity are required for correct motor axon guidance and the expression of specific guidance molecules. Neuron 43:687-701.

Helmbacher F, Schneider-Maunoury S, Topilko P, Tiret L, Charnay P. 2000. Targeting of the EphA4 tyrosine kinase receptor affects dorsal/ventral pathfinding of limb motor axons. Development 127:3313-3324.

Henley J, Poo MM. 2004. Guiding neuronal growth cones using Ca2+ signals. Trends Cell Biol 14:320-330.

Hippenmeyer S, Shneider NA, Birchmeier C, Burden SJ, Jessell TM, Arber S. 2002. A role for neuregulin1 signaling in muscle spindle differentiation. Neuron 36:1035-1049.

Howard MJ. 2005. Mechanisms and perspectives on differentiation of autonomic neurons. Dev Biol 277:271-286.

Huber K. 2006. The sympathoadrenal cell lineage: specification, diversification, and new perspectives. Dev Biol 298:335-343.

Hunter E, Begbie J, Mason I, Graham A. 2001. Early development of the mesencephalic trigeminal nucleus. Dev Dyn 222:484-493.

Karvonen SL, Kallioinen M, Yla-Outinen H, et al. 2000. Occult neurofibroma and increased S100 protein in the skin of patients with neurofibromatosis type 1: new insight to the etiopathomechanism of neurofibromas. Arch Dermatol 136:1207-1209.

Kasemeier-Kulesa JC, Kulesa PM, Lefcort F. 2005. Imaging neural crest cell dynamics during formation of dorsal root ganglia and sympathetic ganglia. Development 132:235-245.

Klein R. 2004. Eph/ephrin signaling in morphogenesis, neural development and plasticity. Curr Opin Cell Biol 16:580-589.

Kruger RP, Aurandt J, Guan KL. 2005. Semaphorins command cells to move. Nat Rev Mol Cell Biol 6:789-800.

Krull CE, Koblar SA. 2000. Motor axon pathfinding in the peripheral nervous system. Brain Res Bull 53:479-487.

Kulesa PM. 2004. Developmental imaging: Insights into the avian embryo. Birth Defects Res C Embryo Today 72:260-266.

Ladher RK, Anakwe KU, Gurney AL, et al. 2000. Identification of synergistic signals initiating inner ear development. Science 290:1965-1967.

Ladher RK, Wright TJ, Moon AM, et al. 2005. FGF8 initiates inner ear induction in chick and mouse. Genes Dev 19:603-613.

Landmesser LT. 2001. The acquisition of motoneuron subtype identity and motor circuit formation. Int J Dev Neurosci 19:175-182.

Le Douarin NM. 2004. The avian embryo as a model to study the development of the neural crest: a long and still ongoing story. Mech Dev 121:1089-1102.

Le Douarin NM, Creuzet S, Couly G, Dupin E. 2004. Neural crest cell plasticity and its limits. Development 131:4637-4650.

Lee VM, Bronner-Fraser M, Baker CV. 2005. Restricted response of mesencephalic neural crest to sympathetic differentiation signals in the trunk. Dev Biol 278:175-192.

Litsiou A, Hanson S, Streit A. 2005. A balance of FGF, BMP and WNT signalling positions the future placode territory in the head. Development 132:4051-4062.

Liu BP, Strittmatter SM. 2001. Semaphorin-mediated axonal guidance via Rho-related G proteins. Curr Opin Cell Biol 13:619-626.

Masuda T, Shiga T. 2005. Chemorepulsion and cell adhesion molecules in patterning initial trajectories of sensory axons. Neurosci Res 51:337-347.

McCabe KL, Manzo A, Gammill LS, Bronner-Fraser M. 2004. Discovery of genes implicated in placode formation. Dev Biol 274:462-477.

McLarren KW, Litsiou A, Streit A. 2003. DLX5 positions the neural crest and preplacode region at the border of the neural plate. Dev Biol 259:34-47.

Meulemans D, Bronner-Fraser M. 2004. Gene-regulatory interactions in neural crest evolution and development. Dev Cell 7:291-299.

Mukouyama YS, Shin D, Britsch S, Taniguchi M, Anderson DJ. 2002. Sensory nerves determine the pattern of arterial differentiation and blood vessel branching in the skin. Cell 109:693-705.

Pareyson D. 2004. Differential diagnosis of Charcot-Marie-Tooth disease and related neuropathies. Neurol Sci 25:72-82.

Piper M, Little M. 2003. Movement through Slits: cellular migration via the Slit family. Bioessays 25:32-38.

Santiago A, Erickson CA. 2002. Ephrin-B ligands play a dual role in the control of neural crest cell migration. Development 129:3621-3632.

Sieber-Blum M, Grim M. 2004. The adult hair follicle: cradle for pluripotent neural crest stem cells. Birth Defects Res C Embryo Today 72:162-172.

Sieber-Blum M, Grim M, Hu YF, Szeder V. 2004. Pluripotent neural crest stem cells in the adult hair follicle. Dev Dyn 231:258-269.

Skovronsky DM, Oberholtzer JC. 2004. Pathologic classification of peripheral nerve tumors. Neurosurg Clin N Am 15:157-166.

Sommer L. 2001. Context-dependent regulation of fate decisions in multipotent progenitor cells of the peripheral nervous system. Cell Tissue Res 305:211-216.

10

Streit A. 2004. Early development of the cranial sensory nervous system: from a common field to individual placodes. Dev Biol 276:1-15.

Teddy JM, Kulesa PM. 2004. In vivo evidence for short- and long-range cell communication in cranial neural crest cells. Development 131:6141-6151.

Vetter ML, Dorsky RI. 2005. Neurogenesis. In: Rao MS, Jacobson M, editors. Developmental Neurobiology. New York: Kluwer Academic/Plenum Pubs. pp 129-150.

Wakamatsu Y. 2004. Understanding glial differentiation in vertebrate nervous system development. Tohoku J Exp Med 203:233-240.

Weinstein BM. 2005. Vessels and nerves: marching to the same tune. Cell 120:299-302.

Wilkinson DG. 2001. Multiple roles of EPH receptors and ephrins in neural development. Nat Rev Neurosci 2:155-164.

Yoshikawa S, Thomas JB. 2004. Secreted cell signaling molecules in axon guidance. Curr Opin Neurobiol 14:45-50.

Young HM, Anderson RB, Anderson CR. 2004. Guidance cues involved in the development of the peripheral autonomic nervous system. Auton Neurosci 112:1-14.

Wong K, Park HT, Wu JY, Rao Y. 2002. Slit proteins: molecular guidance cues for cells ranging from neurons to leukocytes. Curr Opin Genet Dev 12:583-591.

Zou Y. 2004. Wnt signaling in axon guidance. Trends Neurosci 27:528-532.

Development of the Respiratory System and Body Cavities

11

Summary As discussed in Chapter 4, shortly after the three germ layers form during gastrulation, **body folding** forms the endodermal foregut at the cranial end of the embryo, thereby delineating the inner tube of the **tube-within-a-tube body plan**. On day 22 the foregut produces a ventral evagination called the **respiratory diverticulum** or **lung bud**, which is the primordium of the lungs. As the lung bud grows, it remains ensheathed in a covering of splanchnopleuric mesoderm, which will give rise to the lung vasculature and to the connective tissue, cartilage, and muscle within the bronchi. On days 26 to 28 the lengthening lung bud bifurcates into left and right **primary bronchial buds**, which will give rise to the two lungs. In the 5th week a second generation of branching produces three **secondary bronchial buds** on the right side and two on the left. These are the primordia of the future lung lobes. The bronchial buds and their splanchnopleuric sheath continue to grow and bifurcate, gradually filling the pleural cavities. By week 28 the 16th round of branching generates **terminal bronchioles**, which subsequently divide into two or more **respiratory bronchioles**. By week 36 these respiratory bronchioles have become invested with capillaries and are called **terminal sacs** or **primitive alveoli**. Between 36 weeks and birth, the alveoli mature. Additional alveoli continue to be produced throughout early childhood.

During the 4th week, partitions form to subdivide the intraembryonic coelom into pericardial, pleural, and peritoneal cavities. The first partition to develop is the **septum transversum**, a block-like wedge of mesoderm that forms a ventral structure partially dividing the coelom into a thoracic **primitive pericardial cavity** and an abdominal **peritoneal cavity**. Cranial body folding and differential growth of the developing head and neck regions translocate this block of mesoderm from the cranial edge of the embryonic disc caudally to the position of the future diaphragm. Coronal **pleuropericardial folds** meanwhile form on the lateral body wall of the primitive pericardial cavity and grow medially to fuse with each other and with the ventral surface of the foregut mesoderm, thus subdividing the primitive pericardial cavity into a definitive **pericardial cavity** and two **pleural cavities**. The pleural cavities initially communicate with the peritoneal cavity through a pair of **pericardioperitoneal canals** passing dorsal to the septum transversum. However, a pair of transverse **pleuroperitoneal membranes** grow ventrally from the dorsal body wall to fuse with the transverse septum, thus closing off the pericardioperitoneal canals. Therefore, the septum transversum and the pleuroperitoneal membranes form major parts of the future diaphragm.

As discussed in Chapter 6, as a result of folding, the amnion, which initially arises from the dorsal margin of the embryonic disc ectoderm, is carried ventrally to enclose the entire embryo, taking origin from the **umbilical ring** surrounding the roots of the vitelline duct and connecting stalk. The amnion also expands until it fills the chorionic space and fuses with the chorion. As the amnion expands, it encloses the connecting stalk and yolk sac neck in a sheath of amniotic membrane. This composite structure becomes the **umbilical cord**.

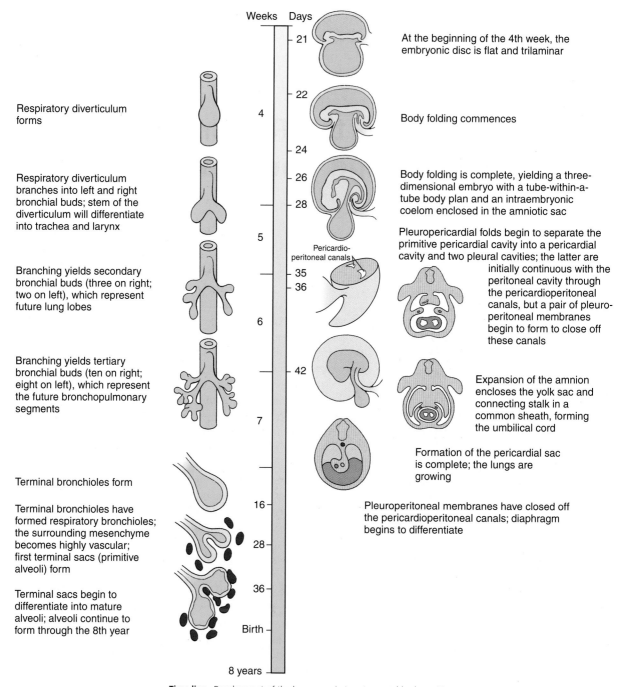

Respiratory diverticulum forms

Respiratory diverticulum branches into left and right bronchial buds; stem of the diverticulum will differentiate into trachea and larynx

Branching yields secondary bronchial buds (three on right; two on left), which represent future lung lobes

Branching yields tertiary bronchial buds (ten on right; eight on left), which represent the future bronchopulmonary segments

Terminal bronchioles form

Terminal bronchioles have formed respiratory bronchioles; the surrounding mesenchyme becomes highly vascular; first terminal sacs (primitive alveoli) form

Terminal sacs begin to differentiate into mature alveoli; alveoli continue to form through the 8th year

Weeks Days

21

22

4

24

26

28

5

Pericardio-
peritoneal canals

35
36

6

42

7

16

28

36

Birth

8 years

At the beginning of the 4th week, the embryonic disc is flat and trilaminar

Body folding commences

Body folding is complete, yielding a three-dimensional embryo with a tube-within-a-tube body plan and an intraembryonic coelom enclosed in the amniotic sac

Pleuropericardial folds begin to separate the primitive pericardial cavity into a pericardial cavity and two pleural cavities; the latter are initially continuous with the peritoneal cavity through the pericardioperitoneal canals, but a pair of pleuro-peritoneal membranes begin to form to close off these canals

Expansion of the amnion encloses the yolk sac and connecting stalk in a common sheath, forming the umbilical cord

Formation of the pericardial sac is complete; the lungs are growing

Pleuroperitoneal membranes have closed off the pericardioperitoneal canals; diaphragm begins to differentiate

Time line. Development of the lungs, respiratory tree, and body cavities.

An 18-year-old construction worker undergoes surgical repair of a broken femur after falling off a roof. The surgery and initial postoperative course are uncomplicated. However, the bedridden patient experiences a prolonged postoperative oxygen requirement despite receiving appropriate respiratory care, including frequent use of incentive spirometry (the patient exhales into this device to maintain lung volumes). He develops increasing cough and shortness of breath, and five nights after surgery he spikes a high fever. The on-call resident orders a chest X-ray that shows a focal consolidation (area of dense lung tissue) in the left lower lobe consistent with a bacterial pneumonia. The patient is started on intravenous antibiotics and receives more intensive respiratory therapy.

The family tells the team that the man has had pneumonia once before, and he has also had several cases of sinusitis. He has a chronic cough that was diagnosed as "asthma," but the cough is not severe enough to prevent him from being physically active. One of the patient's older brothers also has a similar respiratory issue and was found to be sterile after failing to conceive children.

The patient improves on antibiotics and respiratory therapy. After a repeat chest X-ray is done to monitor the pneumonia, the radiologist calls to inform the team that an error was made during the performance of the previous chest X-ray. Apparently the patient has **situs inversus**, and the night radiology technician who performed the previous X-ray mislabeled that film. The radiologist also notes subtle changes at the bases of the patient's lung fields consistent with bronchiectasis (abnormal dilation and inflammation of airways associated with mucous blockage) like that seen in **primary ciliary dyskinesia** (PCD) or cystic fibrosis. The combination of recurrent sinus infections, bronchiectasis, and situs inversus is consistent with the diagnosis of **Kartagener syndrome** (pronounced "KART-agayner"; also see Chs. 3 and 12 for additional discussion of Kartagener syndrome), a variant of PCD. Kartagener syndrome is caused by autosomal recessive mutations in the *DYNEIN AXONEMAL HEAVY CHAIN* 5 (*DNAH5*) gene. Mutations in this gene result in **immotile cilia** in the respiratory tract leading to poor mucus transport and frequent infections. Because cilia are also involved in sperm transport, affected males are sterile. During embryonic development, cilia in the node are involved in determination of the left-right axis (discussed in Ch. 3). Loss of node ciliary function in PCD leads to randomization of laterality, with 50% of affected individuals having situs inversus.

11

Development of Lungs and Respiratory Tree

Development of the lungs begins on day 22 with formation of a ventral outpouching of the endodermal foregut called the **respiratory diverticulum**. (Fig. 11-1). This bud grows ventrocaudally through the mesenchyme surrounding the foregut, and on days 26 to 28, it undergoes a first bifurcation, splitting into right and left **primary bronchial** (or **lung**) **buds**. These buds are the rudiments of the two lungs and the right and left **primary bronchi**, and the proximal end (stem) of the diverticulum forms the **trachea** and **larynx**. The latter opens into the pharynx via the **glottis**, a passageway formed at the original point of evagination of the diverticulum. As the primary bronchial buds form, the stem of the diverticulum begins to separate from the overlying portion of the pharynx, which becomes the **esophagus**. During weeks 5 and 28, the primary bronchial buds undergo about 16 rounds of branching to generate the respiratory tree of the lungs. The pattern of branching of the

lung endoderm is regulated by the surrounding mesenchyme, which invests the buds from the time that they first form. The stages of development of the lungs are summarized in Table 11-1 and the histologic appearance of the human lung during these stages is shown in Figure 11-2.

The first round of branching of the primary bronchial buds occurs early in the 5th week. This round of branching is highly stereotypical and yields three **secondary bronchial buds** on the right side and two on the left. The secondary bronchial buds give rise to the **lung lobes**: three in the right lung and two in the left lung. During the 6th week, a more variable round of branching typically yields 10 tertiary bronchi on both sides; these become the **bronchopulmonary segments** of the mature lung.

By week 16, after about 14 more branchings, the respiratory tree produces small branches called **terminal bronchioles** (Fig. 11-3). Between 16 and 28 weeks each terminal bronchiole divides into two or more **respiratory bronchioles**, and the mesodermal tissue surrounding these structures becomes

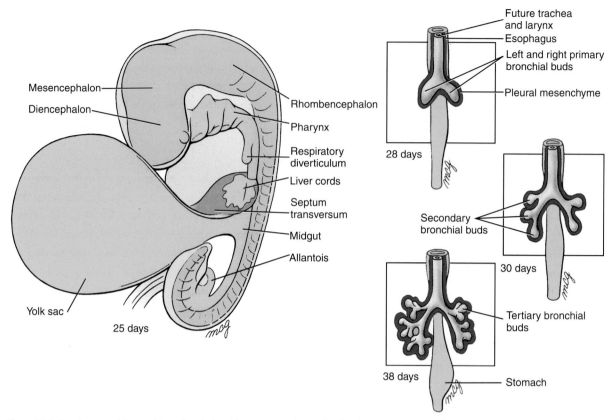

Figure 11-1. Development of the respiratory diverticulum. The respiratory diverticulum first forms as an evagination of the foregut on day 22 and immediately bifurcates into two primary bronchial buds between day 26 and day 28. Early in the 5th week, the right bronchial bud branches into three secondary bronchial buds, whereas the left bronchial bud branches into two. By the 6th week, secondary bronchial buds branch into tertiary bronchial buds (usually about 10 on each side) to form the bronchopulmonary segments.

Table 11-1 Stages of Human Lung Development

Stage of Development	Period	Events
Embryonic	26 days to 6 weeks	Respiratory diverticulum arises as a ventral outpouching of foregut endoderm and undergoes three initial rounds of branching, producing the primordia successively of the two lungs, the lung lobes, and the bronchopulmonary segments; the stem of the diverticulum forms the trachea and larynx.
Pseudoglandular	6 to 16 weeks	Respiratory tree undergoes 14 more generations of branching, resulting in the formation of terminal bronchioles.
Canalicular	16 to 28 weeks	Each terminal bronchiole divides into two or more respiratory bronchioles. Respiratory vasculature begins to develop. During this process, blood vessels come into close apposition with the lung epithelium. The lung epithelium also begins to differentiate into specialized cell types (ciliated, secretory, and neuroendocrine cells proximally and precursors of the alveolar type II and I cells distally).
Saccular	28 to 36 weeks	Respiratory bronchioles subdivide to produce terminal sacs (primitive alveoli). Terminal sacs continue to be produced until well into childhood.
Alveolar	36 weeks to term	Alveoli mature.

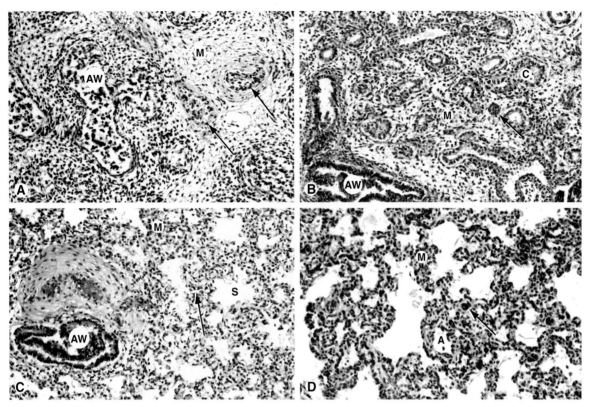

Figure 11-2. Histologic stages of human lung development. *A*, Pseudoglandular stage. *B*, Canalicular stage. *C*, Saccular stage. *D*, Alveolar stage. A, alveolus; AW, airway; C, smooth-walled canaliculus; M, mesenchyme; S, saccule; *Arrows*, part A, pulmonary artery (thick wall) and vein (thin wall); *Arrows*, parts B-D, capillaries.

highly vascularized. By week 28 the respiratory bronchioles begin to sprout a final generation of stubby branches. These branches develop in craniocaudal progression, forming first at more cranial terminal bronchioles. By week 36 the first-formed wave of terminal branches are invested in a dense network of capillaries and are called **terminal sacs (primitive alveoli)**. Limited gas exchange is possible at this point, but the alveoli are still so few and immature that infants born at this age may die of respiratory insufficiency without adequate therapy (discussed in the following "In the Clinic" section of this chapter). Additional terminal sacs continue to form and differentiate in craniocaudal progression both before and after birth. The process is largely completed by 2 years. About 20 to 70 million terminal sacs are formed in each lung before birth; the total number of alveoli in the mature lung is 300 to 400 million. Continued thinning of the squamous

epithelial lining of the terminal sacs begins just before birth, resulting in the differentiation of these primitive alveoli into mature alveoli. An important process of **septation**, which further subdivides the alveoli, occurs after birth. Each septum formed during this process contains smooth muscle and capillaries.

The lung is a composite of endodermal and mesodermal tissues. The endoderm of the respiratory diverticulum gives rise to the mucosal lining of the bronchi and to the epithelial cells of the alveoli. The remaining components of the lung, including the muscle and cartilage supporting the bronchi and the visceral pleura covering the lung, are derived from the splanchnopleuric mesoderm, which covers the bronchi as they grow out from the mediastinum into the pleural space. The lung vasculature is thought to develop via angiogenesis (i.e., sprouting from neighboring vessels; discussed in Ch. 13).

11

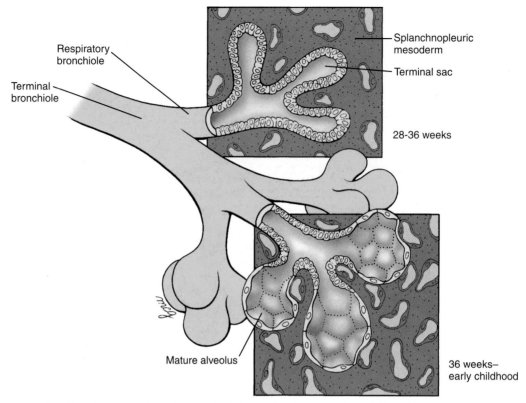

Respiratory
bronchiole

Terminal
bronchiole

Splanchnopleuric
mesoderm

Terminal sac

28-36 weeks

Mature alveolus

36 weeks–
early childhood

Figure 11-3. Maturation of lung tissue. Terminal sacs (primitive alveoli) begin to form between weeks 28 and 36 and begin to mature between 36 weeks and birth. However, only 5% to 20% of all terminal sacs eventually produced are formed before birth. Subsequent septation of the alveoli is not shown.

IN THE CLINIC

DEVELOPMENTAL ABNORMALITIES OF LUNG AND RESPIRATORY TREE

Many lung anomalies result from a failure of the respiratory diverticulum or its branches to branch or differentiate correctly. The most severe of these anomalies, **pulmonary agenesis**, results when the respiratory diverticulum fails to split into right and left bronchial buds and to continue growing. Errors in the pattern of pulmonary branching (**branching morphogenesis**) during the embryonic and early fetal periods result in defects ranging from an abnormal number of pulmonary lobes or bronchial segments to the complete absence of a lung. Finally, defects in the subdivision of the terminal respiratory bronchi or the formation of septae after birth can result in an abnormal paucity of alveoli, even if the respiratory tree is otherwise normal. Some of these types of pulmonary anomalies are caused by intrinsic molecular and cellular defects of branching morphogenesis (see the following "In the Research Lab"

section in this chapter). However, the primary cause of **pulmonary hypoplasia**—a reduced number of pulmonary segments or terminal air sacs—often represents a response to some condition that reduces the volume of the pleural cavity and thus restricts growth of the lungs (for example, protrusion of the abdominal viscera into the thoracic cavity, a condition known as congenital diaphragmatic hernia; discussed in the "In the Clinic" section near the end of the chapter).

Esophageal atresia (a blind esophagus) and **tracheoesophageal fistula** (an abnormal connection between tracheal and esophageal lumina resulting from a failure of the foregut to separate completely into trachea and esophagus; also called **esophagotracheal fistula**) are usually found together and occur in one of 3000 to 5000 births (Fig. 11-4). In addition, both of these defects can be associated with other defects (e.g., esophageal atresia with cardiovascular defects such as tetralogy of Fallot—discussed in Ch. 12; tracheoesophageal fistula with **VATER or VACTERL association**—discussed in Ch. 3). Both esophageal atresia

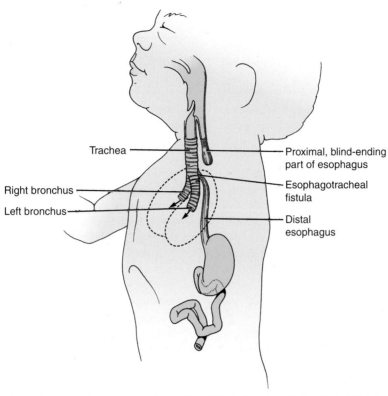

Trachea

Right bronchus

Left bronchus

Proximal, blind-ending part of esophagus

Esophagotracheal fistula

Distal esophagus

Figure 11-4. Diagram of an infant with esophageal atresia and tracheoesophageal fistula shows how the first drink of fluid after birth could be diverted into the newly expanded lungs (arrows).

and tracheoesophageal fistula are dangerous to the newborn because they allow milk or other fluids to be aspirated into the lungs. Hence, they are surgically corrected in the newborn. In addition to threatening survival after birth, esophageal atresia has an adverse effect on the intrauterine environment prior to birth: the blind-ending esophagus prevents the fetus from swallowing amniotic fluid and returning it to the mother via the placental circulation. This leads to an excess of amniotic fluid (**polyhydramnios**) and consequent distention of the uterus.

The cause of esophageal atresia is thought to be a failure of the esophageal endoderm to proliferate rapidly enough during the 5th week to keep up with the elongation of the embryo. However, the cause of tracheoesophageal fistula and the reason why the two defects are usually found together are unknown. In experimental mouse models, disruption of the *Sonic hedgehog* pathway or *Thyroid*

transcription factor-1 causes tracheoesophageal fistula. *Sonic hedgehog* is expressed in the endoderm and is believed to function by controlling proliferation of the surrounding mesoderm—a process important in the development of this region.

LUNG MATURATION AND SURVIVAL OF PREMATURE INFANTS

As the end of gestation approaches, the lungs undergo a rapid and dramatic series of transformations that prepare them for air breathing. The fluid that fills the alveoli prenatally is absorbed at birth, the defenses that will protect the lungs against invading pathogens and against the oxidative effects of the atmosphere are activated, and the surface area for alveolar gas exchange increases greatly. Changes in the structure of the lung take place during the last 2 months, accelerating in the days just preceding a normal term delivery. If a child is born prematurely, the state of development of the lungs is usually the prime factor determining whether he/she will live. Infants born between 26 weeks and term—during the phase of accelerated terminal lung maturation—have a very good chance of survival with appropriate neonatal support. Infants born before 26 weeks (in the canalicular phase of lung development) require intensive respiratory assistance to survive. Even then, they may die or develop lung fibrosis that results in long-term respiratory problems.

Although the total surface area for gas exchange in the lung depends on the number of alveoli and on the density of alveolar capillaries, efficient gas exchange will occur only if the barrier separating air from blood is thin—that is, if the alveoli are thin-walled, properly inflated, and not filled with fluid. The walls of the maturing alveolar sacs thin out during the weeks before birth. In addition, specific alveolar cells (the alveolar type II cells) begin to secrete **pulmonary surfactant**, a mixture of phospholipids and surfactant proteins that reduces the surface tension of the liquid film lining the alveoli and thus facilitates inflation. In the absence of surfactant, the surface tension at the air-liquid interface of the alveolar sacs tends to collapse the alveoli during exhalation. These collapsed alveoli can be inflated only with great effort.

The primary cause of the **respiratory distress syndrome** of premature infants (pulmonary insufficiency accompanied by gasping and cyanosis) is an inadequate production of surfactant. Respiratory distress syndrome not only threatens the infant with immediate asphyxiation, but the increased rate of breathing and mechanical ventilation required to support the infant's respiration can also damage the delicate alveolar lining, allowing fluid and cellular and serum proteins to exude into the alveolus. Continued injury may lead to detachment of the layer of cells lining the alveoli, a condition called **hyaline membrane disease**. Chronic lung injury associated with preterm infants causes a condition termed **bronchopulmonary dysplasia**.

In mothers with a high risk for premature delivery, the fetus can be treated antenatally with steroids to accelerate lung maturation and the synthesis of surfactant. Moreover, amniocentesis can be done in late pregnancy to assess fetal lung maturity. In this test, the sample of amniotic fluid is analyzed with thin-layer chromatography to determine the lecithin-sphingomyelin ratio (L/S; greater than 1.9 = mature; less than 1.5 = immature) and to detect phosphatidylglycerol (presence indicates lung maturity).

Critically ill *newborns* were first successfully treated with **surfactant replacement therapy**—the administration of exogenous surfactant—in the late 1970s. A variety of surfactant preparations are now used for this purpose, some derived from animal lungs or human amniotic fluid, others synthetic. However, experiments indicate that these phospholipid preparations would be more effective if they also included some of the supplementary proteins found in natural surfactant. For example, it has been found that the addition of small amounts of human surfactant proteins enhances surfactant activity. Two of these proteins (A and B) seemingly act by organizing the surfactant phospholipids into tubular structures termed *tubular myelin*, which is particularly effective at reducing surface tension. Although surfactant protein C is not required for tubular myelin formation, it does enhance the function of surfactant phospholipids. Surfactant proteins A and D apparently play important roles in innate host defense of the lung against viral, bacterial, and fungal pathogens.

A fatal disease called **hereditary surfactant protein B deficiency** has been described as an uncommon cause of **respiratory failure** in full-term newborn infants. Alveolar air spaces are filled with granular eosinophilic proteinaceous material and tubular myelin is absent. Even though aggressive medical interventions have been applied in these cases, including surfactant replacement therapy, infants afflicted with this disease typically die within the first year of life. It was found that this disease is an autosomal recessive condition typically characterized by a complete absence or mutation of one of the genes encoding surfactant proteins, *SURFACTANT PROTEIN B* (*SP-B*).

The genetic basis for hereditary *SP-B* deficiency has been examined. In most cases, a **frameshift mutation** in exon 4 of the human *SP-B* gene has been identified. This mutation results in premature termination of translation of the *SP-B* protein. Other mutations of the *SP-B* gene have also been identified that result in synthesis of defective forms of the *SP-B* protein. It has also been demonstrated that effects of *SP-B* deficiency extend beyond the disruption of translation of the *SP-B* gene. The results of studies of null mutations of the *Surfactant B* gene in transgenic mice, for example, show that although the amount of *Surfactant C* or *Surfactant A* mRNA is not affected, precursors of the mature *Surfactant C* protein are not completely processed. In addition, the processing of pulmonary phospholipids is also disrupted. Similar disruptions of *SURFACTANT C* peptide and phospholipid processing have been described in a human infant with *SP-B* deficiency. More than 15 different mutations in the *SP-B* gene have been associated with hereditary *SP-B* deficiency. Mild mutations can cause chronic pulmonary disease in infants. Although these studies have been useful in diagnosis, it is hoped that they will also lead to effective therapies for this usually fatal disease.

IN THE RESEARCH LAB

APPROACHES FOR STUDYING LUNG DEVELOPMENT AND BRANCHING MORPHOGENESIS

Organ Culture

Just after formation of the primary bronchial buds, the lung primordia can be removed from embryonic birds or mice and cultured in media free of serum and other exogenous growth factors. Under these conditions, the lung primordia will grow and branch for a few days. However, in the absence of an intact vascular system, complete development is not possible. With this limitation, it is possible to use these cultured lungs to analyze the roles of growth factors and other agents in the branching process. In one such study, a small peptide that served as a competitive inhibitor of ligand binding to *Integrins* resulted in abnormal morphology of the developing lung primordium. In another study, incubation with monoclonal antibodies to specific sequences of the extracellular matrix protein *Laminin* resulted in reduction of terminal buds and segmental dilation of the explanted lung primordia. In another strategy, lung explants were treated with antisense oligonucleotides, which bind with and inactivate the mRNA of the specific factor of interest. Experiments with antisense oligonucleotides against transcription factors such as *Thyroid transcription factor1* (*Ttf1*) resulted in reduction in the number of terminal branches of the lung primordium. It is possible to cleanly separate the endoderm of the lung buds from the mesoderm and to culture each alone or together and in the presence of purified factors. This can reveal the mechanisms by which these layers and factors interact in vivo.

Transgenic and Gene-Targeting Technologies

Genetic strategies, including the generation of engineered loss-of-function mutations (gene knock outs) and gain-of-function transgenes, have provided important insights into lung development. Recent advances have enabled genes to be deleted only in lung epithelial cells, either in the embryo or the adult, thus bypassing the early lethality of some null mutations. In addition, transgenes can be selected that drive expression of proteins in specific respiratory cells types. Among the examples, a *Surfactant B* gene null mutation was described in the preceding "In the Clinic" section of this chapter. Similar approaches have implicated many transcription factors in the control of lung growth, differentiation, and branching. These include the proto-oncogene *N-myc*, the homeodomain protein *Gata6*, and the Lim homeodomain factor *Lhx4* (previously known as *Gsh4*). Similarly, the homeodomain-containing transcription factor *Thyroid transcription factor1* (*Ttf1*), and the winged helix transcription factors *Foxa1* and *Foxa2* (previously known, respectively, as *Hepatic nuclear factor3α* and *β*, or *Hnf3α*

and *β*), have been shown to be required for the regulation of lung cell genes, including surfactant synthesis. A dramatic result was obtained by the targeted disruption of the function of a *Fibroblast growth factor* (*Fgf*) *receptor* protein in the lung. A transgene consisting of the *Surfactant C* promoter element and a mutant form of the *Fgf receptor* that lacked a kinase sequence was constructed and injected into fertilized eggs to generate transgenic mice. Inclusion of the *Surfactant C* promoter element in the transgene resulted in its expression only in the airway epithelium. The rationale behind the experiment is that formation of a functional *Fgf receptor* requires dimerization of two normal *Fgf* protein monomers. Therefore, the dimerization of the mutant protein produced by the transgene with the endogenous wild-type (normal) *Fgf* protein, resulted in formation of inactive receptors only in the lungs. As a consequence, other tissue of the embryos developed normally, but branching of the respiratory tree in the transgenic pups was completely inhibited. This resulted in formation of elongated epithelial tubes that were incapable of supporting normal respiratory function at birth (Fig. 11-5). Subsequent gene-targeting experiments in mice demonstrated that *Fibroblast growth factor 10* (*Fgf10*) and an isoform of its receptor in the respiratory epithelium, the *Fgf-receptor2*, were critical for formation of both lungs and limbs. Similarly, ablation of *Ttf1* blocked formation of both thyroid and lung.

Genetic strategies have also been used to create models of human pulmonary disease such as **cystic fibrosis**. Mouse mutants in which the c-AMP–stimulated chloride secretory activity of the cystic fibrosis gene is absent or reduced have been created by homologous recombination. These mice express some, but not all, of the abnormal phenotypes characteristic of the human disease. In other experiments, transgenic mice have been created that carry the normal human cystic fibrosis gene to demonstrate that it is nontoxic and, therefore, probably safe to use in human therapy. Currently, various approaches for human gene therapy of cystic fibrosis are being developed with viral- and DNA-based delivery systems. The long-term goal is to insert the cystic fibrosis gene directly to the somatic airway epithelial cells of afflicted infants and children.

Molecular and Cellular Basis of Branching Morphogenesis and Alveolar Differentiation

As discussed earlier in the chapter, the endodermal bronchial buds and subsequent airway branches grow into the mesenchyme surrounding the thoracic gut tube. Deficiencies or abnormalities in the branching of the respiratory tree are the basis of many forms of **pulmonary hypoplasia** (discussed in the preceding "In the Clinic" section of this chapter). Studies over the past several decades have demonstrated that

11

branching **morphogenesis** of the respiratory tree is regulated by reciprocal interaction between the endoderm and surrounding mesoderm. For example, when mesenchyme in the region of the bifurcating bronchial buds is replaced with mesenchyme from around the developing trachea, further branching is inhibited. Conversely, replacement of tracheal mesenchyme with that from the region of the bifurcating bronchial buds stimulates ectopic tracheal budding and branching. Based on experiments such as these, components of the **extracellular matrix** and **growth factors** have both been implicated in the stimulation and inhibition of branching. For example, *Collagens types IV* and *V, Laminin, Fibronectin,* and *Tenascin*—all components of the extracellular matrix—are thought to play either a permissive or a stimulatory role in branching of the bronchial buds. Likewise, regulation of expression of receptors for these matrix components has also been implicated in control of branching morphogenesis.

Many **growth factors** have been implicated in the growth, differentiation, and branching morphogenesis of the lung. Among them are Retinoic acid (RA), *Transforming growth factorβ* (Tgfβ), *Bone morphogenetic proteins* (Bmps), *Sonic hedgehog* (Shh), *Wnts, Fgfs, Epithelial growth factor* (Egf), *Platelet-derived growth factor* (Pdgf), *Insulin-like growth factor* (Igf), and *Transforming growth factorα* (TGFα). These growth factors and their receptors are expressed in specific cell populations during different phases of lung growth and branching, consistent with their postulated roles in this complex process. For example, branching during the **pseudoglandular stage** is apparently influenced in part by the dynamic activity of RA, *Shh, Fgf (especially Fgf10), Bmp,* and *TGFβ* signaling pathways. Thus, experiments have shown that *Fgf10,* produced by the mesenchyme overlying the tips of the outgrowing bronchial buds, promotes both the proliferation of the endoderm and its outward **chemotaxis** (i.e., directed movement according to the presence of so-called chemotactic factors in the cellular environment). On the other hand, *Shh,* produced by the endoderm, promotes the proliferation and differentiation of the overlying mesoderm. Genetic deletion of either *Fgf10* or *Shh* leads to profound inhibition of lung development and branching morphogenesis.

Growth factors such as *Fgfs* and *Egf* not only regulate the early growth and branching of the lung, but also the later formation and maturation of terminal sacs during the saccular stage. Later still *PdgfA* is required for the postnatal formation of alveolar septae–containing myofibroblasts. Like *Ttf1* and *Foxa1/a2* (discussed in the preceding section of this "In the Clinic"), cytokines, glucocorticoids, and thyroxine stimulate surfactant synthesis before birth. It is hoped that these findings will lead to therapeutic stimulation of adequate alveolar formation and differentiation and surfactant synthesis within the lungs of premature infants.

Considerable effort has also been spent in identifying genes that regulate the differentiation of lung progenitor cells into specialized types such as ciliated, secretory (Clara), and neuroendocrine cells. For example, analysis of lungs from mice lacking the gene *Mash1* (a member of the *Notch* pathway; discussed in Ch. 5) have shown that they lack neuroendocrine cells, whereas in *Hes1* (another member of the *Notch* pathway) null mutants, neuroendocrine cells form prematurely and in larger numbers than normal. The gene *Foxj1* (one of the many *Fox* transcription factors) is required for the development of differentiated ciliated cells. The formation of submucosal glands, which are the major source of mucus production in the normal lung, is also regulated genetically. Mice lacking genes controlling the *Ectodysplasin* (*Eda/Edar*) signaling pathway (a gene involved in epithelial morphogenesis; discussed in Ch. 7) do not develop submuscosal glands. These glands are also absent in humans lacking the *EDA* gene.

DROSOPHILA TRACHEAL SYSTEM DEVELOPMENT

The respiratory organ in Drosophila, the tracheal system, consists of a branched network of tubes. Interestingly, given the central role for *Fgf* signaling in vertebrate lung development just discussed, formation of the tracheal system also involves Drosophila orthologs of the *Fgf* signaling system. Three components of this system have been identified during development of the tracheal system: *Branchless,* an *Fgf*-like ligand; *Breathless,* an *Fgf receptor;* and *Sprouty,* an endogenous *Fgf* inhibitor. Although at least 30 other genes are involved in tracheal development, *Branchless* and *Breathless* are used repeatedly to control branch budding and outgrowth. *Sprouty* provides negative feedback regulation by antagonizing *Fgf* signaling, thereby limiting the amount of branching that occurs.

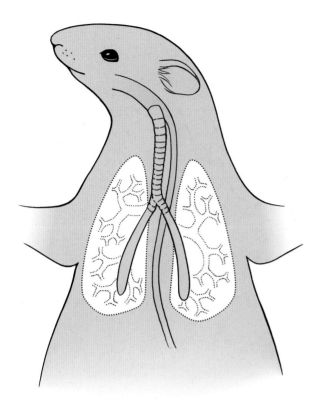

Figure 11-5. Mutation of a *Fibroblast growth factor receptor* specifically expressed in the lungs results in inhibition of branching of the respiratory tree and formation of elongated epithelial tubes that end bluntly. The outline of the lungs and their wild-type branching pattern is shown in stippling.

Partitioning of Coelom and Formation of Diaphragm

At the beginning of the 4th week of development, prior to body folding, the **intraembryonic coelom** forms a horseshoe-shaped space that partially encircles the future head end of the embryo (Fig. 11-6). Cranially, the intraembryonic coelom lies just caudal to the **septum transversum** and represents the future **pericardial cavity**. The two caudally directed limbs of the horseshoe-shaped intraembryonic coelom represent the continuous future **pleural** and **peritoneal cavities**. At about the midtrunk and more caudal levels, the intraembryonic coelom on each side is continuous with the **extraembryonic coelom** or chorionic cavity.

With body folding, changes occur in the position of the intraembryonic coelom. The **head fold** moves

the future pericardial cavity caudally and repositions it on the anterior (ventral) side of the developing head (Fig. 11-7*A*). The septum transversum, which initially constitutes a partition that lies cranial to the future pericardial cavity, is repositioned by the head fold to lie caudal to the future pericardial cavity. The developing heart (discussed further in Ch. 12), which initially lies ventral to the future pericardial cavity, is repositioned dorsally and quickly begins to bulge into the pericardial cavity. Thus, after formation of the head fold, the intraembryonic coelom is reshaped into a ventral cranial expansion (**primitive pericardial cavity**); two narrow canals called **pericardioperitoneal canals** (future **pleural cavities**) that lie dorsal to the septum transversum; and two more caudal areas (future **peritoneal cavities**) where the intraembryonic and extraembryonic coeloms are broadly continuous (Fig. 11-7*B*).

During the 4th and 5th weeks, the continued folding and differential growth of the embryonic axis cause a gradual caudal displacement of the septum transversum. The ventral edge of the septum finally becomes fixed to the anterior body wall at the 7th thoracic level, and the dorsal connection to the esophageal mesenchyme becomes fixed at the 12th thoracic level. Meanwhile, myoblasts (muscle cell precursors) differentiate within the septum transversum. These cells, which will form part of the future diaphragm muscle, are innervated by spinal nerves at a transient, cervical level of the septum transversum—that is, by fibers from the spinal nerves of cervical levels 3, 4, and 5 (C3, C4, C5). These fibers join together to form the paired **phrenic nerves**, which elongate as they follow the migrating septum caudally.

Pericardial Sac is Formed by Pleuropericardial Folds That Grow from Lateral Body Wall in a Coronal Plane

During the 5th week, the pleural and pericardial cavities are divided from each other by **pleuropericardial folds** that originate along the lateral body walls in a coronal plane (Fig. 11-8; see Fig. 11-7*B*). These septae appear as broad folds of mesenchyme and pleura that grow medially toward each other between the heart and the developing lungs. At the end of the 5th week, the folds meet and fuse with the foregut mesenchyme, thus subdividing the primitive pericardial cavity into three compartments: a fully enclosed, ventral **definitive pericardial cavity** and two dorsolateral **pleural cavities**. The latter are still continuous

11

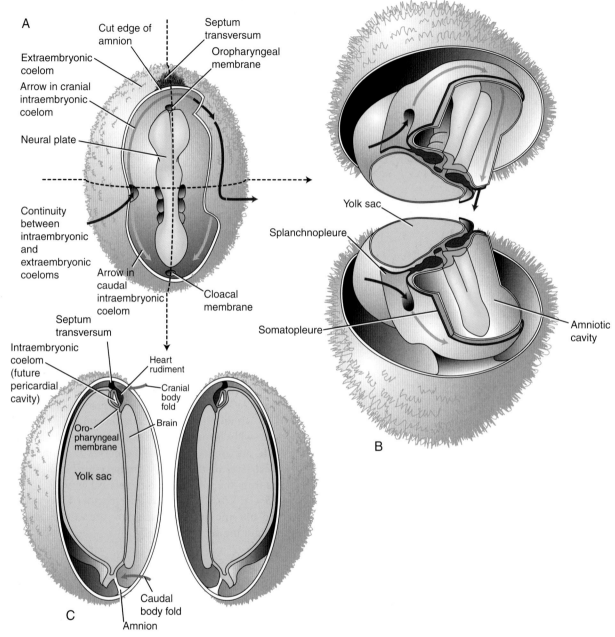

Figure 11-6. The intraembryonic coelom prior to body folding. *A*, At the beginning of the 4th week the intraembryonic coelom forms a horseshoe-shaped space partially encircling the head end of the embryo. Diagram of the epiblast after removal of the amnion showing the position of the neural plate, oropharyngeal and cloacal membranes, and intraembryonic coelom; the latter is continuous with the extraembryonic coelom at about the midtrunk and more caudal levels. *B*, Cranial (top) and caudal (bottom) halves of embryos transected at the level indicated in *A*. Arrows show continuity between the intraembryonic and extraembryonic coeloms. *C*, Midsagittal view through the right side of an embryo at the level indicated in *A*. Arrows show the direction of the head and tail body folds.

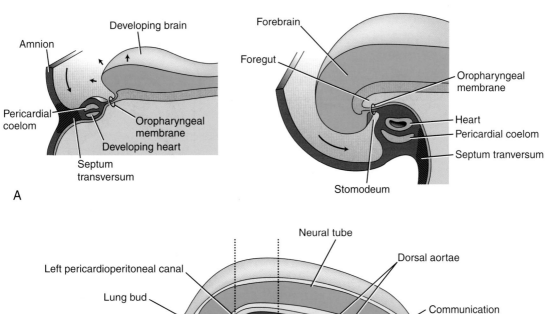

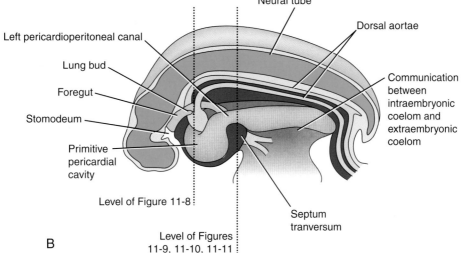

Figure 11-7. Body folding changes the shape of the intraembryonic coelom. *A*, The head end of the embryo prior to (top) and after (bottom) formation of the head fold. *B*, Initial subdivision of the intraembryonic coelom into a primitive pericardial cavity, paired pericardioperitoneal canals, and paired peritoneal cavities. The latter are continuous on each side with the extraembryonic coelom. Subsequent lateral body folding progressively separates the intraembryonic and extraembryonic coeloms as the yolk stalk narrows.

with the more caudal peritoneal cavities through the pericardioperitoneal canals. The name *pericardioperitoneal* is retained for these canals, even though they now provide communication between the pleural cavities and the peritoneal cavities.

As the tips of the pleuropericardial folds grow medially toward each other, their roots migrate toward the ventral midline (see Fig. 11-8*B, C*). By the time the tips of the folds meet to seal off the pericardial cavity, their roots take origin from the ventral midline. Thus, the space that originally constituted the lateral portion of the primitive pericardial cavity is

converted into the ventrolateral part of the right and left pleural cavities.

The pleuropericardial folds are three-layered, consisting of mesenchyme sandwiched between two epithelial layers; all three layers are derived from body wall. The thin definitive pericardial sac retains this threefold composition, consisting of inner and outer serous membranes (the inner **serous pericardium** and the outer **mediastinal pleura**) separated by a delicate filling of mesenchyme-derived connective tissue, the **fibrous pericardium**. The phrenic nerves, which originally run through the portion of the body wall

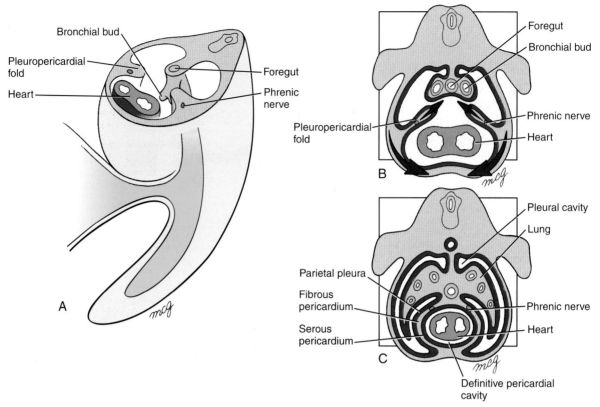

Figure 11-8. Subdivision of the primitive pericardial cavity. *A,* During the 5th week, pleuropericardial folds grow out from the lateral body wall toward the midline, where they fuse with each other and with mesoderm associated with the esophagus. Simultaneously, the roots of these folds migrate ventrally so that they ultimately originate from the ventral body wall. *B,* The phrenic nerves initially embedded in the body wall are swept into these developing partitions. *C,* The pleuropericardial folds with their associated serous membrane form the pericardial sac and transform the primitive pericardial cavity into a definitive pericardial cavity and right and left pleural cavities.

mesenchyme incorporated into the pleuropericardial folds, course through the fibrous pericardium of the adult.

Pleuroperitoneal Membranes Growing from Posterior and Lateral Body Wall Seal Off Pericardioperitoneal Canals

Recall that the **septum transversum** is repositioned by the head fold to lie ventral to the paired **pericardio-peritoneal canals** (Fig. 11-9; see Fig. 11-7*B*). At the beginning of the 5th week, a pair of membranes, the **pleuroperitoneal membranes**, arise along an oblique line connecting the root of the 12th rib with the tips of ribs 12 through 7 (Fig. 11-10). These membranes grow ventrally to fuse with the septum transversum, thus

sealing off the pericardioperitoneal canals. The left pericardioperitoneal canal is larger than the right and closes later. Closure of both canals is complete by the 7th week. The membranes that close these canals are called *pleuroperitoneal membranes* because they do not contact the septum transversum until after the pericardial sac is formed; thus, after they fuse with the septum transversum, they separate the definitive pleural cavities from the peritoneal cavity.

Diaphragm Is a Composite Derived from Four Embryonic Structures

The definitive musculotendinous **diaphragm** incorporates derivatives of four embryonic structures: (1) the septum transversum, (2) pleuroperitoneal membranes,

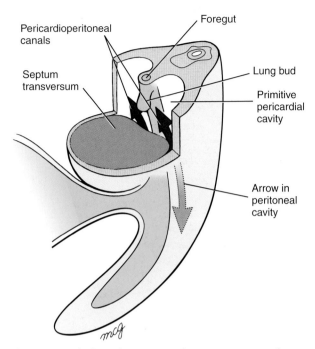

Figure 11-9. In the future thoracic region, the septum transversum forms a ventral partition beneath the paired pericardioperitoneal canals (arrows), which interconnect the primitive pericardial cavity cranially and peritoneal cavities caudally.

(3) mesoderm of the body wall, and (4) esophageal mesenchyme (Fig 11-11A). Some of the myoblasts that arise in the septum transversum emigrate into the pleuroperitoneal membranes, pulling their phrenic nerve branches along with them. Most of the septum transversum then gives rise to the nonmuscular **central tendon** of the diaphragm (Fig. 11-11B).

The bulk of the **diaphragm muscle** within the pleuroperitoneal membranes is innervated by the phrenic nerve. However, the outer rim of diaphragmatic muscle arises from a ring of body wall mesoderm (see Figs. 11-10A, 11-11B); this mesoderm is derived from somatic mesoderm and is invaded by myoblasts arising from the myotomes of the neighboring somites. Therefore, the peripheral musculature of the diaphragm is innervated by spinal nerves from thoracic spinal levels T7 through T12. Finally, mesoderm arising from vertebral levels L1 through L3 condenses to form two muscular bands, the **right** and **left crura** of the diaphragm, which originate on the vertebral column and insert into the dorsomedial diaphragm (see Fig. 11-11B). The right crus originates on vertebral bodies L1 through L3, and the left crus originates on vertebral bodies L1 and L2.

11

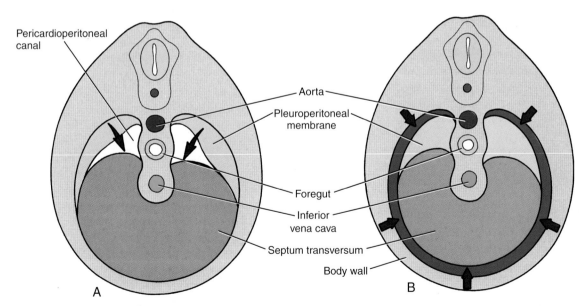

Figure 11-10. A, B, Closure of the pericardioperitoneal canals. Between weeks 5 and 7, a pair of horizontal pleuroperitoneal membranes grow from the posterior body wall to meet the septum transversum *(arrows)* A, thus closing the pericardioperitoneal canals. These membranes form the posterior portions of the diaphragm and completely seal off the pleural cavities from the peritoneal cavity. Arrows in B indicate invasion of the developing diaphram by muscle fibers from the adjacent body wall.

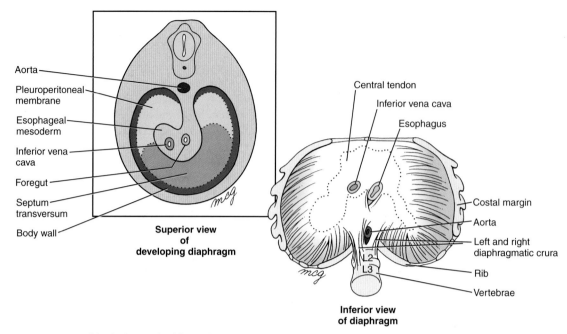

Figure 11-11. Formation of the diaphragm. The definitive diaphragm is a composite structure including elements of the septum transversum, pleuroperitoneal membranes, and esophageal mesenchyme, as well as a rim of body wall mesoderm.

IN THE CLINIC

DIAPHRAGMATIC DEFECTS AND PULMONARY HYPOPLASIA

As discussed earlier in the chapter, **pulmonary hypoplasia** often occurs in response to some conditions that reduce the volume of the pleural cavity and thereby restrict growth of the lungs. In **congenital diaphragmatic hernia**, the developing abdominal viscera bulge into the pleural cavity (Fig. 11-12). If the mass of displaced viscera is large enough, it will stunt growth of the lung on that side. Congenital diaphragmatic hernia occurs in about 1 of 2500 live births. The left side of the diaphragm is involved four to eight times more often than is the right, probably because the left pericardioperitoneal canal is larger and closes later than the right. Diaphragmatic hernias can be surgically corrected at birth and have also rarely been corrected by surgery during fetal life (discussed in Ch. 6). However, if the hernia has resulted in severe pulmonary hypoplasia, the newborn may die of pulmonary insufficiency even if the hernia is repaired. Small congenital hernias sometimes occur in the parasternal region or through the esophageal hiatus, but these usually do not have severe clinical consequences.

If the development of muscle tissue in the diaphragm is deficient, the excessively compliant diaphragm may allow the underlying abdominal contents to balloon or **eventrate** into the pulmonary cavity (Fig. 11-13). This condition can also result in pulmonary hypoplasia, which may be fatal.

OLIGOHYDRAMNIOS AND PULMONARY HYPOPLASIA

As discussed earlier in the chapter, pulmonary hypoplasia can result from failure of proper branching morphogenesis during development of the lungs and respiratory tree, as well as from diaphragmatic defects as just described. Another classic cause of pulmonary hypoplasia is **oligohydramnios**, the condition in which there is an insufficient amount of amniotic fluid. Presumably, oligohydramnios causes pulmonary hypoplasia by reducing the volume of fluid "inhaled" by the fetus, and consequently reducing fluid pressure within the respiratory tree. Compression of the fetal chest by the uterine wall may also play a role. Beginning at about 16 weeks of gestation, a substantial fraction of the amniotic fluid is contributed by the fetal kidneys. Therefore, **bilateral renal agenesis**—failure of both kidneys to form (discussed in Ch. 15)—results in oligohydramnios. Finally, oligohydramnios can result form premature rupture of the amnion.

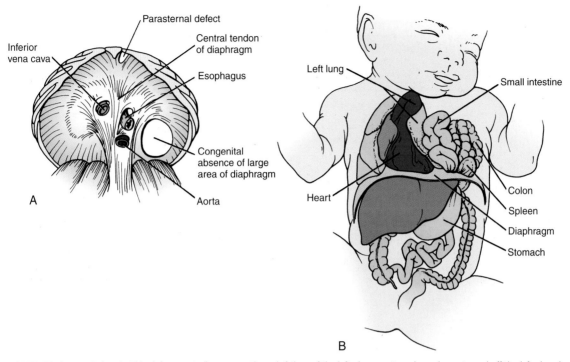

Figure 11-12. Diaphragmatic hernia. This defect most often occurs through failure of the left pleuroperitoneal membrane to seal off the left pleural cavity completely from the peritoneal cavity. *A,* Inferior view. *B,* Abdominal contents may herniate through the patent pericardioperitoneal canal, preventing normal development of the lung on that side.

IN THE RESEARCH LAB

CONGENITAL DIAPHRAGMATIC HERNIA

Little is known about the molecular mechanisms of diaphragm formation and how this process fails to occur, resulting in congenital diaphragmatic hernia (CDH). However, it was recently shown in a screen of fetal mice harboring ENU-induced genetic mutations that CDH resulted from a mutation in the *Fog2* (*Friend of Gata2*; *Gata2* is a transcription factor) gene. In addition, pulmonary hypoplasia occurred early in gestation and *Fog2* was expressed throughout the pulmonary mesenchyme during stages of branching morpho-genesis, suggesting a direct role of *Fog2* in pulmonary development. Screening of DNA from patients with congenital diaphragramatic defects revealed mutations in *FOG2*, demonstrating a role for this gene in development of the diaphragm in both mouse and human.

Additional evidence that *FOG2* is critical for normal diaphragm formation comes from studies that have shown that *Fog2* is an important regulator of *Gata4* in the developing heart, and that both genes are coexpressed during cardiac embryogenesis. Homozygous mice null for *Gata4* also have CDH, suggesting that abnormal regulation of *Gata4* by *Fog2* might also be important for diaphragm development. Furthermore, *Fog2* binds to the ligand-binding domain of *Chicken ovalbumin upstream promoter transcription factor II* (*Coup-tfII*). *Coup-tfII* has been shown to be necessary for *Fog2* to repress the transcription of a *Gata4*. Importantly, mice with tissue-specific mutations of *Coup-TFII* have CDH and *Coup-TFII* is located on human chromosome 15q26.2, a genomic region that is deleted in some CDH patients.

11

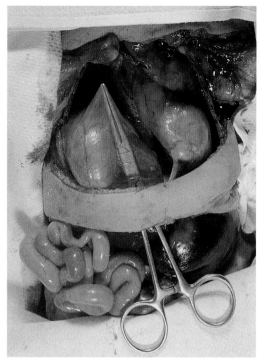

Figure 11-13. Eventration of the diaphragm. Failure of the pleuroperitoneal membranes to differentiate normally during fetal life may allow abdominal organs to dilate the abnormally thin regions of the diaphragm and eventrate into the pleural cavity.

Suggested Readings

Ackerman KG, Herron BJ, Vargas SO, et al. 2005. Fog2 is required for normal diaphragm and lung development in mice and humans. PLoS Genet 1:58-65.

Affolter M, Bellusci S, Itoh N, et al. 2003. Tube or not tube: remodeling epithelial tissues by branching morphogenesis. Dev Cell 4:11-18.

Affolter M, Shilo BZ. 2000. Genetic control of branching morphogenesis during Drosophila tracheal development. Curr Opin Cell Biol 12:731-735.

Breakthroughs in Bioscience. 2004. Bubbles, babies and biology: The story of surfactant. opa.faseb.org/pages/Publications/breakthroughs.htm.

Cardoso WV. 2000. Lung morphogenesis revisited: old facts, current ideas. Dev Dyn 219:121-130.

Cardoso WV. 2001. Molecular regulation of lung development. Annu Rev Physiol 63:471-494.

Cardoso WV, Lu J. 2006. Regulation of early lung morphogenesis: questions, facts and controversies. Development 133:1611-1624.

Chuang PT, McMahon AP. 2003. Branching morphogenesis of the lung: new molecular insights into an old problem. Trends Cell Biol 13:86-91.

Davies JA. 2002. Do different branching epithelia use a conserved developmental mechanism? Bioessays 24:937-948.

del Moral PM, De Langhe SP, Sala FG, et al. 2006. Differential role of FGF9 on epithelium and mesenchyme in mouse embryonic lung. Dev Biol 293:77-89.

Denholm B, Skaer H. 2003. Tubulogenesis: a role for the apical extracellular matrix? Curr Biol 13:R909-R911.

Desai TJ, Chen F, Lu J, et al. 2006. Distinct roles for retinoic acid receptors alpha and beta in early lung morphogenesis. Dev Biol 291:12-24.

Ghabrial A, Luschnig S, Metzstein MM, Krasnow MA. 2003. Branching morphogenesis of the Drosophila tracheal system. Annu Rev Cell Dev Biol 19:623-647.

Hogan BL, Kolodziej PA. 2002. Organogenesis: molecular mechanisms of tubulogenesis. Nat Rev Genet 3:513-523.

Holder AM, Klaassens M, Tibboel D, et al. 2007. Genetic factors in congenital diaphragmatic hernia. Am J Hum Genet 80:825-845.

Ito T, Udaka N, Yazawa T, et al. 2000. Basic helix-loop-helix transcription factors regulate the neuroendocrine differentiation of fetal mouse pulmonary epithelium. Development 127:3913-3921.

Liu X, Driskell RR, Engelhardt JF. 2004. Airway glandular development and stem cells. Curr Top Dev Biol 64:33-56.

Lubarsky B, Krasnow MA. 2003. Tube morphogenesis: making and shaping biological tubes. Cell 112:19-28.

Lung database: www.ana.ed.ac.uk/database/lungbase/lunghome.html.

Maden M. 2004. Retinoids in lung development and regeneration. Curr Top Dev Biol 61:153-189.

Mariani TJ, Kaminski N. 2004. Gene expression studies in lung development and lung stem cell biology. Curr Top Dev Biol 64:57-71.

Nguyen NM, Senior RM. 2006. Laminin isoforms and lung development: all isoforms are not equal. Dev Biol 294:271-279.

Pauling MH, Vu TH. 2004. Mechanisms and regulation of lung vascular development. Curr Top Dev Biol 64:73-99.

Prodhan P, Kinane TB. 2002. Developmental paradigms in terminal lung development. Bioessays 24:1052-1059.

Rosin D, Shilo BZ. 2002. Branch-specific migration cues in the Drosophila tracheal system. Bioessays 24:110-113.

Sudarsan V. 2003. Tube morphogenesis: no pipe dream in Drosophila. Curr Biol 13:R131-R133.

Uv A, Cantera R, Samakovlis C. 2003. Drosophila tracheal morphogenesis: intricate cellular solutions to basic plumbing problems. Trends Cell Biol 13:301-309.

Warburton D, Berberich MA, Driscoll B. 2004. Stem/progenitor cells in lung morphogenesis, repair, and regeneration. Curr Top Dev Biol 64:1-16.

Warburton D, Schwarz M, Tefft D, et al. 2000. The molecular basis of lung morphogenesis. Mech Dev 92:55-81.

White AC, Xu J, Yin Y, et al. 2006. FGF9 and SHH signaling coordinate lung growth and development through regulation of distinct mesenchymal domains. Development 133:1507-1517.

Whitsett JA, Wert SE, Trapnell BC. 2004. Genetic disorders influencing lung formation and function at birth. Hum Mol Genet 13 Spec No 2:R207-R215.

Zelzer E, Shilo BZ. 2000. Cell fate choices in Drosophila tracheal morphogenesis. Bioessays 22:219-226.

Development of the Heart **12**

Summary In response to inductive and permissive signals emanating from the endoderm, ectoderm, and midline mesoderm, cardiogenic precursors form a cardiac primordium within the splanchnic mesoderm at the cranial end of the embryonic disc called the **cardiac crescent**, or **primary heart field**. In response to signals from the underlying endoderm, a subpopulation of cells within the cardiac crescent form a pair **lateral endocardial tubes** through the process of **vasculogenesis**. The cranial and lateral folding of the embryo during the early 4th week causes these tubes to be brought together along the midline in the future thoracic region, where they fuse to form a single **primitive heart tube**, with the adjacent mesoderm differentiating into cardiomyocytes.

Between weeks 4 and 8, the primitive heart tube undergoes a process of looping, remodeling, realignment, and septation that transforms its single lumen into the four chambers of the definitive heart, thus laying down the basis for the separation of pulmonary and systemic circulations at birth.

Lengthening of the primitive heart tube and proper cardiac looping are driven through the addition of cardiac precursor cells by the **secondary heart field**. As the heart tube lengthens, it develops a series of expansions and shallow sulci that subdivide it into primordial heart chambers. Starting at the inflow end, these are the left and right horns of the **sinus venosus**, the **primitive atrium**, the **primitive ventricle**, the **bulbus cordis**, and the **outflow tract**. The bulbus cordis forms much of the right ventricle, whereas the primitive ventricle gives rise to the left ventricle. The outflow tract (the **conotruncus**) will form the **conus arteriosus** and the **truncus arteriosus**, both of which split to become outflow regions of the two ventricles, and the ascending aorta and pulmonary trunk.

Venous blood initially enters the sinus horns through paired, symmetrical **common cardinal veins**. However, as described in Chapter 13, changes in the venous system rapidly shift the entire systemic venous return to the right so that all blood from the body and umbilicus enters the future right atrium through the developing **superior** and **inferior venae cavae**. The left sinus horn becomes the **coronary sinus**, which drains the myocardium. A process of intussusception incorporates the right sinus horn and the ostia of the venae cavae into the posterior wall of the future right atrium, displacing the original right half of the primitive atrium. Meanwhile, the **pulmonary vein** develops in the midline and then shifts to the future left atrium; the trunk of the pulmonary vein is subsequently incorporated by intussusception to form most of the left atrium. In the 5th and 6th weeks, a pair of septa, the **septum primum** and the **septum secundum**, grow to separate the right and left atria. These septa are perforated by a staggered pair of foramina that allow right-to-left shunting of blood throughout gestation. The **bicuspid (mitral)** and **tricuspid atrioventricular valves** also develop from atrioventricular cushion tissue during the 5th and 6th weeks. Meanwhile, the heart undergoes remodeling that brings the future atria and ventricles into correct alignment with each other and also aligns both ventricles with their respective outflow vessels. The bulbus cordis expands to form the right ventricle, and during the 6th week a **muscular ventricular septum** partially separates the ventricles. During the 7th and 8th week, the outflow tract of the heart has completed the process of septation and division, converting it into the separate, helically arranged outflow regions of both ventricles and ascending aorta and pulmonary trunk. During this process, remodeling within the distal conus arteriosus gives rise to the **semilunar valves** of the aorta and pulmonary artery. Complete ventricular septation requires fusion between the muscular interventricular, conotruncal, and atrioventricular septa.

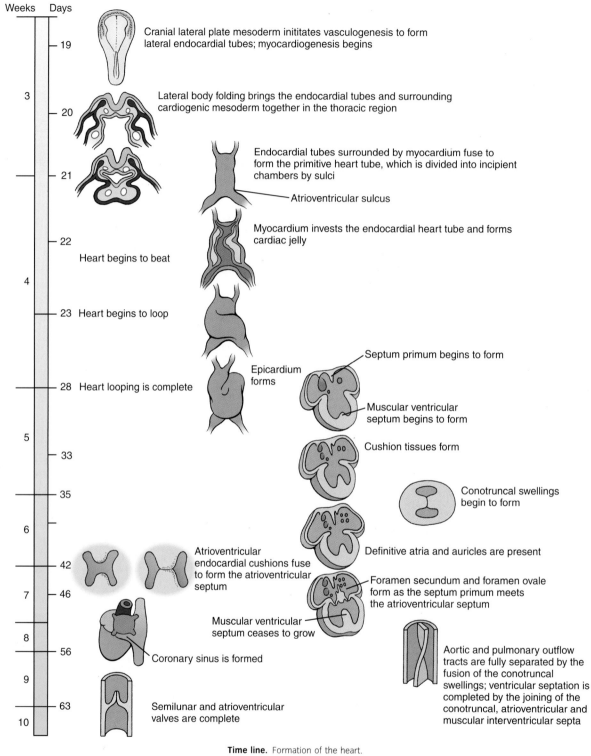

Weeks | Days

19 — Cranial lateral plate mesoderm inititates vasculogenesis to form lateral endocardial tubes; myocardiogenesis begins

3

20 — Lateral body folding brings the endocardial tubes and surrounding cardiogenic mesoderm together in the thoracic region

21 — Endocardial tubes surrounded by myocardium fuse to form the primitive heart tube, which is divided into incipient chambers by sulci

Atrioventricular sulcus

22 — Myocardium invests the endocardial heart tube and forms cardiac jelly

Heart begins to beat

4

23 — Heart begins to loop

Septum primum begins to form

28 — Heart looping is complete

Epicardium forms

Muscular ventricular septum begins to form

5

33 — Cushion tissues form

35 — Conotruncal swellings begin to form

6

Atrioventricular endocardial cushions fuse to form the atrioventricular septum

Definitive atria and auricles are present

42 —

7 — 46

Foramen secundum and foramen ovale form as the septum primum meets the atrioventricular septum

Muscular ventricular septum ceases to grow

Coronary sinus is formed

8

56 —

Aortic and pulmonary outflow tracts are fully separated by the fusion of the conotruncal swellings; ventricular septation is completed by the joining of the conotruncal, atrioventricular and muscular interventricular septa

9

63 — Semilunar and atrioventricular valves are complete

10

Time line. Formation of the heart.

A full-term boy is born to a primigravid (first gestation) mother after an uncomplicated pregnancy. The delivery goes smoothly, with healthy Apgar scores of 8/10 at 1 minute and 9/10 at 5 minutes. Growth parameters (length, weight, and head circumference) are all normal, ranging between the 10th and 25th centiles. The newborn exam is also normal, and the infant is returned to his mother to begin breastfeeding.

The boy initially feeds well, but he becomes sleepy and disinterested in feeding as the day progresses. At 20 hours after birth, he exhibits decreased peripheral perfusion, cyanosis, and lethargy. A pulse oximeter shows oxygen saturation in the low 80% range (normal equals >90%) with increasing **respiratory distress**. Paradoxically, blood oxygen saturation worsens after administration of oxygen. The boy is emergently transferred to the neonatal intensive care unit in worsening shock. There, he is intubated, central intravascular catheters are placed, and he is started on **prostaglandins**.

A chest x-ray shows **cardiomegaly** (enlarged heart) and increased pulmonary vascularity (indicative of increased blood flow). An **echocardiogram** shows a very small left ventricle with a small aortic outflow tract, leading to the diagnosis of **hypoplastic left heart syndrome** (HLHS).

HLHS is a shunt-dependent lesion: survival of these patients depends on maintaining a **patent ductus arteriosus** (PDA) to carry blood from the pulmonary artery to the aorta and out to perfuse the systemic circulation. Supplemental oxygen lowers the resistance to pulmonary blood flow, causing blood to circulate to the lungs instead of crossing the PDA. Thus, administering supplemental oxygen actually decreases blood oxygen saturation. Administration of prostaglandins prevents the physiologic closure of the ductus arteriosus, maintaining systemic perfusion until surgery can be performed. The first-stage surgery, called the Norwood procedure, connects the right ventricular outflow tract to the aorta, with a separate shunt to provide blood flow to the lungs. More surgeries follow at about 6 months and 2 to 3 years of age. Occasionally, heart transplantation is performed. The 5-year survival rate for HLHS is around 70%.

Establishing Cardiac Lineage

The heart is the first functioning organ in humans. It begins beating rhythmically as early as day 22 and pumps blood by days 24 to 25. Amazingly, much of cardiac development, including remodeling and septation, occurs while the heart is pumping blood. This is necessary to provide nutrients and oxygen and dispose of wastes during embryonic and fetal development. Morphologically, the embryonic heart is first identifiable as a single heart tube composed of contractile myocardium surrounding an inner endocardial (endothelial) tube, with an intervening extracellular matrix. The heart is also an asymmetric organ whose left-right patterning is established during gastrulation (left-right patterning is discussed in Ch. 3 and later in this chapter).

Cardiac progenitor cells are derived from intraembryonic mesoderm emerging from the cranial third of the primitive streak during early gastrulation. These progenitors leave the primitive streak and migrate in a cranial-lateral direction to become localized on either side of the primitive streak (Fig. 12-1A, B). *Mesp1* and *Mesp2*, members of the basic HLH family

of transcription factors, are expressed transiently during the primitive streak stage and are required for migration of the cardiac progenitor cells into the cranial region of the embryo. The cardiac progenitor cells eventually become localized within the cranial lateral plate mesoderm on both sides of the embryo, extending and arcing cranial to the developing head fold, forming a **cardiac crescent** (Fig. 12-1C). It is thought that the cardiac cell lineage is specified from mesodermal cells in the cardiac crescent. Cells in the cardiac crescent constitute the so-called **primary heart field**. As discussed later, the primary heart field is not the sole source of cardiogenic cells for the developing heart.

Formation of Primitive Heart Tube

With formation of the intraembryonic coelom, the lateral plate mesoderm is subdivided into somatic and splanchnic layers; the cardiac crescent forms within the splanchnic mesodermal subdivision. During the process of body folding (discussed in Ch.4), the

12

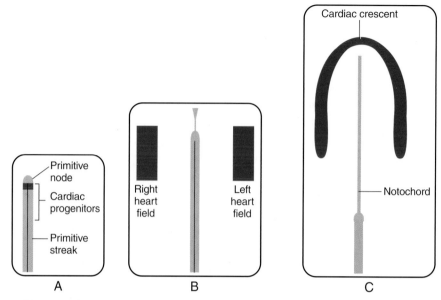

Figure 12-1. Formation of the primary heart field seen in ventral views. *A*, Presumptive location of cardiogenic progenitors in the early primitive streak. *B*, Location of migrating cardiogenic precursors within the mesoderm shortly after gastrulation and during initial specification. *C*, Location of the primary heart field (cardiac crescent) containing specified cardiogenic cells. The crescent-like arrangement of the progenitors is due to their migration pattern, local cardiogenic induction signals, and the development of the body folds.

IN THE RESEARCH LAB

SPECIFICATION OF CARDIAC PROGENITOR CELLS

To what degree cardiac progenitor cells within the epiblast and primitive streak are specified remains unknown. *Activin* and *Tgfβ* produced by the hypoblast of the chick induce cardiogenic properties in some of the overlying epiblast cells (Fig. 12-2*A, B*). Other members of the *Tgfβ* superfamily also play a role in inducing cardiogenic properties in the epiblast of the mouse, including *Nodal* and *Vg1*. During gastrulation, cardiac precursors residing in the primitive streak are uncommitted, but these progenitors become specified to become cardiogenic mesoderm soon after migrating into the lateral plate. Interaction of cranial lateral mesoderm with the endoderm is required for this cardiac specification. The endoderm secretes several signaling molecules—including *Bmp, Fgf, Activin, Insulin-like growth factor 2*, and *Shh*—that promote cell survival and proliferation of cardiogenic cells. One particularly important growth factor is *Bmp2*. Secreted by the endoderm, *Bmp2* is essential for stimulating the expression of early cardiogenic transcription factors such as *Nkx2.5* (*Nkx2 transcription factor related, locus 5*) and *Gata* (a protein that binds to a DNA GATA sequence) within the lateral mesoderm. In the chick embryo, *Bmp2* can induce expression of myocardial cell markers in ectopic regions (i.e., outside their proper position), whereas embryos lacking *Bmp2* fail to develop hearts. However, in mice lacking the *Bmp2* gene, cardiac specification of the mesoderm still occurs although heart development is abnormal. The fact that cardiac specification occurs in the absence of *Bmp2* is likely due to overlapping functions of other *Bmp* family members with *Bmp2*.

Bmp expression occurs in most of the endoderm but its effects on the mesoderm are limited to the lateral mesoderm. Why is this so? The reason is that *Bmp* antagonists and inhibitors are released from midline tissues. The notochord synthesizes and releases *Chordin* and *Noggin*, two molecules that sequester *Bmps* (Fig. 12-2*C*). If *Chordin* activity is blocked or if one forces over expression of *Bmp* in cranial paraxial mesoderm, the medial mesoderm has the capacity to form cardiac cells. In addition, the developing neural plate ectoderm releases *Wnt1* and *Wnt3a*, which further antagonize *Bmp* signaling. For instance if *Wnt* signaling in the endoderm is abrogated in mouse embryos, multiple hearts are generated. Therefore, because of the antagonizing effects of *Chordin/Noggin* and *Wnt* signaling on *Bmp* signaling, *the influence of Bmp on mesoderm is limited to lateral regions.*

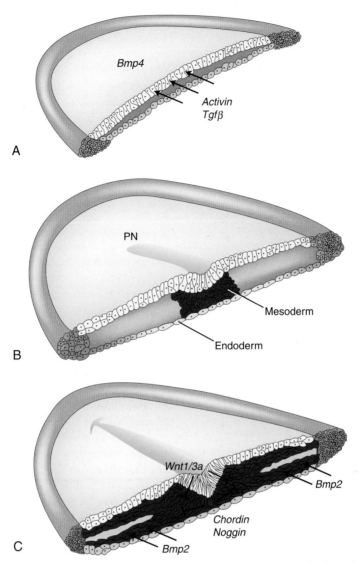

Figure 12-2. Induction of the primary heart field. *A, B,* Prior to and during gastrulation, *Tgfβ* and *Activin* released by the hypoblast induce cardiogenic potential in a subset of epiblast and newly forming mesodermal cells. *C, Bmps,* released from the newly formed endoderm, signal the formation of a cardiogenic lineage from the mesoderm, but their influence is limited to the lateral mesoderm due to the release of *Chordin* and *Noggin* from the notochord and *Wnt1/3a* from the forming neuroectoderm. PN, primitive node.

But why is the cardiogenic region limited to the *cranial* portion of the lateral mesoderm? We know that the caudal lateral plate mesoderm is capable of responding to cardiac specification signals: if it is grafted into the cranial region, it transforms into cardiogenic cells. As discussed earlier in this section, *Wnt1/Wnt3a* and *Chordin/Noggin* inhibit the effects of *Bmps* on mesoderm. Another *Wnt, Wnt8c,* is expressed both in the cranial and caudal mesoderm and it also inhibits *Bmp* effects on the mesoderm. Knowing *Bmp* secretion by the endoderm is required for cardiac mesoderm formation, how can *Bmp* still exert its influence on the cranial lateral mesoderm but not on the caudal lateral plate? The answer is that two other molecules are secreted by the cranial ectoderm that antagonize the negative effects of *Wnt8c* on *Bmp*-driven heart formation. One is *Crescent* (*FrzB2*), a member of the *FrzB* family of *Wnt* receptor antagonists (functions by sequestering *Wnt*); the other is *Dkk-1* (*Dickkopf1*), which binds to and inhibits the *Wnt* coreceptors of the *Lrp* (*Low-density lipoprotein receptor–related protein*) class (Fig. 12-3). Hence, in the absence of *Wnt* signaling, the effect of *Bmp* is to promote the cardiac lineage in the cranial portion of the lateral mesoderm, whereas in the presence of *Wnt* signaling, *Bmp* initiates a hematopoietic (i.e., blood-forming) capacity in the caudal portion of the lateral plate mesoderm.

Several cardiac transcription factors are activated within the cardiac crescent. The earliest transcription factors with limited expression within the cardiac lineage include *Nkx2.5* and the *Gata* family members. *Nkx2.5* is expressed in cardiac progenitor cells soon after the onset of gastrulation under the influence of endodermally derived *Bmp*. Downstream targets of *Nkx2.5* include several other cardiac genes such as *Mef2c*, *Ventricular myosin*, and *Hand1*. A human homolog of *NKX2.5*. has been mapped to chromosome 5q35.2, and mutations in this gene are associated with human congenital heart disease, including atrial septal defects, ventricular septal defects, and defects in the conduction system. *Nkx2.5* knockout mice die *in utero*, but still form a heart, albeit one without left-ventricular markers, with incorrect bending, and with a deranged

cranial-caudal identity. So *Nkx2.5* expression is not solely responsible for dictating the cardiac cell lineage. In Drosophila, *Pannier*, a *Gata* gene, is required for cardiogenesis, and its forced expression results in supernumerary cardiac cells at the expense of other mesoderm. Mice null for *Gata4* have fewer cardiomyocytes, whereas *Gata5* overexpression in fish embryos leads to ectopic *Nkx2.5* expression and formation of ectopic beating cell clusters. Interestingly, *Nkx2.5* and *Gatas* may mutually reinforce cardiac expression of each other, as they contain promoter regions for each other. For example, *Gatas* are needed for sustained *Nkx2.5* expression, and promoters for some of the *Gatas* contain functional *Nkx2.5* binding sites.

In summary, the program of early cardiac specification is quite flexible but it requires the presence of particular **morphogens** that provide a permissive environment for lineage specification. Moreover, no single transcription factor or signaling molecule has been identified that is solely responsible for encoding myocardial specification and differentiation. Rather, it seems that a combination of factors working together are needed to stably specify the cardiac cell lineage.

cranial-most portion of the cardiac crescent swings ventrally and caudally to lie ventral to the newly forming foregut endoderm (Fig. 12-4*A, B*). As the lateral body folds move medially, they bring the right and left sides of the cardiac crescent together, and the two limbs of the crescent fuse in the midline, caudal to the head fold and ventral to the foregut (Figs. 12-4*A-D*, 12-5). This fusion occurs at the site of the anterior intestinal portal and progresses in a cranial-to-caudal direction as the foregut tube lengthens. As the two limbs of the cardiac crescent fuse, a recognizable pair of vascular elements called the **endocardial tubes** develop within each limb of the cardiac crescent (see Figs. 12-4*B, C*, 12-5). These vessels form by a process called **vasculogenesis** (described in Ch. 13). *Vascular endothelial growth factor* (*Vegf*) derived from the cranial endoderm is thought to direct a subset of cells within the cardiac crescent into an endothelial/endocardial cell lineage. These endocardial tubes coalesce into a single tube as the limbs of cardiac crescent join to make the primitive heart tube (see Fig. 12-4*C, D*). If fusion of the cardiac crescent limbs fail, two tube-like structures form rather than one, leading to **cardia bifida** (however, both tubes contract and continue to undergo cardiogenesis, including looping; looping is discussed below). The primitive heart tube harbors progenitors for the atria and ventricles, as well as

endocardium. As the fusion process continues, cell proliferation in the primary heart field continues to add the more caudal segments of the heart, including the atrioventricular canal, atria, and sinus venosus (described later in the chapter). Late in the 3rd week, cranial body folding brings the developing heart tube into the thoracic region (Figs. 12-6, 12-7; also discussed in Chs. 4 and 11).

By day 21, the primitive endocardial tube consists of an endothelium (i.e., endocardium) surrounded by a mass of splanchnic mesoderm containing cardiomyocytic progenitors that invest the fused endocardial tubes to form the **myocardium**, or heart muscle. A thick layer of extracellular matrix, the **cardiac jelly**, is deposited mainly by the developing myocardium, separating it from the fused endocardial tubes (Fig. 12-8). Hence, the primary heart tube is composed of an endocardial tube, invested by cardiac jelly within a myocardial tube. The **epicardium (visceral pericardium)** is formed later by a population of mesodermal cells that are independently derived from splanchnic mesoderm that migrates onto the outer surface of the myocardium (discussed later in the chapter).

A series of constrictions (**sulci**) and expansions form in the primitive heart tube (Fig. 12-9). Over the next 5 weeks as the tubular heart lengthens, these expansions contribute to the various heart chambers.

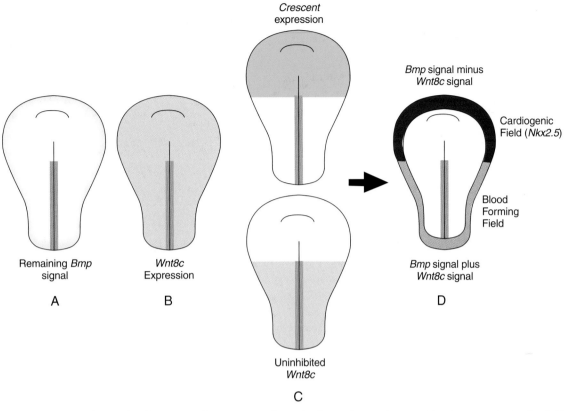

Figure 12-3. Regional specification of cardiogenic mesoderm. *A*, Pattern of *Bmp* signaling on the mesoderm remaining after accounting for *Chordin/Noggin* and *Wnt1/3a* inhibition. *B*, Pattern of *Wnt8c* expression in the mesoderm. *C*, Spatial distribution of *Crescent* expression (a *Wnt* antagonist) in the overlying ectoderm and remaining pattern of uninhibited *Wnt8c* activity in the mesoderm. *D*, Pattern of the cardiogenic marker *Nkx2.5* as a result of *Bmp* signaling in the absence of *Wnt* inhibition. In the presence of *Bmp* and *Wnt8c* signaling, blood-forming fields are primed.

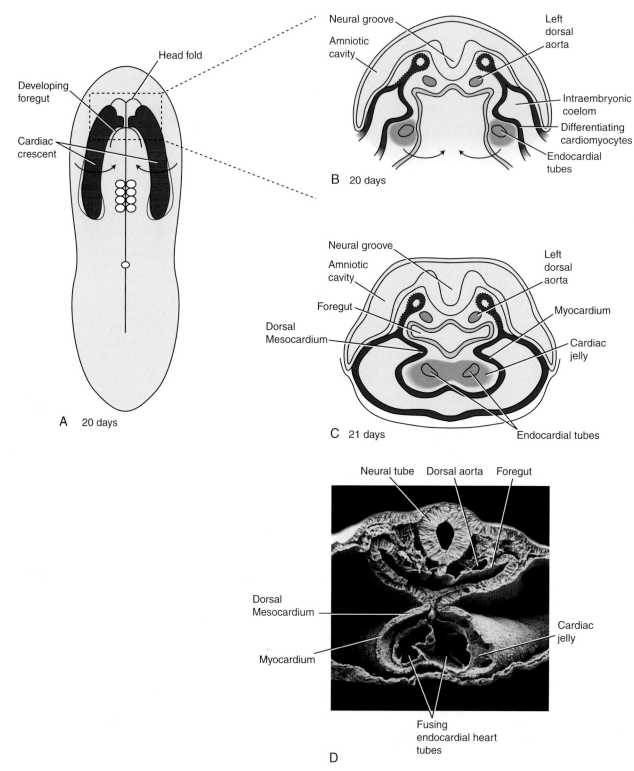

Figure 12-4. Head and lateral body folding at the end of the 3rd week quickly bring the lateral endocardial tubes into the ventral midline in the upper thoracic region, *A, B*, where they fuse to form the primitive heart tube, *C, D*.

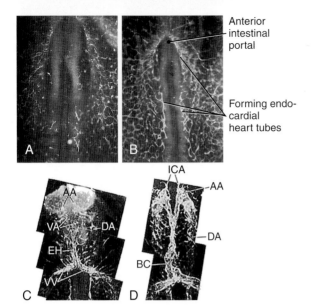

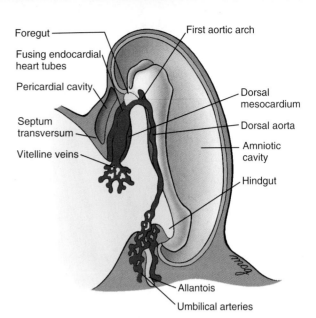

Figure 12-5. Formation of the lateral endocardial heart tubes by vasculogenesis in the chicken embryo. *A, B,* Endocardial progenitor cells aggregate within the horseshoe-shaped cardiogenic area and form short cords that coalesce into a plexus of vessels. These vessels will further consolidate into larger channels to form the endocardial heart tubes. *C,* Two developing endocardial heart (EH) tubes begin fusing to form the primitive heart tube as the lateral body folds meet in the midline to enclose the foregut. Vascular endothelial cords in the dorsal body wall form paired dorsal aortae (DA) both cranial and caudal to the heart tubes. Vitelline veins (VV) are forming just caudal to the heart tubes, and the ventral region of the first aortic arch (VA) is forming just cranial to the heart tubes. *D,* At a slightly later stage, the lateral endocardial tubes have fused and formed a distinct primitive heart tube that is already beginning to show signs of regional specification (seen here as the bulbus cordis, BC). The first aortic arch (AA) loops cranially and dorsally to connect with the cranial ends of the dorsal aortae (DA). The third arch has begun to sprout internal carotid arteries (ICA). The presumptive endothelial and endocardial cells are stained with a specific antibody for endothelial/endocardial cells.

Figure 12-6. Formation of the first aortic arch and dorsal aorta during the 3rd week. The paired dorsal aortae develop in the dorsal mesoderm on either side of the notochord and connect to the fusing endocardial heart tubes while body folding ensues. As the flexion and growth of the head fold carries the primitive heart tube into the cervical and then into the thoracic region (see Fig. 12-7), the cranial ends of the dorsal aortae are pulled ventrally until they form a dorsoventral loop, the first aortic arch. A series of four more aortic arches will develop during the 4th and 5th weeks.

12

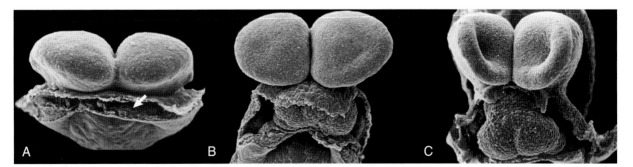

Figure 12-7. *A-C,* Scanning electron micrographs showing how head flexion progressively translocates the developing endocardial tubes from a region just cranial to the neural plate to the thoracic region (arrow in *A,* cardiogenic region).

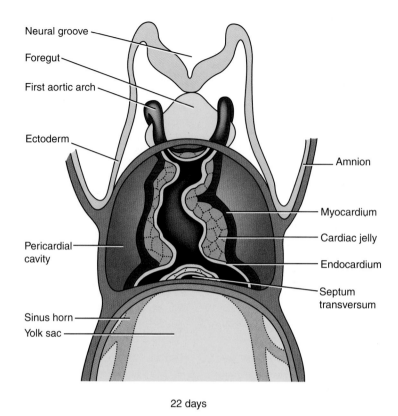

Neural groove

Foregut

First aortic arch

Ectoderm

Amnion

Myocardium

Cardiac jelly

Pericardial cavity

Endocardium

Septum transversum

Sinus horn

Yolk sac

22 days

Figure 12-8. Composition of the primitive heart tube walls. By 22 days, the endocardium of the primitive heart tube is invested by an acellular layer of cardiac jelly and a layer of myocardial cells. The myocardium is derived from a mass of splanchnic mesoderm that encloses the endocardial heart tube. The myocardium then secretes the extracellular cardiac jelly between itself and the endocardium.

Starting at the caudal (inflow) end, the **sinus venosus** consists of the partially confluent left and right **sinus horns** into which the common cardinal veins (discussed later in the chapter) drain. Cranial to the sinus venosus, the next two chambers are the **primitive atrium** and the **primitive ventricle**, which are separated from one another by the **atrioventricular sulcus**. The primitive atrium will form both the right and left atria, and the primitive ventricle will form the definitive left ventricle. The primitive ventricle is separated from the next expansion, the **bulbus cordis**, by the **bulboventricular sulcus**. This segment will form much of the **right ventricle**. Finally, the cranial-most segment, the **outflow tract** (or **conotruncal segment**), forms the distal outflow region for both the left and right ventricles. This segment will be further subdivided into the **conus arteriosus** (or **conus cordis**), which eventually becomes incorporated into the left and right ventricles, and the **truncus arteriosus**, which eventually splits to form the **ascending aorta** and **pulmonary artery**. The truncus arteriosus is connected at its cranial end to a dilated expansion called the **aortic sac**. The aortic sac is continuous with the first aortic arch and, eventually, with the other four aortic arches. The aortic arches form major arteries that transport blood to the head and trunk (discussed in Ch. 13).

The primitive heart tube is initially suspended in the developing pericardial cavity by a **dorsal mesocardium (dorsal mesentery of the heart)** formed by splanchnic mesoderm located beneath the foregut. This dorsal mesocardium promptly ruptures, leaving the heart suspended in the pericardial cavity by its attached vasculature. The region of the ruptured dorsal mesocardium becomes the **transverse pericardial sinus** within the pericardial sac of the definitive

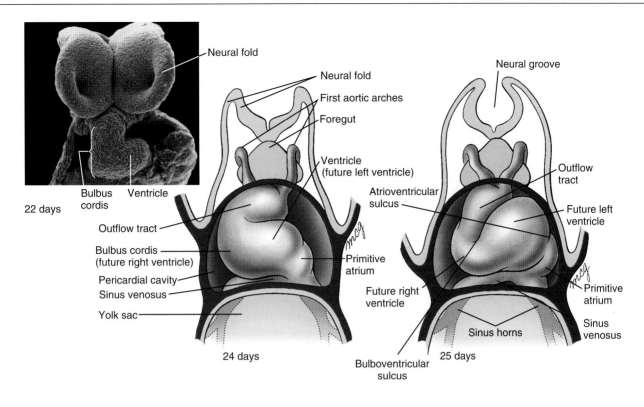

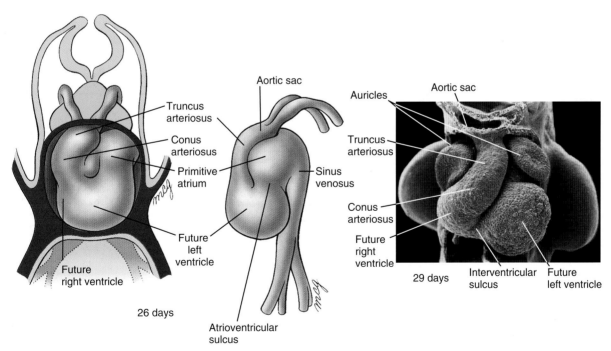

Figure 12-9. Regionalization of the heart tube during its lengthening. As the heart tube lengthens and adds the outflow segment, the looping of the heart tube repositions the bulbus cordis ventrally and to the right and shifts the primitive ventricle to the left and the primitive atrium dorsally and cranially. The bulbus cordis forms much of the right ventricle, whereas the outflow tract will form outflow regions of the right and left ventricles. The primitive ventricle will form most of the definitive left ventricle, and the primitive atrium will give rise to a portion of the atrial wall and auricles of the heart. During this process, deepening sulci increasingly distinguish each segment of the heart tube.

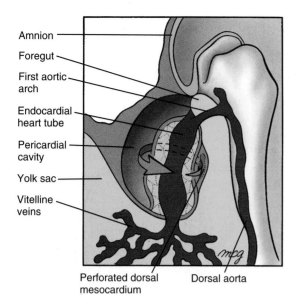

Figure 12-10. Formation of the transverse pericardial sinus of the definitive pericardial cavity by rupture of the dorsal mesocardium early in the 4th week. Arrow passes through the transverse pericardial sinus.

heart (Fig. 12-10), a space separating the cardiac inflow and outflow vessels in adults. During surgery, ligatures are sometimes placed around these vessels to control blood flow.

Not all of the cardiac cells found in the mature heart are derived from the primary heart field (i.e., the initial cardiac crescent). Rather, additional sources of cardiogenic precursors are recruited from the mesoderm immediately adjacent and medial to the initial cardiac crescent (Fig. 12-11). While myocardial cells within developing primitive heart tube continue to proliferate, there is a continued recruitment of cardiac progenitor cells from outside the original cardiac crescent at both the arterial (cranial) pole and venous (caudal) pole. The source of these cells is referred to as the **secondary heart field**. The primitive heart tube lengthens at both ends, particularly the outflow (arterial) end, through the addition of cardiac progenitors from secondary heart field mesoderm. In fact, lineage-tracing studies suggest that in mammals the conotruncus, much of the right ventricle, and a portion of the venous pole are derived from the secondary heart field mesoderm. Interestingly, recent lineage-tracing studies suggest that some cells originating from secondary heart field eventually come to populate all parts of heart including the left ventricle.

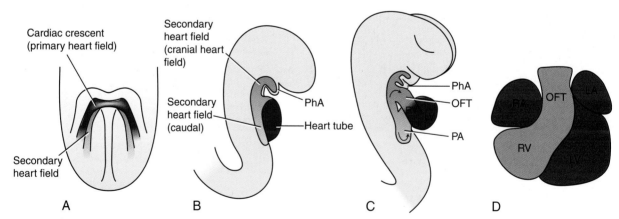

Figure 12-11. The second source of cardiogenic progenitors for the heart, the secondary heart field (shown in light red in *A-D*). *A*, Location of the secondary heart field at the cardiac crescent stage. The secondary heart field is located within the splanchnic mesoderm just medial to primary heart field (cardiac crescent in red). *B*, After formation of the primary heart tube (derived from the primary heart field), the secondary heart field becomes located dorsal to the dorsal mesocardium and runs along the craniocaudal axis. *C*, With rupture of the dorsal mesocardium, the secondary heart field is divided into a caudal segment, responsible for adding to the venous pole of the heart, and a cranial segment, responsible for lengthening the heart tube at the arterial end. *D*, Ventral view of the looped heart showing the contributions of the primary and secondary heart fields. Abbreviations used in the figure are, left atrium (LA), left ventricle (LV), outflow tract (OFT), pharyngeal arch (PhA), primitive atrium (PA), right atrium (RA), and right ventricle (RV).

IN RESEARCH LAB

ROLE OF SECONDARY HEART FIELD IN FORMATION OF OUTFLOW SEGMENT OF HEART

Clonal analysis suggests that cells of the primary heart field and secondary heart field are segregated from a common precursor before the cardiac crescent stage (likely during early gastrulation). At the cardiac crescent stage, cells expressing *Fgf10* and *Isl1* (*Insulin gene enhanced protein1*)—both markers of the secondary heart field—lie just medial to the cardiac crescent. Like the initial cardiac crescent, the secondary heart field is also subjected to the influences of *Bmps* and *Fgfs* released by the foregut (pharyngeal) endoderm that activate cardiogenic transcription factors. However, the more medial location of the secondary heart field at the cardiac crescent stage also positions these cells closer to the negative influence of *Wnts* and *Chordins* emanating from the developing notochord (Fig. 12-12). Therefore, specification of the cardiac cell lineage within the secondary heart field is likely delayed until the initial primitive heart tube is formed and the intervening distance between the secondary heart field and the midline neural tube/notochord increases. As the two limbs of the cardiac crescent move toward the midline during fusion, the secondary heart field cells come into contact with the dorsal surface of the primitive heart tube (future inner curvature of the heart) and end up at both the cranial and caudal ends of the developing dorsal mesocardium (see Fig. 12-11B, C). Secondary heart field cells lying just cranial to the early heart tube and ventral to the developing pharyngeal endoderm assume a *right* ventricular identity, whereas those secondary heart field cells more cranial contribute to the outflow tract myocardium. Those at the caudal end of the heart tube contribute cells to the sinus venosus. The bulk of heart tube lengthening comes from proliferation within the cranial secondary heart field adjacent the developing aortic arch arteries.

GENE MUTATIONS TARGET PRIMARY AND SECONDARY HEART FIELDS

Mutations in particular genes reveal regional sensitivities of the myocardium that reflect the origin of their cardio-myocyte progenitors. For instance in *Tbx5*-deficient mice (*Tbx5* is a T-box transcription family member), the atrium is abnormal and the left ventricle is hypoplastic. Yet, the right ventricle and outflow tract appear normal, suggesting that this mutation mainly targets proliferation and development of cells of the primary heart field. Likewise in *Nkx2.5* null mice, the left ventricle is missing, reflecting a loss of primary heart field–derived cardiomyocytes, whereas the right ventricle is retained (a secondary heart field derivative). *Isl1* is normally expressed in the secondary heart field. Mice null for *Isl1* develop only two heart chambers, the atria and left ventricle. The outflow tract is missing, right ventricular markers are not expressed, and the posterior atrial myocardium is hypoplastic. *Fgf8* is expressed in the ectoderm and pharyngeal endoderm near the arterial pole of the heart tube. Proper *Fgf8* signaling within the secondary heart field is necessary for continued proliferation of secondary heart field cells at the arterial pole. *Fgf8* hypomorphs (a animal with a partial loss-of-function mutation; i.e., *Fgf8* expression in the hypomorph is knocked down but not eliminated completely) die as a result of abnormal outflow tract development. *Tbx1* is a transcription factor expressed in the secondary heart field and interacts genetically with *Fgf8*. Again, loss of *Tbx1* expression in the secondary heart field reduces myocardial cell number in the outflow tract and right ventricle, whereas forced *Tbx1* overexpression in the secondary heart field causes an expansion of the outflow tract. From these studies, it is clear that in addition to a primary heart field (cardiac crescent), a large portion of the definitive heart tube arises from a secondary heart field. As discussed later in the chapter, lengthening of the heart tube by the secondary heart field plays an important role in proper cardiac looping and septation of the heart.

12

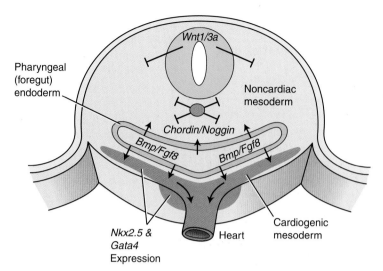

Figure 12-12. Role of growth factors in the lengthening of the heart tube by the secondary heart field. Specification of cardiogenic precursors is similar to that of the primary heart field. The cardiogenic promoting effect of *Bmp* and *Fgf8* released by the endoderm on the splanchnic mesoderm is no longer antagonized by *Wnts* and *Chordin/Noggin* released by midline tissues after the formation of the foregut. As a result, the cardiogenic mesoderm of the secondary heart field begins expressing cardiac markers (e.g., *Nkx2.5* and *Gata4*), proliferates, and drives the lengthening of the heart tube.

Cardiac Looping

On day 23, the primitive heart tube begins to elongate and simultaneously bend into a C-shaped structure, with the bend extending toward the right side. Formation of this bend is not simply a matter of forming a kink in the tube, with the right side of the tubular heart becoming the outer curvature and the left side forming the inner curvature. Rather, it seems that the ventral surface of the tubular heart forms the right outer curvature of the C-shaped heart because the ventral surface is displaced toward the right by torsional forces working along the craniocaudal axis (Fig. 12-13; see Fig. 12-9). With the rupture of the dorsal mesocardium, much of the dorsal side of the straight tubular heart becomes situated on the inner curvature of the C-shaped heart. As the heart tube continues to elongate at both arterial and venous poles, it takes on an S-shaped configuration. In the process, the bulbus cordis is displaced caudally, ventrally, and to the right; the primitive ventricle is displaced to the left; and the primitive atrium is displaceddorsally and cranially (Fig. 12-14; see Figs. 12-9, 12-13). By day 28 the elongation of the heart tube is complete, but there continues to be additional remodeling such that the outflow tract comes to lie between the two presumptive atria

(see Fig. 12-9). The end result of cardiac looping is to bring the four presumptive chambers of the future heart into their correct spatial relationship to each other. The remainder of heart development consists mostly of remodeling these chambers, developing the appropriate septa and valves between them, and forming the epicardium, coronary vasculature, and cardiac innervation and conducting system.

Formation of Primitive Blood Vessels Associated with Endocardial Tube

Many of the major vessels of the embryo, including the paired dorsal aortae, develop at the same time as the endocardial tube. The inflow and outflow vessels of the future heart make connections with the endocardium of the primitive heart even before this tube is translocated into the thorax (see Fig. 12-6). The paired **dorsal aortae**, which form the primary outflow vessels of the heart, develop in the dorsal mesenchyme of the embryonic disc on either side of the notochord. As the flexion and growth of the cephalic fold carries the heart tube into the cervical and then thoracic region

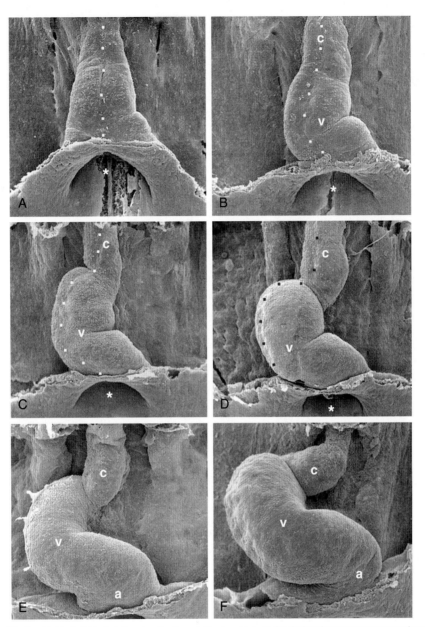

Figure 12-13. Looping of the heart tube. *A*, *B*, Ventral view showing the primitive heart tube in the chick embryo just prior to overt looping. The ventral midline of the primitive heart tube is marked by the dotted line. *C-F*, Cardiac looping is driven in part by cardiac lengthening from the secondary heart field. Note that looping to the right is accompanied by twisting such that the original ventral surface of the primitive heart tube becomes the outer curvature of the looped heart. These forces help drive the formation of atrioventricular and bulboventricular sulci. Several of the cardiac regions are easily identifiable during this process, including the atrium (a), conus arteriosus of the outflow tract (c), and the primitive ventricle (v). The asterisk demarcates the anterior intestinal portal.

12

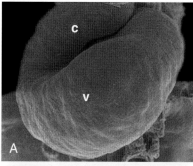

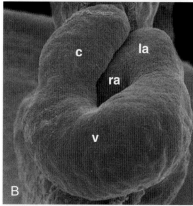

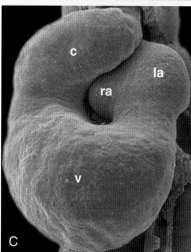

Figure 12-14. *A-C*, position and morphology of the heart regions at progressively later end stages of cardiac looping in the chick embryo. Ventral view of the conal segment of the outflow tract (c), nonseptated ventricle (v), and nonseptated right atrium (ra) and left atrium (la) showing their relative anatomical position near the end of cardiac looping. Note that both atrial and venous poles are now adjacent each other and that the outflow tract is moving leftward and ventral to the atria.

IN THE RESEARCH LAB

MECHANISMS DRIVING CARDIAC BENDING AND LOOPING

Cardiac looping involves two major processes: establishing the directionality of looping, and performing the biomechanical steps that drive the looping itself. Directionality of looping reflects the left-right asymmetry established early during gastrulation (discussed in Ch. 3), which is superimposed on the morphogenetic mechanisms of cardiac looping. In fact, the initial bending of the heart tube into the C-shape is the first morphological evidence of embryonic asymmetry.

The precise mechanisms driving the initial bending and the heart tube's continued looping into an S-shaped tube are still unclear even though considerable effort has gone into identifying the forces responsible for the process. At one time, it was suggested that these processes occur simply because the heart tube, being anchored on both ends, outgrows the length of the primitive pericardial cavity and is forced to bend and loop. However, hearts excised from experimental animals and grown in culture demonstrate an intrinsic ability to bend. Some studies have suggested that the state of hydration of the cardiac jelly controls bending, but when the jelly is removed enzymatically, bending is unaffected. Another suggestion is that bending is induced by hemodynamic forces generated by the circulating blood. Hemodynamic forces are certainly important in heart morphogenesis, but because cultured hearts bend correctly in the absence of blood flow, this suggestion is also ruled out. Other models suggest that remnants of the dorsal mesocardium shorten and force the heart tube to bend. However, the primitive ventricle exhibits signs of bending prior to rupture of the dorsal mesocardium. Alternatively, prior to rupture, the dorsal mesocardium could exert tension on the future inner curvature, providing the biomechanical driving force for bending.

Based on recent studies, another mechanism has been proposed, namely, that asymmetric differences in the extracellular matrix composition within the heart and dorsal mesocardium might exert biomechanical pressure on the heart tube that cause it to bend. One such extracellular matrix molecule is *Flectin*. *Flectin* is a secreted protein having an asymmetric left-right distribution pattern within the cardiac jelly and dorsal mesocardium, and within the secondary heart field in both chick and mouse embryos. Higher levels of *Flectin* are found in the outer curvature of the cardiac jelly and secondary heart field on this same side. In chick embryos, function-blocking antibodies to *Flectin* randomize the direction of heart bending. A positive correlation between *Flectin* protein distribution and cardiac sidedness is also observed in the mouse mutants *iv/iv* (described in Ch. 3) and *inv* (*inversion of embryonic turning mutation*), which exhibit looping anomalies. *Flectin* may be a downstream target of *Pitx2*, because blocking *Pitx2* expression at the early cardiac crescent stage or misexpressing *Pitx2* on the right side randomizes *Flectin* levels and corresponding cardiac bending. How differing *Flectin* levels might drive the bending and looping of the heart tube is unclear, but there is a positive correlation between higher *Flectin* protein levels and higher cell proliferation rates in both the outer curvature of the heart tube and secondary heart field. This suggests that asymmetric myocardial proliferation and growth might help drive bending and looping.

IN THE CLINIC

SIDEDNESS IN HEART LOOPING

As discussed in Chapter 3, abnormal left-right axis determination can lead to development of **heterotaxy** (with an estimated incidence of 3 out of 20,000 live births). The term *heterotaxy* is sometimes used to describe any defect ascribed to abnormal left-right axis formation, be it a reversal of some organs (**situs ambiguous**) or a reversal of all viscera (**situs inversus totalis**). With regard to the heart, this may include abnormal looping, resulting in **dextrocardia** (a right-sided left ventricle as opposed to dextropositioned heart, a shifting of the heart to the right side) (Fig. 12-15*A*, *B*). Proper looping toward the right is a prerequisite for proper cardiac septation, as it is required to bring the primitive left ventricle toward the left, the bulbus cordis (presumptive right ventricle) toward the right, and the conotruncal region to the middle. Because individuals with situs inversus totalis exhibit a reversal in handedness of all organs, they exhibit few problems. In contrast, **visceroatrial heterotaxy syndrome** in humans (where the abdominal viscera and atrial pole are oriented on opposing sides) is associated with structural defects, including common atrium, malalignment of atrioventricular canal and outflow tract, and abnormal venous and arterial vascular connections.

Besides inverted situs, indeterminate left-right axis formation can lead to bilateral left (or right) sidedness, so-called **isomerism**. For example, in the condition called *right atrial isomerism*, both atria have right atrial morphology. Similarly, in *left pulmonary isomerism* both lungs have the lobar and hilar anatomy of the left lung.

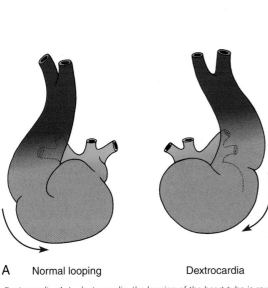
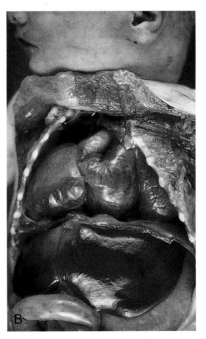

A   Normal looping   Dextrocardia

Figure 12-15. Dextrocardia. *A,* In dextrocardia, the looping of the heart tube is reversed from its normal sinistral looping, producing a heart that is a mirror image of the normal heart. *B,* Infant with dextrocardia.

(see Fig. 12-7), the cranial ends of the dorsal aortae are pulled ventrally until they form a dorsoventral loop, the **first aortic arch** (see Fig. 12-6). A series of four more aortic arches will develop during the 4th and 5th weeks in connection with the pharyngeal arches (Fig. 12-16) (discussed in Chs. 13 and 16). In addition, the craniocaudal flexure facilitates cardiac looping by helping to bring the venous (sinus venosus) and arterial (truncus arteriosus and aortic sac) poles closer to one another in a process called **convergence**.

The inflow to the heart is initially supplied by six vessels; three on each side (see Fig. 12-16). Venous blood from the body of the embryo enters the heart through a pair of short trunks, the **common cardinal veins**, which are formed by the confluence of the paired **posterior cardinal veins** draining the trunk and the paired **anterior cardinal veins** draining the head region (see Fig. 12-16). The yolk sac is drained by a pair of **vitelline veins**, and oxygenated blood from the placenta is delivered to the heart by a pair of **umbilical veins**. The embryonic venous system is discussed in Chapter 13.

IN THE RESEARCH LAB

SUBREGIONS OF HEART ARE SPECIFIED EARLY IN DEVELOPMENT

The chambers of the heart are developmentally, electrophysiologically, and pharmacologically quite distinct. How does this regionalization develop within a single heart tube? Fate mapping studies show that cardiac progenitor cells within the epiblast are topologically organized such that the cardiac inflow progenitors are located more lateral, and the outflow progenitors more medial. Subsequently, during the process of gastrulation, this orientation is converted to a craniocaudal (arterial/venous) topography by the time of the cardiac crescent stage. Interestingly, cells within the early cardiac crescent are still plastic with regard to chamber specification: if caudal cardiac progenitor tissue is substituted for cranial cardiogenic tissue, proper hearts are generated. However, soon afterward, commitment to particular chambers is evident by the expression of chamber-specific myosin isoforms and regulators (Fig. 12-17). *Atrial myosin heavy chain-1 (Mhc1a)* is selectively expressed within atrial cells of the chick

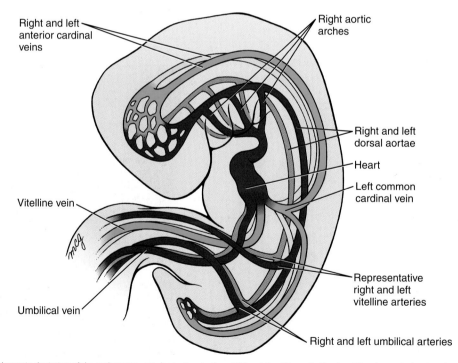

Figure 12-16. Schematic depiction of the embryonic vascular system in the middle of the 4th week. The heart has begun to beat and to circulate blood. The outflow tract is now connected to four pairs of aortic arches and the paired dorsal aortae that circulate blood to the head and trunk. Three pairs of veins—umbilical, vitelline, and cardinal—deliver blood to the inflow end of the heart.

embryo heart. Following formation of the primitive heart chambers, expression of *Mhc1a* is restricted to the primitive atrium (see Fig. 12-17A-C). In contrast, another myosin heavy chain, *Ventricular myosin heavy chain-1* (*Mhc1v*), is expressed by all cells of the differentiating cardiogenic mesoderm (see Fig. 12-17). However, its expression is eventually restricted to the presumptive ventricles of the developing heart (see Fig. 12-17B, C). Early restriction of the expression of atrial- and ventricular-specific myosin genes has also been demonstrated in mice.

Regionalization of the heart is likely an outcome of having at least two separate heart areas within the primary heart field. In mice, clonal analysis suggests that the atrial region becomes clonally distinct (i.e., clones of progenitor cells become restricted to a single compartment) before the rest of the heart. *Irx4*, an *Iroquois* homeoprotein, is expressed only in the cranial portion of the cardiac crescent; later, it is restricted to ventricular cells, where it stimulates the expression of *Mhc1v* and suppresses *Mhc1a* (see Fig. 12-17D-F). *Irx4* is thought to maintain the cranial-caudal phenotype of the heart by suppressing atrial commitment, because loss of *Irx4* expression in mice leads to ectopic expression of atrial markers in the ventricles. *Tbx5* has been linked to atrial lineage determination. Initially expressed in the entire cardiac crescent, *Tbx5* expression becomes limited to the sinus venosus and atria with some expression in the left ventricle (i.e., primary heart field derivatives) (see Fig 12-17E, F). *Tbx5* knockout mice exhibit severe hypoplasia of these chambers, whereas forced expression of *Tbx5* throughout the heart leads to loss of ventricular-specific gene expression, essentially "atrializing" the heart. Mutations in human *TBX5* have been identified in families with **Holt-Oram syndrome**, which includes heart chamber malformations. Once the initial heart tube begins to lengthen and cardiac bending and looping begins, major changes occur in the expression of several chamber/region-restricted transcription factors, with the expression of a number of genes becoming increasingly restricted to atrial and ventricular regions.

Expression of many of the chamber-specific properties depends on many of the same cranial/caudal-patterning influences driving regionalization of the neural ectoderm and paraxial mesoderm. Application of excess retinoic acid during early chick embryo cardiogenesis causes an "atrialization" or "caudalization" of the primitive heart tube, as indicated by ubiquitous expression of *Mhc1a* and *Tbx5* throughout heart tube, whereas retinoic acid antagonists lead to "ventricularization." Atrial gene expression in mice is similarly expanded with retinoic acid treatments *in utero*. A potential mechanism for localized retinoid signaling in embryos is the restricted expression of *Retinaldehyde dehydrogenenase-2* (*Raldh-2*), a limiting enzyme in retinoic acid biosynthesis. Restriction of *Raldh-2* expression to the caudal area of heart is associated with atrial gene expression in both chick and mouse embryos. Mice deficient in *Raldh-2* lack atria and limbs and die in utero.

Coordinated Remodeling of Heart Tube and Primitive Vasculature Produces Systemic and Pulmonary Circulations

At day 22, the primitive circulatory system is bilaterally symmetric: right and left cardinal veins (common, anterior, and posterior) drain the two sides of the body and blood from the heart is pumped into right and left aortic arches and dorsal aortae. The paired dorsal aortae fuse at axial levels T4 to L4 during the 4th week to form a single midline dorsal aorta. The venous system undergoes a complicated remodeling (detailed in Ch. 13), with the result that all systemic venous blood drains into the right atrium through the newly formed superior and inferior venae cavae.

The heart starts to beat on day 22, and by day 24, blood begins to circulate throughout the embryo. Venous return initially enters the right and left sinus horns via the common cardinal veins (Fig. 12-18A). Within the next few weeks, the venous system is remodeled so that all systemic venous blood enters the right sinus horn via the **superior** and **inferior venae cavae** (Fig. 12-18B, C). As venous inflow shifts to the right, the left sinus horn ceases to grow and is transformed into a small venous sac on the posterior wall of the heart (see Fig. 12-18C). This structure gives rise to the **coronary sinus** and the small **oblique vein of the left atrium**. The coronary sinus will receive most of the blood draining from the coronary circulation of the heart muscle.

As the right sinus horn and the venae cavae enlarge to keep pace with the rapid growth of the rest of the heart, the right side of the sinus venosus is gradually incorporated into the right caudal/dorsal wall of the developing atrium, displacing the original right half of

12

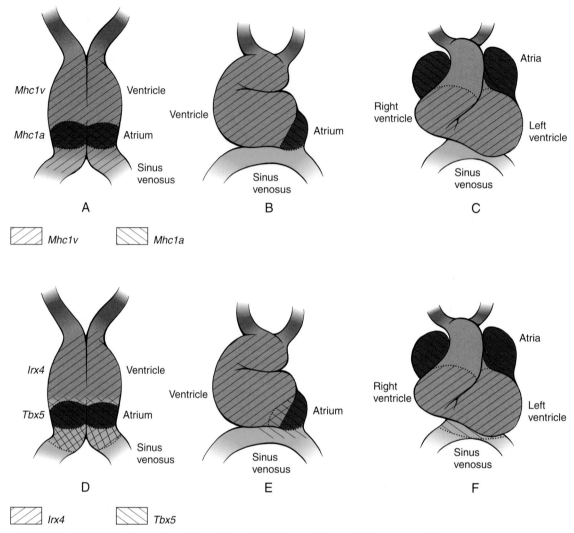

Figure 12-17. Schematic depiction of expression patterns of the myosins *Mhc1a* and *Mhc1v*, and the transcription factors *Irx4* and *Tbx5* during early cardiac chamber specification. *A-C*, As the primitive heart tube forms, *Mhc1a* mRNA is expressed in the atrial end (dark red area), while *Mhc1v* is express throughout the heart tube. As the atrial chamber differentiates and the heart tube folds, *Mhc1a* mRNA expression remains restricted to the primitive atrium, while *Mhc1v* becomes restricted to the ventricle. *D-F*, The expression patterns of the chamber-specific myosins are reflective of specific patterns of transcription factor expression. *Irx4*, a transcription factor driving *Mhc1v* and suppressing *Mhc1a* expression, becomes increasingly restricted to ventricular cells, while *Tbx5*, linked to the atrial phenotype, becomes increasing restricted to the atria and sinus venosus.

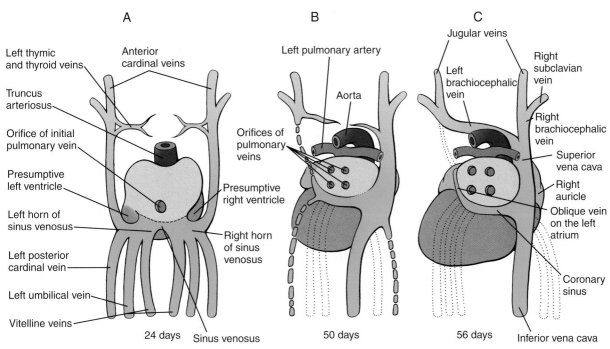

Figure 12-18. Remodeling of the inflow end of the heart between weeks 4 and 8 so that all systemic blood flows into the future right atrium. The left sinus horn is reduced and pulled to the left. It loses its connection with the left anterior cardinal vein and becomes the coronary sinus, draining blood only from the heart wall. The left anterior cardinal vein becomes connected to the right anterior cardinal vein through an anastomosis of thymic and thyroid veins, which form the left brachiocephalic vein. A remnant of the right vitelline vein becomes the terminal segment of the inferior vena cava (discussed in Ch. 13).

the primitive atrial wall farther to the right (Fig. 12-19; see Fig. 12-18). The differential growth of the right sinus venosus also repositions the vestigial left sinus horn (the future coronary sinus) to the right. The portion of the atrium consisting of the incorporated sinus venosus is now called the **sinus venarum**. The original right side of the primitive atrium can be distinguished in the adult heart by the pectinate (comb-like) trabeculation of its wall, which contrasts with the smooth wall of the sinus venarum. In addition, the right atrium develops a small appendage, called the **right auricle**, which is functionally contractile.

Through a process of **intussusception** (folding in of an outer layer) of the right sinus venosus, the openings or **ostia** of the superior and inferior venae cavae and future coronary sinus (former left horn of the sinus venosus) are incorporated into the dorsal wall of the definitive right atrium, where they form the **orifices of the superior and inferior venae cavae** and the **orifice of the coronary sinus** (Fig. 12-20; see Fig. 12-19). As

this occurs, a pair of tissue flaps, the **left** and **right venous valves**, develops on either side of the three ostia. Cranial to the sinuatrial orifices, the left and right valves join to form a transient septum called the **septum spurium**. The left valve eventually becomes part of the septum secundum, one of the septa that contributes to the separation of the definitive right and left atria (discussed later in the chapter). In contrast, the right venous valve remains intact and forms the **valve of the inferior vena cava** and the **valve of the coronary sinus**.

A ridge of tissue called the **crista terminalis** now delimits the trabeculated right atrium from the smooth-walled sinus venarum (Fig. 12-21). The crista terminalis contains the fibers that carry impulses from the primary pacemaker region of the heart (the **sinoatrial node**) to a secondary pacemaker center, the **atrioventricular node**. This fiber tract is part of the conducting system that channels the spread of depolarizing electrical currents through the heart and organizes the contraction of the myocardium (discussed later in the chapter).

12

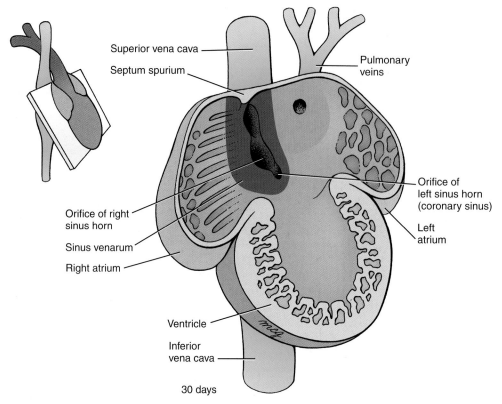

Superior vena cava

Septum spurium

Pulmonary veins

Orifice of left sinus horn (coronary sinus)

Left atrium

Orifice of right sinus horn

Sinus venarum

Right atrium

Ventricle

Inferior vena cava

30 days

Figure 12-19. Initial differentiation of the primitive atrium. During the 5th week, the primitive atrial tissue on the left and right sides is displaced ventrally and laterally to form the trabeculated portion of the atria and auricles of the mature heart. On the right side, the right sinus horn is incorporated into the dorsal wall of the right side of the atrium as the smooth-walled sinus venarum, which will give rise to the definitive right atrium. Meanwhile, a single pulmonary vein develops in the left side of the primitive atrium and then branches twice to produce two right and two left pulmonary veins. The sinus venarum continues to expand within the dorsal wall of the future right atrium.

While the right atrium is being remodeled during the 4th and 5th weeks, the left atrium undergoes a somewhat similar process. During the 4th week, the **pulmonary vein** originates as a midline structure within the caudal **dorsal mesocardium**, which connects the lung anlagen to the dorsal wall of the developing common atrium. From its initial midline position (see Fig. 12-18), the pulmonary vein shifts to the left (see Fig. 12-19) due to asymmetric growth of a projection called the **spina vestibuli** (discussed later in the chapter). The pulmonary vein promptly branches into right and left pulmonary branches, which bifurcate again to produce a total of four pulmonary veins. These veins then grow toward the lungs, where they anastomose with veins developing within the mesoderm investing the bronchial buds (discussed in Ch. 11). During the 5th week, a process of intussusception incorporates the first two branches of the pulmonary vein system into the caudal wall of the left side of the primitive atrium (see Figs. 12-19, 12-20), where they form the smooth wall of the definitive left atrium. The trabeculated left side of the primitive atrium is displaced ventrally and to the left, where it forms a left atrial appendage (the **left auricle**). As a result of intussusception, the pulmonary venous system opens into the left atrium initially through a single large orifice, then transiently through two orifices, and finally through the four orifices of the definitive pulmonary veins (see Fig. 12-21).

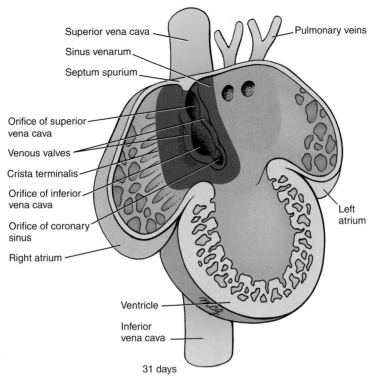

Superior vena cava
Sinus venarum
Septum spurium
Orifice of superior vena cava
Venous valves
Crista terminalis
Orifice of inferior vena cava
Orifice of coronary sinus
Right atrium
Ventricle
Inferior vena cava
Pulmonary veins
Left atrium

31 days

Figure 12-20. Further differentiation of the atrium. Later in the 5th week, the pulmonary vein system begins to undergo intussusception into the dorsal wall of the primitive atrium to form the definitive left atrium.

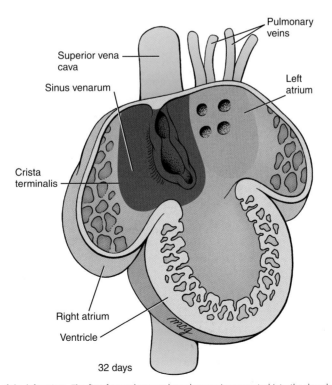

Pulmonary veins
Superior vena cava
Sinus venarum
Left atrium
Crista terminalis
Right atrium
Ventricle

32 days

Figure 12-21. Definitive formation of the left atrium. The first four pulmonary branches are incorporated into the dorsal wall of the left side of the primitive atrium, completing the formation of the smooth-walled part of the future left atrium.

12

Septation of Heart

Partitioning the heart into four chambers is accomplished through the formation of septa (walls) in the primitive atrium, ventricle, and outflow tract. Major events for cardiac septation occur between days 28 and 37 of gestation. Two basic processes play key roles in generating septa. Differential growth and remodeling are responsible mainly for generating the muscular interventricular and interatrial septa, but these processes alone never fully partition the heart chambers. For that, endocardial-derived and neural crest cell–derived cushion tissue is required. In the atrioventricular and outflow tract regions, while cardiac looping continues, extracellular matrix is secreted between the endocardium and myocardium chiefly by the myocardial layer (Fig. 12-22A). This essentially causes the endocardial layer to balloon into the lumen of these

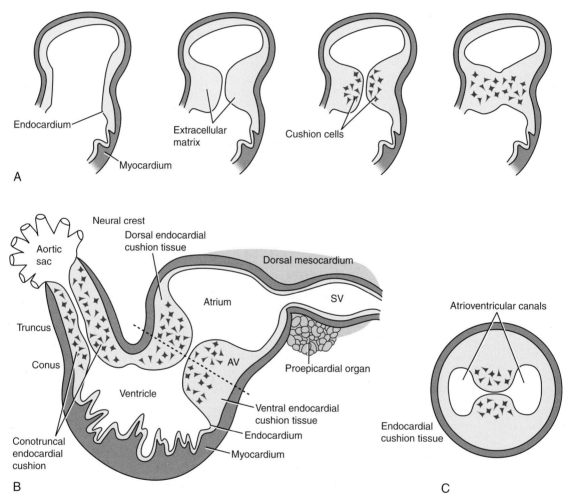

Figure 12-22. Cushion tissue formation. *A,* Steps in the formation of endocardial-derived cushion tissue. The myocardium deposits a unique extracellular matrix between the endocardium and itself at a specific stage in development. This induces an epithelial-to-mesenchymal transformation of the endocardium, resulting in the generation of migrating endocardial cushion cells that are necessary for cardiac septation. *B,* Sites of cushion tissue formation in the heart. Endocardial-derived cushion tissue forms in the atrioventricular region and the outflow tract region (which is also populated by invading neural crest cells; not shown). Eventual fusion of the opposing cushion tissues forms the atrioventricular canals, outflow vessels for the ventricles, and membranous portions of the interatrial and interventricular septa. Dashed line represents the level of the cross section illustrated in *C* and showing the atrioventricular cushion pads and canals.

two regions. Near the completion of cardiac looping, some of the endocardial cells in the atrioventricular and outflow tract regions undergo an **epithelial-to-mesenchymal transformation (EMT)**, generating endocardial-derived mesenchyme that invades this extracellular matrix, proliferates, and differentiates into connective tissue. These mesenchymal-filled bulges (in atrioventricular region) and ridges (along the length of the outflow tract) are often referred to as **cushion tissues** (Fig. 12-22*B*). As discussed later in the chapter, the cushion tissue of the outflow tract not only contains endocardial-derived cells, but these ridges are also invaded by neural crest cells. Thus the cushion tissue of the outflow tract consists of both mesodermally derived mesenchymal cells (**endocardial-derived cushion tissue**) and ectodermally derived mesenchymal cells (**neural crest cell–derived cushion tissue**) (Fig. 12-23; see Fig. 12-22*B*). Proper development of these cushion tissues is essential for completing septation—that is, the generation of the membranous (or fibrous) portion of the interventricular and interatrial septa and the separation of the aorta from the pulmonary artery. These cushion tissues also play a major role in forming the cardiac skeleton of the heart, as well as the atrioventricular valves and semilunar valves.

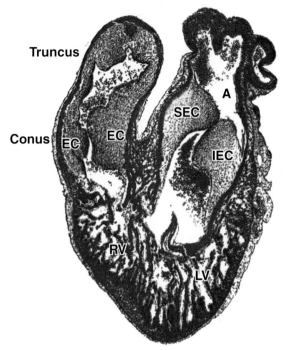

Figure 12-23. Photomicrograph of a sagittal section through a chick embryo heart showing the dorsal and ventral endocardial cushions, also called the superior and inferior endocardial cushion tissue (SEC and IEC, respectively). The endocardial cushion of the outflow tract (EC) is also shown. A, atrium; RV and LV, right and left ventricles, respectively.

IN THE RESEARCH LAB

EPITHELIAL-TO-MESENCHYMAL TRANSFORMATION DURING ENDOCARDIAL CUSHION CELL FORMATION

The epithelial-to-mesenchymal transformation (EMT) of the endocardium can be separated into two major steps: activation (signaling) of the event, which includes the induction and cell-cell separation of a subpopulation of endocardial cells; and (2) delamination and invasion of the endocardial-derived cells into underlying extracellular matrix. Once populating the extracellular matrix, these cells proliferate and differentiate into various connective tissue cell types.

What triggers the EMT of the endocardium and why does this process only occur in the atrioventricular and outflow tract regions of the heart? The answer to this fundamental question is still unclear. Early studies using chick embryos and three-dimensional tissue culture models show that only the atrioventricular and outflow tract myocardium are competent to induce EMT of the endocardium, and that only atrioventricular and outflow tract endocardium are capable of responding. The inducing factor(s) is (are) released into the

extracellular matrix by the myocardium, but the precise nature of this signal is still unclear. One possibility is a multicomponent aggregate referred to as the ES (EDTA soluble) complex. Expression of this complex within the heart is restricted to the atrioventricular and outflow tract regions, and antibodies directed against this complex can block EMT. Another myocardial-secreted molecule, *Versican* (a proteoglycan product of the *Cspg2* gene in mice), is essential for endocardial cushion tissue formation, as mice null for *Versican* lack the initial cushion swellings and do not form cushion cells.

One of the earliest signs of endocardial activation is that a subset of endocardial cells hypertrophy (in this case, the rough endoplasmic reticulum enlarges and Golgi apparatus becomes more prevalent). Soon, this is followed by morphologic signs of cell-cell separation in a subset of endocardial cells and is accompanied by a downregulation of cell-cell adhesion molecules including *N-Cam* (*Neural-Cell adhesion molecule*), *VE-Cadherin* (*Vascular Endothelial-Cadherin*), and *Pe-Cam-1* (*Platelet endothelial-Cell adhesion molecule*). If these cell-cell adhesion molecules are not

12

downregulated, EMT fails. Endocardial EMT also recapitulates many of the same steps as the EMT responsible for gastrulation and neural crest cell formation (discussed in Chs. 3 and 4, respectively). In chick embryos, *Slug* expression is upregulated in a subset of endocardial cells prior to EMT and during early migration of cushion cells in tissue culture, and blocking *Slug* expression prevents EMT of the endocardium. Activated endocardial cells also begin extending filopodia into the extracellular matrix and upregulating invasive cell markers (e.g., *matrix metalloproteinases, serine proteases, hyaluronate synthetases,* and *Rho-associated kinases*). This is soon followed by the transformation of this endocardial subset into mesenchymal cells that migrate and invade the extracellular matrix between the endocardium and myocardium.

There are several growth factors, growth factor receptors, and transcription factors whose expression is required for the initial phase of EMT. Members of the *Tgfβ* family have important roles in initiating endocardial EMT. Adding *Tgfβ1* or *Tgfβ2* to chick embryo cultures of atrioventricular endocardium stimulates EMT. Blocking *Tgfβ2* expression or neutralizing its activity using antibodies inhibits both cell-cell separation and the invasive steps leading to EMT, whereas blocking *Tgfβ3* inhibits EMT only after the cell-cell separation step has occurred. An important role for *TGFβs* in EMT is supported by mouse *Tgfβ* knockout mutants, which exhibit atrioventricular valvular defects, semilunar valvular defects, and atrial septal defects. At least five different *Bmps* (another member of the *TGFβ* family) are also expressed by atrioventricular and outflow tract myocardium. In mice *Bmp2* and *Bmp4* are expressed in the myocardium beneath the atrioventricular and outflow tract endocardium. Using the chick tissue culture model, knocking down *Bmp2* expression significantly reduces endocardial cushion cell migration; in mouse atrioventricular endocardial cultures, *Bmp2* can substitute for the myocardium. The importance of the *Tgfβ* family in the development of the

cardiac cushion tissue and valve formation is also supported by studies showing that disruption of *Bmp* and *Tgfβ* receptor genes (e.g., *Alk3*) results in hypoplastic cushion tissues and valvular defects. A myriad of other growth factors and growth factor receptors have been implicated or shown to have important roles in signaling endocardial EMT, including *Egfs, Fgfs,* and *Vegfs.* Several transcription factors are also important for proper cushion formation and valve development, many of which have been implicated in EMTs and mesenchymal tissue development elsewhere in the embryo, including *Msx1* and *Msx2, Prx1* and *Prx2, Id, Sox4,* and *NF-ATc (Nuclear Factor of activated T cells, isoform c).*

EFFECTS OF HYPERGLYCEMIA AND HYPOXIA ON CUSHION TISSUE FORMATION

Neonates born to diabetic mothers have an almost three-fold increased risk of having congenital heart defects. Because the risk can be reduced by strict maternal glycemic control, hyperglycemia seems to act as a teratogen. In mice, hyperglycemic conditions inhibit the EMT necessary for cushion tissue formation. Hyperglycemia inhibits the release of *Vegf* from the myocardium, a growth factor essential for cushion tissue formation, leading to retention of *Pe-Cam-1* in endocardial cells. As mentioned earlier, endocardial cushion tissue formation requires the turnover of this cell-cell adhesion molecule, among others, prior to the EMT. Experimentally blocking the bioavailability of endogenous *Vegf* mimics the effect of hyperglycemia on endocardial EMT; adding *Vegf* back reverses the deleterious effects of the hyperglycemic conditions. In contrast, hypoxia increases the release of *Vegf* and elevates *Vegf* levels. However, elevated levels of *Vegf* inhibit endocardial cushion formation. Thus, specific levels of *Vegf* are required for EMT and normal endocardial cushion tissue formation.

Septation of Atria and Division of Atrioventricular Canal

A required step in separation of the systemic and pulmonary circulations is the partial separation of the definitive atria and the division of the common atrioventricular canal into right and left canals. The mature interatrial septum is formed by the fusion of two embryonic partial muscular septa, the septum primum and the septum secundum. These septa both have large openings that allow right-to-left shunting of blood throughout gestation. This shunting is required for normal development and expansion of the left atrium and left ventricle, and it permits

oxygenated blood from the umbilicus to bypass the developing pulmonary system and enter the systemic circulation.

On about day 26, while atrial remodeling is in progress, the roof of the atrium develops a depression along the midline at the site beneath the overlying outflow tract. On day 28, this deepening depression results in a crescent-shaped myocardial wedge, called the **septum primum**, which extends into the atrium from the cranial-dorsal wall as the primitive atrial chamber expands (Fig. 12-24). Meanwhile at the venous pole, the dorsal mesocardium sends a projection of cells into the atrium, called the **spina vestibuli** (or **atrial spine**), which joins the septum primum and

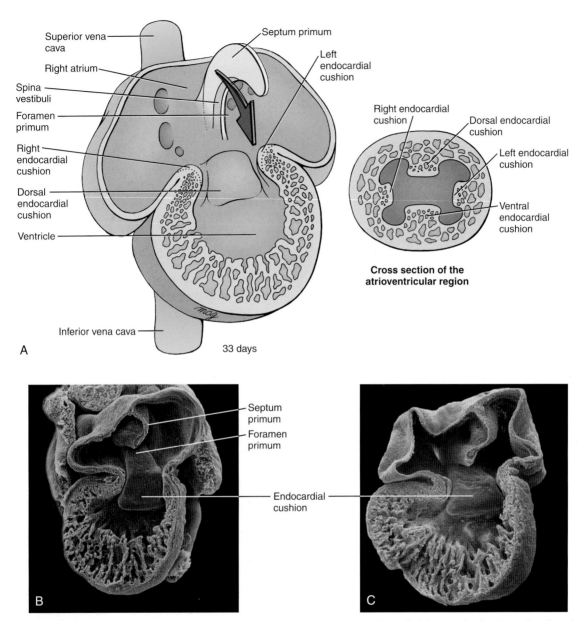

Figure 12-24. *A*, Initial septation of the atria. The spina vestibuli and septum primum form from the roof of the atrial chamber during the 5th week and together grow as a crescent-shaped wedge toward the atrioventricular canal. Simultaneously, the atrioventricular canal is being divided into right and left atrioventricular orifices by the growing dorsal and ventral endocardial cushions. *B, C*, Scanning electron micrographs showing the development of the foramen primum.

contributes to this atrial septum. During the 5th week, the septum primum and spina vestibuli grow toward the atrioventricular canal, thus, gradually separating the nascent right and left atria. The diminishing foramen between the atria is called the **foramen primum** (or **ostium primum**).

As the septum primum elongates by differential growth, two major endocardial-derived cushion tissues—called the **dorsal** (or **superior**) and **ventral** (or **inferior**) **endocardial cushions**—develop around the periphery of the atrioventricular canal (see Figs. 12-22*B*, 12-23, 12-24). At the end of the 6th week,

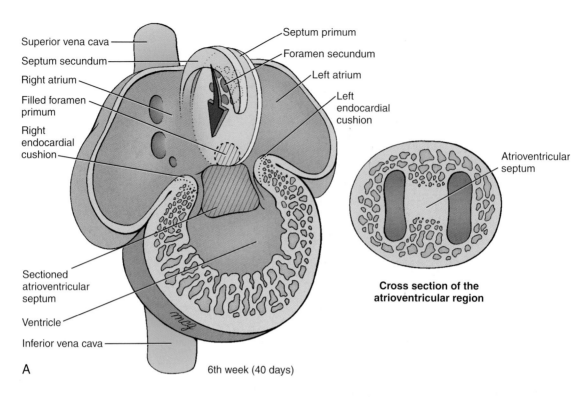

Superior vena cava

Septum secundum

Right atrium

Filled foramen primum

Right endocardial cushion

Septum primum

Foramen secundum

Left atrium

Left endocardial cushion

Atrioventricular septum

Cross section of the atrioventricular region

Sectioned atrioventricular septum

Ventricle

Inferior vena cava

A

6th week (40 days)

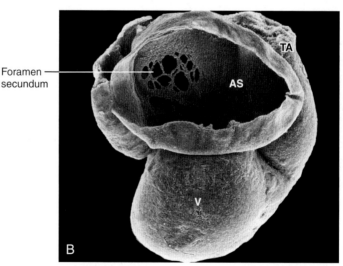

Foramen secundum

TA

AS

V

B

Mid 6th week (38 days)

Figure 12-25. Further septation of the atria. *A,* During the 6th week, the thick septum secundum grows from the roof of the right atrium, and the septum primum fuses with a contribution from the atrioventricular cushion. However, before the foramen primum is obliterated, the foramen secundum forms by coalescence of small ruptures in the septum primum. *B,* Scanning electron micrograph showing the development of the foramen secundum.

the dorsal and ventral cushions meet and fuse, forming the **atrioventricular septum** (or **septum intermedium**) that divides the common atrioventricular canal into **right** and **left atrioventricular canals** (Figs. 12-25A, 12-26, 12-27C). At the end of the 6th week, the growing edge of the atrioventricular septum fuses with septum primum (see Fig. 12-25A). This event obliterates the foramen primum. However, before the foramen primum closes, programmed cell death and cell rearrangement in an area near the dorsal edge of the septum primum creates small perforations that coalesce to form a new foramen, the **foramen secundum** (or **ostium secundum**) (see Fig. 12-25). Thus, a new channel for right-to-left shunting opens before the old one closes.

While the septum primum is lengthening, a second crescent-shaped ridge of tissue forms on the ceiling of the right atrium, just adjacent and to the right of septum primum (see Fig. 12-25A). This **septum secundum** is thick and muscular, in contrast to the thin septum primum. The edge of the septum secundum grows cranial-caudally and ventral-dorsally, but it halts before it reaches the atrioventricular septum, leaving an opening called the **foramen ovale** near the floor of the right atrium (see Fig. 12-26). Therefore, throughout the rest of fetal development, blood that shunts from the right atrium to the left atrium passes through two staggered openings: the foramen ovale near the floor of the right atrium, and the foramen secundum near the roof of the left atrium. This arrangement allows blood to flow from the right atrium to the left atrium, but not in the reverse direction, as the thin septum primum collapses against the stiff septum secundum, effectively blocking blood flow back into the right atrium. This shunt closes at birth because the abrupt dilation of the pulmonary vasculature, combined with the cessation of umbilical flow, reverses the pressure difference between the atria and pushes the flexible septum primum against the more-rigid septum secundum, even during atrial diastole (see the discussion of changes in circulation at birth in Ch. 13).

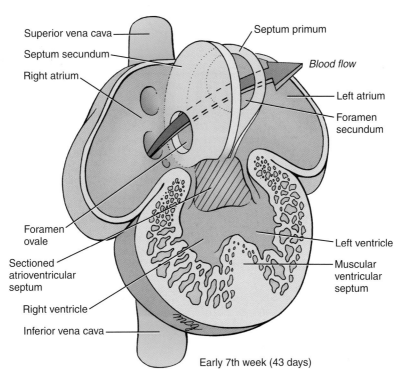

Early 7th week (43 days)

Figure 12-26. Definitive fetal separation of the atria. The septum secundum does not completely close, leaving an opening in this septum called foramen ovale. During embryonic and fetal life, much of the blood entering the right atrium passes to the left atrium via the foramen ovale and the foramen secundum.

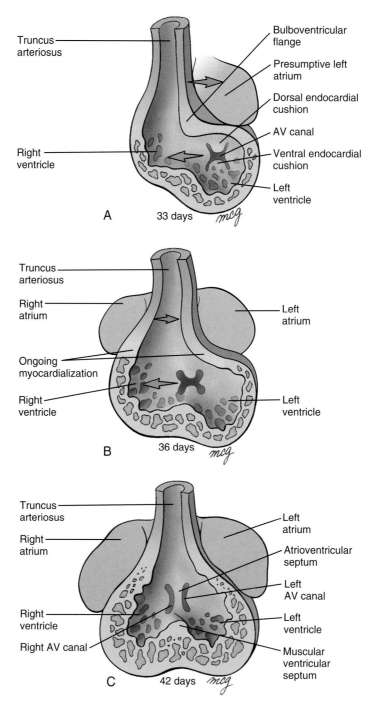

Figure 12-27. *A-C,* Realignment of the heart. As the atrioventricular septum forms during the 5th and 6th weeks, the heart is remodeled to align the developing left atrioventricular canal with the left atrium and ventricle, and the right atrioventricular canal with the right atrium and ventricle. Arrows indicate realignment direction of atrioventricular canal and outflow tract.

Realignment of Primitive Chambers of Developing Heart

Even after cardiac looping is nearly finished, the atrioventricular canal only provides a direct pathway between the future atrium and the future left ventricle (Fig. 12-27A). Moreover, the cranial end of the presumptive right ventricle, but not the presumptive left ventricle, is initially continuous with the outflow tract that gives rise to both the aortic and pulmonary outflow vessels. Proper cardiac tube looping, chamber expansion, and realignment must occur to bring the developing atrioventricular canal into alignment with the right atrium and ventricle, and also to provide the left ventricle with a direct path to the outflow tract. This process is illustrated in Figure 12-27.

The atrioventricular canal initially lies between the left primitive atrium and the future left ventricle. The mechanism by which the right and left atrioventricular canals come into alignment with both the future right and left ventricles is unclear. However, this change may be accomplished by active remodeling of the dorsal bulboventricular sulcus. Here, the dorsal atrioventricular cushion is continuous with the nearby proximal limb of the conotruncal cushion ridge, and the cushion cells in this region are eventually replaced by a subsequent invasion of the surrounding myocardial cells through a process referred to as **myocardialization** (Fig. 12-28). In this process, myocardial cell projections extend into the conal cushions, where it is thought that many of the cushion cells undergo **apoptosis**. Myocardialization also leads to a thinning of the inner curvature, and it has been proposed that this helps reposition the outflow tract toward the left so that it comes to override the atrioventricular canal during the 5th week of development. In addition, evidence suggests that shortening of the outflow tract by apoptotic death of the myocardial tunic and shortening at its distal end generates torsional forces that rotate the outflow tract and position it over the atrioventricular canal. At the same time, the atrioventricular canal is being divided into right and left channels by the growth of the dorsal and ventral endocardial cushions. Thus, by the time the common canal has split into right and left atrioventricular canals, the latter are correctly aligned with their respective atria and ventricles (see Fig. 12-27C).

Once the atrioventricular canals, ventricles, and cardiac outflow tract are all correctly aligned, the stage is set for the remaining phases of heart morphogenesis: completion of atrial septation, septation of the ventricles, septation of the outflow tract into ascending

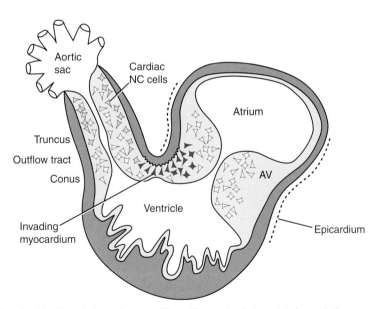

Figure 12-28. Myocardialization of cushion tissue during realignment of the outflow tract and atrioventricular canal. The myocardial wall of the inner curvature thins and sends projections of myocardial cells into the underlying cardiac jelly, replacing the cushion tissue cells. Myocardialization is essential for enabling the remodeling necessary for aligning the atrioventricular septum with the outflow tract.

aorta and pulmonary trunk, and the development of the heart valves, coronary vasculature, and conducting system.

Initiation of Septation of Ventricles

At the end of the 4th week, the ventral bulboventricular sulcus begins to protrude into the cardiac lumen along the interface between the presumptive right and left ventricular chambers as the ventricular chambers expand (Fig. 12-29; see Fig. 12-27). This protrusion, the **muscular interventricular septum**, is thought to form as the expanding walls of the right and left ventricles become more closely apposed to one another. By 7 weeks, expansion of the muscular interventricular septum ceases without joining the atrioventricular septum. If fusion occurred too soon, the left ventricle would be shut off from the ventricular outflow tract.

At the same time that the muscular interventricular septum is forming, the myocardium begins to thicken and myocardial ridges or **trabeculae** form on the inner wall of both ventricles. Trabeculation begins about the 4th week of human gestation, with projections or ridges first forming in the greater

curvature of the heart. These trabecular ridges are transformed into fenestrated trabecular sheets while the outer cardiomyocytes adjacent to the primitive epicardium rapidly proliferate forming an outer compact layer of myocardium (see Fig. 12-29). At this stage the trabecular layer is thicker than the outer compact layer, and the fenestrated nature of the trabeculae is thought to facilitate the delivery of nutrients to the working myocardial cells until the coronary vascular system develops.

The ventral portion of the muscular interventricular septum is trabeculated and is called the **primary ventricular fold** or **septum** . The smooth-walled dorsal part of the septum is called the **inlet septum** because of its proximity to the atrioventricular canals. On the right wall of the muscular interventricular septum, the boundary between the trabeculated primary fold and the inlet septum is marked by a prominent trabecula called the **moderator band** or **septomarginal trabecula** (see Fig. 12-29B). This structure connects the muscular septum with the forming **anterior papillary muscle** attached to the right atrioventricular valve. The moderator band forms as a result of right ventricular chamber expansion at a secondary site located near the

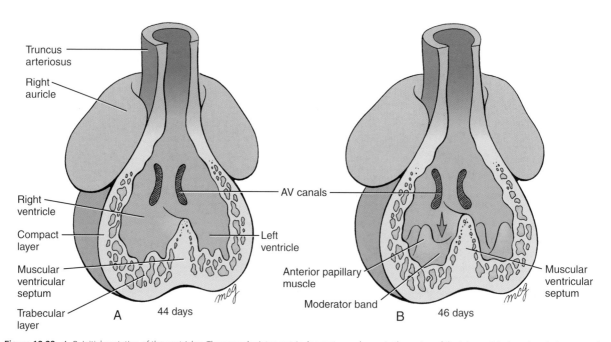

Figure 12-29. *A, B,* Initial septation of the ventricles. The muscular interventricular septum enlarges in the region of the interventricular sulcus between weeks 4 and 7. (See Fig. 12-33 for the completion of ventricular septation.) The arrow indicates the site of right ventricular expansion responsible, in part, for the formation of the moderator band.

atrioventricular canal and dorsal interventricular muscular septum (see *arrow* in Fig. 12-29B). This expansion eventually forms a large part of the mature right ventricular chamber. If expansion of this area is insufficient, the developing tricuspid portion of the atrioventricular canal can remain associated with the interventricular foramen, leading to tricuspid atresia and other valvular anomalies.

Development of Atrioventricular Valves

The atrioventricular valves begin to form between the 5th and 8th weeks. These valve **leaflets** or **cusps** are firmly rooted in the rim of the right and left atrioventricular canals and are thought to arise from proliferation and differentiation of the adjacent endocardial cushion tissues. How the mature valves are formed is not fully understood. However, morphological studies and lineage tracing studies in mice suggest that the bulk of the valve leaflets are derived from endocardial cushion tissue with some possible contribution of epicardial-derived connective tissue. The leaflets are freed from the

12

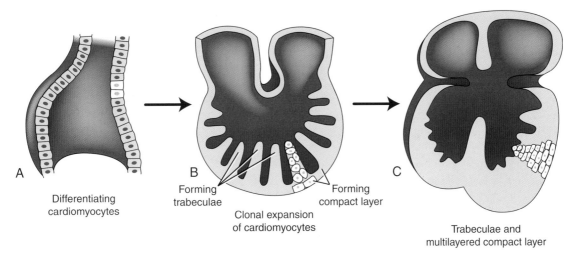

A — Differentiating cardiomyocytes

B — Forming trabeculae / Clonal expansion of cardiomyocytes / Forming compact layer

C — Trabeculae and multilayered compact layer

Figure 12-30. *A-C*, Formation of cardiac trabeculae. Myocardial trabeculae develop from clonal expansion of cardiomyocytes within the myocardial wall and are then subsequently remodeled as the heart increases in size. Clonal expansion of the compact layer into a multilayered myocardium requires an interaction with the developing epicardium.

myocardial wall by remodeling and erosion of the ventricular myocardial wall. This forms ventricular outpockets beneath the valvular primordia and leaves thin strands of cells that form the **chordae tendineae** and small hillocks of myocardium called **papillary muscles** (Fig. 12-31*A-D*). The valve leaflets are designed so that they fold back to allow blood to enter the ventricles from the atria during diastole, but shut to prevent backflow when the ventricles contract during systole (see Fig. 12-31*D*). The left atrioventricular valve has only anterior and posterior leaflets and is called the **bicuspid valve** (**mitral valve**). The right atrioventricular valve usually (but not always) develops a third, small **septal cusp** during the 3rd month; therefore, it is called the **tricuspid valve** (Fig. 12-32; see Fig. 12-31*D*).

Septation of Outflow Tract and Completion of Septation of Ventricles

When the muscular interventricular septum ceases to grow, the two ventricles still communicate with each other, as well as with the expanded base of the conus arteriosus, through the interventricular foramen (Fig. 12-33*A*, *B*). Separation of the outflow tract and ventricles must be coordinated with realignment and rotation of the outflow tract relative to the ventricles if the heart is to function properly. Not surprisingly, a large proportion of cardiac defects are the result of errors in this complex process (discussed later in the chapter).

The cardiac outflow tract is divided by the formation of a pair of endocardial-covered **conotruncal swellings** (or **ridges**) that grow inward along the length of the conotruncal segment. These swellings eventually fuse to form a septum, the **conotruncal septum** (sometimes called **aorticopulmonary septum**), that completely separates the right and left ventricular outflow pathways (Fig. 12-34, see Fig. 12-33). As outlined earlier, both endocardial-derived and neural crest cell–derived cushion cells populate these swellings. The conotruncal swellings separating left and right ventricular outflow tracts run in a spiral along the walls of the outflow tract, rather than running straight. This is required for the right ventricle to connect to the future pulmonary circulation and the left ventricle to connect to the systemic circulation. As a result, the left and right ventricular outflow tracts and, eventually, the aorta and pulmonary trunk twist around each other in a helical arrangement

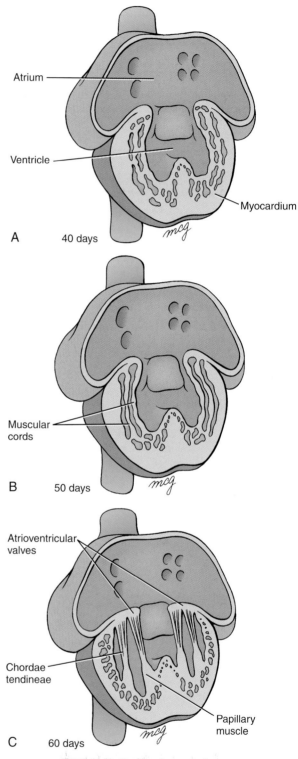

A 40 days

B 50 days

C 60 days

Figure 12-31. See legend on opposite page.

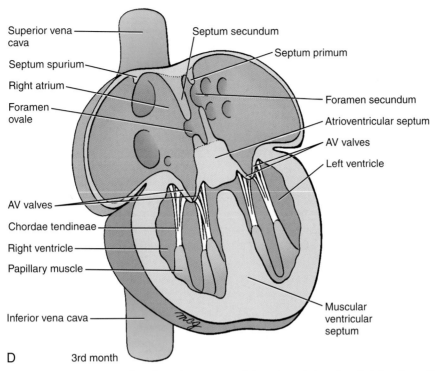

Superior vena cava

Septum spurium

Right atrium

Foramen ovale

AV valves

Chordae tendineae

Right ventricle

Papillary muscle

Inferior vena cava

Septum secundum

Septum primum

Foramen secundum

Atrioventricular septum

AV valves

Left ventricle

Muscular ventricular septum

D   3rd month

Figure 12-31. *A-D,* Development of the atrioventricular valves. The structures of the atrioventricular valves, including the papillary muscles, chordae tendineae, and cusps, are sculpted from the muscular walls of the ventricles. The definitive tricuspid valve within the right ventricle is not completely formed until the development of a septal cusp in the 3rd month.

12

(see Fig. 12-33), an arrangement that is still obvious in the adult. This spiral arrangement is thought to be driven, in part, by rotational and torsional forces on the outflow tract generated as a consequence of cardiac looping.

Formation of the conotruncal septum is complex. Examination of human embryos shows that a mesenchymal wedge of tissue develops between the fourth and sixth aortic arch vessels (separating the future systemic and pulmonary circuits) in the roof of the aortic sac (Fig. 12-35). This tissue extends toward the developing conotruncal swellings and fuses with them. Subsequent fusion of the paired conotruncal swelling then commences from the distal truncus arteriosus and proceeds proximally (upstream of blood flow), partitioning the truncus arteriosus first and then the conus arteriosus. By an unknown mechanism, the conotruncal region is then separated into two distinct vessels (see Fig. 12-34). Separation of the right and left ventricles is completed when the muscular interventricular septum fuses with the conotruncal septum and the ventricular side of the atrioventricular septum. Development of this **membranous ventricular septum** normally occurs between weeks 5 and 8. Failure of complete fusion results in a ventricular septal defect (see the following "In the Clinic" section of this chapter).

Once the conotruncal septum is complete, several modifications also occur in the conus arteriosus. The cushion cells are eventually replaced by a subsequent invasion of the surrounding myocardial cells through the process described earlier as myocardialization. Here, myocardial cells invade the conotruncus septum and ultimately muscularize this region to form the outflow portion of the definitive right and left ventricles. In trisomy 16 mice (a model for Down syndrome in humans), myocardialization fails, increasing the incidence of outflow tract–related septal defects, which are common in patients with **Down syndrome.**

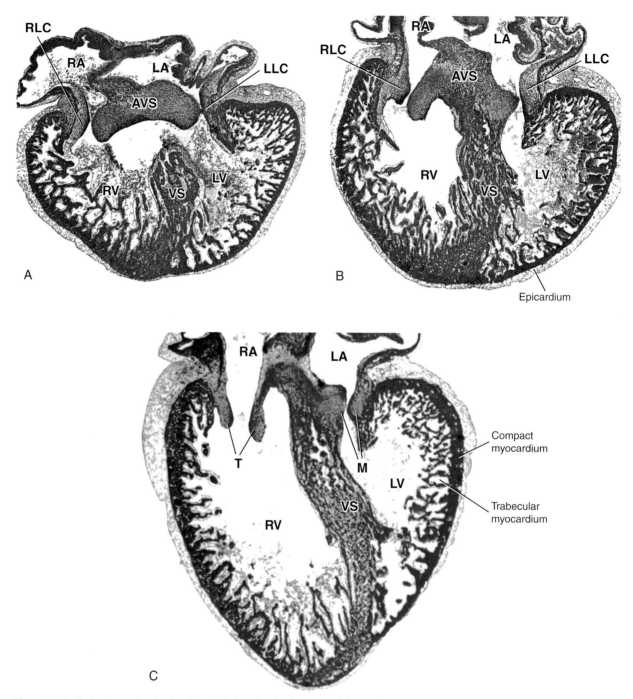

Figure 12-32. Photomicrographs showing atrioventricular valve development and the two layers of myocardium in the chick embryo. Labels on the micrographs indicate the right lateral cushion (RLC), left lateral cushion (LLC), right and left atria (RA and LA, respectively), right and left ventricles (RV and LV, respectively), developing mitral (M) and tricuspid (T) valves, atrioventricular septum (AVS), and interventricular muscular septum (VS).

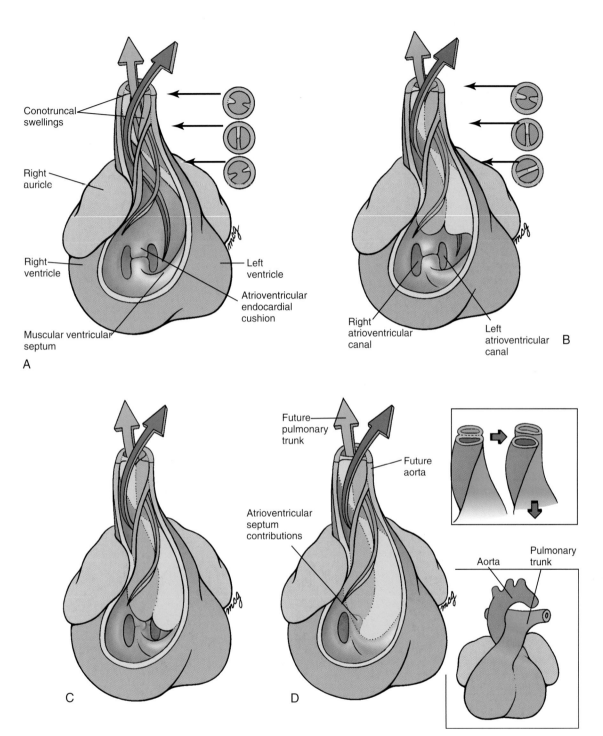

Figure 12-33. Septation of the cardiac outflow tract and completion of ventricular separation. Right oblique view. The cranial-lateral wall of the right ventricle has been removed to show the interior of the right ventricular chamber and the presumptive outflow tracts of both ventricles. *A, B,* Starting in the 5th week, the right and left conotruncal swellings grow out from the walls of the common outflow tract. These swellings are populated by endocardial and neural crest cell–derived cushion cells and develop in a spiraling configuration. They fuse with one another in a cranial-to-caudal direction forming the conotruncal septum, which separates the aortic and pulmonary outflow tracts. *C, D,* By the 9th week, the caudal end of the conotruncal septum has reached the level of the muscular portion of the interventricular septum and the atrioventricular septum. Here it fuses with these others to complete the interventricular septum.

12

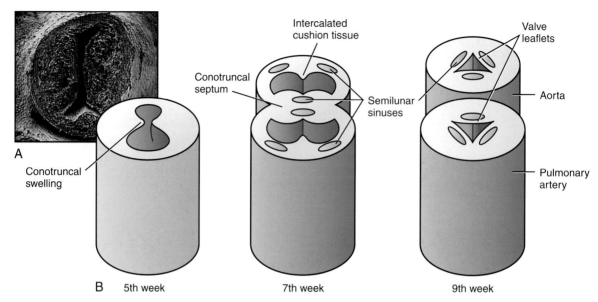

Figure 12-34. *A, B,* Formation of the semilunar valves. During formation of the conotruncal septum, two smaller and shorter intercalated cushion tissues form in the opposite quadrants. In the distal most conal segment, this new cushion tissue is excavated and remodeled within the wall of each new vessel to form two cavities. A similar cavity forms in both the aortic and pulmonary sides of the conotruncal septum. These cavities and the intervening tissue are subsequently remodeled to form the valvular sinuses and semilunar valves.

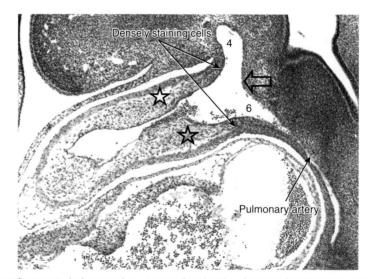

Figure 12-35. Division of the outflow tract in the human embryo. A mesenchymal wedge of tissue (indicated by open arrow) develops between the fourth (labeled 4) and sixth (labeled 6) aortic arch vessels in the roof of the aortic sac and begins separating the future systemic and pulmonary circuits. This septum extends toward the fusing conotruncal ridges (indicated by the stars) and fuses with them. The densely stained cells include migrating cardiac neural crest cells.

Development of Semilunar Valves

During the formation of the conotruncal septum, two additional smaller cushion tissues form in the opposite quadrants of the outflow tract called the **intercalated cushion tissue**. In the distal conal segment, this new cushion tissue is excavated and remodeled to form two cavities (the primordia of the **semilunar sinuses**) at the origin of the future ascending aorta and pulmonary artery (see Fig. 12-34B). Similarly, a cavity forms on both the aortic and pulmonary sides of the conotruncal septum at this same level. These cavities and the intervening tissue serve as the primordia for the **semilunar valves** and valvular sinuses. Although the conotruncal septum and tunics of the aorta and pulmonary vessels contain neural crest cell–derived cells, recent studies in mice show that semilunar valve leaflets are of endocardial-derived cushion tissue origin. However, studies suggest that interactions between endocardial-derived and neural crest cell–derived tissues may be required for proper semilunar valve formation. Development of the semilunar valves is complete by 9 weeks in humans.

IN THE RESEARCH LAB

NEURAL CREST CELL CONTRIBUTION TO OUTFLOW TRACT SEPTATION

The importance of neural crest cells in septation of the heart was first shown in neural crest cell ablation studies performed in chick embryos about 25 years ago. If the cardiac neural crest cell progenitors are removed from experimental animals before neural crest cells begin migrating, cardiac looping is abnormal and conotruncal septation is incomplete. Ablation of cardiac neural crest cells causes persistent truncus arteriosus, tricuspid stenosis, ventricular septal defects, transposition of the great vessels, double outlet right ventricle, and tetralogy of Fallot (see the following "In the Clinic"). Further evidence for a role of neural crest cells in heart development can be found in the frequent association of these cardiac anomalies with defects in development of the pharyngeal arches—structures through which the cardiac neural crest cells normally migrate. Birth defects in humans involving both the outflow tract and pharyngeal arches include **CHARGE syndrome** (coloboma of the eye, heart defects, atresia of the choanae, retarded growth and development, genital and urinary anomalies, and ear anomalies and hearing loss) and **22q11.2 deletion syndrome** (also known as **DiGeorge** or **velocardiofacial syndrome**; these syndromes are discussed later and in Ch. 16).

Neural crest cells contributing to the conotruncal septum are derived from a specific level of the future myelencephalon and are called **cardiac neural crest cells** (Fig. 12-36). Both cell-tracing studies using quail-chick transplantation chimeras and transgenic reporter mice (both discussed in Ch. 5) have revealed that not only do neural crest cells invade the conotruncal swellings, but a subset continues to invade and become localized adjacent the interventricular septum and atrioventricular canal. Moreover, there is some evidence suggesting that after a time, these neural crest cells undergo apoptosis. What their role is in this region is unclear, but it may have something to do with the remodeling necessary for realigning the atrioventricular canal, myocardialization, and separation of atrial and ventricular myocardium from one another. In addition to forming connective tissue and smooth muscle of the conotruncal septa and tunics of the aorta and pulmonary artery, neural crest cells give rise to the parasympathetic postganglionic neurons of the heart (the cardiac ganglia).

As mentioned earlier in the chapter, the loss of neural crest cell–derived mesenchymal cells in the outflow tract leads directly to cardiovascular defects. The loss of neural crest cell–derived mesenchyme in the heart can stem from faulty neural crest cell formation, migration, or proliferation. Perturbation of neural crest cell formation and migration leads to neural crest hypoplasia and an inadequate number of neural crest–derived mesenchymal cells reaching the heart. Several genes have been shown to play important roles in maintaining proper cardiac neural crest cell number and migration. *Splotch* mice, characterized by a mutation of *Pax3*, have a reduced number of neural crest cells reaching the pharyngeal arches and entering the outflow tract. These mice exhibit a phenotype resembling neural crest cell ablation including persistent truncus arteriosus and ventricular septal defects. These heart defects, but not the axial defects associated with *Splotch* mice, are rescued using promoters and enhancers that drive neural crest cell–specific *Pax3* expression in transgenic *Splotch* mice.

Double *Retinoic acid receptor* knockout animals (e.g., *RARα1* and all *RARβ1-3*) display intrinsic defects of the myocardium, but they also exhibit anomalies of heart development similar to those produced by neural crest cell ablation. Lineage-tracing studies of neural crest cells in

12

RARα1/RARβ-deficient mice suggest that neural crest cells themselves do not respond directly to retinoic acid but rather that the effects on cardiac neural crest cells is indirect. Other important molecules for directing or enabling cardiac neural crest cell migration are *Semaphorins*, a family of secreted molecules important in axon guidance as well as in directing neural crest cell migration. *Sema3C* and their receptors, complexes of *Plexins* and *Neuropilins*, are important in targeting cardiac neural crest cells into the pharyngeal arches and outflow tract, as mice lacking *Sema3C* and *Neuropilin* exhibit persistent truncus arteriosus and great vessel defects. In mice, knocking out the *Tgfβ type-II receptor* specifically in neural crest cells results in cardiovascular defects resembling those seen in DiGeorge syndrome. In this case, neural crest cell migration into the outflow tract seems normal. However, their subsequent differentiation into smooth muscle cells and connective tissue fails, resulting in persistent ductus arteriosus and ventricular septal defects.

MANY HEART DEFECTS MAY BE RELATED TO INTERACTIONS BETWEEN SECONDARY HEART FIELD AND NEURAL CREST CELLS

As stated earlier, if cardiac neural crest cells are removed from experimental animals before they migrate, several outflow tract and septal defects occur. However, these embryos exhibit other signs of abnormal cardiac development, including cardiac looping defects and early contractility defects, well before the stage when neural crest cells begin invading the outflow tract. As mentioned earlier, point mutations in *Tbx1* lead to heart defects such as persistent truncus arteriosus and tetralogy of Fallot. *Tbx1* is expressed in endoderm and mesoderm of the secondary heart field, and *Tbx1* deficiency leads to decreased levels of *Fgf8* here. Recent studies in chick embryos suggest that particular levels of *Fgf8* are required for proper secondary heart field cell proliferation. Interestingly, neural crest cell ablation increases *Fgf8* levels in the secondary heart field, resulting in outflow tract defects that can be rectified by adding *Fgf8* antibodies. Therefore, it seems that neural crest cells are required for maintaining specific levels of *Fgf8* within the secondary heart field, levels necessary for proper outflow tract lengthening, cardiac looping, and realignment. Neural crest cells may also regulate the expression of several other genes within the secondary heart field, including *Goosecoid*, *Dlx2* and *Dlx3*, and *Hand1* and *Hand2*. Therefore, abnormal cardiac neural crest cell development can lead to aberrant heart development by means other than only a loss of neural crest cell–derived cushion cells in the heart.

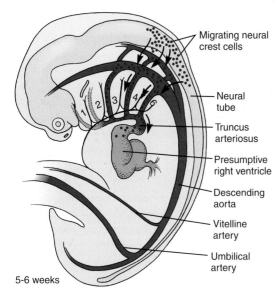

Figure 12-36. Source and migration route of cardiac neural crest cells. Neural crest cells migrate from the hindbrain through pharyngeal arches 3, 4, and 6 and then invade the outflow tract and contribute mesenchymal cells to the conotruncal septum.

Labels in figure:
- Migrating neural crest cells
- Neural tube
- Truncus arteriosus
- Presumptive right ventricle
- Descending aorta
- Vitelline artery
- Umbilical artery
- 5-6 weeks

Development of Pacemaker and Conduction System

The heart is one of the few organs that has to function almost as soon as it forms. The rhythmic waves of electrical depolarization (action potentials) that trigger the myocardium to contract arise spontaneously in the cardiac muscle itself and spread from cell to cell. The sympathetic and parasympathetic neural input to the heart that arises later in development modifies the heart rate but does not initiate contraction. Cardiomyocytes removed from the primitive heart tube and grown in tissue culture will begin to beat in unison if they become connected to one another, and studies with voltage-sensitive dyes indicate that cardiomyocytes may begin to produce rhythmic electrical activity even before the two early endocardial tubes have fused.

In a normally functioning mature heart, the beat is initiated in the **sinoatrial (SA) node** (the **pacemaker)**, which has a faster rate of spontaneous depolarization than the rest of the myocardium. Moreover, the depolarization spreads from the SA node to the rest of the heart along specialized **conduction pathways** that control the timing of contraction of the various regions of the myocardium, ensuring the chambers contract efficiently and in the right sequence. In the primitive heart tube, the cardiomyocytes begin contracting asynchronously. However, pacemaker activity is rapidly taken over by a cluster of cells in the sinoatrial region, which are derived either from the right common cardinal vein or the right sinus venosus. These cells eventually differentiate to form the contractile, pacemaking component of the distinct ovoid SA node located near the left venous valve.

Soon after development of the SA node, cells within the atrioventricular junction adjacent to the endocardial cushion begin to form a secondary pacemaker center, the **atrioventricular (AV) node**, which regulates conduction of the impulses from the atrium to the ventricles and coordinates the contraction of the two ventricles. The main conduction pathway between the SA node and AV node runs through the crista terminalis, although other pathways in the interatrial septum have been found. The development of the AV node is accompanied by the formation of a bundle of specialized conducting cells, the **bundle of His**, which sends one branch into the left ventricle and the other into the right ventricle within the moderator band. This conduction pathway must be carefully avoided during the repair of ventricular septal defects. Branches of **Purkinje fibers** spreading out from the bundles then deliver the depolarization signal to the rest of the ventricular myocardium.

The detailed ontogeny of the cardiac conduction system is unclear. However, it seems that most of the conduction pathway arises from cardiogenic mesoderm and cardiomyocytes, and it is postulated that tissue interactions between neural crest cell–derived cells and the epicardium have, as yet, an undetermined role in the differentiation of the central conducting system and Purkinje system. The myocardial cells of the conducting system are contractile but differentiate into cells specialized for generating and conducting action potentials responsible for mediating rhythmic and wavelike contraction of the heart.

Understanding development of this network is important, as many adults experience arrhythmias, with some anomalies being associated with mutations in developmental control genes having key roles in heart development. For instance, in humans as well as mice, mutations in *NKX2.5* are associated with anomalies of the conduction system. Understanding embryonic development of the conducting system may also shed light on the etiological basis of congenital arrhythmias.

Development of Epicardium and Coronary Vasculature

The progenitor of the epicardium, the **proepicardial organ**, consists of a special group of splanchnic mesodermal cells forming at the posterior dorsal mesocardium/septum transversum junction (Fig. 12-37A; see Fig. 12-22B). These cells migrate as an epithelial sheet of cells over the entire myocardial surface (Fig. 12-37B). Once it covers the surface of the myocardium, this epicardial epithelium deposits and assembles an extracellular matrix between the epicardial epithelium and myocardium. This is followed by an epithelial-to-mesenchymal transformation of the epicardial epithelium, generating a mesenchymal cell population that invades the subepicardial extracellular matrix in much the same way as endocardial-derived cushion tissue is generated. In addition to forming the connective tissue of the epicardium, **epicardial-derived mesenchymal cells** provide the progenitor cells for the coronary endothelium and smooth muscle cells. After initial vasculogenesis, ensuing **angiogenesis** (sprouting from preexisting blood vessels; discussed in Ch. 13) into the myocardial walls seems to be driven by hypoxia resulting from the thickening of the myocardium. The initial vasculogenic and angiogenic processes leading to formation of the coronary vascular network involves many of the same signaling molecules and regulatory events as occur during blood vessel formation elsewhere in the embryo (discussed in Ch. 13). The connection of the developing coronary vasculature to the aorta occurs by invasion of the developing coronary arteries through the wall of the (ascending) aorta. Why only two coronary artery trunks form and how they find their way to the future site of the aortic sinuses is still unclear. However, factors secreted by neural crest cell–derived parasympathetic ganglia may provide important directional cues: developing coronary artery trunks lie close to these ganglia, and in neural crest cell–ablated chick embryos, the coronary trunks arise in abnormal positions.

12

Primitive ventricle

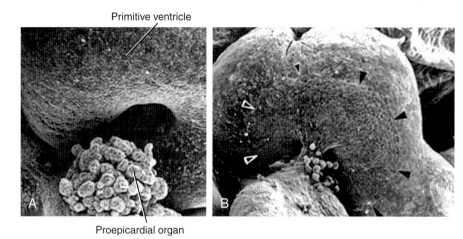

Proepicardial organ

Figure 12-37. *A, B,* The epicardium is formed from migrating cells derived from the proepicardial organ found in the region of the sinus venosus. These cells migrate over and cover the entire myocardium (arrowheads) and eventually form the epicardium and the coronary vessels.

IN THE CLINIC

FREQUENCY AND ETIOLOGY OF CARDIOVASCULAR MALFORMATIONS

Congenital cardiovascular malformations account for about 20% of all congenital defects observed in live-born infants. They occur in about 5 to 8 of every 1000 live births, and the percentage in stillborn infants is probably even higher. In addition, the recurrence risk in siblings with isolated heart malformations is 2% to 5%, indicating that heart defects include a genetic contribution.

Neither the cause nor the pathogenesis of most heart defects is understood. However, progressively more of these defects are being associated with specific genetic errors or environmental teratogens. Overall, about 4% of cardiovascular defects can be ascribed to single-gene mutations; another 6% to chromosomal aberrations such as trisomies, monosomies, or deletions; and 5% to exposure to specific teratogens. The teratogens known to induce heart defects include not only chemicals such as lithium, alcohol, and retinoic acid but also factors associated with certain maternal diseases such as diabetes and rubella (German measles). The etiology of most of the remaining cardiac abnormalities seems to be **multifactorial**—that is, they stem from the interaction of environmental or outside influences with a poorly defined constellation of the individual's own genetic determinants. Thus, individuals may show very different genetic susceptibilities to the action of a given teratogen.

Blood pressure and blood flow, factors unique to the developing cardiovascular system, play important roles in the development of the heart such that perturbations in the pressure relationships among the heart chambers and outflow tracts cause malformations. Such perturbations may be brought about by several kinds of primary defects—by abnormal compliance or deformability of the atrial, ventricular, or outflow tract walls; or by abnormal expansion or constriction of the semilunar valves, ductus arteriosus, and great arteries (discussed in Ch. 13). For example, if ejection of blood from the right ventricle is prevented by pulmonary valvular atresia, the right ventricle becomes hypoplastic and the pulmonary arteries underdeveloped. If blood flow into the right ventricle from the right atrium is prevented by tricuspid atresia, the right ventricle becomes hypoplastic while the left ventricle hypertrophies under the extra workload placed on it to drive blood into the pulmonary circulation through a ventricular septal defect. Excessive interatrial flow can cause a septum secundum defect by enlarging the foramen ovale and eroding septal structures. The resulting increased inflow through the left side of the heart may interfere with the normal formation of the conotruncal septum and prevent development of the ventricular membranous septum.

COMMON HEART MALFORMATIONS
Atrial Septal Defects

In about 6 of 10,000 live-born infants, the septum secundum is too short to cover the foramen secundum completely (or the foramen secundum is too large), so that an **atrial septal defect** persists after the septum primum and septum secundum are pressed together at birth (Fig. 12-38). Septum

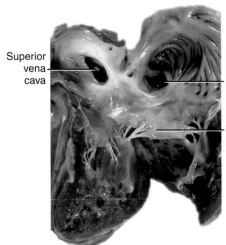

Superior vena cava

Atrial septal defect—foramen ovale and foramen secundum overlap

Tricuspid leaflet

Figure 12-38. Infant heart with atrial septal defect. The foramen secundum and foramen ovale in this heart overlap abnormally and, therefore, could not close at birth, resulting in continued mixing of right and left atrial blood after birth.

secundum defects cause shunting of blood from the left atrium to the right atrium. Infants with this abnormality are generally asymptomatic, but the persistent increase in flow to the right atrium may lead to enlargement of the right atrium and ventricle, resulting in debilitating atrial arrhythmias later in life. Excessive pulmonary blood flow also causes pulmonary hypertension over time, leading to heart failure. Atrial septal defects are mostly detected by echocardiography in childhood, and they may warrant closure either surgically or by an occluding device to prevent the onset of cardiac hypertrophy and pulmonary hyper-tension. An atrial septal defect is associated with almost all documented autosomal and sex chromosome aberrations, and is a common accompaniment of several partial and complete trisomies, including trisomy 21 (Down syndrome).

Persistent Atrioventricular Canal

Persistent atrioventricular canal arises from failure of the dorsal and ventral endocardial cushions to fuse. This defect commonly occurs in **Down syndrome**. The failure of the dorsal and ventral endocardial cushions to fuse can lead to a variety of secondary abnormalities, including incompletion of the septum primum or interventricular septum and malformation of the atrioventricular valves. One physiologic consequence of the defect is persistent left-to-right shunting of blood after birth, the magnitude of which depends on the severity of the defect. Congestive heart failure in infancy is not unlikely if the defect is severe. Atrial septal defects,

malformed mitral valves, and absent interventricular septums can all be corrected surgically.

Ventricular Septal Defects

Ventricular septal defects are one of the most common of all congenital heart malformations, accounting for 25% of all cardiac abnormalities documented in live-born infants and occurring as isolated defects in 12 of 10,000 births (Fig. 12-39). The prevalence of this defect seems to be increasing, a statistic that may represent an actual increase in incidence or may simply reflect the application of better diagnostic methods. A ventricular septal defect can arise from several causes: (1) deficient development of the proximal conotruncal swellings, (2) failure of the muscular and membranous ventricular septa to fuse, (3) failure of the dorsal and ventral endocardial cushions to fuse (atrioventricular septal defect), and (4) insufficient development of the interventricular muscular septum. Whatever the origin of a ventricular septal defect, its most serious consequence is the left-to-right shunting of blood and the consequent increased blood flow to the pulmonary circulation. It can be repaired surgically.

Atrioventricular Valve Defects

Atrioventricular valve defects arise from errors in the remodeling necessary for forming the valve leaflets, chordae tendineae, and papillary muscles from the endocardial cushion tissue and ventricular myocardium. The pathogenesis of **valve atresia**, in which the valvular orifice is completely obliterated, is not understood. If the atrioventricular septum does not form, sometimes the wedging and remodeling required for aligning the atrioventricular canals with the appropriate ventricle fails. As a consequence, a ventricle can end up having a double inlet (having the inflow from both atria). Likewise, malalignment of the outflow tract may lead to a ventricle having a double outlet (having both the aorta and pulmonary artery). In **double-outlet right ventricle malformation**, both the aortic and pulmonary outflow tracts connect to the right ventricle, and this malformation is almost always accompanied by a ventricular septal defect. All arterial blood flow leaves from the right ventricle and there is mixing of oxygenated blood with unoxygenated blood within the right ventricle. Symptoms show up within days after birth and include **cyanosis** (inadequate oxygenation of the blood), heart **murmur**, breathlessness, and (later) poor weight gain. The incidence of this malformation is approximately 1 in 3,000 births, and it can be corrected surgically.

In **tricuspid valve atresia**, the right atrium is cut off from the right ventricle due to abnormal development of the tricuspid valve. As a result, right atrial blood shunts to

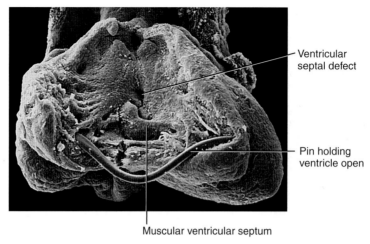

Figure 12-39. Typical ventricular septal defect in a mouse fetus with trisomy 12. Failure of the membranous ventricular septum to fuse with the upper ridge of the muscular septum in this heart has resulted in a ventricular septal defect.

the left atrium through a **persistent foramen ovale**. Moreover, most of the blood that reaches the pulmonary arteries does so by taking a roundabout route through a ventricular septal defect and/or via the aorta and a **persistent ductus arteriosus**. The ductus arteriosus is a connection between the aorta and the pulmonary trunk and normally closes soon after birth (discussed in Ch. 13). As a consequence, the heart is functionally a univentricular heart, as the circulation is driven solely by the left ventricle. Hence, the right ventricle is **hypoplastic** while the left ventricle enlarges (i.e. **hypertrophies**). Over time this leads to cardiac failure.

Semilunar Valvular Stenosis

Semilunar valvular stenosis involves stenosis of either the aortic valve or the pulmonary valve. **Aortic valvular stenosis** leads to **hypertrophy** of the left ventricle, pulmonary hypertension, and eventually cardiac failure. It can be congenital (usually the case if the symptoms appear before age 30), the result of an infection (such as rheumatic fever), or degenerative (a consequence of aging). Collectively, the incidence is 1% to 2% of the population, with a greater frequency in males (4:1, male to female ratio). Congenital valvular stenosis is likely caused by an error in the cavitation and remodeling within the distal conal cushion tissue responsible for forming the aortic semilunar valves, leading to a **bicommissural** (also called bicuspid, that is, with two rather than three leaves) **aortic valve**. A bicommissural valve can be asymptomatic or stenotic from infancy or may become stenotic over time, often due to calcification.

Septation Defects of Outflow Tract

A variety of malformations resulting from errors in the septation of the outflow tract may be caused by abnormal neural crest cell development. In about 1 of 10,000 live-born infants, the conotruncal septa do not form at all, resulting in a **persistent truncus arteriosus** (Fig. 12-40A, B). This malformation necessarily includes a **ventricular septal defect**. The result is that blood from the two sides of the heart mixes in the common outflow tract, mainly in left-to-right shunting toward the pulmonary side, leading to pulmonary hypertension. Left untreated, infants with this defect usually die within the first 2 years. Surgical correction is possible and involves repairing the ventricular septal defect and implanting a valved prosthetic shunt between the right ventricle and the pulmonary arteries.

In about 5 of 10,000 live-born infants, the conotruncal septa develop but do not display the usual spiral pattern. The result is **transposition of the great vessels**, in which the left ventricle empties into the pulmonary circulation and the right ventricle empties into the systemic circulation (Fig. 12-40C, D). Transposition of the great vessels is often fatal unless the ductus arteriosus remains patent or is accompanied by intrinsic atrial or ventricular septal defects or by defects introduced surgically (to establish an interatrial communication), allowing the deoxygenated systemic and the newly oxygenated pulmonary blood to mix. Transposition can be surgically corrected with a favorable prognosis. Nevertheless, it is the leading cause of death in infants with cyanotic heart disease younger than 1 year old.

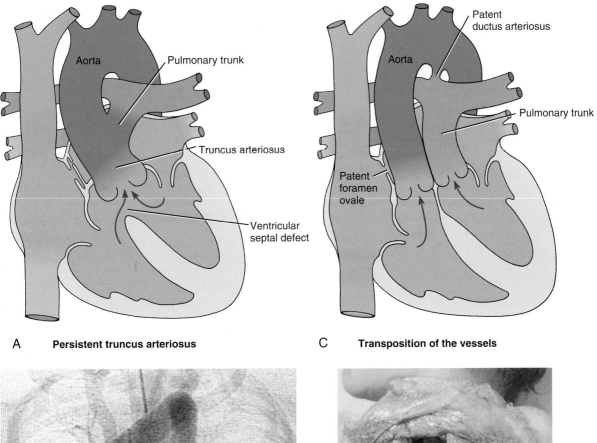

A   **Persistent truncus arteriosus**

C   **Transposition of the vessels**

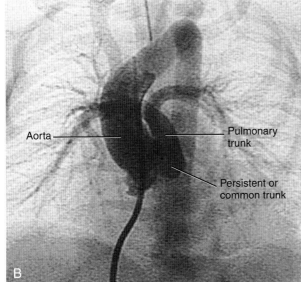

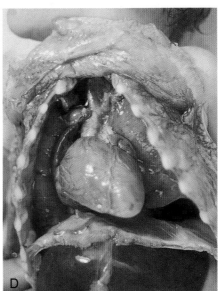

Figure 12-40. *A, B,* Persistent truncus arteriosus (shown in an angiogram in *B*). Incomplete separation of aortic and pulmonary outflow tracts accompanies a ventricular septal defect when the conotruncal septum fails to form. *C, D,* Transposition of the great arteries results from failure of the conotruncal septum to spiral as it separates the aortic and pulmonary outflow tracts.

Tetralogy of Fallot

Many cardiac defects occur together more often than in isolation. In some cases, such associated defects are actually components of the same malformation—as, for example, a ventricular septal defect is a necessary consequence of persistent truncus arteriosus. In other cases, a primary malformation sets off a cascade of effects that leads to other malformations. An example is the pathogenesis of **tetralogy of Fallot**, a syndrome described by Steno of Denmark in 1673 and referred to as *maladie bleue* by Etienne-Louis Arthur Fallot in 1888 (Fig. 12-41). Fallot used the term *tetralogy* to refer to the four classic malformations in this syndrome: (1) **pulmonary stenosis**, (2) **ventricular septal defect**, (3) rightward displacement of the aorta (sometimes called **overriding aorta**), and (4) **right ventricular hypertrophy**. The primary defect is unequal division of the outflow tract, favoring the aorta, with malalignment of the muscular outlet septum with respect to the right and left ventricles. All these defects conspire to raise the blood pressure in the right ventricle, resulting in progressive right ventricular hypertrophy. Tetralogy of Fallot is the most common cyanotic congenital heart malformation, occurring in approximately 1 of 1000 live-born infants. The condition may be corrected surgically by relieving the obstruction of the pulmonary trunk and repairing the ventricular septal defect.

KNOWN GENETIC CAUSES OF HEART MALFORMATIONS

Based on genetic studies in families, many cardiac malformations have been ascribed to single-gene mutations, with continuing progress in identifying more through animal studies and human genetic linkage studies. However, to date only a few have been found that are non–syndrome-associated gene mutations occurring in so-called isolated heart defects. One of the earliest acting of these mutations occurs in *NKX2.5*. This gene plays an important role in specification of the early cardiogenic field, but it is also involved in several subsequent cardiac morphogenic events. Mutations in *NKX2.5* in humans are associated with atrial septal defects and defects in the conduction system. Mutations in *GATA4* have also been found in the human population. These mutations alter the transcriptional activity of *GATA4* and its interaction with other gene products important in cardiac development, including *TBX5*. Mutations in *GATA4* have been linked to atrial septal defects and pulmonary valvular stenosis. Mutations in *CYSTEINE-RICH PROTEIN WITH EGF-LIKE DOMAINS* (*CRELD1*; a cell adhesion molecule) have been found in patients with atrioventricular septal defects.

A number of specific gene mutations have also been identified in syndromes that contain heart defects as a consistent finding. Mutations have been found in various genes causing laterality and cardiac looping defects.

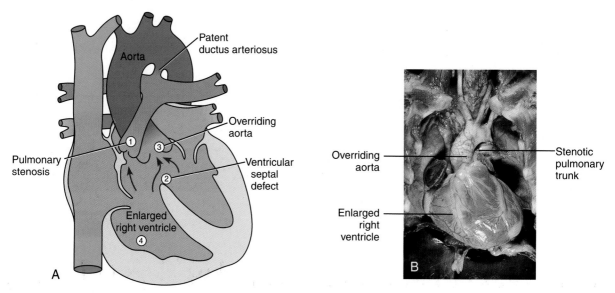

Figure 12-41. Tetralogy of Fallot. *A*, Classically, tetralogy of Fallot is characterized by (1) stenosis (narrowing) of the pulmonary trunk, (2) ventricular septal defect, (3) overriding aorta, and (4) an enlarged right ventricle. A patent ductus arteriosus is also present. *B*, The enlarged right ventricle and overriding aorta are obvious in this case of tetralogy of Fallot.

Mutations in genes encoding axonemal *DYNEINS* are found in patients with **Kartagener syndrome** (discussed in Chs. 3 and 11). **Randomized laterality** and **visceroatrial heterotaxy** occur in patients with mutations in *NODAL*, *LEFTY1*, *LEFTY2*, *CRYPTIC*, and *ACVR2B* (an *Activin* receptor). Patients with **Leopard syndrome** or **Noonan syndrome** both exhibit pulmonary stenosis and conduction anomalies as well as overlapping craniofacial and skeletal anomalies that can be caused by the different mutations in the *PTPN11* gene. This gene encodes a *SHP2* protein, a nonreceptor *Tyrosine phosphatase* involved in intracellular signal transduction (Noonan syndrome is also discussed in Ch. 13). Deletion or mutations in the *JAGGED1* gene (a gene encoding a ligand for *NOTCH* signaling) or *NOTCH2* (a gene encoding for a *NOTCH* receptor) is responsible for **Alagille syndrome** (mentioned in Chs. 3, 5, 13, and 14), and 70% to 95% of these patients exhibit heart defects including stenosis of the pulmonary arteries or valves, septal defects, and tetralogy of Fallot. Mutations of the *CHD7* (*CHROMODOMAIN HELICASE DNA-BINDING PROTEIN 7*) gene on human chromosome 8 have been found in 60% of patients with **CHARGE syndrome** (incidence 1 out of 9,000 to 10,000; also discussed in Chs. 4 and 17), and 75% of these patients exhibit heart defects. Studies in human embryos show neural crest cell–derived mesenchyme is one of the primary tissues expressing this gene.

Most of the 250,000 individuals who suffer sudden death each year in the United States die of **cardiac arrhythmias**. One inborn cause of arrhythmias is **long QT syndrome**, characterized by prolongation of the depolarization (Q) and repolarization (T) intervals diagnosed by electrocardiogram (ECG or EKG). Long QT syndrome predisposes affected individuals to **syncope** (loss of consciousness) and sudden death. Not surprisingly, genetic disruptions underlying this autosomal dominant disease include mutations in *KVLQT1*, *HERG*, *SCN5A*, and other genes that encode **cardiac ion channels**.

22Q11.2 DELETIONS AND HEART MALFORMATIONS

Patients with **22q11.2 deletion syndrome** (also known as **DiGeorge** and **velocardiofacial syndromes**) exhibit congenital anomalies that place them within the neurocristopathy family of defects (discussed in Ch. 4; 22q11.2 deletion syndrome is also discussed in Ch. 13 and 16). They involve at least one element of abnormal neural crest cell development and manifest congenital heart defects as a part of their pathology. These patients have microdeletions within the 22q11.2 region, which occur in 1 out of 10,000 to 20,000 live births. Common heart defects are tetralogy of Fallot, interrupted aortic arch (discussed in Ch. 13), ventricular septal defects, persistent truncus arteriosus, and

vascular rings (discussed in Ch. 13). Therefore, presentation of these types of defects should alert the physician to look for possibility of 22q11.2 deletions and other pathologic conditions that may arise from such deletions. The search is on for genes in this region that may be responsible for the symptoms of these deletions. Several putative genes have been identified including *TBX1*, *UFD1* (*UBIQUITIN FUSION DEGRADATION 1*, a gene regulated by *HAND2*), and *HIRA* (a gene encoding for a protein that interacts with *PAX3*). In the case of *TBX1*, rare mutations have been found in patients with DiGeorge phenotype lacking a 22q11.2 deletion, suggesting that in some cases a single gene can cause DiGeorge syndrome. However, in the vast majority of patients, the loss of multiple linked 22q11.2 genes is likely responsible.

Suggested Readings

Anderson RH, Webb S, Brown NA, et al. 2003. Development of the heart: (2) septation of the atriums and ventricles. Heart 89:949-958.

Anderson RH, Webb S, Brown NA, et al. 2003. Development of the heart: (3) formation of the ventricular outflow tracts, arterial valves, and intrapericardial arterial trunks. Heart 89:1110-1118.

Armstrong EJ, Bischoff J. 2004. Heart valve development: endothelial cell signaling and differentiation. Circ Res 95:459-470.

Ausoni S, Sartore S. 2001. Cell lineages and tissue boundaries in cardiac arterial and venous poles: developmental patterns, animal models, and implications for congenital vascular diseases. Arterioscler Thromb Vasc Biol 21:312-320.

Brand T. 2003. Heart development: molecular insights into cardiac specification and early morphogenesis. Dev Biol 258:1-19.

Buckingham M, Meilhac S, Zaffran S. 2005. Building the mammalian heart from two sources of myocardial cells. Nat Rev Genet 6:826-835.

Farrell MJ, Kirby ML. 2001. Cell biology of cardiac development. Int Rev Cytol 202:99-158.

Firulli AB, Conway SJ. 2004. Combinatorial transcriptional interaction within the cardiac neural crest: a pair of HANDs in heart formation. Birth Defects Res C Embryo Today 72:151-161.

Gittenberger-de Groot AC, Bartelings MM, Deruiter MC, Poelmann RE. 2005. Basics of cardiac development for the understanding of congenital heart malformations. Pediatr Res 57:169-176.

Hutson MR, Kirby ML. 2003. Neural crest and cardiovascular development: a 20-year perspective. Birth Defects Res C Embryo Today 69:2-13.

Kathiriya IS, Srivastava D. 2000. Left-right asymmetry and cardiac looping: implications for cardiac development and congenital heart disease. Am J Med Genet 97:271-279.

Lamers WH, Moorman AF. 2002. Cardiac septation: a late contribution of the embryonic primary myocardium to heart morphogenesis. Circ Res 91:93-103.

Linask KK. 2003. Regulation of heart morphology: current molecular and cellular perspectives on the coordinated emergence

12

of cardiac form and function. Birth Defects Res C Embryo Today 69:14-24.

Lincoln J, Alfieri CM, Yutzey KE. 2004. Development of heart valve leaflets and supporting apparatus in chicken and mouse embryos. Dev Dyn 230:239-250.

Majesky MW. 2004. Development of coronary vessels. Curr Top Dev Biol 62:225-259.

Manner J, Perez-Pomares JM, Macias D, Munoz-Chapuli R. 2001. The origin, formation and developmental significance of the epicardium: a review. Cells Tissues Organs 169:89-103.

Marvin MJ, Di Rocco G, Gardiner A, et al. 2001. Inhibition of Wnt activity induces heart formation from posterior mesoderm. Genes Dev 15:316-327.

Moorman A, Webb S, Brown NA, et al. 2003. Development of the heart: (1) formation of the cardiac chambers and arterial trunks. Heart 89:806-814.

Munoz-Chapuli R, Gonzalez-Iriarte M, Carmona R, et al. 2002. Cellular precursors of the coronary arteries. Tex Heart Inst J 29:243-249.

Person AD, Klewer SE, Runyan RB. 2005. Cell biology of cardiac cushion development. Int Rev Cytol 243:287-335.

Plageman TF, Jr., Yutzey KE. 2005. T-box genes and heart development: putting the "T" in heart. Dev Dyn 232:11-20.

Restivo A, Piacentini G, Placidi S, et al. 2006. Cardiac outflow tract: a review of some embryogenetic aspects of the conotruncal region of the heart. Anat Rec A Discov Mol Cell Evol Biol 288:936-943.

Tomanek RJ, Hansen HK, Dedkov EI. 2006. Vascular patterning of the quail coronary system during development. Anat Rec A Discov Mol Cell Evol Biol 288:989-999.

Sedmera D, Pexieder T, Vuillemin M, et al. 2000. Developmental patterning of the myocardium. Anat Rec 258:319-337.

van den Hoff MJ, Kruithof BP, Moorman AF. 2004. Making more heart muscle. Bioessays 26:248-261.

Webb S, Qayyum SR, Anderson RH, et al. 2003. Septation and separation within the outflow tract of the developing heart. J Anat 202:327-342.

Xavier-Neto J, Rosenthal N, Silva FA, et al. 2001. Retinoid signaling and cardiac anteroposterior segmentation. Genesis 31:97-104.

Yutzey KE, Kirby ML. 2002. Wherefore heart thou? Embryonic origins of cardiogenic mesoderm. Dev Dyn 223:307-320.

Zaffran S, Frasch M. 2002. Early signals in cardiac development. Circ Res 91:457-469.

Development of the Vasculature

13

Summary

Starting on day 17, vessels begin to arise in the splanchnic mesoderm of the yolk sac wall from aggregations of cells called **hemangioblastic aggregates**. From these aggregates two cell lineages arise, primitive **hematopoietic stem cells** and **endothelial precursor cells**. On day 18, **vasculogenesis** (de novo blood vessel formation) commences in the splanchnic mesoderm of the embryonic disc and later in the paraxial mesoderm. In the embryonic disc, endothelial cell precursors differentiate into endothelial cells and organize into networks of small vessels that coalesce, grow, and invade other tissues to form the primary embryonic vasculature. This primitive vasculature is expanded and remodeled by **angiogenesis**. Hematopoiesis begins in the yolk sac and extraembryonic mesoderm. It is later shifted to the liver, where the hematopoietic stem cells are joined by a second source of hematopoietic stems cells arising from intraembryonic splanchnic mesoderm surrounding the dorsal aorta of the gonadal/mesonephric region. Definitive hematopoietic stem cells are programmed within the liver, and they later colonize the bone marrow and other lymphatic organs.

As body folding carries the endocardial tubes into the ventral thorax during the 4th week, the paired dorsal aortae attached to the cranial ends of the tubes are pulled ventrally to form a pair of dorsoventral loops, the **first aortic arches**. During the 4th and 5th weeks, four additional pairs of aortic arches develop in craniocaudal succession, connecting the aortic sac at the distal end of the truncus arteriosus to the dorsal aortae. This aortic arch system is subsequently remodeled to form the system of great arteries in the upper thorax and neck.

The paired dorsal aortae remain separate in the region of the aortic arches but fuse below the level of the fourth thoracic segment to form a single median dorsal aorta. The dorsal aorta develops three sets of branches: (1) a series of ventral branches, which supply the gut and gut derivatives; (2) lateral branches, which supply retroperitoneal structures such as the suprarenal glands, kidneys, and gonads; and (3) dorsolateral intersegmental branches called **intersegmental arteries**, which penetrate between the somite derivatives and give rise to part of the vasculature of the head, neck, body wall, limbs, and vertebral column. The ventral branches, which supply the gastrointestinal tract, are derived from remnants of a network of **vitelline arteries**, which develop in the yolk sac and vitelline duct and anastomose with the paired dorsal aortae. The paired dorsal aortae become connected to the **umbilical arteries** that develop in the connecting stalk and carry blood to the placenta.

The primitive venous system consists of three major components, all of which are at first bilaterally symmetric: the **cardinal system**, which drains the head, neck, body wall, and limbs; the **vitelline veins**, which initially drain the yolk sac; and the **umbilical veins**, which develop in the connecting stalk and carry oxygenated blood from the placenta to the embryo. All three systems initially drain into both sinus horns, but all three undergo extensive modification during development as the systemic venous return is shifted to the right atrium.

The cardinal system initially consists of paired **anterior (cranial)** and **posterior (caudal) cardinal veins**, which meet to form short **common cardinal veins** draining into the right and left sinus horns. However, the posterior cardinals are supplemented and later replaced by two subsidiary venous systems, the **subcardinal** and **supracardinal** systems, which grow caudally from the base of the posterior cardinals in the medial dorsal body wall. All three of these cardinal systems, along with a small region of the right vitelline vein, give rise to portions of the inferior vena cava and its major branches. The supracardinals also form the azygos and hemiazygos systems draining the thoracic body wall. The vitelline venous system gives rise to the liver sinusoids and to the portal

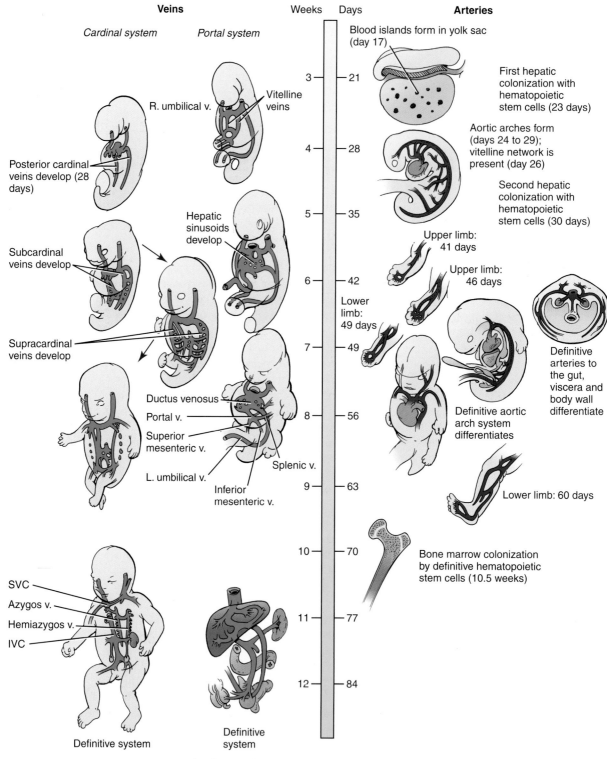

Veins

Weeks Days

Arteries

Cardinal system   *Portal system*

Blood islands form in yolk sac
(day 17)

First hepatic
colonization with
hematopoietic
stem cells (23 days)

R. umbilical v.

Vitelline
veins

3 — 21

Posterior cardinal
veins develop (28
days)

4 — 28

Aortic arches form
(days 24 to 29);
vitelline network is
present (day 26)

Hepatic
sinusoids
develop

5 — 35

Second hepatic
colonization with
hematopoietic
stem cells (30 days)

Subcardinal
veins develop

Upper limb:
41 days

Upper limb:
46 days

6 — 42

Lower
limb:
49 days

Supracardinal
veins develop

7 — 49

Definitive
arteries to
the gut,
viscera and
body wall
differentiate

Ductus venosus

Portal v.

Superior
mesenteric v.

8 — 56

Definitive aortic
arch system
differentiates

L. umbilical v.

Splenic v.

Inferior
mesenteric v.

9 — 63

Lower limb: 60 days

10 — 70

Bone marrow colonization
by definitive hematopoietic
stem cells (10.5 weeks)

SVC

Azygos v.

Hemiazygos v.

IVC

11 — 77

12 — 84

Definitive system

Definitive
system

Time line. Development of the arterial and venous systems.

system, which carries venous blood from the gastrointestinal tract to the liver. Within the substance of the liver, the **vitelline system** also forms the **ductus venosus**, a channel that shunts blood from the umbilical vein directly to the inferior vena cava during gestation.

All three venous systems undergo extensive modification during development. In the cardinal and vitelline systems, the longitudinal veins on the left side of the body tend to regress, whereas those on the right side persist and give rise to the great veins. Thus, a bilateral system that drains into both sinus horns becomes a right-sided system that drains into the right atrium. In contrast, the right umbilical vein disappears, whereas the left umbilical vein persists. However, the left umbilical vein loses its original connection to the left sinus horn and secondarily empties into the ductus venosus.

A dramatic and rapid change in the pattern of circulation occurs at birth as the newborn begins to breathe, the pulmonary vasculature expands, and circulation stops from the placenta to the fetus. Much of the development described in this chapter is focused on the problem of producing a circulation that will effectively distribute the oxygenated blood arriving from the placenta via the umbilical vein to the tissues of the embryo and fetus, yet will be able to convert rapidly at birth to the adult pattern of circulation required by the air-breathing infant.

Clinical Taster   While examining a 14-year-old girl with a history of severe recurrent epistaxis (nosebleeds), an otolaryngologist—ear, nose, and throat (or ENT) specialist—notes several small dilated blood vessels on the mucosa of the nasal passages and mouth. The girl's nosebleeds started at age 11. Recently they have become more frequent and now occur two or three times a week. The bleeding has been severe enough to cause a mild anemia despite treatment with iron.

In addition to nosebleeds, the patient has significant dyspnea (shortness of breath) during exercise that is out of proportion to her degree of anemia. She also has increased heart rate and subtle clubbing of the fingers. A pulse oximeter reading shows a blood oxygen saturation of 88%. The ENT makes a presumptive diagnosis of **hereditary hemorrhagic telangiectasia (HHT)**, also known as **Osler-Weber-Rendu disease**.

The girl is referred for an air-contrast **echocardiogram** that shows air bubbles passing from the right side of the heart to the left, indicating a pulmonary arterial-venous shunt. A CT (computed tomography) angiogram verifies the presence of a right-sided **pulmonary arterial-venous malformation** measuring 7 mm in diameter. Interventional radiology is consulted, and the shunt is corrected using coil embolization (inserting a small coil to clot off the vessel). Following the procedure, the girl's oxygen saturation increases to normal, and her exercise tolerance gradually improves. Genetic testing reveals an inactivating mutation in the **ENDOGLIN** (ENG) gene.

HHT is an autosomal dominant condition characterized by abnormal connections between arteries and veins without intervening capillaries. When small, these abnormalities are called **telangiectases** and occur on the mucosal surfaces of the nose, mouth, and gastrointestinal track, as well as on the fingers. These thin-walled lesions are near the surface and bleed easily. Larger telangiectases, or arterial-venous malformations (AVM), can occur in the lungs, liver, or brain. Besides the morbidity associated with shunting of blood, a variety of other life-threatening complications are associated with AVMs including stroke, abscess, or bleeding in the brain. HHT is caused by mutations in the genes encoding either the *TGFβ*-binding protein *ENDOGLIN* or one type of *TGFβ* receptor (*ACTIVIN A RECEPTOR, TYPE II-LIKE KINASE 1*). Both of these proteins are involved in cell signaling during development of vascular endothelial cells.

13

Formation of Vasculature Begins Early in Third Week

Hematopoietic stem cells (HSC) and endothelial cells are among the first and earliest cell types to differentiate into a functional phenotype in the embryo. In humans, the earliest evidence for blood and blood vessel formation is seen in the extraembryonic splanchnic mesoderm of the yolk sac at about day 17 in the form of hemangioblastic aggregates developing adjacent the endoderm (Fig. 13-1).

Hemangioblastic aggregates subsequently form in the connecting stalk and mesoderm of the chorion. Two cell lineages arise from within the hemangioblastic aggregates (most likely from a single precursor referred to as a hemangioblast), the primitive HSCs and endothelial precursor cells (EPCs). Together they form what are often referred to as blood islands (see Fig. 13-1). Primitive HSCs of the yolk sac form almost exclusively erythropoietic cells (and some pluripotent progenitor cells for megakaryocytes and primitive macrophages) through a process known as hematopoiesis or hemopoiesis

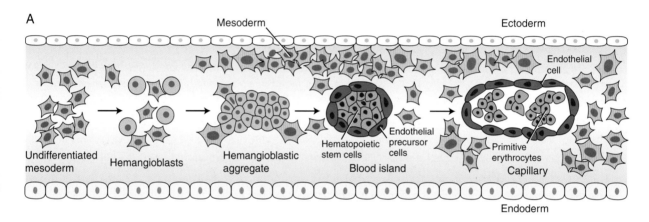

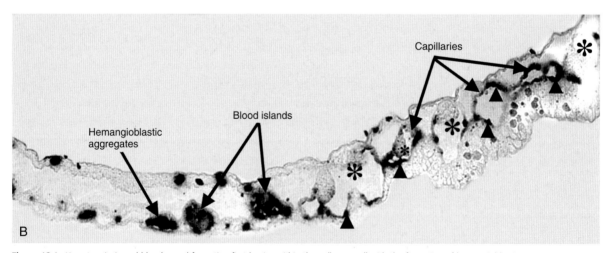

Figure 13-1. Hematopoiesis and blood vessel formation first begins within the yolk sac wall with the formation of hemangioblastic aggregates. *A*, Drawing illustrating the formation of hemangioblastic aggregates and their differentiation into hematopoietic stem cells and endothelial precursor cells within blood islands. Blood islands subsequently form both endothelial cells and primitive erythrocytes. *B*, Expression of *Vegfr2* mRNA, an early marker for hemangioblastic aggregates, within the yolk sac wall of a 15-somite avian embryo. As the blood islands develop, endothelial cells retain *Vegfr2* expression, whereas hematopoietic stem cells progressively lose it.

(blood cell production). Hemangioblasts surrounding the islands of primitive HSCs enter into the EPC lineage, then differentiate into endothelial cells and organize into small capillary vessels through a process called **vasculogenesis** (described in the following section). These small capillaries lengthen and interconnect, establishing an initial primary vascular network. By the end of the 3rd week, this network completely vascularizes the yolk sac, connecting stalk, and chorionic villi.

The yolk sac is the first supplier of blood cells to the embryonic circulation. The cells supplied are predominantly nucleated erythrocytes containing embryonic hemoglobin (**primitive erythrocytes**). By day 60, the yolk sac no longer serves as a hematopoietic organ. Rather, this task is relayed to intraembryonic organs, including the liver, spleen, thymus, and bone marrow. With the onset of a functional circulatory system, primitive HSCs (i.e., those with limited pluripotential) from the extraembryonic mesoderm colonize these organs. The first organ to be colonized is the **liver**. This organ remains the main hematopoietic organ of

the embryo and fetus until initiation of **bone marrow** hematopoiesis near **parturition** (birth). Colonization of the liver primordia by HSCs likely occurs in two waves, the first beginning at about day 23 and the other at about day 30, but these HSCs arise from two different sources (Fig. 13-2; discussed in the following "In the Research Lab"). The shift from generating primitive nucleated erythroblasts to enucleated erythrocytes synthesizing fetal hemoglobin (**definitive erythrocytes**) occurs by 5 weeks of gestation. The liver is where long-term **definitive HSCs** arise that have the potential to generate all the hematopoietic cell lineages of the adult, with both primitive and definitive HSC production overlapping for a time. Evidence suggests that definite HSCs come to colonize the bone marrow and contribute blood cells as early as 10.5 weeks, but the bulk of the hematopoietic burden is still carried by the liver until birth. Thus, the extraembryonic, primitive HSCs serve mainly to provide an early, but necessary, blood supply for the developing embryo until the definitive intraembryonic hematopoietic organs can assume this task.

13

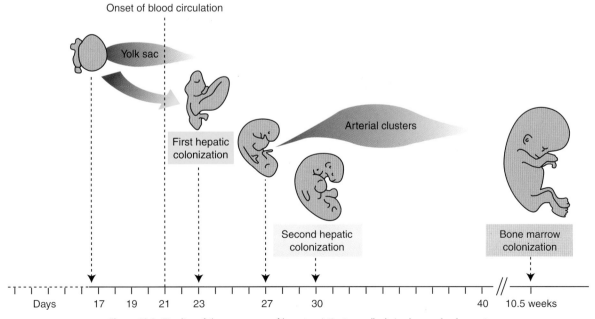

Figure 13-2. Timeline of the appearance of hematopoietic stem cells during human development.

IN THE RESEARCH LAB

SECOND SOURCE OF HEMATOPOIETIC STEM CELLS

Although the initial hematopoietic stem cells (HSCs) colonizing the developing liver arise from the yolk sac, a separate intraembryonic source of HSCs eventually colonizes the liver. Evidence for this second source of HSCs was first garnered using quail-chick transplantation chimeras (discussed in Ch. 5) in which quail embryos were grafted onto chick embryo yolk sacs (after removal of the chick embryo) and allowed to develop. Initially, all blood lineages in the hematopoietic organs including circulating blood were chicken in origin, with quail cells providing the stromal (connective tissue) cells. However, within 5 days of incubation, a mixture of quail- and chick-derived blood cells were found circulating within the embryo, and eventually the majority of cells became quail derived. Hence, the yolk sac gave rise to short-lived HSCs as opposed to long-term definitive HSCs. Therefore, there had to be a second intraembryonic source of HSCs.

Subsequent studies in birds, amphibians, mice, and humans identified densely packed clusters of HSCs adhering to the ventral endothelium of the dorsal aorta in the region of the genital/mesonephric ridge of the embryo (this structure is described in Ch. 15). This region has been termed the **aortic, gonad**, and **mesonephros** (AGM) **region** (or the paraortic splanchnopleure; Figs. 13-3, 13-4). In humans, HSCs are detected within the AGM aorta at 27 days of development as small groups of two or three cells, but by day 35, they increase to thousands of cells that extend into vessels adjacent to the umbilical cord region. These cells express transcription factors and cell surface markers associated with early blood progenitors (e.g., *Gata2, c-Kit, CD34, CD41, CD45*). These AGM-derived HSCs subsequently colonize the liver, expand in numbers, and then disappear from the AGM region by day 40. Although these intraembryonic HSCs could be derived from colonizing primitive HSCs from the yolk sac, evidence suggests they are of separate origin. In vitro assays comparing the hematopoietic potential of the human yolk sac explants and AGM splanchnic mesodermal explants—both established before day 21 (i.e., before onset of circulation)—revealed that both explants showed equal hematopoietic potential. Therefore, in vertebrates (including humans) there are both extraembryonic and intraembryonic sources of HSC progenitor cells.

INTRAEMBRYONIC HEMATOPOIETIC STEM CELLS MAY BE SOURCE OF DEFINITIVE HEMATOPOIETIC STEM CELLS

Studies in mice show that the yolk sac forms primitive HSCs capable of generating primitive erythrocytes, macrophages, and megakaryocytes. These primitive erythrocytes likely serve as a rapidly forming stopgap population of blood cells that fulfill the oxygen needs of the rapidly developing embryo. HSCs capable of generating **definitive myeloid cells** (definitive erythrocytes, macrophages, and granulocytes) appear within the yolk sac. However, studies suggest that these cells must first colonize and interact with the developing liver to acquire long-term myeloid cell–generating capacity. Coincident with the second wave of liver colonization by AGM HSCs, HSCs residing in the liver acquire the capacity to generate the full spectrum of both myeloid and **lymphoid** (i.e., B and T lymphocytes) **progenitor cells**.

Recent studies in humans show a very similar pattern of hematopoietic development. In humans, the liver primordia is colonized by primitive HSCs from the yolk sac, possibly as early as day 23 to 24, with a second wave of HSCs arriving from the AGM region by day 30. In vitro assays of human tissue explants of both yolk sac and AGM mesoderm show that both explants can make myeloid cells. However, only the AGM mesodermal tissue gives rise to T- and B-lymphocytes. Collectively, these studies suggest that the yolk sac and extraembryonic mesoderm generate primitive HSCs necessary for supporting the early cardiovascular needs of the embryo. However, formation of the **definitive HSCs** that subsequently colonize lymphatic organs and bone marrow and become responsible for long-term hematopoiesis requires that HSCs derived from both the yolk sac and AGM region first seed the liver.

Survival and proliferation of HSCs depends on a trophic factor called *Stem cell factor* (*Scf*, or *c-Kit* ligand) and its receptor, *c-Kit* receptor. Mouse mutants completely devoid of the *c-Kit* receptor or its ligand die in utero of anemia between days 14 and 16 of gestation and contain reduced numbers of erythroid progenitors in the fetal liver. In humans, c-KIT receptor protein is expressed in yolk sac HSCs, the AGM splanchnic mesoderm, and liver HSCs during all stages of liver development. However, the expression of its ligand, SCF, is temporally regulated. SCF protein is expressed in HSCs of the AGM region at low levels between days 25 to 34. However, it is well expressed in human liver HSCs by day 34, before the levels drop off in late-stage liver HSCs (i.e., by 45 days). Only weak expression of *SCF* mRNA is detected in the yolk sac (by quantitative RT-PCR) at 32 days of development. Hence, c-KIT receptor signaling by SCF in HSCs coincides with the colonization of AGM HSCs in the liver and the appearance of definitive, long-term HSCs. This supports the idea that SCF/c-KIT signaling is involved in differentiation and proliferation of AGM-derived HSCs in the liver into definitive, long-term HSCs. In addition, SCF expression may serve as a marker for colonization of liver by AGM-derived HSCs.

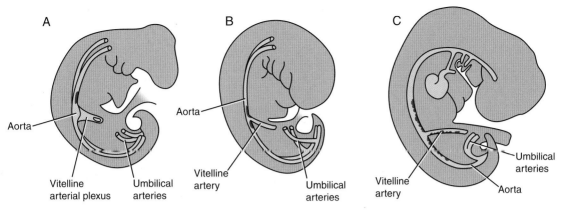

Figure 13-3. A second source of hematopoietic stem cells arises within the splanchnic mesoderm surrounding the aortic, gonad, and mesonephric region (AGM). These cells temporarily reside in the ventral floor of the dorsal aortic of this region. *A,* In humans at about day 27, a small number of hematopoietic stem cells (in red) reside and adhere to the dorsal aorta near the origin of the vitelline artery in the umbilical region. *B,* By day 30, the number of hematopoietic stem cells expands to several thousand. *C,* By day 36, hematopoietic stem cells expand to reside in the ventral floor of the dorsal aorta along almost the entire length of the AGM, and extending into the vitelline artery. By day 40, hematopoietic stem cells are no longer detected in the dorsal aorta.

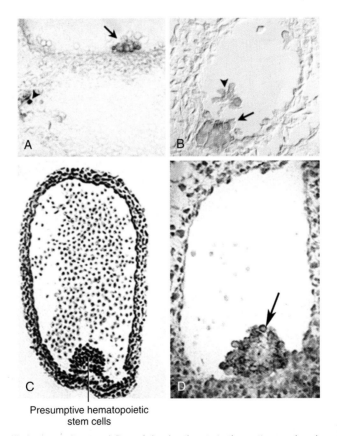

Presumptive hematopoietic
stem cells

Figure 13-4. Hematopoietic stem cell clusters in the ventral floor of the dorsal aorta in the aortic, gonad, and mesonephric region (AGM) of various vertebrates. *A,* Day 3 chick embryo showing *CD41*-positive cells (arrow), a marker for hematopoietic stem cells. *B,* Day 10 mouse embryo immunostained with *CD41* antibody (arrow and arrowhead). *C,* Drawing of a 6- to 15-mm pig embryo dorsal aorta in the AGM. *D,* Day 35 human embryo immunostained with an antibody to *CD45* (arrow), another hematopoietic stem cell marker.

13

Vasculogenesis

On day 18, blood vessels begin developing in the intraembryonic splanchnic mesoderm. Unlike blood vessel formation in the extraembryonic mesoderm and AGM region (discussed in preceding "In the Research Lab"), blood vessel formation within intraembryonic splanchnic mesoderm is not coupled with hematopoiesis. Inducing substances secreted by the underlying endoderm cause some cells of the splanchnic mesoderm to differentiate into EPCs (or **angioblasts**) that develop into flattened endothelial cells and join together to form small vesicular structures. These vesicular structures, in turn, coalesce into long tubes or vessels (Fig. 13-5; see Fig. 12-5A, B). This process is referred to as **vasculogenesis**. These cords develop throughout the intraembryonic mesoderm and coalesce to form a pervasive network of vessels that establishes the initial configuration of the circulatory system of the embryo. This network grows and spreads throughout the embryo by 4 main processes: (1) continued formation, migration, and coalescence of EPCs; (2) **angiogenesis**, the budding and sprouting of new vessels from existing endothelial cords; (3) **vascular intussusception** (nonsprouting angiogenesis), in which existing vessels are split to generate additional vessels; and (4) intercalation of new EPCs into the walls of existing vessels.

Because blood vessels form in the yolk sac on about day 17, but not in the embryonic disc until day 18, it was originally thought that intraembryonic vessels arose mainly because of centripetal extension of the yolk sac vasculature into the embryo proper. However, quail-chick transplantation chimeras (discussed in Ch. 5) provide evidence that almost all of the intraembryonic splanchnic mesoderm has the ability to form blood vessels via vasculogenesis. Furthermore, experiments in which mesoderm is transplanted from one region in the quail embryo to another region in the chick embryo, show that the characteristic branching pattern of the blood vessels in each region is determined by cues from the underlying endoderm and its extracellular matrix. These studies have been facilitated by the availability of antibodies that recognize quail vessels specifically, making it possible to visualize their branching patterns. Although it is clear that the intraembryonic splanchnic mesoderm has the capacity to generate EPCs and undergo vasculogenesis, the intraembryonic somatic mesoderm may not. Studies in avian embryos show that much of this vasculature develops from migrating EPCs derived from the paraxial mesoderm that subsequently form the initial vasculature via vasculogenesis (Fig. 13-6).

IN THE RESEARCH LAB

METHODS FOR VISUALIZING BLOOD VESSEL FORMATION

Much has been learned in recent years regarding blood vessel formation. Classic approaches to the study of vasculogenesis and angiogenesis, including the infiltration of the vasculature with stains such as India ink as well as serial sectioning and three-dimensional reconstruction, have been coupled with genetic and blood flow models to study blood vessel formation and patterning. Modern variants of the former techniques include **microangiography** (the radiologic visualization of injected contrast medium; Fig. 13-7A), the

---

Vasculogenesis

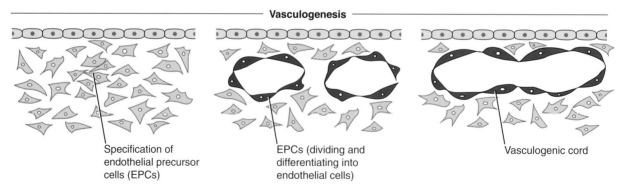

Specification of endothelial precursor cells (EPCs)

EPCs (dividing and differentiating into endothelial cells)

Vasculogenic cord

Figure 13-5. Vasculogenesis begins with the specification of the endothelial precursor cell lineage within the extraembryonic splanchnic mesoderm of the yolk sac, and, later, within the intraembryonic splanchnic mesoderm. Endothelial precursor cells differentiate into endothelial cells and organize into small vascular cords that coalesce to form a primitive embryonic vascular plexus.

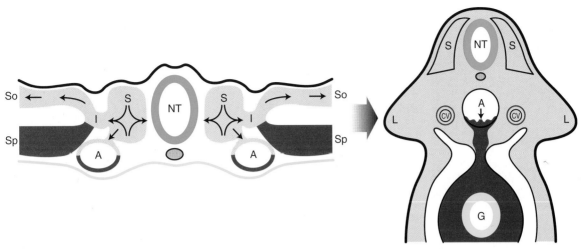

Figure 13-6. Vasculogenesis also occurs in the paraxial mesoderm. In avian embryos, in addition to vasculogenesis in the yolk sac wall and splanchnic mesoderm, the endothelial precursor cell lineage is specified within the paraxial mesoderm. Paraxially derived endothelial precursor cells migrate into distant sites (arrows), differentiate into endothelial cells, and organize a primitive vascular plexus throughout the light red areas. The primitive vasculature derived from endothelial precursor cells of splanchnic mesoderm origin is shown in red. The dorsal aorta may be a chimera of both endothelial precursor cell lineages. Abbreviations: S, somite; NT, neural tube; A, aorta; So, somatopleuric mesoderm; Sp, splanchnic mesoderm; I, intermediate mesoderm; L, limb bud; CV, cardinal vein.

use of transgenic animals expressing a reporter gene driven by cell-type specific promoters (Fig. 13-7*B*), or identification by expression of cell-type–specific antibody markers (Fig. 13-7*C, D*). Alternatively, the vasculature can be perfused with a soluble plastic that is then polymerized to form a solid cast of the vasculature that can be isolated, coated with metal, and examined by scanning electron microscopy (Fig. 13-7*E*). Scanning electron microscopy has also been useful in directly examining development of the vasculature. For this technique, fixed specimens are broken open and then the exposed vascular structures are coated with metal (Fig. 13-7*F*). Recent advances in **magnetic resonance imaging (MRI)** have also made it possible to study embryonic development with this technique, including the developing vasculature (Fig. 13-8).

WHAT INITIATES AND CONTROLS VASCULOGENESIS?

As discussed in Chapter 12 regarding the specification of primary heart field in avian embryos, the inductive effect of endodermally derived *Bmps* in the absence of *Wnt* signaling leads to the cardiogenic cell lineage, whereas *Bmp* signaling coupled with *Wnt8c* signaling enables blood vessel formation in the splanchnic mesoderm. Likewise, *Bmp/Tgfβ* signals emanating from extraembryonic endoderm and *Wnt* signaling in mesoderm prime the extraembryonic mesoderm adjacent to the yolk sac endoderm for blood island formation. In mice, visceral endoderm provides inductive

signals (e.g., *Bmp*, *Vascular endothelial growth factor*, and *Indian hedgehog*) that are necessary for inducing the expression of blood island markers in this mesoderm in tissue culture. However, the precise trigger for forming in vivo hemangioblasts, and eventually the hematopoietic and EPC lineages, is still unclear. Both hematopoietic precursors and EPCs share many of the same early expression markers, so they are closely tied to one another with regard to cell lineage specification.

What is known is that *Vascular endothelial growth factor* (*Vegf*) signaling through the *Vascular endothelial growth factor receptor-2* (*Vegfr2* or *Flk1* in mice and *KDR* in humans) is essential. Knockout mice for *Vegfr2* have a complete absence of HSC and EPC lineages and die in utero. Moreover, homozygote knockout mice for *Vascular endothelial growth factor-A* (*VegfA*) die due to a lack of blood island formation, whereas mice heterozygotic for *VegfA* develop fewer blood islands and die at midgestation due to a lack of subsequent vascular remodeling. Mice lacking *Vascular endothelial growth factor receptor-1* (*Vegfr1*) also die, but the defect seems to be a consequence of abnormal EPC proliferation that results in a disorganized vasculature. *Vegf* is a powerful promoter of vasculogenesis: injecting *Vegf* into embryos at the outset of vasculogenesis can vascularize normally avascular areas (e.g., cartilage-forming areas and cornea). **Hypervascularization** is also

13

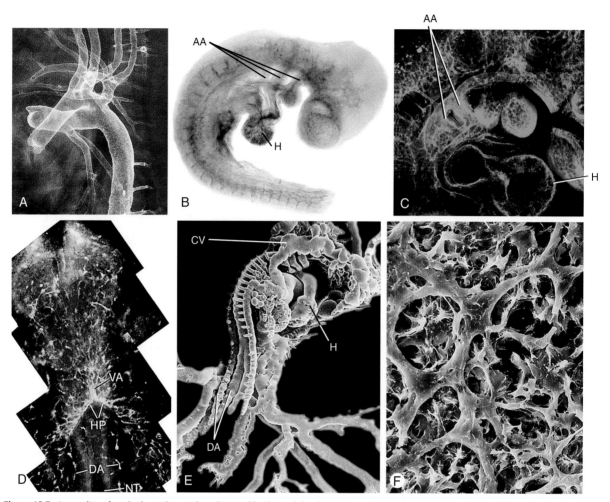

Figure 13-7. A sampling of methods used to study embryonic blood vessel development. *A*, Microangiography (a radiologic technique) showing the major vessels leaving the embryonic heart (not labeled, but to the left of the photo). *B*, Transgenic mouse expressing *LacZ* (a reporter gene that encodes an enzyme that can be detected in various ways) in its vascular system (expression is driven within the vascular system using a *Tie2-Cre* promoter). AA, aortic arches; H, heart. *C*, *Pe-Cam* expression (a protein expressed in the vascular system) detected by immunocytochemical staining; higher magnification of the heart (H) and overlying aortic arches (AA) from an area similar to that shown in the central part of *B*. *D*, Immunocytochemical labeling of vascular precursors in a whole quail embryo during formation of the heart tube; the head end of the embryo is at the top of the photo. The embryo was labeled with an antibody, *QH-1*, that binds to an endothelial precursor cell epitope present in quail (but not in chick). VA, ventral aortae; HP, heart primordia; DA, rudiments of the dorsal aortae; NT, neural tube. *E*, Plastic casting of the entire vasculature of a chick embryo at a later stage than that shown in *D*, viewed with scanning electron microscopy. CV, anterior cardinal vein; DA, dorsal aortae (note the many dorsally directed intersegmental arteries branching from the dorsal aortae); H, heart. *F*, Endothelial cells viewed with scanning electron microscopy.

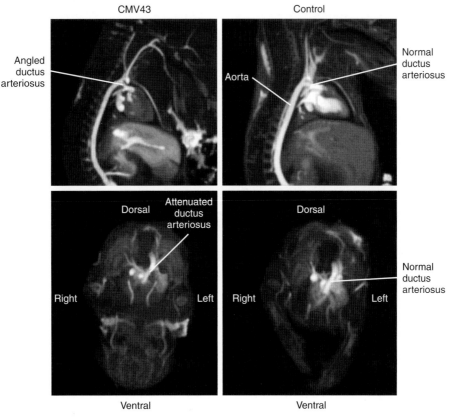

Figure 13-8. Three-dimensional volume rendering of the heart and great vessels from data collected using MRI comparing the morphology of *Connexin-43* (*Cmv43*) knockout mice (left) with normal control littermates (right) at 14.5 days of gestation. Imaging data from a number of organs and tissues was excluded during the rendering of these images to facilitate visualization of the vessels and heart.

observed in transient transgenic gain-of-function quail embryos in which *Vegf* is overexpressed. The coreceptors for *Vegfr2*—*Neuropilin-1* (*Nrp1*) and *Neuropilin-2* (*Nrp2*), a pair of transmembrane receptors belonging to the class III *Semaphorin* family that act as axon repellant factors—are also required. Knockout mice for either *Nrp1* or *Nrp2* die in utero early and are avascular.

Organization of endothelial cells into recognizable blood vessels usually occurs at the site of EPC specification during vasculogenesis. However, as discussed earlier in this chapter, evidence suggests that EPCs can also migrate into and proliferate at distant secondary sites before organizing into blood vessels, in a process distinct from angiogenesis (see Fig. 13-6). Vessels that form through this modified form of vasculogenesis include (in the avian embryo) the posterior cardinal vein and perineural vascular plexus and (in the Xenopus embryo), the bulk of the dorsal aorta and intersegmental vessels.

It was once thought that EPCs were present only in the embryo and fetus. However, evidence suggests that EPCs exist in *adult* bone marrow and peripheral blood. *Vegf, Granulocyte-monocyte colony-stimulating factor, Fgf2,* and *Igf1* all stimulate EPC mobilization and differentiation. The decision of circulating endothelial cells to integrate into blood vessel walls may involve the *Ephrin/EphB* family. *Ephrins* are transmembrane ligands for a family of *EphB receptor-tyrosine kinases* (discussed in Ch. 5) that modulate EPC and endothelial migration and proliferation. In addition, they play important roles in artery/vein specification (discussed below).

ANGIOGENESIS EXPANDS AND REMODELS INITIAL VASCULAR COMPLEX

Once a primary vascular plexus is formed in the embryo, it must be remodeled to accommodate growth of the embryo and develop into a system of arteries and veins. Completion and continual remodeling of blood vessels requires **angiogenesis**. Often, the term *angiogenesis* is inappropriately used interchangeably with *vasculogenesis*. However, angiogenesis is a different process. Angiogenesis is the expansion and remodeling of the vascular system

13

using existing endothelial cells and vessels generated by vasculogenesis (Fig. 13-9). Expansion by angiogenesis occurs by **sprouting** or vascular **intussusception**, a splitting or fusion of existing blood vessels (Figs. 13-9, 13-10, 13-11).

As they do in vasculogenesis, *Vegfs* and their receptors play major roles in angiogenesis: defects in angiogenesis occur in embryos deficient in these molecules. However, another group of *Tyrosine kinase* receptors and ligands act in parallel to promote proper angiogenesis, namely, the *Tie* (*Tyrosine kinase with immunoglobulin-like and EGF-like domains*) *receptor*/*Angiopoietin* group. *Angiopoietin-1* (*Ang1*) and *Tyrosine kinase with immunoglobulin-like and EGF-like domains-2* (*Tie2*) are clearly involved in regulating intussusception of the vasculature, whereas *Ang2*, in cooperation with the stimulatory effects of *Vegf*, stimulates sprouting. Mice lacking the *Tie2* gene or its ligand *Ang1* develop abnormally large and leaky vessels and die in utero. Moreover, these mice exhibit a decrease in endothelial cell number and angiogenic sprouting, as well as a failure of vascular intussusception. *Tyrosine kinase with immunoglobulin-like and EGF-like domains-1* (*Tie1*) knockout mice develop vessels with holes, and the endothelial cells appear necrotic. These results show collectively that *Tie/Ang* signaling along with *Vegf* signaling is essential for expansion and remodeling of blood vessels after the initial primitive vasculature is established by vasculogenesis.

The *Tgfβ* family and *Tgfβ* receptor signaling components—*Alk1, Activin A receptor, Type II-like kinase 5*

protein (*Alk5*), *Tgfβ receptor-II*, and *Endoglin*—play critical roles in vasculogenesis and angiogenesis. Knockout mice for the *Tgfβ* receptors, *Alk1* and *Alk5*, and the *Tgfβ*-binding protein, *Endoglin*, are defective in angiogenic remodeling due to impaired endothelial cell migration and proliferation. They develop abnormal arterial-venous connections, much like that discussed in the "Clinical Taster" for this chapter. Moreover, recruitment of vascular smooth muscle is deficient, leading to poor vascular integrity and vascular instability. *Tgfβ* exhibits both stimulatory and inhibitory effects on endothelial cells. Recent studies suggest that the decision as to whether to continue angiogenesis or mature into a vessel depends on an interplay between the stimulatory effect of *Tgfβ/Alk1* signaling (promoted by *Endoglin*) and the inhibitory effect of *Tgfβ/Alk5* signaling. Stimulatory effect of *Alk1* signaling includes an increased expression of *Id1*, a basic HLH transcription factor that promotes endothelial cell proliferation and migration. In contrast, *Alk5* signaling increases the expression of *Fibronectin*, an extracellular matrix component important in establishing stable vessels. It also promotes expression of *Plasminogen activator inhibitor-1*, a protein that blocks *Plasmin* formation (a protease important in mediating endothelial migration and remodeling). Hence, *Tgfβ*, *Vegf*, and *Tie* signaling all play major roles in mediating angiogenesis.

One of the main driving forces for vascularization by angiogenesis is the need to counteract hypoxia. Low oxygen

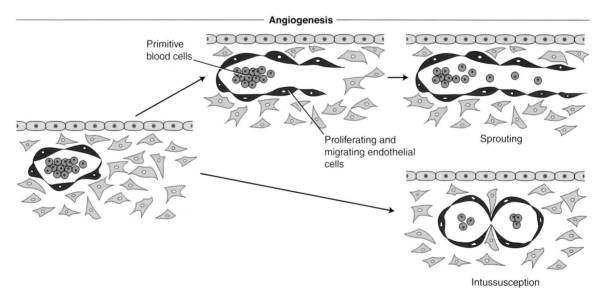

Angiogenesis

Primitive blood cells

Proliferating and migrating endothelial cells

Sprouting

Intussusception

Figure 13-9. The primitive vascular network established through vasculogenesis is expanded and remodeled by angiogenesis. Expansion by angiogenesis occurs by sprouting from existing vessels or by intussusception, a splitting of existing vessels.

saturation leads to stabilization of the transcription factor, *Hypoxia-inducible factor-1α* (*Hif1α*). *Hif1α* upregulates *VegfA* expression and *Nitric oxide synthase* expression. Nitric oxide production dilates existing blood vessels, thereby increasing the permeability and **extravasation** of plasma proteins leading to an increase in the expression and activation of the proteases, *Matrix metalloproteinases* and *Plasmin*. *Matrix metalloproteinases* and *Plasmin* play major roles in promoting proliferation and migration of endothelial cells by activating growth factors and receptors and increasing extracellular matrix turnover, which is necessary for sprouting. Proper vascular development also involves trimming away vessels that are no longer necessary or that would be detrimental should they remain. For example, in its early development the retina initially forms excess vascularity that must be trimmed down later. Experimental **hyperoxia** (i.e., surplus oxygen) in rodents suppresses *Vegf* levels in the retina. Because *Vegf* acts as a survival factor for retinal endothelial cells, hyperoxia resulting from the excess blood supply may drive the pruning of excess vessels by decreasing *Vegf* levels (Fig. 13-12). Hence, the degree of vascularity (i.e., driven either by the formation or pruning of vessels) of a tissue may be mediated by oxygen-dependent regulation of *Vegf* levels.

FORMATION OF ARTERIES VERSUS VEINS

Arteries and *veins* are terms used to describe vessels whose direction of blood flow is either away from heart (artery) or toward the heart (vein). In addition to these differences in directions of blood flow, arteries and veins are very different in their morphology and physiology. So how does a network of interconnecting vessels become designated into one type or the other? Flow dynamics and the physiologic requirements for the various loads placed on the vessels are one of the main considerations thought to drive arterial or venous specification. Based on studies in the chick embryo, where visualization and ready access to the extraembryonic vasculature is possible, it seems that as perfusion of some capillary-sized vessels increases (arterial side), some downstream side branches are disconnected. These disconnected vessels are then remodeled to establish a second, parallel vasculature that connects to vessels leading to the venous pole of the developing heart. Once this occurs, the connection to the arterial side is re-established. Recent studies suggest that endothelial cells in these capillary beds may not all be identical; rather, some may have acquired an arterial or venous specification even before blood flow ensues (discussed later in this section). However, studies also suggest endothelial cells remain

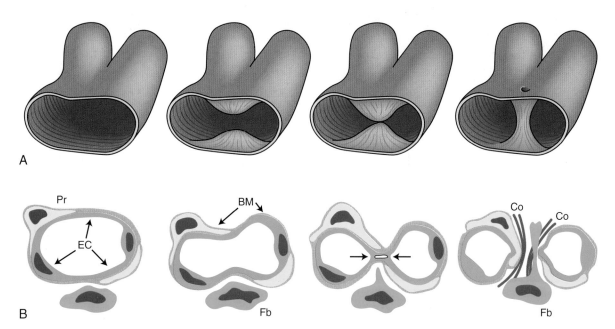

Figure 13-10. Intussusceptive angiogenesis. *A, B,* Drawings illustrating the basic steps of intussusceptive angiogenesis. It begins with the protrusion of opposing capillary endothelial cells (EC) into the lumen. At the point of contact, the endothelial layer and basement membrane (BM) is perforated and invaded by pericytes (Pr, capillary supportive cells) and interstitial fibroblasts (Fb) while the epithelial lining of the newly formed capillaries is reconstituted. Co, collagen.

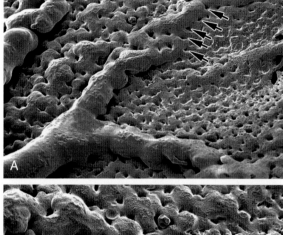

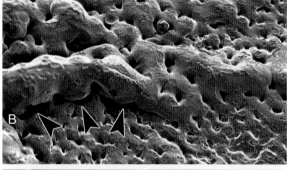

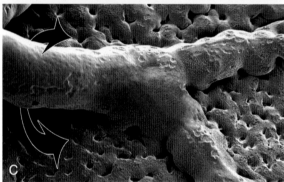

Figure 13-11. Scanning electron micrograph showing branching of chick chorioallantoic membrane vessels by intussusception. *A*, Perforations and pillars penetrate into existing vessels and bridge across the vessel lumen (arrows). *B, C,* Pillars then lengthen and merge (arrowheads) and eventually sever and separate the vessel (curved arrows) from the underlying capillary bed.

somewhat plastic in their ability to integrate into arterial or venous endothelium based on cues present in their local environment.

The factors that direct and guide vessel remodeling are still unclear but several ligands and receptors known to play roles in neuronal guidance (discussed in Chs. 9 and 10) seem to be involved in this process. One such group is the

Eph receptors and their membrane-bound ligands, the *Ephrins*. The binding of *Ephrins* to *EphB* receptors stimulates transduction signals in the *EphB*-expressing cells, but this binding can also transduce a reverse signal into the *Ephrin*-expressing cell. Such interactions and signaling events play important roles not only in the development of the nervous system but also in blood vessel remodeling and the specification of artery or vein phenotype. *EphrinB2* is specifically expressed on the surface of arterial endothelial cells, whereas the *EphB4* receptor is expressed specifically on venous endothelial cells (Fig 13-13). When either *EphrinB2* or *EphB4* is knocked out in mice, the remodeling of primary vascular plexus into arteries and veins fails. How *EphrinB2* and *EphB4* mediate these changes is unclear, but it has been suggested that during angiogenesis, differential expression of these two molecules may restrain cell migration and create tissue boundaries needed to sort out the arterial and venous systems. What is responsible for mediating specific expression of *Ephrins* and *Eph* receptors is unclear. However, it may involve earlier *Tgfβ*-mediated signaling, as *EphrinB2* expression is absent in *Alk1*-deficient mice (a *Tgfβ* receptor).

Another possible set of players that may be important in mediating arterial or venous vessel phenotypes are *Nrp1* and *Nrp2*. As mentioned earlier in this chapter, both *Nrp1* and *Nrp2* are cell-surface receptors for soluble class III *Semaphorins* involved in neuronal guidance. However, *Nrp1* and *Nrp2* also bind specific splice variants of *Vegf*; as a consequence they can mediate *Vegf* signaling in endothelial cells. *Nrp1* is artery specific whereas *Nrp2* expression is restricted to veins (see Fig. 13-13). Hence, vessel-specific *Vegf* signaling, promoting either an arterial or venous vascular phenotype, may depend on whether the endothelial cells expresses *Nrp1* or *Nrp2*.

Yet another group of membrane-bound ligand/receptors important in remodeling the initial vascular complex into arteries and veins are the *Notch* receptors and their ligands. *Notch* proteins (*Notch1-4*) are cell-surface receptors for the membrane-bound ligands *Delta-like 1*(*Dll-1*), *Dll-3*, *Dll-4*, *Jag1*, and *Jag2*, which are important in cell fate decision (discussed in Ch. 5). In mice the *Notch1*, *Notch3*, and *Notch4* receptors and their ligands, *Dll-4*, *Jag1*, and *Jag2*, are expressed in arteries but not veins. Mouse embryos deficient in *Notch1* form an apparently normal initial capillary plexus, but they fail to properly remodel this vasculature. Knockout mice for both *Notch1* and *Notch2* also develop a primitive capillary vasculature, but they exhibit defects in the yolk sac vasculature pattern, fail to develop large vitelline veins, develop abnormal anterior cardinal veins, and have disorganized intersegmental vessels. Likewise, embryos

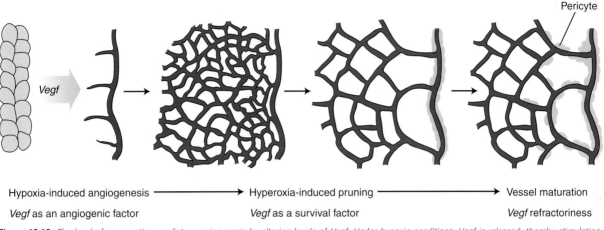

Hypoxia-induced angiogenesis ⟶ Hyperoxia-induced pruning ⟶ Vessel maturation

Vegf as an angiogenic factor *Vegf* as a survival factor *Vegf* refractoriness

Figure 13-12. The level of oxygenation mediates angiogenesis by altering levels of *Vegf*. Under hypoxic conditions, *Vegf* is released, thereby stimulating angiogenesis. Under hyperoxic conditions, *Vegf* levels decrease. Because endothelial cell survival during early angiogenesis requires *Vegf*, the capillaries are pruned or trimmed back under conditions of hyperoxia. Once a vessel matures and is stable, *Vegf* is no longer needed to maintain the vessel.

lacking the *Notch* ligand, *Jag1*, develop a primary capillary plexus, but fail to develop a vitelline or cranial network of vessels. Hence, *Notch* signaling seems to be required for remodeling of the primitive capillary plexus, rather than for its initial development.

Recent studies suggest that *Notch* signaling may have a key role in establishing an arterial or venous identity upstream of *Ephrins/Eph*, possibly even before the formation of the initial vascular complex (see Fig. 13-13). Studies in zebrafish show that inhibiting the *Notch* signaling pathway decreases expression of *EphrinB2* and *Notch3* (both markers of arterial phenotype), resulting in the ectopic expression of venous markers in the dorsal aorta. In contrast, overexpression of active *Notch* decreases the expression of venous markers, but it has no effect on arterial marker expression. Therefore, *Notch* signaling may have an important role in mediating not only vascular remodeling but also arterial/venous specification of EPCs.

IN THE CLINIC

ANGIOMAS

Blood and lymph vessels are stimulated to grow into developing organs by **angiogenic factors**. If vessel growth is not inhibited at the appropriate time or if it is stimulated again later in life, blood or lymph vessels may proliferate until they form a tangled mass that may have clinical consequences. Excessive growth of small capillary networks is called a **capillary hemangioma** or **nevus vascularis**; a proliferation of larger venous sinuses is called a **cavernous**

hemangioma. Hemangioma of infancy is the most common benign tumor of childhood (incidence of about 2.5% in neonates and up to 10% to 12% in 1 year olds; Fig. 13-14). These tumors grow rapidly and consist mainly of endothelial cells with or without lumens, multilayered basement membranes, and fibrous tissue. Hemangiomas differ from some vascular anomalies like **nevus flammeus** that present at birth as **birthmarks** and grow proportionately with the growth of the child. Most cases of hemangioma of infancy pose no immediate or long-term danger. However, they can be potentially life threatening if they grow in vital organs (e.g., in the skull or vertebral canal, where they can lead to nervous system dysfunction, or in airways, where they can obstruct breathing) or are large enough to create a shunt of physiologic significance leading to heart failure. In rare cases, a **hemangiosarcoma** (metastatic angioma) can develop.

Many hemangiomas seem to have a genetic basis to their origin, as they are associated with developmental syndromes resulting from chromosomal anomalies. In the case of hemangioma of infancy, some cases are linked to chromosome region 5q31-33. This region contains genes coding for *FGF4*, *PDGFβ*, and *FMS-RELATED TYROSINE KINASE*, molecules important in blood vessel development. Some hemangiomas are also linked to disregulation of the *TIE/ANG* signaling pathway and to *VEGFR2* mutations. Multiple hemangioblastomas are associated with a rare, dominantly inherited, familial cancer syndrome called **von Hippel-Lindau disease** (incidence 1:36,000) characterized by mutations in a tumor suppressor gene located at chromosome 3p25-26.

13

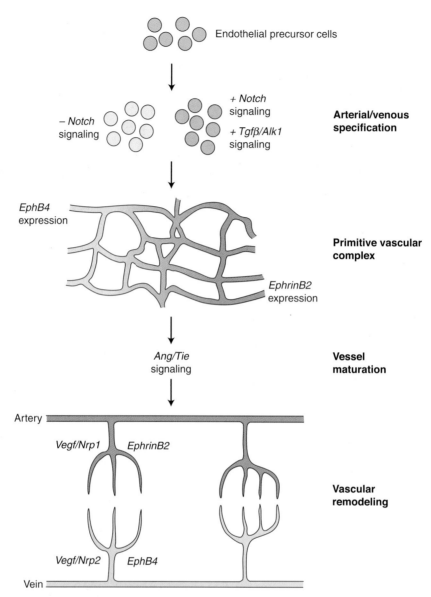

Figure 13-13. Hypothesized model for establishing arterial and venous identity and for the remodeling leading to the formation of two separate types of vessels. *Notch* signaling (by repressing the expression of the venous phenotype) and *Tgfβ/Alk1* signaling both promote the expression of arterial markers in endothelial precursor cells, possibly instilling an arterial identity to these cells before they assemble primitive vessels. This leads to the expression of *EphrinB2* in arterial cords and *EphB4* in the venous cords, which is ultimately responsible for segregating the two vessel groups. In this model, *Ang/Tie* signaling serves to stabilize these vessels and regulate their maturation. Angiogenic growth (mediated by *Vegf/Nrp1* signaling in arterial beds and *Vegf/Nrp2* signaling in venous beds) and remodeling then sculpts these vascular beds into their final configurations.

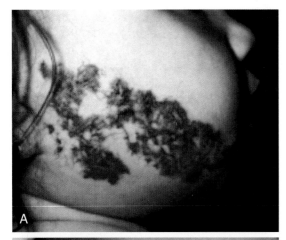

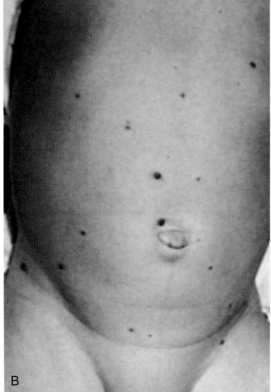

Figure 13-14. Hemangioma of infancy. *A*, Hemangioma of infancy involving the region of the mandible and having airway involvement. This patient was treated with oral corticosteroids, avoiding the need for surgical intervention for an otherwise progressing airway obstruction. *B*, Multifocal hemangiomas in an infant.

These individuals exhibit life-threatening multiple CNS, retinal, and liver hemangioblastomas, renal cell carcinomas, and visceral cysts. Studies show that stromal cells of these tumors produce high levels of *VEGF* and *HIF1α*, which could account for the excessive angiogenesis.

TREATMENT OF CORTICOSTEROID-RESISTANT HEMANGIOMAS IN HUMANS

A clinical application of animal-model studies on blood vessel growth is the development of therapies for treatment of **life-threatening** or **vision-threatening hemangiomas**. Approximately one-third of these endothelial tumors regress in response to corticosteroid therapy (see legend for Fig. 13-14A), but the remainder are insensitive. In a recent clinical trial, *INTERFERON-α2a* was injected subcutaneously into afflicted neonates or infants, resulting in a 50% (or greater) regression of the tumors within about 8 months (in 18 of 20 patients). Moreover, the three-year survival rate increased significantly as compared to the expected survival rate for a nontreated population. *INTERFERON-α2a* is thought to act by interfering with FGF stimulation of angiogenesis.

HEREDITARY HEMORRHAGIC TELANGIECTASIA

As discussed in the Clinical Taster section, mutations in *ALK1* and *ENDOGLIN* have been linked to **hereditary hemorrhagic telangiectasia** (HHT). The most common manifestations of HHT (prevalence 1:5000 to 1:8000) are nosebleeds and small vascular anomalies called telangiectases; however, gastrointestinal bleeding and arterial-venous malformations in the lung, brain, and liver progressively develop. Mice heterozygous for mutations in *Alk1* or *Endoglin* exhibit very similar progressive pathologies, including the development of large arterial-venous shunts. Mutations in human *ALK1* have also been linked to primary **pulmonary hypertension** involving abnormal remodeling of the pulmonary vasculature. Both HHT and some forms of pulmonary hypertension may stem from an improper balance between ALK1 and ALK5 signaling (discussed earlier in the chapter). Endothelial cells from normal healthy patients form extensive, stable, and well-formed vessels in tissue culture, whereas endothelial cells from HHT patients are unable to do so. Interestingly, *ENDOGLIN* also interacts with the actin cytoskeleton. Endothelial cells from HHT patients exhibit a disorganized actin cytoskeleton, but normal actin organization can be restored if normal *ENDOGLIN* is overexpressed in these cells. Endothelial cells with a disorganized, abnormal cytoskeleton are more likely to form vessels prone to vascular instability, hemorrhaging, and vascular disarray.

13

Development of Aortic Arches

The respiratory apparatus of the jawless fishes that gave rise to higher vertebrates consisted of a variable number of gill bars separated by gill slits (Fig. 13-15). Water flowed in through the mouth and out through the gill slits. Each of the gill bars, or **branchial arches**, was vascularized by an **aortic arch artery**, which arose as a branch of the ventral aorta (aortic sac). Gas exchange took place in the gill capillaries, and the dorsal half of each aortic arch conveyed the oxygenated blood to the paired dorsal aortae.

In the human embryo, five pairs of mesenchymal condensations develop on either side of the pharynx, corresponding to branchial arches 1, 2, 3, 4, and 6 of the fish ancestor. The fifth arch never develops at all or forms briefly and then regresses. The mesodermal, ectodermal, and endodermal components of the arches have been modified through evolution so that in humans, they form the structures of the lower face and neck and derivatives of the pharyngeal foregut. Thus, these structures are more appropriately called

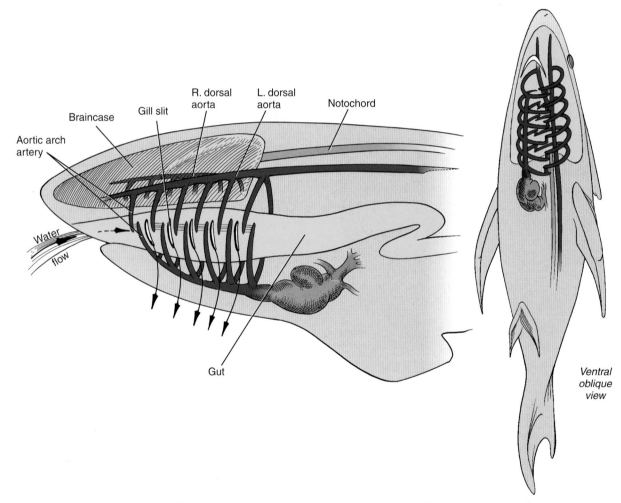

Ventral oblique view

Figure 13-15. Schematic view of the branchial arch artery system of a shark. The pharyngeal arch arteries of humans evolved from the branchial arch arteries of protochordates and fishes. The branchial arch arteries occupy the gill bars and thus enclose the pharynx like a basket. The arteries supply blood to the gills, which extract oxygen from water flowing through the gill slits.

pharyngeal arches than branchial arches. The development of the pharyngeal arches is detailed in Chapter 16; the following discussion is limited to the development of the aortic arch arteries.

Human Aortic Arches Arise in Craniocaudal Sequence and Form a Basket of Arteries around Pharynx

As described in Chapter 12, the first pair of aortic arches is formed between day 22 and day 24. At this point in development, the process of body folding, which carries the forming endocardial tubes into the future thorax, also draws the cranial ends of the attached aortae into a dorsoventral loop (see Fig. 12-6). The resulting first pair of aortic arches lies in the thickened mesenchyme of the first pair of pharyngeal arches on either side of the developing pharynx. Ventrally, the aortic arch arteries arise from the **aortic sac**, an expansion at the cranial end of the truncus arteriosus (Fig. 13-16A). Dorsally, they connect to the left and right dorsal aortae. The dorsal aortae remain separate in the region of the aortic arches, but during the 4th week, they fuse together from the fourth thoracic segment to the fourth lumbar segment to form a midline **dorsal aorta**.

Between days 26 and 29, aortic arches 2, 3, 4, and 6 develop by vasculogenesis and angiogenesis within their respective pharyngeal arches, incorporating EPCs that migrate from the surrounding mesoderm (Fig. 13-17). Neural crest cell–derived mesenchymal cells within the pharyngeal arches also play a significant role in the normal development of the arch arteries, although neural crest cells do not contribute directly to the endothelium of these vessels (see the following "In the Research Lab").

The first two arches regress as the later arches form. The second aortic arch arises in the second pharyngeal arch by day 26 and grows to connect the aortic sac to the dorsal aortae. Simultaneously, the first pair of aortic arches regresses completely (except, possibly, for small remnants that may give rise to portions of the **maxillary arteries**) (Fig. 13-16A, B). On day 28, while the first arch is regressing, the third and fourth aortic arches form. Finally, on day 29 the sixth arch forms, and the second arch regresses except for a small remnant that gives rise to part of the **stapedial artery** (Figs. 13-16B, C, 13-17), which supplies blood to the primordium of the stapes bone in the developing ear (development of the ear is discussed in Ch. 17).

Aortic Arches 3, 4, and 6 Give Rise to Important Vessels of Head, Neck, and Upper Thorax

By day 35, the segments of dorsal aorta connecting the third and fourth arch arteries disappear on both sides of the body, so that the cranial extensions of the dorsal aortae supplying the head receive blood entirely through the third aortic arches (see Fig. 13-16B). The third arch arteries give rise to the right and left **common carotid arteries** (Figs. 13-16B, C, 13-18A) and to the proximal portion of the right and left **internal carotid arteries**. The distal portion of the internal carotid arteries is derived from the cranial extensions of the dorsal aortae, and the right and left **external carotid arteries** sprout from the common carotids (see Fig. 13-16B, C).

By the 7th week, the right dorsal aorta loses its connections with both the fused midline dorsal aorta and the right sixth arch, while remaining connected to the right fourth arch (see Fig. 13-16B, C). Meanwhile, it also acquires a branch, the **right seventh cervical intersegmental artery**, which develops within the right upper limb bud region. The definitive **right subclavian artery** supplying the upper limb is derived from (1) the right fourth arch, (2) a short segment of the right dorsal aorta, and (3) the right seventh intersegmental artery. The region of the aortic sac connected to the right fourth artery is modified to form the branch of the developing aorta called the **brachiocephalic artery** (see Fig. 13-16C).

The left fourth aortic arch retains its connection to the fused dorsal aorta, and with a small segment of the aortic sac it becomes the **aortic arch** (**arch of the aorta** or **ascending aorta**) and the most cranial portion of the **descending aorta**. The remainder of the descending aorta, from the fourth thoracic level caudally, is derived from the fused dorsal aortae. The **left seventh intersegmental artery**, which forms in the paraxial mesoderm and limb region, gives rise to the **left subclavian artery** supplying the left upper extremity (see Fig. 13-16B, C). Development of the **coronary arteries** is discussed in Chapter 12.

The right and left sixth arches arise from the proximal end of the aortic sac, but further development is then asymmetrical (Figs. 13-16B, C, 13-18B). By the 7th week, the distal connection of the right sixth arch with the right dorsal aorta disappears. The left sixth arch, in contrast, remains complete and its distal portion forms the **ductus arteriosus**, which

13

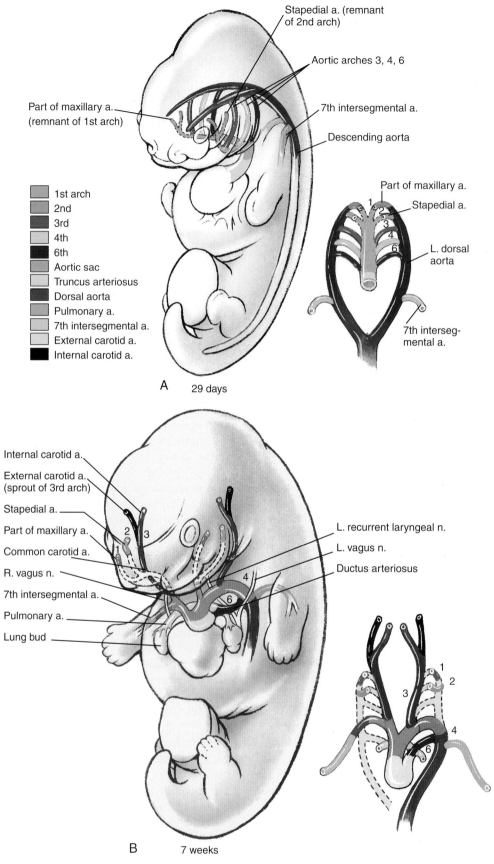

Stapedial a. (remnant of 2nd arch)

Aortic arches 3, 4, 6

Part of maxillary a. (remnant of 1st arch)

7th intersegmental a.

Descending aorta

Part of maxillary a.

Stapedial a.

L. dorsal aorta

7th intersegmental a.

1st arch
2nd
3rd
4th
6th
Aortic sac
Truncus arteriosus
Dorsal aorta
Pulmonary a.
7th intersegmental a.
External carotid a.
Internal carotid a.

A 29 days

Internal carotid a.

External carotid a. (sprout of 3rd arch)

Stapedial a.

Part of maxillary a.

Common carotid a.

R. vagus n.

7th intersegmental a.

Pulmonary a.

Lung bud

L. recurrent laryngeal n.

L. vagus n.

Ductus arteriosus

B 7 weeks

Figure 13-16. Continued next page.

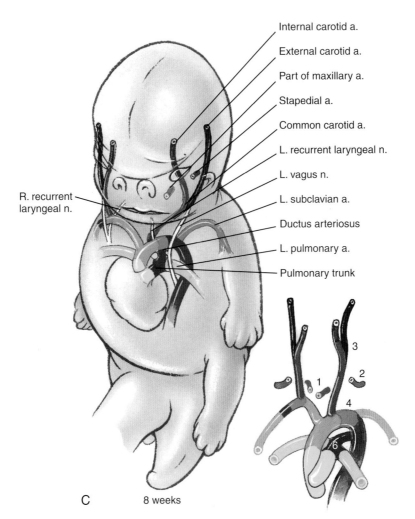

Internal carotid a.

External carotid a.

Part of maxillary a.

Stapedial a.

Common carotid a.

L. recurrent laryngeal n.

L. vagus n.

L. subclavian a.

Ductus arteriosus

L. pulmonary a.

Pulmonary trunk

R. recurrent laryngeal n.

C   8 weeks

Figure 13-16 *Continued.* Development of the aortic system. *A,* The five pairs of aortic arches that form in humans correspond to arches 1, 2, 3, 4, and 6 of evolutionary predecessors. The first arch is complete by day 24 but regresses as the second arch forms on day 26. The third and fourth arches form on day 28; the second arch degenerates as the sixth arch forms on day 29. *B,* Development of the arches in the 2nd month. Note that the arteries arising from the first three pairs of aortic arches are bilateral, whereas vessels derived from arches 4 and 6 develop asymmetrically. The pulmonary arteries initially connect with the base of arch 4 and become secondarily reconnected to the roots of the sixth arches. *C,* 8 weeks. Note the asymmetric development of the recurrent laryngeal branches of the vagus nerve, which innervates the laryngeal muscles. As the larynx is displaced cranially relative to the arch system, the recurrent laryngeal nerves are caught under the most caudal remaining arch on each side. The right recurrent laryngeal nerve therefore loops under the right subclavian artery, whereas the left recurrent laryngeal nerve loops under the ductus arteriosus.

13

allows blood to shunt from the pulmonary trunk to the descending aorta throughout gestation (see Fig. 13-16*B, C*). This bypass closes at birth and is later transformed into the **ligamentum arteriosum**, which attaches the pulmonary trunk to the aorta. Changes in the circulation that take place at birth are discussed in detail near the end of this chapter.

As shown in Figure 13-16*B* and *C*, the asymmetrical development of the left and right sixth arches is responsible for the curious asymmetry of the **left** and **right recurrent laryngeal nerves**, which branch from the vagus nerves. The laryngeal nerves originally arise below the level of the sixth arch and cross under the right and left sixth arches to innervate intrinsic muscles of the larynx. During development, the larynx is translocated cranially relative to the aortic arches. The left recurrent laryngeal nerve becomes caught under the sixth arch on the left side and remains looped

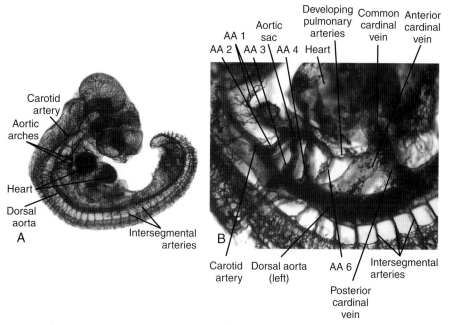

Figure 13-17. Chick embryo vasculature revealed by intravenous injection of ink into a living embryo followed by fixation and clearing of the embryo. *A,* Vasculature of a 3.5-day chick embryo. *B,* Higher magnification of the pharyngeal arch region in a similar embryo. Several of the major aortic arches and vessels are visible, as well as veins entering the atrial pole of the heart.

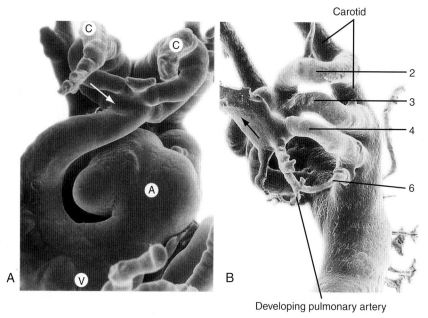

Figure 13-18. *A,* Frontal view of a cast of the aortic arch system. The left and right common carotid arteries (C) are growing toward the viewer from the dorsal segments of the third arches. The third and fourth arches arise from the aortic sac (arrow). V, ventricle; A, primitive atrium. *B,* Inferolateral view of a cast of the aortic arch system. Arches 2, 3, and 4 are fully developed, and the sixth pair is beginning to form. An arrow marks the truncus arteriosus.

under the future ligamentum arteriosum. Because the distal right sixth aortic arch disappears (and because no fifth arch develops), the right recurrent laryngeal nerve becomes caught under the fourth arch, which becomes the right subclavian artery.

Although the pulmonary arteries become connected to the sixth arch arteries and finally to the pulmonary trunk, several classic observations, as well as more recent quail-chick transplantation chimeras (discussed in Ch. 5), suggest that as the primitive pulmonary arteries develop in the splanchnopleuric mesoderm, they are initially connected to the base of aortic arch four as the sixth aortic arches develop. They then establish a secondary connection with the sixth arches before losing their connection with the fourth aortic arches (see Fig. 13-17*B*). In the lungs, the distal ends of the pulmonary arteries then anastomose with the vasculature developing in the mesenchyme surrounding the bronchial buds (discussed in Ch. 11).

IN THE RESEARCH LAB

TISSUE INTERACTIONS DIRECT PHARYNGEAL AORTIC ARCH REMODELING

As discussed in Chapter 16, the mesodermally derived and neural crest cell–derived mesenchyme of the pharyngeal arches is covered on the medial side by endoderm and on the lateral side by ectoderm. Each pharyngeal arch is separated from the adjacent ones by external indentations (pharyngeal ectodermal clefts or grooves) and internal foregut expansions (pharyngeal endodermal pouches), with the ventral floor region of the pharyngeal arches also serving as the site of the secondary heart field (discussed in Ch. 12). Within each of the pharyngeal arches, a pharyngeal arch artery forms that is subsequently remodeled to form the mature great vessels. Quail-chick transplantation chimeras (discussed in Ch. 5) have been used to show that neural crest cells differentiate into the vascular smooth muscle and connective tissue cells forming the tunics of these great vessels. If neural crest cells are ablated or their migration from the neural tube into pharyngeal arches is perturbed, the initial aortic arch vessels still form but the regression and persistence of pharyngeal arch arteries is abnormal: the remaining mesodermally derived mesenchyme is incompetent to sustain continued growth and development of the arteries after blood flow is initiated. Hence, neural crest cells not only provide the mesenchyme for tunics of these vessels, but they also play an important role in patterning of pharyngeal arch arteries.

Based on recent avian and mouse studies, it is becoming clear that tissue-tissue interactions between neural crest cell–derived mesenchyme and the pharyngeal ectoderm and endoderm play key roles in mediating pharyngeal aortic arch development. As mentioned in Chapter 12, particular levels of *Fgf8* signaling modulate proliferation, survival, and differentiation of cells in the secondary heart field. *Fgf8* is specifically expressed in pharyngeal ectoderm and endoderm but not in pharyngeal arch mesoderm or neural crest cell–derived mesenchyme. Yet, it seems that neural crest cells somehow mediate *Fgf8* signaling levels in this region. Not only is heart development sensitive to *Fgf8* signaling within the pharyngeal arches, but pharyngeal vascular development is also dependent on *Fgf8* signaling in both chick and mouse embryos. In mice, *Fgf8* hypomorphs (a animal with a partial loss-of-function mutation; i.e., *Fgf8* expression in the hypomorph is knocked down but not eliminated completely) phenocopy many of the cardiac and aortic arch defects seen in **22q11.2 deletion syndrome** in humans (this syndrome is discussed further in Chs. 4, 12, and 16). If *Fgf8* is specifically knocked out in pharyngeal arch ectoderm of developing mouse embryos, the fourth aortic arch is lost, leading to defects in aorta and subclavian artery development in the absence of cardiac defects. In contrast, loss of *Fgf8* expression in third and fourth pharyngeal arch endoderm leads to defects in both glandular development (e.g., thyroid, parathyroid, and thymus; development of these organs is discussed in Ch. 16) and aortic semilunar valve formation.

Mutations in the transcription factor, *TBX1* (located within the affected 22q11.2 region), in humans can also cause pharyngeal aortic arch defects that phenocopy the full deletion syndrome, including aortic arch anomalies, particularly those involving the fourth aortic arch (e.g., interrupted aortic arch, aberrant origin of the right subclavian artery, and aberrant origin of the right aortic arch). In mice, *Tbx1* is highly expressed in the endoderm of the fourth pouch and overlying the fourth pharyngeal arch; heterozygotic inactivation of *Tbx1* in mice causes the same defects seen in humans with *TBX1* deletion. Complete loss of several different genes expressed in pharyngeal arches causes similar defects, but *Fgf8* and *Tbx1* are the only genes identified to date that do this with a heterozygotic loss.

Endothelins represent a group of regulatory peptides important in blood pressure regulation in adults. During embryonic development, *Endothelins* and their receptors have another important role in mediating neural crest cell development. Knockout mice for the *Endothelin* receptor, *Eta*, or the converting enzyme that proteolytically generates active endothelins, *Endothelin converting enzyme-1* (*Ece1*), have neural crest cell–related defects in cardiac

13

development, pharyngeal arch artery development, and development of enteric ganglia. In the pharyngeal arches, *Endothelin-1* (*Et1*) is expressed by pharyngeal arch ectoderm and endoderm, but not by neural crest cells; *Eta* receptor is expressed only by neural crest cells in the pharyngeal arches. Knocking out either *Ece1* or the *Eta* receptor in mice leads to either the formation of an interrupted aortic arch or an absence of the right subclavian artery. These knockout mice also show altered expression of other genes important in pharyngeal arch development including *Dlx2*, *Dlx3*, *EphA3*, *MsxE*, and *Hand2*. These, and other studies in chick, suggest that even with the loss of *Eta* signaling, neural crest cells still migrate into the pharyngeal arches, and the normal developmental pattern of the initial pharyngeal aortic arch vessels still occurs. However, there seems to be a decrease in the number of neural crest cells within the pharyngeal arches, resulting in hypoplasia and abnormal pharyngeal aortic arch remodeling.

Obviously, pharyngeal aortic arch development is asymmetrical and, therefore, likely under the influence of gene expression responsible for determining sidedness. In mice, *Pitx2c* (an isoform of *Pitx2*) is expressed more prevalently in the left aortic sac, secondary heart field, and pharyngeal arch mesoderm than in the right side. Knockout mice for *Pitx2c* exhibit defects in remodeling of the pharyngeal aortic arch vessels, as well as cardiac defects that might be predicted from a perturbation of secondary heart field sidedness (discussed in Ch. 12). About 30% of these mice have a right aortic arch, about 14% have double aortic arches, and some exhibit double outlet right ventricles. Again, neural crest cell migration seems normal in these mice, and the pharyngeal arch arteries initially have similar amounts of mesenchyme surrounding their endothelia. How *Pitx2c* might mediate asymmetric remodeling of the pharyngeal aortic arch is not known, but it has been suggested that *Pitx2c* may somehow sustain or recruit pharyngeal aortic arch supportive cells to the left side.

Interestingly, innervation of the pharyngeal arches may also have a role in pharyngeal aortic arch development. Knockout mice for *Tgfβ2* exhibit abnormal increases in apoptosis of fourth aortic arch mesenchyme, and they develop an interrupted fourth aortic arch and aberrant right subclavian vessels. Although neural crest cell migration and differentiation into vascular smooth muscle seems normal in these mice, the defects coincide with a loss of fourth pharyngeal arch innervation.

In summary, pharyngeal arch neural crest cells play an important role in maintaining the integrity of particular aortic arch vessels, rather than in the initial formation of the early pharyngeal arch vasculature. Subsequent remodeling events seem to involve complex paracrine interactions between pharyngeal neural crest cells; pharyngeal arch endoderm, ectoderm, and mesoderm; and aortic arch endothelium. These interactions are still not fully understood.

Dorsal Aorta Develops Ventral, Lateral, and Posterolateral Branches

Vitelline Arteries Give Rise to the Arterial Supply of the Gastrointestinal Tract

The blood vessels that arise in the yolk sac wall differentiate to form the arteries and veins of the **vitelline system** (Fig. 13-19). As the yolk sac shrinks relative to the folding embryo, the right and left vitelline plexuses coalesce to form a number of major arteries that anastomose both with the vascular plexuses of the future gut and with the ventral surface of the dorsal aorta. These vessels eventually lose their connection with the yolk sac, becoming the arteries that supply blood from the dorsal aorta to the gastrointestinal tract.

Cranial to the diaphragm, about five pairs of these arteries usually develop and anastomose with the dorsal aorta at variable levels to supply the thoracic esophagus. Caudal to the diaphragm, three pairs of major arteries develop to supply specific regions of the developing abdominal gut. The fields of vascularization of these three arteries constitute the basis for dividing the abdominal gastrointestinal tract into three embryologic regions: the **abdominal foregut, midgut**, and **hindgut**.

The most superior of the three abdominal vitelline arteries, the **celiac artery**, initially joins the dorsal aorta at the seventh cervical level. This connection subsequently descends to the twelfth thoracic level. There the celiac artery develops branches that vascularize not only the abdominal part of the foregut, from the abdominal esophagus to the descending segment of the duodenum, but also the several embryologic outgrowths of the foregut—the liver, pancreas, and gallbladder. The celiac artery also produces a large branch that vascularizes the spleen, which develops within the mesoderm of the dorsal mesogastrium (discussed Ch. 14; the dorsal mesogastrium is the portion of the dorsal mesentery that suspends the stomach).

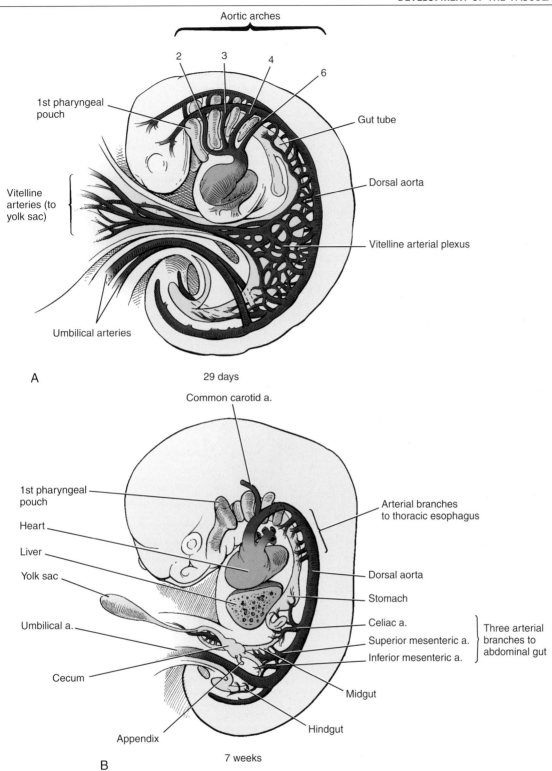

Figure 13-19. Development of the ventral aortic branches supplying the gut tube and derivatives. *A,* In the 4th week, a multitude of vitelline arteries emerge from the ventral surfaces of the dorsal aortae to supply the yolk sac. *B,* After the paired dorsal aortae fuse at the end of the 4th week, many of the vitelline channels disappear, reducing the final number to about 5 in the thoracic region and to 3 (the celiac, superior mesenteric, and inferior mesenteric arteries) in the abdominal region.

13

The second abdominal vitelline artery, the **superior mesenteric artery**, initially joins the dorsal aorta at the second thoracic level; this connection later migrates to the first lumbar level. This artery supplies the developing midgut—the intestine that reaches from the descending segment of the duodenum to a region of the transverse colon near the left colic flexure.

The third and final abdominal vitelline artery, the **inferior mesenteric artery**, initially joins the dorsal aorta at the twelfth thoracic level and later descends to the third lumbar level. It supplies the hindgut: the distal portion of the transverse colon, the descending and sigmoid colon, and the superior rectum. As described in Chapter 14, the inferior end of the anorectal canal is vascularized by branches of the iliac arteries.

Lateral Branches of Descending Aorta Vascularize Suprarenal Glands, Gonads, and Kidneys

The suprarenal (adrenal) glands, gonads, and kidneys are vascularized by lateral branches of the descending aorta. However, as shown in Fig. 13-20 these three organs and their arteries have different developmental histories. The suprarenal glands form in the posterior body wall between the sixth and twelfth thoracic segments and become vascularized mainly by a pair of lateral aortic branches that arise at an upper lumbar level. The suprarenal glands also acquire branches from the renal artery and inferior phrenic artery, but the **suprarenal arteries** developing from these aortic branches remain the major supply to the glands.

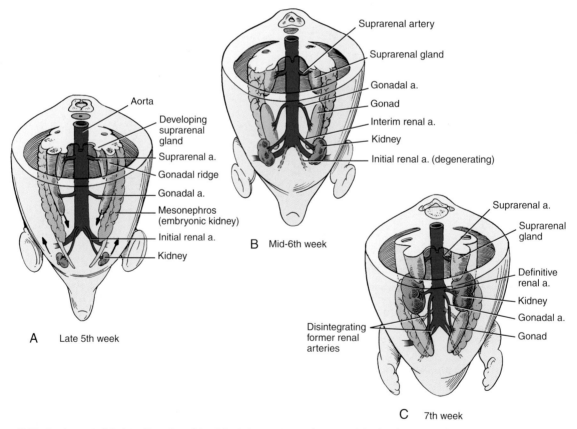

Figure 13-20. Development of the lateral branches of the abdominal aorta. *A,* Lateral sprouts of the dorsal aorta vascularize the suprarenal glands, gonads, and kidneys. During the 6th week, the gonads begin to descend, whereas the kidneys ascend (arrows). *B, C,* The gonadal artery lengthens during the migration of the gonad, but the ascending kidney is vascularized by a succession of new, more cranial aortic sprouts. The suprarenal arteries remain in place.

These glands and their aortic branches develop in place. The presumptive gonads become vascularized by **gonadal arteries** that arise initially at the 10th thoracic level. The gonads descend during development, but the origin of the gonadal arteries becomes fixed at the third or fourth lumbar level. As the gonads (especially the testes) descend further, the gonadal arteries elongate. The definitive kidneys, in contrast, arise in the sacral region and migrate upward to a lumbar site just below the suprarenal glands. As they migrate, they are vascularized by a succession of transient aortic branches that arise at progressively higher levels. These arteries do not elongate to follow the ascending kidneys but instead degenerate and are replaced. The final pair of arteries in this series forms in the upper lumbar region and become the definitive **renal arteries**. Occasionally, a more inferior pair of renal arteries persists as accessory renal arteries. The displacements of the suprarenal glands, gonads, and kidneys as they develop are discussed further in Chapter 15.

Intersegmental Branches Arise from Posterolateral Surface of Descending Aorta and Vascularize Somite Derivatives

At the end of the 3rd week, small posterolateral branches arise by vasculogenesis between the developing somites at the cervical through sacral levels and connect to the dorsal aorta (see Figs. 13-7E, 13-17). In the **cervical, thoracic,** and **lumbar** regions, a dorsal branch of each of these intersegmental vessels vascularizes both the developing neural tube and the epimeres that will form the deep muscles of the neck and back (Fig. 13-21A; epimeres and hypomeres, are discussed in Ch. 8). Cutaneous branches of these arteries also supply the dorsal skin. The ventral branch of each intersegmental vessel supplies the developing hypomeric muscles and associated skin. In the **thoracic** region, these ventral branches become the **intercostal arteries** and their cutaneous branches; in the lumbar and sacral regions, they become the **lumbar** and **lateral sacral arteries**. The short continuation of the dorsal aorta beyond its bifurcation into the common iliac arteries is called the **median sacral artery**.

In the cervical region, the intersegmental branches anastomose with each other to form a more complex pattern of vascularization (Fig. 13-21B-D). The paired **vertebral arteries** arise from longitudinal branches that link together to form a longitudinal vessel, and they secondarily lose their intersegmental connections

to the aorta. The **deep cervical, ascending cervical, superior intercostal, internal thoracic,** and **superior** and **inferior epigastric arteries** also develop from anastomoses of intersegmental arteries.

Umbilical Arteries Initially Join Dorsal Aortae but Shift Their Origin to Internal Iliac Arteries

The right and left **umbilical arteries** develop in the connecting stalk early in the 4th week and are thus among the earliest embryonic arteries to arise. These arteries form an initial connection with the paired dorsal aortae in the sacral region (see Fig. 13-19A). However, during the 5th week, these connections are obliterated as the umbilical arteries develop a new connection with the fifth pair of lumbar intersegmental artery branches called the **internal iliac arteries**. The internal iliac arteries vascularize pelvic organs and (initially) the lower extremity limb bud. As discussed later in the chapter, the fifth lumber intersegmental arteries also give rise to the **external iliac arteries**. Proximal to these branches, the root of the fifth intersegmental artery is called the **common iliac artery** (see Fig. 13-23).

Arteries to Limbs Are Formed by Remodeling of Intersegmental Artery Branches

As indicated above, the arteries to the developing upper and lower limbs are derived mainly from the seventh cervical intersegmental artery and the fifth lumbar intersegmental artery, respectively. These arteries initially supply each limb bud by joining an **axial** or **axis artery** that develops along the central axis of the limb bud (Figs. 13-22, 13-23). In the upper limb, the axis artery develops into the **brachial artery** of the upper arm and the **anterior interosseous artery** of the forearm and thus continues to be the main source of blood for the limb. In the hand, a small portion of the axis artery persists as the **deep palmar arch**. The other arteries of the upper limb, including the **radial, median,** and **ulnar arteries**, develop partly as sprouts of the axis artery.

In the lower limb, in contrast, the axis artery—which arises as the distal continuation of the internal iliac artery—largely degenerates, and the definitive supply is provided almost entirely by the **external iliac artery**, which, as mentioned above, arises as a new

13

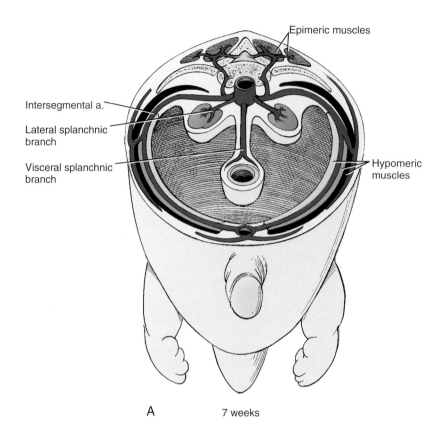

A   7 weeks

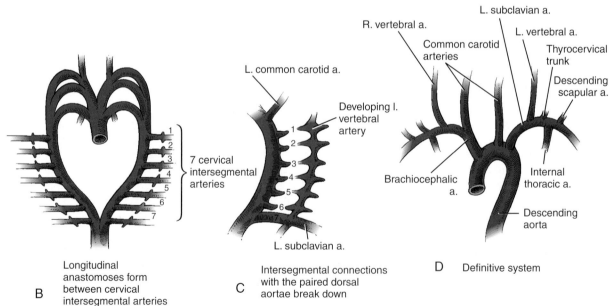

B   Longitudinal anastomoses form between cervical intersegmental arteries

C   Intersegmental connections with the paired dorsal aortae break down

D   Definitive system

Figure 13-21. Development of the arterial supply to the body wall. *A,* Intersegmental artery system in the trunk region. Branches of the paired intersegmental arteries supply the posterior, lateral, and anterior body wall and musculature, the vertebral column, and the spinal cord. *B-D,* The vertebral artery is formed from longitudinal anastomoses of the first through seventh cervical intersegmental arteries.

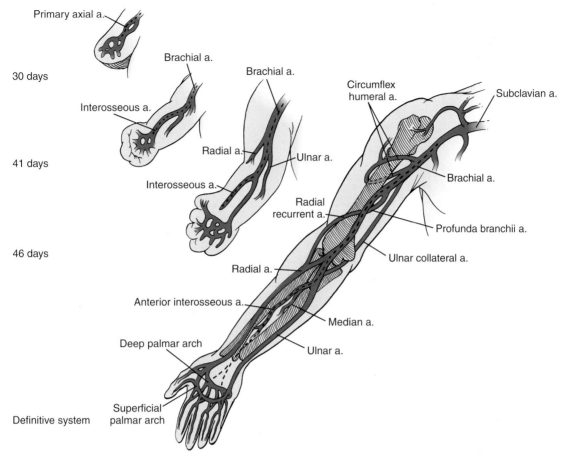

30 days

41 days

46 days

Definitive system

Primary axial a.

Brachial a.

Interosseous a.

Brachial a.

Radial a.

Ulnar a.

Interosseous a.

Radial recurrent a.

Radial a.

Anterior interosseous a.

Deep palmar arch

Median a.

Ulnar a.

Superficial palmar arch

Circumflex humeral a.

Subclavian a.

Brachial a.

Profunda branchii a.

Ulnar collateral a.

Figure 13-22. Development of the arterial system of the upper limb. The seventh cervical intersegmental arteries grow into the limb buds to join the axis arteries of the developing upper limbs. The axis artery gives rise to the subclavian, axillary, brachial, and anterior interosseous arteries and to the deep palmar arch. Other arteries of the upper extremity develop as sprouts of the axis artery.

13

branch of the fifth lumbar intersegmental artery (see Fig. 13-23). The axis artery persists as three remnants: the small **sciatic (ischiadic) artery**, which serves the sciatic nerve in the posterior thigh; a segment of the **popliteal artery;** and a section of the **peroneal (fibular) artery** in the leg. Virtually all other arteries of the lower limb develop as sprouts of the external iliac artery.

IN THE CLINIC

VASCULAR ANOMALIES ARISING FROM ERRORS IN REMODELING OF GREAT VESSELS

The bilaterally symmetric vascular system of the early embryo undergoes an intricate sequence of regressions, remodeling, and anastomoses to produce the adult pattern of great veins and arteries. Regression affects mainly the left

side of the venous system (discussed later in this chapter, see also Ch. 12) and, conversely, the right side of the aortic arch system. As a result, systemic venous return is channeled to the right atrium, whereas the original left fourth aortic arch becomes the arch of the definitive aorta. Congenital vascular malformations can arise at many stages during this process. Vascular malformations can result from the failure of some primitive element to undergo regression, or the inappropriate regression of an element.

FORMATION OF "VASCULAR RINGS" THAT CONSTRICT ESOPHAGUS AND TRACHEA

The aortic arches and dorsal aorta initially form a vascular basket that completely encircles the pharyngeal foregut (see Figs. 13-17, 13-18, 13-19A). In normal development, the regression of the right dorsal aorta opens this basket on the right side so that the esophagus is not encircled by

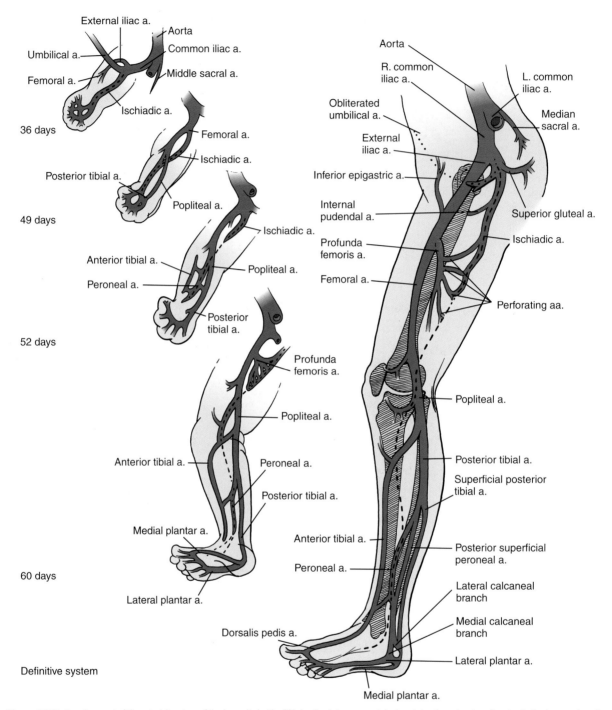

Figure 13-23. Development of the arterial system of the lower limb. The fifth lumbar intersegmental artery joins the axis artery forming in the lower extremity. The only remnants of the axis artery in the lower limb of the adult are the ischiadic artery, a small portion of the popliteal artery, and the peroneal artery.

aortic arch derivatives. However, occasionally the right dorsal aorta persists and maintains its connection with the dorsal aorta, resulting in a **double aortic arch** forming a **vascular ring** that encloses the trachea and esophagus (Fig. 13-24). This ring may constrict the trachea and esophagus, interfering with both breathing and swallowing.

Another malformation that can cause difficulties in swallowing (**dysphagia**) and possibly **dyspnea** (difficulty in breathing) results from the abnormal disappearance of the right fourth aortic arch. If the right fourth arch regresses, the seventh intersegmental artery (future right subclavian artery), which normally connects to the right fourth aortic arch, forms a connection with the descending aorta instead. Therefore, the seventh intersegmental crosses over the midline, usually posterior to the esophagus, forming an **aberrant right subclavian artery** (seen in almost 1% of the general population and almost 40% of **Down syndrome** patients having congenital heart defects; Fig. 13-25). After the great arteries mature, the esophagus may be pinched between the arch of the aorta and the abnormal right subclavian artery. Often this is asymptomatic. However, in some individuals the aberrant right subclavian artery compresses the esophagus, causing dysphagia, and the esophagus may reciprocally compress the right subclavian artery, reducing the blood pressure in the right upper extremity.

Another common aortic arch defect is a **right-sided (right) aortic arch**. In this anomaly, the right dorsal aorta segment between the future right subclavian artery and future thoracic aorta (i.e., the right eighth dorsal aortic segment) is retained whereas the left fourth aortic is lost (Fig. 13-26A). This anomaly is seen in 13% to 35% of the patients with tetralogy of Fallot and about 8% of patients with transposition of the great vessels. In cases of right-sided aortic arch, the ductus arteriosus (ligamentum arteriosum after its postnatal closure) stretches toward the right side either in front or behind the esophagus and trachea. If it passes behind the esophagus, it can constrict the esophagus and trachea causing dysphagia and/or dyspnea.

An **interrupted aortic arch** arises when both the right and left fourth aortic arches are obliterated while the distal right dorsal aorta is retained. After birth, the aorta supplies the head, upper limbs, and body, but the lower body and limbs are supplied by the pulmonary artery (poorly oxygenated blood) via a **patent ductus arteriosus** (Fig. 13-26B).

COARCTATION OF THE AORTA

In its usual form, **coarctation of the aorta** is a congenital malformation in which an abnormal thickening of the aortic wall severely constricts the aorta in the region of the ductus arteriosus. This malformation occurs in approximately 0.3%

13

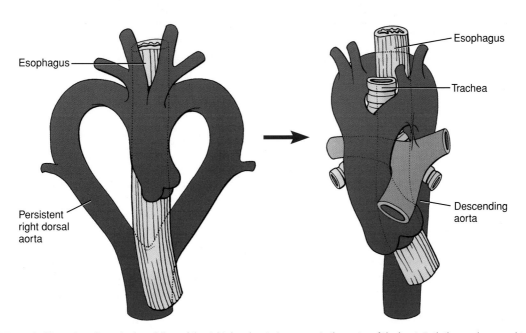

Figure 13-24. A double aortic arch results from failure of the right dorsal aorta to regress in the region of the heart. Both the esophagus and trachea are enclosed in the resulting double arch.

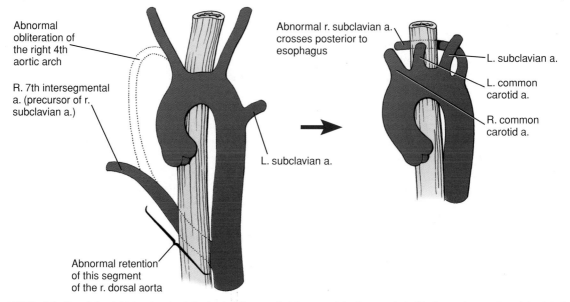

Abnormal
obliteration of
the right 4th
aortic arch

R. 7th intersegmental
a. (precursor of r.
subclavian a.)

Abnormal retention
of this segment
of the r. dorsal aorta

Abnormal r. subclavian a.
crosses posterior to
esophagus

L. subclavian a.

L. common
carotid a.

R. common
carotid a.

L. subclavian a.

Figure 13-25. Retention of the right dorsal aorta at the level of the seventh intersegmental artery coupled with abnormal regression of the right fourth aortic arch may result in an anomalous right subclavian artery that passes posterior to the esophagus.

of all live-born infants. It is more common in males than females and is the most common cardiovascular anomaly in **Turner syndrome**. The pathogenesis of aortic coarctation is not understood, although the malformation may be triggered by genetic factors or by teratogens. Two ideas have been proposed to explain coarctation: 1) abnormal migration of cells into the aortic wall near the ductus arteriosus, and 2) abnormal hemodynamics resulting in abnormal growth of the left fourth aortic arch.

Aortic coarctation occurs most commonly in a juxtaductal position (i.e., adjacent to the ductus arteriosus), but may also occur more proximally (preductal; i.e., upstream) or distally (postductal; i.e., downstream) (Fig. 13-27A, B). **Postductal coarctation** may be asymptomatic in newborn infants if collateral circulation is established from the subclavian, internal thoracic, transverse cervical, suprascapular, superior epigastric, intercostal, and lumbar arteries during the embryonic and fetal period (Fig. 13-27C, D). However, with **preductal coarctation**, collateral circulation does not develop because most of the oxygen- and nutrient-enriched blood from the placenta reaches the lower portion of the body via the **ductus arteriosus**. These infants typically develop problems after birth when the ductus arteriosus closes. This leads to **differential cyanosis**, where the upper part of the body and head are well

perfused but the lower part is cyanotic. The clinical effects of coarctation are variable and depend on the degree of narrowing. Typically, coarctation requires surgical repair in the neonatal period.

As mentioned in Chapters 3, 5, 12, and 14, patients with **Alagille syndrome** exhibit a characteristic facial appearance, paucity of bile ducts, heart defects, vertebral defects, and arterial stenosis (usually pulmonary artery stenosis but sometimes including abdominal coarctation). Mutations in *JAGGED1* and *NOTCH2* have been identified in most of these patients. *Hey2* (or *Herp*) is a basic HLH transcription factor important for mediating *Notch* signaling. In zebrafish, mutants of the *Hey2* homolog, *gridlock*, have defects in the aorta resembling human coarctation. However in mice, *Hey2* knockouts do not develop coarctation of the aorta. Rather, they develop other cardiac anomalies (such as ventricular septal defects). About 10% patients with **Noonan syndrome** (also discussed in Ch. 12) have coarctation of the aorta, a syndrome linked to mutations in the *PTPN11* (a gene encoding a nonreceptor TYROSINE PHOSPHATASE involved in intracellular signal transduction; discussed in Ch. 12). However, in a study of 157 humans with coarctation of aorta (that excluded Noonan patients), a *PTPN11* mutation was found in only a single patient, suggesting mutations in *PTPN11* are not the major cause of isolated coarctation.

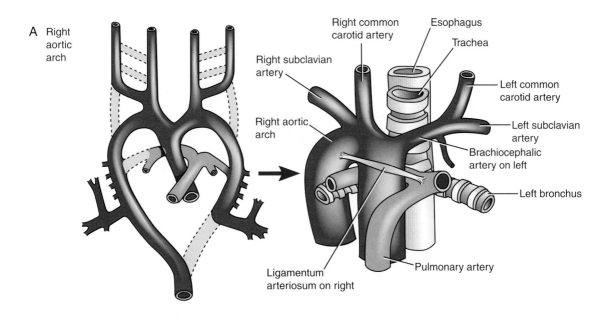

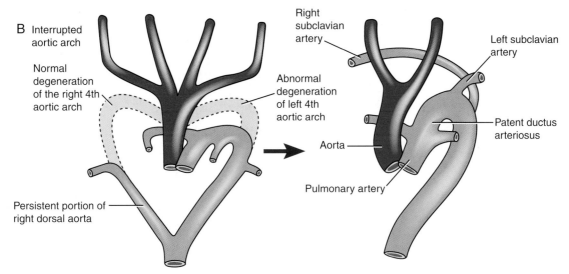

Figure 13-26. *A,* Right aortic arch. The left dorsal aorta downstream from the origin of the left subclavian artery is obliterated, whereas the right side counterpart is retained. Symptoms may occur depending on whether the ligamentum arteriosum passes ventral or dorsal to the esophagus and trachea. *B,* Interrupted aortic arch. Both the right and left fourth aortic arches degenerate (instead of just the right fourth aortic arch degenerating as in normal development), with the distal right dorsal aorta still being retained. After birth, the aorta supplies the head, upper limbs, and body, but the lower body and limbs are supplied by the pulmonary artery (poorly oxygenated blood) via a patent ductus arteriosus.

13

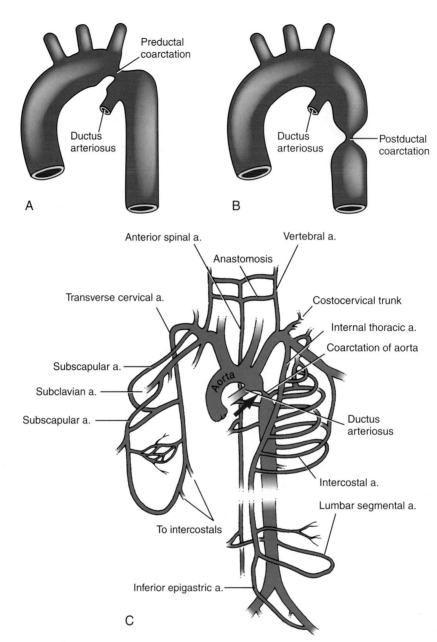

A — Preductal coarctation
Ductus arteriosus

B — Ductus arteriosus — Postductal coarctation

C

Anterior spinal a.
Anastomosis
Vertebral a.
Transverse cervical a.
Costocervical trunk
Internal thoracic a.
Coarctation of aorta
Subscapular a.
Subclavian a.
Aorta
Subscapular a.
Ductus arteriosus
Intercostal a.
Lumbar segmental a.
To intercostals
Inferior epigastric a.

Figure 13-27. *A, B,* Preductal and postductal coarctation of the aorta. *C,* Development of collateral circulation in postductal coarctation of the aorta. The aortic constriction (arrow) partly or completely blocks the flow of blood into the descending aorta. The trunk and lower extremities receive blood through enlarged collaterals that develop in response to the block. Collateral circulation established before birth may utilize internal thoracic arteries or the thyrocervical trunk to deliver blood to the descending aorta via segmental arteries of the trunk.

Continued

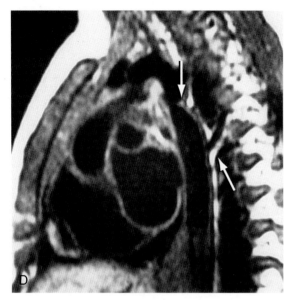

Figure 13-27. Cont'd. *D*, Sagittal magnetic resonance imaging scan in lateral view showing the site of postductal coarctation (top arrow) and a major collateral entering the descending aorta (lower arrow).

Primitive Embryonic Venous System is Divided into Vitelline, Umbilical, and Cardinal Systems

The embryo has three major venous systems that fulfill different functions. The **vitelline system** drains the gastrointestinal tract and gut derivatives; the **umbilical system** carries oxygenated blood from the placenta; and the **cardinal system** drains the head, neck, and body wall. All three systems are initially bilaterally symmetric and converge on the right and left sinus horns of the sinus venosus (Figs. 13-28A, 13-29; see Fig. 12-18). However, the shift of the systemic venous return to the right atrium (discussed in Ch. 12) initiates a radical remodeling that reshapes these systems to yield the adult patterns.

Vitelline System Gives Rise to Liver Sinusoids, Portal System, and a Portion of Inferior Vena Cava

Like the vitelline arteries, the vitelline veins arise from the capillary plexuses of the yolk sac and form part of the vasculature of the developing gut and gut derivatives. Initially, the vitelline system empties into the sinus horns of the heart via a pair of symmetrical **vitelline veins** (see Fig. 13-28A). Right and left vitelline plexuses also develop in the septum transversum and connect to the vitelline veins (Fig. 13-28B). The vessels of these plexuses become surrounded by the growing liver cords and give rise to the **liver sinusoids**, a dense network of anastomosing venous spaces. As the left sinus horn regresses to form the coronary sinus, the left vitelline vein also diminishes. By the 3rd month, the left vitelline vein has completely disappeared in the region of the sinus venosus. The blood from the left side of the abdominal viscera now drains across to the right vitelline vein via a series of transverse anastomoses that have formed both within the substance of the liver and around the abdominal portion of the foregut (Fig. 13-28C).

After the left vitelline vein loses its connection with the heart, the blood from the entire vitelline system drains into the heart via the enlarged right vitelline vein (see Fig. 13-28C). The cranial portion of this vein (the portion between the liver and the heart) becomes the **terminal portion of the inferior vena cava** (IVC) (see Fig. 13-29D, E). Meanwhile, a single oblique channel among the hepatic anastomoses becomes dominant and drains directly into the nascent IVC. As described below, this channel, the **ductus venosus**, is crucial during fetal life because it receives oxygenated blood from the umbilical system and shunts it directly to the right vitelline vein and, hence, the right atrium.

The vitelline veins caudal to the liver regress during the 2nd and 3rd months, with the exception of the portion of the right vitelline vein just caudal to the developing liver and a few of the proximal ventral left-to-right vitelline anastomoses (see Fig. 13-28B). These veins become the main channels of the **portal system**, which drains blood from the gastrointestinal tract to the liver sinusoids. The segment of the right vitelline vein caudal to the liver becomes the **portal vein** and the **superior mesenteric vein** (see Fig. 13-28C, D). Persisting branches collect blood from the abdominal foregut (including the abdominal esophagus, stomach, gallbladder, duodenum, and pancreas) and the midgut. Prominent left-to-right vitelline anastomoses are remodeled to deliver blood to the distal end of the portal vein through two veins: the **splenic vein**, which drains the spleen, part of the stomach, and the greater omentum (discussed in Ch. 14) and the **inferior mesenteric vein**, which drains the hindgut.

13

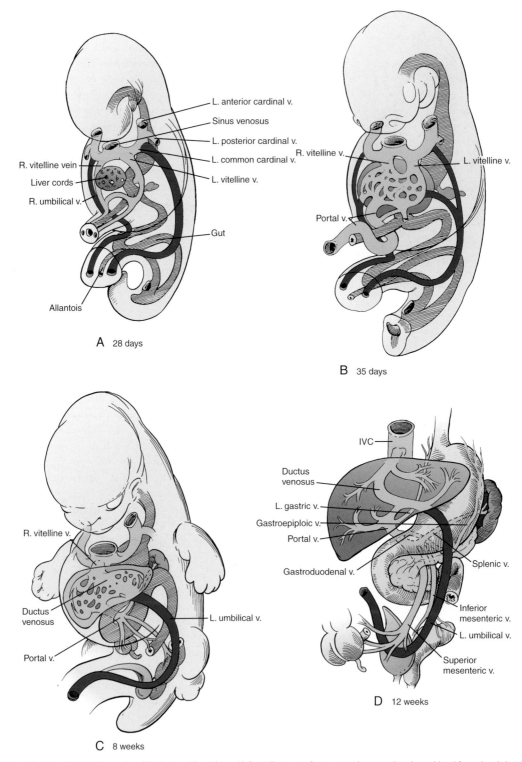

A 28 days

L. anterior cardinal v.
Sinus venosus
L. posterior cardinal v.
L. common cardinal v.
L. vitelline v.
R. vitelline vein
Liver cords
R. umbilical v.
Gut
Allantois

B 35 days

R. vitelline v.
L. vitelline v.
Portal v.

C 8 weeks

R. vitelline v.
Ductus venosus
L. umbilical v.
Portal v.

D 12 weeks

IVC
Ductus venosus
L. gastric v.
Gastroepiploic v.
Portal v.
Gastroduodenal v.
Splenic v.
Inferior mesenteric v.
L. umbilical v.
Superior mesenteric v.

Figure 13-28. *A-D,* Fate of the vitelline and umbilical veins. The right and left vitelline veins form a portal system that drains blood from the abdominal foregut, the midgut, and the upper part of the anorectal canal. The right umbilical vein disappears, but the left umbilical vein anastomoses with the ductus venosus in the liver, thus shunting oxygenated placental blood into the inferior vena cava and to the right side of the heart. IVC, inferior vena cava.

Right Umbilical Vein Disappears and Left Umbilical Vein Anastomoses with Ductus Venosus

In contrast to the vitelline veins in which the left regresses and the right persists, during the second month the right umbilical vein becomes completely obliterated and the left umbilical vein persists (see Fig. 13-28). Concurrently, with formation of the liver and remodeling of vessels in that area, the left umbilical vein loses its connection with the left sinus horn and forms a new anastomosis with the ductus venosus. Oxygenated blood from the placenta thus reaches the heart via the single umbilical vein and the ductus venosus. As described at the end of this chapter, the ductus venosus constricts shortly after birth, eliminating this venous shunt through the liver.

Posterior Cardinal System Is Augmented and Then Superseded by Paired Subcardinal and Supracardinal Veins

As shown in Figure 13-29A, the bilaterally symmetrical cardinal vein system that develops in the 3rd and 4th weeks to drain the head, neck, and body wall initially consists of paired **posterior (caudal)** and **anterior (cranial) cardinal veins**, which join near the heart to form the short **common cardinals** that empty into the sinus horns. The posterior cardinal veins are supplemented and later largely replaced by two additional pairs of veins, the **subcardinal** and **supracardinal** veins, which develop in the body wall medial to the posterior cardinal veins. Like the posterior and anterior cardinals, these two systems are

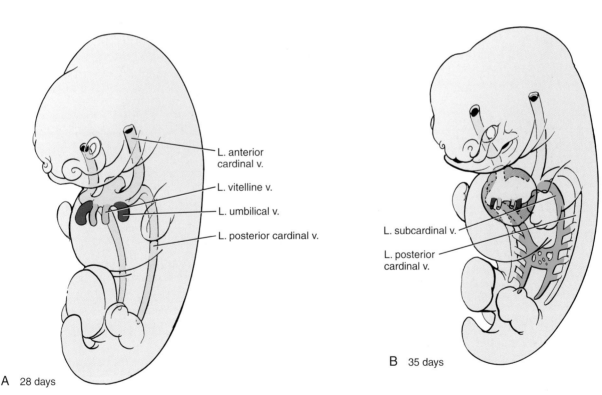

L. anterior cardinal v.

L. vitelline v.

L. umbilical v.

L. posterior cardinal v.

L. subcardinal v.

L. posterior cardinal v.

A 28 days

B 35 days

Figure 13-29. *A–E*, Development of the systemic venous system from the four bilaterally symmetrical cardinal vein systems. These systems are remodeled to drain blood from both sides of the head, neck, and body into the right atrium. The head and neck are initially drained by an anterior cardinal system, and the trunk is drained by a posterior cardinal system. The posterior cardinals are replaced by a set of subcardinal and a set of supracardinal veins. IVC, inferior vena cava; SVC, superior vena cava.

13

Continued

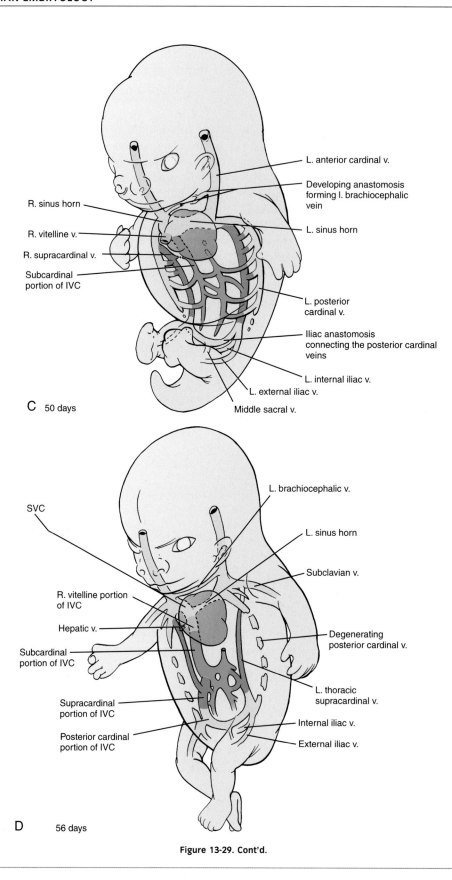

C 50 days

L. anterior cardinal v.

Developing anastomosis forming l. brachiocephalic vein

R. sinus horn

R. vitelline v.

R. supracardinal v.

Subcardinal portion of IVC

L. sinus horn

L. posterior cardinal v.

Iliac anastomosis connecting the posterior cardinal veins

L. internal iliac v.

L. external iliac v.

Middle sacral v.

D 56 days

SVC

L. brachiocephalic v.

L. sinus horn

Subclavian v.

R. vitelline portion of IVC

Hepatic v.

Subcardinal portion of IVC

Degenerating posterior cardinal v.

L. thoracic supracardinal v.

Supracardinal portion of IVC

Posterior cardinal portion of IVC

Internal iliac v.

External iliac v.

Figure 13-29. Cont'd.

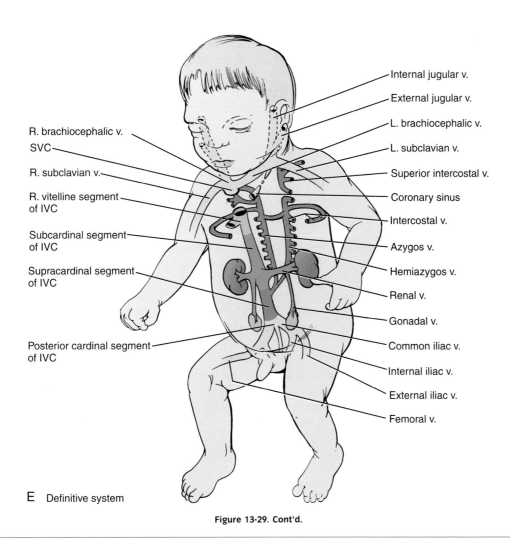

R. brachiocephalic v.
SVC
R. subclavian v.
R. vitelline segment of IVC
Subcardinal segment of IVC
Supracardinal segment of IVC
Posterior cardinal segment of IVC

Internal jugular v.
External jugular v.
L. brachiocephalic v.
L. subclavian v.
Superior intercostal v.
Coronary sinus
Intercostal v.
Azygos v.
Hemiazygos v.
Renal v.
Gonadal v.
Common iliac v.
Internal iliac v.
External iliac v.
Femoral v.

E Definitive system

Figure 13-29. Cont'd.

13

bilaterally symmetrical at first but undergo extensive remodeling during development.

The left and right subcardinal veins sprout from the base of the posterior cardinals by the end of the 6th week and grow caudally in the medial part of the dorsal body wall (see Fig. 13-29B). By the 7th and 8th weeks, these subcardinal veins become connected to each other by numerous median anastomoses and form some lateral anastomoses with the posterior cardinals. However, the longitudinal segments of the left subcardinal vein soon regress, so that by the 9th week, the structures on the left side of the body served by the subcardinal system drain solely through transverse anastomotic channels to the right subcardinal vein. Meanwhile, the right subcardinal vein loses its original connection with the posterior cardinal vein and develops a new anastomosis with

the segment of the right vitelline vein just inferior to the heart to form the portion of the inferior vena cava between the liver and the kidneys (see Fig. 13-29C-E). Through this remodeling process, blood from the organs originally drained by the right and left subcardinal veins now returns to the right atrium via the IVC.

While the subcardinal system is being remodeled, a new pair of veins, the supracardinal veins, sprouts from the base of the posterior cardinals and grow caudally just medial to the posterior cardinal veins (see Fig. 13-29C). These veins drain the body wall via the segmental **intercostal veins**, thus taking over the function of the posterior cardinals. The abdominal and thoracic portions of the supracardinal veins give rise to separate venous components in the adult and, therefore, will be described separately.

While the supracardinals are developing, the posterior cardinals become obliterated over most of their length (see Fig. 13-29C, D). The most caudal portions of the posterior cardinals (including a large median anastomosis) do persist but lose their original connection to the heart and form a new anastomosis with the supracardinal veins. This caudal remnant of the posterior cardinals develops into the common iliac veins and the caudalmost, sacral portion of the IVC. The common iliac veins in turn sprout the internal and external iliac veins, which grow to drain the lower extremities and pelvic organs.

In the abdominal region, the remodeling of the supracardinal system commences with the obliteration of the inferior portion of the left supracardinal vein (see Fig. 13-29D, E). The remaining abdominal segment of the right supracardinal vein then anastomoses with the right subcardinal vein to form a segment of the IVC just inferior to the kidneys.

The thoracic part of the supracardinal system drains the thoracic body wall via a series of **intercostal veins**. The thoracic portions of the supracardinals originally empty into the left and right posterior cardinals and are connected to each other by median anastomoses (see Fig. 13-29C). However, the left thoracic supracardinal vein, called the **hemiazygos vein**, soon loses its connection with the left posterior cardinal vein and left sinus horn and subsequently drains into the right supracardinal system. The remaining portion of the inferior right supracardinal vein also loses its original connection with the posterior cardinal vein and makes a new anastomosis with the segment of the superior vena cava derived from the anterior cardinal vein. The latter, in turn, drains into the heart via a segment representing a small remnant of the right common cardinal vein. The right supracardinal vein is then called the **azygos vein**. Both the hemiazygos and the azygos veins drain into the right atrium via the superior vena cava (see Fig. 13-29D, E).

Figure 13-29E shows the sources of the four portions of the IVC. From superior to inferior, (1) the right vitelline vein gives rise to the terminal segment of the IVC, (2) the right subcardinal vein gives rise to a segment between the liver and the kidneys, (3) the right supracardinal vein gives rise to an abdominal segment inferior to the kidneys, and (4) the right and left posterior cardinal veins plus the median anastomosis connecting them give rise to the sacral segment of the IVC.

Blood Is Drained from Head and Neck by Anterior Cardinal Veins

The left and right anterior cardinal veins originally drain blood into the sinus horns via the left and right common cardinal veins (see Fig. 13-29A-D). However, the proximal connection of the left anterior cardinal vein with the left sinus horn soon regresses, leaving only a small remnant, called the **oblique vein of the left atrium**, lying directly on the heart (see Figs. 13-29E, 12-18). This small remnant collects blood from the left atrial region of the heart and returns it directly to the coronary sinus, which is a vestige of the left sinus horn.

The cranial portions of the anterior cardinal veins in the developing cervical region give rise to the **internal jugular veins;** capillary plexuses in the face become connected with these vessels to form the **external jugular veins**. Simultaneously, a median anastomosis connecting the left and right anterior cardinals develops (see Fig. 13-29C-E). Once the left anterior cardinal vein loses its connection with the heart, all the blood from the left side of the head and neck shunts over to the right anterior cardinal through this anastomosis. The **subclavian vein**, which coalesces from the venous plexus of the left upper limb bud, also empties into the proximal left anterior cardinal vein. The intercardinal anastomosis thus carries blood from the left upper limb as well as the left side of the head and is called the **left brachiocephalic vein** (see Fig. 13-29C-E). The left brachiocephalic vein enters the right anterior cardinal at its junction with the **right brachiocephalic vein**, draining the right upper limb bud and head. The small segment of right anterior cardinal vein between the junction of the right and left brachiocephalic veins and the right atrium becomes the **superior vena cava** (see Fig 13-29E). Thus, by the end of the 8th week, the definitive superior vena cava drains blood from (1) both sides of the head, (2) both upper limbs, and (3) the thoracic body wall (via the azygos vein).

IN THE CLINIC

VENA CAVA ANOMALIES

A relatively rare anomaly called **double inferior vena cava** arises when the caudal portion of the left supracardinal system fails to regress, giving rise to an abnormal left IVC (Fig. 13-30A). The blood entering this vessel ultimately drains either into the right IVC via the left renal vein or into the hemiazygos vein arising from the thoracic part of the supracardinal system.

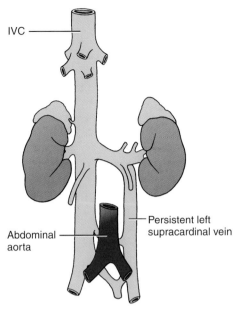

IVC

Abdominal aorta

Persistent left supracardinal vein

A   **Double inferior vena cava**

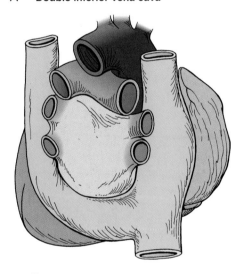

B   **Double superior vena cava**

Figure 13-30. Venous anomalies caused by failure of cardinal veins on the left to undergo normal regression. *A*, Preservation of the left supracardinal vein inferior to the kidney may result in double inferior vena cava. *B*, Preservation of the left anterior cardinal at the level of the heart may result in double superior vena cava (posterior view). The anomalous left superior vena cava empties into the coronary sinus.

Occasionally the left anterior cardinal vein persists and maintains its connection with the left sinus venosus (incidence 0.3% to 0.5% of the general population) resulting in either a **persistent left (double) superior vena cava** (Fig. 13-30*B*) or a **single left superior vena cava**. In 65% of these cases, the left brachiocephalic vein is also missing or very small. With a persistent left superior vena cava, blood from the left side of the head and neck and from the left upper extremity drains through the abnormal left superior vena cava into the coronary sinus. A single left superior vena cava develops when the left anterior cardinal vein persists and the right is obliterated. In this case, the left anterior cardinal vein gives rise to a superior vena cava draining the blood from the entire head and neck, both upper extremities, and the azygos system, directing it into the coronary sinus and right atrium. However in a small subset of double and left superior vena cavas, the left-sided superior vena cava empties directly into the left atrium (more common in cases of heterotaxy).

Development of Lymphatic System

Like blood vessels, lymphatic channels arise by vasculogenesis and angiogenesis from mesodermal precursors. However, lymphatics do not begin to form until about the 5th week. By the end of the 5th week, a pair of enlargements, the **jugular lymph sacs**, develop and collect fluid from the lymphatics of the upper limbs, upper trunk, head, and neck (Fig. 13-31). In the 6th week, four additional lymph sacs develop to collect lymph from the trunk and lower extremities: the **retroperitoneal lymph sac, cysterna chyli**, and paired **posterior lymph sacs** associated with the junctions of the external and internal iliac veins.

The cysterna chyli initially drains into a symmetrical pair of thoracic lymphatic ducts that empty into the venous circulation at the junctions of the internal jugular and subclavian veins. However, during development portions of both of these ducts are obliterated, and the definitive **thoracic duct** is derived from the caudal portion of the right duct, the cranial portion of the left duct, and a median anastomosis.

13

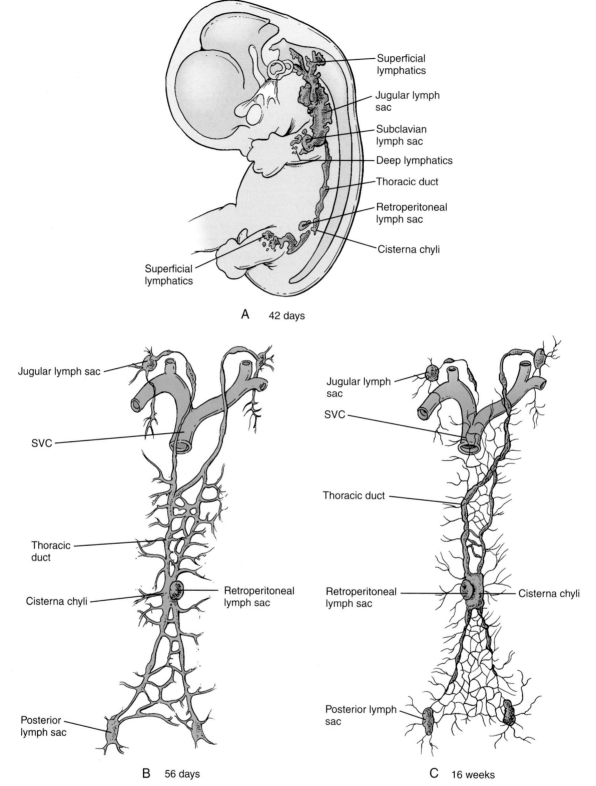

Figure 13-31. Development of the lymphatic system. *A,* Several lymph sacs and ducts develop by lymphangiogenesis and eventually drain fluid from tissue spaces throughout the entire body. *B-D,* The single thoracic duct that drains the cisterna chyli and the posterior thoracic wall is derived from parts of the right and left thoracic ducts and their anastomoses. SVC, superior vena cava.

Continued

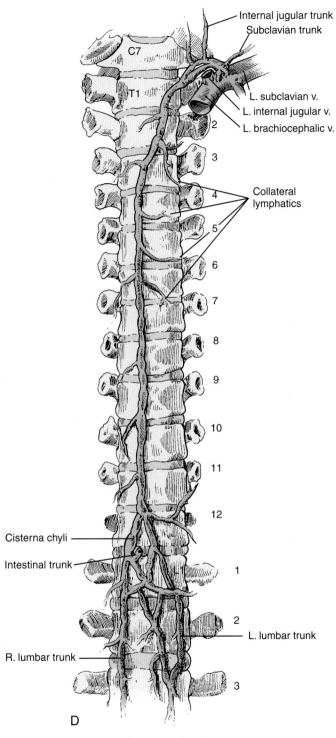

Figure 13-31. Cont'd.

IN THE RESEARCH LAB

MOLECULAR MECHANISMS OF LYMPHATIC DEVELOPMENT

Despite knowing of the existence of the lymphatic system for several centuries, the embryologic origin of this important system is only now becoming clear. In mice, a subset of venous endothelial cells belonging to the cardinal veins migrate out and form the initial lymphatic vessels. These migrating lymphatic endothelial cell precursors express the transcription factor, *Prospero-related homeobox-1* (*Prox1*), homologs of which have been found in humans, chicks, newts, frogs, Drosophila, and zebrafish. Initially, all cardinal vein endothelial cells seem to have lymphatic competency, as indicated by their expression of known lymphatic markers including *Vascular endothelial growth factor receptor-3* (*Vegfr3* or *Flt4*; a receptor for *VegfC* and *VegfD*) and *Lyve1* (a lymphatic specific hyaluronan receptor) (Fig. 13-32). However, only a subset of these endothelial cells are induced (by an unknown mechanism) to begin expressing *Prox1*, form the rudimentary lymphatic sacs, and begin expressing more specific lymphatic markers (e.g., *Nrp2* and *Podoplanin*). When *Prox1* is knocked out in mice, the resulting embryos are unable to develop a lymphatic system. Interestingly in *Prox1*-deficient mice, the migration of these endothelial cells still occurs. However, they never go on to express more definite lymphatic markers. Rather, they retain blood vessel endothelial markers such as *CD34* and *Laminin*. Therefore, *Prox1* is required for lymphatic cell specification in mice, and its expression may represent the master switch in programming lymphatic endothelial cell fate. In fact, ectopic expression of *Prox1* in blood vascular endothelium can redirect vascular endothelial cells into a lymphatic lineage. Although studies in mice show that lymph vessels form via an angiogenic-like process, evidence from avian embryos supports the idea that lymphatic vessels may also arise elsewhere within the embryo by a vasculogenic-like process from lymphangioblastic EPCs.

IN THE CLINIC

LYMPHEDEMA MAY RESULT FROM LYMPHATIC HYPOPLASIA

A major hereditary congenital disorder of the lymphatic system is **hereditary lymphedema** (or primary lymphedemas; a swelling of the lymphatic vasculature) caused by hypoplasia of the lymphatic system. This condition may or may not be associated with other abnormalities. The swelling generally occurs in the legs but, in the case of lymphedema associated with **Turner syndrome**, blockage of lymphatic ducts in the neck and upper trunk may also result in the development of lymph-filled cysts (cystic hygromas). These cysts may disappear if lymphatic drainage improves during subsequent development. **Milroy disease**, a primary lymphedema syndrome, has been linked to mutations in the *VEGFR3* gene. Other, more rare forms of lymphedema have been linked to the *FOXC2* gene, a member of the *Forkhead* family of transcriptions factors. Mutations in *SOX18* (an SRY-related transcription factor) have also been associated with both dominant and recessive inherited forms of lymphedema. Several other potential genes identified from mouse models that develop lymphedemas include *Ang2*, *Nrp2*, *Net*, *Podoplanin*, and *Syk*.

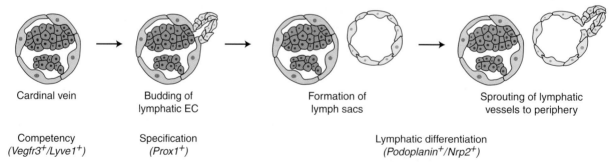

| Cardinal vein | Budding of lymphatic EC | Formation of lymph sacs | Sprouting of lymphatic vessels to periphery |

| Competency (Vegfr3⁺/Lyve1⁺) | Specification (Prox1⁺) | Lymphatic differentiation (Podoplanin⁺/Nrp2⁺) |

Competency
($Vegfr3^+/Lyve1^+$)   Specification
($Prox1^+$)   Lymphatic differentiation
($Podoplanin^+/Nrp2^+$)

Figure 13-32. Postulated steps in generating lymphatic vessels based on mouse studies. Cardinal vein endothelial cells start out competent to form lymphatic vessels as they express the lymphatic markers *Vegfr3* and *Lyve1*. An unknown induction signal initiates lymphangiogenesis in a subset of these endothelial cells and these cells begin expressing *Prox1*. *Prox1*-positive endothelial cells then migrate, form lymphatic sacs, and eventually begin expressing definitive lymphatic differentiation markers (e.g., *Podoplanin*, *Nrp2*).

Dramatic Changes Occur in Circulatory System at Birth

Starting at birth, the systemic and pulmonary circulations are wholly separate and are arranged in series. This arrangement would have been impracticable in the fetus because oxygenated blood enters the fetus via the umbilical vein, and little blood can flow through the collapsed lungs. Therefore, the fetal heart chambers and outflow tracts contain foramina and ducts that shunt the oxygenated blood entering the right atrium to the left ventricle and aortic arch, thus largely bypassing the developing pulmonary circulation. These shunts close at birth, abruptly separating the two circulations.

The transition from fetal dependence on maternal support via the placenta to the relatively independent existence of the infant in the outside world at birth brings about dramatic changes in the pattern of blood circulation within the newborn. In the fetal circulation (Fig. 13-33A), oxygenated blood enters the body through the left umbilical vein. In the **ductus venosus**, this blood mixes with a small volume of deoxygenated portal blood and then enters the IVC, where it mixes with deoxygenated blood returning from the trunk and legs. In the right atrium, this stream of blood, still highly oxygenated, is largely shunted through the foramen ovale to the left atrium. The oxygenated blood entering the fetal right atrium from the IVC and the deoxygenated blood entering from the SVC form hemodynamically distinct streams and undergo very little mixing in the atrium. This separation of streams is accomplished partly by the shape and placement of the valve of the IVC.

In the left atrium, oxygenated blood from the right atrium mixes with the very small amount of blood returning from the lungs via the pulmonary veins. Little blood flows through the pulmonary circulation during fetal life because the vascular resistance of the collapsed fetal lungs is very high. The oxygenated blood in the left ventricle is then propelled into the aorta for distribution first to the head, neck, and arms and then, via the descending aorta, to the trunk and limbs. As blood enters the descending aorta, it mixes with the deoxygenated blood shunted through the ductus arteriosus. This blood consists mainly of the blood entering the right atrium from the superior vena cava and expelled via the right ventricle and pulmonary trunk. Thus, the blood delivered to the head, neck, and arms by the fetal circulation is more highly oxygenated than the blood delivered to the trunk and lower limbs. After the descending aorta has distributed blood to the trunk and lower limbs, the remaining blood enters the umbilical arteries and returns to the placenta for oxygenation.

The fetal circulatory pattern functions throughout the birth process. However, as soon as the newborn infant takes its first breath, major changes convert the circulation to the adult configuration in which the pulmonary and systemic circuits are separate and are arranged in series (Fig. 13-33B). As the alveoli fill with air, the constricted pulmonary vessels open and the resistance of the pulmonary vasculature drops precipitously. In mammalian animal models, **Nitric oxide synthase** levels drastically increase in the pulmonary vasculature at the time of birth, increasing the potential to generate **nitric oxide** and dilate these vessels. The opening of the pulmonary vessels is thought to be a direct response to oxygen, because hypoxia in newborns can cause pulmonary vessels to constrict. At the same time, spontaneous constriction (or obstetrical clamping) of the umbilical vessels cuts off the flow from the placenta.

The opening of the pulmonary circulation and the cessation of umbilical flow create changes in pressure and flow that cause the ductus arteriosus to constrict and the **foramen ovale** to close. When the pulmonary circulation opens, the resulting drop in pressure in the pulmonary trunk is thought to cause a slight reverse flow of oxygenated aortic blood through the **ductus arteriosus**. This increase in local oxygen tension apparently induces the vascular smooth muscle of the ductus arteriosus to contract and restrict blood flow through this vessel. The precise mechanism by which changes in oxygen tension initiate contraction of these cells is still unclear (discussed further in the following "In the Clinic"), but constriction of the ductus arteriosus normally occurs within 24 hours after birth in infants born at term.

The initial closing of the **foramen ovale**, in contrast, is primarily a mechanical effect of the reversal in pressure between the two atria. The opening of the pulmonary vasculature and the cessation of umbilical flow reduce the pressure in the right atrium, whereas the sudden increase in pulmonary venous return raises the pressure in the left atrium. The resulting pressure change forces the flexible septum primum against the more rigid septum secundum, functionally closing the foramen ovale. The septum primum and septum secundum normally fuse by about 3 months after birth.

13

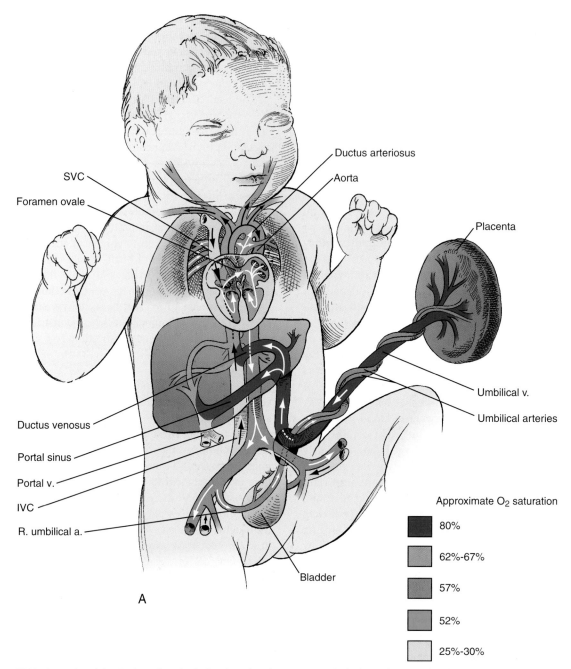

SVC

Foramen ovale

Ductus arteriosus

Aorta

Placenta

Ductus venosus

Portal sinus

Portal v.

IVC

R. umbilical a.

Umbilical v.

Umbilical arteries

Bladder

A

Approximate O$_2$ saturation

80%

62%-67%

57%

52%

25%-30%

Figure 13-33. Conversion of the circulation from the fetal to the air-breathing pattern. At birth, the single circuit of the fetal circulation is rapidly converted to two circuits (pulmonary and systemic) arranged in a series. *A,* Pattern of blood flow in the fetus and placenta just before birth.

Continued

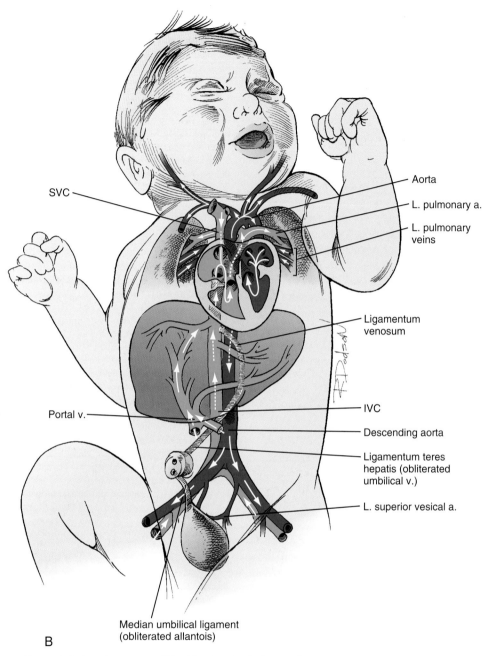

SVC

Aorta

L. pulmonary a.

L. pulmonary veins

Ligamentum venosum

Portal v.

IVC

Descending aorta

Ligamentum teres hepatis (obliterated umbilical v.)

L. superior vesical a.

Median umbilical ligament (obliterated allantois)

B

Figure 13-33. Cont'd. *B*, Pattern of blood flow just after birth. IVC, inferior vena cava; SVC, superior vena cava.

The **ductus venosus** also closes soon after birth. However, rapid constriction of the ductus venosus is not essential to the infant, because blood is no longer flowing through the umbilical vein. *Prostaglandins* (hormones with dilator effects on vascular smooth muscle) seem to play a role in maintaining the patency of the ductus venosus during fetal life, but the signal that brings about the apparently active constriction of this channel after birth is not fully understood. Nevertheless, a normal portal circulation within a few days of birth supplants the hepatic blood flow from the placenta.

IN THE CLINIC

PATENT DUCTUS ARTERIOSUS LEADS TO HEART FAILURE IF NOT CORRECTED

In term infants, the ductus arteriosus constricts in response to a rise in oxygen tension. However, during fetal life the ductus is kept patent, in part, by circulating *Prostaglandins*. Studies in mice show *Prostaglandin E2 receptor subtype-4* is expressed in vascular smooth muscle of the ductus arteriosus. When this receptor is knocked out, the mice develop **patent ductus arteriosus**. Animal models show increases in oxygen levels decrease circulating levels of *Prostaglandins*, signal the release of *Endothelins* (a vasoconstrictor released by endothelial cells), alter K^+ ion channel activity in vascular smooth muscle, and increase intracellular calcium ion levels, all of which promote contraction of vascular smooth muscle in the ductus arteriosus. Interestingly, the importance of increasing oxygen tension in the closure of the ductus arteriosus is supported by the observation that patent ductus arteriosus is more prevalent in patients living under hypoxic conditions (i.e., at high altitudes). For reasons that are unclear, the incidence of patent ductus arteriosus is also higher in cases of **maternal rubella infection**.

Infants who have cardiovascular malformations in which a patent ductus arteriosus is essential to life (see "Clinical Taster" of Ch. 12) may be treated with an infusion of *Prostaglandins* to keep the ductus open until the malformation can be corrected surgically. Conversely, premature infants in whom the ductus arteriosus does not constrict spontaneously are sometimes treated with **Prostaglandin inhibitors** such as **indomethacin**. More recently, **ibuprofen** is being tested as an alternative to indomethacin because it may have fewer side effects. In newborns having a large patent ductus arteriosus, about one third to one half of the blood is shunted from the aorta back into the pulmonary circulation. This means that on its return to the heart from the lungs, the same blood must be pumped back out again by the left ventricle (increasing its work load two to three times). If not corrected, this leads is to progressive pulmonary vasculature obstructive disease, pulmonary hypertension, left atrial dilatation and ventricular hypertrophy, and eventual heart failure. This abnormal blood flow pattern also increases the risk of bacterial **endocarditis**.

Suggested Readings

Adams RH. 2003. Molecular control of arterial-venous blood vessel identity. J Anat 202:105-112.

Baird AM, Gerstein RM, Berg LJ. 1999. The role of cytokine receptor signaling in lymphocyte development. Curr Opin Immunol 11:157-166.

Baron MH. 2003. Embryonic origins of mammalian hematopoiesis. Exp Hematol 31:1160-1169.

Bertolino P, Deckers M, Lebrin F, ten Dijke P. 2005. Transforming growth factor-beta signal transduction in angiogenesis and vascular disorders. Chest 128:585S-590S.

Bohnsack BL, Hirschi KK. 2004. Red light, green light: signals that control endothelial cell proliferation during embryonic vascular development. Cell Cycle 3:1506-1511.

Brauer PR. 2006. MMPs—role in cardiovascular development and disease. Front Biosci 11:447-478.

Bruckner AL, Frieden IJ. 2003. Hemangiomas of infancy. J Am Acad Dermatol 48:477-493; quiz 494-496.

Burri PH, Hlushchuk R, Djonov V. 2004. Intussusceptive angiogenesis: its emergence, its characteristics, and its significance. Dev Dyn 231:474-488.

Dieterlen-Lievre F, Le Douarin NM. 2004. From the hemangioblast to self-tolerance: a series of innovations gained from studies on the avian embryo. Mech Dev 121:1117-1128.

Dor Y, Porat R, Keshet E. 2001. Vascular endothelial growth factor and vascular adjustments to perturbations in oxygen homeostasis. Am J Physiol Cell Physiol 280:C1367-C1374.

Eichmann A, Yuan L, Moyon D, et al. 2005. Vascular development: from precursor cells to branched arterial and venous networks. Int J Dev Biol 49:259-267.

Franco D, Campione M. 2003. The role of Pitx2 during cardiac development. Linking left-right signaling and congenital heart diseases. Trends Cardiovasc Med 13:157-163.

Graham A. 2003. Development of the pharyngeal arches. Am J Med Genet A 119:251-256.

Hong YK, Shin JW, Detmar M. 2004. Development of the lymphatic vascular system: a mystery unravels. Dev Dyn 231:462-473.

Hutson MR, Kirby ML. 2003. Neural crest and cardiovascular development: a 20-year perspective. Birth Defects Res C Embryo Today 69:2-13.

Jain RK. 2003. Molecular regulation of vessel maturation. Nat Med 9:685-693.

Kiserud T. 2005. Physiology of the fetal circulation. Semin Fetal Neonatal Med 10:493-503.

Kurz H, Burri PH, Djonov VG. 2003. Angiogenesis and vascular remodeling by intussusception: from form to function. News Physiol Sci 18:65-70.

le Noble F, Fleury V, Pries A, et al. 2005. Control of arterial branching morphogenesis in embryogenesis: go with the flow. Cardiovasc Res 65:619-628.

Lebrin F, Deckers M, Bertolino P, Ten Dijke P. 2005. TGF-beta receptor function in the endothelium. Cardiovasc Res 65:599-608.

Mavrides E, Moscoso G, Carvalho JS, et al. 2001. The anatomy of the umbilical, portal and hepatic venous systems in the human fetus at 14-19 weeks of gestation. Ultrasound Obstet Gynecol 18:598-604.

McGrath KE, Palis J. 2005. Hematopoiesis in the yolk sac: more than meets the eye. Exp Hematol 33:1021-1028.

Moser M, Patterson C. 2005. Bone morphogenetic proteins and vascular differentiation: BMPing up vasculogenesis. Thromb Haemost 94:713-718.

Oddone M, Granata C, Vercellino N, et al. 2005. Multi-modality evaluation of the abnormalities of the aortic arches in children: techniques and imaging spectrum with emphasis on MRI. Pediatr Radiol 35:947-960.

Patan S. 2004. Vasculogenesis and angiogenesis. Cancer Treat Res 117:3-32.

Rossant J, Howard L. 2002. Signaling pathways in vascular development. Annu Rev Cell Dev Biol 18:541-573.

Scavelli C, Weber E, Agliano M, et al. 2004. Lymphatics at the crossroads of angiogenesis and lymphangiogenesis. J Anat 204:433-449.

Tavian M, Peault B. 2005. Embryonic development of the human hematopoietic system. Int J Dev Biol 49:243-250.

Waldo K, Kirby ML. 1998. Development of the great arteries. In: De la Cruz MV, Markwald RR, editors. Living Morphogenesis of the Heart. Boston, Birkhauser. pp 187-217.

13

Development of the Gastrointestinal Tract

14

Summary The endodermal gut tube created by body folding during the 4th week (discussed in Ch. 4) consists of a blind-ended cranial **foregut**, a blind-ended caudal **hindgut**, and a **midgut** open to the yolk sac through the vitelline duct. As discussed in Chapter 13, the arterial supply to the gut develops through consolidation and reduction of the ventral branches of the dorsal aortae that anastomose with the vessel plexuses originally supplying blood to the yolk sac. About five of these vitelline artery derivatives vascularize the thoracic foregut, and three—the **celiac, superior mesenteric**, and **inferior mesenteric arteries**—vascularize the abdominal gut. By convention, the boundaries of the foregut, midgut, and hindgut portions of the abdominal gut tube are determined by the respective territories of these three arteries. However, these segments and the site of some gastrointestinal organs are already demarcated by specific gene expression patterns observable at even earlier stages.

By the fifth week, the abdominal portion of the foregut is visibly divided into the **esophagus, stomach**, and proximal **duodenum**. The stomach is initially fusiform, and differential growth of its dorsal and ventral walls produces the **greater** and **lesser curvatures**. Meanwhile, **hepatic, cystic**, and **dorsal** and **ventral pancreatic diverticula** bud from the proximal duodenum into the **mesogastrium** and give rise, respectively, to the **liver, gallbladder, cystic duct**, and **pancreas**. In addition, the **spleen** condenses from mesenchyme in the dorsal mesogastrium.

During the sixth and seventh weeks, the stomach rotates around longitudinal and dorsoventral axes so that the greater curvature is finally directed to the left and slightly caudally. This rotation shifts the liver to the right in the abdominal cavity and brings the duodenum and pancreas into contact with the posterior body wall, where they become fixed (i.e., **secondarily retroperitoneal**). This event converts the space dorsal to the rotated stomach and dorsal mesogastrium into a recess called the **lesser sac of the peritoneum**. The pouch of dorsal mesogastrium forming the left lateral boundary of the lesser sac subsequently undergoes voluminous expansion, giving rise to the curtain-like **greater omentum** that drapes over the inferior abdominal viscera.

The midgut differentiates into the distal **duodenum, jejunum, ileum, cecum, ascending colon**, and proximal two thirds of the **transverse colon**. The future ileum elongates more rapidly than can be accommodated by the early peritoneal cavity, so that by the fifth week the midgut is thrown into an anteroposterior hairpin fold, the **primary intestinal loop**, which herniates into the umbilicus during the sixth week. As the primary intestinal loop herniates, it rotates around its long axis by 90 degrees counterclockwise (as viewed from the ventral side) so that the future ileum lies in the right abdomen and the future large intestine lies in the left abdomen. Meanwhile, the cecum and appendix differentiate, and the jejunum and ileum continue to elongate. During the 10th through 12th weeks, the intestinal loop is retracted into the abdominal cavity and rotates through an additional 180 degrees counterclockwise to produce the definitive configuration of the small and large intestines.

The hindgut gives rise to the distal one third of the **transverse colon**, the **descending** and **sigmoid colon**, and **rectum**. Just superior to the cloacal membrane, the primitive gut tube forms an expansion called the **cloaca**. During the 4th to 6th weeks, a coronal **urorectal septum** partitions the cloaca into the **urogenital sinus**, which will give rise to urogenital structures and a **dorsal anorectal canal**. The distal one third of the anorectal canal forms from an ectodermal invagination called the **anal pit**.

Between the 6th and 8th weeks, the lumen of the gut tube becomes solidly filled by epithelium, and then is gradually recanalized. During recanalization, mesodermal extensions project into the lumen and together with the overlying epithelium form

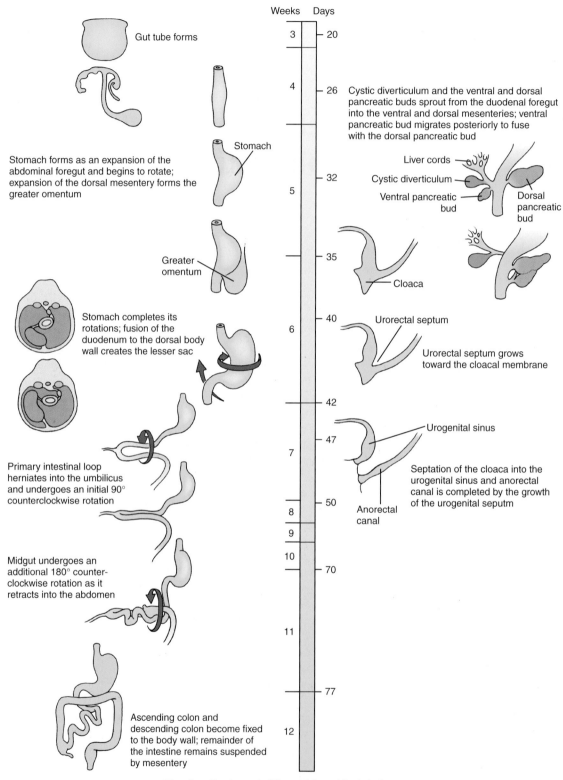

Time line. Development of the gut tube and its derivatives.

Gut tube forms

Stomach forms as an expansion of the abdominal foregut and begins to rotate; expansion of the dorsal mesentery forms the greater omentum

Stomach

Greater omentum

Stomach completes its rotations; fusion of the duodenum to the dorsal body wall creates the lesser sac

Primary intestinal loop herniates into the umbilicus and undergoes an initial 90° counterclockwise rotation

Midgut undergoes an additional 180° counter-clockwise rotation as it retracts into the abdomen

Ascending colon and descending colon become fixed to the body wall; remainder of the intestine remains suspended by mesentery

Weeks | Days
3 | 20
4 | 26
5 | 32
 | 35
6 | 40
 | 42
7 | 47
8 | 50
9 |
10 | 70
11 |
 | 77
12 |

Cystic diverticulum and the ventral and dorsal pancreatic buds sprout from the duodenal foregut into the ventral and dorsal mesenteries; ventral pancreatic bud migrates posteriorly to fuse with the dorsal pancreatic bud

Liver cords
Cystic diverticulum
Ventral pancreatic bud
Dorsal pancreatic bud

Cloaca

Urorectal septum

Urorectal septum grows toward the cloacal membrane

Urogenital sinus

Septation of the cloaca into the urogenital sinus and anorectal canal is completed by the growth of the urogenital seputm

Anorectal canal

the **villi** of the intestines. Cytodifferentiation of the gut epithelium depends on interactions with the underlying mesoderm and is regionally specified based on the cranial-caudal axis and radial axis (lumen to outer tunic) of the gut. Migrating neural crest cells form the **enteric nervous system.**

Clinical Taster A one-week-old infant male is seen in a community health clinic. His mother says that the boy has not been eating well for 48 hours and has been irritable, especially after feeds. Then, beginning last night, he started vomiting a dark greenish liquid consistent with bile. On examination, the infant cries inconsolably and is weak. His heart rate is elevated and his extremities are cool, symptoms of dehydration. His abdomen is somewhat distended. Sips of hydration fluid are returned with bilious vomit.

Intravenous hydration is begun and a nasogastric tube is placed to decompress the abdomen. The infant is transferred by ambulance to the children's hospital, where an upper gastrointestinal tract (upper GI) series is ordered (i.e., sequential X-rays done after ingestion of barium, a radio-opaque liquid used to coat the inside of the digestive system). This study shows markedly delayed gastric emptying and dilation of the duodenum with delayed filling of the jejunum. As the jejunum fills with barium, it takes on an "apple peel" appearance (Fig. 14-1). A subsequent X-ray shows partial filling of the small intestine, which lies predominantly in the right abdomen. The diagnosis of intestinal malrotation with intestinal obstruction is made, and emergency surgery is performed. In the operating room, the surgeons find a midgut volvulus (torsion of the small intestine) with ischemic bowel twisted around a narrow mesenteric pedicle. They untwist the bowel and return it to the abdomen. In 24 hours, they re-examine the bowel and remove a 20 cm necrotic portion. Later, the small intestines are reconnected and the bowel fixed in place so that twisting cannot reoccur.

Intestinal malrotation occurs when the midgut fails to complete its rotation during the 10th through 12th week of development as it returns to the peritoneal cavity from the umbilical herniation. This leaves the small intestine in the right side of the abdomen, tethered to the mesenteric vasculature by a narrowed mesentery. The small bowel can twist around this narrow tether, causing intestinal obstruction and cutting off its circulation, resulting in necrosis. This usually presents in infancy, but cases presenting as late as young adulthood have been reported. The cause of intestinal malrotation is unknown.

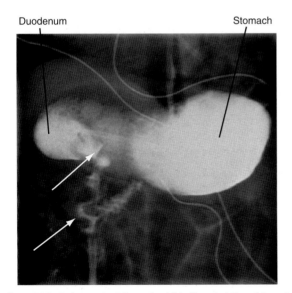

Duodenum · Stomach

Figure 14-1. Barium contrast X-ray of a child with malrotation of the gut, showing a dilated stomach and proximal duodenum, with a volvulus more distally. Note the delayed filling of the affected bowel (arrows).

Body Folding

As described in Chapter 4, the longitudinal and transverse folding of the embryo in the 3rd and 4th weeks converts the flat trilaminar embryonic disc into a trilaminar, elongated cylinder (Fig. 14-2). Because of cranial and caudal body folding, a cranial and caudal endodermal pocket forms (see Fig. 14-2*A-F*). As the cranial and caudal pockets elongate with lengthening of the embryo, the lateral body folds meet in the ventral midline and fuse to generate the elongated body cylinder (see Fig. 14-2*G-H*). The outer layer is the ectoderm (the future skin), which now covers the entire outer surface of the embryo except in the umbilical region, where the yolk sac and connecting stalk emerge. The innermost layer is the endodermal **primary gut tube.** Separating these two layers is a layer of mesoderm that contains the coelom. Thus, the three germ layers bear the same fundamental topologic relation

14

437

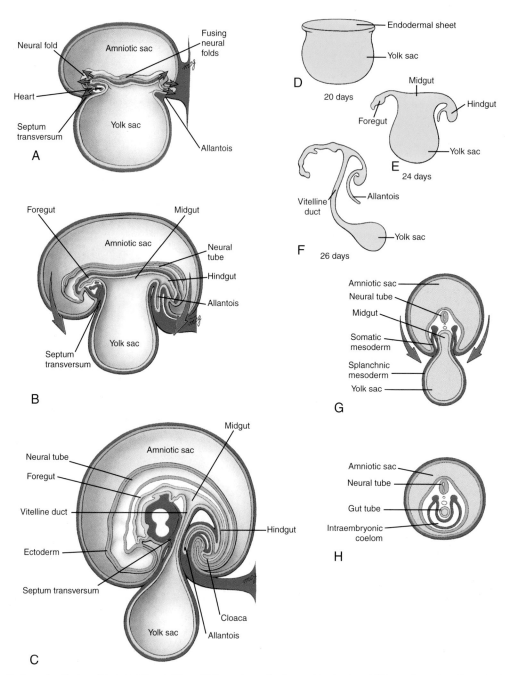

Figure 14-2. The foregut, midgut, and hindgut of the primitive gut tube are formed by the combined action of differential growth and lateral and craniocaudal folding, transforming the embryo from a flat disc to a three-dimensional vertebrate body form. As folding occurs, the embryo grows more rapidly than the yolk sac, the cavity of which remains continuous with the developing gut tube through the narrowing vitelline duct. The septum transversum forms cranial to the cardiogenic area in the germ disc (A), and is translocated to the future lower thoracic region through the folding of the cranial end of the embryo (B, C). The foregut and hindgut are blind-ending tubes that terminate at the oropharyngeal and cloacal membranes, respectively. The midgut is at first completely open to the cavity of the yolk sac (D, E). However, as folding proceeds, this connection is constricted to form the narrow vitelline duct (F). Fusion of the ectoderm, mesoderm, future coelomic cavities, and endoderm from opposite sides is prevented in the immediate vicinity of the vitelline duct (G), but not in the more cranial and caudal regions (H).

to each other after folding as they did in the flat embryonic disc.

Body folding plays an essential role in internalizing the endoderm, as mutations in genes involved in body folding (e.g., *Gata4*, *Sox17*, and *Furin/Spc1*) exhibit not only body folding defects but also endodermal tube defects. By the time body folding is nearly complete, the gut tube consists of cranial and caudal blind-ending tubes, the presumptive **foregut** and **hindgut**, and a central **midgut**, which still opens ventrally to the yolk sac. Cranially, the foregut terminates at the **oropharyngeal membrane** (or buccopharyngeal membrane); caudally, the hindgut terminates at the **cloacal membrane**. Because the embryo and gut tube lengthen relative to the yolk sac and folding continues to convert the open midgut into a tube, the neck of the yolk sac narrows until it becomes the slender vitelline duct. The **vitelline duct** and yolk sac are eventually incorporated into the umbilical cord. Table 14-1 lists the organs and structures that are ultimately derived from the three portions of the gut tube.

During the process of lateral body folding, the endodermal lining of the gut tube becomes surrounded by cells derived from lateral plate splanchnic mesoderm (see Fig. 14-2G-H). This mesoderm condenses and differentiates into the lamina propria, submucosa, muscular walls, vascular elements, and connective tissue of the gastrointestinal tract and organs. Once the basic gut tube regions are formed, various organs develop within specific regions that are delineated by restricted gene expression and tissue-tissue interactions.

Dorsal Mesentery Initially Suspends Abdominal Gut Tube

When the coelom first forms, the gut is broadly attached to the dorsal body wall by mesoderm (Fig. 14-3A). However, in the region of the future abdominal viscera (from the abdominal esophagus to the most proximal part of the future rectum), the mesenchyme within this region of attachment gradually disperses during the 4th week, resulting in formation of a thin,

Table 14-1 Derivatives of Primitive Gut Tube

Regions of Differentiated Gut Tube	Accessory Organs Derived from Gut Tube Endoderm
Foregut	
Pharynx	Pharyngeal pouch derivatives (see Ch. 16)
Thoracic esophagus	Lungs (see Ch. 11)
Abdominal esophagus	
Stomach	
Superior half of duodenum (superior to ampulla of pancreatic duct)	Liver parenchyma and hepatic duct epithelium Gallbladder, cystic duct, and common bile duct Dorsal and ventral pancreatic buds (exocrine cells, endocrine and pancreatic ductal cells)
Midgut	
Inferior half of duodenum	
Jejunum	
Ileum	
Cecum	
Appendix	
Ascending colon	
Right two thirds of transverse colon	
Hindgut	
Left one third of transverse colon	
Descending colon	
Sigmoid colon	
Rectum	Urogenital sinus and derivatives (see Ch. 15)

14

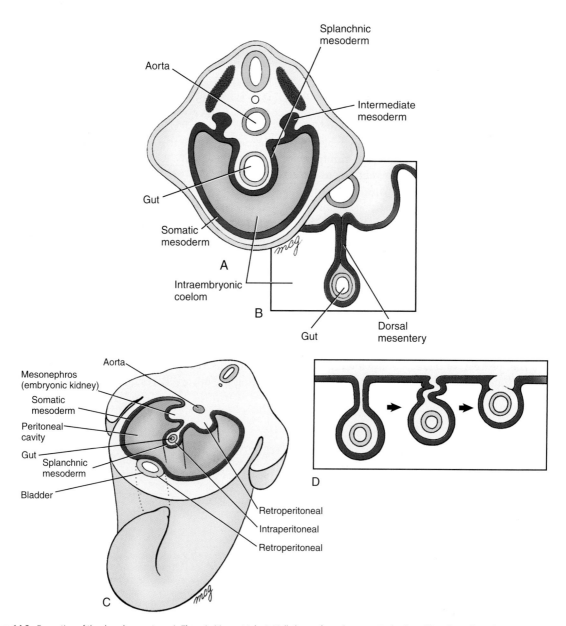

Figure 14-3. Formation of the dorsal mesentery. *A,* The primitive gut tube initially hangs from the posterior body wall by a broad bar of mesenchyme but, *B,* in regions inferior to the septum transversum this connection thins out to form a membranous dorsal mesentery composed of reflected peritoneum. *C,* Viscera suspended within the peritoneal cavity by a mesentery are called intraperitoneal, whereas organs embedded in the body wall and covered by peritoneum are called retroperitoneal. *D,* The mesentery suspending some intraperitoneal organs disappears as both mesentery and organ fuse with the body wall. These organs are then called secondarily retroperitoneal.

bilayered **dorsal mesentery** that suspends the abdominal viscera in the coelomic cavity (Fig. 14-3*B*). Because the abdominal gut tube and its derivatives are suspended in what will later become the **peritoneal cavity,** they are referred to as **intraperitoneal** viscera.

In contrast to the intraperitoneal location of most of the gut tube and its derivatives, some of the visceral organs develop within the body wall and are separated from the coelom by a covering of serous membrane (Fig. 14-3*C*). These organs are said to be **retroperitoneal.** It is important to realize that the designation retroperitoneal means that an organ is located behind the peritoneum from a viewpoint inside the peritoneal cavity—not that it is necessarily located in the *posterior* body wall. Thus, the kidneys are retroperitoneal, but so is the bladder, which develops in the anterior body wall (see Fig. 14-3C).

Further complicating the intraperitoneal/retroperitoneal distinction is that some parts of the gut tube that are initially suspended by mesentery later become fused to the body wall, thus taking on the appearance of retroperitoneal organs (Fig. 14-3D). These organs, which include the ascending and descending colon, duodenum, and pancreas, are said to be **secondarily retroperitoneal.**

At the end of the 4th week, almost the entire abdominal gut tube—the portion within the peritoneal cavity from the abdominal esophagus to the superior end of the developing cloaca—hangs suspended by the dorsal mesentery. Except in the region of the developing stomach, the coelomic cavities in the lateral plate mesoderm on either side of the embryonic disc coalesce during folding to form a single, continuous peritoneal cavity. In the stomach region, the gut tube remains connected to the ventral body wall by the thick septum transversum. By the 5th week, the caudal portion of the septum transversum thins to form the **ventral mesentery** connecting the stomach and developing liver to the ventral body wall (Fig. 14-4).

Three Regions of Primitive Gut

By convention, the boundaries of the foregut, midgut, and hindgut correspond to the territories of the three

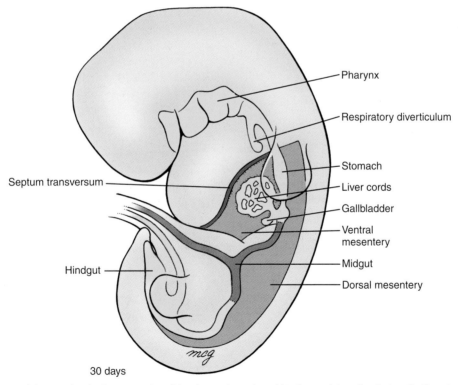

Figure 14-4. Structure of the gut tube. The foregut consists of the pharynx, located cranial to the respiratory diverticulum, the thoracic esophagus, and the abdominal foregut. The abdominal foregut forms the abdominal esophagus, stomach, and about half of the duodenum; it gives rise to the liver, gallbladder, pancreas, and their associated ducts. The midgut forms half of the duodenum, the jejunum and ileum, the ascending colon, and about two thirds of the transverse colon. The hindgut forms one third of the transverse colon, the descending colon, and sigmoid colon and the upper two thirds of the anorectal canal. The abdominal esophagus, stomach, and superior part of the duodenum are suspended by dorsal and ventral mesenteries; the abdominal gut tube excluding the rectum is suspended in the abdominal cavity by a dorsal mesentery only.

arteries that supply the abdominal gut tube. As described in Chapter 13, the gut tube and its derivatives are vascularized by unpaired ventral branches of the descending aorta. These branches develop by a process of consolidation and reduction from the left and right vitelline artery plexuses that arise on the yolk sac, spread to vascularize the gut tube, and anastomose with the dorsal aortae (see Fig. 13-19). About five definitive aortic branches supply the thoracic part of the foregut (the pharynx and thoracic esophagus; development of the pharyngeal part of the foregut is discussed in Ch. 16). Three arteries serve the remainder of the gut tube: the **celiac trunk**, which supplies the abdominal foregut (the abdominal esophagus, stomach, and cranial half of the duodenum and its derivatives); the **superior mesenteric trunk**, which supplies the midgut; and the **inferior mesenteric artery**, which supplies the hindgut. However, studies show that boundaries between the different endodermal segments along the cranial-caudal axis depend on patterns of segmental and homeotic gene expression within the gut that are established before the development of these vessels. For instance, during late-stage mouse gastrulation, *Lhx1 (Lim homeobox-1)*, *Otx1 (Orthodenticle homolog-1)*, *Hesx1 (Homeobox expressed in ES cells-1)*, and *Cerl (Cerebus-like)* are expressed within the cranial definitive endoderm, whereas *Cdx2 (Caudal-type homeobox-1)* expression demarcates the caudal endoderm well before these blood vessels are visible.

IN THE RESEARCH LAB

REGIONALIZATION OF GUT TUBE DEMARCATES SITES OF ORGAN FORMATION

Regionalization of the gut plays an important role in demarcating sites of organ formation. Regional specification of endoderm and its interaction with mesoderm, neural crest cells, and ectoderm play important roles in mediating the development of the pharyngeal arches, pharyngeal vasculature, and organ formation in the cranial region (discussed in Chs. 13 and 16). The following discussion is limited to gastrointestinal development caudal to the pharyngeal arches. Unfortunately, much less is known regarding the patterning of the endoderm of the caudal gastrointestinal tract than that of the pharyngeal region.

How does the early endoderm obtain its cranial-caudal identity? Less is known regarding the regionalization of the early endoderm than is known regarding that of the ectoderm and mesoderm. The ectoderm and mesoderm acquire much of their regional identity during gastrulation through a variety of signaling molecules derived from the primitive streak and organizer (primitive node in humans) (discussed in Ch. 3). These signaling molecules are also likely to be involved in the regionalization of the endoderm. One of the earliest known markers delineating regional differences of the definitive endoderm was discovered from work in Drosophila where the gene *Caudal* was identified and found to be required for gut formation. *Caudal* homologs in vertebrates include *Cdx1*, *Cdx2*, and *Cdx3*. In vertebrates, *Cdx2* is expressed in the caudal endoderm and mesoderm of primitive streak–stage embryos before the expression of most *Hox* genes. Mice null for the *Cdx2* gene die during gastrulation due to anomalies in the extraembryonic tissues; mice haplodeficient for *Cdx2* (i.e., heterozygous mice having one mutant and one wild-type copy of *Cdx2*) exhibit lesions within the colon segment resembling ectopic stomach and small intestinal tissue. Other genes important in early gut regionalization include *Shh*, *Fgfs*, *Bmps*, *Pdx1*, *Pax*, and various *Hox* genes that are discussed later in this section. *Wnt* signaling has also been implicated in early hindgut specification, as mice null for the *Wnt* downstream targets *Tcf4* and *Tcf1* exhibit severe caudal truncations.

As indicated above, the process of regionalizing the gut tube into foregut, midgut, and hindgut is likely initiated by events occurring during gastrulation. However, regionalization of the endoderm is refined by tissue-tissue interactions between the germ layers. The overlying ectoderm and mesoderm provide not only permissive influences but also inductive influences on the endoderm. For instance, in vitro, mouse cranial endoderm in presomitic embryos can be respecified to express caudal endodermal markers through interactions with caudal mesoderm. However, by the early somitic stage, the endoderm is more restricted in its developmental potential. Several transcription factors and morphogens involved in refining the regionalization of the gut have been identified, some of which are illustrated in Figures 14-5 and 14-6.

After initiation of cranial body folding, the endoderm of the ventral foregut is situated adjacent to the caudal cardiogenic mesoderm. In the chick embryo, this cardiogenic mesoderm induces the foregut endoderm to begin expressing hepatic markers (*Albumin* and *Alpha fetoprotein*). In the nonhepatic dorsal foregut endoderm, the expression of hepatic markers is repressed by the overlying dorsal mesoderm and ectoderm. By binding to *Fgfr1* and *Fgfr4* of endodermal cells, *Fgf2* from the cardiogenic mesoderm represses the expression of *Ipf1* (*insulin promoter factor 1*, a marker of pancreas), turns on *Shh* expression (a repressor of pancreas development), and induces expression of hepatic markers. Thus, interactions between mesoderm and

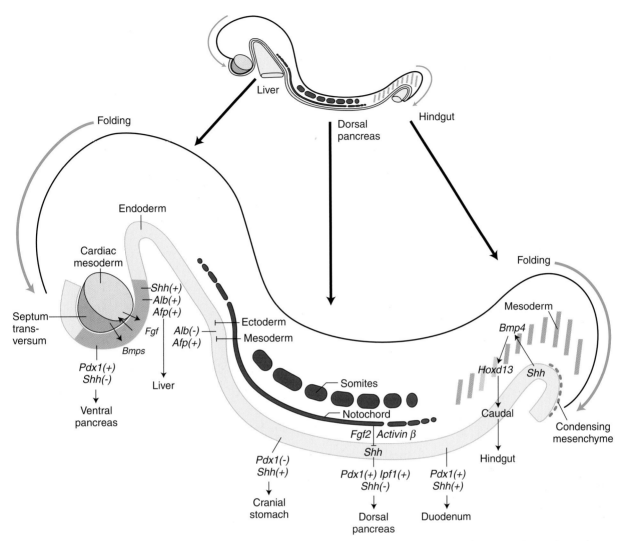

Figure 14-5. Signals and transcription factors important in establishing regional differences in the early developing gastrointestinal tract. The top drawing represents an early mammalian embryo shortly after the initiation of embryonic folding, with areas enlarged below showing some of the signaling events involved in liver, pancreas, and hindgut specification. After initiation of cranial body folding, the endoderm of the ventral foregut is situated adjacent to the caudal cardiogenic mesoderm and septum transversum. Tissue-tissue interactions between the cardiogenic mesoderm and the endoderm, mediated by *Fgf* and *Bmp* signals, induce hepatocytic markers within the endoderm (e.g., *Albumin* and *Alpha fetoprotein*) while suppressing pancreatic development by upregulating *Shh* expression. The homeoprotein pancreatic/duodenal marker, *Pdx1*, promotes pancreatic development. However, in the presence of *Shh*, pancreatic development is repressed. Much of the endoderm expresses *Shh*, but it is repressed by notochordal release of *Fgf 2* and *Activin B* in the future pancreatic region. *Shh* expression within the hindgut endoderm induces *Bmp4* and *Hoxd13* expression within the caudal mesoderm. *Shh/Bmp4* are only capable of inducing *Hoxd13* expression in the caudal gut, possibly due to the caudal restriction of *Cdx2* expression established during gastrulation. *Hoxd13* instills a caudal identity to the hindgut. *Alb, Albumin; Afp, Alpha fetoprotein; Ipf1, insulin promoter factor 1.*

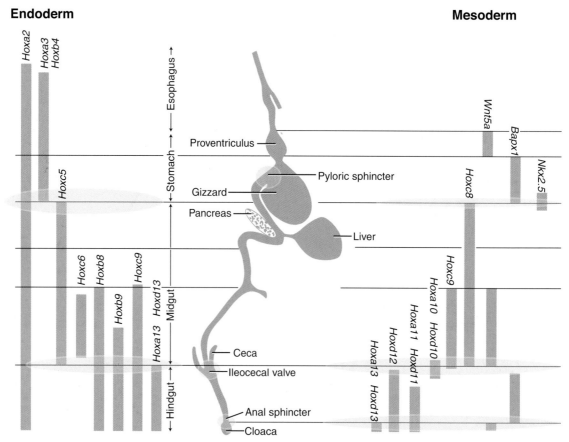

Figure 14-6. *Hox* gene expression boundaries in the endoderm and mesoderm during early chick gut development. Specific combinations of homeobox gene expression can be mapped to specific regions of the gastrointestinal tract, with some combinations demarcating the position of sphincters and organs. The regional expression patterns of mouse homologs are similar.

endoderm play crucial roles in dictating regional organ development.

The endoderm of the forgut and midgut forms many sections of the gastrointestinal tract including the esophagus, stomach, pancreas, and duodenum. The pancreatic-promoting transcription factor, *Pdx1* (*Pancreas and duodenal homeobox gene 1*), is expressed in the early stomach, and in the dorsal and ventral prepancreatic and preduodenal endoderm (see Fig. 14-5). *Shh* is expressed along the entire length of these endodermal regions until day 10.5 of development, except at the site of pancreatic bud formation. Perturbation of *Shh* signaling within the *Pdx1*-expressing endoderm results in the ectopic expression of *Insulin* in the stomach and duodenun, suggesting that *Shh* normally represses expression of pancreatic cell fate in all *Pdx1*-positive endoderm.

This endoderm is in contact with the notochord until the fusion of the two dorsal aortae within the midline intervenes.

An interaction between the notochord and endoderm is required for proper pancreatic development: for example, removal of the notochord in chick embryos results in loss of pancreatic markers. Additional studies in several species show that the notochord specifically represses the expression of *Shh* in the prepancreatic endoderm, thereby removing the repressive effect of *Shh* on *Pdx1* (see Fig. 14-5). The notochord represses *Shh* expression specifically at the prepancreatic level by releasing *Fgf2* and *Activin B*, both of which inhibit endodermal *Shh* expression, thereby promoting pancreatic development (i.e., by removing the repression of *Shh* on *Pdx1*, which when expressed promotes pancreas development). Although coculturing pancreatic endoderm with notochord results in expression of pancreatic markers in prepancreatic endoderm, this does not hold true when notochord is cocultured with nonpancreatic endoderm, suggesting that the notochord provides a permissive environment (i.e., by reducing *Shh* levels) rather than inducing pancreatic development.

The subsequent separation of the notochord from the pancreatic endoderm by the fusing dorsal aortae also places the pancreatic endoderm under the influence of endothelial cells. Recent in vivo and in vitro studies in *Xenopus* and mice suggest that dorsal aortic endothelial cells also influence pancreatic cell fate specification.

Hox genes are also expressed within gut endoderm and play important roles in regional specification and development of the gut (see Figs. 14-5, 14-6). In the chick, *Hoxa* gene expression is regionally restricted, demarcating boundaries of the midgut and hindgut, with *Hoxd13* expression being limited to the caudal-most hindgut mesoderm. Interactions between the hindgut endoderm and mesoderm seem to be responsible for restricting *Hoxd13* expression. *Hoxd13* instills caudal identity to the hindgut, because when missexpressed in more cranial mesoderm of chick embryos, the stomach endoderm is transformed into intestinal endoderm. *Hox* genes also play major roles in demarcating regions of the gastrointestinal tract, particularly specifying sites of sphincter formation that separate the gut segments (see Fig. 14-6). Mice null for both *Hoxa13* and *Hoxd13* have severe muscular defects in the anal sphincter, and mice null for both *Hoxd4* and *Hoxd13* lack ileocecal sphincters and form abnormal pyloric and anal sphincters.

Development of Abdominal Foregut

Formation and Rotation of Stomach

The stomach first becomes apparent during the early part of the 4th week, as the foregut just caudal to the septum transversum expands slightly. On about day 26, the thoracic foregut begins to elongate rapidly. Over the next 2 days, the presumptive stomach, now much farther removed from the lung buds, expands further into a fusiform (Latin, "spindle-shaped") structure that is readily distinguished from the adjacent regions of the gut tube (Fig. 14-7). During the 5th week, the dorsal wall of the stomach grows faster than the ventral wall, resulting in the formation of the **greater curvature of the stomach.** Concurrently, deformation of the ventral stomach wall forms the **lesser curvature of the stomach.** By the end of the 7th week, the continual differential expansion of the superior part of the greater curvature results in the formation of the **fundus** and **cardiac incisure**.

During the 7th and 8th weeks, the developing stomach undergoes a 90-degree rotation around its craniocaudal axis so that the greater curvature lies to the left and the lesser curvature lies to the right (see Fig. 14-7D). As shown in Figure 14-7E differential thinning of the right side of the **dorsal mesogastrium** (the portion of the dorsal mesentery attached to the stomach) is thought to play a role in this rotation. The right and left vagus plexuses, which originally run through the mesoderm on either side of the gut tube, thus rotate to become posterior (dorsal) and anterior (ventral) vagal trunks in the region of the stomach. However, fibers of the left and right vagal plexuses mix to some degree, so that the more caudal anterior and posterior vagal trunks contain fibers from each of these more cranial plexuses. The stomach also rotates slightly around a ventrodorsal axis so that the greater curvature faces slightly caudally, and the lesser curvature slightly cranially (see Fig. 14-7D).

The rotations of the stomach bend the presumptive duodenum into a C shape and displace it to the right until it lies against the dorsal body wall, to which it adheres, thus becoming secondarily retroperitoneal. The rotation of the stomach and the fusion of the duodenum create an alcove dorsal to the stomach called the **lesser sac of the peritoneal cavity** (see Fig. 14-8). The rest of the peritoneal cavity is now called the **greater sac.** The lesser sac enlarges because of progressive expansion of the dorsal mesogastrium connecting the stomach to the posterior body wall. The resulting large, suspended fold of mesogastrium, called the **greater omentum**, hangs from the dorsal body wall and the greater curvature of the stomach and drapes over more inferior organs of the abdominal cavity (see Fig. 14-8C). The portion of the lesser sac directly dorsal to the stomach is now called the **upper recess of the lesser sac**, and the cavity within the greater omentum is called the **lower recess of the lesser sac.** The lower recess is obliterated during fetal life as the anterior and posterior folds of the greater omentum fuse together.

14

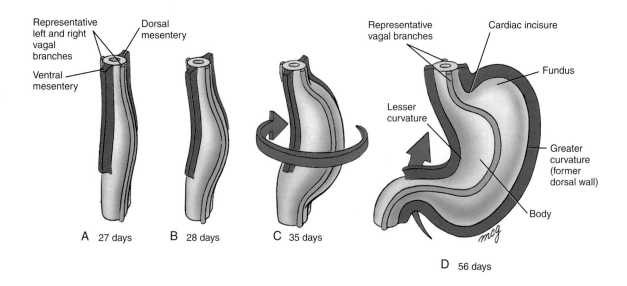

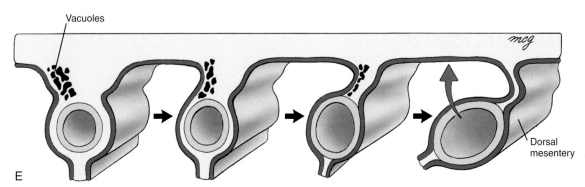

Figure 14-7. Rotations of the stomach. *A-C,* Oblique frontal views. *D,* Direct frontal view. The posterior wall of the stomach expands during the 4th and 5th weeks to form the greater curvature. During the 7th week, the stomach rotates clockwise on its longitudinal axis (when viewed from above). *E,* The rotation of the stomach around its longitudinal axis commences with vacuolization of the right side of the thick mesenchymal bar that initially suspends the stomach from the posterior body wall. Curved arrows indicate directions of movements; straight arrows (*E*) indicate a series of changes over time.

Development of Liver and Gallbladder

On about day 22, a small endodermal thickening, the **hepatic plate**, forms on the ventral side of the duodenum. Over the next few days, cells in this plate proliferate and form the **hepatic diverticulum**, which grows into mesenchymal cells that will give rise to the inferior region of the septum transversum (Fig. 14-9). The hepatic diverticulum gives rise to ramifying cords of **hepatoblasts** (the liver primordial cells). Hepatoblasts express several genes that are specific to hepatocytes, but hepatoblasts are cytologically undifferentiated at this stage. Under the influence of *Notch* signaling and other regulatory proteins (discussed in the following "In the Research Lab"), hepatoblasts become **hepatocytes** (parenchyma), **bile canaliculi** of the liver, or **hepatic ducts.** In contrast, the mesoblastic **supporting stroma** of the liver develops from the septum transversum and splanchnic mesoderm originating near the stomach, as well as from endothelial precursor cells (that develop into the **sinusoidal endothelium** of the liver) of unknown origin. Cardiogenic mesoderm,

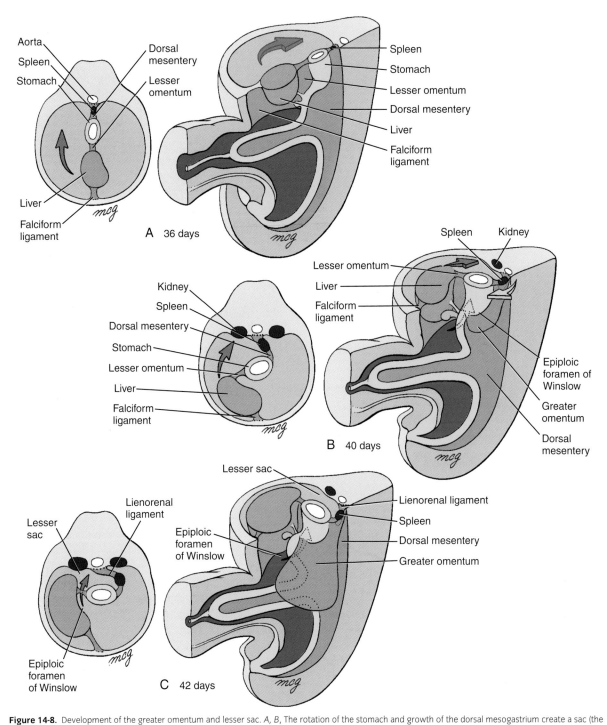

Figure 14-8. Development of the greater omentum and lesser sac. *A, B,* The rotation of the stomach and growth of the dorsal mesogastrium create a sac (the greater omentum) that dangles from the greater curvature of the stomach. *B, C,* When the duodenum swings to the right, it becomes secondarily fused to the body wall, enclosing the space posterior to the stomach and within the expanding cavity of the greater omentum. This space is the lesser sac of the peritoneal cavity. The remainder of the peritoneal cavity is now called the greater sac. The principal passageway between the greater and lesser sacs is the epiploic foramen of Winslow. Curved arrows indicate directions of movements.

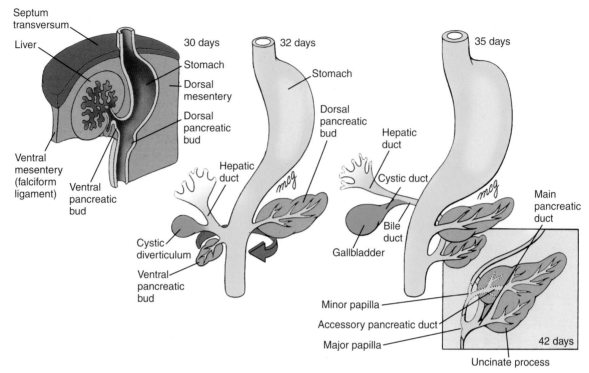

Figure 14-9. Development of the liver, gallbladder, pancreas, and their duct systems from endodermal diverticula of the duodenum. The liver bud sprouts during the 4th week and expands in the ventral (anterior) mesentery. The cystic diverticulum and ventral pancreatic bud also grow into the ventral mesentery, whereas the dorsal pancreatic bud grows into the dorsal mesentery. During the 5th week, the ventral pancreatic bud migrates around the posterior side (former right side) of the duodenum to fuse with the dorsal pancreatic bud. The main duct of the ventral bud ultimately becomes the major pancreatic duct, which drains the entire pancreas.

endothelium, and the septum transversum mesenchymal cells emit growth factor signals (including *Vegfs*, *Bmps*, and *Fgfs*) that are required for liver parenchymal development (discussed in the following "In the Research Lab").

As discussed in Chapter 13, the liver is a major early **hematopoietic organ** of the embryo. Hematopoietic stem cells originating from the yolk sac wall (and later from the aortic, gonad, and mesonephric region) colonize the embryonic liver, expand their numbers, and diversify before populating other hematopoietic organs. Hepatic progenitors along with the hepatic stromal cells generate a hematopoietic microenvironment necessary for adult-type hematopoiesis. As the hematopoietic function is shifted to the peripheral organs, hepatocytes begin upregulating the expression of numerous genes related to mature liver function (e.g., those associated with amino acid metabolism and detoxification). Throughout embryonic and

fetal development, hepatocytes proliferate (mainly mediated by autocrine mechanisms). This proliferation gradually slows and is arrested with postnatal development. From then on, migration and proliferation of hepatocytes requires extraneous growth factors including *Egf* and *Hepatocyte growth factor* (*Hgf*).

By day 26, a distinct endodermal thickening forms on the ventral side of the duodenum just caudal to the base of the hepatic diverticulum and buds into the ventral mesentery (see Fig. 14-9). This **cystic diverticulum** will form the **gallbladder** and **cystic duct.** No sooner does the cystic diverticulum form than cells at the junction of the hepatic and cystic ducts proliferate and form the **common bile duct.** As a result, the developing cystic duct is carried away from the duodenum. The gallbladder and cystic duct develop from histologically distinct populations of duodenal cells.

IN THE RESEARCH LAB

HEPATOBLAST SPECIFICATION AND FATE

As discussed earlier in the chapter, cardiogenic mesoderm plays a significant role in specifying liver formation and hepatic gene expression within the foregut endoderm (see Fig. 14-5). However, additional signals promoting liver formation originate from the mesoderm of the septum transversum. As discussed in earlier chapters, *Bmp* signaling has major role in the development of lateral plate mesoderm and this is true for the liver as well. *Bmp4* is expressed in the septum transversum (see Fig. 14-5); in mice lacking *Bmp4*, the liver bud fails to grow or express *Albumin*. As discussed earlier in the chapter, *Fgfs* from the adjacent cardiogenic region stimulate *Albumin* expression in the endodermal liver primordia. In explant cultures of the liver primordia, *Noggin* (an antagonist of *Bmps*) inhibits this *Fgf*-induced *Albumin* expression. Although *Bmps* alone are insufficient to induce hepatic development, blocking *Bmp* signaling with *Noggin* increases the expression of the pancreatic marker *Pdx1* in this endoderm. Therefore, *Bmps* may contribute to *Fgf*-mediated endodermal patterning by promoting the liver phenotype and repressing the pancreatic phenotype. What downstream targets are invoked by *Fgfs* and *Bmps* to induce hepatoblast lineage and growth are unclear but may include *Gata4*, *Hnf3* (Hepatic nuclear factor-3), and *C/EBP* (CAAT-enhancer binding proteins).

Wnt signaling has also been implicated in liver development and is required for bile duct lineage specification in mice. Zebrafish with mutations in the gene *Prt*, exhibit defective hepatic specification and lack expression of hepatic markers. This gene encodes a *Wnt2b* homolog, called *Wnt2bb*, that is expressed within the lateral plate mesoderm involved in liver development in the zebrafish. In mice, the *Wnt2bb* homolog is *Wnt13*. *Wnt13* is expressed immediately adjacent the cardiogenic mesoderm of the foregut. In mice and Xenopus, the *secreted Frizzled-related protein 5* gene (a *Wnt* inhibitor) is also expressed in the nascent liver primordia. Because of the importance of the *Wnt* family in mediating cell proliferation and specification in other developing organ systems, it has been suggested that spatial and temporal waves of *Wnt* signaling and inhibition may be necessary for proper endodermal patterning of liver primordia.

Much more needs to be learned regarding the cell fate decision of hepatoblasts as to whether they take on a hepatocytic or bile-ductal cell fate. A number of factors have been implicated in mediating cell determination of these two lineages. Like the segregation of neuronal and glial precursor cells from the neuroepithelium (discussed in Ch. 9),

Notch signaling seems to have a role in mediating the decision as to whether a hepatoblast becomes a hepatocyte or bile duct lining cell (**cholangiocytes**). As discussed in Chapters 3, 5, 12, and 13, mutations in the *NOTCH* ligand *JAGGED1* (or in the receptor *NOTCH2*) are associated with autosomal dominant **Alagille syndrome.** These patients exhibit a paucity of bile ducts. Double heterozygotic mice for a *Jagged1* and *Notch2* null mutation lack intrahepatic bile ducts at birth and mimic Alagille syndrome. Recent studies in mice also show that *Jagged1* is expressed in cells adjacent to *Notch2*-positive epithelium at the site of biliary differentiation, and that *Notch2* represses the hepatocyte lineage. Hence, *Jagged1/Notch2* interactions likely have critical roles in hepatocytes/cholangiocyte determination.

A major change in liver functions occurs near birth as the burden of hematopoiesis is shifted away from the liver, and the liver begins taking on the metabolic and detoxifying burdens. One group of transcription factors important in mediating these functions is the *Hepatic nuclear factor (Hnf)* family. *Hnfs* activate specific liver genes. Mice with the *Hnf4α* gene deleted from the liver primordium using a cre-lox system (discussed in Ch. 5) develop small livers that lack organized epithelia and fail to express almost all liver-specific genes. However, forced expression of *Hnf4α* in fibroblast cultures does not induce liver-specific gene expression even though the fibroblasts take on an epithelial-like morphology. This suggests other cell lineage–determining factors must be in place before *Hnfs* can initiate liver-specific gene expression

Another transcription factor that activates several liver genes and is involved in the functional change to mature liver function is *C/EBPα* (*C/EBP* is discussed earlier in this section). *C/EBPα*-deficient mice die at birth because of hypoglycemia. Although the liver tissue appears normal, hepatocytes are deficient in their ability to store glycogen and lipids. Other molecules implicated in late fetal liver maturation are *Oncostatin M* and *Glucocorticoids*. *Oncostatin M* stimulates the expression of hepatic differentiation markers, promotes liver-like morphology, and induces liver-specific gene expression in liver progenitor explant cultures. Glucocorticoids alone are capable of inducing most of the cellular responses typical of the liver differentiation promoted by *Oncostatin M*, suggesting that they work together to promote liver maturation. Other factors involved in liver maturation likely include *Hgf* (upregulated on hepatic injury and hepatic regeneration) and *Tgfβ* (which may inhibit hepatocyte proliferation and promote differentiation).

The liver is unique in that, in the adult, mature hepatocytes can regenerate the liver if it is partially removed.

14

This regeneration is thought to be the result of proliferation of mature hepatocytes rather than of proliferation of hepatic progenitor cells. Embryologically, hepatocytes and bile ductal cells are thought to arise from common precursor, the **hepatoblast**. Stem cell isolation and characterization studies performed using fetal mouse livers show a single **hepatic stem cell** forms both hepatocytes and cholangiocytes. In culture, these stem cells can generate canaliculi-like and bile duct–like structures. Moreover, when transplanted into adult mice, they can differentiate into liver parenchymal cells. Whether adult livers in mice or humans contain hepatoblast stems cells is unknown.

Development of Pancreas

On day 26, another duodenal bud begins to grow into the dorsal mesentery just opposite the hepatic diverticulum. This endodermal diverticulum is the **dorsal pancreatic bud** (Fig. 14-10, see Fig. 14-9). Over the next few days, as the dorsal pancreatic bud elongates into the dorsal mesentery, another endodermal diverticulum, the **ventral pancreatic bud**, sprouts into the ventral mesentery just caudal to the developing gallbladder (see Figs. 14-9, 14-10). By day 32, the main duct of the ventral pancreatic bud becomes connected to the proximal end of the common bile duct.

Once specified, the pancreatic endoderm thickens, forming a multilayered solid bud within the duodenal portion of the gastrointestinal tract that continues to proliferate into the closely apposed mesoderm. The branching of this bud occurs differently from the classic branching of other organs such as the developing lung (Fig. 14-11*A*). Rather than expanding and folding the epithelium, epithelial clusters form, followed by the appearance of intraepithelial microlumens. These soon coalesce to generate continuous lumens, forming an epithelial tree draining exocrine products into the duodenum (see Fig. 14-11*B*). The **pancreatic exocrine cells** that produce digestive enzymes, the **pancreatic ductal cells** that transport the digestive enzymes, and the **pancreatic endocrine cells** in the **islets of Langerhans** that produce insulin, glucagon, and somatostatin all differentiate from the endoderm of the pancreatic buds. As the endocrine cell lineage proliferates within the endodermal epithelium, these cells delaminate and subsequently aggregate into islets, where they continue to proliferate throughout the embryonic period. Although several transcriptional factors and signaling molecules have been identified leading to the specification of exocrine and endocrine cell lineages, virtually nothing is known regarding the cellular mechanisms responsible for allocating endodermal cells to a ductal lineage.

Interactions with the mesoderm play an essential role in growth and differentiation of the pancreas, and the expression of several growth-promoting transcription factors expressed within the mesoderm are important in this. *Isl1 (Insulin gene enhancer protein-1)* is expressed by mesoderm surrounding the dorsal pancreatic bud. If *Isl1* is knocked out in mice, pancreatic mesenchyme is almost completely lost, and the expression of the pancreatic marker *Pdx1* is greatly reduced. *Fgf10* is also expressed in pancreatic mesoderm and *Fgf10* knockout mice have hypoplastic dorsal and

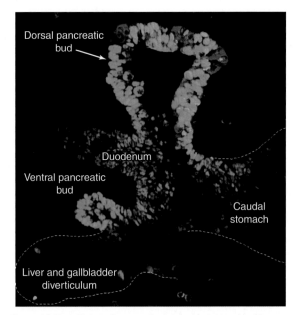

Figure 14-10. Initiation of pancreatic development in a day 10 mouse embryo. Pancreatic development begins with the formation of endodermal buds projecting into the splanchnic mesoderm near the stomach-duodenal border. *Pdx1* is expressed (seen here by immunostaining in green) in both the dorsal and ventral pancreatic bud endoderm. *Glucagon*-positive cells are also detected at this early stage (cells in red) within the pancreatic endodermal buds.

A Epithelial branching

B Microlumen fusion

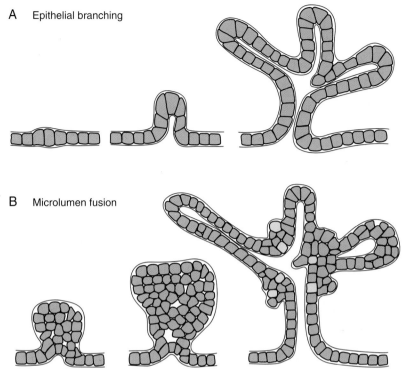

Figure 14-11. Diagrammatic representation of basic branching mechanisms for the formation of tubular glands. *A,* Classic branching mechanism whereby the expanding epithelium is thrown into epithelial folds. *B,* Branching mechanism whereby a proliferating single-layered epithelium is converted into multiple layers and becomes stratified. This is followed by the formation of microlumens that coalesce within the epithelium to form branched lumens. The formation of an endocrine cell lineage within the epithelium is indicated in yellow.

ventral pancreatic buds. Mice lacking *Pbx1 (Pre-B-cell leukemia transcription factor-1)*, another transcriptional marker for pancreatic endoderm, exhibit severe hypoplasia of dorsal pancreas and loss of acinar development. However, this defect can be rescued in culture by wild-type mesoderm.

While the common bile duct and ventral pancreatic bud are branching, proliferating, and differentiating, the mouth of the common bile duct and ventral pancreatic bud migrate posteriorly around the duodenum toward the dorsal mesentery (see Fig. 14-9). By the early 6th week, the ventral and dorsal pancreatic buds lie adjacent in the plane of the dorsal mesentery. Late in the 6th week, the two pancreatic buds fuse to form the definitive pancreas. The dorsal pancreatic bud gives rise to the **head, body**, and **tail** of the pancreas, whereas the ventral pancreatic bud gives rise to

the hook-like **uncinate process.** Like the duodenum, the pancreas fuses to the dorsal body wall and becomes secondarily retroperitoneal.

When the ventral and dorsal pancreatic buds fuse, their ductal systems also become interconnected (see Fig. 14-9). The proximal end of the duct connecting the dorsal bud to the duodenum usually degenerates, leaving the ventral pancreatic duct, now called the **main pancreatic duct**, as the only conduit for the dorsal pancreas into the duodenum. The main pancreatic duct and the common bile duct meet and empty their secretions into the duodenum at the **major duodenal papilla** or **ampulla of Vater.** In some individuals, the proximal dorsal pancreatic duct persists as an **accessory pancreatic duct** that empties into the duodenum at a **minor duodenal papilla** (see Fig. 14-9).

14

IN THE CLINIC

ABNORMAL FORMATION AND ROTATION OF VENTRAL PANCREAS

Occasionally, the pancreas forms a complete ring encircling the duodenum, a condition known as **annular pancreas**. As shown in Figure 14-12, this abnormality probably arises when the two lobes of a bilobed ventral pancreatic bud (a normal variation) migrate in opposite directions around the duodenum to fuse with the dorsal pancreatic bud. An annular pancreas compresses the duodenum and may cause gastrointestinal obstruction **(duodenal stenosis)**. Interestingly, *Indian hedgehog* null mice have an overgrowth of the ventral pancreas and develop an annular pancreas. *Hedgehog* signaling may restrict pancreatic size, as *Shh* null mice exhibit large increases in pancreatic size (and annular pancreas in some genetic backgrounds). *Shh* null mice also display gut malrotations and imperforate anus, defects seen with annular pancreas in humans. Studies are in progress examining what potential role *Hedgehog* signaling may have in the development of diabetes mellitus, pancreatitis, and pancreatic cancer.

IN THE RESEARCH LAB

NOTCH SIGNALING AND PANCREATIC CELL LINEAGE DETERMINATION

With the expansion and branching of the pancreatic buds, the pancreatic epithelium consists of convoluted sheets of epithelium that uniformly expresses *Pdx1*. From this epithelium arise exocrine cells and endocrine cells. As in hepatic cell specification (discussed in an earlier "In the Research Lab" in this chapter), *Notch* signaling also plays an important role in mediating pancreatic cell specification, determining which cells activate the endocrine lineage within the pancreatic epithelium. One downstream target of *Notch* signaling in the pancreatic endoderm is *Hes1* (*Hairy and enhancer-of-split-like-1*). This transcription factor downregulates the proendocrine bHLH transcription factor *Neurogenin-3* (*Ngn3*), a member of *Neurogenin/NeuroD* family (Fig. 14-13). *Ngn3* is transiently expressed within scattered cells of the pancreatic endoderm during the budding stage and later in early *Glucagon*-positive cells. Mice lacking *Ngn3* not only fail to develop pancreatic endocrine cells but also lack intestinal enteroendocrine cells and gastric endocrine cells. Moreover, *Pdx1* promoter-driven *Ngn3* expression in mice generates massive amounts of *Glucagon*-secreting endocrine cells in the gut. In the

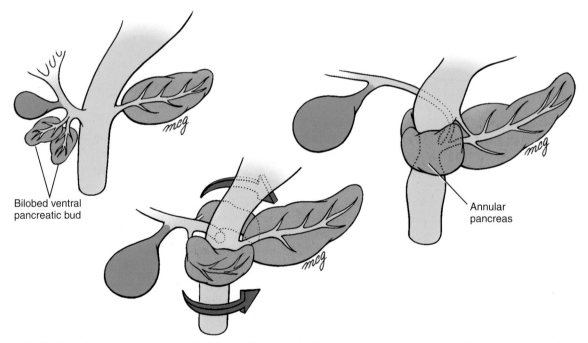

Figure 14-12. The ventral pancreas may consist of two lobes. If the lobes migrate around the duodenum in opposite directions to fuse with the dorsal pancreatic bud, an annular pancreas is formed.

Bilobed ventral pancreatic bud

Annular pancreas

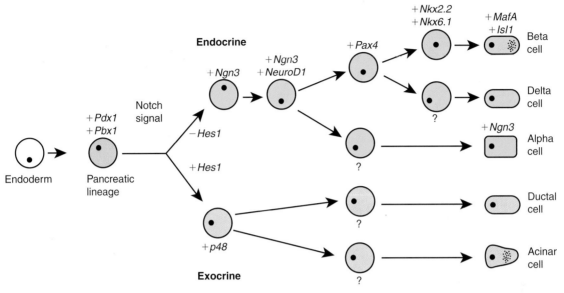

Figure 14-13. Illustration showing our basic understanding of the transcription factors expressed along various steps in the cell lineage pathway responsible for specifying various cell types derived from pancreatic endoderm.

chick, ectopic *Ngn3* expression induces the formation of *Glucagon-* and *Insulin*-secreting cells within endoderm outside the pancreatic endoderm. Finally, introducing the expression of *Ngn3* in cultured human pancreatic ductal cells induces endocrine marker expression. Hence, *Ngn3* is a proendocrine transcription factor that, in the absence of *Notch* signaling, is sufficient to initiate the endocrine pathway in pancreatic epithelium.

Cells in which *Ngn3* expression is repressed by *Notch* signaling (i.e., via expression of *Hes1*) become part of the *exocrine* pancreas. Other members of the bHLH family, particularly the *p48* subunit of the *Ptf1a (Pancreas specific transcription factor-1a)* complex, are thought to drive the differentiation of the exocrine pancreas (see Fig. 14-13). Mice lacking *p48* do not develop acini or ductal epithelia, whereas pancreatic islets still form within the adjacent mesenchyme. What controls *p48* expression in the pancreatic primordia is still unclear.

Glucagon-synthesizing cells are the first endocrine cells to form within the endoderm, appearing early in the pancreatic bud stage (see Fig. 14-10). For a long time, it was thought these cells were the precursors of both **alpha cells** (*Glucagon* producing) and **beta cells** (*Insulin* producing). However, recent experiments in mice using the cre-lox silencing elements for the *Glucagon* hormone allele and for the *Insulin* allele show that both alpha and beta cell lines

develop independently. Whereas *Ngn3* seems to preferentially drive alpha cell specification of the endoderm, studies suggest *Nkx2.2* and *Nkx6.1* act downstream with *Ngn3* to promote beta cell specification (see Fig. 14-13). Knockout mice for *Nkx2.2* generate equal numbers of endocrine precursor cells as compared to their wild-type littermates but fail to activate the *Insulin* gene, suggesting they have a deficiency in beta-cell differentiation. Moreover, these endocrine precursors no longer express *Nkx6.1*. Knockout mice for *Nkx6.1*, a transcription factor specifically expressed in adult beta-islet cells, generate small numbers of *Insulin*-producing cells but fail to maintain or increase their numbers during subsequent development. *Pax4* knockout mice have a complete lack of both beta and delta cell types and develop diabetes at birth, suggesting that *Pax4* works downstream of *Ngn3* but upstream of *Nkx2.2* and *Nkx6.1*. However, recent evidence shows that activating *Notch* signaling in *Pax4*-positive progenitor cells can redirect early endocrine progenitors toward a ductal fate, suggesting that early pancreatic endocrine cells maintain a degree of developmental plasticity.

NeuroD1, a transcription fact or whose expression closely follows *Ngn3* expression and can be activated by *Ngn3*, is expressed in all endocrine cells of pancreas after their specification and differentiation. *NeuroD1* plays an important role in mediating the expression of differentiated endocrine

14

products of the islet (e.g., *Insulin*). Mice lacking the *NeuroD1* gene develop the normal complement of islet cell types but the beta cell number is gradually reduced by apoptosis. Mutations in *NEUROD1* in humans are associated with **maturity-onset diabetes of the young**, where the β-cells become insensitive to blood glucose levels and/or are unable to synthesize adequate amounts of *Insulin*. Mutations in *NEUROD1* are also associated with human **type II diabetes**. Another transcription factor that may be involved in beta cell specification is *MafA (v-Maf Musculoaponeurotic fibrosarcoma oncogene homolog A)*. *MafA* expression in the early pancreas is limited to beta cells, is a strong activator of the *Insulin* promoter, and seems to function downstream of *Nkx6.1*.

IN THE CLINIC

REGULATION OF NUMBER OF ISLET CELLS

The number of islet cells that develop in the pancreas is generally set during fetal life but can be influenced by such factors as **intrauterine growth restriction** (IUGR; discussed in Ch. 6) due to vascular insufficiency, maternal diabetes, and fetal malnutrition. Embryonic and fetal islet cells, like those in the adult, respond to elevated blood glucose levels with compensatory hyperplasia. This fetal maladaptation is frequently seen in neonates born to diabetic mothers. Such hyperplasia, called **congenital hyperinsulinism** (sometimes referred to by the term nesidioblastosis, "nesidio" is Greek for *islet*), can occur locally or diffusely throughout the pancreas and lead to life-threatening decreases in blood glucose levels (i.e., **hypoglycemia**). Hyperinsulinemia is typically treated by diazoxide therapy until the hyperinsulinemia is resolved or by partial or near-total pancreatectomy. Some forms of congenital hyperinsulinism are associated with specific gene mutations or recessive disorders of the *SULPHONYLUREA RECEPTOR*, but the majority are nonfamilial and of unknown cause.

Before birth, islet cells are generated through the proliferation and differentiation of pancreatic progenitor cells. As just discussed, the number of islets generated within the developing pancreas is amenable to the need for maintaining proper glucose levels during embryonic and fetal period. However, the capacity to generate more islet cells after birth is greatly reduced. Nevertheless, the islet cell population can still increase, albeit very slowly and with limited capacity, at least until adolescence. Recent studies in adult mice show that new beta islet cells arise from preexisting beta cells rather than from an unidentified resident pancreatic progenitor cells. Therefore, if human adult pancreatic beta cells share this proliferative capacity, the hope is that new therapeutic strategies for human **type I diabetes** (where beta cells have been destroyed or are nonfunctional) could be developed.

Development of Spleen

As the dorsal mesogastrium of the lesser sac begins its expansive growth at the end of the 4th week, a mesenchymal condensation develops in it near the body wall. This condensation differentiates during the 5th week to form the **spleen**, a vascular lymphatic organ (see Fig. 14-8). Smaller splenic condensations called **accessory spleens** may develop near the hilum of the primary spleen. It is important to remember that the spleen is a mesodermal derivative, not a product of the gut tube endoderm like most of the intra-abdominal viscera. The rotation of the stomach and growth of the dorsal mesogastrium translocate the spleen to the left side of the abdominal cavity. The rotation of the dorsal mesogastrium also establishes a mesenteric connection called the **renal-splenic ligament** between the spleen and the left kidney. The portion of the dorsal mesentery between the spleen and the stomach is called the **gastrosplenic ligament.**

The spleen initially functions as a hematopoietic organ and only later acquires its definitive lymphoid character. During the **preliminary stage** of its development, until 14 weeks, the spleen is strictly hematopoietic. From 15 to 18 weeks (the **transformation stage**), the organ develops its characteristic lobular architecture. The **stage of lymphoid colonization** then commences as T-lymphocyte precursor cells begin to enter the spleen. Starting at 23 weeks, B-cell precursors arrive and form the **B-cell regions** of the definitive spleen.

Derivatives of Ventral Mesentery

As the liver enlarges, the caudal portion of the septum transversum and the ventral mesentery are modified to form a number of membranous structures, including the serous coverings of the liver and the membranes that attach the liver to the stomach and to the ventral body wall. As described in Chapter 11, the central tendon of the diaphragm forms from the **septum transversum.** By the 6th week, the enlarging liver makes contact with the septum transversum and the portion of the ventral mesentery covering the liver begins to split apart (Fig. 14-14). The caudal portion of the ventral mesentery covering almost the entire surface of the liver becomes **visceral peritoneum.** However, at the cranial end, the liver tissue makes direct contact with the developing central tendon of the diaphragm and thus has no peritoneal covering. This zone becomes the **bare area of the liver** (see Fig. 14-14). Around the margins of the bare area, the peritoneum covering the inferior surface of the peripheral diaphragm makes a fold or reflection onto the surface of the liver. Because this reflection encircles the bare area like a crown, it is called the **coronary ligament.** The direct contact between the liver and the diaphragm in the bare area results in the formation of anastomoses between hepatic portal vessels and the systemic veins of the diaphragm.

The narrow sickle-shaped flap of ventral mesentery attaching the liver to the ventral body wall differentiates into the membranous **falciform ligament** (see Fig. 14-14; also see Fig. 14-8). The free caudal margin of this membrane carries the umbilical vein from the body wall to the liver. The portion of the ventral mesentery between the liver and the stomach thins out to form a translucent membrane called the **lesser omentum.** The caudal border of the lesser omentum, connecting the liver to the developing duodenum, is called the **hepatoduodenal ligament** and contains the portal vein, the proper hepatic artery and its branches, and the hepatic, cystic, and common bile ducts. The region of the lesser omentum between the liver and the stomach is called the **hepatogastric ligament.**

When the stomach rotates to the left and the liver shifts into the right side of the peritoneal cavity, the lesser omentum rotates from a sagittal into a coronal (frontal) plane. This repositioning reduces the communication between the greater and lesser sacs of the peritoneal cavity to a narrow canal lying just posterior to the lesser omentum. This canal is called the **epiploic foramen of Winslow** (see Fig. 14-8).

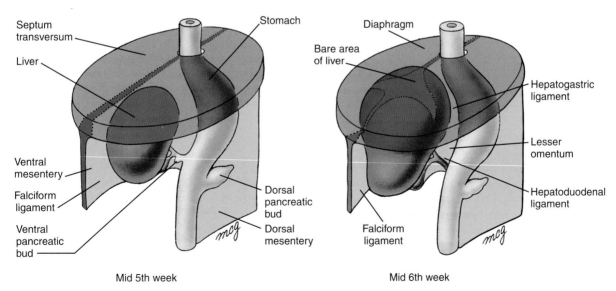

Septum transversum
Liver
Ventral mesentery
Falciform ligament
Ventral pancreatic bud
Stomach
Dorsal pancreatic bud
Dorsal mesentery

Mid 5th week

Diaphragm
Bare area of liver
Hepatogastric ligament
Lesser omentum
Hepatoduodenal ligament
Falciform ligament

Mid 6th week

Figure 14-14. Formation of the liver and associated membranes. As the liver bud grows into the ventral mesentery, its expanding crown makes direct contact with the developing diaphragm. The ventral mesentery that encloses the growing liver bud differentiates into the visceral peritoneum of the liver, which is reflected onto the diaphragm. This zone of reflection, which encircles the area where the liver directly contacts the diaphragm (the bare area), becomes the coronary ligament. The remnant of ventral mesentery connecting the liver with the anterior body wall becomes the falciform ligament, whereas the ventral mesentery between the liver and lesser curvature of the stomach forms the lesser omentum.

Development of Midgut

Primary Intestinal Loop

By the 5th week, the presumptive ileum, which can be distinguished from the presumptive colon by the presence of a cecal primordium at the junction between the two, begins to elongate rapidly. The growing ileum lengthens much more rapidly than the abdominal cavity itself, and the midgut is, therefore, thrown into a dorsoventral hairpin fold called the **primary intestinal loop** (Fig. 14-15A). The cranial limb of this loop will give rise to most of the ileum; the caudal limb will become the ascending colon and transverse colon. At its apex, the primary intestinal loop is attached to the umbilicus by the vitelline duct, and the superior mesenteric artery runs down the long axis of the loop. By the early 6th week, the continuing elongation of the midgut, combined with the pressure resulting from the dramatic growth of other abdominal organs (particularly the liver), forces the primary intestinal loop to herniate into the umbilicus (Fig. 14-15B,C).

As the primary intestinal loop herniates into the umbilicus, it also rotates around the axis of the superior mesenteric artery (i.e., around a dorsoventral axis) by 90 degrees counterclockwise as viewed from in front. Thus, the cranial limb moves caudally and to the embryo's right, and the caudal limb moves cranially and to the embryo's left (see Fig. 14-15B). This rotation is complete by the early 8th week. Meanwhile, the midgut continues to differentiate. The lengthening jejunum and ileum are thrown into a series of folds called the **jejunal-ileal loops**, and the expanding cecum sprouts a wormlike **vermiform appendix** (Fig. 14-15C).

During the 10th week, the midgut retracts into the abdomen. The mechanism responsible for the rapid retraction of the midgut into the abdominal cavity during the 10th week is not understood but may involve an increase in the size of the abdominal cavity relative to the other abdominal organs. As the intestinal loop reenters the abdomen, it rotates counterclockwise through an additional 180 degrees, so that now the retracting colon has traveled a 270-degree circuit relative to the posterior wall of the abdominal cavity (Fig. 14-15D, E; see Fig. 14-15 C). The cecum consequently rotates to a position just inferior to the liver in the region of the right iliac crest. The intestines have completely returned to the abdominal cavity by the 11th week.

After the large intestine returns to the abdominal cavity, the dorsal mesenteries of the ascending colon and descending colon shorten and fold, bringing these organs into contact with the dorsal body wall, where they adhere and become secondarily retroperitoneal (see Fig. 14-3D). The cecum is suspended from the dorsal body wall by a shortened mesentery soon after it returns to the abdominal cavity. In the case of ascending and descending colons, the shortening and folding of the mesenteries is probably related to the relative lengthening of the lumbar region of the dorsal body wall. The transverse colon does not become fixed to the body wall but remains an intraperitoneal organ suspended by mesentery. The most inferior portion of the colon, the sigmoid colon, also remains suspended by mesentery. Figure 14-16 summarizes the final disposition of the gastrointestinal organs with respect to the body wall.

IN THE CLINIC

ABNORMAL ROTATION AND FIXATION OF MIDGUT

As described in this chapter, the normal-handed asymmetry of the midgut is based on a relatively intricate series of rotations and fixations. Not surprisingly, errors in one or more of these steps lead to a varied spectrum of anomalies in humans.

Rotational Defects of Midgut

The anomaly called **nonrotation of the midgut** arises when the primary intestinal loop fails to undergo the normal 180-degree counterclockwise rotation as it is retracted into the abdominal cavity (Fig. 14-17). The earlier 90-degree rotation may occur normally. The result of this error is that the original cranial limb of the primary intestinal loop (consisting of presumptive jejunum and ileum) ends up on the right side of the body, and the original caudal limb of the primary intestinal loop (consisting mainly of presumptive colon) ends up on the left side of the body. Therefore, this condition is sometimes called **left-sided colon**. The cecum and the most proximal region of the large intestine may or may not fuse to the dorsal body wall to become secondarily retroperitoneal.

In **reversed rotation of the midgut**, the primary intestinal loop undergoes the initial 90-degree counterclockwise rotation normally, but the second 180-degree rotation occurs *clockwise* instead of counterclockwise, so the net rotation of the midgut is 90 degrees clockwise (Fig. 14-18). This rotation brings the regions of the midgut and hindgut into their normal spatial relationships, with one important exception: the duodenum lies ventral to the transverse colon instead of dorsal to it. The duodenum thus does not become

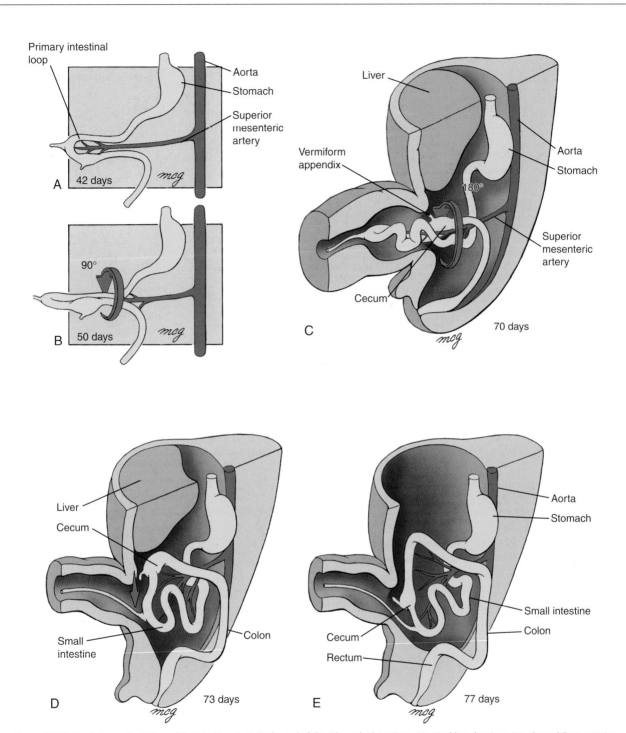

Figure 14-15. Herniation and rotations of the intestine. *A, B,* At the end of the 6th week, the primary intestinal loop herniates into the umbilicus, rotating through 90 degrees counterclockwise (in frontal view). *C,* The small intestine elongates to form jejunal-ileal loops, the cecum and appendix grow and, at the end of the 10th week, the primary intestinal loop retracts into the abdominal cavity, rotating an additional 180 degrees counterclockwise. *D, E,* During the 11th week, the retracting midgut completes this rotation as the cecum is positioned just inferior to the liver. The cecum is then displaced inferiorly, pulling down the proximal hindgut to form the ascending colon. The descending colon is simultaneously fixed on the left side of the posterior abdominal wall. The jejunum, ileum, transverse colon, and sigmoid colon remain suspended by mesentery.

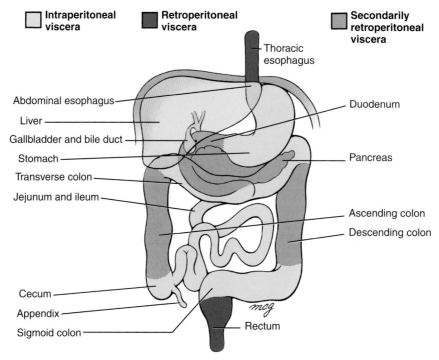

Intraperitoneal viscera ☐   **Retroperitoneal viscera** ■   **Secondarily retroperitoneal viscera** ▨

- Thoracic esophagus
- Abdominal esophagus
- Liver
- Gallbladder and bile duct
- Stomach
- Transverse colon
- Jejunum and ileum
- Cecum
- Appendix
- Sigmoid colon
- Duodenum
- Pancreas
- Ascending colon
- Descending colon
- Rectum

Figure 14-16. Intraperitoneal, retroperitoneal, and secondarily retroperitoneal organs of the abdominal gastrointestinal tract.

secondarily retroperitoneal, whereas the region of the transverse colon underlying it does.

In **mixed rotations of the midgut** (also called **malrotations**), only the cephalic limb of the primary intestinal loop undergoes the initial 90-degree rotation, whereas only the caudal limb undergoes the later 180-degree rotation (Fig. 14-19). The result of this mixed or uncoordinated behavior of the two limbs is that the distal end of the duodenum becomes fixed on the right side of the abdominal cavity, and the cecum becomes fixed near the midline just inferior to the pylorus of the stomach. This abnormal position of the cecum may cause the duodenum to be enclosed by a band of thickened peritoneum and leaves the small intestines tethered, on the right, by a narrow mesentery that increases the risk of developing an intestinal obstruction.

Volvulus of Intestines

A significant fraction of all cases of intestinal obstruction are caused by abnormal rotation or fixation of the midgut. Specific regions of the intestine, such as the duodenum, may be pinned against the dorsal body wall by bands of abnormal mesentery (called **Ladd's bands**), resulting in constriction and obstruction. Alternatively, malrotation may leave much of the midgut suspended from a single point of attachment on the dorsal body wall. Such freely suspended coils are prone to torsion or **volvulus**, which can lead to acute obstruction (Fig. 14-20). As described in this chapter's "Clinical Taster," **bilious vomiting** is a common symptom of intestinal volvulus.

Intestinal volvulus may also compress part of the intestinal vasculature. If the arterial supply to part of the gut is restricted or cut off, intestinal ischemia or infarction may occur, resulting in a segment of necrotic or stenotic bowel. A volvulus may also compress lymphatic vessels, inhibiting lymphatic drainage and leading to **venous mucosal engorgement** and consequent **gastrointestinal bleeding**.

The presence of a rotational abnormality is usually signaled during infancy or childhood by the sudden onset of acute abdominal pain, vomiting, or gastrointestinal bleeding, or by intermittent vomiting or failure to thrive. Occasionally, such an abnormality remains clinically silent until adulthood. Definitive diagnosis involves barium swallow or barium enema in conjunction with X-rays. Volvulus must be treated surgically.

DEFECTS OF THE UMBILICUS AND ANTERIOR ABDOMINAL WALL

Meckel's Diverticulum

The **vitelline duct** normally regresses between the 5th and 8th weeks (discussed in Ch. 6), but in about 2% of live-born infants it persists as a remnant of variable length and location (Fig. 14-21). Most often, it is observed as a 1- to

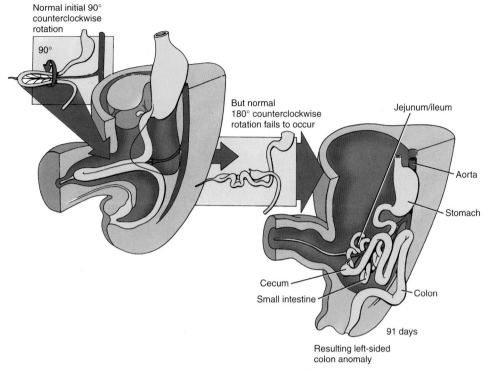

Figure 14-17. Nonrotation of the gut (also called left-sided colon).

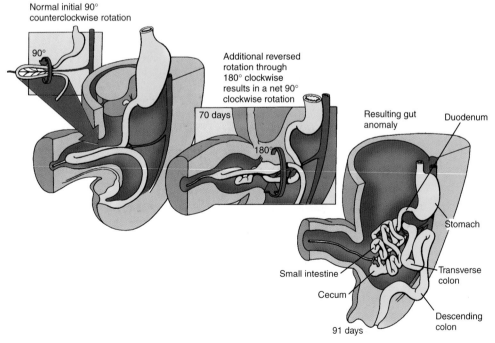

Figure 14-18. Reversed rotation of the gut. The net rotation is 90 degrees clockwise, so the midgut viscera are brought to their normal locations in the abdominal cavity but the duodenum lies anterior to the transverse colon.

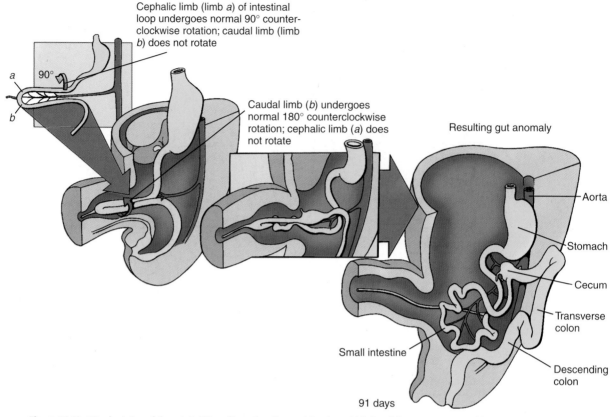

Cephalic limb (limb *a*) of intestinal loop undergoes normal 90° counter-clockwise rotation; caudal limb (limb *b*) does not rotate

Caudal limb (*b*) undergoes normal 180° counterclockwise rotation; cephalic limb (*a*) does not rotate

Resulting gut anomaly

a

90°

b

Aorta

Stomach

Cecum

Transverse colon

Small intestine

Descending colon

91 days

Figure 14-19. Mixed rotation of the gut. In this malformation, the cranial and caudal limbs of the primary intestinal loop rotate independently.

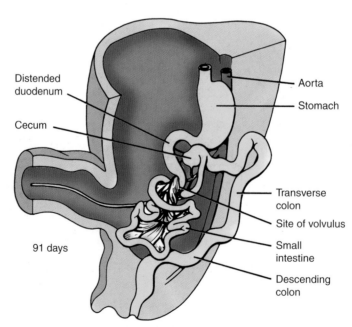

Distended duodenum

Cecum

Aorta

Stomach

Transverse colon

Site of volvulus

Small intestine

Descending colon

91 days

Figure 14-20. Volvulus. Volvulus may occur as suspended regions of the gut twist around themselves, constricting the intestine and/or compromising its blood supply.

5-cm intestinal diverticulum projecting from the antimesenteric wall of the ileum within 100 cm of the cecum (see Fig. 14-21A). In other cases, part of the vitelline duct within the abdominal wall persists, forming an open **omphalomesenteric fistula**, an **omphalomesenteric cyst** (or enterocyst), or an **omphalomesenteric ligament** (or **fibrous band**) connecting the small bowel to the umbilicus (see Fig. 14-21B-D). These conditions are known collectively as **Meckel's diverticulum** in honor of J.F. Meckel, who first discussed the embryologic basis of the abnormality in the early 19th century. Meckel's diverticulum is seen in about 2% of the general population and is about twice as common in males as in females.

Most cases of Meckel's diverticulum are asymptomatic. However, it is estimated that 15% to 35% of individuals who have Meckel's diverticulum develop symptoms of intestinal obstruction, gastrointestinal bleeding, or peritonitis—many before 10 years of age. Meckel's diverticulum complications can manifest as a consequence of bowel obstruction caused by the trapping of part of the small bowel by a fibrous band representing a remnant of the vitelline vessels connecting the diverticulum to the umbilicus. Symptoms may closely mimic appendicitis, involving periumbilical pain that later localizes to the right lower quadrant. Up to 60% of Meckel's diverticula harbor abnormal tissue, usually pancreatic or gastric. In the latter case, patients may develop bleeding ulceration of the gut. Mortality in untreated cases is estimated to be 2.5% to 15%.

The facts about Meckel's diverticulum can be remembered using the "rule of twos": it occurs in 2% of the population and is 2 times more common in males; 2% of individuals with Meckel's diverticulum have medical symptoms, usually by 2 years of age; it is usually present 2 feet proximal to the terminal ileum and is usually 2 inches long; and it contains 2 types of abnormal lining.

Umbilical Hernia, Omphalocele, and Gastroschisis

The terms used to describe defects of the anterior abdominal wall in which the abdominal contents protrude are often used inconsistently in the literature. Here, they are divided into three groups: **umbilical hernia**, **omphalocele**, and **gastroschisis**.

An **umbilical hernia** consists of a small protrusion of bowel through the umbilical ring, which is covered by skin. It is often more apparent when the infant cries or strains. More than 95% of umbilical hernias close spontaneously by 5 years of age. Umbilical hernia can occur as an isolated defect but it is commonly associated with syndromes (e.g., **Beckwith Wiedemann syndrome**).

Omphalocele (discussed in Ch. 4; see Fig. 4-3A) also involves herniation of bowel or other viscera through the umbilical ring, which is covered by a thin avascular membrane that may rupture. In contrast to an umbilical hernia, in extreme cases, an omphalocele can involve a large herniation consisting of the entire bowel and liver, with the umbilical cord inserting into the apex of the omphalocele. Omphalocele occurs in about 2.5 of 10,000 births, and it is often associated with chromosome abnormalities or other malformation syndromes. Several possible explanations for omphalocele exist. Recall that during the 6th to 10th weeks of development, the midgut undergoes a physiologic herniation into the developing umbilical cord. One possibility is that the herniated bowel does not fully retract into the abdominal cavity during the 10th week, and thus remains herniated. Another possibility is that lateral body folding and fusion fails to occur properly during the 4th to the 8th weeks, creating a body wall weakness that allows the bowel to later herniate as it grows. A third possibility is that incomplete migration and differentiation may occur of the mesoderm that normally forms the connective tissue of the skin and hypaxial musculature of the ventral body wall, again resulting in a body wall weakness. Mutations in multiple genes in mice—including a serine/threonine protein kinase called *Omphalocele kinase-1*, which is expressed in the ventral body wall (ectoderm and mesoderm)—result in formation of omphalocele.

Gastroschisis is a defect of the anterior abdominal wall in which bowel protrudes without a covering sac between the developing rectus muscles just lateral to, and usually to the right of, the umbilicus (discussed in Ch. 4; see Fig. 4-3B). In gastroschisis, the umbilical ring closes normally. The cause of gastroschisis, like that of omphalocele, is unclear, but the two defects likely share some of the same mechanisms postulated above. Gastroschisis differs from omphalocele in being less often associated with other abnormalities, and it has not been correlated with chromosomal anomalies. The incidence of this defect is about 1 in 10,000 births.

Other defects of the anterior body wall include ectopia cordis, isolated protrusion of the heart through the body wall, and a constellation of five defects called **pentalogy of Cantrell** (supraumbilical abdominal wall defect, diaphragmatic hernia (discussed in Ch. 11), pericardial defect, sternal cleft, and intracardiac anomaly).

14

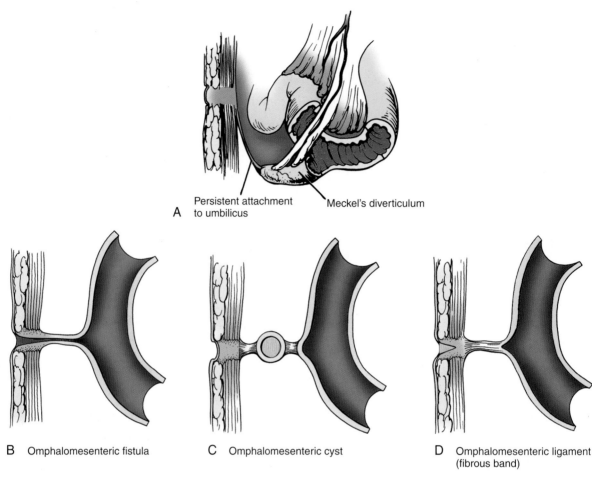

A Persistent attachment to umbilicus — Meckel's diverticulum

B Omphalomesenteric fistula

C Omphalomesenteric cyst

D Omphalomesenteric ligament (fibrous band)

Figure 14-21. Meckel's diverticulum. *A*, A typical Meckel's diverticulum is a finger-like projection of the ileum. A Meckel's diverticulum may form: *B*, a patent fistula connecting the umbilicus with the ileum; *C*, an isolated cyst suspended by ligaments; or *D*, a fibrous band connecting the ileum and anterior body wall at the level of the umbilicus.

Cytodifferentiation of Endodermal Epithelium of Gut

The gastrointestinal tract is composed of the endoderm forming the epithelial lining of the lumen, the splanchnic mesoderm forming the smooth muscle and connective tissue tunics, and the ectoderm. The latter form the most cranial and caudal luminal linings (derived, respectively, from the stomodeum and proctodeum; the stomodeum is discussed in Ch. 16 and the proctodeum is discussed later in the chapter)

and enteric nervous system (derived from neural crest cells; discussed later in the chapter). As evident from the previous discussion, the orientations cranial-caudal, dorsal-ventral, and right-left (manifested mainly by the turning and looping of the gut and positioning of the stomach) reflect the final regionalization of organs and orientation of the adult intestinal tract. Superimposed on the cranial-caudal axis is another axis, the **radial axis**, with the establishment of the glandular epithelium of the gastrointestinal tract. Early in development, much of the endodermal lining of the gastrointestinal tract remains uniform in morphology until epithelial-mesenchymal interactions, dictated by regionalization signals, direct endodermal differentiation. Many of the major morphologic changes and cytodifferentiation events occur during the midgestation (fetal) period.

Initially, the gastrointestinal epithelium is pseudostratified but is converted into a simple columnar epithelium in a wave beginning at the stomach and progressing toward the colon. Early in the 2nd month, the lumen of the gastrointestinal tract is temporarily occluded or nearly so (Fig. 14-22). Occlusion of the lumen has been attributed to a rapid proliferation of the epithelium. However, recent morphologic studies in humans suggest that convergent extension of the epithelium, much like what occurs during gastrulation and neurulation (discussed in Chs. 3 and 4), may be responsible. Over the next two weeks vacuoles develop within the base of the thickened epithelial layer and coalesce until the gut tube is fully **recanalized.** In humans, the initial vacuolization of the epithelium seems to be mediated through epithelial apoptosis. Stenosis or duplication of the digestive tract may result from incomplete recanalization. Meanwhile, mesodermal expansions project into the region of vacuolization. Together with the overlying epithelium, they form the villi of the intestines, the length of which depends on the cranial-caudal level

of the intestines. In the intestines, formation of villi is accompanied by endodermal invagination into the mesoderm, forming crypts. In the stomach, villi do not form but the endoderm does invaginate into the mesoderm, forming pits (future gastric glands). Finally, in the 9th week, the definitive mucosal epithelium differentiates from the endodermal lining of the regenerated gut lumen.

Cytodifferentiation of the endodermal epithelium along the radial axis (i.e., base of the pit/crypts to the tip of the villi) depends on interactions with the underlying mesoderm and occurs late in development. As epithelial cells of the gastrointestinal tract undergo rapid turnover during our lifetime, they must be replaced by stem cells that retain this radial axial influence. These stem cells produce progenitors for **enterocytes** (absorptive cells), **enteroendocrine cells** (regulatory peptide-secreting cells), **Paneth cells** (antimicrobial peptide-secreting cells), and **goblet** or **mucus cells** (Fig. 14-23). Enterocytic, goblet, and enteroendocrine cells continue to proliferate, differentiate, and mature while migrating up the villus to the tip, where they are eventually extruded into the lumen (a two- to three-day journey). Paneth cells reside at the base of the crypt (for about 21 days before dying and being removed by

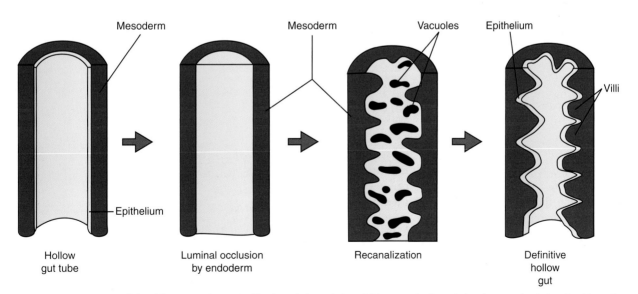

Mesoderm Mesoderm Vacuoles Epithelium

Epithelium Villi

Hollow gut tube

Luminal occlusion by endoderm

Recanalization

Definitive hollow gut

Figure 14-22. Formation of the definitive gut lumen. Proliferation of the endodermal lining completely occludes the gut tube during the 6th week. Recanalization is completed by week 9. During recanalization, projections of underlying mesoderm into the regions bordering the epithelial vacuoles drive villi development.

14

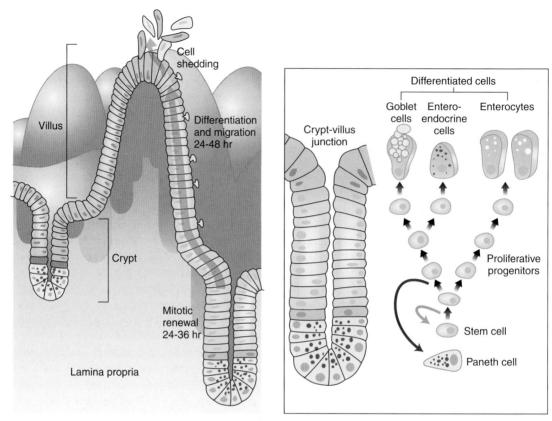

Figure 14-23. Cytodifferentiation of the endodermal epithelium of the small intestines. Epithelial cells of the gastrointestinal tract undergo rapid turnover and must be replaced by stem cells. These stem cells produce the progenitors for enterocytes, enteroendocrine cells, Paneth cells, and goblet cells. Enterocytic, goblet, and enteroendocrine cells continue to proliferate, differentiate, and mature while migrating up the villus, where they are shed into the lumen at the tip. Paneth cells reside at the base of the crypt. In the small intestines, the stem cells reside in the region about the 4th cell position from the base of the crypt because Paneth cells occupy the base. Committed progenitor cells differentiate near the crypt/villus border and migrate toward the villus tips (or in the case of Paneth cells toward the bottom of the crypt). Hence, various stages in the life of a gastrointestinal epithelial cell are arranged along the radial (crypt-to-villus) axis of the gut.

phagocytosis). In the small intestines, the stem cells reside in the region located at about the fourth cell position from the base of the crypt because Paneth cells occupy the base. Therefore, committed progenitor cells differentiate near the crypt/villus junction and migrate toward the villus tips (or in the case of Paneth cells, toward the bottom of the crypt). (In the colon, the stems cells reside and proliferate in the bottom two thirds of the crypts because there are no Paneth cells in this region.) Hence, various stages in the life of a gastrointestinal epithelial cell are arranged along the radial (crypt-to-villus) axis of the gut.

IN THE RESEARCH LAB

DIFFERENTIATION OF GASTROINTESTINAL TRACT EPITHELIUM

The position of cells along the radial axis is one of the important factors mediating cellular differentiation. As discussed in Chs. 5, 9, and 13, *Ephrins* and their receptors play essential roles in mediated cell migration and establishing boundaries. These ligands and receptors are also expressed within the intestinal epithelium. *EphB2* and *EphB3* receptors and their ligands, *EphrinB1* and *EphrinB2*, are expressed in an inverse gradient along the radial axis, with the *Ephrins* being most concentrated in the villus and villus/crypt border, and their receptors being more prominent within the proliferating region (Fig.14-24). This spatial relationship suggests a role for mediating the migration of epithelial cells along the radial axis: *EphB2/EphB3* double knockout mice lose the proliferative/differentiation boundary, and ectopic proliferating epithelial cells can be found along the entire villus. In normal adults, *EphB3* receptor expression is restricted to the columnar cells found in the base of the crypt where Paneth cells usually reside. However, in *EphB3* null mice, Paneth cells are found distributed throughout the crypt/villus unit. Experiments further suggest that the expression patterns of the *Ephrins* and *Ephrin* receptors within the gut are regulated by *β-Catenin/Tcf* transcriptional activity. Thus, a *Wnt* signaling gradient may control gut epithelial cell positioning along the radial axis by mediating *Ephrin* signaling.

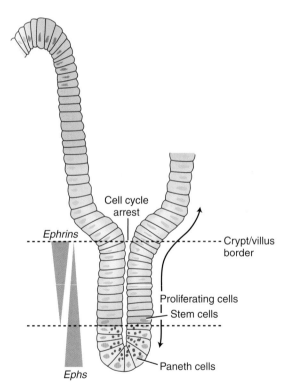

Figure 14-24. *Ephrins* and their receptors are expressed in an inverse gradient along the radial axis, with *Ephrins* being most concentrated in the crypt/villus border and their receptors, *EphB2* and *EphB3*, being more prominent within the proliferating region and base of the crypt. This spatial relationship is important in mediating the migration of epithelial cells along the radial axis. Arrows indicate the direction of cell migration.

What particular *Wnts* might drive gut epithelial proliferation and migration and what their sources might be is unclear. Several different *Wnts* are expressed within the intestinal epithelium and mesoderm along the cranial-caudal axis including *Wnt4*, *Wnt5a*, and *Wnt11*. What mediates the levels of these *Wnts* or their signaling along the radial axis is unknown, but *Shh* and *Ihh* have been suggested as possible antagonists of *Wnt* signaling. The growth factors *Tgfβ* and *Bmps* have also been implicated in limiting *Wnt* signaling, as *Tgfβ* and *Bmp* signaling inhibits *β-Catenin/Tcf4* transactivation by sequestering *β-Catenin* through *Smad* binding (activated through *Tgfβ* and *Bmp* receptor signaling).

As discussed in an earlier "In the Research Lab" in this chapter, *Notch* signaling increases *Hes1* expression, thereby repressing endocrine lineage specification in the pancreatic endoderm. *Hes1* is also expressed within the intestinal precursor population. As would be predicted, *Hes1* null mice have an increase in the number of secretory cells within the gut epithelium at the expense of enterocytes. However, in mice deficient in *Math1*, a bHLH transcription factor repressed by *Hes1*, the intestinal epithelium is almost entirely composed of enterocytes, almost the complete opposite phenotype that would be predicted from the *Hes1* knockout phenotype. Why this occurs is unclear but it has been hypothesized that at this point, two cell types are present within the intestinal epithelium (Fig. 14-25). In one, *Notch* signaling increases *Hes1* expression that then represses *Math1* expression (this cell takes on an enterocyte lineage). In the other, because of a lack of *Hes1*, *Math1* expression increases, and the cell type becomes committed to a multipotent secretory progenitor cell lineage (e.g., goblet, Paneth, or enteroendocrine cell).

FAULTY WNT SIGNALING AND β-CATENIN TURNOVER IS OFTEN A PRELUDE TO COLON CANCER

As described in Chapter 5, *Wnt* signaling is initiated by the binding to the *Frizzled* family of receptors and the coreceptors *Lrp5* or *Lrp6*. In the absence of *Wnt*, *β-Catenin* is constantly being degraded by a complex containing *Adenomatous polyposis coli (APC)* protein, *Axin*, and *Gsk3* (Fig. 14-26). When bound to this complex, *β-Catenin* becomes phosphorylated, and this phosphorylation targets *β-Catenin* for ubiquination-mediated proteosomal destruction. However, in the presence of *Wnt*, the action of this destruction complex is blocked, and consequently *β-Catenin* levels accumulate. With increasing levels of free cytoplasmic *β-Catenin*, *β-Catenin* enters the nucleus and binds to the *Tcf4/Lef* family of transcription factors, driving the transcription of many other genes (the so-called canonical pathway).

14

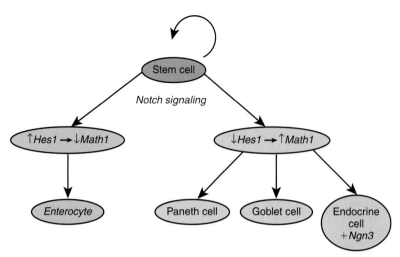

Figure 14-25. The role of *Notch* signaling in cell lineage specification of intestinal epithelial cells. Experiments suggest that *Notch* signaling increases *Hes1* expression, which in turn represses *Math1* expression. These cells then take on an enterocyte lineage. Other cells deficient in *Hes1* increase *Math1* expression and become committed to a multipotent secretory progenitor cell lineage (e.g., goblet, Paneth, or enteroendocrine cell).

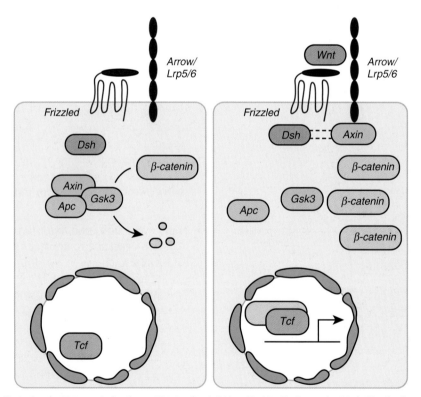

Figure 14-26. Diagram illustrating the *Wnt* canonical pathway. *Wnt* signaling is initiated by *Wnt* binding to the *Frizzled* family of receptors and coreceptors, *Lrp5* or *Lrp6*. In the absence of *Wnt*, *β-Catenin* is constantly being degraded by a complex composed, in part, by *Apc*, *Axin*, and *Gsk3* (left cell). However, in the presence of *Wnt* signaling cell on (right), the action of this destruction complex is blocked, and as a consequence *β-Catenin* levels accumulate. With increasing levels of free *β-Catenin*, *β-Catenin* enters (right cell) the nucleus and binds to the *Tcf/Lef* family of transcription factors, enabling the transcription of many other genes.

The *Wnt/β-Catenin/Tcf4* cascade is critical for maintaining the proliferative compartment within the gut epithelium and in patterning the glandular phenotype along the radial axis. The distribution pattern of *β-Catenin* and *Tcf4* within the gut epithelium coincides with the primary site of epithelial proliferation: *β-Catenin* accumulates within the nucleus of epithelial cells at the bottom third of the small intestinal crypt, where the levels of *Tcf4* are also the highest. *Wnt* signaling imposes continual proliferation (maintenance) of crypt epithelial cells, and in the absence of *Wnt* signaling, these cells go into cell cycle arrest and initiate differentiation. Thus, knockout mice for *Tcf4* are unable to maintain an intestinal epithelial progenitor population. Therefore, *Wnt* signaling, through actions of the *Tcf4/Lef* family of transcription factors, mediates the switch between proliferation, maintenance, and differentiation of the epithelial cells. The switch itself depends on strict radial axis controls.

Familial adenomatous polyposis patients have one mutant copy of *APC*. Moreover, detectable *APC* mutations are found in about 80% of spontaneous cases of colorectal cancers, suggesting that *APC* is a key regulator of both forms of colorectal cancers (other cases of colorectal cancers are associated with mutations in *β-Catenin* or *Axin*). Any decrease in the functional levels of *APC* increases the level of *β-Catenin* within the cytoplasm and nucleus, ultimately mimicking the effects of positive *Wnt* signaling. In the case of intestinal epithelial cells, this leads to inappropriate cell proliferation and malignant transformation. Candidate target genes for constitutive *Wnt* signaling associated with colorectal cancers include the cell cycle genes (e.g., *C-Myc*, *Cyclin D*), *MATRIX METALLOPROTEINASES*, growth factors, and angiogenic factors. *APC* can also function as a nuclear-cytoplasmic shuttle and hence mutations in *APC* might alter *β-Catenin* entry into the nucleus.

Development of Outer Intestinal Wall and Its Innervation

As described earlier in the chapter, the gut tube consists of an endodermally derived epithelium covered by splanchnopleuric mesoderm. The mesodermal layer develops into multiple layers including the lamina propria, muscularis mucosa, submucosa, and circular and longitudinal muscular layers. Innervation of these layers is via the **enteric nervous system** (also discussed in Ch. 10) composed collectively of sympathetic and parasympathetic components that are patterned around the radial axis. The enteric nervous system eventually becomes arranged in two general layers, the inner **Meissner's plexus** (between submucosa and smooth muscle layer) and **Auerbach's plexus** (on the outer portion of the smooth muscle tunic).

Studies suggest that endodermal *Shh*, in cooperation with *Ihh*, directly mediates smooth muscle development of the gastrointestinal tract and indirectly mediates neuronal patterning via its effect on *Bmp4* expression within the mesenchyme. In chick embryos, all gastrointestinal mesoderm has the potential to form smooth muscle. *Shh* emanating from the endoderm inhibits the expression of *Smap (Smooth muscle activating protein)* in the adjacent mesoderm (Fig. 14-27), thereby restricting smooth muscle tunic formation to the outermost radial axis of the gut tube. Consequently, the mesoderm nearest the endoderm forms lamina propria and submucosa. *Shh* developmental signals are often relayed through *Bmps*. *Bmp4* is expressed between the epithelium and developing smooth muscle layer. Alone, however, *Bmp4* is incapable of inhibiting *Smap* expression. But mice deficient in *Shh* have thinner circular smooth muscle tunics and exhibit a larger number of enteric neurons distributed throughout the mesenchymal wall, some of which can even be found within the gut epithelium. The latter effect is thought to the result of a loss in *Bmp4* signaling, as transgenic mice expressing *Noggin* (a *Bmp* antagonist) in neurons show a similar effect on enteric ganglia. The effect of knocking out *Shh* on the development of smooth muscle suggests either that the regulation of smooth muscle cell proliferation and differentiation involves additional signaling molecules or that *Hedgehogs* initiate the formation of the smooth muscle cell lineage within the splanchnic mesoderm but then later restricts their differentiation adjacent to the epithelium.

The **enteric nervous system**, which provides the intrinsic innervation of the gastrointestinal tract, consists of glia, interconnected afferent and efferent neurons, and interneurons. The enteric nervous system functions to regulate gut peristalsis, blood flow, secretion, absorption, and endocrine processes. It is also unique in the capacity to exhibit integrative neuronal activity in the absence of the central nervous system.

14

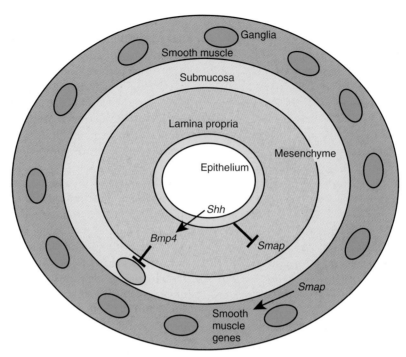

Figure 14-27. Schematic representation of the differentiation of the gut wall along the radial axis. Studies suggest that *Shh* emanating from the endoderm inhibits the expression of *Smap* (*Smooth muscle activating protein*) in the adjacent mesoderm, thereby restricting smooth muscle tunic formation to the outermost radial axis of the gut tube. As a consequence, the mesoderm nearest the endoderm forms lamina propria and submucosa. *Bmp4*, induced by *Shh* within the lamina propria and submucosa, limits enteric neuronal cell differentiation to the outer region of the gut wall.

Hence, it is sometimes referred to as "the brain" of the gastrointestinal tract, or "the second brain" of the body.

Postganglionic sympathetic fibers originate from the sympathetic chain ganglia or paraortic ganglia and follow the gastrointestinal vascular supply to enter the wall of the gastrointestinal tract. The parasympathetic postganglionic fibers originate from ganglia found within the wall of the gastrointestinal tract. Cells forming the enteric parasympathetic ganglia and glia originate from a subset of migrating neural crest cells that begin colonizing the human gut at its cranial end starting about week 7, and at its rectal end starting about week 12. Neural crest cells arising from the occipitocervical levels (somites 1 to 7) are the source of the vagal (parasympathetic) neurons and glia and eventually populate the gut's entire length (Fig. 14-28). Studies in chick and mouse embryos show sacral enteric ganglionic neurons and glia arise from neural crest cells formed caudal to somite pair 28 in birds and somite pair 24 in mice, and that this subset of cells colonizes the hindgut after the arrival of the vagal neural crest cells. Although sacral-derived neural crest cells align themselves with the vagal nerve plexus, experiments show that sacral neural crest cell migration and differentiation is normal even when vagal neural crest cells are ablated. Hence, sacral neural crest cells can innervate the hindgut independent of vagal innervation. Neural crest cells arising from the neural tube immediately caudal to the vagal neural crest cells have been suggested as a possible source of enteric cells populating the foregut. Because of the complexity of the enteric nervous system, the frequency of gut motility disorders, and the side effects of many neuropharmaceutical drugs on the gastrointestinal tract physiology, the enteric nervous system is the subject of intense investigation.

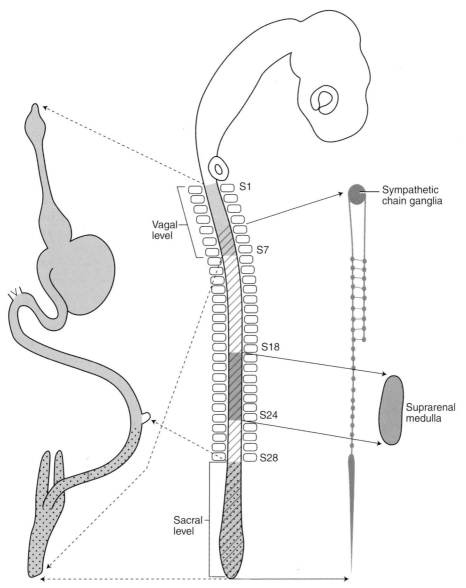

S1

Vagal
level

S7

Sympathetic
chain ganglia

S18

Suprarenal
medulla

S24

S28

Sacral
level

Figure 14-28. The origin of neural crest cells forming the enteric nervous system in the chick embryo. Postganglionic sympathetic fibers innervating the enteric nervous system are derived from neurons located within the sympathetic chain. These neurons and glia originate from neural crest cells arising from the dorsal neural tube at axial levels beginning at somite level 5 and extending into the sacrum (hatched). The origin of neural crest cells forming the suprarenal medulla are shown in purple. Vagal postganglionic neurons and glia are derived from neural crest cells arising at somite levels 1 to 7 (tan, no stippling), whereas sacral enteric ganglionic neurons and glia arise from neural crest cells caudal to somite pair 28 in chickens (tan, stippled).

14

IN THE CLINIC

HIRSCHSPRUNG DISEASE

Disorders of **enteric nervous system** in humans can be divided into two major groups: those characterized by an abnormal number of ganglia (Hirschsprung), or those characterized by abnormal neuronal differentiation (intestinal neuronal dysplasia). In **Hirschsprung disease** (1 in 5000 live births; also known as **congenital aganglionic megacolon**), there is a complete or partial obstruction of intestine due to total absence of both **myenteric** and **submucosa ganglia**. This leads to abnormal dilation or distention of a variable length of the colon, and increased wall thickness due to muscular hypertrophy in the intestine proximal to the aganglionic segment. The enlarged bowel (i.e., megacolon) in patients with Hirschsprung disease is essentially a secondary symptom caused by the obstruction and lack of peristalsis in the colon segment distal to the dilation (Fig. 14-29). Removal of the constricted distal segment remains the only effective treatment for the disease, and refinement of the surgical approaches to Hirschsprung disease have led to decreased mortality.

The first sign of Hirschsprung disease is usually a delay in the passage of meconium (usually meconium is passed within 48 hours), the material filling the lower bowel of newborn infants. This may be accompanied by other symptoms such as constipation, vomiting, abdominal pain, and distention. These patients are at risk for life-threatening complications such as intestinal infection (enterocolitis) or rupture of the cecum. Most individuals with Hirschsprung disease are diagnosed during their first year of life. Barium enema examinations show the nonperistaltic segment usually involves the sigmoid colon and rectum, although it may vary in length from a small portion of the rectum to the entire large intestine and part of the ileum. Diagnosis of Hirschsprung disease is made by suction biopsy of the rectal mucosa, with histopathology demonstrating an absence of enteric ganglia.

Hirschsprung disease occurs as an isolated, sporadic defect or in the context of a syndrome, and can be inherited as a familial trait or as part of a chromosomal imbalance. The latter is seen in about 12% of Hirschsprung disease patients, with trisomy 21 being the most common. A family history of Hirschsprung disease is positive in about 7% of cases, and about 15% of Hirschsprung disease cases are associated with at least one other congenital anomaly. The genetic causes of Hirschsprung disease are heterogeneous and involve multiple factors, with evidence for both low penetrance and sex dependence, that vary with regard to the length of the aganglionic segment. The male-to-female ratio of Hirschsprung disease is 4:1 for short segmental ganglionic agenesis but is more equal in frequency between the sexes as the length of the segment involved becomes longer. Hirschsprung disease (also discussed in the following "In the Research Lab") is associated with multiple gene mutations and occurs as part of at least 10 syndromes.

IRRITABLE BOWEL SYNDROME

The **enteric nervous system** is composed of the neurons and glia of the **myenteric** and **submucosal plexuses** of the gastrointestinal tract. The enteric nervous system can control enteric reflexes independently from input by extrinsic autonomic neurons, but it is also connected to the brain. The enteric nervous system is known to affect the central nervous system and to have a marked impact on mood. This is illustrated by the fact that vagal nerve stimulation is used in treatment-resistant depression. In some cases, the reciprocal relationship between the enteric nervous system and the brain may be significant in the pathogenesis of **irritable bowel syndrome**. Irritable bowel syndrome is characterized by changes in the normal patterns of peristalsis, secretion, and sensation, which may be the result of molecular alterations intrinsic to the bowel. The amount of mucosal *Serotonin*, the expression of *Tryptophan hydroxylase-1*, and the expression of the *Serotonin transporter* are significantly reduced in the colon of irritable bowel syndrome patients. Whether these are primary defects or secondary adjustments to disease remains to be established. It will be of interest to know if these changes in *Serotonin* homeostasis in irritable bowel syndrome patients are limited to the bowel, or if they also occur in the central nervous system.

INFANTILE HYPERTROPHIC PYLORIC STENOSIS

Infantile hypertrophic pyloric stenosis (1 to 3 in 1000 live births) is characterized by the development of pyloric hypertrophy and a gastric outlet obstruction, which classically presents with projectile vomiting in the first two months postnatally. Abnormal thickening of the circular pyloric circular muscle can often be palpated on physical examine (described as the "olive"). The cause of stenosis is an abnormal innervation of the pylorus, analogous to that occurring in Hirschsprung disease. Some studies suggest neurons in this region fail to express *Nitric oxide synthase*, as mice null for the gene coding this enzyme exhibit pyloric stenosis and an enlarged stomach. In addition, *Bmps* have been implicated in mediating smooth muscle cell proliferation and differentiation here, as altering levels of *Bmp4* signaling in this region alters the thickness of the muscular tunic as well as development of the enteric nervous system in chick embryos.

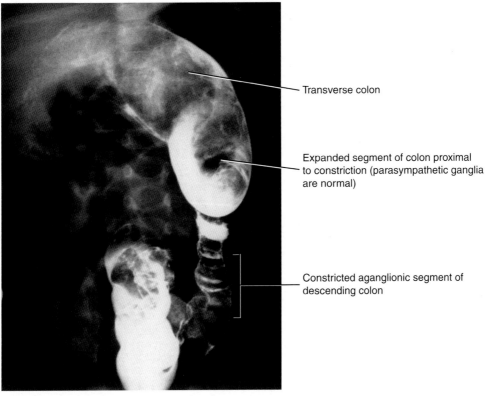

Transverse colon

Expanded segment of colon proximal to constriction (parasympathetic ganglia are normal)

Constricted aganglionic segment of descending colon

Figure 14-29. Radiograph after a barium enema showing the constricted inferior gastrointestinal tract of an individual with Hirschsprung disease. The adjacent, more proximal, region of the tract with normal autonomic innervation is distended.

IN THE RESEARCH LAB

HIRSCHSPRUNG DISEASE AND NEURAL CREST CELL DEFECTS

The absence of enteric ganglia within the gut is recognized as the main cause of the Hirschsprung disease and is generally attributed to a failure of neural crest cell migration, proliferation, and differentiation, either before or after arriving within the gut wall. Defects in any of the developmental mechanisms required for neural crest cell morphogenesis could, therefore, result in congenital megacolon. Several studies in chick, mice, and humans support this hypothesis.

Many Hirschsprung-related mutations in humans are found in genes coding for *RET*. The *RET* proto-oncogene, which has been mapped to human chromosome 10q11.2, encodes a TYROSINE KINASE that serves as a receptor for members of the GLIAL CELL-DERIVED NEUROTROPHIC FACTOR (GDNF) ligand family. During embryogenesis of vertebrates, *Ret* is expressed in the developing renal system and in all cell lineages of the peripheral nervous system. Premigratory vagal and sacral neural crest cells express *Ret*, and it is required for normal enteric nervous system development in mice and humans. *Ret*-positive neural crest cells, when injected into stomachs of mice having aganglionic intestines, colonize and reconstitute the enteric nervous system. In vitro, the ligand for *Ret*, *Gndf*, is a chemoattractant for vagal neural crest cells. Studies suggest that *Gndf* gradients within the gut direct vagal neural crest cell migration in a cranial-to-caudal direction and promote directional neurite outgrowth.

RET mutations have been identified in 50% of familial and 15% to 20% of sporadic Hirschsprung disease cases including large deletions, microdeletions, insertions, nonsense, missense, and splicing mutations. Haploinsufficiency is the most likely mechanism in Hirschsprung disease. This is in contrast to **multiple endocrine neoplasia type 2**, in which *RET* mutations lead to constitutive dimerization and activation of *RET* and, therefore, to malignant transformation. Although severe *RET* mutations may lead to phenotypic

14

expression with haploinsufficiency, hypomorphic *RET* mutations may require a mutation in an additional pertinent gene (e.g., *Endothelin*; discussed later in this section).

The *lethal spotted* and *piebald* lethal mouse mutants are characterized by mutations of the *Endothelin-3 gene (Et3)* and the gene encoding its G protein-coupled receptor, the *Endothelin-B receptor (Etb)*. These mice lack enteric ganglia and exhibit Hirschsprung disease. In mice, null mutations for the *Et3* gene or its receptor, *ETB*, also result in agangliosis of the distal colon, but these mice have normal proximal gut innervation. This suggests that *Et3* signaling is required for late stages of gut colonization by neural crest cells. The lack of ganglia in *lethal spotted* mice is thought to be due to a premature exit from the cell cycle and premature differentiation of enteric neural crest cells, resulting in an inability to generate enough progenitors to colonize gut. Mutations in *ETB*, which maps to human chromosome 13q22, have been found in about 5% of isolated Hirschsprung disease in humans (i.e., in the absence of other congenital anomalies). Patients with **Waardenburg type 4 syndrome** have **Hirschsprung disease**, accompanied by pigmentary anomalies and sensorineural deafness. Patients with homozygous mutations in *ET3* or *ETB* present with complete Waardenburg type 4 phenotype, including Hirschsprung disease, whereas heterozygotes for *ET3* or *ETB* may only have isolated Hirschsprung disease. Waardenburg type 4 symptoms are also observed in some patients with mutations in *SOX10*, which directly regulates *RET* expression. In mice, RET has shown to be important in the survival of early neural crest cells and for glial fate determination of enteric neural crest cells.

Recent studies suggest that interactions between the independent gene loci of *RET* and *ETB* are necessary for normal formation of the enteric nervous system in humans and mice. Individuals carrying an *RET* mutation have a significantly higher risk of developing Hirschsprung disease if they also have a hypomorphic mutation (i.e., a partial loss-of-function mutation) in *ETB*. Mice heterozygotic null for *Ret* and having a loss-of-function mutation for *Etb* develop Hirschsprung disease without exhibiting defects in renal development or pigmentation that are otherwise often seen in isolated *Ret* and *Et3/Etb* mutations. Recent studies suggest *Et3*

signaling cooperates with *Gndf* (the *Ret* ligand) in promoting the proliferation of undifferentiated enteric neuronal progenitors. In gut tissue explants, exogenous *Et3* limits the chemoattractant effect of *Gndf* on enteric neural crest cells, but *Et3* has no effect on neural crest cell migration in the absence of *Gdnf*. Thus, a balance between *Ret* and *Et3/Etb* signaling pathways seems to be required for normal colonization of the gut.

Splotch mutant mice harbor mutations of *Pax3*, a transcription factor that plays an important role in neural tube and musculoskeletal development. In addition to the neural tube defects that these mice exhibit, homozygotes of several well described *Pax3* mutations exhibit severe defects of neural crest cell migration and/or differentiation, including cardiovascular defects (discussed in Ch. 12), hearing loss, pigmentation defects, and Hirschsprung disease. Among these, mutations arising from chromosomal deletions are most severe. In humans, deletions or mutations in the human homolog of *Pax3* cause **Waardenburg type 1 syndrome.** These patients have pigmentation and auditory system defects, but lack Hirschsprung disease, suggesting that there is redundancy of *Pax3* function in humans that is not present in mice.

Other genes implicated in the development of neural crest cells and the enteric nervous system include: *Netrin* and *Netrin* receptors; *Semaphorin3a*; *Neurotrophin-3* and its receptor, *TrkC* (promoting survival and differentiation of enteric neurons and glia needed for formation of myenteric and submucosal plexuses); *Bmp* signaling molecules (mediating *Neurotrophin-3* signaling and *Gdnf*-driven expansion of the enteric precursor pool, and promoting intrinsic primary afferent enteric neuron development); *Mash1* (a bHLH transcription factor required for forming enteric neurons containing *Serotonin* and *Nitric oxide synthase*); *Phox2a* and *Phox2b* (paired box homeodomain transcription factors; *Phox2b* when knocked out leads to loss of all peripheral autonomic nerves); *Hand2* (necessary for differentiation of enteric neurons); *Brain-derived neurotrophic factor; Persephin* (a neurotrophic factor of the *Gdnf* family); *Artemin* (another neurotrophic factor of the *Gdnf* family); and *Smad interacting protein-1*.

Development of Hindgut

The portion of the primitive hindgut tube lying just deep to the cloacal membrane forms an expansion called the **cloaca.** A slim diverticulum of the cloaca called the **allantois** extends into the connecting stalk (see Fig. 14-2). Between the 4th and 6th weeks, the

cloaca is partitioned into a dorsal **anorectal canal** and a ventral **urogenital sinus** by the formation of a coronal partition called the **urorectal septum** (Fig. 14-30). The urogenital sinus gives rise to the bladder, pelvic urethra, and a lower expansion, the phallic segment. As discussed in Chapter 15, in the male, the pelvic urethra becomes the membranous and prostatic

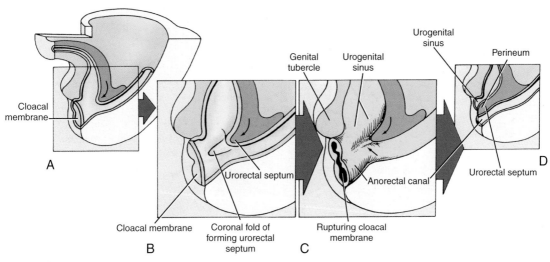

Figure 14-30. *A-D,* Subdivision of the cloaca into a ventral primitive urogenital sinus and a dorsal anorectal canal between 4 and 6 weeks. The urorectal septum dividing the cloaca is formed by mesodermal folds growing in a coronal plane from the surrounding urogenital sinus and hindgut. As the tip of the urorectal septum approaches the cloacal membrane dividing the cloaca into the urogenital sinus and anorectal canal, the cloacal membrane ruptures, thereby opening the urogenital sinus and dorsal anorectal canal to the exterior. The tip of urorectal septum forms the perineum.

urethra, and the phallic segment becomes the penile urethra. In the female, the pelvic urethra becomes the membranous urethra, and the phallic segment contributes to the vestibule of the vagina. All of these urogenital structures are thus lined with an epithelium derived from endoderm.

The urorectal septum is often described as forming from two integrated mesodermal septal systems: a cranial fold (called the *Tourneux fold*) growing toward the cloacal membrane, and a pair of lateral folds (called the *Rathke folds*) growing toward the midline of the cloaca. However, closer examination of mouse, rat, and human embryos suggests that the urorectal septum is formed by the fusion and wedging of the mesoderm surrounding the allantois and hindgut (see Fig. 14-30). As the human embryo grows and caudal body folding continues, the tip of this urorectal septum approaches the cloacal membrane, dividing the cloaca into a ventral urogenital sinus and dorsal anorectal canal (see Fig. 14-30B, C). Whether the urorectal septum in humans descends toward the cloacal membrane (composed of opposing ectoderm and endoderm) by actively growing or descends passively due to caudal body folding is unclear. Before the urorectal septum has an opportunity to fuse with the cloacal membrane, the cloacal membrane ruptures (about week 8), thereby opening the urogenital sinus and

dorsal anorectal canal to the exterior. Eventually, the urorectal septum completely separates the urogenital sinus and anorectal canal from one another, and its tip forms the future perineum (Fig. 14-31; see Fig. 14-30 C-D). Meanwhile, mesoderm adjacent to

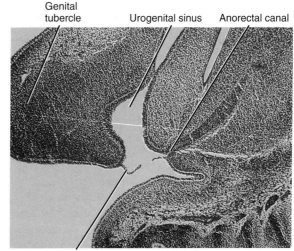

Figure 14-31. Human cloacal separation. Light micrograph of a sagittal section through the caudal region of an 18-mm human embryo (50 to 51 days) just after rupture of the cloacal membrane.

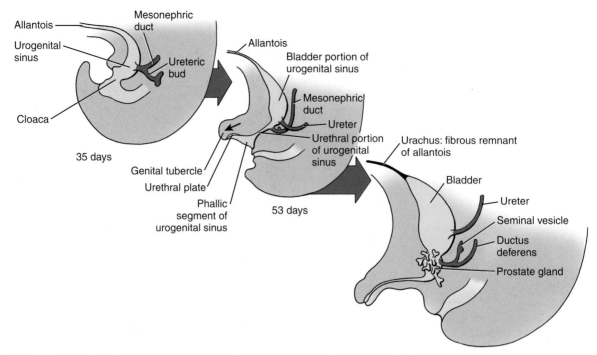

Figure 14-32. Fate of the allantois and urogenital sinus. The urogenital sinus is subdivided into a bladder, pelvic urethral region, and phallic segment. Normally, the allantois becomes occluded to form the urachus (or median umbilical ligament) of the adult. With the rupture of the cloacal membrane, the roof of the phallic segment forms a urethral plate of endodermal cells that lengthen as the genital tubercle grows.

the phallic segment of the urogenital sinus expands, generating the **genital tubercle** that eventually forms the phallus. With the rupture of the cloacal membrane, the floor of the phallic segment is lost, whereas the roof of the phallic segment expands along the lower surface of the genital tubercle as the genital tubercle enlarges (Fig. 14-32). This endodermal extension forms the **urethral plate** (or **urethral membrane;** Figs. 14-32, 14-33). As discussed in Chapter 15, this plate forms the penile urethra in males and vaginal vestibule in females. **Urogenital folds** (or **cloacal folds**) then form on either side of this plate through an expansion of mesoderm underlying the ectoderm.

Soon after the formation of the anorectal orifice, the anorectal walls become opposed to one another and an ectodermal plug, the **anal membrane**, forms that temporarily obliterates the distal end of the anorectal canal (see Figs. 14-31, 14-33). Meanwhile, the mesenchyme around the anal membrane proliferates forming a raised border surrounding the anal membrane that creates an **anal pit** or **proctodeum** (see Fig. 14-33). The anal membrane breaks down in the 8th week. The former location of this membrane is marked in

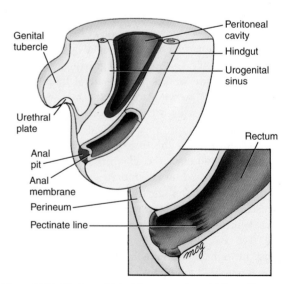

Figure 14-33. The lower third of the anorectal canal is formed by an ectodermal invagination called the anal pit. The border between the cranial end of the anal pit and the caudal end of the rectum is demarcated by mucosal folds called the pectinate line in the adult.

the adult by an irregular folding of mucosa within the anorectal canal, called the **pectinate line.** Hence, the cranial two thirds of the anorectal canal is derived from the distal part of the hindgut (lined with endodermally derived epithelium); the inferior one third of the anorectal canal is derived from the anal pit (lined with ectodermally derived epithelium). The vasculature of the anorectal canal is consistent with this dual origin: superior to the pectinate line, the canal is supplied by branches of the inferior mesenteric arteries and veins serving the hindgut; inferior to the pectinate line, it is supplied by branches of the internal iliac arteries and veins. Anastomoses between tributaries of the superior rectal vein and tributaries of the inferior rectal vein within the mucosa of the anorectal canal may later swell into hemorrhoids if the normal portal blood flow into the inferior vena cava is restricted.

IN THE CLINIC

HINDGUT ABNORMALITIES AND ASSOCIATED ABDOMINAL WALL DEFECTS

In a series of abnormalities ranging from **epispadias** (the urethral opening is on the dorsum of the genital tubercle rather than on its ventral side; discussed in Ch. 15) to **exstrophy of the bladder** or **cloaca**, hindgut structures can remain open to the anterior surface of the body through a defect in the anterior body wall. In exstrophy of the bladder, the bladder is revealed by an abdominal wall defect; in exstrophy of the cloaca, the lumina of both the bladder and the anorectal canal are exposed. The abdominal wall defect in these conditions may be a secondary effect of anomalous development of the cloacal membrane. According to one idea, the primary defect is that the cloacal membrane is abnormally large, so that when it breaks down it produces an opening too wide to permit normal midline fusion of the tissue layers on either side of it. An alternative theory posits an inability to reduce the size of cloacal membrane at its superior and lateral sides because of insufficient tissue proliferation and migration in the infraumbilical region. Coupled with the membrane's subsequent rupture, this could also lead to exstrophy of the bladder, epispadias, or cloacal exstrophy depending on the degree and timing of the deficiencies. Epispadias may also arise if the genital tubercle develops from the urorectal septum rather than from mesoderm adjacent the phallic segment of the urogenital sinus. Exstrophy of the bladder with epispadias is the most common anomaly of those discussed in this section, occurring in approximately 1 of 40,000 births. Exstrophy of the cloaca is much less frequent, occurring in about 1 of 200,000 births. All these malformations are about twice as common in males as in females.

URACHAL ANOMALIES

Normally, the allantois and the superior end of the presumptive bladder undergo regression between the 4th and 6th weeks, at the same time that the urorectal septum is partitioning the cloaca into the urogenital sinus and a dorsal anorectal canal. The allantois and the constricted bladder apex are transformed into a ligamentous band, the **urachus** or **median umbilical ligament**, that runs through the subperitoneal fat from the bladder to the umbilicus. This band is about 5 cm long and 1 cm wide in the adult (see Fig. 14-32).

In a very small number of individuals (with an incidence of about three per million), part or all of the allantois and bladder apex remains patent, resulting in a **patent urachus (urachal fistula)**, **umbilical urachal sinus**, **vesicourachal diverticulum**, or **urachal cyst** (Fig. 14-34). Symptoms include leakage of urine from the umbilicus, urinary tract infections, and peritonitis resulting from perforation of the patent urachus. These conditions may be life threatening. The initial symptoms of infection, as with Meckel's diverticulum, are easily confused with those of appendicitis.

See Chapter 15 for a discussion of defects of the anal opening.

14

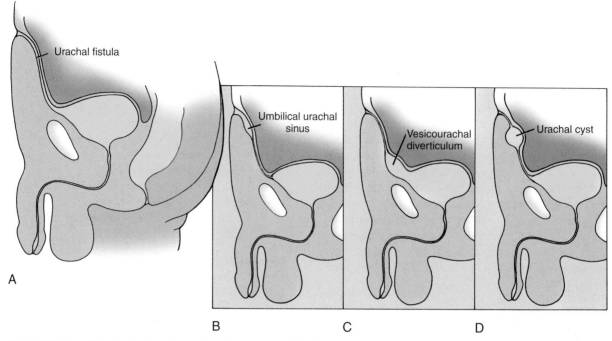

Figure 14-34. Fate of the allantois. Normally, the allantois becomes occluded to form the urachus or median umbilical ligament of the adult. Very rarely, parts of the allantois may remain patent, producing a urachal fistula, *A;* umbilical urachal sinus, *B;* vesicourachal diverticulum, *C;* or urachal cyst, *D.*

Suggested Readings

Amiel J, Lyonnet S. 2001. Hirschsprung disease, associated syndromes, and genetics: a review. J Med Genet 38:729-739.

Bai Y, Chen H, Yuan ZW, Wang W. 2004. Normal and abnormal embryonic development of the anorectum in rats. J Pediatr Surg 39:587-590.

Beck F, Tata F, Chawengsaksophak K. 2000. Homeobox genes and gut development. Bioessays 22:431-441.

Burns AJ. 2005. Migration of neural crest-derived enteric nervous system precursor cells to and within the gastrointestinal tract. Int J Dev Biol 49:143-150.

Cleaver O, Krieg PA. 2001. Notochord patterning of the endoderm. Dev Biol 234:1-12.

Coates MD, Mahoney CR, Linden DR, et al. 2004. Molecular defects in mucosal serotonin content and decreased serotonin reuptake transporter in ulcerative colitis and irritable bowel syndrome. Gastroenterology 126:1657-1664.

de Santa Barbara P, van den Brink GR, Roberts DJ. 2002. Molecular etiology of gut malformations and diseases. Am J Med Genet 115:221-230.

de Santa Barbara P, van den Brink GR, Roberts DJ. 2003. Development and differentiation of the intestinal epithelium. Cell Mol Life Sci 60:1322-1332.

Fukuda K, Yasugi S. 2002. Versatile roles for sonic hedgehog in gut development. J Gastroenterol 37:239-246.

Gariepy CE. 2004. Developmental disorders of the enteric nervous system: genetic and molecular bases. J Pediatr Gastroenterol Nutr 39:5-11.

Gershon MD, 1998. The Second Brain. Harper Collins Pubs, New York. p. 312.

Gershon MD. 2003. Serotonin and its implication for the management of irritable bowel syndrome. Rev Gastroenterol Disord 3 Suppl 2:S25-S34.

Gershon MD. 2004. Review article: serotonin receptors and transporters—roles in normal and abnormal gastrointestinal motility. Aliment Pharmacol Ther 20 (Suppl) 7:3-14.

Gershon MD, Ratcliffe EM. 2004. Developmental biology of the enteric nervous system: pathogenesis of Hirschsprung's disease and other congenital dysmotilities. Semin Pediatr Surg 13:224-235.

Gregorieff A, Clevers H. 2005. Wnt signaling in the intestinal epithelium: from endoderm to cancer. Genes Dev 19:877-890.

Harmon EB, Ko AH, Kim SK. 2002. Hedgehog signaling in gastrointestinal development and disease. Curr Mol Med 2:67-82.

Holemans K, Aerts L, Van Assche FA. 2003. Lifetime consequences of abnormal fetal pancreatic development. J Physiol 547:11-20.

Jensen J. 2004. Gene regulatory factors in pancreatic development. Dev Dyn 229:176-200.

Kamiya A, Gonzalez FJ, Nakauchi H. 2006. Identification and differentiation of hepatic stem cells during liver development. Front Biosci 11:1302-1310.

Kinoshita T, Miyajima A. 2002. Cytokine regulation of liver development. Biochim Biophys Acta 1592:303-312.

Kruger GM, Mosher JT, Bixby S, et al. 2002. Neural crest stem cells persist in the adult gut but undergo changes in self-renewal, neuronal subtype potential, and factor responsiveness. Neuron 35:657-669.

Lammert E, Cleaver O, Melton D. 2003. Role of endothelial cells in early pancreas and liver development. Mech Dev 120:59-64.

Le Douarin NM. 2004. The avian embryo as a model to study the development of the neural crest: a long and still ongoing story. Mech Dev 121:1089-1102.

Lemaigre F, Zaret KS. 2004. Liver development update: new embryo models, cell lineage control, and morphogenesis. Curr Opin Genet Dev 14:582-590.

Lewis SL, Tam PP. 2006. Definitive endoderm of the mouse embryo: Formation, cell fates, and morphogenetic function. Dev Dyn 235:2315-2329.

Logan CY, Nusse R. 2004. The Wnt signaling pathway in development and disease. Annu Rev Cell Dev Biol 20:781-810.

Matsumoto A, Hashimoto K, Yoshioka T, Otani H. 2002. Occlusion and subsequent re-canalization in early duodenal development of human embryos: integrated organogenesis and histogenesis through a possible epithelial-mesenchymal interaction. Anat Embryol (Berl) 205:53-65.

Murtaugh LC, Melton DA. 2003. Genes, signals, and lineages in pancreas development. Annu Rev Cell Dev Biol 19:71-89.

Nebot-Cegarra J, Fabregas PJ, Sanchez-Perez I. 2005. Cellular proliferation in the urorectal septation complex of the human embryo at Carnegie stages 13-18: a nuclear area-based morphometric analysis. J Anat 207:353-364.

Newgreen D, Young HM. 2002. Enteric nervous system: development and developmental disturbances—part 1. Pediatr Dev Pathol 5:224-247.

Newgreen D, Young HM. 2002. Enteric nervous system: development and developmental disturbances—part 2. Pediatr Dev Pathol 5:329-349.

Penington EC, Hutson JM. 2003. The absence of lateral fusion in cloacal partition. J Pediatr Surg 38:1287-1295.

Pla P, Larue L. 2003. Involvement of endothelin receptors in normal and pathological development of neural crest cells. Int J Dev Biol 47:315-325.

Plaza-Menacho I, Burzynski GM, Groot JW, Eggen BJ, Hofstra RM. 2006. Current concepts in RET-related genetics, signaling and therapeutics. Trends Genet 22:627-636.

Puri P, Shinkai T. 2004. Pathogenesis of Hirschsprung's disease and its variants: recent progress. Semin Pediatr Surg 13:18-24.

Radtke F, Clevers H. 2005. Self-renewal and cancer of the gut: two sides of a coin. Science 307:1904-1909.

Roberts DJ. 2000. Molecular mechanisms of development of the gastrointestinal tract. Dev Dyn 219:109-120.

Sukegawa A, Narita T, Kameda T, Saitoh K, Nohno T, Iba H, Yasugi S, Fukuda K. 2000. The concentric structure of the developing gut is regulated by Sonic hedgehog derived from endodermal epithelium. Development 127:1971-1980.

Wang DZ, Olson EN. 2004. Control of smooth muscle development by the myocardin family of transcriptional coactivators. Curr Opin Genet Dev 14:558-566.

Wells JM, Melton DA. 1999. Vertebrate endoderm development. Annu Rev Cell Dev Biol 15:393-410.

Wilson ME, Scheel D, German MS. 2003. Gene expression cascades in pancreatic development. Mech Dev 120:65-80.

Zumkeller W. 1999. Nesidioblastosis. Endocr Relat Cancer 6:421-428.

14

Development of the Urogenital System

15

Summary   As important to survival on dry land as the lungs, the **urinary system** maintains the electrolyte and water balance of the body fluids that bathe the tissues in a salty, aqueous environment. The development of this system involves the transient formation and subsequent regression or remodeling of vestigial primitive systems, thereby providing a glimpse of evolutionary history (another glimpse is provided by the development of the pharyngeal arches discussed in Ch. 16). Copulatory organs of the **genital system** developed to ensure efficient fertilization. They display morphologic variations among species. The degree of such variations is quite prominent and likely reflects divergent modes of copulatory behaviors and copulation physiology on land and in water. The development of the genital system is closely integrated with the primitive urinary organs in both males and females, as they share similar common tubular structures enabling both uresis and gamete transport. Therefore, this chapter describes both the development of the urinary and genital systems.

The **intermediate mesoderm** on either side of the dorsal body wall gives rise to three successive nephric structures of increasingly advanced design. The intermediate mesoderm, also known as the **nephrotome**, forms a segmental series of epithelial buds. In the cervical region, these structures presumably represent a vestige of the **pronephroi**, or primitive kidneys, which develop in some lower vertebrates. As these cranial pronephroi regress in the 4th week, they are succeeded by a pair of elongated **mesonephroi**, which develop in the thoracic and lumbar regions. The mesonephroi are functional, having complete, though simple **nephrons**. The mesonephroi are drained by a pair of **mesonephric (wolffian) ducts**, which grow caudally to open into the posterior wall of the primitive urogenital sinus. By the 5th week, a pair of **ureteric buds** sprouts from the distal mesonephric ducts and induce the overlying sacral intermediate mesoderm to develop into the **metanephroi**, or definitive kidneys.

As described in the preceding chapter, the cloaca (the distal expansion of the hindgut) is partitioned into a dorsal anorectal canal and a ventral urogenital sinus. The latter is continuous with the allantois, which projects toward the umbilical cord. The expanded superior portion of the urogenital sinus becomes the bladder, whereas its inferior portion gives rise (in males) to the **pelvic urethra (membranous** and **prostatic)** and **penile urethra** and (in females) to the **pelvic urethra (membranous)** and **vestibule of the vagina**. During this period, the openings of the mesonephric ducts are translocated down onto the pelvic urethra by a process that also emplaces the openings of ureters on the bladder wall.

By the 6th week, the **germ cells** migrating from the yolk sac begin to arrive in the mesenchyme of the dorsal body wall. The arrival of germ cells in the area just medial to the mesonephroi at the 10th thoracic segment induces cells of the mesonephros and adjacent coelomic epithelium to become **somatic support cells** that invest the germ cells. Somatic support cells will differentiate into **Sertoli cells** in the male and **follicle cells** (or granulosa cells) in the female. During the same period, a new pair of ducts, the **müllerian (paramesonephric) ducts**, form in the dorsal body wall just lateral to the mesonephric ducts.

The sexual differentiation of genetic males begins at the end of the 6th week, when a specific gene on the Y chromosome *(SRY)* is expressed in the somatic support cells. Embryos in which this gene is not expressed develop as females. The product of this gene, called the **SRY protein**, initiates a developmental cascade that leads to the formation of the testes, the male genital ducts and associated glands, the male external genitalia, and the entire constellation of male secondary sex characteristics. The SRY protein exerts autonomous control of somatic support cell development into **pre-Sertoli cells**. Pre-Sertoli cells then recruit mesonephric mesenchymal cells into the gonadal ridge and these cells give rise to **Leydig cells, myoepithelial cells,** interstitial

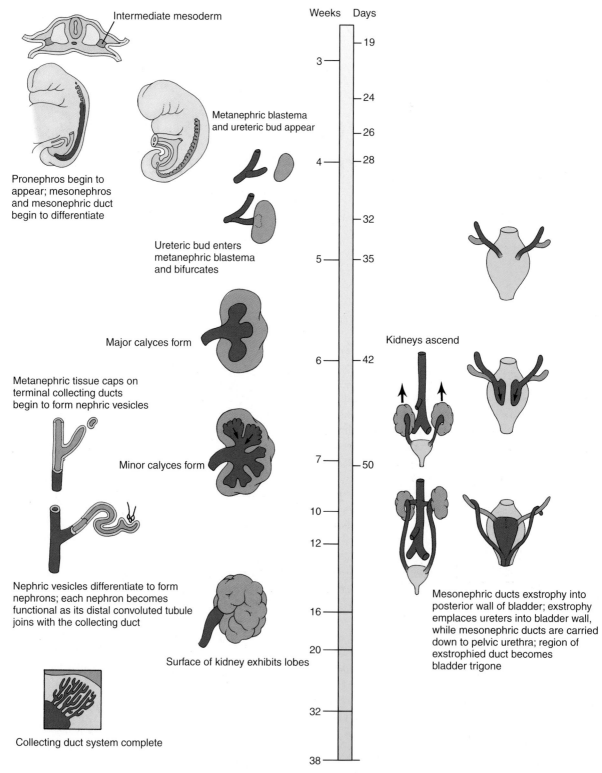

Intermediate mesoderm

Pronephros begin to appear; mesonephros and mesonephric duct begin to differentiate

Metanephric blastema and ureteric bud appear

Ureteric bud enters metanephric blastema and bifurcates

Major calyces form

Metanephric tissue caps on terminal collecting ducts begin to form nephric vesicles

Minor calyces form

Nephric vesicles differentiate to form nephrons; each nephron becomes functional as its distal convoluted tubule joins with the collecting duct

Surface of kidney exhibits lobes

Collecting duct system complete

Kidneys ascend

Mesonephric ducts exstrophy into posterior wall of bladder; exstrophy emplaces ureters into bladder wall, while mesonephric ducts are carried down to pelvic urethra; region of exstrophied duct becomes bladder trigone

Weeks   Days

3 — 19

— 24

— 26

4 — 28

— 32

5 — 35

6 — 42

7 — 50

10

12

16

20

32

38

Time line. Development of the urinary system.

Weeks

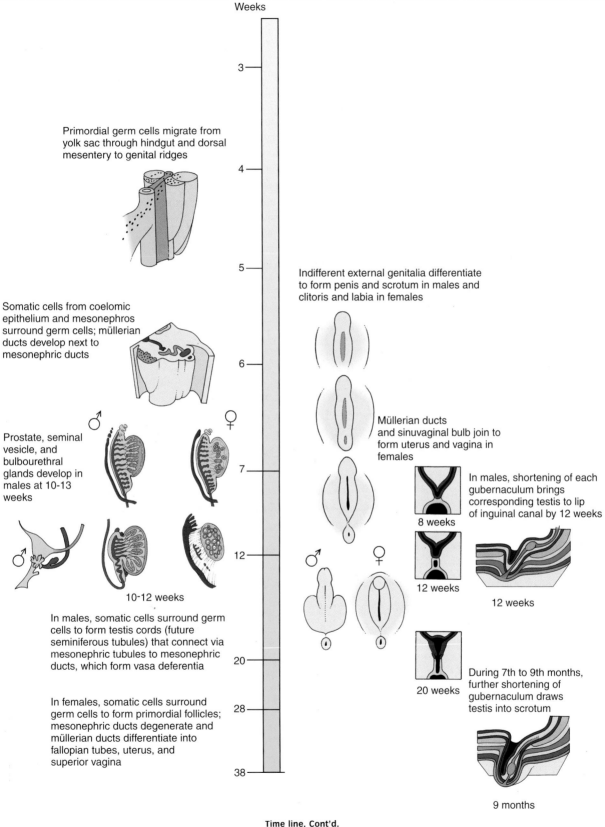

Primordial germ cells migrate from yolk sac through hindgut and dorsal mesentery to genital ridges

Somatic cells from coelomic epithelium and mesonephros surround germ cells; müllerian ducts develop next to mesonephric ducts

Prostate, seminal vesicle, and bulbourethral glands develop in males at 10-13 weeks

10-12 weeks

In males, somatic cells surround germ cells to form testis cords (future seminiferous tubules) that connect via mesonephric tubules to mesonephric ducts, which form vasa deferentia

In females, somatic cells surround germ cells to form primordial follicles; mesonephric ducts degenerate and müllerian ducts differentiate into fallopian tubes, uterus, and superior vagina

Indifferent external genitalia differentiate to form penis and scrotum in males and clitoris and labia in females

Müllerian ducts and sinuvaginal bulb join to form uterus and vagina in females

8 weeks

12 weeks

In males, shortening of each gubernaculum brings corresponding testis to lip of inguinal canal by 12 weeks

12 weeks

20 weeks

During 7th to 9th months, further shortening of gubernaculum draws testis into scrotum

9 months

Time line, Cont'd.

15

cells, and endothelial cells. Differentiating Sertoli cells then envelop the germ cells and together with the myoepithelial cells organize into **testis cords** (future **seminiferous tubules**). The deepest portions of the somatic support cells in the developing gonad, which do not contain germ cells, differentiate into the **rete testis**. The rete testis connects with a limited number of mesonephric tubules and canalizes at puberty to form conduits connecting the seminiferous tubules to the mesonephric duct. These nephric tubules become the **efferent ductules** of the testes, and the mesonephric ducts become the **vasa deferentia** (singular, **vas deferens**). The müllerian ducts degenerate. During the 3rd month, the distal vas deferens sprouts the **seminal vesicle**, and the **prostate** and **bulbourethral glands** grow from the adjacent pelvic urethra. Simultaneously, the indifferent external genitalia (consisting of paired **urethral** and **labioscrotal folds** on either side of the **urethral plate** and an anterior **genital tubercle**) differentiate into the **penis** and **scrotum**. Late in fetal development, the testes descend into the scrotum through the **inguinal canals**.

Because genetic females lack a Y chromosome, they do not produce SRY protein. Hence, the somatic support cells do not form Sertoli cells but rather differentiate into follicle cells that surround the germ cells to form **primordial follicles** of the ovary. The mesonephric ducts degenerate, and the müllerian ducts become the genital ducts. The proximal portions of the müllerian ducts become the **fallopian tubes** (or **oviducts**). Fusion of the distal portions of the ducts gives rise to the **uterus** and possible contributions to the cranial **vagina**; the caudal portion of the vagina is thought to develop from a pair of endodermal **sinuvaginal** bulbs that develop from the posterior wall of the urogenital sinus. The indifferent external genitalia develop into the female external genitalia: the **clitoris** and the paired **labia majora** and **minora**.

Clinical Taster

A couple, expecting a boy based on prenatal ultrasound, is surprised when told by the delivery room nurse that they, instead, have a baby girl. Then some confusion seems to ensue among the caregivers. Later, a doctor from the nursery arrives and informs the family that their child has "ambiguous genitalia," with an enlarged clitoris that was likely confused with a penis on the ultrasound. She tells them that the genitals look more like a girl's than a boy's, with a separate urethra and vagina, but that there is partial fusion of the labia with what may be testes being palpable in the groin area. She explains that further testing will be needed to determine the infant's sex.

The family is visited by several doctors over the next two days, including specialists in urology, endocrinology, and genetics. They hear, variously, that the child should be "thought of as a girl," or that the child is "a boy but may need to be raised as a girl." They hear terms that are new to them like "intersex" and "undervirilized." A battery of tests is done. These include laboratory tests on blood that show normal testosterone and luteinizing hormone levels and an ultrasound that shows no cervix, uterus, or fallopian tubes. Gonads, likely testes, are found in the inguinal canal. Later in the week, they find out that their child has a "Y" chromosome (46,XY) and is, therefore, genetically, a boy. Further tests (such as measuring androgen response in skin fibroblasts) confirm the diagnosis of androgen insensitivity syndrome (AIS). Males with AIS (also know as testicular feminization) have mutations in the *Androgen receptor* gene and are unable to respond appropriately to testosterone during development.

Options for sex assignment are presented to the baby's parents. One is male sex assignment. Although this choice would be consistent with the karyotype, it would involve multiple surgeries in childhood and adolescence, along with testosterone treatment (the response to androgens is usually not completely absent). Another would be female sex assignment, which involves estrogen therapy along with surgery in childhood or puberty to remove the gonads, enlarge the vaginal opening, and reduce the size of the clitoris. With either option, there is the risk that the child will be uncomfortable with their gender identity later in life. Given all the uncertainties, the parents find it difficult to commit to a gender assignment and decide on a third option: to make a temporary assignment of female, but to wait to do surgery until she is old enough to make her own decisions.

Three Nephric Systems Develop

As discussed in Chapter 3, the mesoderm formed on either side of the midline during gastrulation differentiates into three subdivisions: the paraxial mesoderm, **intermediate mesoderm** (also called the **nephrotome**), and lateral plate mesoderm (Fig. 15-1). The fates of the paraxial and lateral plate mesoderm are discussed in other chapters. The intermediate mesoderm gives rise to the nephric structures of the embryo, portions of the suprarenal glands, the gonads, and the genital duct system. During embryonic development, three sets of nephric systems develop in craniocaudal succession from the intermediate mesoderm. These are called the **pronephros, mesonephros**, and **metanephros** (or definitive kidneys). Formation of the pronephric kidney (i.e., pronephros) lays the foundation for the induction of the mesonephric kidney (i.e., mesonephros), and it in turn lays the foundation for the induction of the metanephric kidney (i.e., metanephros). Hence, formation of a pronephric kidney is really the start of a developmental cascade leading to the formation of the definitive kidney.

Formation of Pronephros

Early in the 4th week, intermediate mesoderm along the fifth to seventh cervical axial levels gives rise to a small duct generated by epithelialization of some of the intermediate mesoderm. This duct is called the **mesonephric duct** (or **wolffian duct**). The mesonephric ducts first appear as a pair of solid longitudinal rods that condense within the intermediate mesoderm beginning in the pronephric region (Figs. 15-2A, 15-3). These rods grow in a caudal direction owing to the proliferation and migration of the cells at their caudal tips. Meanwhile, intermediate mesoderm ventromedial and adjacent to the mesonephric duct, condenses and reorganizes into a series of epithelial buds (see Fig. 15-2). These buds, which quickly become hollow, constitute the **pronephros** (plural, pronephroi; derived from the Greek for "first kidney") because they resemble the functional embryonic pronephroi of some lower vertebrates. In humans, these units do not differentiate into functional excretory structures but instead cease developing and disappear by day 24 or 25.

As the mesonephric ducts develop and extend caudally, they induce the formation of **mesonephric tubules** from mesenchyme in the more caudal intermediate mesoderm, thereby initiating mesonephros formation (Fig. 15-2B, C). As the ducts grow into the lower lumbar region, they diverge from the intermediate mesoderm and grow toward and fuse with the ventrolateral walls of the cloaca on day 26 (Figs. 15-4A, see Fig. 15-2). This region of fusion will become a part of the posterior wall of the future bladder. As the rods fuse with the cloaca, they begin to cavitate at their distal ends to form a lumen, and this canalization progresses cranially. At its caudal end, the mesonephric

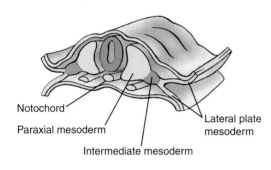

Notochord

Paraxial mesoderm

Lateral plate mesoderm

Intermediate mesoderm

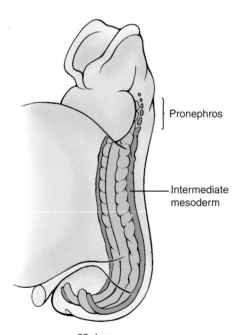

Pronephros

Intermediate mesoderm

23 days

Figure 15-1. The intermediate mesoderm gives rise to paired, segmentally organized buds from the cervical to the sacral region. The pronephros is initially formed early in the 4th week in the cervical region.

15

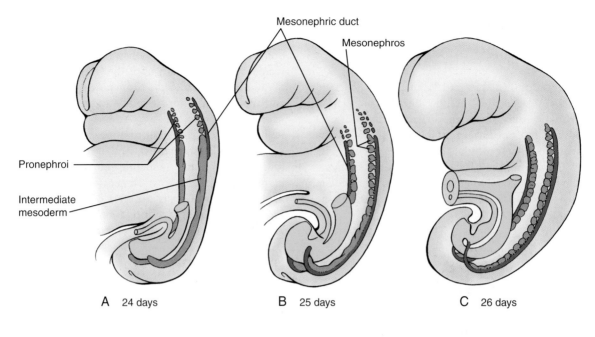

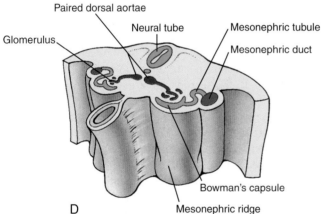

Figure 15-2. Development of the pronephros and mesonephros. *A*, A pair of pronephroi form along the fifth to seventh cervical segments, but these quickly degenerate during the 4th week. The mesonephric ducts first appear on day 24. *B, C*, Mesonephric tubules form in craniocaudal sequence throughout the thoracic and lumbar regions. The more cranial pairs regress as caudal pairs form, and the definitive mesonephroi contain about 20 pairs, confined to the first three lumbar segments. *D*, The mesonephroi contain functional nephric units consisting of glomeruli, Bowman's capsules, mesonephric tubules, and mesonephric ducts.

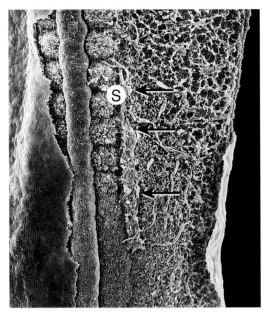

Figure 15-3. Scanning electron micrograph showing a growing mesonephric duct (arrows) just adjacent to the somites (S) on one side of an embryo. The duct is elongating in a cranial-to-caudal direction.

duct induces the evagination of the ureteric bud (see Fig. 15-4).

Development of Mesonephros

Early in the 4th week, mesonephric tubules begin to develop within intermediate mesoderm adjacent the mesonephric duct on either side of the vertebral column, from the upper thoracic region to the third lumbar level (see Fig. 15-2B, C). About 40 **mesonephric tubules** are produced in craniocaudal succession; thus, several form in each segment. Because the gonads begin developing just medial to the mesonephric ridge, this region is sometimes collectively referred to as the **urogenital ridge**. As the more caudal tubules differentiate, the more cranial ones regress, so there are never more than about 30 pairs in the mesonephroi. By the end of the 5th week, the cranial regions of the mesonephroi undergo massive regression, leaving only about 20 pairs of tubules occupying the first three lumbar levels. The mesonephric tubules differentiate into excretory units resembling an abbreviated version of the adult metanephric nephron (see Fig. 15-2D; discussed later) with the medial end of the tubule forming a cup-shaped sac, called a **Bowman's capsule**, which wraps around a knot of capillaries called a **glomerulus** to form a **renal corpuscle**.

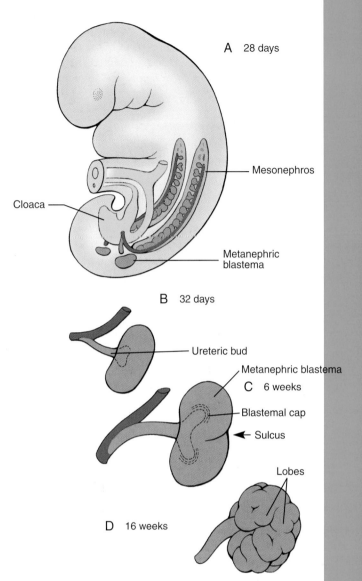

Figure 15-4. Origin of the metanephric kidneys. *A*, A metanephric blastema develops from intermediate mesoderm on each side of the body axis early in the 5th week. *B*, Simultaneously, each mesonephric duct sprouts a ureteric bud that grows into each metanephric blastema. *C*, By the 6th week, the ureteric bud bifurcates and the two growing tips (ampullae) induce cranial and caudal lobes in the metanephros. *D*, Additional lobules form during the next 10 weeks in response to further bifurcation of the ureteric buds.

The lateral tip of each developing mesonephric tubule fuses with the mesonephric duct, thus opening a passage from the excretory units to the cloaca. The mesonephric excretory units are functional between about 6 and 10 weeks and produce small amounts of urine. After 10 weeks, they cease to function and then

15

regress. As discussed later, the mesonephric ducts also regress in the female. However, in the male the mesonephric ducts, plus a few modified mesonephric tubules, persist and form important elements of the male genital duct system.

FORMATION OF NEPHRIC LINEAGE

Few genes have been found, thus far, that affect the initial specification of nephric development. One of the earliest genes expressed in the nephrogenic intermediate mesoderm is *Pax2*. Mice deficient in *Pax2* still form a mesonephric duct in the pronephric and mesonephric regions, but the mesonephric ducts fail to extend into metanephric region. Therefore, the metanephric kidney does not develop (because it is dependent on branching from the lower mesonephric duct). When double knockout mice for *Pax2* and *Pax8* (another *Pax* family member expressed in the intermediate mesoderm) are generated, the intermediate mesoderm does not form any portion of the mesonephric duct or express the nephric markers *Lim1* and *Ret* (both required for subsequent metanephric kidney development). Apparently, in the absence of these two *Pax* genes, many of the pronephric and mesonephric progenitor cells within the intermediate mesodermal cells undergo apoptosis. *Pax2* expression is a particularly potent initiator of nephron development: ectopic nephric structures can be induced almost anywhere within the intermediate mesoderm, including the gonadal ridge of chick embryos, when *Pax2* is ectopically expressed by viral transfection of mesoderm at the midprimitive streak stage. Hence, *Pax2* expression is able to specify a nephric lineage in almost any intermediate mesodermal derivative.

What tissue interactions are responsible for inducing the nephric lineage within intermediate mesoderm is unclear, but this lineage seems to depend on the somitic field because *Pax2* and *Lim1* expression is lost in chick embryos if the intermediate mesoderm is separated from the somites. Moreover, one can induce ectopic pronephric tissue within the intermediate and lateral plate mesoderm by grafting somites into ectopic locations. Ectoderm may also have a role in specifying or maintaining nephric capacity within intermediate mesoderm, as removal of the overlying ectoderm decreases the expression of *Pax2*, *Lim1*, and *Sim1* (another marker of nephrogenic mesoderm) within the intermediate mesoderm and this mesoderm loses its nephrogenic capacity. Therefore, secreted factors from adjacent tissues are needed to induce and maintain nephrogenic mesoderm.

Development of Metanephros

The definitive kidneys, or **metanephroi**, are composed of two functional components, the excretory portion and the collecting portion. These two portions are derived from different sources of intermediate mesoderm (Table 15-1). Development of the metanephric kidney involves epithelial tube formation and elongation, tubular branching, cell condensation, mesenchymal-to-epithelial conversion, angiogenesis, and the specification and differentiation of numerous specialized cell types.

Formation of the metanephros kidney begins with the induction and formation of a pair of new structures, the **ureteric buds**, within the intermediate mesoderm of the sacral region. Ureteric buds sprout from the distal portion of the mesonephric ducts on about day 28 (see Fig. 15-4A). By day 32, each ureteric bud penetrates a portion of the sacral intermediate mesoderm called the **metanephric blastema**, and the bud begins to bifurcate (see Fig. 15-4B). As the ureteric bud branches, each new growing tip (called an **ampulla**) acquires a caplike aggregate of metanephric blastemal tissue, giving the metanephros a lobulated appearance. By the middle of the 6th week, the developing metanephros consists of two lobes separated by a sulcus. By the end of the 16th week, 14 to 16 lobes have formed (see Fig. 15-4C, D). Morphologic evidence of the initial branching of the ureteric bud is eventually obscured as the sulci between the lobes are filled in.

The ureters and the collecting duct system of the kidneys differentiate from the ureteric bud; the **nephrons** (the definitive urine-forming units of the kidneys) differentiate from the metanephric blastema. Like the nephrons and mesonephric duct of the mesonephric kidney, the differentiation of each of these primordia depends on inductive signals from one another (see the following "In the Research Lab").

Table 15-1 Structures Composing the Collecting and Excretory Portions of the Metanephric Kidney

Collecting Portion (Ureteric Bud)	Excretory Portion (or Nephron) (Metanephric Blastema)
Ureter	Bowman's capsule
Renal pelvis	Proximal convoluted tubule
Major and minor calyces	Loop of Henle
Collecting ducts	Distal convoluted tubule
Collecting tubules	

Specifically, the metanephric mesenchyme induces the ureteric bud to grow and branch to form the **collecting ducts** and **tubules**, whereas the tips of the ureteric buds induce the mesenchyme to condense and convert into an epithelial vesicle (Fig. 15-5). Several hours of direct contact with a ureteric bud ampulla are required to induce nephron differentiation in blastema tissue. If the ureteric bud is abnormal or missing, the kidney does not develop. Conversely, **reciprocal inductive signals** from the metanephric blastema regulate the orderly branching and growth of the bifurcating tips of the ureteric buds. The number of nephrons formed ultimately depends on growth and branching of the ureteric bud, formation of mesenchymal condensations, and conversion to epithelial tubules.

In the mature kidney, urine produced by the nephrons flows through a collecting system consisting of collecting tubules, collecting ducts, minor calyces, major calyces, the renal pelvis and, finally, the ureter. This system is entirely the product of the ureteric bud. The ureteric bud undergoes an exact sequence of bifurcations (Fig. 15-6), and the expanded major and minor calyces arise through phases of intussusception in which previously formed branches coalesce.

When the ureteric bud first contacts the metanephric blastema, its tip expands to form an initial ampulla that will give rise to the **renal pelvis**. During the 6th week, the ureteric bud bifurcates four times, yielding 16 branches. These branches then coalesce to form two to four **major calyces** extending from the renal pelvis.

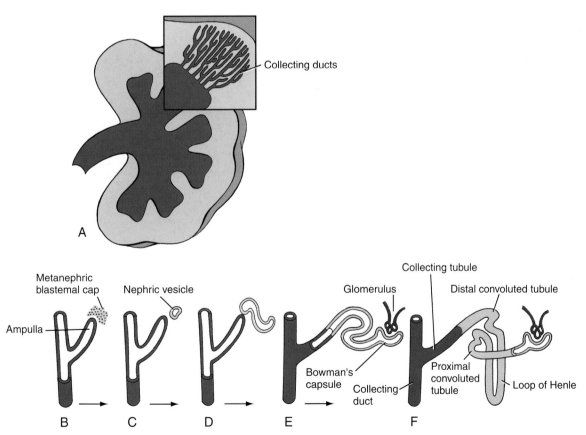

Figure 15-5. Development of the renal collecting system and nephrons. *A*, The ureteric buds continue to bifurcate until the 32nd week, producing 1 to 3 million collecting tubules and ducts. *B-F*, The tip of each collecting tubule induces the development of a metanephric blastemal cap, which differentiates into a nephric vesicle. This vesicle ultimately forms a Bowman's capsule and the proximal and distal convoluted tubules and loops of Henle. Functional nephric units (of the type shown in *E*) first appear in distal regions of the metanephros at 10 weeks.

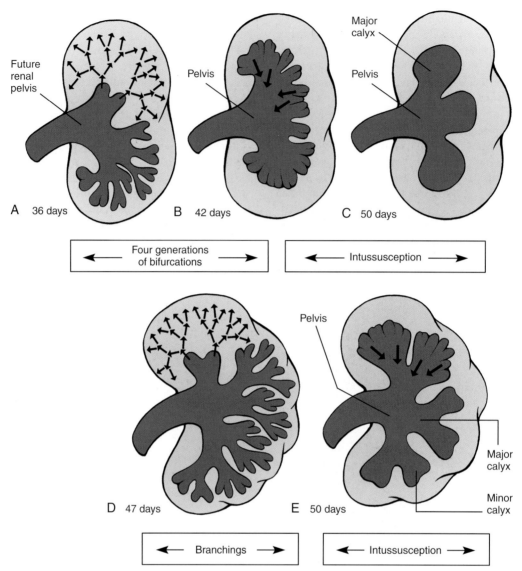

Figure 15-6. Development of the renal pelvis and calyces. *A–C,* The first bifurcation of the ureteric bud forms the renal pelvis, and the coalescence of the next 4 generations of bifurcations produces the major calyces. *D, E,* The next 4 generations of bifurcation coalescese to form the minor calyces of the renal collecting system.

By the 7th week, the next four generations of branches also coalesce, forming the **minor calyces**. By 32 weeks, approximately 11 additional generations of bifurcation have formed 1 to 3 million branches, which will become the future collecting tubules and ducts of the kidney (see Fig. 15-5A). The definitive morphology of the collecting ducts is created by variations in the pattern of branching and by a tendency for distal branches to elongate.

Each nephron originates as an epithelial (nephric) vesicle within the blastemic cap surrounding the ampulla of a collecting tubule (see Fig. 15-5B). Formation of nephron involves several stages (see Fig. 15-5B-F). First, the nephric vesicle develops into a comma-shaped structure and then forms an S-shaped tubule. The S-shaped tubule fuses with the ureteric duct, and eventually the two lumina become continuous forming the so-called uniferous tubule. Meanwhile, the renal corpuscle segment of the nephric tubule forms the outer (parietal) layer of Bowman's capsule and glomerular epithelial cells (**podocytes**) that surround the glomerular tuft of capillaries forming within the adjacent stroma. While the renal corpuscle is forming, the lengthening nephric tubule forms the remaining elements of the nephron: the proximal convoluted tubule, descending and ascending limbs of the loop of Henle, and distal convoluted tubule. The definitive nephron with its renal corpuscle is also called a **metanephric excretory unit**. The medulla of the kidney also begins to take shape as the growing nephron tubules and interstitial tissue develops. **Nephrogenesis** is complete by birth in humans.

Morphogenesis of the renal vascular supply during the development of the nephron and collecting systems is poorly understood. Organ cultures and interspecies grafting experiments show that angiogenesis is likely the major mechanism responsible for the development of the renal vasculature, including the glomerular capillaries. However, the prevascular metanephric mesenchyme expresses vasculogenic markers (e.g., *Vegf*, *Vegfr*, *Tie2*), and if fetal mouse kidney tissue is grafted into the mouse anterior eye chamber, this tissue can form capillaries within the graft, suggesting that it has vasculogenic capacity.

During the 10th week, the tips of the distal convoluted tubules begin connecting to the collecting tubules, and the metanephroi become functional. Blood plasma from the glomerular capillaries is filtered in the renal corpuscle to produce a dilute glomerular filtrate, which is concentrated and converted to urine by the activities of the convoluted tubules and the loop of Henle. The urine passes down the collecting system into the ureters and thence into the bladder. Even though the fetal kidneys produce urine throughout the remainder of gestation, their main function is not to clear waste products out of the blood—that task is handled principally by the placenta. Instead, fetal urine is important because it supplements the production of amniotic fluid. Fetuses with **bilateral renal agenesis** (complete absence of both kidneys) do not make enough amniotic fluid (**oligohydramnios**) and hence are confined to an abnormally small amniotic space. This results in a condition called **Potter sequence** (described in the following "In the Clinic").

Figure 15-7 shows the structure of the definitive fetal kidney. This architecture reflects the events of the first 10 weeks of renal development, that is, in

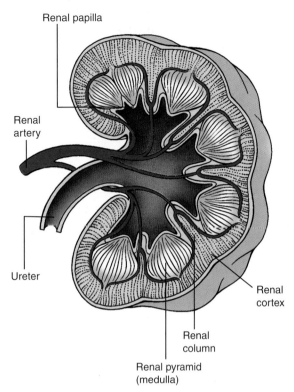

Figure 15-7. The definitive renal architecture of the metanephros is apparent by the 10th week.

weeks 5 to 15 of development. The kidney is divided into an inner medulla and an outer cortex. The cortical tissue contains the nephrons, whereas the medulla contains collecting ducts and loops of Henle. Each minor calyx drains a tree of collecting ducts within a **renal pyramid**, which converge to form the **renal papilla**. The renal pyramids of the kidney are separated by zones of nephron-containing cortical tissue called **renal columns** or **columns of Bertin**. Thus, in the definitive kidney, the cortical tissue not only covers the outside of the kidney, but it also forms piers projecting toward the pelvis. Nevertheless, nephrons in the cortical tissue all arise from cortical regions of the primary lobes of the metanephric blastema.

The autonomic nervous system of the kidney, which regulates blood flow and secretory function, arises from neural crest cells that invade the metanephroi early in their development. Further aspects of the development of the autonomic nervous system of the abdomen and pelvis are discussed in Chapter 10.

IN THE RESEARCH LAB

FACTORS EXPRESSED IN METANEPHRIC MESODERM REGULATE INDUCTION OF BUDDING AND BRANCHING OF THE URETERIC BUD

What induces the formation of the ureteric bud and specifies its location along the mesonephric duct? It seems that both the induction and location of the ureteric bud largely depends on the nephrogenic mesenchyme of the intermediate mesoderm. Formation of ureteric bud from the mesonephric duct is induced by signals emanating from the adjacent mesoderm and involves the *Ret* receptor, its coreceptor, *Gfrα*, and its ligand, *Gdnf*. *Ret* and *Gfrα* are expressed within the mesonephric duct, whereas the ligand, *Gdnf*, is found within the metanephric mesenchyme (Fig. 15-8). Misexpression of *Gdnf* elsewhere within the intermediate mesoderm is sufficient to induce ectopic ureteric buds, and mice deficient in either *Ret* or *Gdnf* exhibit bilateral renal agenesis. Therefore, faults in the tissue-tissue interactions between the metanephric mesoderm and mesonephric duct mediated through *Ret* signaling may be responsible for formation of duplex kidneys or for renal agenesis.

Experiments suggest that the cranial-caudal positioning of ureteric bud formation may be the result of a repression of nephrogenic determinants within the more cranial regions of the intermediate mesoderm. *Forkhead* genes are one group of transcription factors that seem to be involved. *Foxc1* and *Foxc2* expression is normally restricted to the cranial end of nephrogenic mesoderm. When *Foxc1* is knocked out in mice or *Foxc1/Foxc2* null heterozygotes are generated, ectopic ureteric buds form over a broad span of the mesonephric duct. A similar phenotype is seen in mice deficient in *Slit2*, or its receptor, *Robo2* (pathfinding signaling molecules; discussed further in Ch. 10). *Foxc1/Foxc2* and *Slit2/Robo2* may repress *Gdnf* expression in the more cranial regions, because *Slit2* expression occurs in a cranial-caudal gradient within the mesenchyme that is the inverse of that of *Gdnf* expression.

Bmp4 is another extracellular signaling molecule implicated in restricting ureteric bud development. *Bmp4*-deficient mice develop ectopic ureteric buds and double ureters. *Bmp4* is normally expressed in the mesoderm surrounding the mesonephric duct and ureteric buds but not in the mesonephric duct itself. Experiments suggest that *Bmp4* inhibits *Ret* signaling within the mesonephric duct, rather than altering *Gdnf* levels released from the mesoderm, because *Bmp4* can block the effect of ectopic *Gdnf* on ureteric bud formation in metanephric organ cultures.

Other factors important in the formation and budding of the ureteric bud are *Eya1* (discussed further in Ch. 17) and the *Hox11* group of homeotic genes. Mutants deficient in these genes fail to turn on *Gdnf* and do not develop ureteric buds. Hence, the induction and position of the ureteric bud seem to depend on a balance between mesodermally mediated activation and negative regulation of *Ret* signaling within the mesonephric duct. Several malformations can arise if the ureteric buds sprout from incorrect sites along the mesonephric duct, as the resulting ureters will be incorrectly emplaced into the dorsal wall of the developing bladder.

SIGNALS FROM URETERIC BUD INDUCE NEPHROGENIC MESODERM TO CONDENSE WHILE MESODERM DRIVES CONTINUAL URETERIC BRANCHING AND GROWTH

As the ureteric bud grows and branches into metanephric mesoderm, it induces the adjacent mesenchyme to condense around the tips of the ureteric branches. These condensations serve as the primordia of the nephrons. However, reciprocal signaling from the metanephric mesenchyme is necessary for the continual expansion and branching of ureteric buds to form the ureter, calyces, and collecting tubules and ducts.

One of the first genes identified as important in ureteric bud branching in humans was the **WT1 (WILMS TUMOR SUPPRESSOR 1)** gene (not to be confused with *Wnt1*, a *Wingless* family member). Mutations in *WT1* are associated with several renal and gonadal malformations and are the most common cause (although rare) of children's kidney tumors. **Wilms tumors** (nephroblastoma) affect about 1:10,000 children. Inactivating mutations in the tumor suppressor gene, *WT1*, are responsible for 10% to 15% of these neoplasms. Tumors are typically diagnosed in children at 3 or 4 years of age and, fortunately, can be treated chemotherapeutically, with a cure rate of about 80% to 90%. *WT1* is encoded on human chromosome 11p13, and mutations in *WT1* lead to malformations of the urinary and genital systems.

WT1 is essential for normal urogenital development. *WT1* is upregulated in the metanephric mesenchyme as it condenses, and it continues to be expressed during the mesenchymal-to-epithelial transition responsible for forming the nephric epithelial vesicles. Mice lacking the *Wt1* gene fail to induce ureteric buds even though *Gdnf* is still expressed within the metanephric mesenchymal cap, suggesting that *Wt1* operates independently of *Gdnf* signaling. Closer examination of *Wt1* knockout mice reveals that waves of apoptosis occur within the metanephric mesenchyme, beginning about the time the mesenchyme begins to condense. Although the precise role for *Wt1* in renal development is still unclear, it may make the mesenchymal population receptive to ureteric

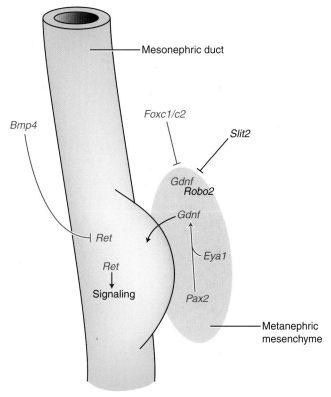

Figure 15-8. Positioning of ureteric bud formation is mediated by *Ret* signaling. Expression of *Ret* within the mesonephric duct epithelium is restricted to caudal portions of the duct by *Bmp4* released from cranial urogenital ridge mesenchyme. Mesenchymal expression of the *Ret* ligand, *Gdnf*, requires *Pax2* expression in the urogenital ridge but is restricted to the metanephric region by the cranial expression of *Foxc1*, *Foxc2*, and *Slit2* in the mesenchyme. The receptor for *Slit2* and *Robo2* is expressed in the urogenital ridge mesenchyme.

bud induction signals that are necessary for maintaining the mesenchymal population. Therefore, the inability to maintain a condensing mesenchymal cap adjacent the ureteric buds may be the reason for failed ureteric bud growth and branching.

Another factor necessary for maintaining the population of condensing mesenchyme is the *Wingless* family member *Wnt4*. *Wnt4* is expressed within the early condensing blastemal mesenchyme. In organ cultures, *Wnt4* can induce nephron differentiation in the absence of ureteric bud epithelium. *Emx2* (*Empty spiracles homolog-2*) knockout mice (a transcription factor expressed in the ureteric bud) fail to activate *Wnt4* expression within metanephric mesenchymal condensations. In these mice, although the ureteric bud forms and begins invading the metanephric mesenchymal, it does not branch, apparently due to apoptotic death of *Wnt4*-dependent

adjacent mesenchyme. Therefore, initiation and maintenance of *Wnt4* expression in the metanephric mesenchymal cap is also required for nephron differentiation.

So what does the ureteric bud release that mediates *Wnt4* expression in the mesenchyme? Recent evidence suggests that it is *Wnt9b* (Fig. 15-9). In mice deficient in *Wnt9b*, the ureteric bud undergoes an initial branching but the mesenchyme fails to condense, resulting in renal agenesis. *Wnt9b* is expressed by ureteric buds, and in explant cultures, *Wnt9b* can substitute for the ureteric bud in promoting nephrogenesis. Several *Frizzled* family members (*Wnt* receptors) are also expressed in metanephric mesenchymal. However, their role in mediating *Wnt* signaling during renal development is still unclear. Collectively, these observations are consistent with the idea that interactions between the ureteric bud and metanephric mesenchyme are mediated in

15

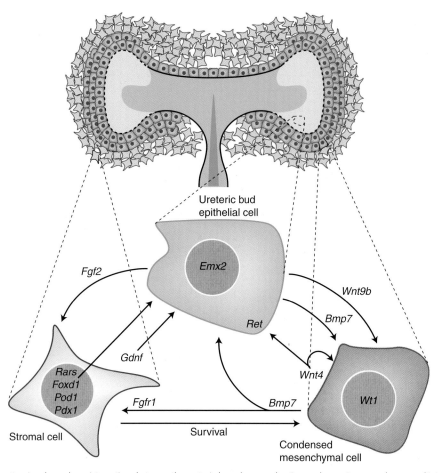

Figure 15-9. Kidney patterning depends on interactions between the ureteric branches, condensing nephrogenic mesenchyme, and interstitial stromal cells. *Wt1* expression is upregulated in the metanephric mesenchyme, making the mesenchyme receptive to ureteric bud induction. *Wnt4* released by the condensed mesenchyme induces continual ureteric bud branching and growth. *Wnt9b*, expressed by ureteric buds, promotes Wnt4 expression within the condensing mesenchyme; *Wnt4* is necessary for maintaining the survival of this mesenchyme and for subsequent nephron differentiation. Stromal cells express *Foxd1*, *Pod1*, and *Pdx1* and the retinoic acid receptors, *RARα* and *RARβ2*, necessary for balancing stromal and nephron progenitor specification and survival. The growth factors *Fgf2* and *Bmp* promote stromal cell differentiation at the expense of the nephron mesenchymal population. Moreover, retinoic acid signaling in stromal cells is required for maintaining *Ret* expression in the ureteric buds.

part by *Wnt* signaling, and that this signaling is essential for maintaining the mesodermal cap.

Kidney developmental patterning not only depends on interactions between the ureteric branches and condensing nephrogenic mesenchyme but also involves interactions with the interstitial stromal cells surrounding the condensing mesenchyme (see Fig. 15-9). Stromal cells specifically express *Foxd1* (also called *Bf2*), *Pod1*, and *Pdx1*. Mice with null

mutations for these genes develop small and dysmorphic kidneys with nephron and branching defects. All three knockout mice ectopically express *Ret* along the entire ureteric epithelium rather than just at the ureteric tips (i.e., ampullae). This expanded *Ret* expression may be responsible for the branching defects seen in these mice, as similar defects are generated when *Ret* is misexpressed. Studies suggest that *Foxd1*, *Pod1*, and *Pdx1* may also regulate the balance between stromal and nephron progenitor specification. For instance in mouse metanephric explant cultures, the stromal-promoting growth factors, *Fgf2* and *Bmp7*, increase the number of *Foxd1*-positive cells at the expense of the nephron population.

Another stromal signaling factor important in kidney patterning is retinoic acid. The *Retinoic acid receptors, Rarα* and *Rarβ2*, are expressed exclusively within the stromal compartment of the developing kidney (see Fig. 15-9). In mouse embryos deficient in both the *Rarα* and *Rarβ2*, the expression of *Ret* is not initiated in the tips of ureteric buds, resulting in renal agenesis. Moreover, these receptor-deficient mice exhibit ectopic expression of *Foxd1*, *Pod1*, and *Pbx1* within the ureteric epithelium. Interestingly, normal renal development can be rescued if *Ret* expression is restored in the mice. Because *Rarα*, *Rarβ2*, *Foxd1*, *Pod1*, and *Pbx1* are all normally expressed exclusively within the stromal compartment, these experiments imply essential signals influencing ureteric bud *Ret* expression emanate from the stroma.

INFLUENCES BETWEEN URETERIC BUD AND METANEPHRIC BLASTEMA INDUCE FORMATION OF NEPHRON THROUGH MESENCHYMAL-TO-EPITHELIAL CONVERSION OF BLASTEMA

The mesenchyme adjacent the tip of the branching ureteric bud is surrounded by extracellular matrix that rapidly changes in composition in response to inductive influences of the ureteric bud. The interaction of the mesenchyme with ureteric bud not only induces the transformation of mesenchymal cap into an epithelium but also rescues the adjacent mesenchyme from apoptosis. Initially, the mesenchyme adjacent the bud is surrounded by extracellular matrix containing interstitial *Collagens* (type I and type III), *Fibronectin*, and *Syndecans*. However, with induction, *Collagen type I* and *type III* are replaced by *Collagen type IV*, *Fibronectin* is replaced by *Laminin*, and the mesenchyme begins expressing *Heparan sulfate proteoglycans*. As the condensing mesenchyme forms, it increases its expression of *Ncam*, *Cadherin-11*, and *Syndecan-1* (as well as *Wnt4*), but these begin to disappear as *R-Cadherin*, *Cadherin-6*, and then *E-Cadherin* levels increase and the mesenchyme begins to take on the organization of an epithelium. Concurrent with the changes leading to cell polarization and epithelial formation is an upregulation of *Integrin α6* and *α8* expression.

What is responsible for driving the conversion from a mesenchyme to an epithelium is unclear but as discussed earlier, ureteric bud–induced expression of *Wnt4* is required. During the condensation phase, *Wnt4* expression increases and is maintained as the mesenchyme is converted into a comma-shaped epithelium and then an S-shaped epithelium. If *Wnt4* is knocked out in mice, the mesenchyme begins condensing, but rather than organizing into an epithelium, it undergoes apoptosis. Tissue culture experiments show that *Wnt4* is also necessary for epithelial conversion and not the condensation step. *Cadherin* switching plays an important role in establishing epithelial cell polarity. Intracellularly, *Cadherins* interact with the cytoskeleton through a network of *α-, β-,* and *γ-Catenins*. As cells switch toward *Cadherin* types associated with organizing an epithelium, *β-Catenin* becomes localized to lateral cell surfaces. Therefore, in addition to mediating *β-Catenin* transcriptional activity, *Wnt* signaling within the nephrogenic mesenchyme likely alters *Cadherin* activity necessary for the mesenchymal-to-epithelial conversion.

IN THE CLINIC

RENAL AGENESIS AND DYSPLASIA

Kidneys may fail to develop on one or both sides due to faulty tissue-tissue interactions between the ureteric bud and nephrogenic and stromal mesenchyme. Infants with **bilateral renal agenesis** are stillborn or die within a few days of birth. In contrast, infants with **unilateral renal agenesis** usually live because the remaining kidney undergoes compensatory hypertrophy. Although the relative frequencies of unilateral and bilateral renal agenesis are difficult to determine because unilateral renal agenesis often goes undetected, autopsy data suggest that unilateral renal agenesis is about four to eight times more common than bilateral renal agenesis.

Renal agenesis is typically associated with other congenital defects. The kidneys contribute to the production of amniotic fluid. Therefore, bilateral renal agenesis results in **oligohydramnios**, or insufficient amniotic fluid (also discussed in Ch. 6). Oligohydramnios can result in a spectrum of abnormalities called **Potter sequence**. These include deformed limbs; wrinkly, dry skin; and an abnormal facies (in this context, *facies* means "facial appearance") consisting of wide-set eyes with infraorbital skin creases, beak nose, recessed chin, and low-set ears.

15

Renal agenesis is often associated with a spectrum of ipsilateral genitourinary abnormalities, including defects in structures derived from the mesonephric duct in males and Müllerian duct in females. Failure of mesonephric duct development leads to absence of both the vas deferens and kidney, because the kidney develops from an outgrowth of this duct, which in the male is the progenitor of the vas deferens (discussed later). This can occur bilaterally or unilaterally.

Abnormal kidneys may arise from abnormal inductive interactions. In some cases, subtle defects in the interaction between ureteric bud and metanephric blastema result in hypoplasia or dysplasia of the developing kidney. The small number of nephrons in a hypoplastic kidney results either from inadequate branching of the ureteric bud or from an inadequate response by the metanephric cap tissue. In cases of renal dysplasia, the nephrons themselves develop abnormally and consist of primitive ducts lined by undifferentiated epithelium sheathed within thick layers of connective tissue. The genetic causes for some of these renal anomalies are beginning to be identified. Mutations in *PAX2* are associated with dominant transmission of renal hypoplasia and dysplasia (seen in **renal-coloboma syndrome**). Mutations in *EYA1* (a transcription factor required for *GDNF* expression and, hence, ureteric bud development) and *SIX1* (*SINE OCULIS HOMEOBOX HOMOLOG 1*; a transcription factor that interacts with *EYA1*) causes **BOR (branchio-oto-renal) syndrome** (discussed in the "Clinical Taster" for Ch. 17). In addition to renal anomalies, *EYA1* haploinsufficient individuals also develop pharyngeal cleft cysts and have both outer and inner ear defects.

MUTATIONS CAUSING NEPHRON PATHOLOGIES

The glomerular and tubular systems of the nephron are composed of highly specialized cell types responsible for waste secretion. Initial filtration occurs between capillary and podocyte cells at the glomerulus. Defects in podocyte foot processes surrounding capillaries and defects in the basement membrane separating the two usually result in excessive protein loss into the urine (**proteinuria**).

In animal models, mutations in several genes and gene targets have been identified that are associated with deficient glomerular formation and function. *Pdgfs* and their receptors have an important role in renal corpuscle development. Initially, *Pdgf* and *Pdgf receptors* are expressed throughout the nephronic mesenchyme, stromal cells, and vascular cells but later become restricted to the intraglomerular **mesangial cells** (essential pericytes of glomerular capillaries). If either the *Pdgfb* ligand or *Pdgfrβ* receptor is knocked out in mice, the glomeruli lack mesangial cells and fail to form normal capillary tufts. Glomerular formation is initiated and the endothelial and podocyte lineages are present: they just do not organize properly in the absence of mesangial cells.

Mice lacking the gene encoding *Integrin α3* exhibit severe kidney anomalies resulting in defects in the later stages of nephrogenesis. Although the number of nephrons formed is the same as in wild-type mice, the capillary beds surrounding the proximal convoluted tubules are abnormal, the glomerular basement membrane is disorganized, and the podocytes fail to form foot processes.

Post-transcriptional modifications of *Wt1* mRNA lead to the production of up to 24 different isoforms of *Wt1* as a result of alternative mRNA splicing, the presence of multiple start codons, or RNA editing. Alterations in the ratio of two alternative splice variants of the *Wt1* gene—*Wt1(-Kts)* and *Wt1(+Kts)*, each of which having a different DNA binding site and different transcriptional activity—can lead to abnormal glomerular development. For instance, a heterozygous point mutation causing a decrease in levels of *WT1(+KTS)* is associated with **Frasier syndrome**. These patients develop **renal mesangial sclerosis** (abnormal thickening of the glomerular basement membrane and mesangial extracellular matrix) with progressive renal failure and streaked gonads (*WT1* has a key role in early gonadal development, as discussed later in the chapter; streaked, also called streak, gonads are undeveloped) in addition to Wilms tumors.

Heterozygous mutations in *WT1* are also linked to **Denys-Drash syndrome**. These patients exhibit genitourinary malformations including sexual ambiguity as well as podocytic underdevelopment and glomerular nephropathy caused by diffuse mesangial sclerosis leading to end-stage renal failure. In this case, the mutation is restricted to the *WT1* locus whereby a missense mutation results in the replacement of arginine for tryptophan at residue 394 in the zinc-finger domain of the WT1 protein. Other mutations occurring within this zinc finger domain have also been identified in children with Denys-Drash syndrome. In adults, WT1 expression in the kidney is restricted to glomerular podocytes. WT1 regulates *PODOCALYXIN*, an integral membrane protein connected to the cytoskeleton of podocytes and thought to maintain podocyte three-dimensional shape. Mutations in the *WT1* gene cause glomerulopathy-associated syndromes like Denys-Drash and Frasier, possibly by misregulating PODOCALYXIN expression.

Abnormalities of the eyes and brain may also occur in patients with Wilms' tumor, but these anomalies may be explained by the disruption of other genes located in close proximity to the mutated *WT1* gene on chromosome 11. For example, the **WAGR syndrome** is characterized by Wilms tumor, aniridia, genital abnormalities, and mental retardation. **Aniridia** refers to the absence of the iris of the eye. In this syndrome, aniridia is caused by a hemizygous deletion of the *PAX6* transcription factor. In contrast, the genitourinary malformations are caused by a hemizygous deletion of the *WT1* gene.

Human mutations in the genes coding for NEPHRIN (*NPHS1*, a podocyte membrane slit protein) or PODOCIN (*NPHS2*), or the loss of COLLAGEN TYPE IV in the basement membrane (as seen in Alport syndrome), can all lead to defects in glomerular function in humans. In mice, the *Kriesler* gene (or *MafB*) mediates glomerular *Nephrin* and *Podocin* expression levels and is required for normal podocyte development. *Kriesler* mutant mice exhibit glomerular defects and proteinuria.

Mutations in the *LMX1B* gene are responsible for **nail-patella syndrome**, which is characterized by skeletal anomalies and glomerular dysfunction. LMXB1 expression is involved in transcriptional regulation of *COLLAGEN TYPE α3(IV)* (or GOODPASTURE ANTIGEN), *COLLAGEN TYPE α4(IV)*, and *NPHS2* genes; it thus links together nail-patella syndrome, Alport, and congenital nephritic syndrome (caused by mutation in the *NPHS1* gene).

CONGENITAL POLYCYSTIC KIDNEY DISEASE

Autosomal dominant polycystic kidney disease (**ADPKD**) is a common genetic disease associated with formation of cysts in the kidneys as well as in ductal epithelia in the liver, pancreas, testis, and ovary. Mutations in the genes encoding *POLYCYSTIN1* (*PDK1*) and *POLYCYSTIN2* (*PDK2*) account for 85% and 15% of ADPKD, respectively. The precise roles of the *POLYCYSTIN1* and *POLYCYSTIN2* proteins have not yet been elucidated. However, *POLYCYSTIN1* seems to be required for normal elongation and maturation of tubular structures during renal development. It may also function as a mechanosensory channel in primary cilia. These functions may be related to *PDK1*'s ability to modulate *Wnt* signaling by stabilizing endogenous *β-Catenin* levels and altering *β-Catenin/Tcf*-dependent gene expression.

Autosomal recessive polycystic kidney disease (**ARPKD**) is associated with genes involved in mediating ciliary function. ARPKD is caused by mutations in the *PKHD1* gene, which encodes the protein POLYDUCTIN (also called FIBROCYSTIN). This protein is necessary for the proper assembly and function of cilia. Patients in whom the gene is mutated slowly develop renal, hepatic, and biliary cysts. Mutations in *HNFβ1* and *TG737/POLARIS*, two other genes with ties to ciliary assembly and function, are also associated with polycystic kidney disease. What role cilia have in maintaining normal renal, hepatic, and biliary structures is unknown.

Ascent of Kidneys

Between the 6th and 9th weeks, the kidneys ascend to a lumbar site just below the suprarenal glands, following a path just on either side of the dorsal aorta (Fig. 15-10). The mechanism responsible for this ascent is not understood, although the differential growth of the lumbar and sacral regions of the embryo may play a role. As described in Chapter 13, the ascending kidney is progressively revascularized by a series of arterial sprouts from the dorsal aorta (see Fig. 13-20), and the original renal artery in the sacral region disappears.

Several anomalies can arise from variations in this process of ascent. Occasionally, one or more of the transient inferior renal arteries fails to regress, resulting in the presence of **accessory renal arteries**. Rarely, a kidney completely fails to ascend, remaining as a **pelvic kidney** (see Fig. 15-10*C*). The inferior poles of the two metanephroi may fuse during the ascent, forming a U-shaped **horseshoe kidney** that crosses over the anterior (ventral) side of the aorta. During ascent, this kidney becomes caught under the inferior mesenteric artery and, therefore, does not reach its normal site (see Fig. 15-10*D*). The right kidney usually does not rise as high as the left kidney because of the presence of the liver on the right side, although this is not always the case.

Contributions of Hindgut Endoderm to Urinary Tract

As discussed in Chapter 14, the cloacal region of the hindgut is partitioned by the urorectal septum into a ventral **urogenital sinus** and a dorsal **anorectal canal** (Fig. 15-11; see also Fig. 14-32). The urogenital sinus consists of an expanded cranial presumptive **bladder**, a narrow neck that becomes the **pelvic urethra**, and a **phallic segment** that expands beneath the growing **genital tubercle** (see Fig 15-11). In males, the pelvic urethra becomes the **membranous** and **prostatic urethra**, and the phallic segment

15

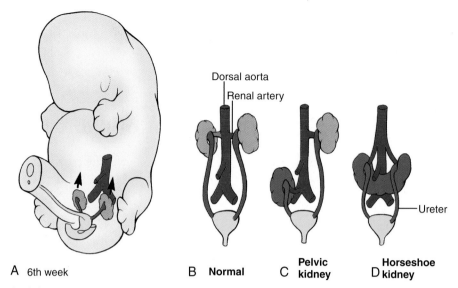

A 6th week   **B** **Normal**   **C** **Pelvic kidney**   **D** **Horseshoe kidney**

Figure 15-10. Normal and abnormal ascent of the kidneys. *A, B,* The metanephroi normally ascend from the sacral region to their definitive lumbar position between the 6th and 9th weeks. *C,* Infrequently, a kidney may fail to ascend, resulting in a pelvic kidney. *D,* If the inferior poles of the metanephroi make contact and fuse before ascent, the resulting horseshoe kidney catches under the inferior mesenteric artery.

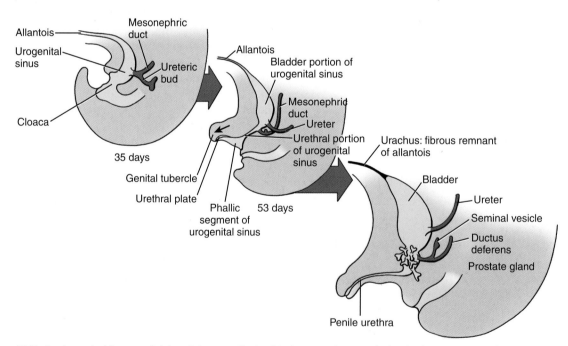

Figure 15-11. Development of the urogenital sinus. Between weeks 4 and 6, the urorectal septum divides the cloaca into a ventral urogenital sinus and a dorsal anorectum. The superior part of the urogenital sinus, continuous with the allantois, forms the bladder. The constricted pelvic urethra at the base of the future bladder forms the membranous urethra in females, and the membranous and prostatic urethra in males. The distal expansion of the urogenital sinus forms the vestibule of the vagina in females, and the penile urethra in males.

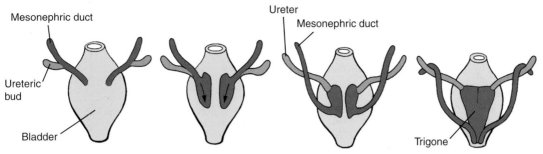

Figure 15-12. Exstrophy of the mesonephric ducts and ureters into the bladder wall. Between weeks 4 and 6, the root of the mesonephric duct exstrophies into the posterior wall of the developing bladder. This process brings the openings of the ureteric buds into the bladder wall, whereas the opening of the mesonephric duct is carried inferiorly to the level of the pelvic urethra. The triangular region of exstrophied mesonephric duct incorporated into the posterior bladder wall forms the trigone of the bladder.

contributes to the **penile urethra**. In females, the pelvic urethra becomes the **membranous urethra**, and the phallic segment contributes to the **vestibule of the vagina**.

Concurrently with the septation of the cloaca by the urorectal septum, the distal portions of the mesonephric ducts and attached ureteric ducts become incorporated into the posterior wall of the presumptive bladder by a process called **exstrophy** (Fig. 15-12). Exstrophy refers to the eversion of a hollow organ. It begins as the mouths of the mesonephric ducts flare into a pair of trumpet-shaped structures that begin to expand, flatten, and blend into the bladder wall. The cranial portion of this trumpet expands and flattens more rapidly than the caudal part, so that the mouth of the narrow portion of the mesonephric duct appears to migrate caudally along the posterior bladder wall. This process incorporates the distal ureters into the wall of the bladder and causes the mouths of the narrow part of the mesonephric ducts to migrate caudally until they open into the pelvic urethra just below the neck of the bladder. The triangular area of exstrophied mesonephric duct on the posteroinferior wall of the bladder is called the **trigone** of the bladder. The mesodermal tissue of the trigone is later overgrown by endoderm from the surrounding bladder wall, but the structure remains visible in the adult bladder as a smooth triangular region lying between the openings of the ureters, laterally and superiorly, and the opening of the pelvic urethra, inferiorly. Splanchnic mesoderm associated with the hindgut forms the smooth muscle of the bladder wall in the 12th week.

IN THE CLINIC

URINARY TRACT ANOMALIES

About 1% of all newborns have a developmental abnormality of the urinary tract. Most of these anomalies do not cause clinical problems. However, about 45% of all cases of childhood renal failure result from anomalous development of the ureteric bud or metanephric mesenchyme. Development of each of these anlagen is dependent on inductive signals from the other. Thus, abnormalities in one anlage often result in abnormal development of the other.

Duplicated Ureter

The ureteric bud normally does not bifurcate until it enters the substance of the metanephric blastema. Occasionally, however, it bifurcates prematurely, resulting in a Y-shaped **bifid ureter** (Fig. 15-13). The undivided caudal end of the ureter attaches normally to the bladder. Typically, the branch attached to its caudal pole drains most of the kidney. One of the branches occasionally ends blindly. A bifid ureter is often, but not always, asymptomatic. Although the two branches of the Y arise from the same ureteric bud, the contractions of their muscular walls seem to be asynchronous. Therefore, urine may reflux from one branch into the other, resulting in stagnation of urine and predisposing the individual to infections of the ureter.

Occasionally, a mesonephric duct sprouts two ureteric buds, which penetrate the metanephric blastema independently (Fig. 15-14). The more cranial bud induces formation of the cranial pole of the kidney, and the caudal bud induces the formation of the caudal pole. As the mesonephric duct undergoes exstrophy into the posterior

15

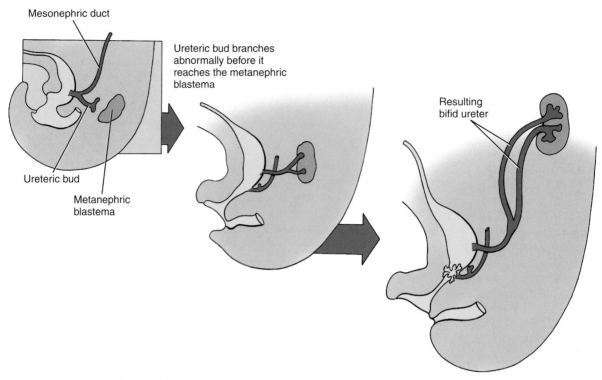

Mesonephric duct

Ureteric bud branches abnormally before it reaches the metanephric blastema

Resulting bifid ureter

Ureteric bud

Metanephric blastema

Figure 15-13. A bifid ureter forms when the ureteric bud bifurcates before entering the metanephric blastema.

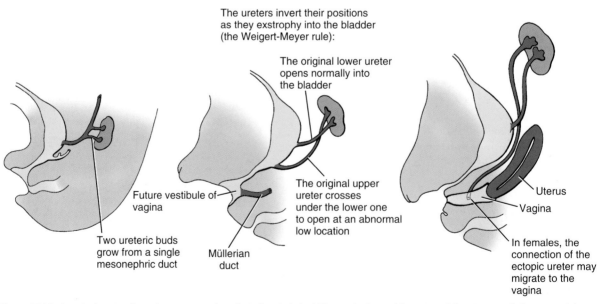

The ureters invert their positions as they exstrophy into the bladder (the Weigert-Meyer rule):

The original lower ureter opens normally into the bladder

Future vestibule of vagina

The original upper ureter crosses under the lower one to open at an abnormal low location

Uterus

Vagina

Two ureteric buds grow from a single mesonephric duct

Müllerian duct

In females, the connection of the ectopic ureter may migrate to the vagina

Figure 15-14. An ectopic ureter forms from an anomalous "extra" ureteric bud. The mechanisms of formation of the trigone and placement of the vas deferens and ureters on the posterior wall of the primitive urogenital sinus were largely deduced from the Weigert-Meyer rule (see text).

wall of the bladder, the caudal ureteric bud is incorporated into the bladder wall in the normal manner. However, the cranial bud is carried caudally along with the descending mesonephric duct (recall that the exstrophy is a craniocaudal process) and may form its final connection with any derivative of the distal mesonephric duct, pelvic urethra, or urogenital sinus (see Fig. 15-14). The caudal ureteric bud thus forms a normal, or **orthotopic**, ureter connected to the bladder, whereas the cranial bud forms a caudal **ectopic** ureter. Because the normal ureter drains the caudal pole of the kidney and the ectopic ureter drains the cranial pole, the two ureters cross each other. This crossing of the normal and ectopic ureters, called the **Weigert-Meyer rule**, is part of the evidence from which the mechanism of mesonephric duct exstrophy was deduced.

In males, an ectopic ureter may drain into the prostatic urethra, the ejaculatory duct, the vas deferens, or the seminal vesicle. These ectopic ureters thus always open superior to the sphincter urethra muscle and do not result in incontinence, although they may cause painful urination or recurrent infections. In females, ectopic ureters often connect to the vestibule, the vagina (see Fig. 15-14) or, less often, the uterus. These **extrasphincteric outlets** of the ectopic ureter result in continuous dribbling of urine unless surgically corrected. Anomalous insertion of the ureter within the bladder can also be a problem because the valve mechanism for preventing reflux of urine to the kidney fails to develop. Reflux predisposes individuals to urinary tract infection.

Development of Suprarenal Gland

The **suprarenal (adrenal) gland** is a crucial component of the hypothalamic-pituitary-suprarenal axis that is responsible for coordinating mammalian stress response and metabolism. Initially, formation of the suprarenal gland is closely tied to that of the gonads, as both arise from a common region of intermediate mesoderm lying adjacent the developing kidney. Segregation of the suprarenal and gonadal primordia occurs when primordial germ cells enter the gonadal region. By the 9th week, the suprarenal primordia are completely enclosed by a capsule. As might be expected, the specification of the suprarenal primordia depends on many of the same transcription factors and signaling molecules as those involved in kidney and gonadal development (e.g., *Wt1* and *Wnt4*).

During the 5th week of development, the coelomic epithelium adjacent to the developing gonadal ridge proliferates and a subset of these cells delaminates and enters the underlying mesoderm (Fig. 15-15). These delaminating cells differentiate into large acidophilic cells forming the **fetal suprarenal cortical cells**. A second wave of delaminating cells subsequently migrates, proliferates, and forms a thinner **definitive cortex** that almost completely surrounds the fetal cortex. Ultrastructurally, cells of both fetal and

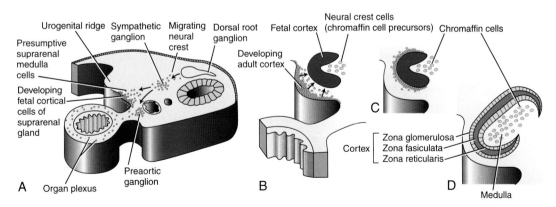

Figure 15-15. Suprarenal gland development. During the 5th week of development, the coelomic epithelium adjacent the developing gonadal ridge proliferates and a subset of cells delaminate and enter the underlying mesoderm, forming the fetal suprarenal cortical cells. A second wave of delaminating cells migrates and forms a thinner definitive cortex surrounding the fetal cortex. By the 2nd postnatal month, the fetal cortex rapidly regresses and the remaining definitive cortical cells organize into the zona glomerulosa, zona fasiculata, and zona reticularis layers seen in the adult suprarenal gland. Before being cordoned off by the forming suprarenal capsule, neural crest cells migrate into the medullary region and differentiate into chromaffin cells.

15

definitive cortical layers exhibit cytologic characteristics of steroid-producing cells. During the second trimester, the fetal cortical layer grows rapidly in size and begins secreting **dehydroepiandrosterone (DHEA)**, a hormone converted by the placenta to **estradiol**, which is essential for maintaining pregnancy. Moreover, products from the fetal suprarenal cortex influence the maturation of the lungs, liver, and digestive tract and may regulate **parturition**. By the second postnatal month, the fetal cortex rapidly regresses and the remaining definitive cortical cells then organize into the **zona glomerulosa, zona fasciculata**, and **zona reticularis** layers seen in the adult suprarenal gland.

Before being cordoned off by the formation of the suprarenal capsule, neural crest cells migrate into the suprarenal medullary region adjacent the developing fetal cortex. These neural crest cells differentiate into **chromaffin cells**, which are specialized postganglionic sympathetic neurons innervated by preganglionic sympathetic fibers that release *Epinephrine* and *Norepinephrine* upon sympathetic stimulation.

IN THE CLINIC

CONGENITAL ADRENAL HYPERPLASIA

Congenital adrenal (suprarenal) hyperplasia (CAH) is usually caused by a genetically determined deficiency of the suprarenal cortical enzymes necessary for the synthesis of **glucocorticoids**. This deficiency leads to **adrenocorticotropic hormone**–driven hyperplasia of the suprarenal cortex. The most common form of CAH (an incidence of 1:15,000 live births) results from a deficiency in 21-HYDROXYLASE (encoded by the *CYP21A2* gene). This deficiency causes a reduction in cortisol production by the suprarenal cortex, resulting in an accumulation of 17-hydroxyprogesterone that, in turn, results in suprarenal hyperplasia and excess production of suprarenal androgens (these are negatively regulated by the presence of cortisol). Excessive levels of suprarenal androgens masculinize the external genitalia of XX individuals during their in utero development, leading to female pseudohermaphrodism (discussed later; also see Fig. 6-16). During childhood, excessive levels of suprarenal androgens accelerate skeletal maturation. In the salt-wasting form of 21-HYDROXYLASE deficiency, insufficient aldosterone secretion can lead to life-threatening **hyponatremia** (low blood sodium).

Mutations in *DAX1* gene (discussed later in the chapter with respect to gonadal development) can also lead to CAH. These patients (most often males) exhibit suprarenal insufficiency, skin hyperpigmentation, and delayed puberty.

Genital System Arises with Urinary System

Sex determination and manifestation begins with genetic sex determination (i.e., 46,XX or 46,XY) that occurs at fertilization (discussed in Ch. 1). The sexual genotype is responsible for directing gonadal development (i.e., testis versus ovary). This in turn directs reproductive tract (internal organs) and external genitalia development. Interestingly, genotypic, gonadal, and phenotypic sex assignments may be discordant (i.e., resulting in pseudohermaphrodism). Although steady progress has been made in our understanding of the molecular and developmental mechanisms responsible for sex determination and genital development, approximately 75% of the genetic alterations responsible for human sex reversal are still unresolved.

In both sexes, formation and differentiation of the gonads begins with the arrival of primordial germ cells in the intermediate mesoderm. As discussed in Chapter 1, primordial germ cells normally migrate from the yolk sac via the dorsal mesentery to populate the mesenchyme of the posterior body wall in an area near the tenth thoracic level during the 5th week (Fig. 15-16A). There, they move to the area adjacent the coelomic epithelium, located just medial and ventral to the developing mesonephric kidney. In response, the coelomic epithelium proliferates, thickens, and together with the primordial germ cells, forms a pair of **genital ridges** (Fig. 15-16B, C, Fig. 15-17).

During the 6th week, cells from the coelomic epithelium form aggregates of somatic supporting cells that completely invest the germ cells (see Fig. 15-16C). **Somatic support cells** are essential for germ cell development within the gonad; if these cells do not invest the germ cells, the germ cells degenerate. After the 6th week, these somatic support cells pursue different fates in males and females.

Also during the 6th week, a new pair of ducts, the **müllerian ducts** (or **paramesonephric ducts**), begin to form just lateral to the mesonephric ducts in both male and female embryos (see Fig. 15-16B, C). These ducts arise by the craniocaudal invagination of a ribbon of thickened coelomic epithelium extending from the third thoracic segment caudally to the posterior wall of the urogenital sinus. The caudal tips of the müllerian ducts then grow to connect with the developing pelvic urethra just medial to the openings of the right and left mesonephric ducts. The tips of the two müllerian ducts adhere to each other just before they

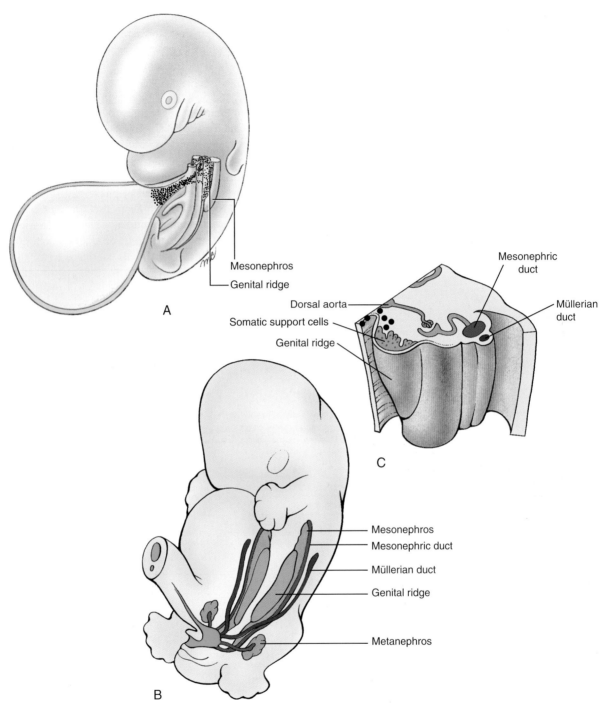

Figure 15-16. Formation of the genital ridges. *A, B,* During the 5th and 6th weeks, the genital ridges form in the posterior abdominal wall just medial to the developing mesonephroi in response to colonization by primordial germ cells (black dots) migrating from the yolk sac. *C,* The primordial germ cells induce the coelomic epithelium lining the peritoneal cavity, as well as cells of the mesonephros, to proliferate and form the somatic support cells.

15

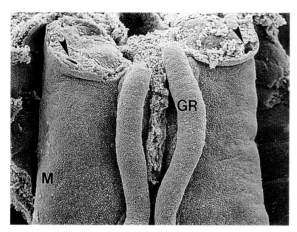

Figure 15-17. Scanning electron micrographs showing the relationship between the developing genital ridges (GR) and the mesonephroi (M). Arrowheads: Mesonephric ducts seen in cross section.

contact the developing pelvic urethra. The cranial ends of the müllerian ducts form funnel-shaped openings into the coelom. The further development of the müllerian ducts in the female is discussed later in the chapter.

At the end of the 6th week, the male and female genital systems appear indistinguishable, although subtle cellular differences may already be present. In both sexes, germ cells and somatic support cells are present in the presumptive gonads, and complete mesonephric and müllerian ducts lie side by side. The **ambisexual** or **bipotential phase** of genital development ends at this point. From the 7th week on, the male and female systems pursue diverging pathways. Table 15-2 lists the homologous male and female adult reproductive cells and organs derived from these embryonic progenitors.

Table 15-2 Adult Derivatives and Vestigial Remnants of Embryonic Male and Female Reproductive Structures

Presumptive Anlagen	Male Structure	Female Structure
Indifferent gonad	Testis	Ovary
Primordial germ cell	Spermatogonia	Oocytes
Somatic support cell	Sertoli cells	Follicle cells
Stromal cells	Leydig cells	Thecal cells
Gubernaculum	Gubernaculum testis	Round ligament of the ovary Round ligament of uterus
Mesonephric tubules	Efferent ducts of testis Paradidymis	Epoöphoron Paroöphoron
Mesonephric duct	Appendix of epididymis Epididymis Vas deferens Seminal vesicle Ejaculatory duct	Appendix vesiculosa Duct of epoöphoron Gartner's duct
Müllerian duct	Appendix of testis	Fallopian tubes Uterus
Urogenital sinus	Prostatic and membranous urethra Prostatic utricle Prostatic gland Bulbourethral glands	Membranous urethra Vagina Urethral/paraurethral glands Greater vestibular glands
Sinus tubercle	Seminal colliculus	Hymen
Genital tubercle	Glans penis Corpus cavernosa of penis Corpus spongiosum of penis	Glans clitoris Corpus cavernosa of clitoris Bulbospongiosum of vestibule
Urogenital folds and urethral plate	Penile urethra/ventral penis	Labia minora
Labioscrotal folds	Scrotum	Labia majora

Initiating Male Versus Female Development

As detailed in Chapter 1, genetic females have two X sex chromosomes, whereas genetic males have an X and a Y sex chromosome. Although the pattern of sex chromosomes determines the choice between male and female developmental paths, the subsequent phases of sexual development are controlled not only by sex chromosome genes but also by hormones and other factors, most of which are encoded on **autosomes**.

A single sex-determining factor seems to control a cascade of events leading to male development. This sex-determining transcription factor is encoded by the **SRY (*Sex-determining region of the Y chromosome*) gene**. When this transcription factor is expressed in the somatic support cells of the indifferent presumptive gonad, male development is triggered. This step is called **primary sex determination**. If the factor is absent or defective, female development occurs. Thus, femaleness has been described as the basic developmental path for the human embryo. However, it should be emphasized that claiming ovarian development and femaleness is a passive (i.e., default), rather than active, process, is a gross oversimplification.

Male Genital Development Begins with Differentiation of Sertoli Cells

The first event in male genital development is the expression of SRY protein within the somatic support cells of the XY gonad (Fig. 15-18). Under the influence of this factor, somatic support cells begin to

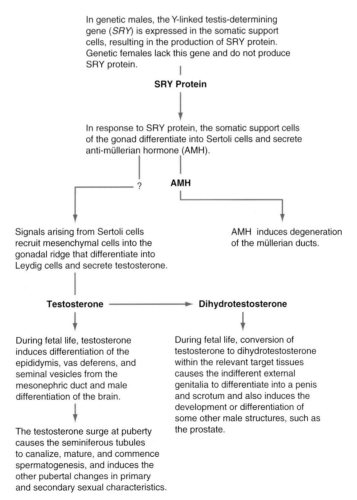

In genetic males, the Y-linked testis-determining gene (*SRY*) is expressed in the somatic support cells, resulting in the production of SRY protein. Genetic females lack this gene and do not produce SRY protein.

SRY Protein

In response to SRY protein, the somatic support cells of the gonad differentiate into Sertoli cells and secrete anti-müllerian hormone (AMH).

? **AMH**

Signals arising from Sertoli cells recruit mesenchymal cells into the gonadal ridge that differentiate into Leydig cells and secrete testosterone.

AMH induces degeneration of the müllerian ducts.

Testosterone → **Dihydrotestosterone**

During fetal life, testosterone induces differentiation of the epididymis, vas deferens, and seminal vesicles from the mesonephric duct and male differentiation of the brain.

The testosterone surge at puberty causes the seminiferous tubules to canalize, mature, and commence spermatogenesis, and induces the other pubertal changes in primary and secondary sexual characteristics.

During fetal life, conversion of testosterone to dihydrotestosterone within the relevant target tissues causes the indifferent external genitalia to differentiate into a penis and scrotum and also induces the development or differentiation of some other male structures, such as the prostate.

Figure 15-18. Summary of the differentiation cascade of the male genital system development.

15

differentiate into Sertoli cells and envelop the germ cells (Fig. 15-19). If *SRY* is absent (i.e., in XX gonads), somatic support cells will differentiate into ovarian follicle cells that envelop the germ cells.

SRY is a single-copy gene found only in genetic males and located on the Y chromosome. The *SRY* gene, a transcription factor, is activated only for a short period within gonadal somatic cells and likely upregulates testis-specific genes and/or represses ovarian genes (discussed in the following "In the Research Lab"). *SRY* expression is first detected between days 41 to 44 post-ovulation and remains detectable there until day 52.

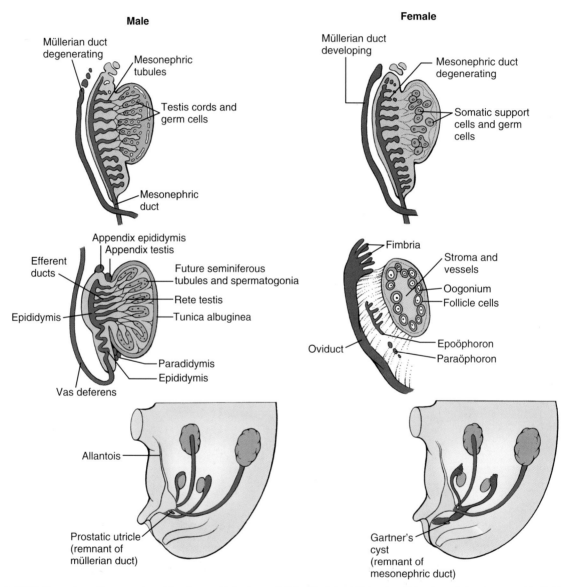

Figure 15-19. Comparison of human male and female gonadal development at the tissue level. The male and female genital systems are virtually identical through the 7th week. In the male, SRY protein produced by the pre-Sertoli cells causes the somatic support cells to differentiate into Sertoli cells. Sertoli cells, together with myoepithelial precursor cells, then organize into testis cords and rete testis tubules. AMH produced by the Sertoli cells causes the müllerian ducts to regress. Leydig cells also develop, which in turn produce testosterone, the hormone that stimulates development of the male genital duct system.

During the 7th week, the differentiating Sertoli cells, together with interstitial cells of the gonad, organize to form **testis cords**, enclosing germ cells in the center of these cords (see Fig. 15-19). At puberty, the testis cords become canalized and differentiate into a system of **seminiferous tubules**. In the region adjacent the mesonephros and devoid of germ cells, Sertoli cells organize into a set of thin-walled ducts called the **rete testis**. The rete testis, which connects the seminiferous tubules with a limited number of mesonephric tubules, canalizes at puberty to form a conduit connecting the seminiferous tubules to the mesonephric ducts. The mesonephric ducts later develop into the **epididymis, spermatic ducts** or **vasa deferentia** (singular, vas deferens), and **seminal vesicles** in the male (discussed later).

During the 7th week, the testes begin to round up, reducing their area of contact with the mesonephros (see Fig. 15-19). As the testes continue to develop, the coelomic epithelium is separated from the testis cords by an intervening layer of connective tissue called the **tunica albuginea.**

Development of Male Gametes

Although the mechanism has not been elucidated, it is clear that direct cell-to-cell contact between Sertoli cells and primordial germ cells within the gonadal ridge plays a key role in the development of the male gametes. This interaction occurs shortly after the arrival of the primordial germ cells in the region of the presumptive genital ridge. It has the immediate effect of inhibiting further mitosis of the germ cells and preventing them from entering meiosis. No further development of the germ cells occurs until about 3 months postnatal, when they differentiate into type A spermatogonia. The rest of the remaining phases of male gametogenesis—further mitosis, differentiation into type B spermatogonia, meiosis, and spermatogenesis—are delayed until puberty (discussed in Ch. 1).

IN THE RESEARCH LAB

SOX9 GENE IS LIKELY A PRIMARY TARGET OF SRY EXPRESSION

Much of what we have learned regarding the molecular and cellular mechanisms involved in gonad development stems from analyses of mouse mutants and **genotype-phenotype correlations** with humans having disorders in sexual development. Several genes are required for the early formation of the indifferent gonad including *Wt1, Steroidogenic factor-1* (*Sf1*), *Emx2, Lim homeobox protein-9* (*Lhx9*), and *Gata-binding protein-4* (*Gata4*). Several of these genes, in addition to being necessary for initial formation of the indifferent gonad, are also required for subsequent expression of *Sry* and *Sry*-targeted genes (Fig. 15-20). For instance, mutations in *WT1* and *SF1* in humans results in malformed gonads and ambiguous genitalia.

The current thought regarding male sex determination is that *SRY* expression has to reach a certain threshold level at the appropriate time during development to render the somatic support cells competent to enter the pre-Sertoli cell lineage. Although the *SRY* gene is instrumental in sex determination, it is still unclear as to whether *SRY* activates a male sex–activating cascade or stifles a male repressor program during the critical period of gonadal sex determination. Unfortunately, we still have not identified *SRY*-specific target genes. The SRY protein binds to minor grooves in DNA via its HMG box motif, and this induces DNA bending and conformational changes that expose binding sites for several other transcriptional regulators. This makes it difficult to identify particular targets of *SRY* specifically involved in driving sex determination.

The *Sox9 (Sry-related HMG box-9)* gene seems to be one key target of *Sry* expression. In XY mice, *Sox9* is upregulated just after the expression of *Sry* in pre-Sertoli cells (Fig. 15-21A, see Fig. 15-20). XY mice with a conditional knock out for *Sox9* lack testis cords, do not form Sertoli cells, and express female-specific markers within the gonad. Expression of *SOX9* in XX gonads can also lead to testicular development. Humans with heterozygotic mutations inactivating *SOX9* develop **campomelic dysplasia** (a severe limb long-bone defect discussed in Ch. 8 and described in Table 18-2; *Sox9* has an important role in cartilage development, as discussed in Ch. 8). Almost 75% of XY patients with campomelic dysplasia also exhibit some degree of sex reversal (i.e., female development), whereas XX patients exhibiting camptomelic dysplasia have normal gonads. Moreover, XX individuals with chromosomal duplications in the *SOX9* gene develop as males. These observations strongly suggest that many of *SRY* effects on sex determination are conveyed through activation of *SOX9*.

SERTOLI CELLS ARE MAIN ORGANIZER OF TESTES

Generally testes development proceeds slightly in advance of that of the ovaries. The size of the male gonad increases relative to the female gonad during the early stages of gonad differentiation. A sort of "community effect" seems to be involved in male gonadal development whereby a sufficient number of Sertoli cells are required to proceed along the male pathway.

15

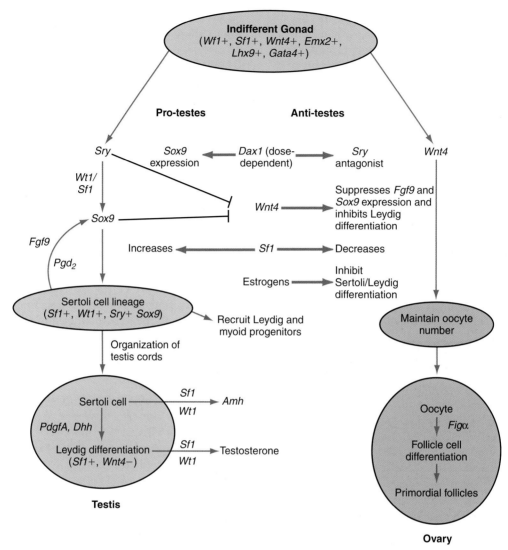

Figure 15-20. Comparison of male and female gonadal determination at the cellular and molecular levels. Expression of *Sry* gene in the indifferent gonad initiates a cascade of events that are "pro-testis," including initiating *Sox9* expression and increasing *Sf1* expression. Female gonadal development is promoted by "anti-testes" factors, including *Wnt4*. *Dax1* expression can be both "pro-testes" or "anti-testes" depending on dosage, but regardless, it is essential for normal testis development. Expression of the *Sry* gene results in Sertoli cell differentiation, and these cells then recruit other cells and organize the testis cords. In the absence of the *Sry* gene, the somatic support cells differentiate into follicle cells under the influence of the oocytes. Together with the oocytes, the follicle cells organize into primordial ovarian follicles.

Primordial germ cells respond very differently to the gonadal environment depending on sex. Upon entering the gonad, primordial germ cells proliferate. In males, the primordial germ cells become surrounded by pre-Sertoli cells and enter mitotic arrest. In females, the primordial germ cells continue mitosis a bit longer and then enter meiosis and quickly arrest. These arrested meiotic germ cells apparently induce the differentiation of follicle cells because in their absence, follicle cells never form. Why germ cells in males do not begin meiosis is unclear, but they may be protected from the effects of retinoic acid generated within the mesonephros when they are surrounded by Sertoli cells (Sertoli cells express an enzyme that metabolizes retinoic acid). But what directs male primordial germs cells into mitotic arrest is unknown, but may include *Prostaglandin D2 (Pdg2)* and the protein encoded by the *tdl* gene (see Chapter 1).

Time

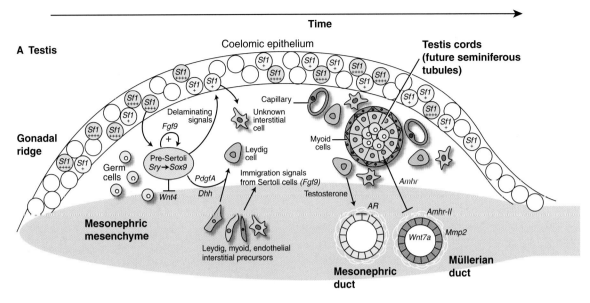

A Testis

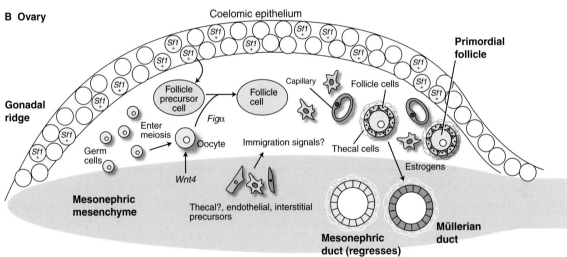

B Ovary

Figure 15-21. Overview of the transcription factors, growth factors, and origin of various cell types responsible for forming the male, *A*, and female, *B*, gonads. *AR, Androgen receptor.*

Sertoli cells act as the main organizing center for testis development because they direct lineage specification and differentiation of other cells within the gonad. In mice, pre-Sertoli cells begin expressing *Sry* and are capable of initiating the recruitment of other non-*Sry* expressing cells into the Sertoli cell lineage. Pre-Sertoli cells produce *Fgf9*, which mediates Sertoli cell precursor proliferation and maintains *Sox9* expression in these cells (discussed later in the chapter), and *Pgd2*, which further upregulates *Sox9* expression, possibly reinforcing male gonadal development once it is initiated (see Fig. 15-20).

What is the origin of the initial Sertoli cell population? Lineage-tracing studies in mice show that the earliest Sertoli cell precursors delaminate from the coelomic epithelium of the genital ridge, rather than arising from the mesonephric/gonadal ridge mesenchyme (although additional pre-Sertoli cells may be recruited from the mesonephros by pre-Sertoli cells within the gonadal ridge). Moreover, these experiments found that an unidentified interstitial cell population of unknown function also delaminates from the same epithelium. Studies suggest that these two epithelial-derived lineages are set apart by differences in the degree of *Sf1* expression.

Sf1 encodes a nuclear hormone receptor protein and is expressed in the forming suprarenal gland and early somatic cells of both early XX and XY gonads. In XX mice, gonadal expression of *Sf1* soon decreases, but in XY mice it is retained in early Sertoli and Leydig cells (where it promotes anti-Müllerian hormone production by Sertoli cells and testosterone production by Leydig cells). Studies in mice suggest that a proliferating, highly expressing *Sf1* subset of coelomic epithelial cells delaminates first, and that these give rise to pre-Sertoli cells (see Fig. 15-21A). In the absence of *Sry*, these delaminating cells do not differentiate into Sertoli cells but rather take on a follicle cell lineage (Fig. 15-21B). Newly formed pre-Sertoli cells, now expressing *Sry* and *Fgf9*, then signal low–*Sf1*-expressing coelomic epithelial cells to divide, delaminate, and generate interstitial cells (see Fig. 15-21A). These results are consistent with observations showing that mutations in *SF1* result in XY gonadal dysgenesis in humans, and that dose-dependent levels of *Sf1* mediate temperature-dependent sex determination of the bipotential (indifferent) gonads in some vertebrates (e.g., in some reptiles and birds).

The coelomic epithelium is not the only source of somatic cells within the developing gonad. Cells are recruited into the gonadal ridge from the mesonephros by signals emanating from *Sf1*-positive pre-Sertoli cells (the nature of which is unknown; see Figs. 15-20, 15-21A). These immigrating cells are thought to serve as precursors for the peritubular myoepithelial cells, Leydig cells, endothelial cells, and supportive cells that are critical for gonadal development. The myoepithelial progenitors, together with the Sertoli cells and germ cells, then organize into epithelial testis cords.

SEX REVERSAL

Recent work in mammalian sex reversal (a condition in which an XX individual develops as a male or an XY individual develops as a female; the incidence is thought to be as high as 1:20,000 in humans) has led some to hypothesize the existence of a "Z" gene that acts as an inhibitor of the male pathway. This gene would normally be expressed in females but blocked by the *Sry* protein in males. In XX sex-reversal cases, both copies of the Z would be mutated, leading to activation of male cascade (e.g., enabling activation of *Sox9* transcription). In XY sex-reversal cases, mutations in *Sry* or elsewhere in the genome (*Sry* mutations are found in less than 15% of cases) would lead to inappropriate activation of the Z gene, resulting in repression of the male cascade. A candidate fitting the definition of a Z gene may have been found in a chromosomal region linking failed horn development in goats with intersexuality. Transcripts from the candidate chromosomal region coding this gene have been reported to exhibit a sex-specific expression pattern within the gonads, and this region is currently being sequenced. Other genes having "Z-type" anti-male activity may exist, much like the anti-male activities of *Wnt4* (*Wnt4* expression inhibits Leydig cell differentiation in female gonads; discussed later in the chapter).

IN THE CLINIC

HERMAPHRODITES

True **hermaphrodites** (i.e., individuals having sex chromosomes, genitalia, and/or secondary sex characteristics that are a mixture of both male and female; also called **intersex individuals**) may be chromosomal males (46,XY), chromosomal females (46,XX), or mosaics (e.g., 45,X/46,XY; 46,XX/47,XXY; or 46,XX/46,XY). The mosaic cases of hermaphrodism are the easiest to explain: In these individuals, ovarian tissue develops from cells without a Y chromosome, whereas testicular tissue develops from cells with a Y chromosome. There is evidence that hermaphrodites with a 46,XX karyotype may also be mosaics. Apparently, the X chromosome in some cells of these individuals carries a fragment of the short arm of the Y chromosome, including the sex-determining region. This fragment was likely acquired by abnormal crossing over early in cleavage.

46,XY hermaphrodites are difficult to explain, as only 15% of these individuals have mutations in *SRY*. The cause may be mutations in other essential genes (e.g., the presumptive Z gene) in the testis pathway that handicap testis development.

The gonads of true hermaphrodites are usually streak-like, composite ovotestes containing both seminiferous tubules and follicles. However, in about 20% of cases, an individual has an ovary or ovotestis on one side and a testis on the other. A Fallopian tube and single uterine horn may develop on the side with the ovary. A few true hermaphrodites have ovulated and conceived, although none is known to have carried a fetus to term. A vas deferens always develops in conjunction with a testis. The testis is usually immature, but spermatogenesis is occasionally detectable. Most true hermaphrodites are reared as males because a phallus is usually present at birth.

Anti-müllerian Hormone and Male Genital Development

As pre-Sertoli cells begin their morphologic differentiation in response to *Sry*, they also begin secreting a glycoprotein hormone called ***Anti-müllerian hormone (Amh)*** or ***Müllerian-inhibiting substance (Mis)***. *Amh* is member of *Tgfβ* family and is expressed specifically by Sertoli cells, beginning in humans at about week 8, causing the müllerian ducts to regress rapidly between the 8th and 10th weeks (see Figs. 15-18, 15-19). Nevertheless, small müllerian duct remnants can be detected in the adult male, including a small cap of tissue associated with the testis, called the **appendix testis**, and an expansion of the prostatic urethra, called the **prostatic utricle** (see Fig. 15-19). In female embryos, as described later, the müllerian ducts do not regress.

Amh signaling acts indirectly through interactions with the *Amh receptor–type II (Amhr-II)* receptor (also known as *Misr-II*) on mesenchymal cells surrounding the müllerian duct, rather than directly on the epithelium of the duct (see Fig. 15-21). Upon receptor activation, mesenchyme-to-epithelial signaling induces müllerian duct regression. Continued epithelial-to-mesenchyme signaling is important for maintaining *Amhr-II* expression in the mesenchyme, because in the absence of *Wnt7a* expression within the duct epithelium, *Amhr-II* expression is lost and müllerian derivatives are inappropriately retained in the male. *AMH* and *AMHR-II* gene mutations have been identified in human males and result in features typical of **persistent müllerian duct syndrome** (discussed below) including **cryptorchidism** (undescended testis) or ectopic testes with inguinal hernias.

Recently, another *Amh* receptor group, the *Amh receptor–type I (Amhr-I)* receptor group, has been identified based on *Amh* being a *Tgfβ/Bmp* family member. Studies have found *Alk2*, *Alk3* (or *Bmpr1a*), and *Alk6* also serve as *Amhr-I receptors*. When these receptors are knocked out in mice or if their signaling is blocked within the müllerian duct mesenchyme, *Amh*-induced müllerian duct regression is lost.

Differentiation of Testis Leydig Cells

In the 9th or 10th week, **Leydig cells** differentiate from mesonephric mesenchymal cells recruited by pre-Sertoli cells (see Figs. 15-18, 15-20, 15-21). These endocrine cells produce the male sex steroid hormone, **testosterone**, which promotes survival of the mesonephric duct,

15

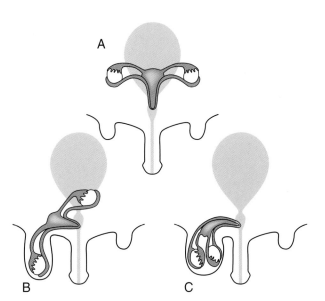

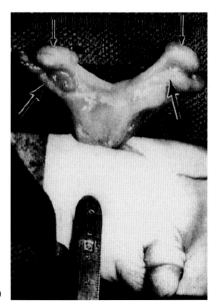

Figure 15-22. Persistent müllerian duct syndrome. In 46, XY individuals with mutations in *AMH* or *AMH RECEPTOR* genes, the müllerian ducts fail to regress. These individuals develop müllerian derivatives, in addition to those from the mesonephric duct. These individuals have a cervix, uterus, and Fallopian tubes, as well as vasa deferentia and male external genitalia. The phenotype varies in that the female organs are in their normal position, but the testes may lie either in the normal position for ovaries (i.e., within the broad ligament, *A*), one testis may lie within the inguinal hernial sac *(B)*, or both testes may lie within same inguinal sac *(C)*. *D*, Phenotype typical of the scenario shown in *A*. The lower two arrows point to the Fallopian tubes, and the upper two arrows indicate the position of the testes within the broad ligament.

necessary for development of the male reproductive tract and later for the development of secondary sexual characteristics. At this early stage of development (up to 12 weeks), testosterone secretion is regulated by the peptide hormone **chorionic gonadotropin**, secreted by the placenta. Later in development, pituitary gonadotropins of the male fetus take over control of synthesizing the masculinizing sex steroids (androgens). Leydig cell number and testosterone levels peak by 14 to 18 weeks of gestation under control of the placental chorionic gonadotropin. Luteinizing hormone receptors on Leydig cells begin appearing at 12 weeks, and there is a concomitant increase in expression of steroidogenic enzymes released by these cells at this time. But after 16 weeks, the number of Leydig cells and levels of steroidogenic enzymes begin falling as gonadotropin control shifts to the pituitary. Pituitary gonadotropin release begins during the 2nd and 3rd trimester. Mutations affecting Leydig cell differentiation and function, or in genes involved in testosterone synthesis, generally lead to male pseudohermaphrodism (discussed later in this chapter).

Two distinct populations of Leydig cells are responsible for androgen biosynthesis during fetal and postnatal life. Fetal Leydig cells generate testosterone necessary for stimulating male organ development

(i.e., to make the epididymis, seminal vesicles, and vas deferens from the mesonephric duct). From testosterone, Leydig cell *5α-Reductase* generates **dihydrotestosterone**, needed to induce male urethra, prostate, penis, and scrotum (discussed later in the chapter) and for testicular descent into scrotum (see Fig. 15-18). However, fetal Leydig cells eventually regress and degenerate late in fetal and early postnatal life. At puberty, a new population of adult Leydig cells differentiates from Leydig progenitor cells residing within peritubular interstitium. Androgens produced by this set of Leydig cells play a major role in masculinizing the brain, mediating male sexual behavior, and initiating spermatogenesis.

IN THE RESEARCH LAB

DIFFERENTIATION OF LEYDIG CELLS

Once Leydig progenitors immigrate into the developing gonad, paracrine interactions between Leydig progenitors and Sertoli cells play a central role in fetal and adult Leydig cell differentiation. Both *Desert hedgehog* (*Dhh*) and *PdgfA* are released by fetal Sertoli cells; their receptors, *Patched1* (*Ptch1*) and *Pdgfrα*, are expressed by fetal Leydig cells (see

Figs. 15-20, 15-21). More than 90% of XY mice with null mutations for *Dhh* are pseudohermaphrodites, and mice deficient in *Pdgfα* exhibit abnormal Leydig cell differentiation. Similar phenotypes (including blind vaginas and underdeveloped mesonephric duct derivatives and prostate glands) are found in XY humans with *DHH* mutations.

Less is known regarding the differentiation of adult Leydig cells. Although the growth factors *Dhh* and *Pdgf* seem to be involved as in fetal differentiation of Leydig cells, several hormones are also involved in adult Leydig cell differentiation. In addition, testicular macrophages are somehow required for adult Leydig cell development. If testicular macrophages are absent from the testicular interstitium, Leydig cells fail to develop, suggesting that these macrophages provide essential growth and differentiation factors for Leydig cells. However, the nature of these signals is still unclear.

Mesonephric Ducts and Accessory Glands of Male Urethra Differentiate in Response to Testosterone

Between 8 and 12 weeks, the initial secretion of testosterone stimulates mesonephric ducts to transform into a system of organs—the epididymis, vas deferens, and seminal vesicle—that connect the testes with the urethra. These mesonephric derivatives are distinguishable by their morphologies and specific pattern of gene expression even though they are contiguous (see the following "In the Research Lab").

The bulk of the mesonephric duct differentiates into the spermatic duct called the **vas deferens** (see Fig. 15-19). The most cranial end of each mesonephric duct degenerates, leaving a small remnant called the **appendix epididymis**, and the region of the mesonephric duct adjacent to the presumptive testis differentiates into the convoluted **epididymis**. During the 9th week, 5 to 12 mesonephric tubules in the region of the epididymis make contact with the cords of the future rete testis. However, it is not until the 3rd month that these **epigenital mesonephric tubules** actually unite with the presumptive rete testis. The epigenital mesonephric tubules are thereafter called the **efferent ductules**, and they will provide a pathway from the seminiferous tubules and rete testis tubules to the epididymis. Meanwhile, the mesonephric tubules at the caudal pole of the developing testis (called the **paragenital mesonephric tubules**) degenerate, leaving a small remnant called the **paradidymis**.

The three accessory glands—the seminal vesicle, prostate, and bulbourethral gland—of the male genital system all develop near the junction between the mesonephric ducts and the pelvic urethra (Fig. 15-23). The glandular **seminal vesicles** sprout during the 10th week from the mesonephric ducts near their attachment to the pelvic urethra. The portion of the vas deferens (mesonephric duct) between each seminal vesicle and the urethra is thereafter called the **ejaculatory duct**.

The **prostate gland** also begins to develop in the 10th week as a cluster of endodermal evaginations that bud from the pelvic urethra. These presumptive prostatic outgrowths are induced by the surrounding mesenchyme, the inductive activity of which probably depends on the conversion of secreted testosterone to dihydrotestosterone. The prostatic outgrowths initially form at least five independent groups of solid prostatic cords. By 11 weeks, these cords develop a lumen and glandular acini, and by 13 to 15 weeks (just as testosterone concentrations reach a high level), the prostate begins its secretory activity. The mesenchyme surrounding the endoderm-derived glandular portion of the prostate differentiates into the smooth muscle and connective tissue of the prostate.

As the prostate is developing, the paired **bulbourethral glands** (or **Cowper's glands**) sprout from the urethra just inferior to the prostate. As in the prostate, the mesenchyme surrounding the endodermal glandular tissue gives rise to the connective tissue and smooth muscle of this gland.

Eventually, the secretions of the seminal vesicles, prostate, and bulbourethral glands all contribute to the seminal fluid protecting and nourishing the

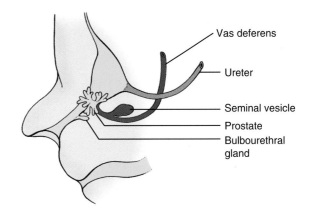

Figure 15-23. Development of the seminal vesicles, prostate, and bulbourethral glands. These glands are induced by androgens between the 10th and 12th weeks.

15

spermatozoa after ejaculation. It should be noted that these secretions are not necessary for sperm function; spermatozoa removed directly from the epididymis can fertilize oocytes.

IN THE RESEARCH LAB

DEVELOPMENT OF THE EPIDIDYMUS, VAS DEFERENS, AND SEMINAL VESICLES

The mesonephric duct requires testosterone for retention and subsequent differentiation; otherwise, it regresses. Interestingly, testosterone acts via paracrine interactions, rather than being delivered by the vasculature to the mesonephric duct, as unilateral castration in male rabbits results only in unilateral regression of the mesonephric duct (hence, testosterone may be transported down the lumen of the mesonephric duct by diffusion). Testosterone binds the *Androgen receptor* (also known as the *Dihydrotestosterone receptor*), which is expressed by the mesenchyme adjacent to the mesonephric duct. Mice lacking the *Androgen receptor* exhibit agenesis of mesonephric duct derivatives and develop female external genitalia. Abnormal mesonephric duct development also occurs in humans having mutations in the *ANDROGEN RECEPTOR* that lead to male pseudohermaphrodism (discussed in a later ''In the Clinic'' of this chapter).

As mentioned earlier, the mesonephric duct forms different structures along its cranial-caudal length. Development of these mesonephric-derived structures depends on regionally specific epithelial-mesenchymal interactions that are initiated by the adjacent mesenchyme. For instance, in vitro studies show that the cranial mesonephric duct, which normally develops into the epididymis, can be redirected toward seminal vesicle development when recombined with seminal vesicle mesenchyme. Moreover, the continued growth of the surrounding mesenchyme also requires reciprocal interaction with the mesonephric duct. These interactions likely involve regional expression of several growth factors (Fig. 15-24). For instance, mice deficient in the growth factors *Gdf7* (*Growth and differentiation factor 7*) or *Fgf10* all exhibit defects in the epididymis and seminal vesicle development.

The cranial-caudal expression of *Hox* genes also plays an important role in the differentiation of the various segments of the mesonephric duct. In XY mice, *Hoxa9* and *Hoxd9* are expressed in the epididymis and vas deferens, *Hoxa10* and *Hoxd10* are mainly expressed in the caudal epididymis and throughout the vas deferens, *Hoxa11* is expressed only in the vas deferens, and *Hoxa13* and *Hoxd13* are expressed in the caudal vas deferens and region of the developing seminal vesicle (see Fig. 15-24). Mutations or disruptions in the expression of these genes can lead to homeotic transformation. For example, if *Hoxa11* expression is lost, the vas deferens is transformed into an epididymal-like cytoarchitecture; if *Hoxa10* is lost, the distal epididymis and proximal vas deferens exhibit epididymal-like cytoarchitecture.

IN THE CLINIC

CYSTIC FIBROSIS TRANSMEMBRANE CONDUCTANCE REGULATOR IS REQUIRED FOR VAS DEFERENS DEVELOPMENT

Disorders of mesonephric duct development are quite common. For example, the incidence of human **congenital bilateral aplasia of the vas deferens** (**CBAVD**) ranges from 1:1,000 to 1:10,000 and is responsible for 1% to 2% of male infertility and almost 10% of obstructive **azoospermia** (absence of spermatozoa in semen due to duct blockage, rather than to absence of spermatozoa production, which is called nonobstructive azoospermia). CBAVD is characterized by an absence of the body and tail of the epididymis, vas deferens, and seminal vesicle. Mutations in both alleles of **Cystic fibrosis transmembrane conductance regulator** (*CFTR*; the gene that when mutated causes cystic fibrosis; further discussed in Ch. 11) are found in approximately 80% of CBAVD cases. This ion transporter is required for vas deferens development: a high proportion of males suffering from cystic fibrosis also exhibit CBAVD and are infertile. Isolated CBAVD in some male patients who do not exhibit the cystic fibrosis lung phenotype, is caused by abnormal splicing of the *CFTR* mRNA in the vas deferens but not in the lungs.

IN THE RESEARCH LAB

DEVELOPMENT OF PROSTATE GLAND

The prostate gland develops from the pelvic urethra. When testicular-generated androgens increase, they induce an outgrowth of solid endodermal buds from the urethral epithelium into the urogenital mesenchyme. Like the mesenchyme surrounding the mesonephric duct, *Androgen receptors* are expressed within the surrounding urogenital mesenchyme, and it seems that an unknown substance is released by the mesenchyme that signals prostatic epithelial development. Not only are androgens required to initiate prostatic development, they maintain its growth and development during the embryonic, fetal, and neonatal period. Prostatic development relies heavily on conversion

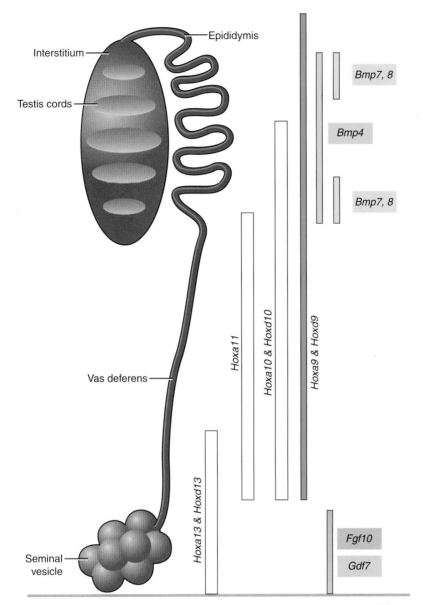

Figure 15-24. Male mesonephric duct differentiation. Under the influence of testosterone, the mesonephric duct forms different structures along its cranial-caudal length, the nature of which depends on regionally specific epithelial-mesenchymal interactions. In mice, restricted expression of several growth factors (including *Bmps*, *Gdf7*, and *Fgf10*) and *Hox* genes within the mesenchyme play major roles in mediating the regional characteristics taken by the mesonephric duct. Mutations or disruptions in the expression of these genes can lead to homeotic transformation of the mesonephric duct derivatives.

15

of testosterone to 5α-dihydrotestosterone by the enzyme *5α-Reductase*, as it binds the *Androgen receptor* more efficiently than does testosterone. Mice lacking *Androgen receptors* do not develop a prostate and are feminized externally, although they do develop testes.

The nature of the factor, or factors, released by androgen-stimulated prostatic mesenchyme that are

responsible for initiating prostatic bud formation is unknown. However, studies in rat and mouse embryos show that once initiated, *Shh* is released from the urethral epithelium and increases expression of *Nkx3.1* in the epithelium and *Hoxa13* and *Hoxd13* in the adjacent mesenchyme, both necessary for normal prostatic development (Fig. 15-25). Continual growth and elongation of the prostatic epithelium is

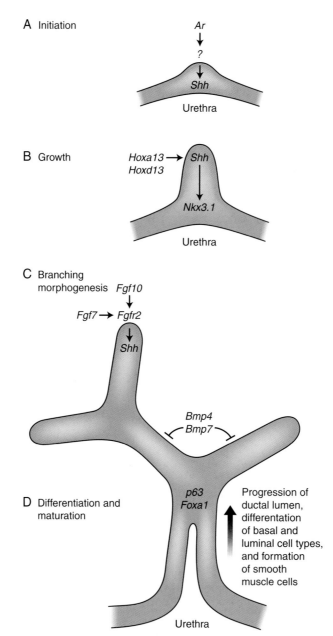

Figure 15-25. Prostatic gland development. When 5α-dihydrotestosterone binds androgen receptors (*Ar*), the prostatic mesenchyme releases unidentified signaling molecules that induce an outgrowth of endodermal prostatic buds into the urogenital mesenchyme. In rat embryos, the prostatic bud releases *Shh*, increasing epithelial *Nkx3.1* and mesenchymal *Hoxa13* and *Hoxd13* expression. *Fgf7* mediates continual growth and elongation of the prostatic epithelium. *Fgf10* released from the mesenchyme and *Fgf* signaling within the epithelium maintain *Shh* expression; however, *Shh* expression is tempered by a negative feedback caused by mesenchymal *Fgf* expression. Inhibitory effects of *Bmp4* and *Bmp7* released by the mesenchyme mediate branching of the ductal epithelium. Subsequent differentiation of the prostate epithelium occurs in a proximal-to-distal progression and is mediated by the expression of several transcription factors including *p63* and *Foxa1*.

mediated by *Fgf7* and *Fgf10*, which are released from the mesenchyme, and *Fgfr2* receptor signaling in the epithelium. This signaling maintains *Shh* expression and is essential for prostate gland development, as mice deficient in *Fgf10* fail to develop a prostate or seminal vesicles. The positive effects of *Fgf* on *Shh* expression are tempered by a negative feedback loop, as *Shh* released from the epithelium downregulates mesenchymal *Fgf* expression. The growth-inhibitory effect of *Bmp4* and *Bmp7* mediates branching of the ductal epithelium. Subsequent differentiation of the prostate epithelium occurs in a proximal-to-distal progression and is mediated by the expression of several transcription factors including *p63* (a tumor suppressor gene with homology to *p53*) and *Foxa1*.

In Absence of Y Chromosome, Female Development Occurs

The basic developmental pathway of the gonad results in ovarian development. Expression of *SRY* diverts the developmental pathway of the gonad toward the testis pathway by initiating the differentiation of Sertoli cells. In the female embryo, the XX **somatic support cells** do not contain a Y chromosome or the *SRY* gene. Therefore, they differentiate as **follicle cells** instead of Sertoli cells. Sertoli cells are responsible for the production of *AMH* and the differentiation of all other cell types in the testis. In their absence, neither AMH nor testosterone is produced. Therefore, male genital ducts and accessory sexual structures are not stimulated to develop. Instead, the müllerian ducts persist and are stimulated to differentiate into the Fallopian tube, uterus, and upper vagina (Fig. 15-26).

Formation of Ovarian Primordial Follicles

In genetic females, the somatic support cells delaminating from the coelomic epithelium do not differentiate into Sertoli cells as they do in males, but rather surround clusters of primordial germ cells. In the male, Sertoli cells inhibit further germ cell development before meiosis begins. In the female, the germ cells go on to differentiate into oogonia, proliferate, and enter the first meiotic division to form primary oocytes (see Fig. 15-26; see Fig. 15-21). These

Female

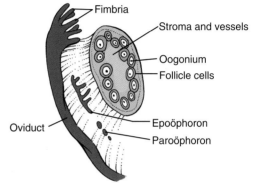

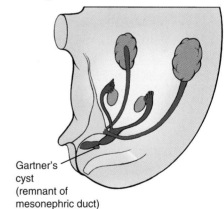

Figure 15-26. Human female gonadal development at the tissue level. In the absence of *SRY*, the somatic support cells differentiate into follicle cells. These cells surround the oocytes to form primordial follicles, which tend to localize to the outer cortical region of the ovary. The mesonephric ducts and mesonephric tubules disappear except for remnants such as the epoöphoron, the paroöphoron, and Gartner's cysts. The Müllerian ducts continue to develop to form the oviducts, uterus, and cranial part of the vagina. See Figure 15-19 for a comparison of female and male gonadal development.

15

meiotic oocytes stimulate adjacent somatic support cells to differentiation into follicle cells (or granulosa cells) that then surround individual oocytes and form **primordial follicles** within the ovary. These follicles become generally localized to the cortical region of the ovary. The medullary region of the ovary is devoted to developing the vasculature, nerves, and connective tissue of the organ. Follicle cells then arrest further oocyte development until puberty, at which point individual oocytes resume gametogenesis in response to each monthly surge of gonadotropins (discussed in Ch. 1).

IN THE RESEARCH LAB

FEMALE GONADOGENESIS IS NOT A SIMPLE MATTER OF DEFAULT

In the absence of *SRY* and thus pre-Sertoli cells, the primordial germ cells begin meiotic division. Once primordial germ cells in females enter their first meiotic division, they are committed to the oocyte lineage. These oocytes provide a key stimulus for the differentiation of follicle cells from somatic support cells generated by delamination of the coelomic epithelium (see Figs. 15-20, 15-21). Recruitment and differentiation of these follicle cells is driven and dependent on an oocyte-released factor called *FIGα (FACTOR IN GERMLINE ALPHA)*. *FIGα* activates the **folliculogenesis** program in the ovary. Without *FIGα*, primordial follicles never form and oocytes regress soon after birth. *FIGα* also stimulates the formation of the **zona pellucida** in the primordial follicle.

By now it must be evident why development of the female gonad is sometimes described as the "default" path for the human embryo in the absence of the *SRY* gene. However, this is an oversimplification. Although little is known regarding "pro-ovarian" pathways, a number of "pro-ovarian" genes have been identified. For instance, *Wnt4* seems to play an active role in promoting oocyte development. As discussed earlier in this chapter, *Wnt4* is essential for the development of the mesonephric and metanephric kidneys, but studies in knockout mice also show that *Wnt4* is crucial for normal female sexual development. *Wnt4* is initially expressed in the mesonephric and genital ridge mesenchyme and is required for the initial formation of the müllerian duct in both sexes. As the gonads develop, *Wnt4* is downregulated in the testis (most likely by pre-Sertoli cell expression of *Fgf9*) but is retained in the ovary (possibly by a synergistic effect between *WNT 4* and *R-SPONDIN1*—a gene found mutated in some cases of human XX sex reversal that codes for a secreted molecule that may activate or maintain *WNT* signaling). Studies show XX mice null for *Wnt4* have less than 10% of the normal number of oocytes found in their wild-type and heterozygotic littermates. Moreover, this loss in oocytes compromises the interstitial cell population of the gonad, including follicle cells. In these mice, the loss is not the result of a failure of germ cell migration into the gonadal ridge but rather seems to be a direct effect of a need for *Wnt4* to maintain the female germ line (see Figs. 15-20, 15-21).

In addition to "pro-ovarian" activities, *Wnt4* also exhibits "anti-testis" activities. XX mice lacking *Wnt4* develop ectopic Leydig-like cells that produce testosterone, and as such, retain and masculinize the mesonephric ducts. In contrast, gonads of *Wnt4* XY knockout mice develop normally. In wild-type XY mice, *Sry* and *Sox9* expression suppresses *Wnt4* expression, thereby providing an environment conducive for Leydig cell differentiation in males (see Figs. 15-20, 15-21). In *Fgf9* null mice, *Wnt4* fosters ovarian development by promoting primordial follicle development while repressing Leydig cell precursor development in XX individuals.

Dax1 (Dosage sensitive sex reversal, adrenal hypoplasia congenita-critical region of the X chromosome, gene 1) is described as being an ovarian-promoting factor because it can act as an "anti-testis" factor. The human *DAX1* gene is found on the X chromosome. When the *DAX1*-containing portion of the X chromosome is duplicated in XY individuals, *DAX1* leads to sex reversal. In this case, *DAX1* may antagonize *SRY*, because if *Dax1* and *Sry* expression are both driven from the *Sry* promoter in XX mice, 100% of the offspring develop as females, whereas in XX transgenic mice expressing the *Sry* gene with the normal genetic complement of *Dax1*, the XX mice develop as males. These observations suggest that *Dax1* acts as an "anti-testis" gene rather than as an ovarian-determining gene (see Fig. 15-20).

In XX mice, knocking out *Dax1* has little effect on ovarian development but in XY mice, surprisingly, it leads to testis dysgenesis. Closer examination of the phenotype in *Dax1* knockout XY mice shows these mice exhibit abnormal testis cord development even though they have normal levels of *Sry* and have Sertoli and germ cells. However, *Dax1* XY knockout mice seem to have lower levels of *Sox9* and fewer peritubular myoepithelial cells, and they exhibit compromised migration and/or development of Leydig cells. This shows that *Dax1* expression is also a critical "pro-testis" factor (see Fig. 15-20). How *Dax1* operates as both a "pro-testis" and "anti-testis" factor is unclear, but it is speculated that particular levels of *Dax1* are required within a narrow window of time for normal gonadogenesis to occur (Fig. 15-27). If *Dax1* levels are higher than normal (e.g., through gene duplication) or lower than normal (e.g., the result of an inactivating mutation) during this

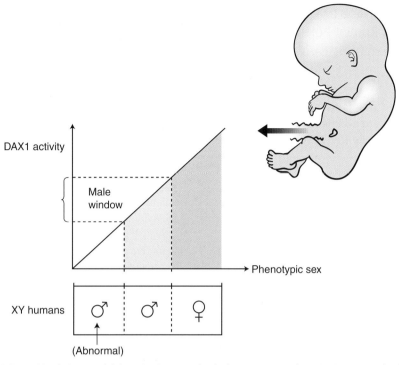

Figure 15-27. Window of DAX1 activity during gonadal determination. DAX1 has both "anti-testis" and "pro-testis" activities but how it operates is unclear. Particular levels of DAX1 may be required within a narrow window of time for normal gonadogenesis to occur. For example, in an XY individual, the testes would be formed if the DAX1 dose/activity was within a "window." If DAX1 levels were higher than normal (e.g., through gene duplication) or lower than normal (e.g., because of an inactivating mutation) during this critical period, abnormal testis development would occurs. The male window is shown in blue and the female window is shown in pink. Abbreviations: ♀ represents a male phenotype; ♂ represents a female phenotype.

critical period, abnormal testis development occurs. Much more needs to be learned regarding the regulation of *Dax1*, its target genes, and its dosage-dependent effects to understand its precise role in sex determination and in the etiology of sex reversal.

Steroids and steroid receptors also play an important role in female gonadogenesis. Ovaries in mice lacking both estrogen receptors, *Erα* and *Erβ*, express Sertoli cell markers and develop what resemble seminiferous tubules and Sertoli cells within their gonads during postnatal development. XX mice lacking the gene coding for *Aromatase* (a key enzyme in the conversion of androgens into estrogens) also begin expressing *Sox9* and markers for Sertoli and Leydig cells. Interestingly,

early postnatal treatment with 17β-estradiol in *Aromatase*-deficient mice reduces the number of Sertoli and Leydig cells in these ovaries and increases folliculogenesis of the existing follicles (these mice still express estrogen receptors). Surprisingly, male mice lacking estrogen receptors also exhibit defects in testis development. The testes are reduced in size with few intact seminiferous tubules, and there is a reduction in the number of germ cells. Whether these effects represent a reversal of later steps in gonad formation (a regression) or are the result of abnormalities in initial gonadal development is unclear. However, what is clear is that the estrogenic environment plays a key role in gonadal development.

15

Müllerian Ducts Give Rise to Fallopian Tubes, Uterus, and Cranial Portion of Vagina, while Mesonephric Ducts Degenerate

In the absence of *Sry* and subsequent expression of male pathway genes, the female gonads form primordial follicles and **thecal cells** (the Leydig cell homolog in females). The stromal thecal cells, which do have steroidogenesis activity, express only low levels of the genes necessary for synthesizing testosterone. Because mesonephric ducts and mesonephric tubules require testosterone for their development, they rapidly disappear in the female except for a few vestiges. Two remnants, the **epoöphoron** and **paroöphoron**, are found in the mesentery of the ovary, and a scattering of tiny remnants called **Gartner's cysts** cluster near the vagina (Fig. 15-28C; see also Fig. 15-26). The müllerian ducts, in contrast, develop uninhibited.

Recall that the distal tips of the growing müllerian ducts adhere to each other just before they contact the posterior wall of the pelvic urethra. The wall of the pelvic urethra at this point forms a slight thickening called the **sinusal tubercle** (Fig. 15-28A). As soon as the fused tips of the müllerian ducts connect with the sinusal tubercle, the müllerian ducts begin to fuse from their caudal tips cranially, forming a short tube with a single lumen (Fig. 15-28B, C). This tube, called the **uterovaginal canal** or **genital canal**, becomes the uterus and possibly contributes to the cranial portion of the vagina (the latter idea is controversial and is discussed in the following paragraph). The unfused, cranial portions of the müllerian ducts become the fallopian tubes (or oviducts or uterine tubes), and the funnel-shaped cranial openings of the müllerian ducts become the infundibula of the fallopian tubes.

The formation of the vagina is poorly understood. While the uterovaginal canal is forming during the 3rd month, the endodermal tissue of the sinusal tubercle in the posterior urethra continues to thicken, forming a pair of evaginating swellings called the **sinuvaginal bulbs** that fuse to form a solid block of tissue called the **vaginal plate** (see Fig. 15-28). The vaginal plate is thought to give rise to the inferior portion of the vagina, whereas the caudal region of the uterovaginal canal is thought to form the upper vagina. The lower end of the developing vagina lengthens between the 3rd and 4th month, and its junction with the urogenital sinus is thought to translocate caudally until it comes to rest on the posterior wall of the urogenital sinus (see Fig. 15-28C). The vaginal plate is then canalized by a process of **desquamation** (cell shedding), forming the vaginal lumen. However, an endodermal membrane temporarily separates the lumen of the vagina from the base of the urogenital sinus (the latter forms the **vestibule of the vagina**). This barrier degenerates partially after the 5th month, but its remnant persists as the vaginal **hymen**.

It should be noted that some studies suggest that the entire vagina arises from a downward growth of both mesonephric and Müllerian ducts, and that the sinuvaginal bulbs are really derivatives of persistent caudalmost segments of the mesonephric duct. Three-dimensional reconstructions of vaginal development in wild-type androgen-responsive and androgen-insensitive mice support this view and suggest that vaginal development is under androgen-dependent negative control by the mesonephric ducts (thereby explaining why patients with **androgen insensitivity syndrome** develop a shortened vagina). As such, the mucous membrane lining the vagina would be derived from the mesoderm rather than from the endodermal epithelium of the urogenital sinus. Further investigation is necessary to better understand the morphogenetic steps responsible for the development of the lower female reproductive tract.

IN THE RESEARCH LAB

MÜLLERIAN DUCT DEVELOPMENT AND REGIONALIZED EXPRESSION OF HOX GENES

In females, the mesonephric duct regresses due to a lack of male androgens. In contrast, the müllerian duct proliferates and differentiates in a cranial-caudal progression, forming the fallopian tube, uterus, and upper vagina. During this time, the single-layered müllerian duct epithelium differentiates into distinct morphologies ranging from ciliated columnar epithelium in the fallopian tube to stratified squamous epithelium in the vagina. It should not be surprising, given the müllerian and mesonephric duct share much of the same mesenchyme, that *Hox* gene expression plays a key role in mediating the regional characterization of structures found along the cranial-caudal axis of the female reproductive tract. Similar to those described for the mesonephric duct earlier in the chapter, *Hox* deficiencies can lead to homeotic transformations within müllerian ducts. For example, in mice, *Hoxa10* deficiency transforms the cranial part of uterus into fallopian tube–like structures and reduces fertility.

Wnt7a expression is also important for proper *Hox* expression and radial axis patterning of müllerian ducts.

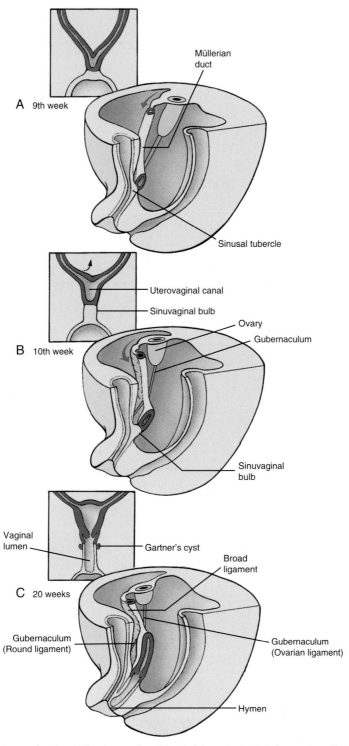

Figure 15-28. Formation of the uterus and vagina. *A,* The uterus and cranial end of the vagina begin to form as the müllerian ducts fuse together near their attachment to the posterior wall of the urogenital sinus. *B, C,* The ducts then zip together in a cranial direction between the 3rd and 5th months. As the müllerian ducts are pulled away from the posterior body wall, they drag a fold of peritoneal membrane with them, forming the broad ligaments of the uterus. *A-C,* The caudal end of the vagina is thought to form from the sinuvaginal bulbs on the posterior wall of the urogenital sinus.

15

Female mice deficient in *Wnt7a* show dramatic caudal transformation of the reproductive tract whereby Fallopian tubes are absent and the uterus exhibits the cytoarchitecture of the vagina. Normal mesenchymal expression of *Hoxa10* and *Hoxa11* in these regions is lost in these mice, suggesting that *Wnt7a* is required for maintaining normal *Hox* expression in this region. In addition, *Wnt7a*-deficient mice exhibit abnormal myometrial patterning and lack uterine glands.

IN THE CLINIC

ANOMALIES OF UTERUS

The incidence of müllerian duct anomalies has been difficult to assess but is thought to be about 1% of normal fertile women and about 3% of women with repeated miscarriages. The majority of women with müllerian duct anomalies can usually conceive but they have higher rates of spontaneous abortion, premature delivery, and **dystocia** (difficult or abnormal delivery).

Many anomalies related to the development of the uterus and vagina are attributable to abnormal fusion or regression of the caudal portion of the müllerian duct (Fig. 15-29). At about 9 weeks of development, the müllerian ducts fuse at their inferior (caudal) margin, forming a single lumen uterovaginal canal. Incomplete fusion of the lower segments of the müllerian ducts leads to development of a duplicated uterus with or without a duplicated vagina. Failed regression of the uterine septum (a transient structure resulting from müllerian duct fusion) can lead to the development of a bicornate uterus (two uterine bodies with a single cervical portion), a septated uterus (accounts for approximately 55% of müllerian duct anomalies), or atresia of the cervix. A unicornuate uterus (approximately 20% of müllerian duct anomalies) results if one of the entire müllerian ducts regress or if one fails to elongate during development. In cases of congenital absence of the vagina (incidence of 1 in 4000 to 5000 female births), the entire uterus may also be missing, as tissue-tissue interactions responsible for inducing the vagina and for uterine differentiation may be absent.

DIETHYLSTILBESTROL CAUSES SEVERAL REPRODUCTIVE ANOMALIES

Diethylstilbestrol (DES) was the first synthetic estrogenic compound orally administered to pregnant women to prevent miscarriage (from years 1947 to 1971). It became evident that young women born of DES-treated mothers had significantly higher risks of developing **clear cell adenocarcinoma of the vagina**, a rare cancer usually found in women 50 years and older. In addition, in utero exposure to DES increased the risk of reproductive tract anomalies, including uterine anomalies and **vaginal adenosis** (transformation of stratified squamous epithelium to a columnar type, a possible precursor step toward

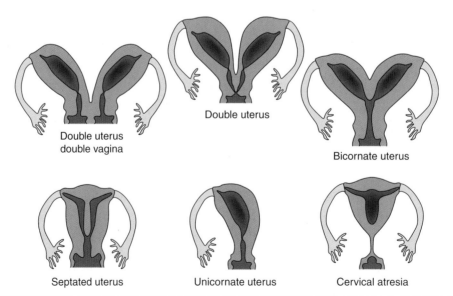

Double uterus
double vagina

Double uterus

Bicornate uterus

Septated uterus

Unicornate uterus

Cervical atresia

Figure 15-29. Anomalies of the uterus and vagina. Many anomalies related to the development of the uterus and vagina are attributable to abnormal fusion or regression of the caudal portion of the müllerian duct.

development of adenocarcinoma), whereas males exposed to DES in utero exhibited such anomalies as cryptorchidism, hypospadias (condition where penile urethra opens on the ventral surface of the penis), and testicular hypoplasia.

DES binds to the estrogen receptor, $Er\alpha$, with much higher affinity than its endogenous ligand, 17β-estradiol, and it seems to have a much longer half-life. Therefore, it is a strong estrogen. In mice, DES has similar teratogenic effects on female reproductive development as described in humans. These defects closely resemble those observed in *Hox* and *Wnt7a* mutants. In mice, DES treatment represses *Hoxa10*, *Hoxa11*, and *Wnt7a* expression during the critical period of uterine and vaginal development. Moreover, DES alters the expression pattern of the tumor suppressor gene *p63* within the epithelium of these reproductive organs, providing a link for the increase in adenocarcinomas seen in DES-exposed women.

Development of External Genitalia

The early development of the external genitalia is similar in males and females. As discussed in Chapter 14, the urorectal septum completely separates the urogenital sinus and anorectal canal from one another. Meanwhile, mesoderm anterior and cranial to the **phallic segment** of the urogenital sinus expands, generating the **genital tubercle**, which eventually forms the **phallus** (Fig. 15-30). With the rupture of the cloacal membrane, much of the floor of the phallic segment of the urogenital sinus is lost, whereas the roof of the phallic segment expands along the lower surface of the genital tubercle as the genital tubercle enlarges (Fig. 15-31A, see 15-30). This endodermal extension forms the **urethral plate** (or **urethral membrane**).

Early in the 5th week, a pair of swellings called **urogenital folds** (or **cloacal folds**) develops on either side of the urethral plate through an expansion of mesoderm underlying the ectoderm (see Fig. 15-31A). Inferiorly, these folds meet and join the genital tubercle. Similarly, there is an expansion of underlying mesoderm flanking the anal membrane forming the **anal folds**. A new pair of swellings, the **labioscrotal swellings**, then appears on either side of the urethral folds (see Fig. 15-31A).

The appearance of the external genitalia is similar in male and female embryos through the 12th week, and embryos of this age are difficult to sex on the basis of their external appearance. See Table 15-2 (page 502) for the adult derivatives of the embryonic external genital structures.

In Males, Urethral Groove Becomes Penile Urethra, and Labioscrotal Swellings Form Scrotum

During the 6th week, a **urethral groove** forms along the ventral surface of the genital tubercle from extensions of the urethral plate and urogenital folds as the genital tubercle elongates (Fig. 15-31B). Initially, the urethral groove and urethral folds extend only a part of the way along the shaft of the elongating phallus. Distally, the urethral groove terminates but the urethral plate continues to grow and extend distally as a solid, multilayered cord. As the phallus elongates, the urethral folds grow toward one another and fuse in the midline, beginning proximally in the perineal region and extending distally toward the glans penis. This converts the urethral groove into a tubular **penile urethra**. Exactly how the human urethra forms within the glans penis is unclear. However, recent studies in mice show that the solid urethral plate extends to the very tip of the glans penis and then canalizes to form the **glans urethra** and **external penile meatus** (see Fig. 15-31B). **Hypospadias** results from failure of formation or fusion of the urethral folds (penile hypospadias) or abnormal canalization of the urethral plate within the glans penis (glans hypospadias).

Starting in the 4th month, the effects of dihydrotestosterone on the male external genitalia become readily apparent (see Fig. 15-31B). The perineal region separating the urogenital sinus from the anus begins to lengthen. The labioscrotal folds fuse at the midline to form the **scrotum**, and the urethral folds fuse to enclose the **penile urethra**. The penile urethra is completely enclosed by 14 weeks.

In Females, Genital Tubercle Does Not Lengthen, and Labioscrotal and Urethral Folds Do Not Fuse

In the absence of dihydrotestosterone in female embryos, the genital tubercle does not lengthen, and the labioscrotal and urethral folds do not fuse across the midline (Fig. 15-31C). The phallus bends inferiorly, becoming the **clitoris**, and the phallic portion of the urogenital sinus becomes the **vestibule of the vagina**. The urethral folds become the **labia minora**, and the labioscrotal swellings become the **labia majora**.

15

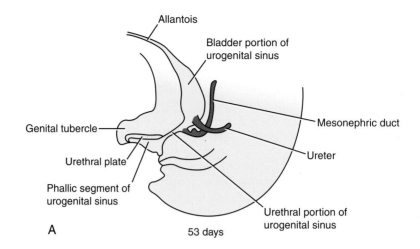

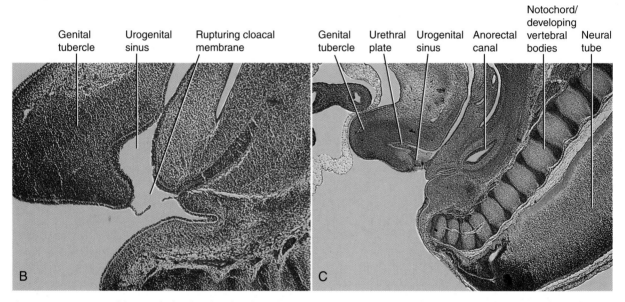

Figure 15-30. Formation of the genital tubercle and urethra plate. *A*, The urogenital sinus is subdivided into the bladder, pelvic urethral region, and phallic segment. With the rupture of the cloacal membrane, the roof of the phallic segment forms a urethral plate of endodermal cells that lengthen as the genital tubercle grows. *B*, Light micrograph of a sagittal section through the caudal region of the 18 mm human embryo (50 to 51 days) just after the initial rupture of the cloacal membrane. *C*, Light micrograph of a sagittal section through the caudal region of a 21 mm human embryo (52-53 days) showing the genital tubercle and elongating urethral plate.

IN THE RESEARCH LAB

FORMATION OF EXTERNAL GENITALIA

The role of the distal end of the urethral plate epithelium in promoting the outgrowth of the genital tubercle is in some ways akin to that of the apical epidermal ridge of the limb bud (discussed in Ch. 18). In mice, if the distal (ventral) urethral plate is removed, the genital tubercle is hypoplastic. *Shh* is released by the entire urethral plate, whereas *Bmp7* and *Fgf8* are released by the distal urethral plate adjacent to the site of the forming genital tubercle (Fig. 15-32). In *Shh* null mice, genital tubercle development is arrested at the initial outgrowth phase, showing that *Shh* has a key role in early genital tubercle and urethral development. *Shh* is required to maintain *Fgf8* expression within urethral plate as well as *Bmp4* and *Wnt5a* within the genital tubercle mesenchyme. *Shh*-dependent expression of *Fgf8* is required for genital tubercle growth, as anti-*Fgf8* inhibits tubercle outgrowth

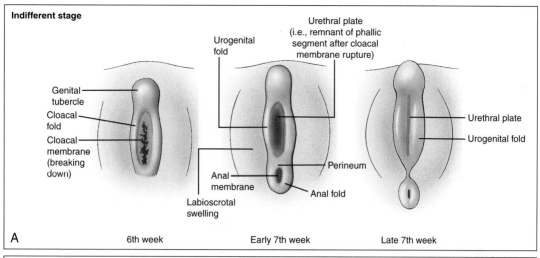

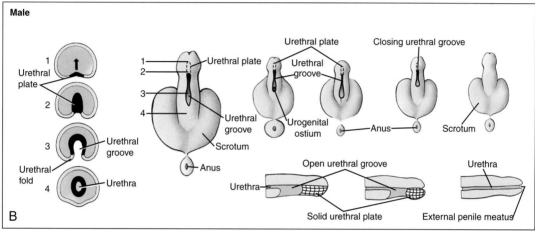

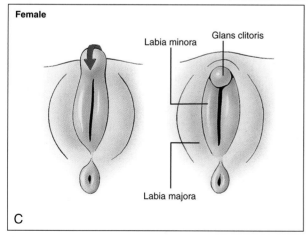

Figure 15-31. Formation of the external genitalia in males and females. *A,* The external genitalia form from a pair of labioscrotal folds, a pair of urogenital folds, and an anterior genital tubercle. Male and female genitalia are morphologically indistinguishable at this stage. *B,* In males, the urogenital folds fuse and the genital tubercle elongates to form the shaft and glans of the penis. Fusion of the urethral folds encloses the phallic portion of the urogenital sinus to form the penile urethra. The distal urethra is formed by canalization of a solid endodermal extension of the urethral plate into the glans. The labioscrotal folds fuse to form the scrotum. *C,* In females, the genital tubercle bends inferiorly to form the clitoris, and the urogenital folds remain separated to form the labia minora. The labioscrotal folds form the labia majora.

15

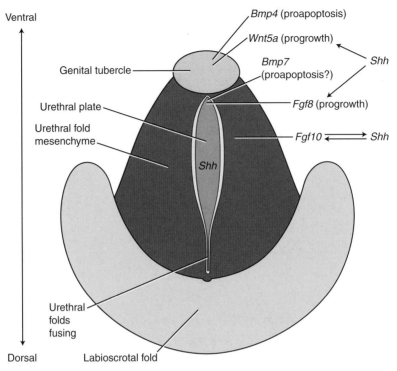

Figure 15-32. Growth factors and transcription factors involved in external genitalia development. After rupture of the cloacal membrane, the urethral plate is bordered by the genital tubercle ventrally (anteriorly) and the urethral folds laterally. *Shh* signaling from the urethral plate upregulates *Bmp4* and *Wnt5a* expression in the genital tubercle mesenchyme, and *Fgf8* in the distal urethral epithelium. This expression pattern balances apoptosis and proliferation necessary for proper growth of the genital tubercle and urethral plate. The penile urethra subsequently forms by proximal-to-distal fusion of the urethral folds. *Shh* emanating from the urethral plate also signals the adjacent bilateral mesenchyme to express *Fgf10*. *Fgf10* expression must be maintained by *Shh* if the urethral folds are to fuse properly.

in explant cultures, which can be restored with exogenous *Fgf8*. One of the targets of *Fgf8* is *Bmp4*. *Bmp4* is expressed in the mesenchyme of the genital tubercle, and *Fgf8* upregulates this expression. Conditional knockouts for the *Bmp4* receptor, *Bmpr1a*, or overexpression of the *Bmp* antagonist, *Noggin*, results in genital tubercle hyperplasia and hypospadias. Higher than normal levels of *Bmp4* expression increase apoptosis within genital tubercle mesenchyme, and knocking out *Noggin* causes genital tubercle hypoplasia. Interestingly, human mutations in *NOGGIN* are associated with feminization of the external genitalia in XY individuals. Collectively, these observations suggest that normal genital tubercle and urethral development requires a proper balance between apoptosis and proliferation, mediated through epithelial-mesenchymal interactions involving *Fgf* and *Bmp* signaling.

Shh from the urethral plate also upregulates *Hoxa13* and *Hoxd13* expression within the genital tubercle mesenchyme. The expression of these two *Hox* genes is required for the development of the early cloaca and genital tubercle, because these structures fail to develop in double knockout mice for these two genes (likely reflecting their importance in hindgut development). Interestingly, deficits in human *HOXA13* expression are seen in a dominant autosomal disorder causing **hand-foot-genital syndrome**, which is characterized by malformed distal limbs and hypospadias.

Hypospadias is a common defect, suggesting that closure of the urethral folds is very sensitive to perturbations. *Shh* is not only involved in early stages of genital tubercle development but may also have a role in the formation of the penile urethra. *Fgf10* null mice exhibit severe glans dysgenesis and urethral defects, whereas initial genital tubercle development seems normal (Fig. 15-33). *Fgf10* is expressed in the urethral fold mesenchyme adjacent to the *Shh*-expressing urethral plate, and antibodies directed against *Shh* can alter *Fgf10* expression in the genital tubercle mesenchyme (see Fig. 15-32). This suggests that *Shh* not only has an important role in early genital tubercle development but also in regulating

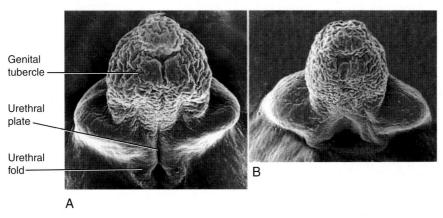

Figure 15-33. Scanning electron micrographs of external genitalia and urethral development. *A*, Wild-type mouse. *B*, *Fgf10* gene mutation leads to severe defects in urethra formation.

Fgf10 expression, which is important in the closure of urethra later in development. *Ephrins* and their receptors have also been implicated as playing a role in this process, as mice deficient in *EphrinB2* and *EphB2/EphB3* signaling exhibit faulty urethral closure.

Although both *5α-reductase* and *Androgen receptors* are expressed in females, females do not develop male external genitalia due to their low levels of testosterone. Even though the early steps of genital tubercle and urethral plate formation occur in females, the lack of dihydrotestosterone means that the genital tubercle and urethral plate do not lengthen and grow to any great extent, nor do the urethral folds fuse. Unfortunately, little is known regarding the molecular embryology of the later stages of female external genitalia development that are responsible for the formation of the clitoris, labia, and vestibule.

Suspension of Mesonephric-Gonadal Complex within Abdomen

As the mesonephric-gonadal complex becomes more segregated from the adjacent intermediate mesoderm, it remains anchored by two ligaments, the **cranial suspensory ligament** and the **gubernaculum** (or **caudal genito-inguinal ligament**). The cranial suspensory ligament runs from the cranial portion of the mesonephric-gonadal complex to the diaphragm (Fig. 15-34). The gubernaculum was first described by John Hunter in 1762 and given the name gubernaculum (Latin: rudder or helm) as "it connects the testis with the scrotum, and directs its course in its descent." The gubernaculum is attached to the caudal portion of the male and female mesonephric-gonadal complex and extends to the peritoneal floor where it is attached to the fascia between the developing external and internal oblique abdominal muscles in the region of the labioscrotal swellings.

Development of Inguinal Canals

A slight evagination of the peritoneum, called the **vaginal process** or **processus vaginalis**, develops on three sides of each gubernaculum, forming a nearly annular, blind-end cavity. The **inguinal canal** is a caudal evagination of the abdominal wall that forms when the vaginal process grows inferiorly, pushing out a sock-like evagination consisting of the various layers of the abdominal wall (Fig. 15-35).

The first layer encountered by the vaginal process is the transversalis fascia, lying just deep to the transversus abdominis muscle. This layer will become the internal spermatic fascia of the spermatic cord. The vaginal process does not encounter the transversus abdominis muscle itself, because this muscle has a large hiatus in this region. Next, the vaginal process picks up the fibers and fascia of the internal oblique muscle. These become the cremasteric fascia of the spermatic cord. Finally, the vaginal process picks up a thin layer of external oblique

15

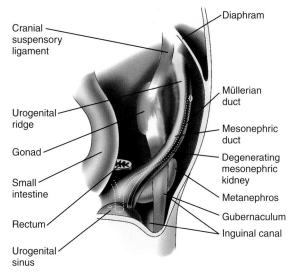

Figure 15-34. At the indifferent gonad stage, two ligaments, a cranial suspensory ligament and the gubernaculum, anchor the mesonephric-gonadal complex. The cranial suspensory ligament runs from the cranial portion of the mesonephric-gonadal complex to the diaphragm. The gubernaculum is attached to the caudal portion of the gonad and extends to the peritoneal floor, where it is attached to the fascia between the developing external and internal oblique abdominal muscles in the region of the labioscrotal swellings.

muscle, which will become the external spermatic fascia. As the vaginal process elongates, it hollows out the inguinal canals and the labioscrotal swellings, providing a cavity into which the testes descend in the male. The superior ring of the canal is called the **deep ring of the inguinal canal** (see Fig. 15-35E). The inferomedial rim of the canal formed by the point of eversion of the external oblique muscle is called the **superficial ring of the inguinal canal**. In females, the vaginal process remains rudimentary and normally degenerates during development.

Descent of Testes

During embryonic and fetal life, the testes and the ovaries both descend from their original position at the 10th thoracic level, although the testes ultimately descend much farther. In both sexes, the descent of the gonad depends on the ligamentous gubernaculum. The gubernaculum condenses during the 7th week within the subserous fascia of a longitudinal peritoneal fold on either side of the vertebral column (see Fig. 15-34). Between the 7th and 12th weeks

(the intra-abdominal phase), the extrainguinal portions of the gubernacula shorten and in males, pull the testes down to the vicinity of the deep inguinal ring within the plane of the subserous fascia while the cranial suspensory ligament regresses (see Fig. 15-35). The gubernacula shorten mainly by swelling at their base; this serves the secondary purpose of enlarging the inguinal canal.

The testes remain in the vicinity of the deep ring from the 3rd to the 7th month but then enter the inguinal canal in response to renewed shortening and migration of the gubernacula (the inguinal-scrotal phase). The testes remain within the subserous fascia of the **vaginal process** through which they descend toward the scrotum (see Fig. 15-35). The increased abdominal pressure created by the growth of the abdominal viscera also aids the movement of the testes through the canal. By the 9th month, just before normal term delivery, the testes have completely entered the scrotal sac and the gubernaculum is reduced to a small ligamentous band attaching the caudal pole of the testis to the scrotal floor. **Cryptorchidism** (undescended testes) is a common condition and is a risk factor for development of malignancy within the gonad (discussed in the following "In the Clinic").

Within the 1st year after birth, the cranial portion of the vaginal process is usually obliterated, leaving only a distal remnant sac, the **tunica vaginalis**, which lies ventral to the testis (Figs. 15-36A, 15-37). During infancy, this sac wraps around most of the testis. Its lumen is normally collapsed, but under pathologic conditions, it may fill with serous secretions, forming a **testicular hydrocele** (Fig. 15-36B, D).

As mentioned earlier, it is not rare for the entire vaginal process to remain patent, forming a connection between the abdominal cavity and the scrotal sac. During childhood, loops of intestine may herniate into the vaginal process, resulting in an **indirect inguinal hernia** (Fig. 15-36C). Repair of these hernias is one of the most common childhood operations.

IN THE RESEARCH LAB

DESCENT OF TESTES

As discussed earlier in this chapter, the process of testicular descent occurs in two distinct and sequential phases: the intra-abdominal phase and the inguinoscrotal phase. Although hormonal control of testicular descent is still not

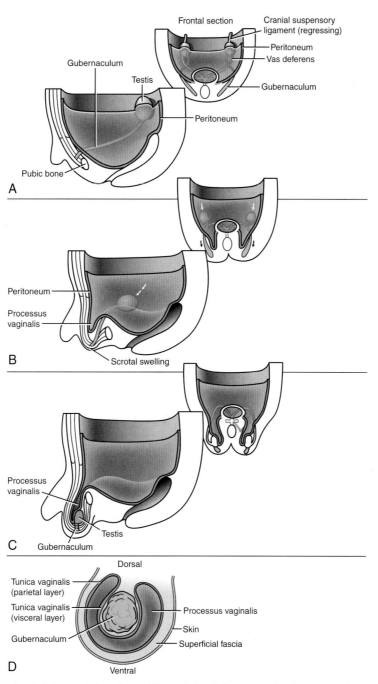

Figure 15-35. Descent of the testes. *A–C,* Between 7th week and birth, shortening of the gubernaculum testis causes the testes to descend from the tenth thoracic level into the scrotum. The testes pass through the inguinal canal in the anterior abdominal wall. *D,* Cross section of the gubernaculum showing the layers of the tunica vaginalis and processus vaginalis at the level of the labioscrotal swelling.

Continued

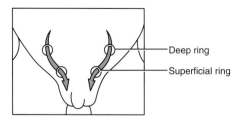

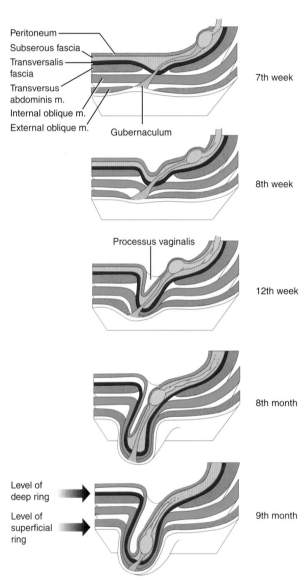

E

Figure 15-35, cont'd. *E,* After the 8th week, a peritoneal evagination called the processus vaginalis forms just ventral to the gubernaculum and pushes out sock-like extensions of the transversalis fascia, the internal oblique muscle, and the external oblique muscle, thus forming the inguinal canal. The inguinal canal extends from the base of the everted transversalis fascia (the deep ring) to the base of the everted external oblique muscle (the superficial ring). After the vaginal process has evaginated into the scrotum, the gubernaculum shortens and simply pulls the gonads through the canal. The gonads always remain within the plane of the subserous fascia even though it bulges into the abdominal cavity and later the processus vaginalis.

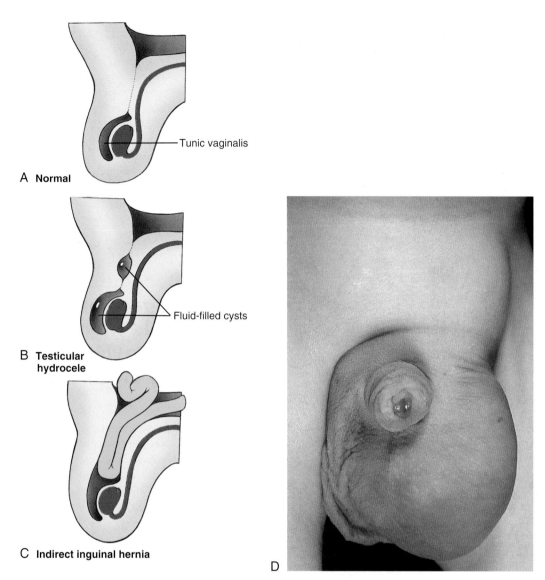

A **Normal**

Tunic vaginalis

B **Testicular hydrocele**

Fluid-filled cysts

C **Indirect inguinal hernia**

D

Figure 15-36. Normal and abnormal development of the processus vaginalis. *A,* The proximal end of the processus vaginalis normally disintegrates during the 1st year after birth, leaving a distal remnant called the tunica vaginalis. *B,* Some proximal remnants may remain, and these and the tunica vaginalis may fill with serous fluid, forming testicular hydroceles in pathologic conditions or subsequent to injury. *C,* If the proximal end of the processus vaginalis does not disintegrate, abdominal contents may herniate through the inguinal canal into the scrotum. This condition is called congenital inguinal hernia. *D,* Infant with a testicular hydrocele.

15

completely understood, androgens and pituitary hormones clearly play essential roles in mediating the second stage of descent. In the absence of testosterone generated by Leydig cells or in the case of nonfunctional or absent *Androgen receptors,* testicular descent is arrested at the inguinoscrotal stage.

Much less is known regarding the crucial first stage of testes descent, but it is increasingly recognized that factors released by the testes play key roles. Leydig cells generate a factor called *Insulin-like factor-3* (*Insl3*) or *Relaxin-like factor.* Mice lacking *Insl3* exhibit bilateral cryptorchidism, with their testes remaining adjacent the kidneys. This cryptorchidism is rectified if *Insl3* is overexpressed in pancreatic beta cells of these *Insl3* null mice. Moreover, if *Insl3* is misexpressed in female mice, their ovaries descend. Steroid hormones like estradiol and diethylstilbestrol can downregulate *Insl3*

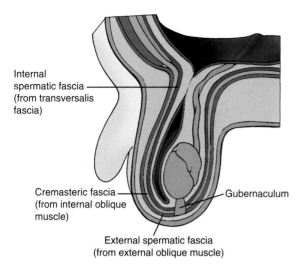

Internal spermatic fascia (from transversalis fascia)

Cremasteric fascia (from internal oblique muscle)

Gubernaculum

External spermatic fascia (from external oblique muscle)

Figure 15-37. The three extruded layers of abdominal wall pushed into the scrotum by the evaginating processus vaginalis from three layers of spermatic fascia. These three layers enclose the tunica vaginalis and the testis in a common compartment.

expression in Leydig cells, thereby providing an explanation of why in utero exposure of male embryos to excess androgens causes cryptorchidism. One target of *Insl3* is a novel G-protein–coupled receptor referred to as *Lgr8* (*Leucine-rich repeat-containing protein-coupled receptor 8*). Mutations in *Lgr8* lead to cryptorchidism in mice, and a mutation in this gene has been identified in a case of human cryptorchidism.

Another possible player in testes descent may be the innervation of the genital region. The genitofemoral nerve innervates the region that includes the spermatic cord in the male and the round ligament in the female. This nerve seems to have a role in mediating shortening of the gubernacula, because if this nerve is severed, cryptorchidism results. *Calcitonin gene–related peptide* (*Cgrp*) is the principal neurotransmitter released by this nerve. Because it can restore normal descent in animals with severed genitofemoral nerves, *Cgrp* may stimulate gubernacular smooth muscle contraction, mediate the direction of gubernacular migration, and help pull the testes toward the scrotum.

IN THE CLINIC

CRYPTORCHIDISM

Cryptorchidism is the failure of both testes or a single testis to descend into the scrotum. Although many infants may be cryptorchid at birth, most spontaneously correct themselves by 3 months of age. Cryptorchidism is very common, having an incidence of 1% to 4% of live male births. Many patients with this condition respond to treatment with human chorionic gonadotropin or gonadotropin-releasing hormone. If a testis has not descended by 4 to 6 months, it is brought down surgically (**orchiopexy**). Patients with cryptorchid testes have a higher risk of developing testicular cancer and an extremely high risk of becoming irreversibly infertile. As the normal male testicular environment is usually 3 to 5 degrees cooler than the abdominal temperature, the higher abdominal temperature reduces the number of adult type A spermatogonia available for spermatogenesis and promotes transformation of germ cells into carcinoma cells, if the descent is delayed beyond 1 to 2 years of age.

Ovaries Become Suspended in Broad Ligament of Uterus and Are Held High in Abdominal Cavity by Cranial Suspensory Ligaments

Like the male embryo, the female embryo develops a gubernaculum and a rudimentary inguinal canal (Fig. 15-38). In females, the gubernaculum does not swell or shorten. Nevertheless, it causes the ovaries to descend during the 3rd month and to be swept out into a peritoneal fold called the **broad ligament of the uterus** (see Fig. 15-38; see Fig. 15-28). This translocation occurs because during the 7th week, the gubernaculum becomes attached to the developing müllerian ducts, where these two structures cross each other on the posterior body wall. As the müllerian ducts zip together from their caudal ends, they sweep out the broad ligaments and simultaneously pull the ovaries into these peritoneal folds.

In the absence of male hormones, the female gubernaculum remains intact and grows in step with the rest of the body. The inferior gubernaculum becomes the **round ligament of the uterus**, connecting the fascia of the labia majora to the uterus, and the superior gubernaculum becomes the **round ligament of the ovary**, connecting the uterus to the ovary. Also, in the absence of androgens, the cranial suspensory ligament persists and anchors the ovary high in the abdomen.

As in males, the vaginal process of the inguinal canal is normally obliterated. However, it occasionally remains patent and may become the site of an **indirect inguinal hernia**.

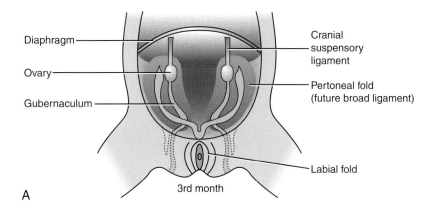

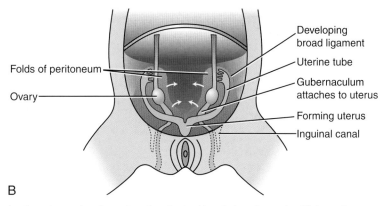

Figure 15-38. *A, B,* In females, the gubernaculum does not swell or shorten. Nevertheless, the ovaries still descend to some extent during the 3rd month and are swept out into a peritoneal fold called the broad ligament of the uterus (see Fig. 15-28). This translocation occurs because the gubernaculum becomes attached to the developing müllerian ducts. As the müllerian ducts zip together from their caudal ends, they sweep out the broad ligaments and simultaneously pull the ovaries into these peritoneal folds. As a consequence, the remnant of the female gubernaculum connects the labia majora with the wall of the uterus and is then reflected laterally, attaching to the ovary.

Continued

IN THE CLINIC

PSEUDOHERMAPHRODISM

Many congenital defects of sexual development are caused by mutations or chromosomal anomalies affecting autosomes or sex chromosomes. Not surprisingly, mutations of the sex-determining region of the Y chromosome have drastic effects, as do deletions or duplications of the sex chromosomes. However, most genital system malformations arise from alterations in autosomal genes.

A pseudohermaphroditic individual is one whose gonads and sex chromosomes are discordant with secondary sex characteristics, which include the genital tract and external genitalia. Genetic males (46,XY) with feminized genitals are

called **male pseudohermaphrodites**, and genetic females (46,XX) with virilized genitals are called **female pseudohermaphrodites**. Pseudohermaphrodism is usually caused either by abnormal levels of sex hormones or by anomalies in the sex hormone receptors.

Male Pseudohermaphrodism

In genetically male fetuses, any deficiency in androgen action will tend to allow autonomous female development to proceed, resulting in some degree of genital feminization. Which structures show feminization depends on which of the male sex steroids are affected by the deficiency. Male pseudohermaphroditism affecting the external genitals may be caused by 5α-REDUCTASE deficiency. Mutations that reduce or disable this enzyme have little consequence in

15

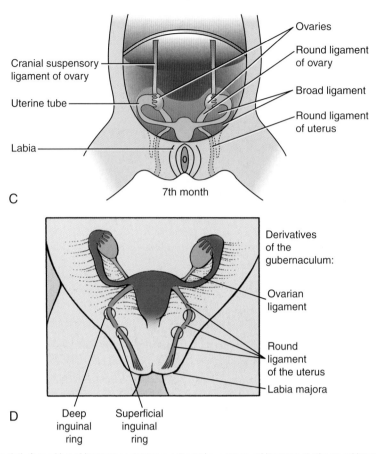

Figure 15-38. cont'd, *C*, Completly formed broad ligament containing ovaries and ovarian round ligament. *D*, The round ligament of the uterus (remnant of the gubernaculum) exits the abdominal cavity via the deep and superficial inguinal rings and connects to the base of the labia majora.

females, but in males the resulting absence of dihydrotestosterone results in severe penoscrotal hypospadias and genitalia that seem to be female at birth. These individuals have normal testes located either within the inguinal canals or in the labioscrotal swellings. The testes produce AMH and testosterone at the appropriate times, so müllerian duct derivatives are absent and the mesonephric ducts differentiate into vasa deferentia. In male pseudohermaphrodites of this type, the sudden rise of testosterone at puberty may cause a dramatic differentiation of the external genitalia and accessory glands into typically male structures. The urethral folds and labioscrotal swellings may fuse completely, and the genital tubercle may differentiate into a penis. These former pseudohermaphrodites may be fertile and produce offspring. The normal testosterone levels during fetal life and after puberty are thought to result in normal male differentiation of the brain and, hence, a sense of male gender identity.

Male pseudohermaphroditism may be caused by **testosterone deficiency**. Mutations that affect enzymes required for the synthesis of testosterone—such as *20, 22-Desmolase, 17-hydroxylase, Steroid 17,20-desmolase,* and *17β-Hydroxysteroid dehydrogenase*—cause a deficiency or absence of testosterone. The resulting pseudohermaphroditism affects all structures that depend on androgens for their differentiation. The mesonephric ducts do not differentiate, the testes do not descend, and both the external genitalia and gender identity are female. Because testosterone levels do not rise at puberty, feminization is not reversed and the individual may continue to resemble a normal female. However, because testes develop and produce AMH, the müllerian ducts degenerate.

Although not restricted to individuals with pseudohermaphroditism, one common manifestation of male pseudohermaphroditism is **hypospadias**, the condition in which the urethra opens onto the ventral surface of the penis. Hypospadias occurs in about 0.5% of all live births. In simple cases, a single anomalous opening is found on the underside of the glans or shaft (Fig. 15-39*A, B*). In more severe cases, the penile urethra has multiple openings or is

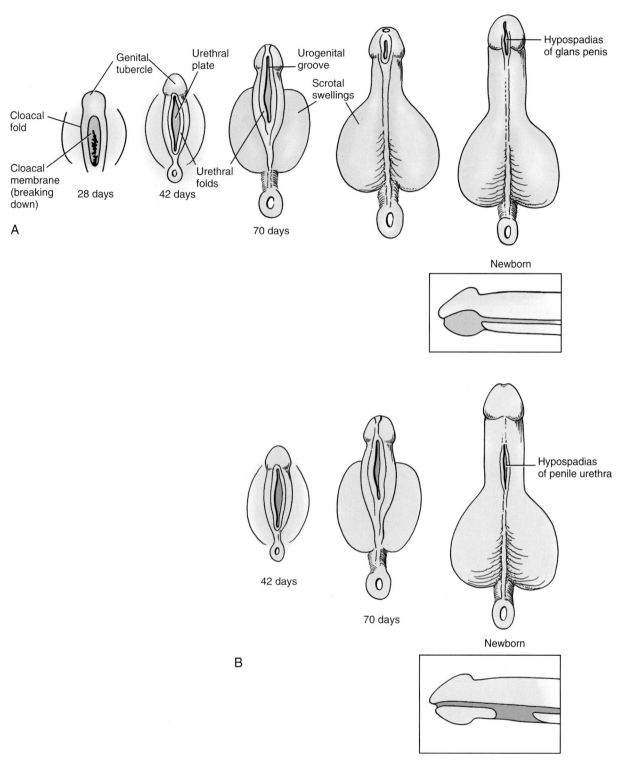

Figure 15-39. Hypospadias. *A-C,* The severity and morphology of hypospadias depend on the extent and location of the anomalous opening into the penile urethra. *D,* Infant with penoscrotal hypospadias.

Continued

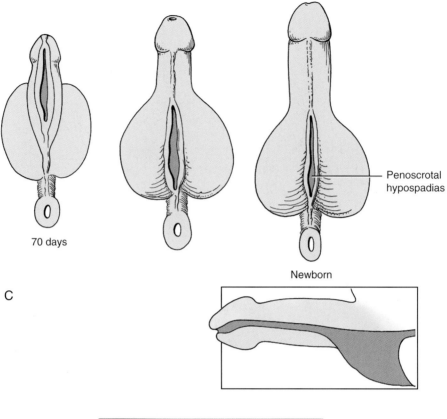

70 days

Penoscrotal
hypospadias

Newborn

C

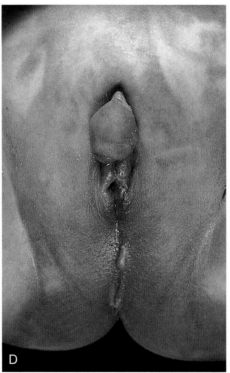

D

Figure 15-39. cont'd.

not enclosed at all. Hypospadia of the glans is influenced by multiple factors, but its direct cause is probably defective canalization of the solid distal urethral plate. Openings on the penile shaft represent failures of the urethral folds to fuse completely.

A more complex condition, **penoscrotal hypospadias**, results when the labioscrotal swellings as well as the urethral folds fail to fuse (Fig. 15-39C, D). If the labioscrotal folds fuse partially, the urethra will open through a hole between the base of the penis and the root of the scrotum. In the most severe form of the defect, the labioscrotal folds do not fuse at all and the urethra opens into the bottom of a depression in the perineum. This condition is usually accompanied by restricted growth of the phallus, so that the genitals seem to be female at birth.

If ANDROGEN RECEPTORS are disabled or absent, the male fetus may have normal or high levels of male steroid hormones, but the target tissues do not respond and development proceeds as though androgens were absent. This condition is called **androgen insensitivity syndrome** (also called **testicular feminization syndrome**). As in cases of primary testosterone deficiency, testes are present and AMH is produced, so the müllerian ducts regress, although a blind-ending vagina may form. The phenotype is usually female but can range from a complete female genital morphology (Fig. 15-40) to an ambiguous type (discussed in the "Clinical Taster" in this chapter) to a male phenotype with infertility.

Mutations in the SRY DNA-binding domain of human SRY are found in cases of **Swyer syndrome**, where there is total

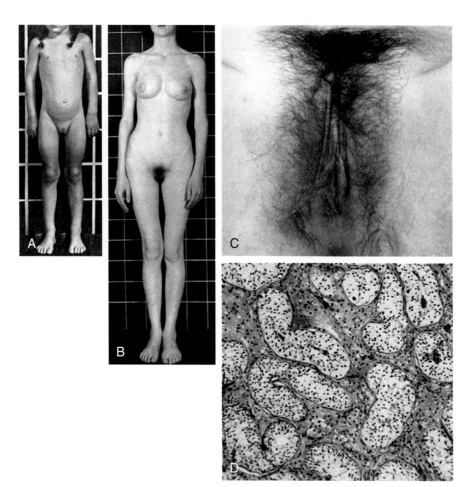

Figure 15-40. Patients with androgen insensitivity syndrome having 46,XY karyotypes and female external genitalia. A, Eleven-year-old patient. B, Seventeen-year-old patient. C, Photograph showing normal female external genitalia in patient in B. D, Photomicrograph of the cytoarchitecture of the testis removed from the inguinal canal of the patient in B showing Sertoli cell–lined seminiferous tubules. Germ cells are missing and the interstitial cells are hypoplastic.

15

gonadal dysgenesis (neither testes or ovaries) in XY individuals. These individuals are phenotypically female and have a female reproductive tract, but they do not enter puberty. Individuals with Swyer syndrome are usually treated with estrogen and progesterone to facilitate development of secondary sexual characteristics and engender a menstrual cycle. The streaked gonads are removed because they have a tendency to develop cancer. Although these individuals cannot generate ova, they may be able to become pregnant by embryo transfer into the uterus.

Female Pseudohermaphroditism

Female pseudohermaphrodites are genetic females who possess ovaries but whose genitalia are virilized by exposure to abnormal levels of virilizing sex steroids during fetal development. In most cases, the virilizing androgens are produced by congenital hyperplastic suprarenal glands. Some cases have apparently been caused by the administration of virilizing progestin compounds to prevent spontaneous abortion. Whatever the cause, the external genitalia of female pseudohermaphrodites exhibit clitoral hypertrophy and fusion of the urethral and labioscrotal folds. However, because testes and AMH are absent, the vagina, uterus, and fallopian tubes develop normally.

Failure to Enter Puberty

When a boy or girl fails to undergo the developmental changes associated with puberty, the cause is usually a deficiency of the appropriate sex steroids normally secreted by the gonads—testosterone in males and estrogen in females. Increased levels of pituitary gonadotrophic hormones stimulate the pubertal surge in sex steroid production. Hypogonadism may thus be caused by a defect either in the gonads themselves or in the hypothalamus and pituitary.

In **primary hypogonadism**, the hypothalamus and pituitary are normal and produce high levels of circulating gonadotropins, but the gonad does not respond with an increased production of sex steroids. Most cases of primary hypogonadism are associated with one of two major chromosomal anomalies, although a few cases are of unknown (idiopathic) origin.

In males, primary hypogonadism is usually a component of **Klinefelter syndrome**, which occurs in about 1 of 500 to 1000 live male births. Klinefelter syndrome is caused by a variety of sex chromosome anomalies involving the presence of an extra X chromosome. As discussed in Chapter 1, the extra X chromosome is acquired by nondisjunction during gametogenesis or early cleavage. The most common karyotype of Klinefelter syndrome is 47,XXY. Other individuals with Klinefelter syndrome are mosaics: either mosaics of cells with normal male karyotype (46,XY) and cells with an abnormal karyotype (e.g., 47,XXY; 48,XXYY; 45,X; and 47,XXY), or mosaics of cells with a female 46,XX karyotype and cells with an abnormal 47,XXY karyotype. In all cases, the primary defect is a failure of the Leydig cells to produce sufficient amounts of male steroids, which results in small testes and **azoospermia** (lack of spermatogenesis) or **oligospermia** (low sperm count). Many of these individuals also exhibit **gynecomastia** (development of breasts in males) and **eunuchoidism** (slender habitus, elongated extremities, and sparse hair).

Primary hypogonadism in females is usually associated with **Turner syndrome**. This condition occcurs in 1 of 5000 live female births. The cause is a 45,X karyotype or 45,X/46,XX mosaicism. In addition to the failure of normal sexual maturation at puberty, Turner syndrome is characterized by a range of anomalies, including short stature and webbed neck, coarctation of the aorta (discussed in Ch. 13), and cervical lymphatic cysts.

Secondary hypogonadism is caused by defects of hypothalamus or anterior pituitary gland. Individuals with **secondary hypogonadism** have depressed levels of gonadotropins as well as depressed levels of sex steroids. Most often, the cause is an insufficient secretion of gonadotropin-releasing hormone by the hypothalamus, as in **Kallmann syndrome** (discussed in Ch. 9) and the **fertile eunuch syndrome** in males. A variety of secondary hypogonadotropic disorders in males and females show autosomal recessive inheritance.

DEFECTIVE PARTITIONING OF CLOACA

In as many as 1 of 5000 infants, the urorectal septum is incomplete. Depending on the location and size of the defect, a wide range of malformations involving cloacal derivatives and their connections with the ureters and genital ducts may result. A few of the more common examples are described in the following paragraphs (some are also discussed in Ch. 14).

Fistulas

If the caudal portions of the urorectal septal folds fail to grow and fuse, the caudal part of the cloaca is not separated into urogenital sinus and anorectal canal, resulting in abnormal **rectourethral fistulas** (Fig. 15-41). In males, these connections usually take the form of a narrow **rectoprostatic urethral fistula** connecting the rectum to the prostatic urethra (see Fig. 15-41). In females, the situation is complicated by the presence of the müllerian ducts. Most often, the müllerian ducts attach to the pelvic

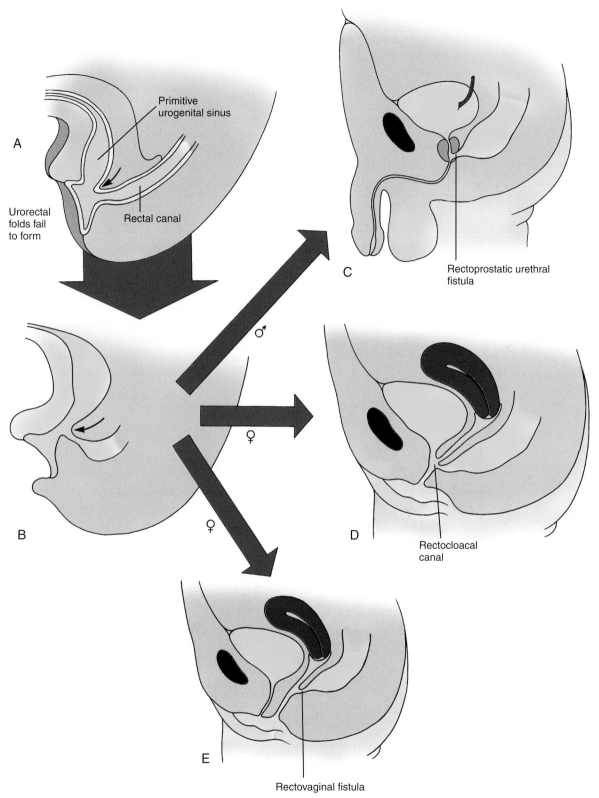

A — Primitive urogenital sinus

A — Urorectal folds fail to form — Rectal canal

C — Rectoprostatic urethral fistula

D — Rectocloacal canal

E — Rectovaginal fistula

Figure 15-41. *A-E,* Failure of the caudal folds of the urorectal septum to form results in characteristic anomalous development of the urogenital and lower gastrointestinal tracts in males and females.

urethra just cranial to the rectourethral fistula. The caudal undivided region of the cloaca thus becomes a common outlet for the urethra, the vagina, and the rectum, and is called a **rectocloacal canal** (see Fig. 15-41D). Occasionally, the uterovaginal canal incorporates the rectourethral fistula while migrating to a more caudal position on the posterior wall of the cloaca. In these cases, the vagina and urethra open separately into the vestibule, but the rectum communicates with the vagina through a **rectovaginal fistula** (see Fig. 15-41E; 15-43C, D). This fistula may be located high or low in the vagina. If the rectourethral fistula is originally located at the vaginal-cloacal junction low, the resulting **anovestibular fistula** will open into the vestibule of the vagina.

Sometimes the entire length of the folds forming the urorectal septum fail to fuse causing a more severe defect with the formation of an abnormal communication between the rectum and bladder called a **rectovesical fistula** (Fig. 15-42). In females, this anomaly may interfere with the normal fusion of the inferior ends of the müllerian ducts, resulting in separate bilateral vaginas and uterae that empty directly into the bladder.

If the caudalmost portion of the urorectal septal folds fuse separately but do not align properly with the cranial portion of the folds, then the distal end of the cloaca may be correctly partitioned, but a fistula will persist cranially (Fig. 15-43). The result in males is a **rectourethral fistula** connecting the prostatic urethra to the rectal canal (Fig. 10-43B). In this situation, the penile urethra and the anal canal empty through their normal channels, but the penile urethra is frequently stenotic, causing urine to exit preferentially through a urorectal fistula and the anorectal canal.

In females, the urogenital opening of the fistula is incorporated by the descending uterovaginal canal, resulting in a high **rectovaginal fistula** connecting the rectum to the vagina (see Fig. 15-43C, D). However, the urethra and vagina open normally to the outside.

Anal Malformations

Abnormal development of the urorectal septum can cause the rectum to end blindly in the body wall (Fig. 15-44A). This condition is called **anal agenesis** or **atresia**. The rectum usually ends cranial to the pelvic diaphragm and is usually accompanied by a fistula. Occasionally, the anorectal canal forms normally, but the anal membrane separating the ectodermal and endodermal portion of the anus is abnormally thick. This thickened anal membrane may fail to rupture or may rupture incompletely, resulting in an **imperforate anus** or **anal stenosis**, respectively (Fig. 15-44B).

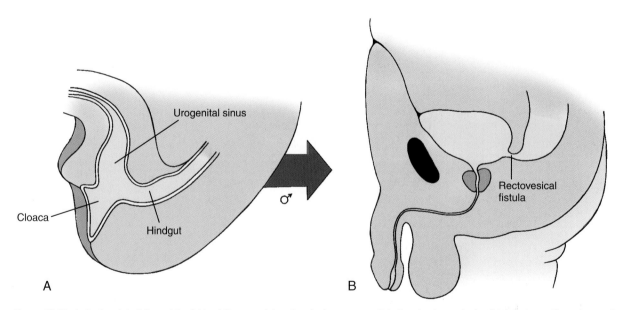

A

B

Figure 15-42. *A, B,* Complete failure of the folds of the urorectal septum to fuse may result in the development of a fistula between the rectum and the bladder, shown in this case with anal atresia.

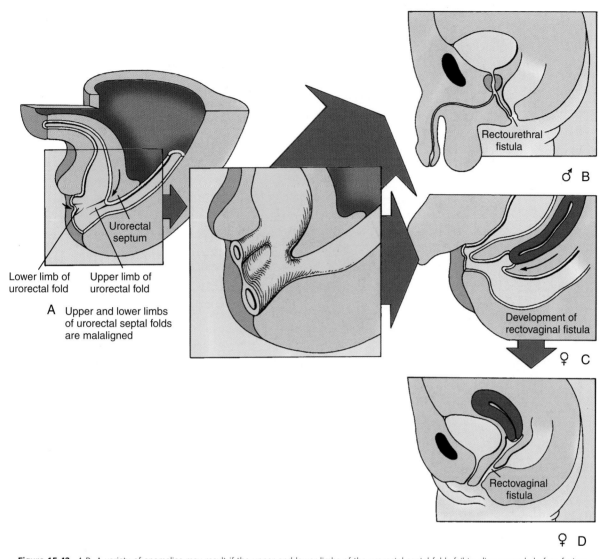

Lower limb of
urorectal fold

Upper limb of
urorectal fold

Urorectal
septum

A Upper and lower limbs
of urorectal septal folds
are malaligned

Rectourethral
fistula

♂ B

Development of
rectovaginal fistula

♀ C

Rectovaginal
fistula

♀ D

Figure 15-43. *A-D,* A variety of anomalies may result if the upper and lower limbs of the urorectal septal folds fail to align properly before fusing.

Excessive dorsal fusion of urogenital folds may partly or completely cover the anus. This condition, called **covered anus**, usually occurs in males because the genital folds do not normally fuse at all in females. The resulting malformation is called **anocutaneous occlusion** if the anus is completely covered. In some cases, a defect in the perineal mesoderm just anterior to the anus results in the development of a displaced anterior anal opening, a condition called **anteriorly displaced** or **anterior ectopic anus**.

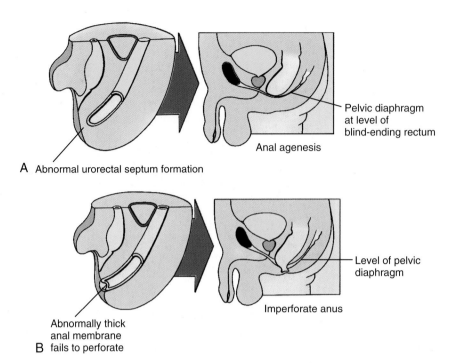

A Abnormal urorectal septum formation

Pelvic diaphragm at level of blind-ending rectum

Anal agenesis

Level of pelvic diaphragm

Imperforate anus

Abnormally thick anal membrane
B fails to perforate

Figure 15-44. *A*, Anal agenesis resulting from failure of proper urorectal septum formation. *B*, Imperforate anus may occur in cases where an abnormally thick anal membrane fails to rupture.

Suggested Readings

Barasch J. 2001. Genes and proteins involved in mesenchymal to epithelial transition. Curr Opin Nephrol Hypertens 10:429-436.

Boletta A, Germino GG. 2003. Role of polycystins in renal tubulogenesis. Trends Cell Biol 13:484-492.

Bouchard M. 2004. Transcriptional control of kidney development. Differentiation 72:295-306.

Brennan J, Capel B. 2004. One tissue, two fates: molecular genetic events that underlie testis versus ovary development. Nat Rev Genet 5:509-521.

Britt KL, Findlay JK. 2003. Regulation of the phenotype of ovarian somatic cells by estrogen. Mol Cell Endocrinol 202:11-17.

Cummings AM, Kavlock RJ. 2004. Function of sexual glands and mechanism of sex differentiation. J Toxicol Sci 29:167-178.

Dressler G. 2002. Tubulogenesis in the developing mammalian kidney. Trends Cell Biol 12:390-395.

Dressler G.R. 2006. The cellular basis of kidney development. Annu Rev Cell Dev Biol 22:509-529.

Drews U, Sulak O, Schenck PA. 2002. Androgens and the development of the vagina. Biol Reprod 67:1353-1359.

Gattone VH, 2nd, Goldowitz D. 2002. The renal glomerulus and vasculature in 'aggregation' chimeric mice. Nephron 90:267-272.

Hannema SE, Hughes IA. 2006. Regulation of Wolffian duct development. Horm Res 67:142-151.

Hudson BG, Tryggvason K, Sundaramoorthy M, Neilson EG. 2003. Alport's syndrome, Goodpasture's syndrome, and type IV collagen. N Engl J Med 348:2543-2556.

Hutson JM, Hasthorpe S. 2005. Abnormalities of testicular descent. Cell Tissue Res 322:155-158.

Hynes PJ, Fraher JP. 2004. The development of the male genitourinary system. I. The origin of the urorectal septum and the formation of the perineum. Br J Plast Surg 57:27-36.

Hynes PJ, Fraher JP. 2004. The development of the male genitourinary system: II. The origin and formation of the urethral plate. Br J Plast Surg 57:112-121.

Ivell R, Hartung S. 2003. The molecular basis of cryptorchidism. Mol Hum Reprod 9:175-181.

Kanai Y, Hiramatsu R, Matoba S, Kidokoro T. 2005. From SRY to SOX9: mammalian testis differentiation. J Biochem (Tokyo) 138:13-19.

Karihaloo A, Nickel C, Cantley LG. 2005. Signals which build a tubule. Nephron Exp Nephrol 100:e40-e45.

Keegan CE, Hammer GD. 2002. Recent insights into organogenesis of the adrenal cortex. Trends Endocrinol Metab 13:200-208.

Kim Y, Capel B. 2006. Balancing the bipotential gonad between alternative organ fates: a new perspective on an old problem. Dev Dyn 235:2292-2300.

Kuure S, Vuolteenaho R, Vainio S. 2000. Kidney morphogenesis: cellular and molecular regulation. Mech Dev 92:31-45.

Lee SB, Haber DA. 2001. Wilms tumor and the WT1 gene. Exp Cell Res 264:74-99.

Loffler KA, Koopman P. 2002. Charting the course of ovarian development in vertebrates. Int J Dev Biol 46:503-510.

Ludbrook LM, Harley VR. 2004. Sex determination: a 'window' of DAX1 activity. Trends Endocrinol Metab 15:116-121.

Martinez-Frias ML, Bermejo E, Rodriguez-Pinilla E, Frias JL. 2001. Exstrophy of the cloaca and exstrophy of the bladder: two different expressions of a primary developmental field defect. Am J Med Genet 99:261-269.

Miller A, Hong MK, Hutson JM. 2004. The broad ligament: a review of its anatomy and development in different species and hormonal environments. Clin Anat 17:244-251.

Morrish BC, Sinclair AH. 2002. Vertebrate sex determination: many means to an end. Reproduction 124:447-457.

Nievelstein RA, van der Werff JF, Verbeek FJ, et al. 1998. Normal and abnormal embryonic development of the anorectum in human embryos. Teratology 57:70-78.

Ozisik G, Achermann JC, Meeks JJ, Jameson JL. 2003. SF1 in the development of the adrenal gland and gonads. Horm Res 59 (Supp. 1):94-98.

Sariola H, Saarma M. 1999. GDNF and its receptors in the regulation of the ureteric branching. Int J Dev Biol 43:413-418.

Scholz H, Kirschner KM. 2005. A role for the Wilms' tumor protein WT1 in organ development. Physiology (Bethesda) 20:54-59.

Shah MM, Sampogna RV, Sakurai H, et al. 2004. Branching morphogenesis and kidney disease. Development 131:1449-1462.

Sinisi AA, Pasquali D, Notaro A, Bellastella A. 2003. Sexual differentiation. J Endocrinol Invest 26:23-28.

Thomson AA. 2001. Role of androgens and fibroblast growth factors in prostatic development. Reproduction 121:187-195.

Tilmann C, Capel B. 2002. Cellular and molecular pathways regulating mammalian sex determination. Recent Prog Horm Res 57:1-18.

Troiano RN, McCarthy SM. 2004. Mullerian duct anomalies: imaging and clinical issues. Radiology 233:19-34.

Vaiman D, Pailhoux E. 2000. Mammalian sex reversal and intersexuality: deciphering the sex-determination cascade. Trends Genet 16:488-494.

Veitia RA, Salas-Cortes L, Ottolenghi C, et al. 2001. Testis determination in mammals: more questions than answers. Mol Cell Endocrinol 179:3-16.

Viger RS, Silversides DW, Tremblay JJ. 2005. New insights into the regulation of mammalian sex determination and male sex differentiation. Vitam Horm 70:387-413.

Vise PD, Woolf AS, Bard JBL. 2003. The Kidney. From Normal Development to Congenital Disease. New York: Academic Press.

Visser JA. 2003. AMH signaling: from receptor to target gene. Mol Cell Endocrinol 211:65-73.

Wagner KD, Wagner N, Schedl A. 2003. The complex life of WT1. J Cell Sci 116:1653-1658.

Wilhelm D, Koopman P. 2006. The makings of maleness: towards an integrated view of male sexual development. Nat Rev Genet 7:620-631.

Yamada G, Satoh Y, Baskin LS, Cunha GR. 2003. Cellular and molecular mechanisms of development of the external genitalia. Differentiation 71:445-460.

Yamada G, Suzuki K, Haraguchi R, et al. 2006. Molecular genetic cascades for external genitalia formation: an emerging organogenesis program. Dev Dyn 235:1738-1752.

Yao HH. 2005. The pathway to femaleness: current knowledge on embryonic development of the ovary. Mol Cell Endocrinol 230:87-93.

Yin Y, Ma L. 2005. Development of the mammalian female reproductive tract. J Biochem (Tokyo) 137:677-683.

15

Development of the Pharyngeal Apparatus and Face

16

Summary The skeleton of the head and pharynx is made up of the **neurocranium**—the bones that support and protect the brain and sensory organs (the olfactory organs, eyes, and inner ears)—and the **viscerocranium**—the bones of the face and pharyngeal arches. The neurocranium can be subdivided into the cranial base (the bones underlying the brain), cranial vault (the bones covering the brain), and sensory capsules (the bones encapsulating the sensory organs). There are two types of bone in the head. One type, **endochondral bone**, forms from a cartilaginous intermediate and ossifies through the process of **endochondral ossification** (discussed in Ch. 8). The bones of the skull formed by endochondral ossification are collectively called the **chondrocranium**; this portion of the skull is the first to form in the embryo. The other type of bone develops from an ossification directly in the mesenchyme through the process of **intramembranous ossification** (discussed in Ch. 8); this type of bone is known as **membrane** or **dermal** bone. The jaws and the skull vault are formed almost entirely of membrane bone. Many of the skeletal structures in the head are unusual in that they are formed from **neural crest cells** rather than from mesoderm, as they are in the rest of the body.

In humans, five pairs of **pharyngeal arches** (also called *branchial arches*) form on either side of the pharyngeal foregut, starting on day 22. Because of their evolutionary history from ancestors with 6 arches, these arches correspond to numbers 1, 2, 3, 4, and 6. Each arch has an outer covering of ectoderm, an inner covering of endoderm, and a core of mesenchyme derived from paraxial and lateral plate mesoderm and neural crest cell–derived ectomesenchyme. Each arch contains a cartilaginous supporting element, an aortic arch artery (discussed in Ch. 13), and an arch-associated cranial nerve (consisting of cranial nerves V, VII, IX, and X; discussed in Ch. 10). The pharyngeal arches are separated externally by ectoderm-lined **pharyngeal clefts** (also called **grooves**) and internally by endoderm-lined **pharyngeal pouches**.

The skeletal elements in arches 1 to 4 are derived from neural crest cells, whereas the muscles and endothelial cells are derived from the mesoderm. The first arch (and more cranially associated mesenchyme) initially forms the transient **Meckel's** and **palatopterygoquadrate cartilages**, which ultimately give rise to the **malleus** and **incus** of the middle ear, respectively. The second arch initially forms **Reichert's** cartilage, and later the **stapes, stylohyoid**, and the **upper rim** of the **body** of the **hyoid**. The third arch forms the **lower rim** of the **body** of the **hyoid**. The mesoderm of the first arch forms the **muscles of mastication**, and the mesoderm of the second arch forms the **muscles of facial expression**. The mesoderm in arches 3, 4, and 6 forms the intrinsic muscles of the larynx. The muscles derived from each pharyngeal arch are innervated by a corresponding cranial nerve. The extraocular muscles form from the most rostral paraxial mesoderm and prechordal plate mesoderm. These are innervated by the oculomotor (III), trochlear (IV), and abducens (VI) nerves.

The human face is formed between the 4th and 10th weeks by the fusion of five **facial prominences**: the **frontonasal prominence**, a pair of **maxillary prominences**, and a pair of **mandibular prominences**. During week 5, a pair of thickened ectodermal **nasal (olfactory) placodes** develop on the frontonasal prominence and then invaginate to form the nasal pits and simultaneously divide part of the frontonasal prominence into the **medial** and **lateral nasal processes**. The facial primordia merge to form the **face**; defects in this mergence result in **facial clefts**. During normal development, the medial nasal processes merge to generate the bridge of the **nose**, the **philtrum**, and the **primary palate**; the lateral nasal processes give rise to the side of the nose;

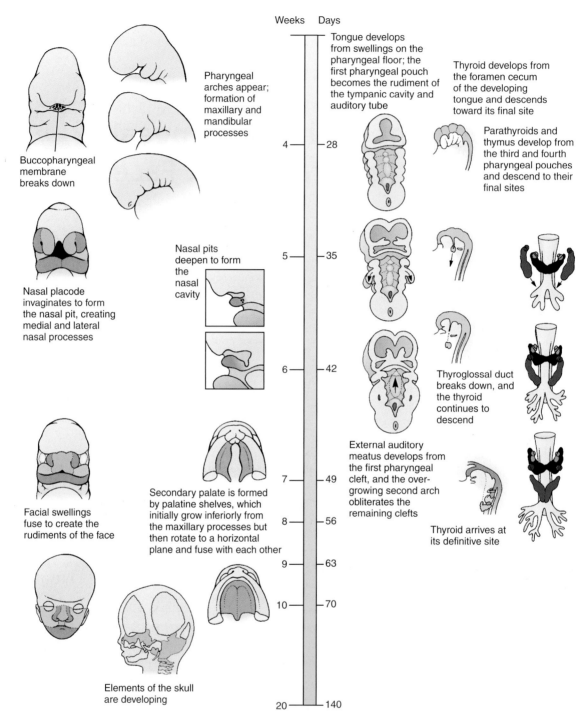

Buccopharyngeal membrane breaks down

Nasal placode invaginates to form the nasal pit, creating medial and lateral nasal processes

Facial swellings fuse to create the rudiments of the face

Elements of the skull are developing

Pharyngeal arches appear; formation of maxillary and mandibular processes

Nasal pits deepen to form the nasal cavity

Secondary palate is formed by palatine shelves, which initially grow inferiorly from the maxillary processes but then rotate to a horizontal plane and fuse with each other

Weeks   Days

4 — 28

5 — 35

6 — 42

7 — 49

8 — 56

9 — 63

10 — 70

20 — 140

Tongue develops from swellings on the pharyngeal floor; the first pharyngeal pouch becomes the rudiment of the tympanic cavity and auditory tube

External auditory meatus develops from the first pharyngeal cleft, and the over-growing second arch obliterates the remaining clefts

Thyroid develops from the foramen cecum of the developing tongue and descends toward its final site

Parathyroids and thymus develop from the third and fourth pharyngeal pouches and descend to their final sites

Thyroglossal duct breaks down, and the thyroid continues to descend

Thyroid arrives at its definitive site

Time line. Development of the head, neck, and pharyngeal apparatus.

and the maxillary processes generate much of the cheek. The mandibular processes form the lower jaw. The **secondary palate** is formed from shelves that grow out from the maxillary swellings.

Each of the pharyngeal pouches gives rise to an adult structure. The first pouch becomes the **tympanic cavity** and **auditory (eustachian) tube**. The second pouch gives rise to the **palatine tonsils**. The third pouch forms the **thymus gland** and **inferior parathyroid glands**, and the fourth pouch forms the **superior parathyroid glands**. The thymus and parathyroid glands migrate to their final position.

The **thyroid gland** forms as a midline, ventral endodermal evagination of the pharynx; its point of evagination is marked in the adult by the **foramen cecum** on the upper surface of the tongue. This primordium of the thyroid gland elongates after its evagination, detaches from the pharyngeal endoderm, and finally migrates to its definitive location just inferior and ventral to the larynx.

The tongue develops from endoderm-covered swellings on the floor of the pharynx. The anterior two thirds of the tongue mucosa is derived from first-arch swellings, whereas the posterior one third receives contributions from the third and fourth arches. Most tongue muscles, in contrast, are formed from myocytes arising from somites. For this reason, the motor and sensory nerve fibers of the tongue are carried by separate sets of cranial nerves.

With the exception of the first pharyngeal cleft (the cleft separating the first and second pharyngeal arches), which forms the **external auditory meatus**, all other pharyngeal clefts are obliterated by overgrowth of the second pharyngeal arch, although they occasionally persist as abnormal cervical cysts or fistulae.

Clinical Taster An 18-year-old woman was taken to the emergency room complaining of a "heart attack." She was noticeably sweaty, out of breath, and experiencing chest pain. The symptoms began an hour earlier while she was jogging. She became especially alarmed when her jogging mate said, "I can see your heart beating in your neck!"

A normal ECG, normal laboratory tests, and improvement without therapy ruled out a heart attack. The physical findings of costochondritis (inflammation of the rib joints) provided a likely cause for the chest pain, which, in turn, led to a panic attack. However, the ER physician continued to hear inspiratory stridor (a sound made by partial obstruction of a large airway) well after the panic attack had subsided. This, combined with the visible arterial pulsations at the base of the patient's neck, suggested a vascular anomaly. The doctor also noticed that the woman had minor craniofacial anomalies, including low-set abnormally shaped ears, retrognathia (a setback jaw), a short philtrum (the structure between the upper lip and nose), and a broad nasal tip. In addition, the patient had a bifid uvula and hypernasal speech, suggestive of palatal dysfunction.

Magnetic resonance angiography (MRA) done one week later revealed a **cervical aortic arch** (CAA) that was impinging on, and partially obstructing, the trachea, causing stridor during deep inhalation. CAA results from abnormal development of the aortic arches, with regression of the left fourth aortic arch and enlargement of the left third aortic arch. Normally, as discussed in Chapter 13, the left fourth aortic arch persists and contributes to the arch of the aorta. CAA and related vascular anomalies, especially when accompanied by craniofacial defects and velopharyngeal insufficiency (dysfunction of the palate and pharynx; "velo" refers to palate), commonly occur in chromosome **22q11.2 deletion syndrome** (also known as **velocardiofacial** or **DiGeorge syndrome**). Genetic testing confirmed this deletion. 22q11.2 deletion syndrome is characterized by a wide range of abnormalities, often subtle in infancy (Fig. 16-1), affecting the craniofacial and pharyngeal arch neural crest cell derivatives.

16

Origin of Skull

There are two types of bones in the head—those formed through ossification of a cartilaginous intermediate are known as **endochondral bones** and those formed through direct ossification in the mesenchyme are known as **membrane** or **dermal bones** (discussed in Ch. 8). In humans, dermal bones, with the exception of part of the **clavicle**, are found only in the head.

The cranial skeleton of fishes is composed of (1) the **chondrocranium**, which encloses the brain and helps to form the **sensory capsules** that support and protect the olfactory organs, eyes, and inner ears; (2) an external armor of **membrane (dermal) bones;** and (3) the **visceral skeleton** or **viscerocranium** that supports the gill bars and jaws (Fig. 16-2A). The bones of the chondrocranium (as the name indicates) are preformed in cartilage and ossify by the process of **endochondral**

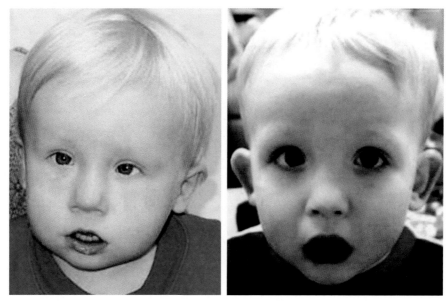

Figure 16-1. Two unrelated children with the characteristic, but subtle, facial appearance of 22q11.2 deletion syndrome, including prominent nose with rounded tip and hypoplastic alae nasi, reduced midface, small mouth and chin, unusually shaped ears, and small palpebral fissures (eye openings).

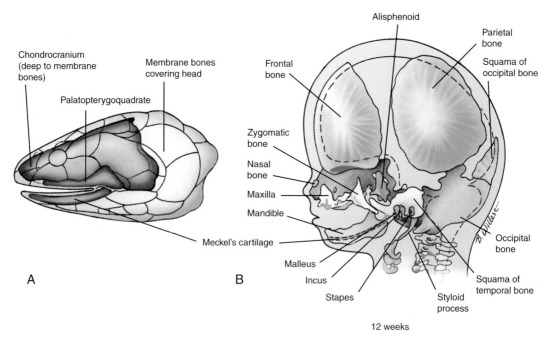

Figure 16-2. The evolutionary origin of the human skull from the pharyngeal arch skeleton, braincase, and dermal bones of primitive vertebrates. *A, B,* The expanding brain in the line of fishes leading to humans was housed in a cranium formed partly by the chondrocranium (purple) and partly by membrane bones (blue). In humans, the chondrocranium forms the cranial base, whereas the skull vault is formed by membrane bones. Membrane bones also form a large part of the highly modified facial skeleton of humans. The cartilaginous viscerocranium is shown in green.

ossification (this process is in contrast to **intramembranous ossification** in which mesenchymal cells ossify directly without first forming cartilage; these processes are discussed in Ch. 8). These three components of the cranial skeleton of fishes can still be distinguished in the genesis of the human skull (Fig. 16-2*B*). Thus, in humans the bones of the head can be divided into the **neurocranium** and **viscerocranium.** The **neurocranium** encompasses the bones surrounding and protecting the brain and sensory organs—the endochondral bones of the cranial base and sensory organs, and the dermal bones of the skull vault (see Fig. 16-2*B*). The **viscerocranium** encompasses the bones of the face and pharyngeal arches.

In humans, the **chondrocranium** is defined as that portion of the skull formed by endochondral ossification. The chondrocranium develops from three pairs of cartilaginous precursors present in our early ancestors—the **prechordal cartilages (trabeculae cranii), hypophyseal cartilages**, and **parachordal cartilages** (Fig. 16-3). These cartilages contribute to the cranial base and, together with cartilaginous capsules that develop around the otic and nasal pits, help to protect the brain and sensory organs.

The caudalmost pair of elements, the parachordal cartilages, is derived from the occipital sclerotomes plus the first cervical sclerotome and are, therefore, modified vertebral elements derived from mesoderm (discussed in Ch. 8). The parachordal cartilages form the base of the occipital bone (see Fig. 16-2*B*, 16-3). The hypophyseal cartilages fuse to form the body of the sphenoid bone, and the prechordal cartilage gives rise to the ethmoid bone, which together with the nasal and turbinate bones, encapsulates the nasal cavity (see Figs. 16-2*B*, 16-3). The **otic capsules** of humans are descended from primitive otic capsule ossification centers, which will fuse with the parachordal cartilages to form a single mass called the **periotic** or **petromastoid bone.** Two cartilages develop around the eye (derived from the **optic capsules**; see Fig. 16-3). These are the **orbitosphenoid (ala orbitalis)** and the **alisphenoid (ala temporalis)** (see Fig. 16-2*B*). They will ultimately contribute to the greater and lesser wings of the sphenoid (see Fig. 16-3).

The membrane-bone armor that covers the skull of our piscine ancestors (bony fishes) is represented in humans by the membrane bones of the skull, consisting of the flat bones of the **cranial vault**, or **calvaria**, as well as many bones of the face (Fig. 16-4, see 16-2*B*). The mesenchyme from which they develop is derived from neural crest cells and mesoderm (discussed in a later "In the Research Lab" section of this chapter).

The bones of the cranial vault do not complete their growth during fetal life. The soft, fibrous sutures that join them at birth permit the skull vault to deform as it passes through the birth canal and also allow it to continue growing throughout infancy and childhood. Six large, membrane-covered **fontanelles** occupy the areas between the corners of cranial vault bones at birth (see Fig. 16-4). The **posterior and anterolateral fontanelles** close by 3 months after birth, whereas the **anterior and posterolateral fontanelles** normally close during the second year. Palpation of the anterior fontanelle can be used to detect elevated intracranial pressure or premature closure of the skull sutures.

IN THE CLINIC

HOLOPROSENCEPHALY

Holoprosencephaly is the most common developmental defect of the forebrain, affecting 1 in 16,000 births. It results from a disturbance in early patterning of the forebrain (Fig. 16-5). The spectrum of phenotypes is wide, but in its most severe form only a single cerebral lobe forms (and hence the name of the condition) rather than paired right and left hemispheres. Defects of the olfactory nerves, olfactory bulbs, olfactory tracts, basal olfactory cortex, and associated structures including the limbic lobe, hippocampus, and mammillary bodies are also found. The corpus callosum is sometimes affected; the hindbrain is usually normal.

The forebrain defects are accompanied by a spectrum of facial abnormalities that often but not always (for example, following mutation of the *ZIC2* gene; see next paragraph) reflect the severity of the forebrain defect. Facial anomalies typical of holoprosencephaly include a flat nose, ocular hypotelorism (closely spaced eyes), deficient philtrum or cleft lip, high arched or cleft palate, and microcephaly (small skull). Particularly severe cases involve dramatic defects of the facial structures arising from the frontonasal prominence, most notably the nasal placodes (development of the face is discussed in detail later in this chapter). Failure of the medial nasal processes to form results in agenesis of the intermaxillary process and the reduction or absence of other midfacial structures such as the nasal bones, nasal septum, and ethmoid. The consequence may be cebocephaly (a single nostril; see Fig. 16-5) and, at the most extreme, cyclopia (a single eye). Mild cases of holoprosencephaly are characterized by relatively minimal midface anomalies and by trigonocephaly, a triangular skull

16

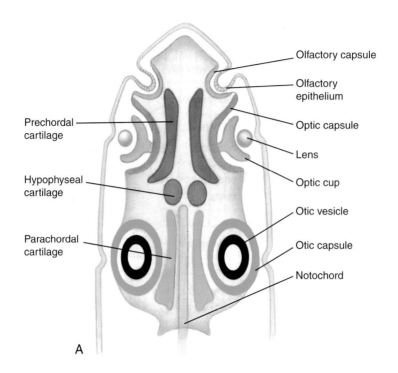

Olfactory capsule

Olfactory epithelium

Optic capsule

Lens

Optic cup

Otic vesicle

Otic capsule

Notochord

Prechordal cartilage

Hypophyseal cartilage

Parachordal cartilage

A

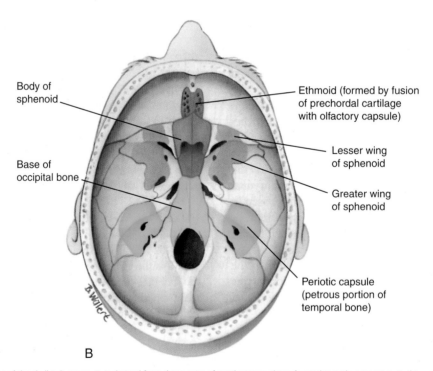

Body of sphenoid

Base of occipital bone

Ethmoid (formed by fusion of prechordal cartilage with olfactory capsule)

Lesser wing of sphenoid

Greater wing of sphenoid

Periotic capsule (petrous portion of temporal bone)

B

Figure 16-3. The base of the skull in humans, *B*, is derived from three pairs of cartilaginous plates formed in early ancestors, *A*, the prechordal, hypophyseal, and parachordal cartilages. The sensory organs are also protected by sensory capsules.

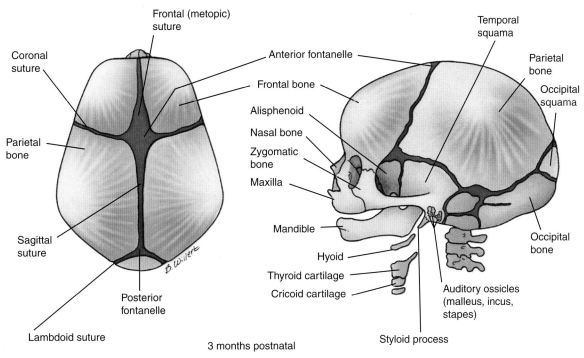

Figure 16-4. The brain in humans is mostly enclosed by the dermal bones of the cranial vault, which are separated by sutures and fontanelles. These bones do not fuse together until early childhood. The unfused sutures allow the cranium to deform during birth and to expand during childhood as the brain grows.

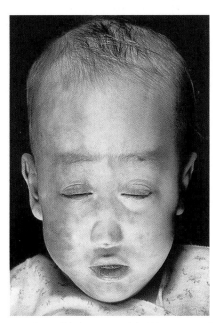

Figure 16-5. A infant with holoprosencephaly. This spectrum of malformations ranges in severity from minor midfacial defects to extremely devastating malformations. In this infant, there is a narrowing of the upper face and a single nostril.

shape that develops as a result of premature closure (synostosis) of the suture between the frontal bones and causes compression of the growing cerebral hemispheres. Occasionally, the presence of a single, central incisor and the loss of the maxillary midline frenum are the only indications of a holoprosencephalic phenotype.

At least twelve genetic loci have been implicated in holoprosencephaly in humans, and mutations in 7 genes in these loci have been identified. Of these, 3 are components of the *SONIC HEDGEHOG* signaling pathway (*SHH*, *PTC1*, and *GLI2*). The others are the *TERATOCARCINOMA-DERIVED GROWTH FACTOR 1* (*TDGF1/CRIPTO*) and the transcriptional factors *ZIC2* (which can modulate the *SHH* pathway), *SIX3*, and *TRANSFORMING GROWTH FACTOR INTERACTING FACTOR* (*TGIF*).

Emphasizing the importance of the *Shh* pathway, *Shh-/-* mutant mice exhibit cyclopia with a proboscis. Likewise, loss of factors involved in *Shh* signaling such as *Dispatched*, needed for the transport of *Shh* out from the cell, and *Sil*, an intracellular factor needed to activate the *Smo* receptor, result in holoprosencephalic phenotypes in mice. *Shh* signaling is initially required in the prechordal plate region to divide the single midline eye primordium in the forebrain

16

549

into eye (*Pax6*-expressing) and non-eye (non-*Pax6* expressing) territories. *Shh* signaling is also required at later stages of facial development: application of *Shh*-blocking antibodies in the developing chick frontonasal prominence results in hypotelorism. *Tgif* modulates *Nodal* signaling, which is needed for the establishment of the prechordal plate and, hence, acts at a very early stage of facial midline patterning.

Holoprosencephaly is also a component in 5% of **Smith-Lemli-Opitz syndrome** patients. The syndrome affects about 1 in 9000 births (live and stillborn). This syndrome is the result of a mutation in the *DHCR7* gene, which encodes 7-DEHYDROCHOLESTEROL REDUCTASE, an enzyme involved in the penultimate step of cholesterol synthesis. The holoprosencephalic phenotype is caused by abnormalities in the cells receiving the *SHH* signal, not by alterations in the cholesterol modification of *SHH* (i.e., not by activity). This is demonstrated by the fact that two cholesterol synthesis inhibitors that induce holoprosencephaly, the plant alkaloids cyclopamine and jervine, target the responding cell by inhibiting the function of *Smo* receptors. Environmental agents are also associated with holoprosencephaly and include maternal exposure to **alcohol** and excess **vitamin A**, as well as **maternal diabetes**. Infants of diabetic mothers have a risk of holoprosencephaly that may be as high as 1%.

Conversely, there are syndromes that have hypertelorism (wide-set eyes) as a component. This is seen in **craniofrontonasal dysplasia**, resulting from mutations in *EFNB1* (*EPHRIN-B1*), and **Greig cephalopolysyndactyly**, which results from mutations in *GLI3* (again, a component of the *SHH* pathway). The heterozygous *extra-toes* mice (*Gli3* mutants) also have an enlarged frontal bone. Greig cephalopolysyndactyly and the *extra-toes* mutant are likely caused by excess *Shh* signaling, as *Gli3* is a repressor of *Shh* signaling. Furthermore, misexpression of *Shh* in the developing chick frontonasal prominence results in increased cell proliferation and, consequently, in expansion of the medial-lateral axis of the face.

CRANIOSYNOSTOSIS

Craniosynostosis, the premature closure of sutures, affects approximately 1 in 2500 children and occurs in many syndromes, including **Crouzon, Apert, Pfeiffer, Muenke**, and **Saethre-Chotzen syndromes**. Sutures, which occur where two membrane bones meet, contain the progenitor cells that will give rise to new bone cells, the osteoblasts. These are the sites of membrane bone growth. Long-term fate mapping studies in mice have shown that the coronal and sagittal sutures arise at neural crest cell-mesoderm interfaces. The coronal suture is derived from mesoderm and separates the neural crest cell-derived frontal bone and the mesoderm-derived parietal bone. The sagittal suture is formed from neural crest cells and separates the two mesodermally derived parietal bones.

In craniosynostosis, the sagittal and coronal sutures are most commonly affected. Closure at one suture causes increased growth at other sutures, thereby deforming the brain and skull. This is shown in Figure 16-6A. Here, the coronal suture has closed, so the head cannot grow in length, and now the developing brain forces growth along the other sutures. The result is a skull deformity, with possible changes in neurologic function and intracranial pressure. Craniosynostosis syndromes involve mutations in three *FGF RECEPTORS*, *FGFR1*, *2*, and *3*; two transcription factors, *TWIST* and *MSX2*; and one ligand, *EPHRIN-B1* (*EFNB1*). Analysis of the *FGF RECEPTOR* mutations has shown that these are gain of function (i.e., these mutations result in an increase in *FGF* signaling). *FGFs* are expressed in the osteoblastic front of membrane bones (Fig. 16-6B) and have two roles. Low levels of *FGFs* promote cell proliferation through *FGFR2*, whereas high levels promote osteoblast differentiation through *FGFR1*. Therefore, the rate of osteogenesis is carefully controlled by balancing the level of *FGF* signaling (Fig. 16-6C). Increased signaling accelerates osteoblast differentiation, resulting in synostosis (the closure) of the sutures. Curiously, *FGFR2* and *3* mutations are usually inherited as spontaneous new mutations through the paternal lineage, increasing in frequency with paternal age. One such mutation in *FGFR2* (a mutation that causes **Apert syndrome**) increases clonal expansion of male germ cells. The *EFNB1* mutation causes **craniofrontonasal dysplasia**, which is characterized in part by the early fusion of the coronal suture. This is an unusual X-linked syndrome in that heterozygote females show more severe phenotypes than hemizygous males. In mice, *Efnb1* is expressed in the coronal suture. Therefore, in heterozygote females, the suture will consist of a mixture of cells that either express one copy of the functional *EFNB1* gene or express the mutated nonfunctional EFNB1 protein. *EFNB1* encodes a ligand that functions to prevent cell mixing, and it is thought that loss of one copy of the gene produces abnormal cell mixing between the tissue interfaces at the coronal suture. In contrast, in the hemizygous males, none of the cells in the coronal suture express a functional *EFNB1* gene, and, consequently, such abnormal cell mixing will not occur.

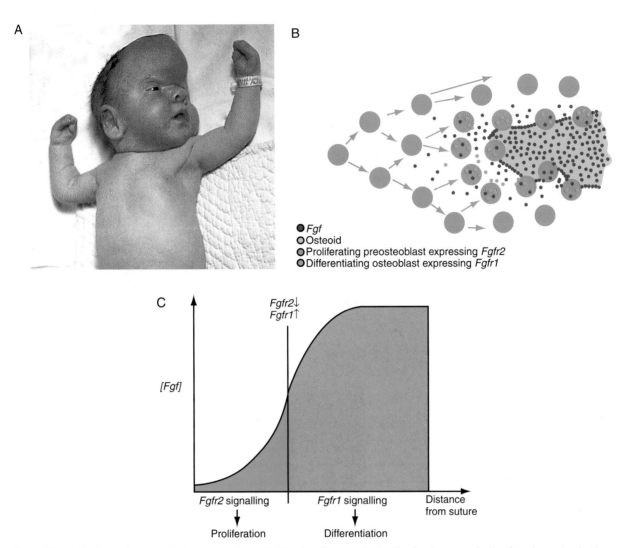

Figure 16-6. *A*, Craniosynostosis occurring in Apert syndrome. In this infant, the coronal suture has fused prematurely; therefore, the cranium has been forced to adopt a "tower skull" (acrocephalic) shape to accommodate the growing brain. *B*, Diagram showing expression of *Fgfs* and *Fgfr1* and *2* in a suture. *C*, Bone growth is controlled by balancing the level of *Fgf* signaling, with a low dose increasing proliferation and a high dose promoting bone differentiation. Therefore, increased *Fgf* signaling that occurs in many craniosynostotic syndromes causes premature suture closure.

Development of Pharyngeal Arches

The pharyngeal arches evolved from the gill arches of jawless fishes and have been evolutionarily conserved. These arches form during the embryogenesis of all vertebrates. In jawed vertebrates, the first arch gives rise to the lower jaw. The remaining arches form the gills in modern fishes and many structures of the face and neck in humans.

Pharyngeal Apparatus

In human embryos, there are 5 pairs of pharyngeal arches numbered 1, 2, 3, 4, and 6. Arch 5 either never forms in humans or forms as a short-lived rudiment and promptly regresses. Arches 4 and 6 cannot be seen externally (Fig. 16-7). Like so many other structures in the body, the pharyngeal arches form in craniocaudal succession: the first arch forms on day 22; the second and third arches form sequentially on

16

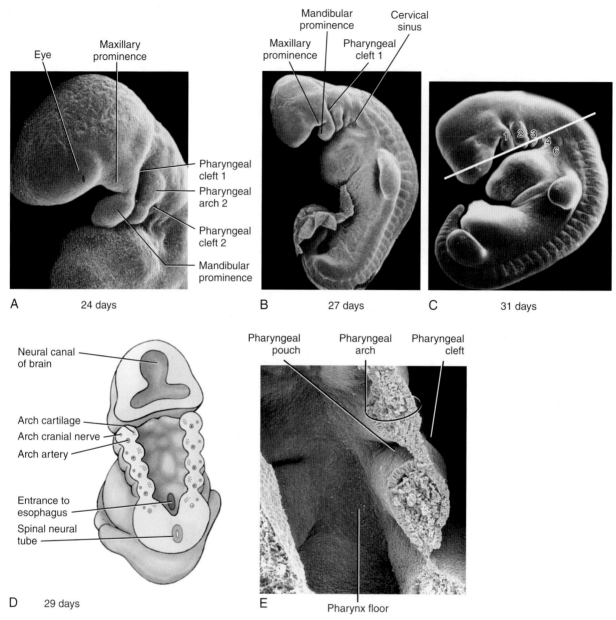

Figure 16-7. Formation of the pharyngeal arches. The pharyngeal arches form in craniocaudal sequence during the 4th and 5th weeks. *A*, By day 24, the first two arches have formed. *B*, By day 27, the first three arches have formed, as have the maxillary and mandibular prominences. *C*, By the early 5th week, all five arches have formed. The dashed line indicates the plane of the section shown (at a slightly earlier stage) in part *D*. *D*, Schematic cross section through the pharyngeal arches, showing the cartilage, artery, and cranial nerve in each arch. *E*, Scanning electron micrograph of a section similar to that shown in *D*.

day 24; and the fourth and sixth arches form sequentially on day 29. This craniocaudal sequence of development is clearly seen in some human syndromes where the more caudal arch derivatives are more severely affected than those from the more cranial arch—this is typified by **22q11.2 syndrome** (discussed in the last "In the Clinic" in this chapter).

Each pharyngeal arch consists of a mesenchymal core (mesoderm and neural crest cell ectoderm) lined on the outside with ectoderm and on the inside with endoderm (see Fig. 16-7D, F). Each arch contains: (1) a central cartilaginous skeletal element (derived from neural crest cells); (2) striated muscle rudiments (derived from head mesoderm) innervated by an arch-specific cranial nerve; and (3) an aortic arch artery (discussed in Ch. 13).

The pharyngeal arches of human embryos initially resemble the gill arches of fish, except that they never become perforated to form gill slits. Instead, the external **pharyngeal clefts** or **grooves** between the arches remain separated from the apposed, internal **pharyngeal pouches** by thin **pharyngeal membranes**. These membranes are two layered, consisting of ectoderm and endoderm.

Pharyngeal Arch Cartilages and Origin of Skeletal Elements

The cartilages that form within the pharyngeal arches develop from neural crest cells originating from the midbrain and hindbrain regions. As discussed in Chapter 4, neural crest cells arise from the neural folds and migrate ventrolaterally. In the trunk region, their migration occurs mainly through active neural crest cell movement. In the head, migration also involves active neural crest cell movement. But in contrast to trunk neural crest cells, migration of head neural crest cells also involves a passive component in which ventral displacement of the surrounding tissue also translocates neural crest cells ventrally.

Figure 16-8 and Table 16-1 illustrate and summarize, respectively, the skeletal elements derived from the pharyngeal arch cartilages.

The first pharyngeal arch has two prominences associated with it: the **mandibular** and **maxillary prominences** (or **swellings;** see Fig. 16-7A-C), which give rise to the lower and part of the upper jaw, respectively. Although the maxillary prominence was long thought to develop from branching of the first arch, it is now known that the maxillary prominence arises from mesenchyme cranial to the first arch. Each

maxillary and mandibular prominence contains a transient central cartilaginous element. The central cartilage of the maxillary prominence is the **palatopterygoquadrate bar**, and the central cartilage of the mandibular prominence is **Meckel's cartilage** (see Fig. 16-8). Both the maxillary and mandibular prominences are formed largely from neural crest cells that migrate from the neural folds of the midbrain (mesencephalon) and cranial hindbrain (metencephalon) (discussed later in this chapter).

Most of **Meckel's cartilage** disappears, either being resorbed or becoming encapsulated by the developing mandibular bone. However, the proximal part forms the **malleus, sphenomandibular ligament**, and the **anterior ligament of the malleus** (see Fig. 16-8). The maxillary cartilage (palatopterygoquadrate bar) forms the **incus** and a small bone called the **alisphenoid** located in the orbital wall (see Fig. 16-8). These derivatives become surrounded by the maxilla, zygomatic, and squamous portion of the temporal bones, which together with the mandible, are all membrane bones. Therefore, the majority of the facial skeletal structures are derived from bones of dermal origin.

The second pharyngeal arch cartilage forms from neural crest cells that migrate from neural folds at the level of rhombomere 4 of the hindbrain (rhombomeres are discussed further in Ch. 9; see Fig. 16-12). After the jaws evolved, the second-arch cartilages were recruited as bracing elements to help support the jaws and attach them to the neurocranium. The human second-arch cartilage is called **Reichert's cartilage.** This arch will ultimately form the **stapes** of the middle ear, the **styloid process** of the temporal bone, the fibrous **stylohyoid ligament**, and the **lesser horns (cornua)** and **upper rim** of the **body** of the **hyoid** bone (see Fig. 16-8). The hyoid bone is stabilized by muscle attachments to the styloid process and mandible; through its muscular attachments to the larynx and the tongue, it functions in both swallowing and vocalization.

The third pharyngeal arch cartilage is formed from neural crest cells that migrate from the caudal hindbrain (myelencephalon). Ossification of this cartilage occurs endochondrally to form the **greater horns** (cornua) and **lower rim** of the **body** of the **hyoid** bone (see Fig. 16-8).

The fourth and sixth pharyngeal arches together give rise to the larynx, consisting of the **thyroid, cuneiform, corniculate, arytenoid**, and **cricoid** cartilages (see Fig. 16-8). Recent neural crest cell fate mapping studies in mice have shown that these cartilages arise from neural crest cells, with the mesodermal boundary forming at the tracheal cartilages. The **epiglottal**

16

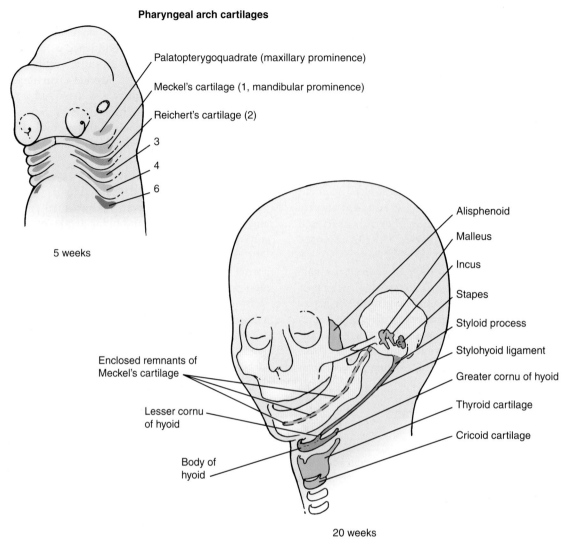

Pharyngeal arch cartilages

Palatopterygoquadrate (maxillary prominence)

Meckel's cartilage (1, mandibular prominence)

Reichert's cartilage (2)

3

4

6

5 weeks

Alisphenoid

Malleus

Incus

Stapes

Styloid process

Stylohyoid ligament

Greater cornu of hyoid

Thyroid cartilage

Cricoid cartilage

Enclosed remnants of
Meckel's cartilage

Lesser cornu
of hyoid

Body of
hyoid

20 weeks

Figure 16-8. Fate of the pharyngeal arch cartilages. These cartilages give rise to the alisphenoid (a small bone of the orbit), elements of the jaw skeleton, three auditory ossicles, and the hyoid and laryngeal skeleton.

cartilages do not form until the 5th month, long after the other pharyngeal arch cartilages have formed. These cartilages arise in the fourth-arch area, but their precise origin is unknown.

Development of Temporomandibular Joint

In all jawed vertebrates except mammals, the jaw joint is formed from endochondral bones that develop from the maxillary and mandibular cartilages, even though other portions of the jaw may be made of membrane bones. However, among the immediate ancestors of mammals, a second, novel jaw articulation developed between two membrane bones: the temporal and mandible. As this new **temporomandibular joint (TMJ)** became dominant, the bones of the ancient endochondral jaw articulation shifted into the adjacent middle ear and joined with the preexisting stapes to form the unique three-ossicle auditory mechanism of mammals.

The components and cavities of the TMJ are established by week 14 of gestation. The TMJ consists of a synovial joint between the **mandibular condyle** and the **glenoid blastema** (associated with the temporal bone), which are separated by an **interarticular disc**. The joint forms from week 9, starting with development of the condylar process on the mandible.

Table 16-1 Derivatives of the Pharyngeal Arches and Their Tissues of Origin

Pharyngeal Arch	Arch Artery[a]	Skeletal Elements	Muscles	Cranial Nerve[b]
1	Terminal branch of maxillary artery	Derived from arch cartilages (originating from neural crest cells): From maxillary cartilage: alisphenoid, incus From Meckel's cartilage: malleus Derived by direct ossification from arch dermal mesenchyme: maxilla, zygomatic, squamous portion of temporal bone, mandible (originate from neural crest cells)	Muscles of mastication (temporalis, masseter, and pterygoids), mylohyoid, anterior belly of the digastric, tensor tympani, tensor veli palatini (originate from head mesoderm)	Maxillary and mandibular division of trigeminal nerve (V)
2	Stapedial artery (embryonic), corticotympanic artery (adult)	Stapes, styloid process, lesser horns and upper rim of hyoid (derived from the second-arch [Reichert's] cartilage; originate from neural crest cells)	Muscles of facial expression (orbicularis oculi, orbicularis oris, risorius, platysma, auricularis, frontalis, and buccinator), posterior belly of the digastric, stylohyoid, stapedius (originate from head mesoderm)	Facial nerve (VII)
3	Common carotid artery, root of internal carotid	Lower rim and greater horns of hyoid (derived from the third-arch cartilage; originate from neural crest)	Stylopharyngeus (originates from head mesoderm)	Glossopharyngeal nerve (IX)
4	Arch of aorta (left side), right subclavian artery (right side); original sprouts of pulmonary arteries	Laryngeal cartilages (derived from the fourth-arch cartilage; originate from neural crest cells)	Constrictors of pharynx, cricothyroid, levator veli palatini (originate from occipital somites 2 to 4)	Superior laryngeal branch of vagus nerve (X)
6	Ductus arteriosus; roots of definitive pulmonary arteries	Laryngeal cartilages (derived from the sixth-arch cartilage; originate from neural crest cells)	Intrinsic muscles of larynx (originate from occipital somites 1 and 2)	Recurrent laryngeal branch of vagus nerve (X)

[a]Aortic arch artery development is discussed in Chapter 13.
[b]Cranial nerve development is discussed in Chapter 10.

16

One week later, the condylar cartilage has formed and the blastema of the temporal bones has started to develop. At this time, the condylar cartilage and temporal bone are separated by the condensation of the interarticular disc. Cavitation starts at week 10 in two waves: first between the condylar process and interarticular disc, forming the **inferior joint space;** and then (1 week later) between the disc and temporal bone, forming the **superior joint space**.

The condylar cartilage is distinct from endochondral cartilages in that it arises within the periosteum of a membrane bone. It is one of several cartilages, termed **secondary cartilages**, to develop in this way during facial growth. Secondary cartilages have unique properties, including that they grow in response to mechanical stimulation. Unlike some of the other facial secondary cartilages, the condylar cartilage persists postnatally and plays a significant role in postnatal growth of the lower jaw.

Origin of Vascular Supply

As discussed in detail in Chapter 13, the aortic arch artery system initially takes the form of a basket-like arrangement of five pairs of arteries that arise from the expansion at the end of the truncus arteriosus called the **aortic sac.** These arteries connect the paired ventral aorta with the paired dorsal aortae (Fig. 16-9).

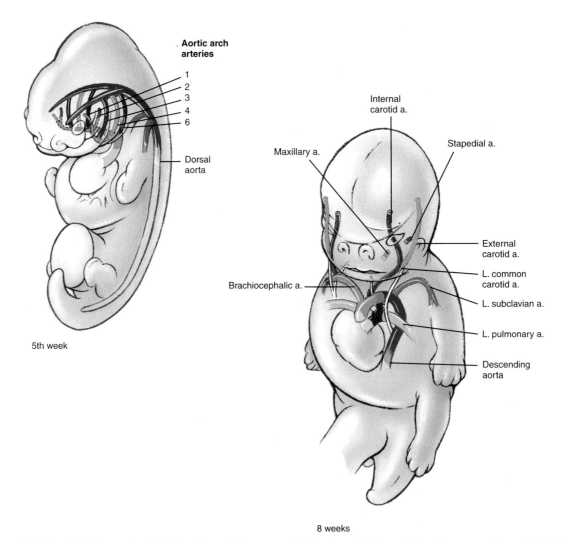

Figure 16-9. Fate of the pharyngeal arch arteries. These arteries are modified to form definitive arteries of the upper thorax, neck, and head (discussed in Ch. 13).

This system is remodeled to produce the great arteries of the thorax and the branches that supply the head and neck (illustrated in Figure 16-9 and summarized in Table 16-1; see Ch. 13 for details of this remodeling).

As discussed in Chapter 13, arterial blood reaches the head via paired vertebral arteries that form from intersegmental artery anastomoses and via the **common carotid arteries**. The common carotid arteries branch to form the **internal** and **external carotid arteries**. The internal carotid and vertebral arteries supply the brain and the external carotid arteries supply the face. The common carotids and the roots of the internal carotids are derived from the third-arch arteries, whereas the distal portions of the internal carotids are derived from the cranial extensions of the paired dorsal aortae. The external carotid arteries sprout de novo from the common carotids. The endothelium of the head vasculature and aortic arch arteries is derived from paraxial mesoderm.

Origin and Innervation of Musculature

The musculature of the pharyngeal arches is derived from the cranial head mesoderm. This includes the first five (so-called occipital) somites and the unsegmented mesoderm located rostral to these somites (paraxial mesoderm). Myoblasts for each pharyngeal arch, and also the precursors of the extraocular muscles, arise at discrete locations within this unsegmented mesoderm. The muscles that form in each pharyngeal arch are innervated by a cranial nerve branch that is specific to that arch, and they maintain their relationship in the adult. This close relationship has been conserved since the evolution of jawed fishes; along with the pharyngeal pouches, it defines a conserved segmental organization for the pharyngeal arch system. Figure 16-10 shows the muscles derived from the pharyngeal arches and Figure 16-11 shows the innervation of these muscles; Table 16-1 summarizes the muscles formed in each pharyngeal arch and their innervation.

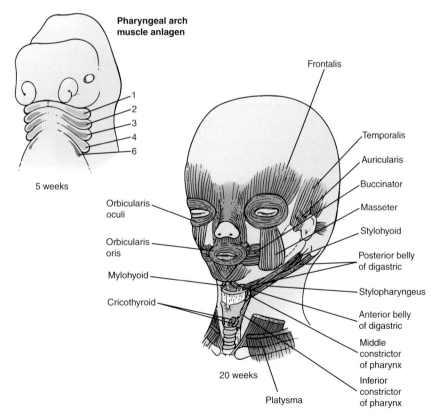

Figure 16-10. Fate of the pharyngeal arch musculature. The pharyngeal arch muscles develop from cranial paraxial mesoderm and occipital somites. The myoblasts of the sixth arch become the intrinsic laryngeal muscles (not shown).

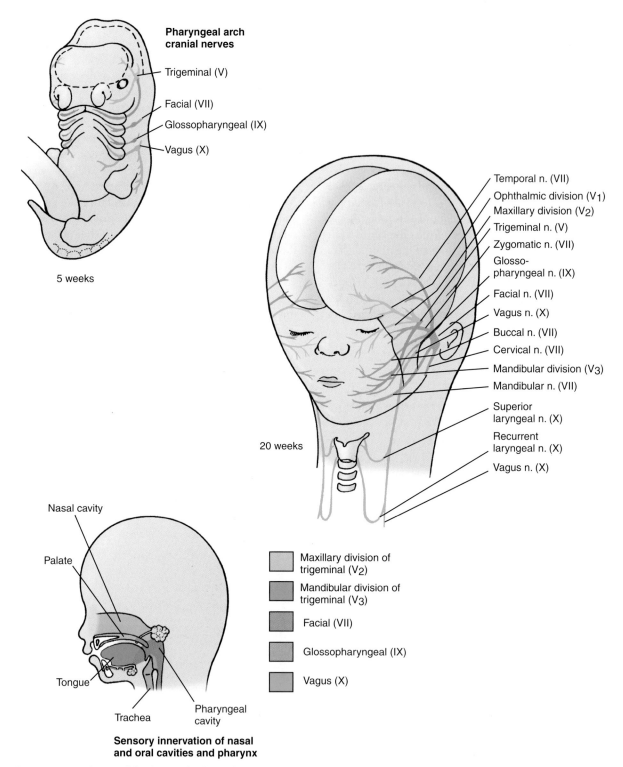

Pharyngeal arch cranial nerves

- Trigeminal (V)
- Facial (VII)
- Glossopharyngeal (IX)
- Vagus (X)

5 weeks

- Temporal n. (VII)
- Ophthalmic division (V1)
- Maxillary division (V2)
- Trigeminal n. (V)
- Zygomatic n. (VII)
- Glosso-pharyngeal n. (IX)
- Facial n. (VII)
- Vagus n. (X)
- Buccal n. (VII)
- Cervical n. (VII)
- Mandibular division (V3)
- Mandibular n. (VII)
- Superior laryngeal n. (X)
- Recurrent laryngeal n. (X)
- Vagus n. (X)

20 weeks

- Nasal cavity
- Palate
- Tongue
- Trachea
- Pharyngeal cavity

Maxillary division of trigeminal (V2)

Mandibular division of trigeminal (V3)

Facial (VII)

Glossopharyngeal (IX)

Vagus (X)

Sensory innervation of nasal and oral cavities and pharynx

Figure 16-11. Distributions of the pharyngeal arch cranial nerves. The muscles that develop in each pharyngeal arch are served by the cranial nerve that originally innervates that arch. The sensory innervation of the nasal and oral cavities and pharynx is also diagrammed.

In the first arch, paraxial mesoderm originating beside the metencephalon (rhombomere 2) gives rise to the **muscles of mastication** (the **temporalis, masseter**, and **medial** and **lateral pterygoids**), as well as to the **mylohyoid, anterior belly of the digastric, tensor tympani**, and **tensor veli palatini** muscles. Branches of the **trigeminal (V) nerve** innervate all of these muscles.

In the second arch, paraxial mesoderm gives rise to the **muscles of facial expression**, including the **orbicularis oculi, orbicularis oris, risorius, platysma, auricularis, frontalis**, and **buccinator** muscles, as well as to the **posterior belly of the digastric**, the **stylohyoid**, and the **stapedius** muscles. The muscle primordia of this arch migrate to their final position in the head and are innervated by the **facial (VII) nerve**.

In the third arch, paraxial mesoderm gives rise to a single muscle: the long, slender **stylopharyngeus**, which originates on the styloid process and inserts into the wall of the pharynx. This muscle raises the pharynx during vocalization and swallowing, and it is innervated by the **glossopharyngeal (IX) nerve**.

Muscles originating in the fourth and sixth arches are the **superior, middle**, and **inferior constrictors** of the pharynx, the **cricothyroid**, and the **levator veli palatini**, which function in vocalization and swallowing. These muscles are innervated by the **vagus (X) nerve**.

To summarize, four of the cranial nerves arising in the hindbrain supply branches to the pharyngeal arches and their derivatives (see Fig. 16-11; the cranial nerves are discussed in detail in Ch. 10): (1) The maxillary and mandibular prominences (derivatives of the cranial mesenchyme and first arch) are innervated, respectively, by the **maxillary** and **mandibular branches** of the **trigeminal** nerve (cranial nerve V); (2) the second arch is innervated by the **facial** nerve (cranial nerve VII); (3) the third arch is innervated by the **glossopharyngeal** nerve (cranial nerve IX); and (4) the fourth and sixth arches are innervated by the **superior laryngeal** and **recurrent laryngeal** branches of the **vagus** nerve (cranial nerve X).

In addition to muscles arising from the pharyngeal arches, myoblasts from the myotomes of the occipital somites coalesce beside somite 4 and extend ventrally as an elongated column, the **hypoglossal cord**, eventually becoming located ventral to the caudal region of the pharynx. Some of these myoblasts shift dorsally to form the **intrinsic laryngeal musculature** (i.e., the lateral **cricoarytenoids, thyroarytenoids**, and **vocalis** muscles), which are mainly devoted to vocalization.

Like the muscles originating in the fourth and sixth arches, these muscles are innervated by the **vagus nerve**. However, most of the myoblasts of the hypoglossal cord remain ventral and shift cranially. These will form the **intrinsic** and **extrinsic musculature** of the tongue. All of these muscles except one (the palatoglossus, which is innervated by the vagus nerve; discussed later in the chapter in the section on development of the tongue) are innervated by the **hypoglossal** nerve (cranial nerve XII).

Additional Cranial Nerve Innervation

As discussed in more detail in Chapter 10, in addition to the cranial nerves just discussed, seven other cranial nerves innervate structures that develop in association with the pharyngeal apparatus. Six **extraocular muscles** (derived from mesoderm that migrates to surround the developing eyes) are innervated by cranial nerves: (1) four muscles (**inferior oblique, medial rectus, superior rectus**, and **inferior rectus**) are innervated by the **oculomotor nerve** (cranial nerve III; originates from the mesencephalon); one muscle (**superior oblique**) is innervated by the **trochlear nerve** (cranial nerve IV; originates from the hindbrain); and one muscle (**lateral rectus**) is innervated by the **abducens nerve** (cranial nerve VI; originates from the hindbrain). One other important group of muscles is innervated by the remaining cranial nerve: the **accessory nerve** (cranial nerve XI) innervates the neck muscles (**sternocleidomastoid, trapezius**).

Three **sensory organs** are innervated by cranial nerves: (1) the **olfactory nerve** (cranial nerve I; originates from the nasal placode and is associated with the telencephalon) innervates the olfactory epithelium of the developing nasal cavities; (2) the **optic nerve** (cranial nerve II; originates from the sensory layer of the optic cup and is associated with the diencephalon) innervates the developing retina of the eye; (3) the **vestibulocochlear nerve** (cranial nerve VIII; originates from the otic placode and is associated with the hindbrain) innervates the developing inner ear.

Many Cranial Nerves Are Mixed Nerves

As discussed in Chapter 10, the various cranial nerves carry different combinations of somatic motor, autonomic, and sensory fibers. In the trunk, nerves are mixed, but in the head, cranial nerves can be either mixed (V, VII, IX, and X), predominantly sensory (I, II, and VIII), or motor (III, IV, VI, XI, and XII). However, in all cases, the somatic motoneurons have

16

their cell bodies in the brain, whereas the cell bodies of the sensory neurons are located in cranial nerve ganglia. In the trunk, the sensory neurons are always derived from neural crest cells, but in the head, some sensory neurons (V, VII, VIII, IX, and X) are derived from 2 populations—neural crest cells, as in the trunk, and special areas of ectoderm known as **neurogenic ectodermal placodes**. These placodes are discussed in detail in Chapter 10.

The sensory innervation of the face is provided by the ophthalmic, maxillary, and mandibular divisions of the trigeminal nerve, as would be expected from the fact that the dermis in this region develops from neural crest cells that migrate into the first pharyngeal arch and frontonasal prominence of the face (see Fig. 16-11). The sensory innervation of the dorsal side of the head and neck is provided by the second and third cervical spinal nerves. The sensory innervation of the mouth, pharynx, and larynx is provided by cranial nerves V, VII, IX, and X, as illustrated in Figure 16-11.

IN THE RESEARCH LAB

HINDBRAIN IS SEGMENTED

As discussed in Chapter 9, the developing brain is initially subdivided into the prosencephalon, mesencephalon, and rhombencephalon, and the latter is transiently subdivided into distinct segments called rhombomeres (r). Each rhombomere expresses a unique combination of transcription factors. Of particular relevance are those of the *Hox* gene family, which are expressed in nested patterns along the cranial-caudal axis of the hindbrain, with their rostral limit corresponding to a rhombomere boundary (Fig. 16-12A). The *Hox* genes are needed for the development of specific rhombomeres. For example, *Hoxa1* is necessary for the development of r4 and 5, as both are severely reduced or absent in mice in which *Hoxa1* is inactivated. *Hoxb1* is specifically expressed in r4. Genetic inactivation of *Hoxb1* in mice and zebrafish results in the transformation of r4 to r2. Conversely, when *Hoxb1* is misexpressed in r2 in chick, r2 acquires r4 characteristics.

One important aspect of hindbrain segmentation is that it provides the framework for establishing neuronal patterning within the developing pharyngeal arches: the motor nuclei of cranial nerves V, VII, and IX, arise in a 2-segment (i.e., rhombomere) periodicity, with each of their nerves innervating

one pharyngeal arch (see Fig. 16-12A). Thus, cranial nerve V innervates pharyngeal arch 1, cranial nerve VII innervates pharyngeal arch 2, and cranial nerve IX innervates pharyngeal arch 3 (cranial nerves X and XII innervate pharyngeal arches 4 and 6). When *Hoxb1* function is lost in mice, the motoneurons that arise from r4 behave like those that arise from r2, migrating in a pattern characteristic of r2 neurons. In a converse experiment in chick in which *Hoxb1* is overexpressed in r2, r2 motoneurons migrate into the second arch instead of towards their usual first arch targets.

Hindbrain segmentation also plays a role in keeping different neural crest cell populations apart so that hindbrain neural crest cells migrate in register in three segmental streams: a stream derived from r1 and r2, a stream from r4, and a stream from r6, r7 (Fig. 16-12B; note that in addition to the three streams of hindbrain neural crest cells, there is a cranial stream of neural crest cells arising from the midbrain and caudal forebrain). Formation of the three hindbrain streams is achieved in part by the fact that comparatively few neural crest cells originate from r3 and r5; those that do migrate cranially or caudally into the adjacent neural crest cell streams (see Fig. 16-12B). Separation of the first (those from r1 and r2) and second (those from r4) hindbrain neural crest cell streams is extremely important, as these are characterized by the absence and presence, respectively, of *Hoxa2* expression: specifically, r2 neural crest cell progeny downregulate *Hoxa2* expression as they start to migrate, and *Hoxa2* expression in the presumptive r1 neural crest cells is inhibited by *Fgf8* signaling from the isthmus (a constricted zone consisting of the caudal midbrain and cranial hindbrain) (Fig. 16-13A). If *Hoxa2* is mutated in mice, the second pharyngeal arch is homeotically transformed into the first pharyngeal arch. Thus, second arch derivatives such as the stapes and styloid process are absent and are replaced by an ectopic tympanic ring, malleus, and incus, usually derivatives of the first pharyngeal arch (Fig. 16-13B). Conversely, overexpression of *Hoxa2* in the first pharyngeal arch in both chick and Xenopus transforms the first pharyngeal arch into a second pharyngeal arch. Hence, the absence or presence of *Hoxa2* determines first versus second pharyngeal arch identity.

RETINOIC ACID ACTS IN NORMAL AND ABNORMAL DEVELOPMENT OF HEAD AND NECK

Retinoic acid (RA), the biologically active derivative of vitamin A (retinol), is needed for development and segmentation of the caudal pharyngeal arches. But when it is given in excess, it acts as a potent craniofacial **teratogen**, especially affecting pharyngeal arches 1 and 2 in which it

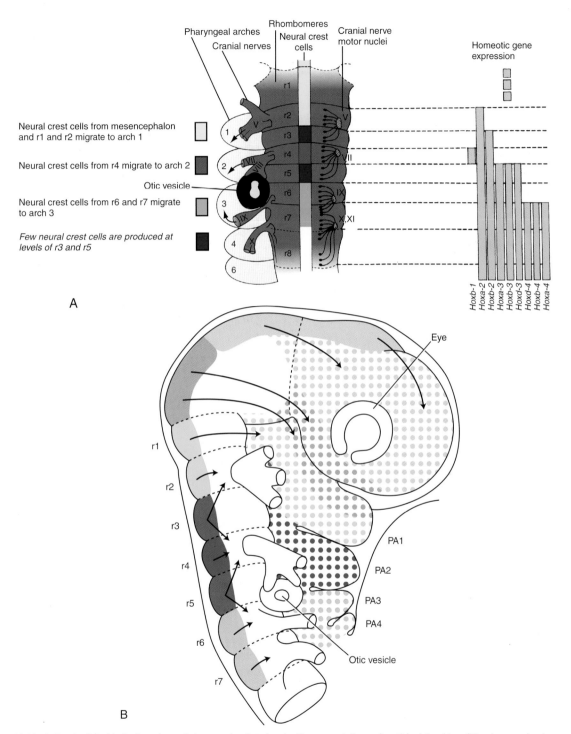

Figure 16-12. *A*, Sketch of the hindbrain region and pharyngeal arches showing the segmentation and spatial relationships of the pharyngeal arches, cranial nerves, cranial nerve motor nuclei, rhombomeres, and rhombomere-specific neural crest cell derivatives. Rhombomeres are associated with the expression of specific combinations of *Hox* genes, which in most cases (see text for important exceptions) are also expressed by their neural crest cell derivatives. The *Hox* code expressed by each rhombomere is illustrated by the colored vertical bars on the right. *B*, Routes of migration of the head neural crest cells (arrows). PA1 to PA4, pharyngeal arches 1 to 4; r1 to r7, rhombomeres 1 to 7.

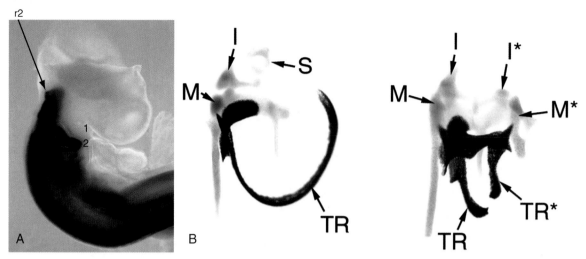

Figure 16-13. *Hoxa2* determines second arch identity. *A*, Whole mount in situ hybridization showing the expression of *Hoxa2* in a developing chick embryo. *Hoxa2* is specifically expressed in the second (2) and more caudal pharyngeal arches, but not in the first (1) pharyngeal arch mesenchyme. r2 indicates the position of rhombomere 2 of the hindbrain. *B*, Loss of *Hoxa2* function in mice (wild-type on left; mutant on right) results in loss of the stapes (S), styloid process, and the lateral horn of the hyoid—all derivatives of the second arch. In contrast, first arch structures—the malleus (M), incus (I), and tympanic ring (TR)—are duplicated (duplicated member indicated by asterisk).

causes hypoplasia. Isotretinoin (Accutane or 13-*cis*-retinoic acid), a drug used to treat a severe form of acne, can cause such hypoplasia when embryos are exposed during gastrulation and early organogenesis (i.e., exposure during early pregnancy). The developmental sensitivity to RA is explained by the gradient of RA that forms across the hindbrain during development owing to the differential expression of RA-synthesizing enzymes, *Raldh1-4*, and RA-catabolizing *Cytochrome P450* enzymes (*Cyp2A1*, *B1*, and *C1*). *Raldh2* is expressed in the mesoderm underlying the developing caudal hindbrain, whereas the catabolic enzyme *Cyp26C1* is expressed in the mesoderm underlying the presumptive cranial hindbrain and midbrain (Fig 16-14).

The gradient of RA patterns the hindbrain. RA acts by binding to the ligand-dependent transcription factors *RAR* and *RXR*, which act as heterodimers to activate RA-sensitive genes. Two RA target genes are *Hoxa1* and *Hoxb1*, which contain **RETINOIC ACID RESPONSE**

ELEMENTS (RAREs) in their **enhancers**. Ectopic application of retinoic acid to developing chick embryos, for example, transforms rhombomeres 2/3 to rhombomeres 4/5. Conversely, loss of RA as in *Raldh2* knockout mice or in vitamin A (VAD)–deficient quails results in the cranialization of the hindbrain, such that the normal expression of *Hoxa-1* and *Hoxa-2* in the neuroepithelium caudal to r4 is abolished.

The endoderm, which is required for pharyngeal arch segmentation, is also a direct target of RA signaling. The role of the endoderm in pharyngeal arch segmentation is highly conserved and occurs even in amphioxus, in which embryos form pharyngeal arches but lack neural crest cells. Loss of RA signaling downregulates *Tbx1*, a transcription factor implicated in **22q11.2 syndrome** (discussed elsewhere in this chapter), *Pax9* (another type of transcription factor), and *Fgf8* expression. All of these are needed for normal pharyngeal arch development and patterning.

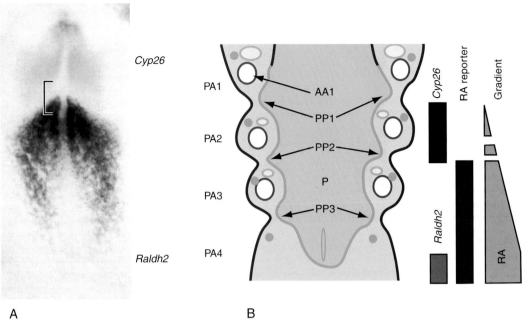

Figure 16-14. A gradient of retinoic acid patterns the hindbrain. *A*, Whole mount in situ hybridization showing the expression of *Raldh2*, a retinoic acid–producing enzyme, and *Cyp26*, a retinoic acid–degrading enzyme, in the early chick embryo. *Raldh2* is expressed caudally (dark blue), whereas *Cyp26* (light blue) is expressed cranially. The region where neither is expressed (marked by the bracket) is the presumptive mid-hindbrain; thus, there is a gradient of retinoic acid signaling across the cranial-caudal axis of the hindbrain. *B*, Sketch illustrating the gradient of retinoic acid signaling (RA), as shown by the expression of a retinoic acid reporter gene (RA reporter). AA1, aortic arch 1; PP1-3, pharyngeal pouches 1-3; P, pharynx; PA1-4, pharyngeal arches 1-4.

Development of Face

The basic morphology of the face is established between the 4th and 10th weeks by the development and fusion of five prominences: the **frontonasal prominence** overlying the forebrain, **plus** the two **maxillary prominences** and two **mandibular prominences** associated with the first pharyngeal arches (Fig. 16-15). The mesenchyme in the frontonasal prominence arises from neural crest cells derived from the midbrain and forebrain, whereas the maxillary and mandibular prominences receive neural crest cell contributions from both the midbrain and hindbrain (see Fig. 16-12). The spectrum of congenital facial defects known as **facial clefts**—including cleft lip and cleft palate—result from the failure of some of these facial processes to grow and fuse correctly. These relatively common congenital anomalies are discussed in the following "In the Clinic" section of this chapter.

All five facial swellings form by the end of the 4th week. These initially surround the primitive oral cavity, the **stomodeum**, which is separated from the gastrointestinal tract by the **oropharyngeal (buccopharyngeal** or **oral) membrane** (see Fig. 16-15C). During the 5th week, the paired maxillary prominences enlarge and grow ventrally and medially. Simultaneously, a pair of ectodermal thickenings, called the **nasal** or **olfactory placodes** (also called **nasal discs** or **nasal plates**) form on the frontonasal prominence and begin to enlarge (see Fig. 16-15C). In the 6th week, the ectoderm at the center of each nasal placode invaginates to form an oval **nasal pit**, dividing the frontonasal prominence into the **lateral** and **medial nasal processes** (Fig. 16-16A, B). The groove between the lateral nasal process and the adjacent maxillary prominence is called the **nasolacrimal groove (naso-optic furrow)** (Fig. 16-16C). During the 7th week, the ectoderm at the floor of this groove invaginates into the underlying

16

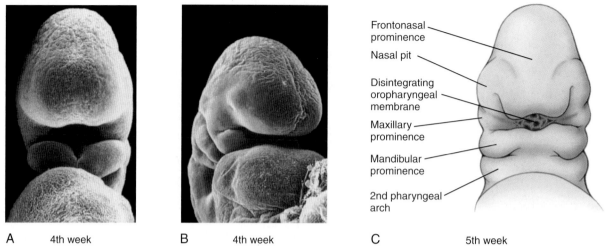

A   4th week   B   4th week   C   5th week

Figure 16-15. Origin of the human face and mouth. The face develops from five primordia that appear in the 4th week: the frontonasal prominence, the two maxillary prominences, and the two mandibular prominences. The oropharyngeal membrane breaks down in the 5th week to form the opening to the oral cavity. *A, C,* ventral views; *B,* oblique view.

mesenchyme to form a tube called the **nasolacrimal duct** and **lacrimal sac**. This duct is invested by bone during the ossification of the maxilla. After birth, it functions to drain excess tears from the conjunctiva of the eye into the nasal cavity.

During the 6th week, the medial nasal processes migrate toward each other and fuse to form the primordium of the bridge and septum of the nose (see Fig. 16-16*A*, *B*). By the end of the 7th week, the inferior tips of the medial nasal processes expand laterally and inferiorly and fuse to form the **intermaxillary process** (Fig. 16-16*C*, *D*). The tips of the maxillary prominences grow to meet the intermaxillary process and fuse with it. The intermaxillary process gives rise to the **philtrum** (Fig. 16-16*E*) and **primary palate** containing four incisor teeth.

Although the two mandibular prominences seem to be separated by a fissure midventrally (see Fig. 16-16*A*), they actually form in continuity with each other like the rest of the pharyngeal arches. The transient intermandibular depression is filled in during the 4th and 5th weeks by proliferation of mesenchyme, creating the primordium of the lower lip (see Fig. 16-16*B*, *C*). Meanwhile, during the 5th week, rupture of the oropharyngeal membrane occurs to form a broad, slit-like embryonic mouth (see Fig. 16-16*C*, *D*). The mouth is reduced to its final width during the 2nd month as the fusion of the lateral portions of the maxillary and mandibular swellings creates the cheeks (see Fig. 16-16*E*).

IN THE RESEARCH LAB

OUTGROWTH OF FACIAL PROMINENCES IS REGULATED BY EPITHELIAL-MESENCHYMAL INTERACTIONS

Outgrowth of the facial primordia is controlled by epithelial-mesenchymal interactions; thus, if the epithelium is removed, the facial prominences are truncated. These interactions are mediated by growth factors that commonly signal elsewhere (e.g., *Shh* and members of the *Bmp*, *Fgf*, and *Wnt* families). During development of the lower jaw, an additional growth factor, *Endothelin1*, also plays a key role. These growth factors control cell proliferation and/or survival. Furthermore, they differentially regulate homeobox-gene expression, thereby regulating patterning of the facial prominences (discussed below).

Endothelin1 (Et1) is a small peptide. Genetic inactivation of *Et1*, its receptor, or the enzyme involved in its activation *(Ece1)* results in severe hypoplasia of the lower jaw, together with cardiac and aortic arch remodeling abnormalities. *Et1* also regulates the expression of the homeobox gene *Dlx*, with loss of *Et1* function resulting in a transformation of facial structures similar to those found in the *Dlx5/6* mutants (discussed below).

Bmp4 and *Fgf8*, which are expressed in complementary domains in the epithelium of the lower jaw, seem to be the most important of the *Bmp* and *Fgf* families. These factors have antagonistic effects typified by their opposing effects on the positioning of the odontogenic field: *Fgf8* promotes the expression of *Pax9*, a marker of the early odontogenic

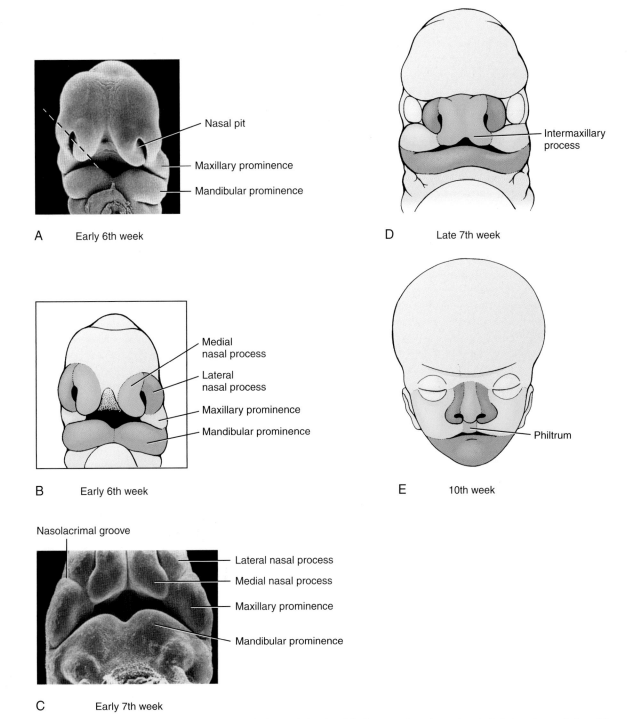

Figure 16-16. Development of the face. *A, B,* In the 6th week, the nasal placodes of the frontonasal prominence invaginate to form the nasal pits and the lateral and medial nasal processes. Dashed line in *A* indicates section level shown in Figure 16-19. *C, D,* In the 7th week, the medial nasal processes fuse at the midline to form the intermaxillary process. *E,* By the 10th week, the intermaxillary process forms the philtrum of the upper lip.

mesenchyme, whereas *Bmp4* inhibits *Pax9* expression (tooth development is discussed in detail in Ch. 7). *Bmp4* also regulates the expression of *Msx1*, a homeobox-containing gene essential for outgrowth. *Wnt5a* is expressed in the neural crest cell–derived ectomesenchyme, with highest levels of expression in the distal facial prominences. In *Wnt5a*-deficient mice the face is truncated. Outgrowth of the facial prominences has some parallels with the limbs: in both regions, the epithelium, *Fgf8*, and *Wnt5a* are essential for normal outgrowth (limb development is discussed in detail in Ch. 18).

PATTERNING OF FACIAL PROMINENCES IS REGULATED BY EPITHELIAL-MESENCHYMAL INTERACTIONS

Facial development requires the integration of multiple reciprocal and changing tissue interactions among neural crest cells, mesoderm, ectoderm, and endoderm, with each tissue playing specific roles. Transplantation of neural crest cells between different species has shown that the facial morphology is determined by the neural crest cell donor. Thus, if duck neural crest cells are transplanted into a quail host, or vice versa, the resulting structures are characteristic of the donor neural crest cells (Fig. 16-17A, B). The donor neural crest cells also establish the temporal pattern of gene expression in the overlying ectoderm and the development and patterning of ectodermally derived structures such as feathers (Fig. 16-17C). The ectoderm then signals back to the mesenchyme to coordinate facial outgrowth (as discussed above). However, facial morphology is not determined solely by neural crest cells: some aspects of neural crest cell gene expression are plastic. Thus, if small groups of neural crest cells or single neural crest cells are transplanted into an ectopic environment, gene expression is altered according to the new location. However, if the mesoderm is also included in the transplant, neural crest cells maintain their gene expression according to their original location, demonstrating a role for the mesoderm in neural crest cell patterning.

The ectoderm also has patterning ability, illustrated by the fact that the odontogenic epithelium can induce tooth development in nonodontogenic mesenchyme (discussed in Ch. 7) and that the **frontonasal ectodermal zone**, a region in the frontonasal prominence characterized by the juxtaposition of *Shh* and *Fgf8* expression, can induce duplicated distal beak structures when transplanted ectopically. Finally, the endoderm is essential for facial development: ablation of endoderm results in loss of facial structures, whereas transplantation of endoderm causes the formation of ectopic facial structures. Strikingly, the orientation and identity of the skeletal structures is determined by the region of endoderm that is transplanted and its orientation in the host.

Recent studies of "Darwin's finches" from the Galapagos Islands have identified two candidate genes that may determine facial morphology. Expression of the growth factor *Bmp4*, which controls mesenchymal cell proliferation and chondrogenesis, is highest in the finches with the broadest and deepest beaks, the ground finches. In contrast, the facial primordia of finches with long and slender beaks, the cactus finches, have higher levels of the intracellular signaling factor *Calmodulin kinase II*, which promotes distal outgrowth.

DLX CODE PATTERNS THE FIRST PHARYNGEAL ARCH

Members of the *Hox* gene family (*A, B, C, D*) are not expressed in the first pharyngeal arch or in ectomesenchyme cranial to it and, therefore, cannot pattern the facial primordia. Rather, this patterning role is thought to be controlled by the related homeobox-containing genes *Msx1, 2, Dlx1-6* (note *Dlx7* is now called *Dlx4*), *Gsc1, Lhx6/7,* and *Barx1*, with the combinatorial expression of these factors determining facial structures. Until recently, gene inactivation studies have failed to provide evidence in support of this model: inactivation of single genes result in loss/malformation of structures with no evidence of transformation. However, the *Dlx* family of genes, related to the *distalless* homolog in Drosophila, have now emerged as key players in patterning. All members of the *Dlx* family are expressed in nested domains in the mandibular prominence (Fig. 16-18A). *Dlx1* and *2* are also expressed in the maxillary prominence (see Fig. 16-18A). Loss of a single member of the *Dlx* family (*Dlx1, 2, 5, 6*) affects the development of a subset of facial structures: for example, in *Dlx1*-deficient mice, the palatine, pterygoid, maxillary, and squamosal bones are affected. Strikingly, loss of both *Dlx5* and *6* results in a homeotic transformation such that part of the mandibular prominence is replaced with skeletal structures normally formed in the maxillary prominence. Specifically, the proximal part of the dentary bone is absent and is replaced with an ectopic maxilla, ala temporalis, jugal, squamosal, and palatine bones (Fig. 16-18B). These bones are mirror image duplications of their endogenous counterparts, suggesting that there is a signaling center controlling patterning of the surrounding structures between the maxillary and mandibular prominences. This transformation is also associated with transformation of overlying structures: there is an additional set of vibrissae in the transformed mandibular prominence, and ectopic rugae also form in association with the ectopic palatine bone.

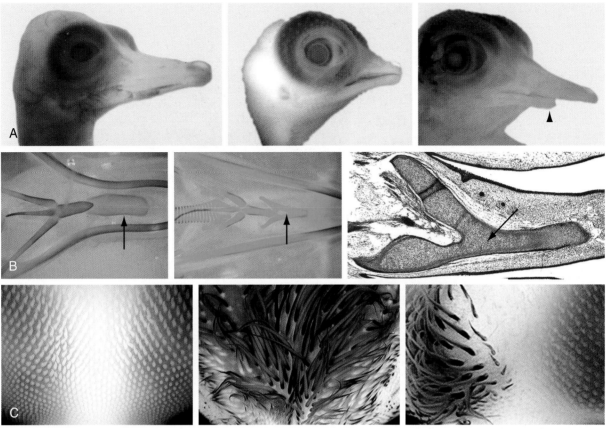

Figure 16-17. Neural crest cells control patterning of the facial primordia. *A,* Length and shape of the jaws in a duck (left), quail (center), and transplantation chimera in which neural crest cells that contribute to the lower jaw were transplanted from a quail to a duck (right). Note that the lower jaw length in the chimera mimics that of the quail (arrow) and is shorter than that of the duck. *B,* Bones of the lower jaw stained to highlight cartilage in a duck (left) and quail (center). The entoglossum bone (arrows) is a supporting bone for the tongue. In the duck, this bone is broad and flat, whereas in the quail, it is spear shaped. In a duck embryo in which quail neural crest cells were transplanted (right), the entoglossum mimics the shape of the quail entoglossum (i.e., it is spear shaped, as seen in histologic section; adjacent sections, not shown, revealed that the entoglossum was derived entirely from quail neural crest cells). *C,* Head skin patches show feathers in duck (left), quail (center), and chimeric embryos (right). The feathers, which are ectodermally derived, also develop according to the time table and pattern of the donor neural crest cells, as shown in a duck embryo in which quail neural crest cells were transplanted on the left side of the figure showing the chimera (right panel). The difference in pigmentation between duck and quail feathers is due to the presence of neural crest cell–derived quail melanocytes.

16

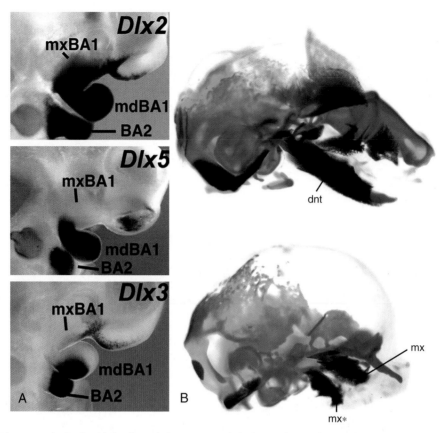

Figure 16-18. *Dlx* code patterns the first branchial arch. *A*, Whole mount in situ hybridization showing the nested expression of members of the *Dlx* family in the mandibular (mdBA1) and maxillary prominences (mxBA1). *B*, The loss of both *Dlx5* and *6* in mice results in derivatives of the mandibular prominence being transformed into derivatives of the maxillary prominence (top = wild-type; bottom = double knock out). Namely, Meckel's cartilage and the dentary bone (dnt) are replaced by an ectopic maxilla (mx∗) and other maxillary derived bones (not shown). mx, position of normal maxilla.

Development of Nasal and Oral Cavities

Figure 16-19 illustrates the process by which the nasal pits give rise to the nasal passages. At the end of the 6th week, as the medial nasal processes start to merge, the dorsal region of the deepening nasal pits fuse to form a single, enlarged ectodermal nasal sac lying superoposterior to the intermaxillary process (see Fig. 16-19*A*, *B*). From the end of the 6th week to the beginning of the 7th week, the floor and posterior wall of the nasal sac proliferate to form a thickened, platelike fin, or keel, of ectoderm separating the nasal sac from the oral cavity. This structure is called the **nasal fin** (see Fig. 16-19*B*). Vacuoles develop in the nasal fin and fuse with the nasal sac, thus enlarging the sac and thinning the fin to a thin membrane called the **oronasal membrane**, which separates the sac from the oral cavity (see Fig. 16-19*C*). This membrane ruptures during the 7th week to form an opening called the **primitive choana** (see Fig. 16-19*D*, *E*). The floor of the nasal cavity at this stage is formed by a posterior extension of the intermaxillary process called the **primary palate** (see Fig. 16-19*E*).

At this point the nasal and oral cavity are continuous but these will be separated by the formation of the palatal shelves. During the 7th and 8th weeks, the medial walls of the maxillary prominences produce

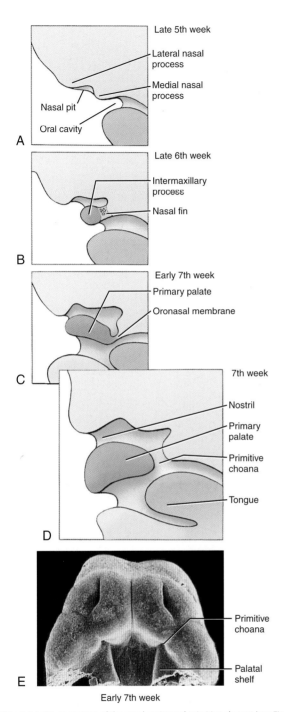

A

Late 5th week
Lateral nasal process
Medial nasal process
Nasal pit
Oral cavity

B

Late 6th week
Intermaxillary process
Nasal fin

C

Early 7th week
Primary palate
Oronasal membrane

D

7th week
Nostril
Primary palate
Primitive choana
Tongue

E

Primitive choana
Palatal shelf

Early 7th week

Figure 16-19. Formation of the nasal cavity and primitive choana (see Fig. 16-16A for orientation of the sections). A, B, The nasal pits invaginate to form a single nasal cavity separated from the oral cavity by a thick partition called the nasal fin. C-E, The nasal fin thins to form the oronasal membrane, which breaks down completely to form the primitive choana. The posterior extension of the intermaxillary process forms the primary palate.

a pair of thin medial extensions called the palatine shelves (Figs. 16-20A, B). At first, these shelves grow downward, parallel to the lateral surfaces of the tongue. However, at the end of the 7th week, they rotate rapidly upward into a horizontal position and then fuse with each other and with the primary palate to form the secondary palate (Fig. 16-20C, D). The rotation of the palatine shelves has been ascribed to the rapid synthesis and hydration of *Hyaluronic acid* within the extracellular matrix of the shelves, and the alignment of the elevated shelves in a horizontal plane may be determined by the orientation of *Collagen* and mesenchymal cells. Fusion occurs near the middle of the palatine shelves and proceeds both anteriorly and posteriorly. The central region, where the primary palate and secondary palate meet, is marked by the incisive foramen (see Fig. 16-20D). Growth and lowering of the mandibular primordium are also important for palatal shelve elevation as they lower the tongue, which initially fills the oral cavity (see Fig. 16-20A). Therefore, cleft palate can be secondarily associated with defects in lower jaw development (see the following "In the Clinic").

Intramembranous mesenchymal condensations in the anterior portion of the secondary palate form the bony **hard palate**. In the posterior portion of the secondary palate, myogenic mesenchyme condenses to give rise to the musculature of the soft palate.

While the secondary palate is forming, ectoderm and mesoderm of the frontonasal prominence and the medial nasal processes proliferate to form a midline **nasal septum** that grows down from the roof of the nasal cavity to fuse with the upper surface of the primary and secondary palates along the midline (see Fig. 16-20). The nasal cavity is now divided into two **nasal passages** that open into the pharynx behind the secondary palate through an opening called the **definitive choana** (see Fig. 16-20D).

IN THE CLINIC

FACIAL CLEFTING

As described earlier in this chapter, the face is created by the growth and fusion of five facial swellings. Complete or partial failure of fusion between any of these swellings results in a **facial cleft**, which may be unilateral or bilateral, and is a component of more than 300 syndromes. The two most common types of facial cleft are **cleft lip** (Figs. 16-21, 16-22; also see Fig. 4-10, which shows the much rarer median cleft lip), which usually results from failure of the

16

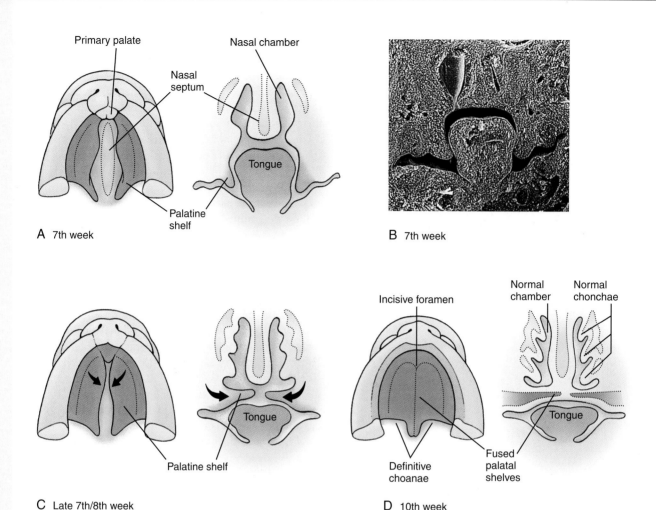

Figure 16-20. Formation of the secondary palate and nasal septum. The secondary palate forms from palatine shelves that grow medially from the maxillary swellings. During the same period, growth of the nasal septum separates the left and right nasal passages. The palatine shelves at first grow inferiorly on either side of the tongue *(A, B)* but then rapidly rotate upward to meet in the midline *(C)*, where they fuse with each other and with the inferior edge of the nasal septum *(D)*.

maxillary prominence to fuse with the intermaxillary process, and **cleft palate** (see Fig. 16-22), which results from the failure of the two palatine shelves to fuse with each other along the midline. Although cleft lip and cleft palate often occur together, the two defects differ in their distribution with respect to sex, familial association, race, and geography. Therefore, they probably have different etiologies. Cleft lip is more prevalent in males, whereas cleft palate occurs more frequently in females. The latter is attributable to the 1-week delay in palatal shelve elevation in females, which occurs at week 8 as compared to week 7 in males.

Cleft lip has been ascribed to underdevelopment of the mesenchyme of the maxillary prominence and medial nasal process, which would result in their inadequate contact. The resulting cleft may range in length from a minor notch in the vermilion border of the lip, just lateral to the philtrum, to a cleft that completely separates the lateral lip from the philtrum and nasal cavity. The depth of clefting also varies: some clefts involve just the soft tissue of the lip; others divide the lateral portion of the maxillary bone from the premaxillary portion (the portion bearing the incisors) and from the primary palate. Clefts of this type often result in deformed, absent, or supernumerary teeth.

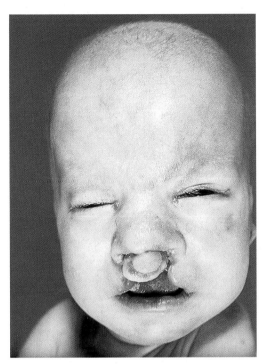

Figure 16-21. Bilateral cleft lip. This malformation results from failure of the medial nasal processes to fuse with the maxillary swellings.

Any of several pathogenetic factors might account for the underdevelopment of the maxillary prominence and medial nasal process in cleft lip. These include inadequate migration or proliferation of neural crest cell ectomesenchyme, and excessive cell death during the developmental modeling of the maxillary prominence and nasal placode. Although the etiology of the defect is generally multifactorial, a number of common drugs—including the anticonvulsant phenytoin (Dilantin), vitamin A, and some vitamin A analogs, particularly isotretinoin—have been shown to induce cleft lip in experimental animals. Vitamin A and its analogs are notorious for their ability to cause facial defects.

In cleft palate, failure of the palatine shelves to fuse during the 7th to 10th weeks may result from a variety of errors. These include inadequate growth of the palatine shelves (neural crest cell migration, proliferation, or excess apoptosis), failure of the shelves to elevate at the correct time, an excessively wide head, failure of the shelves to fuse, and secondary rupture after fusion. Cleft palate may also occur as a secondary consequence of mandibular dysplasias. During normal development, the mandibular primordium grows, thereby lowering the tongue relative to the palatal shelves and allowing them to elevate. If the first pharyngeal arch does not develop appropriately, the tongue will not be lowered and will physically obstruct palatal shelf elevation. This secondary cleft palate resulting from a smaller lower jaw (**microagnathia**) and occurring with **glossoptosis** (backward displacement of the tongue) is referred to as **Pierre Robin sequence** and is often seen as part of syndromes like **Stickler** and **Treacher Collins syndromes**. However, most cases are multifactorial in etiology involving both genetic susceptibility and environmental factors, as emphasized by the 24% to 25% concordance of cleft lip and palate in identical twins. Teratogens such as phenytoin, vitamin A and its analogs, and some corticosteroid anti-inflammatory drugs also can cause cleft palate in sensitive individuals.

Several mutations in humans have now been linked to cleft lip and palate. These include mutations in *MSX1* and more recently, the cell adhesion molecule *POLIO VIRUS RECEPTOR RELATED-1 (PVR1, NECTIN-1)* and the transcription factor *INTERFERON REGULATORY FACTOR 6 (IRF6)*. Mutations in the latter are responsible for **van der Woude syndrome**, which is the most common combined cleft lip and palate syndrome. *IRF6* and *PVR1* are expressed in the palatal shelf epithelium, including the medial edge epithelium (the point of palatine shelf fusion) of the elevated palatal shelves, whereas *MSX1* is expressed in the underlying mesenchyme. In addition, the T-box transcription factor *TBX22* has been linked to the **X-linked cleft palate plus ankylogossia syndrome**.

Development of Sinuses

At birth, the ratio of the volume of the facial skeleton to the volume of the cranial vault is about 1:7. During infancy and childhood, this ratio steadily decreases, mainly as a result of the development of teeth (discussed in Ch. 7) and the growth of the four pairs of **paranasal sinuses: the maxillary, ethmoid, sphenoid**, and **frontal sinuses**. These sinuses develop from invaginations of the nasal cavity that extend into the bones. Two of the sinuses appear during fetal life (maxillary and ethmoid) and the other two (sphenoid and frontal) appear after birth. Specifically, the *maxillary* sinuses form during the 3rd fetal month as invaginations of the nasal sac that slowly expand within the maxillary bones. The resulting cavities are small at birth but expand throughout childhood. The *ethmoid* sinuses form during the 5th fetal month as invaginations of the middle meatus of the nasal passages (the space underlying the middle nasal concha) and grow into the ethmoid bone. These sinuses do not complete their growth until puberty. The *sphenoid* sinuses

16

571

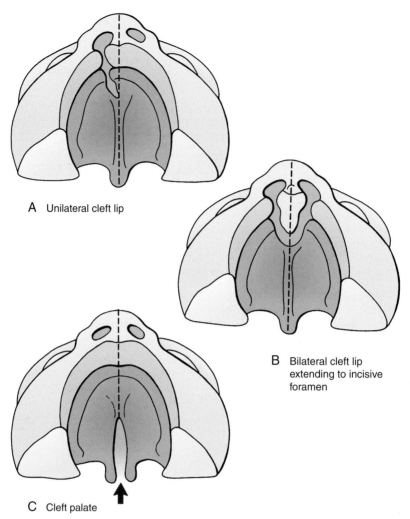

A   Unilateral cleft lip

B   Bilateral cleft lip extending to incisive foramen

C   Cleft palate

Figure 16-22. Cleft lip and cleft palate. *A, B,* Cleft lip. The cleft may involve the lip only, or extend dorsally along one or both edges of the primary palate. *C,* Cleft palate results from failure of the palatine shelves to fuse properly during development of the secondary palate.

actually represent extensions of the ethmoid sinuses. These extensions enlarge within the sphenoid bones throughout infancy and childhood. The *frontal* sinuses do not form until the 5th or 6th postnatal year and expand throughout adolescence. Each frontal sinus actually consists of two independent spaces that develop from different sources. One forms by the expansion of the ethmoid sinus into the frontal bone, and the other develops from an independent invagination of the middle meatus of the nasal passage. Because these cavities never coalesce, they drain independently.

Fate of Pharyngeal Clefts

As described earlier, the pharyngeal arches are separated by pharyngeal clefts externally and by pharyngeal pouches internally (Fig. 16-23*A*; see Fig. 16-7*D, E*). The first pharyngeal cleft and pouch, located between the first and second pharyngeal arches, participate in the formation of the ear: the first cleft becomes the **external acoustic meatus** and the **external part of the tympanic membrane.** The first pouch expands to form a cavity called the **tubotympanic recess,** which differentiates to become the

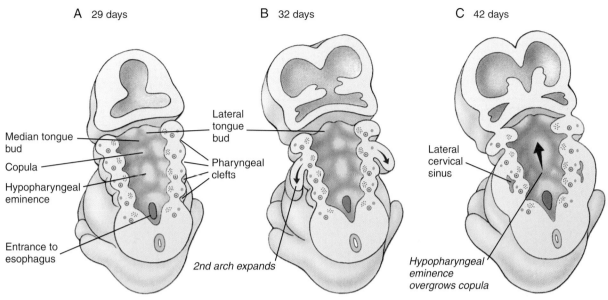

A 29 days   **B** 32 days   **C** 42 days

Median tongue bud
Copula
Hypopharyngeal eminence
Entrance to esophagus
Lateral tongue bud
Pharyngeal clefts
2nd arch expands
Lateral cervical sinus
Hypopharyngeal eminence overgrows copula

Figure 16-23. Fate of the pharyngeal clefts. The first pharyngeal cleft forms the external auditory meatus. The second pharyngeal arch expands and fuses with the cardiac eminence to cover the remaining pharyngeal clefts, which form the transient lateral cervical sinus.

tympanic cavity of the middle ear and the **auditory (eustachian) tube**. The development of these structures is covered in more detail in Chapter 17.

The remaining three pharyngeal clefts are normally obliterated during development. During the 4th and 5th weeks, the rapidly expanding second pharyngeal arch overgrows these clefts and fuses caudally with the cardiac eminence enclosing the clefts in a transient, ectoderm-lined **lateral cervical sinus** (Fig. 16-23B, C). This space normally disappears rapidly and completely.

However, the lateral cervical sinus occasionally persists on one or both sides in the form of a **cervical cyst** located just anterior to the sternocleidomastoid muscle (see sites *b* and *c* in Fig. 16-24). A completely enclosed cyst may expand to form a palpable lump as its epithelial lining desquamates or if it becomes infected. Occasionally, the cyst communicates either with the skin via an **external cervical fistula** or with the pharynx via an **internal cervical fistula** (Fig. 16-24A, B). Internal cervical fistulae most commonly open into the embryonic derivative of the second pouch, the **palatine tonsil**. Less often, they communicate with derivatives of the third pouch. Rarely, a cervical cyst has both internal and external fistulae (see Fig. 16-24B). Cysts of this type may be diagnosed by the drainage of mucus through the small opening of the external fistula on the neck on the anterior border of the sternocleidomastoid muscle (see Fig. 16-24C). Cervical cysts are usually of minor clinical importance but may require resection if they become seriously infected.

Infrequently, duplication of the first pharyngeal cleft results in formation of an ectoderm-lined **first-cleft sinus** or **cervical aural fistula** located in the tissues anterior to the external acoustic meatus (the so-called preauricular area; see site *a* in Fig. 16-24C). A fully enclosed first-cleft sinus may become apparent as a swelling just anterior to the auricle or external ear. Alternatively, it may drain to the exterior through a cervical aural fistula, which usually opens into the external auditory canal. Depending on its position, a first-cleft cyst or fistula may threaten the facial nerve if it becomes infected and may require resection. **Periauricular** (or preauricular) pits, sinuses, or fistulae may also arise due to the defects in fusion of the periauricular hillocks during formation of the outer ear.

Pharyngeal Arches Give Rise to Tongue

At the end of the 4th week, the floor of the pharynx consists of the five pharyngeal arches and the

16

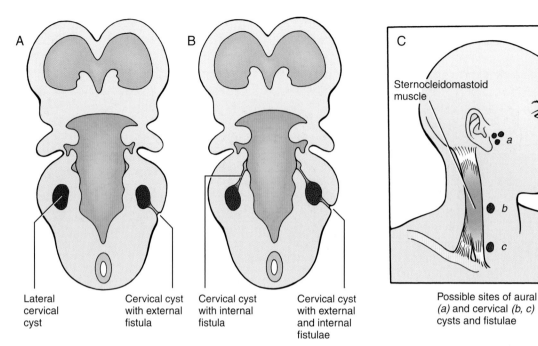

A — Lateral cervical cyst — Cervical cyst with external fistula

B — Cervical cyst with internal fistula — Cervical cyst with external and internal fistulae

C — Sternocleidomastoid muscle — Possible sites of aural (a) and cervical (b, c) cysts and fistulae

Figure 16-24. Abnormal cysts produced by the lateral cervical sinus or first pharyngeal cleft. The lateral cervical sinus occasionally persists in the form of an abnormal lateral cervical cyst. *A, B,* Such cysts may be isolated or may connect to the skin of the neck by an external cervical fistula, or to the pharynx by an internal fistula, or both. *C,* Lateral cervical cysts are located just medial to the anterior border of the sternocleidomastoid muscle. Anomalous derivatives of the first pharyngeal cleft known as aural (or preauricular) cysts may form anterior to the ear.

intervening pharyngeal pouches. The development of the tongue begins late in the 4th week when the first arch forms a median swelling called the **median tongue bud** or **tuberculum impar** (Fig. 16-25A). An additional pair of lateral swellings, the **distal tongue buds** (also called **lateral lingual swellings**), develop on the first arch early in the 5th week and rapidly expand to overgrow the median tongue bud (Fig. 16-25A-D). These swellings continue to grow throughout embryonic and fetal life and form the anterior two thirds of the tongue.

Late in the 4th week, the second arch develops a midline swelling called the **copula** (see Fig. 16-25A). This swelling is rapidly overgrown during the 5th and 6th weeks by a midline swelling of the third and fourth arches called the **hypopharyngeal eminence**, which gives rise to the posterior one third of the tongue (see Fig. 16-25A). The **epiglottis** develops just posterior to the hypopharyngeal eminence (see Fig. 16-25D). The hypopharyngeal eminence expands mainly by the growth of third-arch endoderm, whereas the fourth arch contributes only a

small region on the most posterior aspect of the tongue. Thus, the bulk of the tongue mucosa is formed by the first and third arches. During its development the ventral surface of the tongue is initially attached to the floor of the mouth. This attachment eventually regresses in the anterior region, thereby freeing the anterior part of the tongue, but more posteriorly it persists as the **frenulum**. If regression fails to occur, the resulting defect is called **ankyloglossia** (tongue-tie). Table 16-2 summarizes the developmental origins of the parts of the tongue.

The surface features of the definitive tongue reflect its embryonic origins. The boundary between the first-arch and third-arch contributions—roughly, the boundary between the anterior two thirds and posterior one third of the tongue—is marked by a transverse groove called the **terminal sulcus** (see Fig. 16-25D). The line of fusion between the right and left distal tongue buds is marked by a midline groove, the **median sulcus**, on the anterior two thirds of the tongue. A depression called the **foramen cecum** is visible where the median sulcus intersects

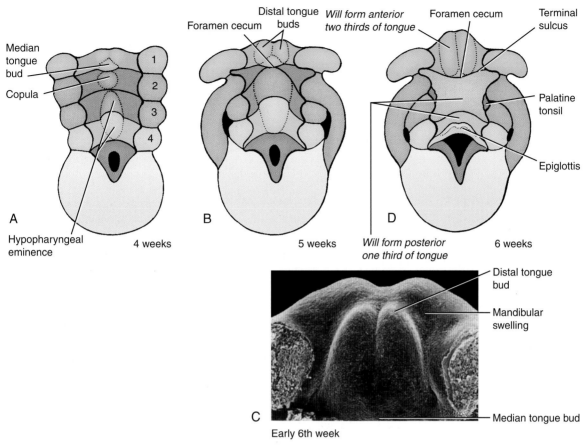

Figure 16-25. *A-D,* Development of the tongue mucosa from the endoderm of the pharyngeal floor. The mucosa of the anterior two thirds of the tongue develops mainly from the distal tongue buds (lateral lingual swellings) of the first pharyngeal arch, whereas the mucosal lining of the posterior one third of the tongue is formed by the hypopharyngeal eminence of the third and fourth arches, which overgrows the copula of the second arch.

the terminal sulcus (see Fig. 16-25*B, D*). As discussed in the next section, this depression is the site of origin of the thyroid gland.

All the muscles of the tongue except the **palatoglossus** are formed by mesoderm derived from the myotomes of the occipital somites, and the proliferation of this mesoderm is responsible for most of the growth of the tongue primordia. The innervation of the tongue muscles is consonant with their origin: all the muscles except the palatoglossus are innervated by the **hypoglossal nerve**, which is the cranial nerve associated with the occipital somites; the palatoglossus is innervated by the **pharyngeal plexus of the vagus nerve**.

The mucosal covering of the tongue is derived from pharyngeal arch endoderm and is innervated by sensory branches of the corresponding four cranial nerves (V, VII, IX, and X; see Table 16-2 and Fig. 16-11).

Thus, the tongue mucosa is innervated by different nerves from those of the tongue musculature (most of the tongue musculature as stated in the previous paragraph is innervated by cranial nerve XII). The general sensory receptors on the anterior two thirds of the tongue are supplied by a branch of the mandibular nerve (cranial nerve V3) called the **lingual nerve**. The taste buds of the anterior two thirds of the tongue are supplied by a special branch of the facial nerve (cranial nerve VII) called the **chorda tympani**. In contrast, the vallate papillae (a row of large taste buds flanking the terminal sulcus) and the general sensory endings over most of the posterior one third of the tongue are supplied by the **glossopharyngeal nerve** (cranial nerve IX). The small area on the most posterior aspect of the tongue that is derived from the fourth pharyngeal arch and the epiglottis receives

16

Table 16-2 Development of the Tongue from Pharyngeal Arches 1 through 4 and the Occipital Somites

Embryonic Precursor	Intermediate Structure	Adult Structure	Innervation
Pharyngeal arch 1	Median tongue bud	Overgrown by lateral lingual swellings	Lingual branch (sensory) of mandibular division of trigeminal nerve (V)
	Lateral lingual swellings	Mucosa of anterior two thirds of tongue	Chorda tympani from facial nerve (VII; innervating arch 2) (innervates all taste buds except vallate papillae)
Pharyngeal arch 2	Copula	Overgrown by other structures	
Pharyngeal arch 3	Large, ventral part of hypopharyngeal eminence	Mucosa of most of posterior one third of tongue	Sensory branch of glossopharyngeal nerve (IX) (also supplies vallate papillae)
Pharyngeal arch 4	Small, dorsal part of hypopharyngeal eminence	Mucosa of small region on dorsal side of posterior one third of tongue	Sensory fibers of superior laryngeal branch of vagus nerve (X)
Occipital somites	Myoblasts	Intrinsic muscles of tongue	Hypoglossal nerve (XII)
Head mesoderm	Myoblasts	Palatoglossus muscle	Pharyngeal plexus of vagus nerve (X)

sensory innervation from the **superior laryngeal** branch of the vagus nerve (cranial nerve X).

Development of Thyroid Gland

Figure 16-26 illustrates the embryogenesis of the **thyroid gland**. The gland primordium first forms late in the 4th week as a small, solid mass of endoderm proliferating at the apex of the foramen cecum on the developing tongue. The thyroid primordium descends through the tissues of the neck at the end of a slender **thyroglossal duct**. The thyroglossal duct breaks down by the end of the 5th week, and the isolated thyroid, now consisting of lateral lobes connected by a well-defined isthmus, continues to descend, reaching its final position just inferior to the cricoid cartilage by the 7th week. Studies of the ability of the embryonic thyroid to incorporate iodine into thyroid hormones and to secrete these hormones into the circulation show that this gland begins to function as early as the 10th to the 12th week in human embryos.

Normally, the only remnant of the thyroglossal duct is the foramen cecum itself. However, occasionally, a portion of the duct persists either as an enclosed **thyroglossal cyst** or as a **thyroglossal sinus** communicating with the surface of the neck. Rarely, a fragment of the thyroid becomes detached during the descent of the gland and forms a patch of ectopic thyroid tissue, which may be located anywhere along the route of descent.

Development of Pharyngeal Pouches

Figures 16-27 and 16-28 summarize the origin and migration of structures that arise from the pharyngeal pouches. The fate of the first pharyngeal pouch, which differentiates into the tympanic cavity and auditory tube, is discussed in Chapter 17.

The palatine tonsils arise from the endoderm lining the second pharyngeal pouch (located between the second and third arches). Development of these tonsils begins early in the 3rd month as the epithelium of the second pouch proliferates to form solid endodermal buds, or ledges, growing into the underlying mesenchyme, which will give rise to the tonsillar stroma. The central cells of the buds later die and slough, converting the solid buds into hollow **tonsillar crypts** that are infiltrated by lymphoid tissue. However, the definitive lymph follicles of the tonsil do not form until the last 3 months of prenatal life.

Similar lymphatic tonsils, called **pharyngeal tonsils**, develop in association with mucous glands of the pharynx. The major pharyngeal tonsils are the **adenoids, tubal tonsils** (associated with the auditory tubes), and **lingual tonsils** (associated with the posterior regions of the tongue). Minor intervening patches of lymphoid tissue also form.

The third pharyngeal pouch gives rise to the thymus and inferior parathyroid glands. The two thymic primordia arise at the end of the 4th week in the form of endodermal proliferations at the end of ventral elongations of the third pharyngeal pouches.

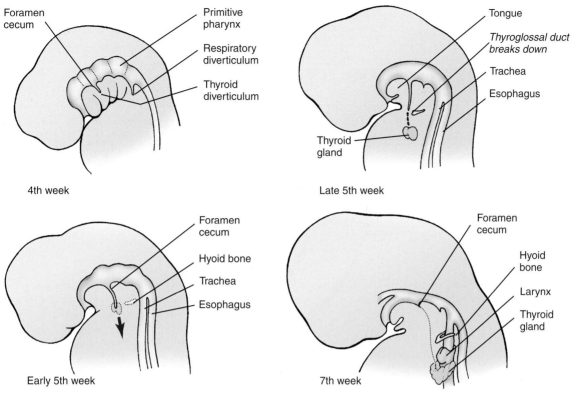

Figure 16-26. The thyroid originates as an endodermal proliferation at the tip of the foramen cecum of the developing tongue and migrates inferiorly to its final site anterior and inferior to the larynx. Until the 5th week, the thyroid remains connected to the foramen cecum by the thyroglossal duct. The gland reaches its final site in the 7th week.

These endodermal proliferations form hollow tubes that invade the underlying mesenchyme and later transform into solid, branching cords. These cords are the primordia of the polyhedral thymic lobules.

Between the 4th and 7th weeks, the thymus glands lose their connections with the pharynx and migrate caudally and medially to their definitive location inferior and ventral to the developing thyroid and just dorsal to the sternum. There they are joined via connective tissue to form a single, bilobate thymus gland. At this point the thymus is still epithelial but it quickly becomes infiltrated by neural crest cells to form septa and the capsule. During the 3rd month lymphocytes and dendritic cells infiltrate the thymus, and by 12 weeks each thymic lobule is 0.5 to 2 mm in diameter and has a well-defined cortex and medulla. The whorl-like **Hassall's corpuscles** in the medulla are thought to arise from the ectodermal cells of the third pharyngeal cleft. Hassall's corpuscles produce signals necessary for the development of

regulatory T cells. The loosely organized **epithelial reticulum** is thought to be of endodermal origin. As with the thyroid gland, ectopic remnants of the thymus are occasionally left along the route of migration.

The thymus is highly active during the perinatal period and continues to grow throughout childhood, reaching its maximum size at puberty. After puberty, the gland involutes rapidly and is represented only by insignificant fatty vestiges in the adult.

The rudiments of the **inferior parathyroid glands (parathyroids III)** form in the dorsal portion of the third pouch and the rudiments of the **superior parathyroid glands (parathyroids IV)** form in the fourth pouch early in the 5th week. They detach from the pharyngeal wall and migrate inferiorly and medially, coming to rest by the 7th week. The inferior parathyroid glands lie on the dorsal side of the inferior end of the thyroid lobes, whereas the superior parathyroid glands are in a position slightly superior to the inferior parathyroid glands. Thus, the superior parathyroids

16

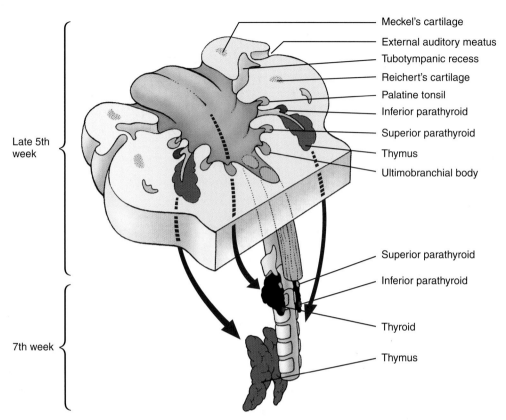

Figure 16-27. Development of the pharyngeal pouch derivatives. All of the pharyngeal pouches give rise to adult structures. These are the tubotympanic recess (pouch 1), the palatine tonsils (pouch 2), the inferior parathyroid glands and thymus (pouch 3), the superior parathyroid glands (pouch 4), and the ultimobranchial (telopharyngeal) body (inferior part of pouch 4 or a hypothetical pouch 5). The parathyroids, thymus primordia, and ultimobranchial bodies separate from the lining of the pharynx and migrate to their definitive locations within the neck and thorax.

arise more inferiorly on the pharynx than the inferior parathyroids, and the two glands switch position during their descent; their names reflect their final relative positions.

During the 5th week, a minor invagination forms just caudal to the fourth pharyngeal pouch. This invagination has been described by many embryologists as a **fifth pharyngeal pouch**. Almost immediately after they appear, these invaginations become populated by cells that form the rudiments of the paired **ultimobranchial bodies**. The cellular origins and composition of the ultimobranchial bodies are unclear, but studies show that neural crest cells infiltrate this structure. These rudiments immediately detach from the pharyngeal wall and migrate medially and caudally to implant into the dorsal wall of the thyroid gland, where they become dispersed within the thyroid.

The ultimobranchial bodies may contribute follicle cells to the thyroid, but it is clear that the calcitonin-producing **C cells (parafollicular cells)** of the thyroid are derived from neural crest cells.

Development of Salivary Glands

Three pairs of salivary glands develop in humans: the **parotid, submandibular**, and **sublingual** glands. The parotid gland develops from a groove-like invagination of ectoderm that forms in the crease between the maxillary and mandibular swellings during week 6. This groove differentiates into a tubular duct that sinks into the underlying mesenchyme towards the ear.

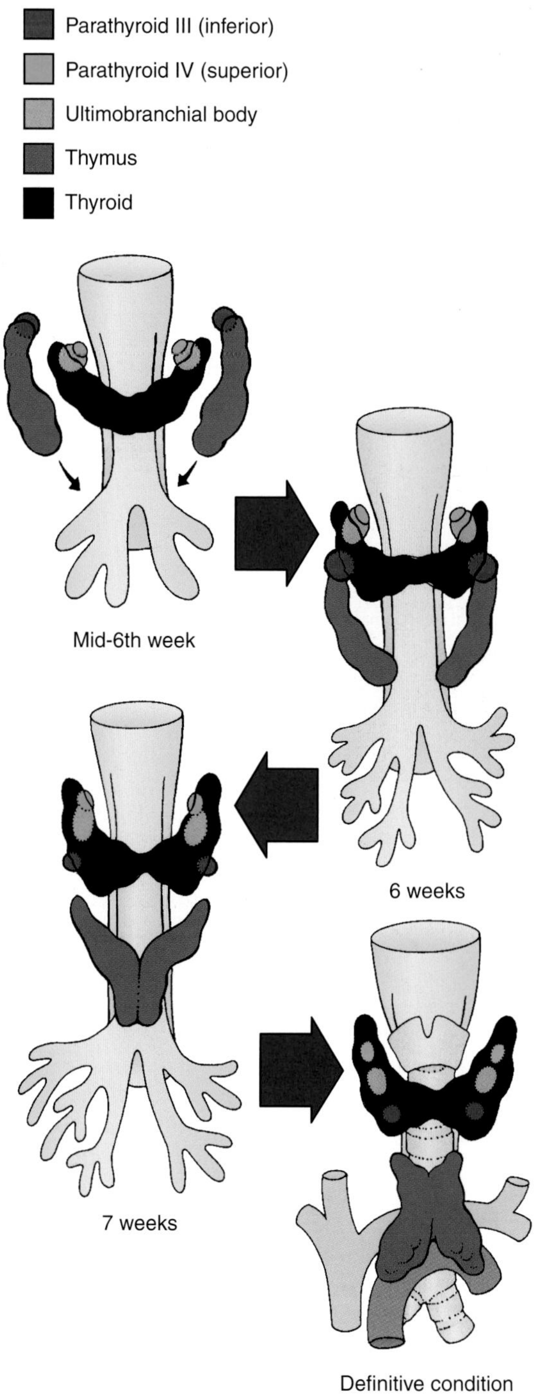

Parathyroid III (inferior)

Parathyroid IV (superior)

Ultimobranchial body

Thymus

Thyroid

Mid-6th week

6 weeks

7 weeks

Definitive condition

Figure 16-28. Migration of pharyngeal pouch derivatives. The parathyroid glands and the ultimobranchial bodies migrate inferiorly to become embedded in the posterior wall of the thyroid gland. The two parathyroids exchange position as they migrate: parathyroid III becomes the inferior parathyroid, whereas parathyroid IV becomes the superior parathyroid.

The invaginating duct maintains a ventral opening at the angle of the primitive mouth. As the cheek portions of the maxillary and mandibular swellings fuse, this opening is transferred to the inner surface of the cheek. The blind dorsal end of the tube differentiates to form the parotid gland, whereas the stem of the tube becomes the **parotid** or **Stensen's duct**. Similar invaginations of the endoderm in the floor of the oral cavity and in the paralingual sulci on either side of the tongue give rise to the submandibular and sublingual salivary glands, respectively.

Development of the salivary glands is dependent on epithelial-mesenchymal interactions. Therefore, it is not surprising that some syndromes such as autosomal dominant **lacrimoauriculodentodigital (LADD) syndrome** (the result of a mutation in *FGF10*) encompass both the salivary glands and other tissues dependent on epithelial-mesenchymal interactions for their development (i.e., lacrimal glands, distal limb, teeth, and ears).

IN THE CLINIC

CAUSES OF CRANIOFACIAL ANOMALIES

It has been estimated that the various kinds of **craniofacial anomalies**—including malformations of the frontonasal process, clefting defects, calvarial malformations, and anomalies of the pharyngeal arch derivatives—account for approximately one third of all congenital defects. Most craniofacial anomalies have a multifactorial etiology, although in some types a clear genetic basis can be demonstrated, as, for example, in **Treacher Collins syndrome** (discussed in the next section of this chapter), which is inherited as an autosomal dominant trait. A number of teratogens are also known to cause craniofacial malformations. Probably the most clinically significant craniofacial teratogen is **alcohol**. Drugs such as the anticonvulsant **hydantoin** and the oral antiacne drug **isotretinoin** (Fig. 16-29) can also cause craniofacial anomalies in humans, as can **toluene, cigarette smoking, ionizing radiation,** and **hyperthermia**. Finally, many craniofacial abnormalities are associated with cardiac abnormalities that are explained by the migration of neural crest cells through the fourth and sixth pharyngeal arches to form the aorticopulmonary septum and the requirement for cranial neural crest cells in the remodeling of the aortic arches (discussed in Ch. 13). Recent studies have also illustrated a common role of the endoderm in development of the face and aortic arches.

16

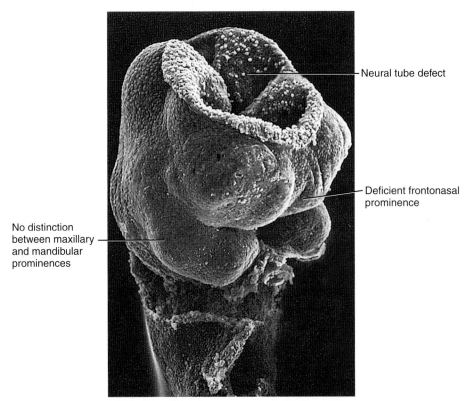

Neural tube defect

Deficient frontonasal prominence

No distinction between maxillary and mandibular prominences

Figure 16-29. Mouse embryo treated with the teratogen isotretinoin (an analog of vitamin A) exhibiting a neural tube defect and first pharyngeal arch and frontonasal prominence abnormalities. Isotretinoin has been implicated in malformations of the skull, face, central nervous system, lungs, cardiovascular system, and limbs of human infants born to mothers ingesting it during the first 3 months of pregnancy.

CRANIOFACIAL SYNDROMES

Not surprisingly, errors in the development of the numerous pharyngeal arch and pouch elements that contribute to the human head and face can cause various malformations. After cleft lip and cleft palate, the most common group of facial malformations are the defects caused by underdevelopment of the first and second arches. An example of these defects is a **lateral cleft**, in which incomplete fusion of the maxillary and mandibular prominences in the cheek region results in a cleft extending back from the corner of the mouth occasionally as far as to the tragus of the auricle.

Lateral clefting can occur as part of a group of more extensive deformities collectively known as **hemifacial microsomia** (*microsomia* is from the Greek for "small body"). In this condition, the lateral cleft of the face usually is not large, but the posterior portion of the mandible, the temporomandibular joint, the muscles of mastication, and the outer and middle ear may all be underdeveloped. **Goldenhar**

syndrome is a particularly severe member of this group, including defects of the eye (scleral dermoids and coloboma of the eyelids) and vertebral column. This entire group of disorders is also referred to as **oculoauriculovertebral spectrum (OAVS)**.

Another group of syndromes is classified as **mandibulofacial dysostosis** and involves generalized underdevelopment of the first pharyngeal arches, resulting in defects of the eye, ear, midface, palate, and jaw. The autosomal-dominant **Treacher Collins syndrome** is a member of this group. The gene for Treacher Collins syndrome, *TCOF1*, has been identified. It encodes a nucleolar phosphoprotein called *Treacle*. *Treacle* is expressed in the neural folds as neural crest cells are forming and emigrating, and later in the pharyngeal arches. Although its precise cellular function is unclear, it is thought to regulate microtubule dynamics, as well as to function in ribosomal DNA gene transcription. Analysis of mutant mice, has shown that there is increased apoptosis of the neural crest precursors and decreased proliferation of the neural crest cells. No migratory defects have been observed.

In addition to these defects of the face (including eye, ear, midface, palate, and jaw), there are defects that extend into the pharyngeal arch derivatives and encompass abnormalities of the neck, heart, thymus, and parathyroid glands. The complex of congenital malformations known as **DiGeorge anomaly** falls into this group and is characterized by a triad of malformations: (1) minor craniofacial defects, including **micrognathia** (small jaw), low-set ears, auricular abnormalities, cleft palate, and hypertelorism; (2) total or partial agenesis of the derivatives of the third and fourth pharyngeal pouches (the thymus and parathyroid glands); and (3) cardiovascular anomalies, including persistent truncus arteriosus and interrupted aortic arch. DiGeorge anomaly is seen in **22q11.2 deletion syndrome**, which is phenocopied by loss of neural crest cells. Consequently, it was originally thought that the primary defect in 22q11.2 deletion syndrome was in neural crest cells. However, genetic studies characterizing the function of each gene that is deleted in the crucial 22q11.2 chromosomal region do not support this original view. These studies have shown that two genes in the deleted region are directly involved: *Tbx1* and *Crkl*. *Tbx1* is a T-box transcription factor expressed in the pharyngeal endoderm and mesoderm, but *not* in neural crest cells. *Crkl* is a ubiquitously expressed gene encoding a receptor adaptor protein. Homozygous *Tbx1*-mutant mice recapitulate the 22q11.2 deletion syndrome phenotype. Studies in which the *Tbx1* gene has been inactivated in either the mesoderm or endoderm show that *Tbx1* is needed in both tissues. However, heterozygous *Tbx1*-mutant mice do not recapitulate the 22q11.2 deletion phenotype, demonstrating that loss of one functional allele of *TBX1* in humans may not result in the abnormalities characteristic of 22q11.2 deletion syndrome. Recent studies have provided an explanation: if one copy of *Tbx1* and one copy of *Crkl*, are deleted in mice, then the resultant phenotype encompasses those seen in the face and pharyngeal arch derivatives of 22q11.2 deletion syndrome patients. This shows that 22q11.2 deletion syndrome is a **contiguous gene syndrome** (i.e., requires deletion of multiple, contiguous genes to manifest the phenotype). Interestingly, loss of *Tbx1* and both *Tbx1* and *Crkl* has been linked to increased retinoic acid signaling in the cranial pharyngeal arches. As discussed above, retinoic acid is a potent teratogen that induces craniofacial malformations.

Suggested Readings

Abzhanov A, Kuo WP, Hartmann C, et al. 2006. The calmodulin pathway and evolution of elongated beak morphology in Darwin's finches. Nature 442:563-567.

Arnold JS, Werling U, Braunstein EM, et al. 2006. Inactivation of Tbx1 in the pharyngeal endoderm results in 22q11DS malformations. Development 133:977-987.

Baldini A. 2005. Dissecting contiguous gene defects: TBX1. Curr Opin Genet Dev 15:279-284.

Begemann G, Meyer A. 2001. Hindbrain patterning revisited: timing and effects of retinoic acid signaling. Bioessays 23:981-986.

Chai Y, Maxson RE, Jr. 2006. Recent advances in craniofacial morphogenesis. Dev Dyn 235:2353-2375.

Cobourne MT. 2004. The complex genetics of cleft lip and palate. Eur J Orthod 26:7-16.

Dixon J, Jones NC, Sandell LL, et al. 2006. Tcof1/Treacle is required for neural crest cell formation and proliferation deficiencies that cause craniofacial abnormalities. Proc Natl Acad Sci U S A 103:13403-13408.

Dixon J, Trainor P, Dixon MJ. 2007. Treacher Collins syndrome. Orthod Craniofac Res 10:88-95.

Francis-West PH, Robson L, Evans DJ. 2003. Craniofacial development: the tissue and molecular interactions that control development of the head. Adv Anat Embryol Cell Biol 169:III-VI, 1-138.

Graham A, Okabe M, Quinlan R. 2005. The role of the endoderm in the development and evolution of the pharyngeal arches. J Anat 207:479-487.

Guris DL, Duester G, Papaioannou VE, Imamoto A. 2006. Dose-dependent interaction of Tbx1 and Crkl and locally aberrant RA signaling in a model of del22q11 syndrome. Dev Cell 10:81-92.

Hall BK. 1999. The Neural Crest in Development and Evolution. New York: Springer.

Helms JA, Cordero D, Tapadia MD. 2005. New insights into craniofacial morphogenesis. Development 132:851-861.

Hilliard SA, Yu L, Gu S, et al. 2005. Regional regulation of palatal growth and patterning along the anterior-posterior axis in mice. J Anat 207:655-667.

Le Douarin NM, Kalcheim C. 1999. The Neural Crest. 2nd Ed. Cambridge: Cambridge University Press. p. 445.

Le Douarin NM, Creuzet S, Couly G, Dupin E. 2004. Neural crest cell plasticity and its limits. Development 131:4637-4650.

Lumsden A. 2004. Segmentation and compartition in the early avian hindbrain. Mech Dev 121:1081-1088.

Maity T, Fuse N, Beachy PA. 2005. Molecular mechanisms of Sonic hedgehog mutant effects in holoprosencephaly. Proc Natl Acad Sci U S A 102:17026-17031.

Mark M, Ghyselinck NB, Chambon P. 2004. Retinoic acid signaling in the development of branchial arches. Curr Opin Genet Dev 14:591-598.

Matsuoka T, Ahlberg PE, Kessaris N, et al. 2005. Neural crest origins of the neck and shoulder. Nature 436:347-355.

Morriss-Kay GM, Wilkie AO. 2005. Growth of the normal skull vault and its alteration in craniosynostosis: insights from human genetics and experimental studies. J Anat 207:637-653.

Noden DM, Trainor PA. 2005. Relations and interactions between cranial mesoderm and neural crest populations. J Anat 207:575-601.

16

Opperman LA. 2000. Cranial sutures as intramembranous bone growth sites. Dev Dyn 219:472-485.

Paylor R, Lindsay E. 2006. Mouse models of 22q11 deletion syndrome. Biol Psychiatry 59:1172-1179.

Rice DP. 2005. Craniofacial anomalies: from development to molecular pathogenesis. Curr Mol Med 5:699-722.

Roessler E, Muenke M. 2003. How a Hedgehog might see holoprosencephaly. Hum Mol Genet 12(Spec No 1):R15-R25.

Trainor PA. 2005. Specification of neural crest cell formation and migration in mouse embryos. Semin Cell Dev Biol 16:683-693.

Trainor PA, Krumlauf R. 2001. Hox genes, neural crest cells and branchial arch patterning. Curr Opin Cell Biol 13:698-705.

Trainor PA, Melton KR, Manzanares M. 2003. Origins and plasticity of neural crest cells and their roles in jaw and craniofacial evolution. Int J Dev Biol 47:541-553.

Walker MB, Trainor PA. 2006. Craniofacial malformations: intrinsic vs extrinsic neural crest cell defects in Treacher Collins and 22q11 deletion syndromes. Clin Genet 69:471-479.

Wallis D, Muenke M. 2000. Mutations in holoprosencephaly. Hum Mutat 16:99-108.

Wilkie AO, Bochukova EG, Hansen RM, et al. 2006. Clinical dividends from the molecular genetic diagnosis of craniosynostosis. Am J Med Genet A 140(23):2631-2639.

Zhang Z, Huynh T, Baldini A. 2006. Mesodermal expression of Tbx1 is necessary and sufficient for pharyngeal arch and cardiac outflow tract development. Development 133:3587-3595.

Development of the Ears and Eyes

17

Ear Development

Summary   The ear is a composite structure with multiple embryonic origins. The external and middle ears arise from the first and second pharyngeal arches and the intervening pharyngeal cleft and pouch. The inner ear, in contrast, develops from an ectodermal otic placode that appears on either side of the neural tube at the level of the future hindbrain. At the end of the 3rd week, this **otic placode** invaginates and then pinches off to form an **otic vesicle (otocyst)** within the head mesenchyme. The otic vesicle rapidly differentiates into three subdivisions: a slender **endolymphatic duct**, the expanded **pars superior**, and a tapered **pars inferior**. From the 4th to the 7th weeks, the pars superior differentiates to form the three **semicircular canals** and the **utricle**. The pars inferior elongates and coils to form the **cochlear duct** distally and the **saccule** proximally. All of these otic vesicle derivatives collectively constitute the **membranous labyrinth**. The otic placode also gives rise to the sensory ganglia of the **vestibulocochlear (statoacoustic) nerve** (cranial nerve VIII). In addition, neural crest cells contribute to the vestibulocochlear nerve and its glial cells. From weeks 9 to 23, the mesenchymal condensation that surrounds the membranous labyrinth, called the **otic capsule**, first chondrifies and then ossifies to form a **bony labyrinth** within the petrous part of the temporal bone.

The first pharyngeal pouch lengthens to form the **tubotympanic recess**, which differentiates into the tympanic cavity of the middle ear and the **auditory (eustachian) tube**. Three auditory ossicles, the **malleus, incus**, and **stapes**, develop in the mesenchyme adjacent to the tympanic cavity. The malleus and incus are formed from the first pharyngeal arch mesenchyme, whereas the stapes is a second arch derivative. In the last month of gestation, the mesenchyme around the ossicles regresses and the tympanic cavity expands to enclose the ossicles. As a consequence, the ossicles are ensheathed by the endoderm that lines the tympanic cavity.

The **auricle (pinna)** of the external ear develops from six **auricular hillocks**, which appear during the 6th week on the lateral edges of the first and second pharyngeal arches. The first pharyngeal cleft lengthens to form the primordium of the **external auditory canal**. The ectoderm lining the canal subsequently proliferates to form a **meatal plug** that completely fills the inner portion of the canal. The definitive canal is formed by recanalization of this plug during the 26th week. The tympanic membrane is derived from the pharyngeal membrane that separates the first pharyngeal pouch and cleft. It develops as a three-layered structure, consisting of an external layer of ectoderm, a middle layer of ectoderm derived from **neural crest cells**, and an inner layer of endoderm. The definitive tympanic membrane is formed during the recanalization of the external auditory meatus.

Eye Development

Summary   The eyes first appear early in the 4th week in the form of a pair of lateral grooves, the **optic sulci**, which evaginate from the forebrain neural groove to form the **optic vesicles**. As soon as the distal tip of the optic vesicle reaches the surface ectoderm, it invaginates, transforming the optic vesicle into a goblet-shaped **optic cup** that is attached to the forebrain by a narrower, hollow **optic stalk**. The adjacent surface ectoderm simultaneously thickens to form a **lens placode**,

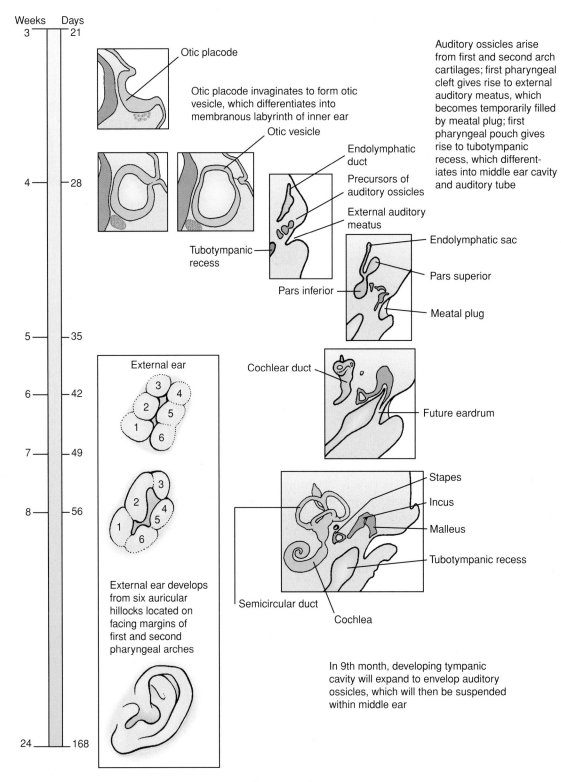

Weeks / Days

Otic placode

Otic placode invaginates to form otic vesicle, which differentiates into membranous labyrinth of inner ear

Otic vesicle

Endolymphatic duct

Precursors of auditory ossicles

External auditory meatus

Tubotympanic recess

Pars inferior

Endolymphatic sac

Pars superior

Meatal plug

Auditory ossicles arise from first and second arch cartilages; first pharyngeal cleft gives rise to external auditory meatus, which becomes temporarily filled by meatal plug; first pharyngeal pouch gives rise to tubotympanic recess, which differentiates into middle ear cavity and auditory tube

External ear

Cochlear duct

Future eardrum

Stapes

Incus

Malleus

Tubotympanic recess

Semicircular duct

Cochlea

External ear develops from six auricular hillocks located on facing margins of first and second pharyngeal arches

In 9th month, developing tympanic cavity will expand to envelop auditory ossicles, which will then be suspended within middle ear

Time line. Ear development.

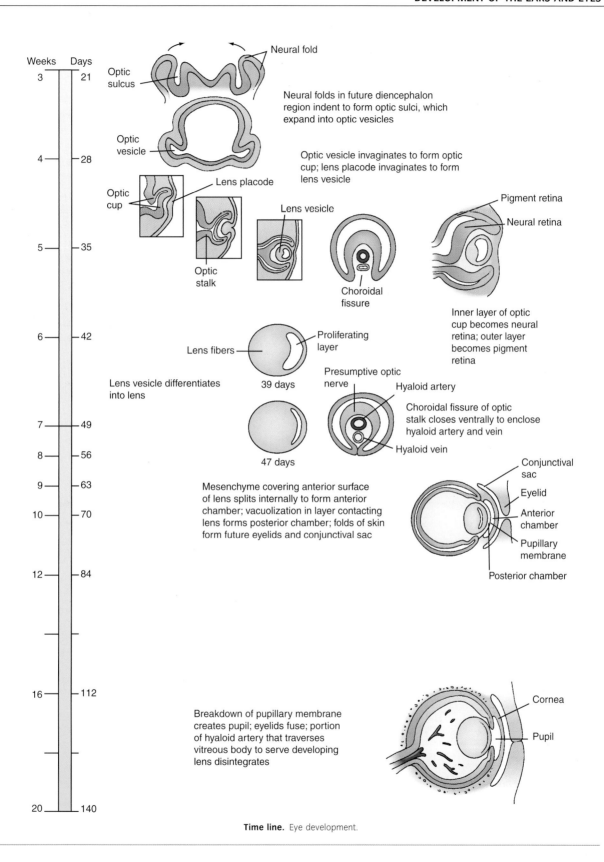

Weeks Days

3 — 21

Neural fold

Optic sulcus

Neural folds in future diencephalon region indent to form optic sulci, which expand into optic vesicles

Optic vesicle

4 — 28

Optic vesicle invaginates to form optic cup; lens placode invaginates to form lens vesicle

Optic cup

Lens placode

Optic stalk

Lens vesicle

Choroidal fissure

Pigment retina

Neural retina

5 — 35

Inner layer of optic cup becomes neural retina; outer layer becomes pigment retina

6 — 42

Lens fibers

Proliferating layer

39 days

Lens vesicle differentiates into lens

Presumptive optic nerve

Hyaloid artery

Choroidal fissure of optic stalk closes ventrally to enclose hyaloid artery and vein

Hyaloid vein

7 — 49

47 days

8 — 56

9 — 63

10 — 70

Mesenchyme covering anterior surface of lens splits internally to form anterior chamber; vacuolization in layer contacting lens forms posterior chamber; folds of skin form future eyelids and conjunctival sac

Conjunctival sac

Eyelid

Anterior chamber

Pupillary membrane

Posterior chamber

12 — 84

16 — 112

Breakdown of pupillary membrane creates pupil; eyelids fuse; portion of hyaloid artery that traverses vitreous body to serve developing lens disintegrates

Cornea

Pupil

20 — 140

Time line. Eye development.

17

which invaginates and pinches off to become a hollow **lens vesicle**. Posterior cells of the lens vesicle form long, slender, anteroposteriorly oriented **primary lens fibers**. Anterior cells develop into a simple epithelium covering the face of the lens and give rise to the **secondary lens fibers**, which make up most of the mature lens.

The inner wall of the optic cup (the former **optic disc**) gives rise to the **neural retina**, whereas the outer wall gives rise to the thin, melanin-containing **pigmented epithelium**. The differentiation of the neural retina takes place between the 6th week and the 8th month. Six types of neuronal cells and one glial (Müller) cell are produced in the outer layer of the neural retina, which is proliferative, forming three layers in the mature retina: the **ganglion cell layer**; an **inner nuclear layer** containing the amacrine, horizontal, and bipolar cells; and an **outer nuclear layer** containing the rods and cone photoreceptors. Axons from the neural retina grow through the optic stalk to the brain, converting the optic stalk to the **optic nerve**.

Blood is supplied to the developing lens and retina by a terminal branch of the ophthalmic artery, the **hyaloid artery**, which enters the optic vesicle via a groove called the **choroidal fissure**. The portion of the artery that traverses the vitreous body to reach the lens degenerates during fetal life as the lens matures; the remainder of the artery becomes the **central artery of the retina**.

As the optic vesicle forms it is enveloped by a sheath of mesenchyme that is derived from neural crest cells and head mesoderm. This sheath differentiates to form the two coverings of the optic cup: the thin inner vascular **choroid** and the fibrous outer **sclera**. The mesenchyme overlying the developing lens splits into two layers to enclose a new space called the **anterior chamber**. The inner wall of the anterior chamber, overlying the lens, is called the **pupillary membrane**. Deep layers of this wall undergo vacuolization to create a new space, the **posterior chamber**, between the lens and the thin remaining pupillary membrane. Early in fetal life, the pupillary membrane breaks down completely to form the **pupil**. The rim of the optic cup differentiates to form the **iris** and **ciliary body**. Mesoderm adjacent to the optic cup differentiates in the 5th and 6th weeks to form the **extrinsic ocular muscles**. The connective tissue components of the extrinsic ocular muscles are derived from neural crest cells. The eyelids arise as folds of surface ectoderm and are fused from the 8th week to about the 5th month.

Clinical Taster

A 2-year-old boy with **profound hearing loss** is admitted to the pediatric service for fever and vomiting. Urinalysis showed leukocytes and bacteria. He is diagnosed with pyelonephritis (urinary tract infection with kidney involvement) and started on intravenous antibiotics.

The boy's hearing loss was detected by a local Department of Health newborn hearing screening program and verified with a sedated _b_rainstem _a_uditory _e_voked _r_esponse (BAER). His hearing loss was determined to be both **conductive** (caused by abnormalities of the external or middle ear) and **sensorineural** (caused by defects of the cochlea or cranial nerve VIII). He had been using hearing aids since 4 months of age.

A renal ultrasound done on admission showed small, dysplastic kidneys and hydronephrosis (dilation of the ureter and renal pelvis) on the right side. Later that night, while researching the differential diagnosis of hearing loss and kidney abnormalities, the medical student on call finds the description of _b_ranchio-_o_to-_r_enal (BOR) syndrome. Intrigued by this possibility, the student returns to the patient's bedside and finds that the boy has cup-shaped ears, preauricular pits, and small cysts over the sternocleidomastoid muscle (Fig. 17-1A). These cysts are later determined to be pharyngeal (branchial) cysts (persisting rudiments of the pharyngeal apparatus, as discussed in Ch. 16). During his hospital stay, the patient has a thin-cut CT (computed tomography) of the temporal bone that shows malformations of the middle ear bones and hypoplastic cochlea.

As suspected by the medical student, the combination of pharyngeal (branchial) arch, otic (ear), and renal (kidney) abnormalities seen in the patient suggests the diagnosis of BOR. Also known as Melnick-Frasier syndrome, BOR is most often caused by mutations in the _EYES ABSENT HOMOLOG 1_ (_EYA1_) gene. As the name suggests, mutations in the Drosophila homolog of this gene (_Eya_) affect the eyes (Fig. 17-1B). Humans with _EYA1_ mutations rarely have abnormalities of the eyes, likely due to functional redundancy of multiple _EYA_ genes (there are four _EYA_ homologs present in humans) during eye development.

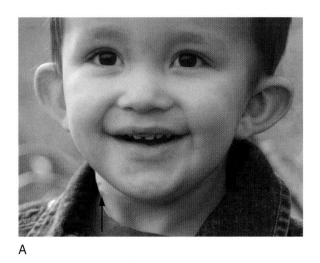

A

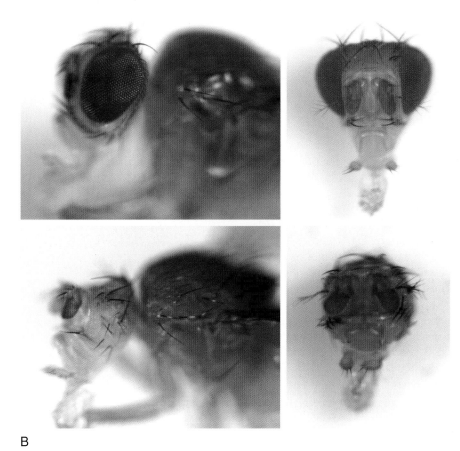

B

Figure 17-1. The role of *Eya1* in embryonic development. *A*, Boy with branchio-oto-renal syndrome (mutation in the *EYA1* gene). Note the cup-shaped ears and branchial cysts (arrow). Preauricular pits and tags (not shown in this case) sometimes accompany the syndrome. *B*, Wild-type Drosophila adult (top) and *Eya1* mutant (bottom) showing the head in lateral (left) and on-front (right) views. Note the total absence of the eyes in the mutant (reddish-orange structures in the wild-type Drosophila).

17

Ear Development

The ear can be divided into three parts, the external, middle, and inner ear, each of which has distinct tissue origins. The external ear consists of the **pinna** (or **auricle**) and **external auditory canal** (ear canal). The middle ear contains the auditory ossicles—the **malleus, incus**, and **stapes**—arranged in a chain in the **tympanic cavity**. The external and middle ear capture and carry the sound waves to the inner ear. The inner ear consists of the **cochlea** and **vestibular apparatus.** The three **semicircular canals**, the **utricle**, and the **saccule** compose the vestibular apparatus. The cochlea perceives sound waves, whereas the vestibular apparatus perceives orientation, movement, and gravity and is necessary for balance. The derivatives of the inner ear are collectively known as the **membranous labyrinth**. Innervated by the **vestibulocochlear nerve** (cranial nerve VIII), the inner ear receives contributions from neural crest cells in the form of melanocytes and Schwann cells.

Development of Inner Ear

All of the inner ear derivatives arise from ectoderm. Late in the 3rd week, a thickening of the surface ectoderm called the **otic placode** or **otic disc** appears next to the hindbrain (Fig. 17-2A, B). During the 4th week, the otic placode gradually invaginates to first form an **otic pit** and then a closed, hollow **otic vesicle** or **otocyst** (Fig. 17-2C-G; see Fig. 17-2B), which is connected briefly to the surface by a stem of ectoderm. Young neurons delaminate from the ventral otocyst to form the **statoacoustic (vestibulocochlear) ganglion** (see Fig. 17-2C).

By day 28, the dorsomedial region of the otic vesicle begins to elongate, forming an **endolymphatic appendage** (Fig. 17-3A; see Fig. 17-2G). Shortly thereafter, the rest of the otic vesicle differentiates into an expanded **pars superior** and an initially tapered **pars inferior** (Fig. 17-3B, C). The endolymphatic appendage elongates over the following week, and its distal portion expands to form an **endolymphatic sac** that is connected to the pars superior by a slender **endolymphatic duct** (see Fig. 17-3C).

During the 5th week, the ventral tip of the pars inferior begins to elongate and coil, forming the **cochlear duct**, which is the primordium of the cochlea (Fig. 17-3D, E). The pars inferior also gives rise to the saccule, which is connected to the cochlea by a narrow channel called the **ductus reuniens**. During the 7th week, cells of the cochlear duct differentiate to form the **spiral organ of Corti** (the structure that contains the sensory **hair cells** responsible for transducing sound vibrations into electrical impulses). The sensory hair cells in the different regions of the cochlea are activated by different sound wave frequencies.

Beginning late in the 5th week, flattened bilayered discs grow dorsally and laterally from the pars superior (see Fig. 17-3D). In the center of the discs, the epithelial walls meet and in these regions the epithelium regresses leaving the anlagen of the semicircular canals. The semicircular canals are oriented perpendicularly to each other and consist of **anterior, posterior**, and **lateral semicircular canals** (see Fig. 17-3D, E). A small expansion called the **ampulla**, which houses the sensory cells, forms at one end of each semicircular canal (see Fig. 17-3E).

The morphogenesis of the mouse inner ear closely resembles that of the human. Figure 17-4 shows the morphogenesis of the mouse inner ear over a 7-day period of embryogenesis, using an injection procedure in which the cavity of the otocyst is filled with paint and the head of the embryo is cleared. This approach provides a more three-dimensional view of the developing inner ear. Because the embryo can be turned and photographed in various orientations, the relationships of the three semicircular canals can be readily understood (Fig. 17-5A; see Fig. 17-4).

IN THE RESEARCH LAB

INDUCTION AND PATTERNING OF RUDIMENTS OF INNER EAR

The otic placode is induced by *Fgf* signaling from the mesoderm together with signals such as *Wnts* and *Fgfs* from the hindbrain. Overexpression of *Fgfs* is sufficient to induce formation of ectopic otic vesicles in chick embryos, whereas in the double *Fgf3/Fgf10* mouse mutant, the otic placode does not form. *Fgf8* (expressed by the endoderm in chick and by all three germ layers in mouse) induces the expression of *Fgfs* in the mesoderm.

Once the placode has formed it invaginates to form the otic vesicle or otocyst, which now must become specified into its different regions (i.e., vestibular structures and the cochlea). The ventral otic vesicle forms the cochlea and saccule, whereas the dorsal otic vesicle forms the remainder of the vestibular structures. This is achieved by the differential expression of homeobox genes. *Pax2* is expressed in the ventral otocyst and is essential for development of the cochlea (Figs. 17-6, 17-7). In contrast,

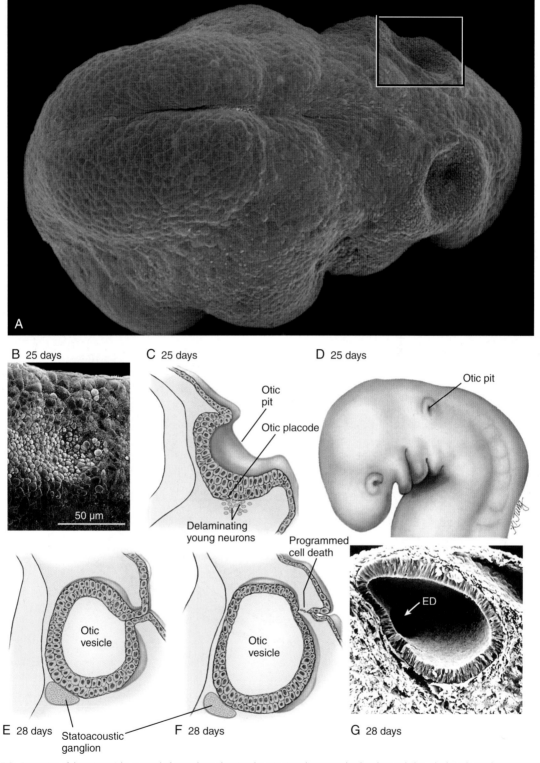

Figure 17-2. Formation of the otic vesicle. *A*, Head of an embryo showing the otic pits adjacent to the rhombencephalon. The box shows the orientation of the image in part *B*. *B*, The otic placode appears in the surface ectoderm late in the 3rd week. *C, D*, By day 25, the placode invaginates to form the otic pit. *E-G*, By the end of the 4th week, continued invagination forms the otic vesicle, which quickly detaches from the surface ectoderm. ED, endolymphatic duct.

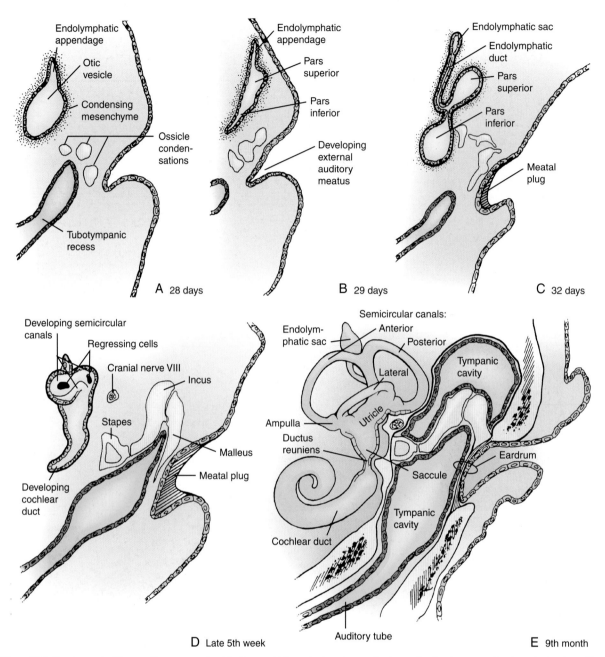

Figure 17-3. Development of the ear. The components of the inner, middle, and external ears arise in coordination from several embryonic structures. The otic vesicle gives rise to the membranous labyrinth of the inner ear and to the ganglia of cranial nerve VIII. *A, B,* The superior end of the otic vesicle forms an endolymphatic appendage, and the body of the vesicle then differentiates into pars superior and pars inferior regions. *C-E,* The endolymphatic appendage elongates to form the endolymphatic sac and duct; the pars superior gives rise to the three semicircular canals and the utricle; and the pars inferior gives rise to the saccule and also coils to form the cochlear duct. Simultaneously, the three auditory ossicles arise from mesenchymal condensations formed by the first and second pharyngeal arches, the first pharyngeal pouch enlarges to form the tubotympanic recess (the future middle ear cavity), and the first pharyngeal cleft (the future external auditory meatus) becomes filled with a transient meatal plug of ectodermal cells. Finally, in the 9th month, the tubotympanic cavity expands to enclose the auditory ossicles, forming the functional middle ear cavity. The definitive eardrum is derived from the first pharyngeal membrane and is thus composed of pharyngeal cleft ectoderm, and pharyngeal pouch endoderm, plus neural crest cells (ectoderm) that infiltrate the space between the cleft ectoderm and pouch endoderm, therefore, the definitive ear drum is a three-layer structure derived from two germ layers.

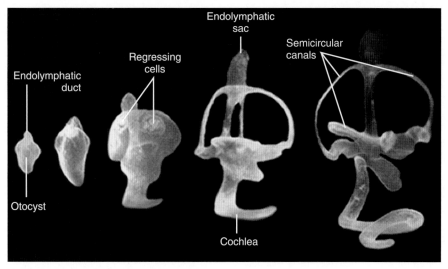

Figure 17-4. Morphogenesis of the mouse inner ear over a 7-day period in embryogenesis, revealed by filling the cavity of the developing otocyst with opaque paint.

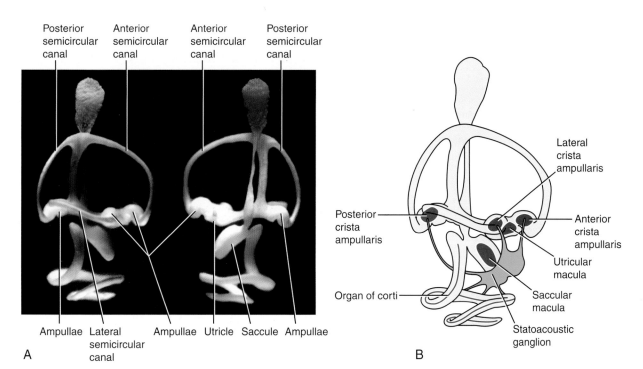

Figure 17-5. Morphology of the inner ear. *A*, Paint-filled otocysts shown in lateral (left) and medial (right) views. *B*, Diagram illustrating the six prosensory regions in the developing inner ear.

17

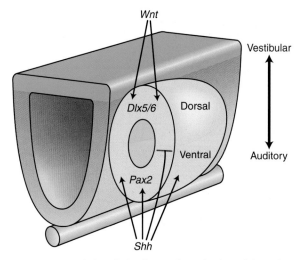

Figure 17-6. Signals from the hindbrain and notochord specify homeobox gene expression in the dorsal and ventral regions of the otic vesicle. The dorsal part of the hindbrain secretes *Wnt* and the notochord and floor plate secrete *Shh*.

the homeobox genes *Hmx2/3*, *Dlx5/6*, and *Nkx5-1* are expressed in the dorsal otocyst and are required for the development of the vestibular apparatus (see Figs. 17-6, 17-7). Loss of function of some homeobox genes (e.g., *Otx1* and *Hmx3*) leads to more limited defects, such as the loss of the lateral canal (see Fig. 17-7).

Experimental manipulations in which the otocyst (or adjacent structures) has been rotated at different stages of development have shown that the cranial-caudal axis is specified first, followed by the medial-lateral axis. These analyses, together with analysis of knockout mice, have also shown that signals from the hindbrain and notochord control homeobox gene expression. *Shh* signaling from the notochord and floor plate controls *Pax2* expression, whereas *Wnt* signaling from the dorsal neural tube controls the expression of *Dlx5* and *6* (see Fig. 17-6). In the absence of *Shh*, the cochlea duct and saccule do not form. Again emphasizing the importance of hindbrain signals, double knockout of *Hoxa1* and *Hoxb1*, which results in the loss of rhombomere 5, affects the development and morphogenesis of the entire inner ear.

Inner ear hair cells, specialized mechanotransducers, arise in six prosensory regions within the developing otic vesicle (see Fig. 17-5B). In the cochlea the prosensory region forms the **organ of Corti**. In the saccule and utricle, it forms the **maculae**, and in the semicircular canals it forms the **cristae**. The maculae are responsible for detecting gravity and linear acceleration. The cristae detect angular acceleration. All of these sensory regions are innervated by the **statoacoustic ganglion** of the **vestibulocochlear nerve** (cranial nerve VIII). The vestibular structures are innervated by the **vestibular branch**, whereas the cochlea is innervated by the **spiral (cochlear) branch**. The latter synapse in the auditory nuclei,

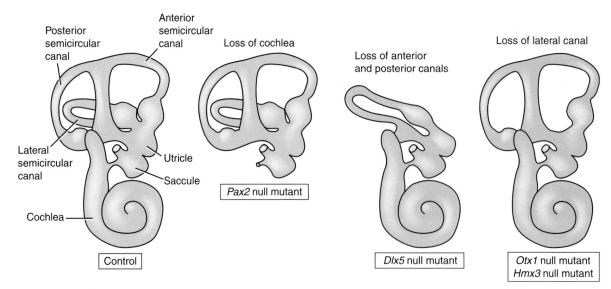

Figure 17-7. Development of the vestibular structures and cochlea is differentially controlled by homeobox genes, as revealed in knockout mice.

which develop in the alar plate of the brainstem (development of the brainstem is discussed in Ch. 9).

There are two types of hair cells in the organ of Corti, the **outer hair cells** and **inner hair cells**, which differ in their physiologic and morphologic properties. There is one row of inner hair cells and three rows of outer hair cells (Fig. 17-8). About 95% of the sensory nerve fibers to the cochlea innervate the inner hair cells, which are, therefore, the primary transducers of signals to the brain. In contrast, outer hair cells receive about 80% of the motor input to the cochlea. The outer hair cells change their length exceptionally rapidly in response to sound (a process known as **electromotility**), which amplifies the sound waves, increasing sensitivity. This ability has been attributed to a unique membrane protein called *Prestin*, and, in fact, nonsyndromic deafness in humans can result from mutations in the gene encoding *PRESTIN*.

In the organ of Corti, the **stereocilia** (specialized microvilli) of the hair cells project into an acellular gelatinous matrix called the **tectorial membrane**, which is necessary for hair cell function (see Fig. 17-8C). The tectorial membrane consists of *Collagens* (*Types II, V, IX,* and *XI*) and ear-specific noncollagenous proteins such as *α-* and *β-Tectorin*. In both the maculae and cristae, the hair cells are also overlain (i.e., capped) by an acellular matrix; this is called the **otoconial membranes** in the maculae and the **cupula** in the cristae. Hair cells are surrounded by endolymph. In the cochlea, the endolymph has a high K^+ concentration that is necessary for hair cell function. The vestibular sensory organs are functional at birth, but the organ of Corti does not become fully differentiated and functional until after birth.

Beginning in the 9th week of development, the mesenchyme surrounding the membranous labyrinth chondrifies to form a cartilage called the **otic capsule**. Transplantation experiments have shown that the otic vesicle induces chondrogenesis in this mesenchyme and that the shape of the vesicle controls the morphogenesis of the capsule. During the 3rd to 5th months, the layer of cartilage immediately surrounding the membranous labyrinth undergoes vacuolization to form a cavity called the **perilymphatic space**. The perilymphatic space is filled with a fluid called **perilymph**, which communicates with the cerebrospinal fluid. Around the cochlea these spaces are known as the **scala vestibuli** and **scala tympani** (see Fig. 17-8B). The otic capsule ossifies between 16 and 23 weeks to form the **petrous portion** of the **temporal bone** (Fig. 17-9; see Fig. 16-3). Continued ossification later produces the **mastoid portion** of the temporal bone. The bony enclosure that houses the membranous labyrinth and the perilymph is called the **bony labyrinth.**

IN THE RESEARCH LAB

FORMATION OF SENSORY CELLS

The prosensory regions containing the presumptive hair cells express a number of factors including *Bmp4, Sox2, Islet1, Ids1, 2,* and *3,* and *Fgf10.* The transcription factor *Sox2* is essential for development of the prosensory region, whereas the *Ids* inhibit hair cell differentiation by binding to basic helix-loop-helix (bHLH) proteins (bHLH proteins are discussed in Ch. 5 in the context of *Notch* signaling, Ch. 8 in the context of muscle differentiation, Ch. 10 in the context of neuronal differentiation, and Ch. 14 in the context of intestine development) and preventing them from binding to DNA. The prosensory region then gives rise to hair cells and the supporting cells that surround them. The proneural gene *Atoh* (also known as *Math1*), a bHLH transcription factor, is essential for hair cell development, whereas, *Hes1* and *5* (the hairy and enhancer of split transcription factors), are required for the development of supporting cells. Consequently, in *Atoh* mutant mice, hair cells do not develop, whereas in *Hes1* or *5* mouse mutants, there are excess hair cells. In addition, overexpression of *Atoh1* can induce the formation of ectopic hair cells. Specification of a hair cell versus a supporting cell from a common precursor is achieved by **lateral inhibition**. The presumptive hair cell expresses the *Notch* ligands *Jagged 2* and *Delta 1,* which activate *Notch* signaling in the adjacent cells (the presumptive supporting cells). *Notch* activation results in the release of the intracellular *Notch* fragment, N^{ICD}, which enters the nucleus to induce the expression of *Hes1* and *5* (Fig. 17-10). The *Hes* proteins inhibit *Atoh* activity, thereby preventing hair cell differentiation and allowing cells to develop as supporting cells. Thus, following loss of *Notch* signaling (e.g., as a result of loss of the *Notch* receptor or the ligands that activate the receptor) there are excess hair cells. This is strikingly illustrated in the ***mind bomb*** zebrafish mutant, which has defective *Notch* signaling. In this mutant, all prosensory cells differentiate as hair cells and there is a total absence of supporting cells.

Specialized microvilli called **stereocilia** develop on each hair cell. Stereocilia consist of parallel dense bundles of actin filaments and are the mechanosensors of the hair cell. There are between 50 to 200 interconnected stereocilia on each hair cell. They are arranged in a "staircase" pattern at one edge of the cell, with stereocilia in adjacent rows of the "staircase" being interconnected by fibrous **tip links**

17

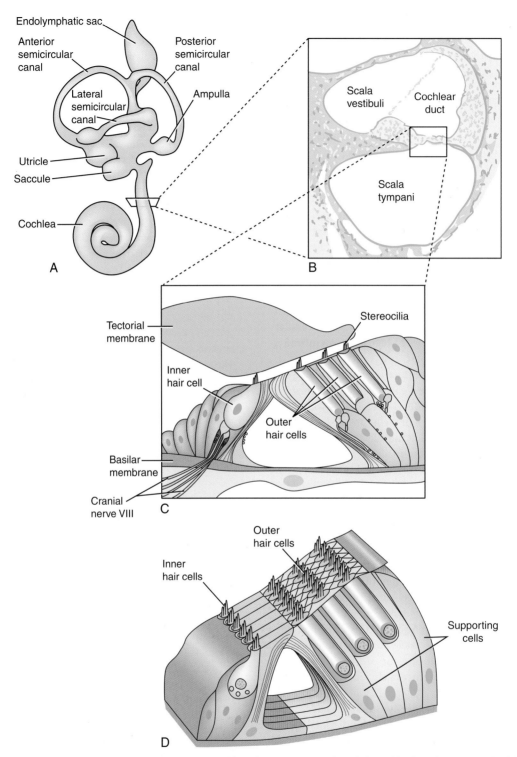

Figure 17-8. Development of the organ of Corti. *A,* The membranous labyrinth. *B,* Cross section through the cochlea (boxed in *A*). *C,* Details of the organ of Corti (boxed in *B*). *D,* The tectorial membrane has been removed to show a more three-dimensional view of the organ of Corti.

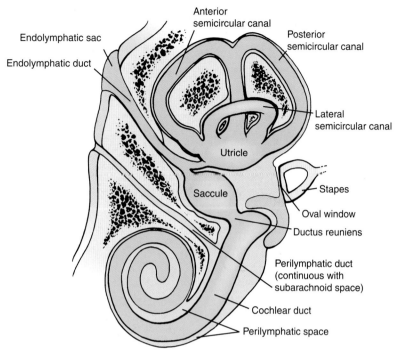

Figure 17-9. The definitive membranous labyrinth is suspended in the fluid-filled perilymphatic space within the bony labyrinth of the petrous portion of the temporal bone. The perilymphatic space is connected to the subarachnoid space by the perilymphatic duct. The membranous labyrinth itself is filled with endolymph.

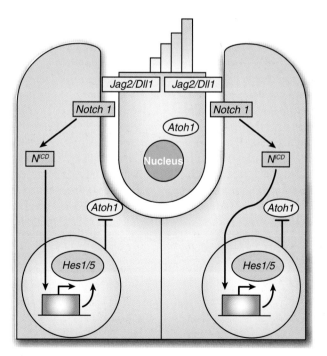

Figure 17-10. Specification of hair cells (top center) and supporting cells (bottom sides) is determined by lateral inhibition involving *Notch* signaling.

17

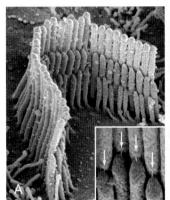
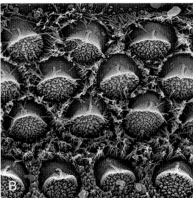
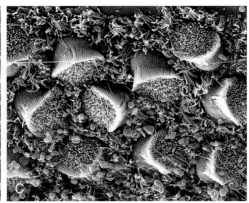

Figure 17-11. Hair cells of the inner ear. *A,* The "staircase" structure of the stereocilia on the inner ear hair cells. Inset shows the tip links (arrows) that interconnect stereocilia in adjacent rows of the "staircase." *B, C,* The orientation of the hair cells is determined by the planar polarity pathway as shown by the randomization of hair cells in mice mutant for the *Celsr1* gene (*C*), as compared to wild-type mice (*B*).

(Fig. 17-11*A*). In the cochlea, the stereocilia on the different hair cells are all orientated in the same direction. The ordered and repetitive pattern of stereocilia formation is essential for hearing and is achieved by signaling via the **planar cell polarity (PCP) pathway**. As discussed in Chapter 4, in Drosophila the PCP pathway is mediated by *Frizzled* receptors and determines the aligned orientation of the sensory bristles in the thorax, hairs in the wings, and ommatidia in the developing eye. Such orientation of structures is also seen in vertebrates—for example, to ensure that all cilia in the respiratory tract or in the oviduct beat in the same orientation. However, the most striking and intricate example in vertebrates is the precisely controlled orientation of the inner ear hair cell stereocilia. Many components of the Drosophila PCP pathway have been conserved in vertebrates. Therefore, the stereocilia are misorientated when components of the PCP pathway, such as the transmembrane proteins *Vangl2* (*Van gogh-like 2)* or *Flamingo* (*Celsr1*), are mutated in mice (Fig. 17-11*B, C*). Likewise, double gene inactivation of the *Frizzled 3* and *6* receptors results in defects in hair cell polarity.

IN THE CLINIC

Total or partial **hearing loss** occurs in more than 1 in 1000 live births and places a significant burden on health care and special education programs. The prevalence of individuals who have hearing loss or who are **deaf** rises to 1 in 500 by adulthood. **Conductive hearing loss** is the result of malformations in the external and/or middle ear, whereas **sensorineural hearing loss** can arise from defects in the inner ear, **vestibulocochlear nerve** (cranial nerve VIII), or the auditory regions of the brain. About half of all hearing loss has genetic causes, with the other half attributed to environmental factors. The latter include in utero viral infections (e.g., **cytomegalovirus** and **rubella**) and neonatal exposure to **aminoglycoside antibiotics** (e.g., **gentamycin** and **tobramycin**).

Hearing loss and deafness due to genetic causes can be **nonsyndromic**, that is, occurring as an isolated defect, or **syndromic**, that is, occurring in conjunction with other anomalies. To date more than 150 chromosomal loci have been linked to nonsyndromic hearing loss, and gene mutations have been identified in more than 50 of them. Although syndromic hearing loss is less common (constituting about 10% to 15% of all cases), more than 300 genetic syndromes have been described in which hearing loss occurs as a component finding. Whether caused by inherited or environmental factors, hearing loss may be present at birth or soon afterward (**congenital** or **prelingual** hearing loss, such as in **Usher syndrome type I**), or it may be associated with age-dependent or progressive loss of hearing (**postlingual**, as in the case of mutations in the transcription factors *POU4F3* and *EYA4*). Prelingual hearing loss is associated with greater disturbances in the development of communication. In addition, hearing loss occurs naturally with aging, a condition called **presbycusis**.

MALFORMATIONS OF INNER EAR: SENSORINEURAL HEARING LOSS

Sensorineural hearing loss and balance dysfunction can result from various structural malformations or the improper functioning of inner ear structures, including the cochlea and vestibular system. These **vestibulocochlear dysplasias** range from complete absence of the membranous labyrinth **(labyrinthine aplasia)** to partial absence or underdevelopment of specific inner ear structures such as the cochlea **(cochlear hypoplasia)**. In addition to relatively gross malformations of inner ear components, hearing loss can also result from more subtle dysplasias that affect only a single cell type (e.g., disruption of stereocilia organization in individuals with mutations in *Cadherin 23*, also known as *Otocadherin*). Examples of a range of inner ear defects are discussed below.

An example of a syndrome characterized by vestibulocochlear dysplasias is **CHARGE syndrome** (coloboma of the eye, heart defects, atresia of the choanae, retarded growth and development, genital and urinary anomalies, and ear anomalies and hearing loss), often caused by mutations in *CHD7* (discussed in Ch. 12). Inner ear defects commonly range from labyrinthine aplasia (sometimes called **Michel aplasia**) to reduction in the number of cochlear turns (less than 2.5 turns) and/or semicircular canal defects (collectively often referred to as **Mondini dysplasia**). Hearing loss in CHARGE syndrome can also result from defects in development of the middle ear, and external ear abnormalities are a cardinal feature of the syndrome.

An inner ear dysplasia that enlarges the bony canal that transmits the endolymphatic duct (i.e., the vestibular aqueduct; Figure 17-12) is a common cause of sensorineural hearing loss and vestibular anomalies. **Large vestibular aqueduct** (LVA; also called enlarged vestibular aqueduct or EVA) can be diagnosed radiographically (i.e., thin-cut CT) and is associated with **Pendred syndrome**. The responsible gene encodes ***PENDRIN***, a chloride-iodide transporter protein.

Hair cells play an essential role in both hearing and balance. Many genes affect the development and function of hair cells and when mutated, result in hearing loss and vestibular dysfunction. These include genes that encode **stereocilia** cytoskeletal components (e.g., *ACTIN, DIAPHANOUS 1, ESPIN, HARMONIN, SANS, WHIRLIN*), intracellular motors that control actin assembly (e.g., *MYO6, MYO7a, MYO15A*), and cell adhesion components (e.g., *CADHERIN 23, PROTOCADHERIN 15*) (Fig. 17-13). Alternatively, the gene may be necessary for hair cell survival (e.g., *POU3F4*).

The sensitivity of stereocilia to gene mutations is illustrated by **Usher syndrome type 1**, an autosomal recessive disorder characterized by **sensorineural hearing loss** and **retinitis pigmentosa**. This syndrome can be caused by mutations in one of several of the genes listed in the preceding paragraph (i.e., *MYO7A, HARMONIN, CADHERIN 23, SANS, PROTOCADHERIN 15*). Analysis of the relevant mouse mutants, which are also all characterized by deafness, has shown that the stereocilia are disorganized and do not have the normal "staircase" pattern. Auditory hair cell function also requires contact of the stereocilia with the overlying **tectorial membrane**. Mutation in *α-TECTORIN*, a key constituent of this membrane (see Fig. 17-13), results in an autosomal dominant nonsyndromic hearing disorder, and analysis of *α-Tectorin* mutant mice has shown that the tectorial membrane is not attached to the sensory hair cells.

Signaling through the **ion channels** in hair cells and the maintenance of hair cell integrity requires high K^+ levels in the endolymphatic fluid. This is achieved by recycling the K^+ that enters the activated hair cells via gap junctions to the **stria vascularis**. From here, K^+ is transported back into the lymph by the channel proteins *KCNQ1* and *KCNE1* (see Fig. 17-13). Defects in K^+ recycling can result in hearing loss. For example, mutations in several **connexin proteins** (*CX26, CX30, CX31*), which are components of **gap junctions**, have been identified in many patients with deafness. In fact, mutations in the gene encoding *CX26*, which is expressed in the nonsensory epithelium between the organ of Corti and the stria vascularis (see Fig. 17-13), are responsible for between 20% to 30% of cases of prelingual nonsyndromic deafness, making it the most common known cause of hereditary congenital deafness. Mutation in *KCNQ1* can cause **Jervell and Lange-Nielsen syndrome**, characterized by prelingual sensorineural hearing loss and cardiac arrhythmia (**long QT syndrome**; also discussed in Ch. 12); the latter can result in sudden death.

Finally, a number of deafness syndromes are the result of mutations affecting **mitochondrial** function and can be caused by mutations in mitochondrial DNA (which, because we inherit all our mitochondria from our mothers, are **maternally inherited**). One such condition is caused by mutations in the *MTRNR1* gene that encodes the mitochondrial 12S ribosomal RNA and causes late-onset sensorineural hearing loss. However, hearing loss in individuals carrying *MTRNR1* mutations may be precipitated suddenly by treatment with **aminoglycoside antibiotics** because of the increased sensitivity the mutation confers to the **ototoxic** effects of these drugs.

17

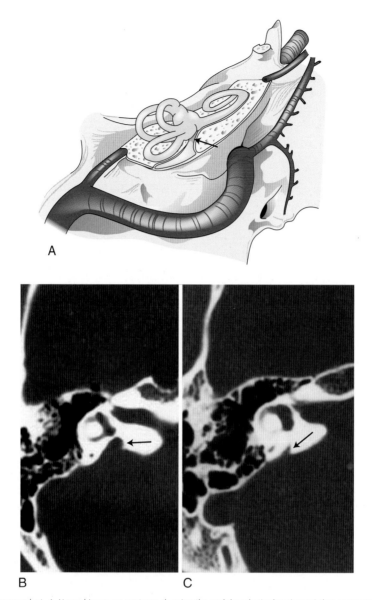

Figure 17-12. Large vestibular aqueduct. *A*, Normal inner ear anatomy showing the endolymphatic duct (arrow) that connects the endolymphatic sac to the vestibule, passing through the bony vestibular aqueduct. *B*, Large vestibular aqueduct (arrow) shown by axial CT of the temporal bone. *C*, Normal caliber of the bony aqueduct (arrow) is less than 1.5 mm. Bone appears as a white signal.

Development of Middle Ear

As discussed in chapter 16, the first pharyngeal pouch elongates to form the **tubotympanic recess**, which subsequently differentiates to form the expanded **tympanic cavity** of the middle ear and the slender **auditory (eustachian) tube**, which connects the tympanic cavity to the pharynx. Cartilaginous precursors of the three **auditory ossicles** condense in the mesenchyme near the tympanic cavity (see Fig. 17-3). The **malleus** and **incus** arise from the first pharyngeal arch, whereas the **stapes** arises from the second pharyngeal arch. The developing ossicles remain embedded in the mesenchyme adjacent to the tympanic cavity until

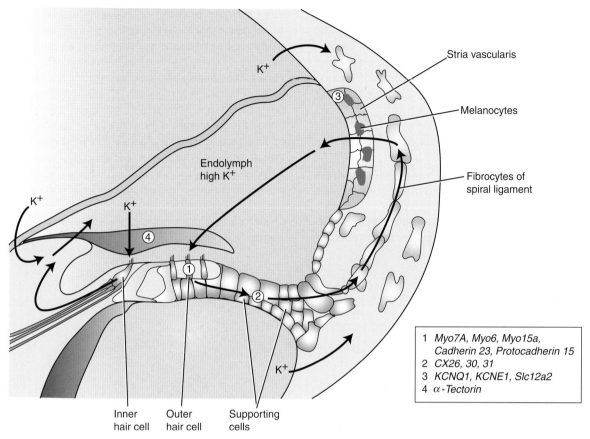

Stria vascularis

Melanocytes

Fibrocytes of
spiral ligament

Endolymph
high K+

K+

K+

K+

K+

K+

1	*Myo7A, Myo6, Myo15a, Cadherin 23, Protocadherin 15*
2	*CX26, 30, 31*
3	*KCNQ1, KCNE1, Slc12a2*
4	*α-Tectorin*

Inner
hair cell

Outer
hair cell

Supporting
cells

Figure 17-13. Hearing loss can result from mutations of the many different genes expressed in the inner ear.

the 8th month of gestation. During the 9th month of development, the mesenchyme surrounding the auditory ossicles is removed, and the tympanic cavity expands to enclose them (see Fig. 17-3E). Therefore, the endoderm that lines the tympanic cavity jackets the ossicles and also forms transient endodermal mesenteries that suspend the ossicles in the cavity until their definitive supporting ligaments develop.

There are two muscles associated with the ossicles—the **tensor tympani** and the **stapedius**—both of which form in the 9th week from first- and second-pharyngeal arch mesoderm, respectively. Reflecting their developmental origin, the tensor tympani muscle is innervated by the **trigeminal nerve** (cranial nerve V), whereas the **stapedius** muscle is innervated by the **facial nerve** (cranial nerve VII).

Meanwhile, the pharyngeal membrane separating the tympanic cavity from the external auditory meatus (derived from the first pharyngeal cleft) develops into the **tympanic membrane** or **eardrum**

(see Fig. 17-3E). The tympanic membrane is composed of an outer lining of ectoderm, an inner lining of endoderm, and an intervening layer called the **fibrous stratum.** The intervening layer is derived from infiltrating **neural crest cells.**

During the 9th month, the suspended auditory ossicles assume their functional relationships with each other and with the associated structures of the external, middle, and inner ears. The ventral end of the malleus becomes attached to the eardrum, and the foot plate of the stapes becomes attached to the **oval window,** a small fenestra in the bony labyrinth (see Figs. 17-3E, 17-9). Sonic vibrations are transmitted from the eardrum to the oval window by the articulated chain of ossicles and from the oval window to the cochlea by the fluid filling the perilymphatic space. The cochlea transduces these vibrations into neural impulses. The ossicles are not totally free to vibrate/move in response to sound until 2 months after birth.

17

During the 9th month, the tympanic cavity expands into the mastoid part of the temporal bone to form the **mastoid antrum**. The **mastoid air cells** in the mastoid portion of the temporal bone do not form until about 2 years of age, when the action of the sternocleidomastoid muscle on the mastoid part of the temporal bone induces the mastoid process to form.

Development of External Ear

The external ear consists of the funnel-shaped **external auditory meatus** and the **auricle (pinna)**. The precursor of the external auditory meatus develops by an invagination of the first pharyngeal cleft during the 6th week. However, the ectodermal lining of the deep portion of this tube later proliferates, producing a solid core of tissue called the **meatal plug** that completely fills the medial end of the external auditory meatus by week 26 (see Fig. 17-3C, D). Canalization of this plug begins almost immediately and produces the medial twothirds of the definitive meatus (see Fig. 17-3E). The meatus does not achieve its final length until the age of 9 or 10 years. The **tympanic membrane** is derived from the pharyngeal membrane that separates the first pharyngeal pouch and cleft. It develops as a three-layered structure, consisting of an external layer of ectoderm, a middle layer of ectoderm derived from infiltrating neural crest cells, and an inner layer of endoderm. The definitive tympanic membrane is formed during the recanalization of the external auditory meatus.

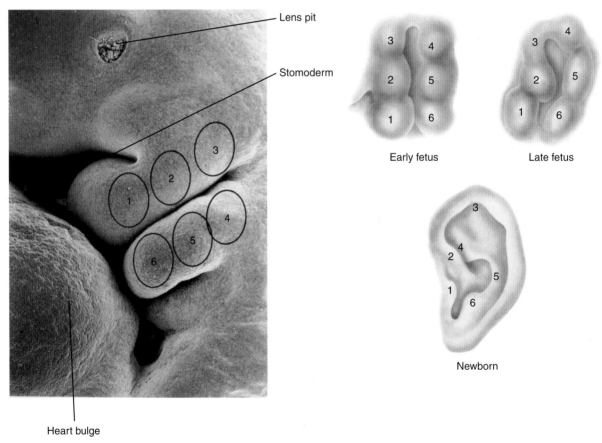

Figure 17-14. Differentiation of the auricle. The auricle develops from six auricular hillocks, which arise on the apposed surfaces of the first and second pharyngeal arches.

The auricle develops from six **auricular hillocks** that arise during the 5th week on the first and second pharyngeal arches (Fig. 17-14). From ventral to dorsal, the hillocks on the first pharyngeal arch are called the **tragus, helix**, and **cymba concha** (or 1 to 3, respectively), and the hillocks on the second arch are called the **antitragus, antihelix**, and **concha** (or 4 to 6, respectively). These names indicate which hillocks eventually form each part of the pinna. During the 7th week, the auricular hillocks begin to enlarge, differentiate, and fuse to produce the definitive form of the auricle. As the face develops, the auricle is gradually translocated from its original location low on the side of the neck to a more lateral and cranial site.

IN THE CLINIC

As mentioned earlier in the chapter, hearing loss may be sensorineural or conductive. **Conductive hearing loss** is caused by structural abnormalities of the middle or external ear that impede conduction of sound to the inner ear.

Besides potential impact on hearing, malformations of the external and middle ear have important clinical implications. These defects are common as a whole and not only have a significant cosmetic impact on patients, they may also be indicative of a more widespread syndrome.

MALFORMATIONS OF EXTERNAL AND MIDDLE EAR: CONDUCTIVE HEARING LOSS

Defects of the external ear (i.e., the **pinna** or **auricle**) result from abnormal growth and morphogenesis of one or more of the auricular hillocks derived from the first and second pharyngeal arches. Suppressed growth of all the hillocks results in **microtia** (small auricle; Fig. 17-15A, B) or **anotia** (absence of the auricle; Fig. 17-15C). Overgrowth of the hillocks results in **macrotia** (large auricle). Accessory hillocks may also form, producing ectopic **preauricular tags** (Fig. 17-15D), which may or may not be accompanied by **preauricular pits**. Defects of the external auditory meatus include **atresia** and **stenosis**.

Significant malformations of the external ear should raise suspicions about potential abnormalities elsewhere in the

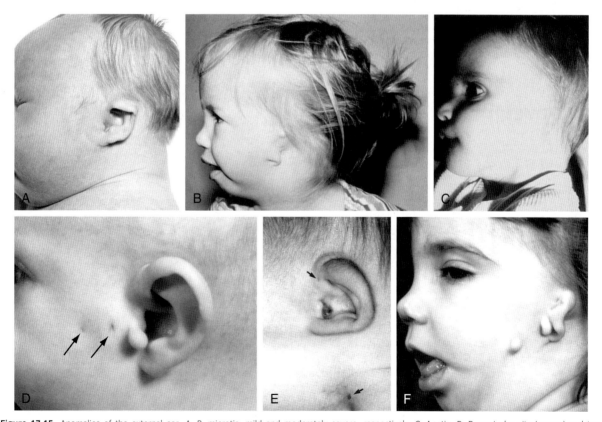

Figure 17-15. Anomalies of the external ear. *A, B,* microtia, mild and moderately severe, respectively. *C,* Anotia. *D,* Preauricular pits (arrows) and tag. *E,* External ear of a boy with BOR syndrome. The upper arrow indicates a preauricular pit and the lower arrow indicates a cervical fistula. *F,* Girl with hemifacial microsomia showing preauricular tags.

17

body. From 20% to 40% of children with microtia/anotia will have additional defects that could suggest a syndrome. For example, microtia occurs in several single gene disorders, including **branchio-oto-renal** (BOR; Fig. 17-15E; *also discussed in Ch. 15*), **CHARGE** (also discussed in Chs. 4 and 12), and **Treacher Collins syndromes**, as well as in **trisomy 21** (also discussed in Ch. 1, 5, 9, 12, 14, and 18) and **18** (also discussed in Chs. 8 and 9). Microtia can also occur following prenatal exposure to **alcohol** or **isotretinoin**. Microtia and preauricular tags (and, more rarely, pits) occur in **oculoauriculovertebral spectrum** (OAVS) (Fig. 17-15F; also discussed in Ch. 16). Macrotia can occur in **Fragile X syndrome**, the most common cause of mental retardation in males. This syndrome is caused by trinucleotide repeat expansions in the *FMR1 (FRAGILE X MENTAL RETARDATION 1)* gene. Atresia or stenosis of the external auditory meatus can suggest deletion of the long arm of chromosome 18.

Defects of the middle ear result from abnormal formation or ossification of the middle ear ossicles, the malleus, incus, and stapes, derived from neural crest cells populating the first and second pharyngeal arches. Suppressed growth of these neural crest cells results in **ossicle hypoplasia** or **aplasia** and **fixation**. These defects occur in association with skeletal dysplasias such as **achondroplasia** (*FGFR3* mutation; discussed in Chs. 5 and 8) and **osteogenesis imperfecta** (multiple *COLLAGEN* mutations), or in various syndromes such as **BOR**, **Treacher Collins**, and **OAVS** (see Fig. 17-15).

Eye Development

The eye develops from several embryonic tissue layers. The ectoderm gives rise to the lens and part of the cornea. The neuroectoderm forms the pigmented epithelium and the neural retina. Neural crest cells contribute to the stroma of the cornea, the ciliary and iris muscles, and the vascular choroid layer together with the fibrous sclera. The mesoderm contributes to the cornea and forms the angioblasts of the choroid layer.

Formation of Optic Cup

The first morphologic evidence of the eye is the formation of the **optic sulcus** in the future diencephalic region of the prosencephalic neural groove (forebrain) at 22 days (Fig. 17-16A-D). By the time that the cranial neuropore closes on day 24, the **optic stalk** is evident (Fig. 17-16E, F) and the optic primordia have developed into lateral evaginations of the neural tube called **optic vesicles** (see Fig. 17-16E, F). The walls of the

optic vesicles are continuous with the neuroepithelium of the future brain, and the cavity or **ventricle** within the optic vesicle is continuous with the neural canal. As the optic vesicle forms, it becomes surrounded by a layer of mesenchyme derived from neural crest cells and head mesoderm. Fate mapping studies in birds and mice have revealed that this mesenchyme gives rise to many ocular tissues, such as the sclera, ocular muscles, connective tissue, and cartilage together with vascular and endothelial cells. The extraocular mesenchyme begins to form on day 24 and completely envelops the optic vesicle by day 26. By day 24 the distal part of the optic vesicle, the **optic disc**, contacts the overlying surface ectoderm. At about this time, the optic cup becomes patterned along its planar axes (see below and in the "In the Research Lab" of Ch. 9).

On about day 32, the optic disc invaginates, converting the optic vesicle into a goblet-shaped **optic cup** (Fig. 17-16G, H). Simultaneously, the ventral part of the optic stalk invaginates to form the **choroidal fissure.** Blood vessels later enter the optic cup through the choroidal fissure (Fig. 17-17), following which the two lips of the fissure fuse together (see Fig. 17-17C). Upon closing of the fissure, the primitive ciliary epithelium secretes aqueous fluid, establishing intraocular pressure.

IN THE RESEARCH LAB

FORMATION OF EYE FIELD

Eye development starts with the formation of a single eye field in the cranial neural plate during gastrulation and neurulation. At the neural plate stage, the morphogen *Sonic hedgehog (Shh)* is secreted by the underlying prechordal plate and is essential for separating the initially single eye field into two individual **optic primordia**; failure of *Shh* signaling results in the persistence of a single eye field and the formation of both **holoprosencephaly** (discussed in Ch. 16) and **cyclopia** (single, midline eye). Furthermore, several transcription factors, which regulate normal eye development, are specifically expressed in the eye field. For example, the homeobox gene *Rx/Rax* is expressed in the eye field in both mice and humans. When deleted in mice, it leads to arrest of eye development at the neural plate stage. This results in **anophthalmia** (absence of the eye) or **microphthalmia** (small eye). Similarly, mutations in the homeobox gene *Sox2* in humans, again a transcription factor expressed in the eye field, result in bilateral anophthalmia. Moreover, ectopic expression of the transcription factor *Pax6*, which is expressed in the developing eyes of model

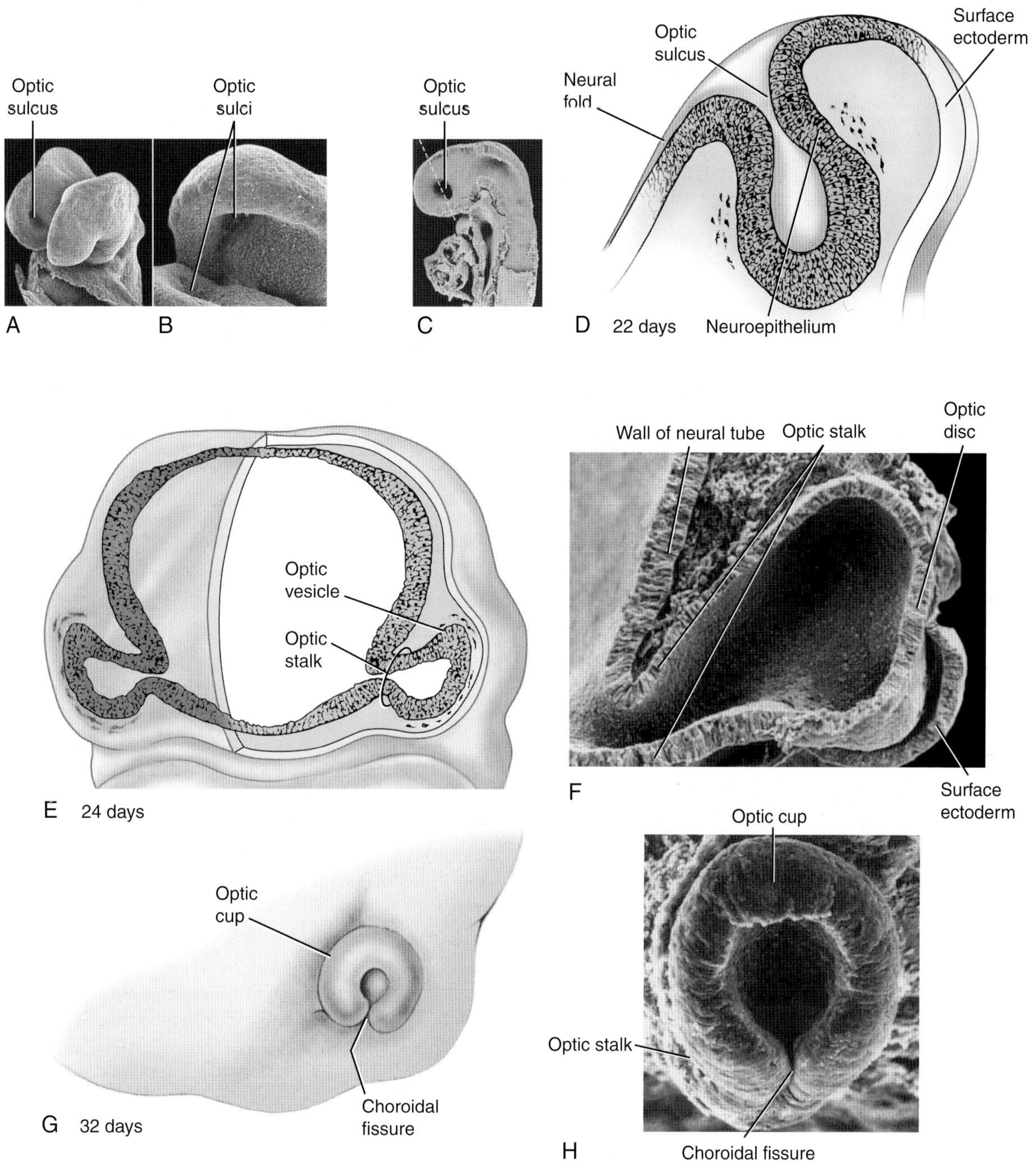

Figure 17-16. Formation of the optic sulcus, vesicle, and cup. *A, B,* Formation of the optic sulcus in the forming forebrain during neurulation. *B* is an enlargement of *A. C, D,* The optic vesicle begins to form as an evagination of the diencephalic neural folds on day 22, before the cranial neuropore has closed. The dashed line indicates the level of the section shown in *D. E, F,* By day 24, the optic vesicles lie adjacent to the surface ectoderm. *G, H,* During the 5th week, the optic vesicle invaginates to become the optic cup, and the choroidal fissure forms on the inferior surface of the optic cup and stalk.

17

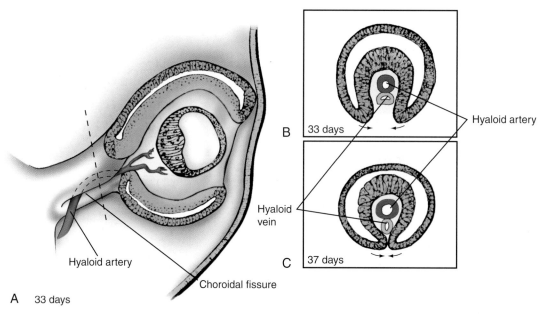

Figure 17-17. Vascularization of the lens and retina. *A*, As the lens vesicle detaches from the surface ectoderm, it becomes vascularized by the hyaloid vessels, which gain access to the lens through the choroidal fissure. *B, C,* During the 7th week, the edges of the choroidal fissure fuse together, enclosing the hyaloid artery and vein in the hyaloid canal. When the lens matures, the vessels serving it degenerate, and the hyaloid artery and vein become the central artery and vein of the retina.

organisms as diverse as Drosophila and mouse, results in the formation of ectopic eyes. These and other findings support the idea that progressive patterning of the neural plate, and subsequently of the eye field, is regulated by a feedback network of eye-field transcription factors. Table 17-1 lists several genes regulating different aspects of eye development in vertebrates.

Formation of Lens

As soon as the optic vesicle contacts the surface ectoderm, the ectoderm apposed to it thickens to form a **lens placode** (Fig. 17-18C). Shortly thereafter, the lens placode invaginates to form a **lens pit** (Fig. 17-18A, B, D, E). By day 33 the placode separates from the surface ectoderm, becoming a hollow **lens vesicle** surrounded by a basal lamina (lens capsule) (Fig. 17-18F). Mesodermally derived mesenchymal cells migrate into the **lentiretinal space** between the lens vesicle and the inner wall of the expanding optic cup and secrete a gelatinous matrix called the **primary vitreous body** (see Fig. 17-18E, F). Beginning on day 37, the cells of the posterior (deep)

wall of the lens vesicle differentiate to form long, anteroposteriorly oriented **primary lens fibers**, which express crystallins (α, β, and γ) necessary for the transparency of the lens (Fig. 17-19). Elongation of these cells transforms the lens vesicle into a rounded **lens body**, obliterating the cavity of the lens vesicle by the 7th week. Anterior lens epithelial cells closest to the cornea remain proliferative throughout life. They migrate peripherally to the lens equator, giving rise to future secondary fetal and adult cortical lens fibers (lens bow). Secondary lens fibers start to be formed from the 6th week.

IN THE RESEARCH LAB

FORMATION AND MORPHOGENESIS OF LENS

Until recently, the optic vesicle was thought to induce the lens placode. More recent experiments have shown that lens formation can occur in the absence of the optic vesicle and that it depends on a complex series of interactions with other tissues that take place long before the optic vesicle is formed. Lens induction starts at gastrulation, when signals from definitive endoderm, adjacent neuroepithelium, and

Table 17-1 Molecules regulating morphogenesis of ocular tissues (selected examples)

Gene	Role
Eye field, Optic vesicle	
Rx	Transcription factor, mutations result in anophthalmia in humans and mice
Pax6	Transcription factor, loss of function results in microphthalmia and anophthalmia in rodents
Otx2	Transcription factor, loss of function results in missing forebrain, microphthalmia, and cyclopia in mouse
Six6	Transcription factor, regulates proliferation of eye field in frog; haploinsufficiency causes anophthalmia in humans
Six3	Transcription factor, mutations are associated with holoprosencephaly in humans; loss of forebrain when mutated in mouse; overexpression results in ectopic eye formation in zebrafish
Retinoic acid signaling	Vitamin and morphogen, deficiency results in microphthalmia in mouse; vitamin A deficiency might cause developmental eye defects such as coloboma in humans
Shh	Secreted protein, mutations can result in holoprosencephaly and cyclopia in humans and other vertebrates
Neural retina	
Pax6	Transcription factor, required for survival and multipotency of retinal progenitor cells in mouse and chick
Chx10	Transcription factor, regulates progenitor cell differentiation; loss of function causes microphthalmia and congenital cataract in humans and ocular retardation in mouse
Sox2	Transcription factor, mutation causes microphthalmia in humans and mouse; functions to maintain neuronal progenitor identity
Notch	Transmembrane protein, regulates multipotency and proliferation of retinal progenitors
Pigmented epithelium	
Otx2	Transcription factor, required for pigmented epithelium specification and differentiation in vertebrates
Mitf	Transcription factor, required for pigmented epithelium specification and differentiation in vertebrates
Rx3	Transcription factor, required for earliest pigmented epithelium specification in zebrafish
Optic stalk	
Pax2	Transcription factor, loss of function results in optic nerve coloboma in mouse and humans
Shh	Secreted protein, required for optic stalk and fissure formation in mouse, chick, and zebrafish
Vax1	Transcription factor, loss of function results in optic nerve coloboma in mouse; required for optic stalk differentiation
HesX1	Transcription factor, mutations in humans can cause septo-optic dysplasia
Lens	
Six3	Transcription factor, sufficient and required for lens formation in mouse
Pax6	Transcription factor, expression in lens ectoderm is required for lens induction in mouse
FoxE3	Transcription factor, mutations cause anterior segment dysgenesis in humans and lens defects in "Dysgenetic lens" mice
Fgf pathway	Secreted protein, required for lens induction and differentiation
Pitx3	Transcription factor, recessive mutation in mouse ("Aphakia") results in absence of lens and microphthalmia
Prox1	Transcription factor, required for lens fiber differentiation in mouse
Anterior segment	
Pitx2	Transcription factor, mutations result in anterior segment defects and glaucoma in humans (Axenfeld-Rieger anomaly)
Pitx3	Transcription factor, mutations result in anterior segment defects in humans (Axenfeld-Rieger anomaly)
Retinoic acid signaling	Vitamin and morphogen, loss of function results in cornea, eyelid, and conjunctiva defects in mouse
Foxc1, Foxc2	Transcription factor, mutations result in anterior segment defects and glaucoma in humans (Axenfeld-Rieger anomaly) and mouse
Cyp1B1	Enzyme, mutations result in Rieger anomaly and congenital glaucoma in humans and abnormal development of iridocorneal angle in mouse
Pax6	Transcription factor, mutations result in aniridia and Peters anomaly in humans, and anterior segment defects in mouse

17

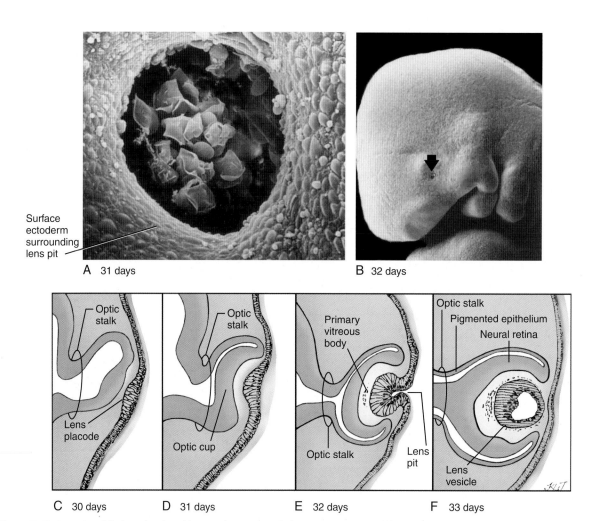

Figure 17-18. Formation of the lens placode and lens vesicle. Contact with the optic cup is necessary for maintenance and development of the lens placode, although other influences are more important in its induction. *A-F,* During the 5th week, the lens placode begins to invaginate to form the lens pit (arrow in *B*). The invaginating lens placode eventually pinches off of the surface ectoderm to form a lens vesicle enclosed in the optic cup (*E, F*).

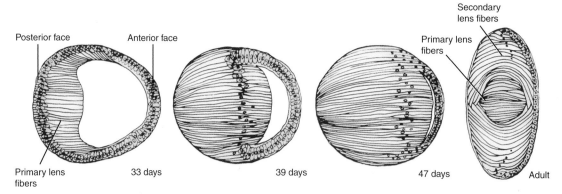

Figure 17-19. Differentiation of the lens. The lens develops rapidly in the 5th to 7th weeks as the cells of its posterior wall elongate and differentiate to form the primary lens fibers. Secondary lens fibers begin to form in the 3rd month.

heart mesoderm initiate the process. Interestingly, head ectoderm adjacent to the normal lens-forming region and competent to form lens is actually inhibited from forming the lens by signals secreted from migrating cranial neural crest cells. Even though the optic cup does not induce the lens placode, several experiments indicate that it does influence the growth, differentiation, and maintenance of the developing lens. If the portion of the optic cup in contact with the ectoderm is removed, the lens eventually degenerates.

Studies using null mutations in mice have demonstrated that several genes are required for induction and maintenance of the lens placode, including *Pax6*, *Bmp4*, and *Bmp7*. Using conditional mutagenesis, *Pax6* has been specifically knocked out in the lens ectoderm, resulting in an absence of all lens structures and in a failure of the optic vesicle to invaginate properly. The latter result shows that signals from the lens are required for the appropriate morphogenesis of the optic vesicle. This has also been demonstrated by experiments in which the lens ectoderm has been removed.

Several different growth factor families and transcription factors regulate differentiation of lens fibers. These include, respectively, *Fgfs*, *Tgfβs*, and *Wnts*, and *Maf* and *Prox-1*. For example, once the lens vesicle has formed, *Fgf* from the retina induces cells in the posterior region of the lens to differentiate. Lower levels of *Fgf* signaling maintain proliferation in the anterior lens epithelium. The homeobox gene *FoxE3* also maintains proliferation, whereas *Prox1*, which is expressed at the equatorial zone, induces cell-cycle exit by switching on the expression of the cell cycle inhibitors $p27^{kip1}$ and $p57^{kip2}$ and the *Crystallin* genes.

Malformations of the anterior segment of the eye can be induced by teratogens in animal models. These malformations include a failure of the lens to undergo separation from the surface ectoderm, resulting in a persistent lens stalk and leading to an arrest of lens development (aphakia). Several genes regulating lens vesicle separation have been identified in mouse (e.g., *FoxE3*, *Pitx3*, and *AP-2α*). Lens defects are also associated with corneal abnormalities, showing that signals from the lens are important for initiating differentiation of the overlying ectoderm and mesenchyme. Conversely, corneal abnormalities can lead to secondary lens defects.

Formation of Neural Retina and Pigmented Epithelium

The two walls of the optic cup give rise to the two layers of the retina: the thick pseudostratified inner wall of the cup develops into the **neural retina**, which contains the light-receptive **rods** and **cones** plus associated neural processes, and the thin outer wall of the cup becomes the cuboidal melanin-containing **pigmented epithelium** (Fig. 17-20; see Fig. 17-18*F*). These two walls are initially separated by a narrow **intraretinal space.** The intraretinal space between the neural retina and pigmented epithelium disappears by the 7th week. However, the two layers of the retina never fuse firmly, and various types of trauma—even a simple blow to the head—can cause **retinal detachment** (that is, the mechanical separation of these two layers).

Melanin first appears in the cells of the developing pigmented epithelium on day 33. Soon afterwards, the basal lamina of the pigmented epithelium, **Bruch's membrane**, develops. Differentiation of the neural retina begins at the end of the 6th week, as the layer of retinal progenitor cells adjacent to the intraretinal space (which is homologous to the proliferative neuroepithelium lining the neural tube; discussed in Chs. 4 and 9) begins to produce waves of cells that migrate inward toward the vitreous body. By the 6th week, the progenitor cells form two cellular embryonic retinal layers: an **outer neuroblastic layer** and an **inner neuroblastic layer.** By the 9th week, two additional membranes develop to cover the two surfaces of the neural retina. An **external limiting membrane** is interposed between the pigmented epithelium and the proliferative zone of the neural retina, and the inner surface of the retina is sealed off by an **internal limiting membrane** (see Fig. 17-20*B*).

The definitive cell layers of the mature neural retina arise from the inner and outer neuroblastic layers (see Fig. 17-20*B*). Six major cell classes of neurons and one glial cell type are produced in an evolutionary conserved order: **ganglion cells, cone photoreceptors**, and **horizontal cells** are born early, **amacrine cells** and **rod photoreceptors** are born next, and **bipolar cells** and **Müller glia** are born last. Reflecting their final location in the inner nuclear layer, the inner neuroblastic layer gives rise to horizontal cells, amacrine cells, bipolar cells, and Müller glia. The rods and cones, which form the outermost layer of the mature neural retina, are derived from the outer neuroblastic layer. The axons of the ganglion cells form the definitive **fiber layer** that lines the inner surface of the retina and courses to the developing optic nerve (see Fig. 17-20*B*, *C*). By the 16th week, the developing neuropil (i.e., the network of neuronal processes within the wall of the neural retina) becomes organized into

17

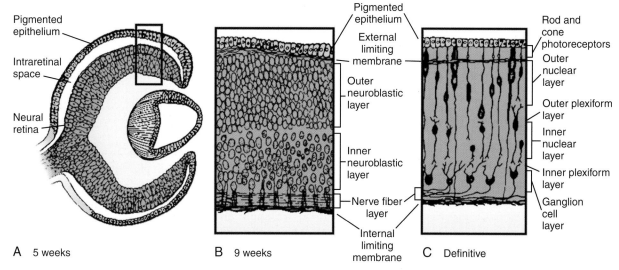

Figure 17-20. Differentiation of the inner layer of the optic cup to form the neural retina. *A*, At 5 weeks, the neural retina consists of a thickened pseudostratified columnar epithelium similar to that of the wall of the neural tube. *B*, By 9 weeks, the neural retina is subdividing into outer and inner neuroblastic layers, a nerve fiber layer, and external and internal limiting membranes. *C*, The definitive layers of the neural retina develop during late fetal life.

inner and outer plexiform layers between the nuclear layers (see Fig. 17-20C). All the cell layers of the definitive retina are apparent by the 8th month.

Cellular differentiation progresses in a wave from inner to outer layers and from the central to peripheral retina. Macular differentiation occurs around the 6th month when cone precursor cells and multiple rows of ganglion cells accumulate in the central macular area. At 7th months, the central macular depression or **primitive fovea** forms. Several months postpartum the **fovea centralis**, the region of the eye with the highest visual acuity, contains only a dense population of cone photoreceptors. This region is also avascular, reducing light scattering within the eye.

There are two types of photoreceptors, rods and cones. Rods are required for vision in low light; cones function in daylight and are necessary for color vision. There are three types of cones, each of which express distinct pigments and responds to one of the three different color wavelengths. S-cones respond to short wavelengths (blue light), M-cones respond to a medium wavelength (green), and L-cones respond to longer wavelengths (red). **Color blindness** is due to the absence of one or more types of cone. **Protanopes** lack L-cones, **deuteranopes** lack M-cones, and **tritanopes** lack S-cones. Retinoid signaling and the *THYROID HORMONE RECEPTOR TRβ2*

are needed for cone differentiation. Consequently, homozygous mutations in *TRβ2* in humans result in S-cone monochromacy (complete color blindness). The genes encoding the photoreceptors are located on the X chromosome and, therefore, color blindness is a frequent occurrence in males (> 2%).

IN THE RESEARCH LAB

PATTERNING OF EYE

As the optic cup forms, it becomes specified into the pigmented epithelium, the neural retina, and the optic stalk (Fig. 17-21; see Fig. 17-18F). These distinct regions are characterized by the differential expression of transcription factors necessary for their specification (see Fig. 17-21). The neural retina expresses *Chx10*, *Pax6*, *Six6*, and *Rx*, the pigmented epithelium expresses *Mitf* and *Otx2*, and the optic stalk expresses *Pax2* (see Fig. 17-21C). Initially, all optic cup cells are equally competent to form the different regions of the eye; subsequent differentiation is induced by the surrounding tissues (see Fig. 17-21D). Signaling from the surface ectoderm, possibly mediated by *Fgfs*, specifies the neural retina (e.g., induces *Chx10* expression), whereas signals from the extraocular mesenchyme, such as the *Tgfβ* family member *Activin A*, specify the pigmented epithelium (i.e., induce *Mitf* expression). *Shh* signals from the midline

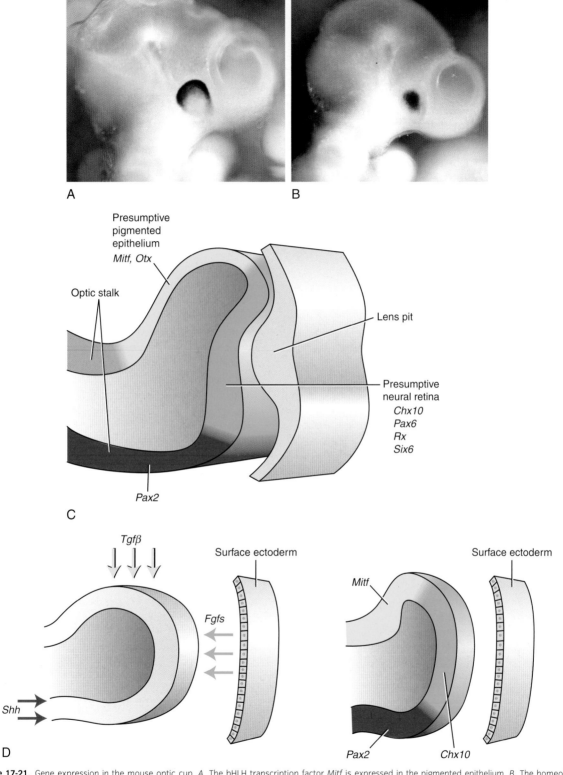

Figure 17-21. Gene expression in the mouse optic cup. *A,* The bHLH transcription factor *Mitf* is expressed in the pigmented epithelium. *B,* The homeobox transcription factor *Chx10* is expressed in the neural retina. *C,* Expression of transcription factors in different regions of the optic cup and stalk. *D,* Patterning of the different regions of the optic vesicle and stalk involves growth factor signaling (arrows) from adjacent tissues.

tissues specify the optic stalk (i.e., induce *Pax2* expression). In the absence of these signals, the eye will not differentiate appropriately. For example, if the ectoderm (the source of *Fgfs*) is removed, the neural retina develops as pigmented epithelium. The boundary between the optic stalk and neural retina is maintained by antagonistic interactions between *Pax2* and *Pax6*, which repress the expression of each other.

DIFFERENTIATION OF PIGMENTED EPITHELIUM

The transcription factors *Mitf* and *Otx2* are required for specification of the pigmented epithelium in the optic cup. Both genes have been shown to activate melanogenic genes such as *Trp1* and *Tyrosinase*. *Mitf* is expressed specifically in the pigmented epithelium (see Fig. 17-21A). In *Mitf* and *Otx1/2* mouse mutants, the pigmented epithelium is respecified to form an ectopic neural retina.

REGULATION OF PROLIFERATION AND DIFFERENTIATION OF RETINAL PROGENITOR CELLS

Several signals have been identified that regulate **proliferation** of retinal progenitor cells. For example, the homeobox transcription factor *Chx10* is specifically expressed in the neural retina (see Fig.17-21B) and is required for retinal proliferation. This effect is mediated by regulators of the cell cycle (*Cyclin D1*, *p27*). Other factors controlling proliferation are *Notch-Delta* signaling, *Fgf*, *Igf*, *Wnt2b*, *Hes1*, *Hdac* (*Histone deacetylase*), *Rx*, and *Sonic hedgehog*.

Lineage studies have shown that neural retinal cells are multipotential, and in some instances can give rise to all cell types. However, at any one time, the competence of the progenitors is generally restricted to a few cell types. For example, early progenitors predominantly produce ganglion cells, whereas "older" progenitors mainly generate rod photoreceptors. This restricted competence is not determined by environmental signals and reflects an intrinsic behavior of the neural progenitors. If "older" progenitors are placed in a "younger" environment, they differentiate according to their original fate.

Differentiation starts centrally in the fovea and is induced by *Fgf* signals from the optic stalk. Subsequently, a wave of *Shh* and *Fgf* expression induces differentiation in the periphery. The balance of proliferation versus neuronal differentiation is controlled by various basic helix-loop-helix (bHLH) transcription factors. *Hes1* and *5* are activated by *Notch* signaling, and they function to maintain proliferation. Therefore, the activity of *Notch* signaling favors the production of the non-neuronal Müller glia cells (normally the last to be born). In contrast, other bHLH factors such as *Mash1*, *Ngn2*, and *Math5* are necessary for the differentiation of the neuronal cell types. *Math5* is required for ganglion cell development, *Mash1* is required for bipolar cell development, and *NeuroD* is required for amacrine and rod formation. The loss of one cell type (e.g., loss of ganglion cells in the *Math5* mutant) is accompanied by the increase in another cell type (in this case amacrine and cone cells). Differentiation is also controlled by homeobox genes. *Pax6* regulates the expression of *Ngn2*, *Mash1*, and *Math5*. Therefore, in the absence of *Pax6*, many of the neuronal derivatives are affected, and only one cell type (amacrine cells) is generated. In contrast, the homeobox gene *Chx10* is required for bipolar cell development, whereas in *Prox1* mutants, horizontal cells do not form. Although specific genes are required for the development of various neuronal subtypes, gain of function does not necessarily result in the converse effect. Furthermore, the expression of a particular gene (e.g., *Math5*) does not necessarily commit the progenitor to a particular cell lineage (e.g., in this case ganglion cells). It is possible that the combination of homeobox gene and bHLH gene expression determines the progenitor fate.

Following differentiation, there are autoregulatory mechanisms to control the number of each neuronal cell type. If amacrine cells are ablated in frogs or goldfish, they are replaced with new amacrine cells from retinal progenitors. Similarly, the number of retinal ganglion cells (RGCs) seems to be regulated by this autoregulatory feedback. RGCs express *Shh* after they have differentiated, and loss of function of *Shh* increases the number of RGCs. It is thought that high levels of *Shh*, for example produced by several RGCs, will inhibit further RGC differentiation, favoring the development of other cell types. In this way, development of one cell type (an RGC in this example) will promote the differentiation of the next cell type (cone, in this example).

Formation of Optic Nerve

The nerve fibers that emerge from the retinal ganglion cells in the 6th week travel along the inner wall of the optic stalk to reach the brain. The stalk lumen is gradually obliterated by growth of these fibers, and by the 8th week the hollow optic stalk is transformed into the solid **optic nerve** (cranial nerve II). Just before the two optic nerves enter the brain, they join to form an X-shaped structure called the **optic chiasm.** Within the chiasm, about half the fibers from each optic nerve cross over to the contralateral (opposite) side of the brain. The resulting combined bundle of ipsilateral and contralateral fibers on each side then grows back to the lateral geniculate body of the thalamus (discussed in Ch. 9), where the fibers synapse starting in the 8th week. More than one million nerve fibers grow from each retina to the brain. The mechanism of axonal pathfinding that allows each of these axons to map to the correct point in the lateral geniculate body is discussed in Chapter 9. The glial cells around the optic nerve arise from the inner layer of the optic stalk, which is of neuroectodermal origin. Myelinization of the optic nerve begins at the optic chiasm around 7 months and continues towards the eye.

Vascularization of Optic Cup and Lens

There are two sources of vascularization to the eye: the **choroid** layer around the eye (see the next section of this chapter) and the transient **hyaloid artery**. This artery develops from a branch of the ophthalmic artery and gains access to the lentiretinal space via the choroidal fissure on the ventral surface of the optic stalk. The hyaloid artery vascularizes the developing retina and initially also vascularizes the lens vesicle (see Fig. 17-17). Branches of the hyaloid artery extend over the lens and are known as the **tunica vasculosa lentis**. The lips of the choroidal fissure fuse by day 33, enclosing the hyaloid artery and its accompanying vein in a canal within the ventral wall of the optic stalk (see Fig. 17-17B, C). The hyaloid vasculature is maximally developed at approximately 10 weeks of gestation. When the lens matures during fetal life and ceases to need a blood supply, the portion of the hyaloid artery that crosses the vitreous body degenerates and is removed by macrophages (end of 4th month). However, even in the adult, the course of this former artery is marked by a conduit through the vitreous body called the **hyaloid canal.** The proximal portion of the hyaloid artery becomes the **central artery of the retina**, which supplies blood to the retina. Vascularization of the retina starts as the hyaloid artery is regressing and is predominant during the final trimester. Formation of this vascular plexus begins at the optic head and extends into the periphery following the wave of neuronal differentiation.

Formation of Choroid, Sclera, and Anterior Chamber

During weeks 6 and 7, the mesenchymal capsule that surrounds the optic cup differentiates into two layers: an inner, pigmented, vascular layer called the **choroid**, and an outer, fibrous layer called the **sclera** (Fig. 17-22). The choroid layer is homologous in origin with the pia mater and arachnoid membranes investing the brain (the leptomeninges), and the sclera is homologous with the dura mater. The choroid is pigmented and develops from neural crest cell–derived mesenchyme (stromal cells, melanocytes, and pericytes) and mesoderm (endothelial cells). The primitive blood vessels/spaces give rise to the embryonic choriocapillaris (i.e., the capillaries forming the inner vascular layer of the choroid) at around 2 months of gestation and supply blood to the retinal epithelium.

The tough sclera supports and protects the delicate inner structures of the eye. The anterior sclera begins as a condensation of mesenchymal tissue that is continuous with the cornea. By approximately 12 weeks, the mesenchymal condensation has reached the optic nerve.

Formation of Cornea

Late in the 6th week, the mesenchyme surrounding the optic cup invades the region between the lens and the surface ectoderm, thus forming a complete mesenchymal jacket around the optic cup (see Fig. 17-22A). The mesenchyme differentiates into a thin inner epithelium overlying the cornea called the **corneal epithelium** or **corneal endothelium**. An **acellular postepithelial layer** or **stroma** forms between the corneal epithelium and the corneal ectoderm, and by the 8th week, these two layers are clearly apparent. The stroma consists of a matrix of *Collagen* fibers, *Hyaluronic acid* (which binds water causing the matrix to swell), and *Glycosaminoglycans*. Mesenchymal cells rapidly invade the stroma and convert it to a cellular **stromal layer (substantia propria).** *Hyaluronidase* removes the *Hyaluronic acid* reducing the matrix volume. *Thyroxine* (circulated from the thyroid gland) also induces the dehydration of the stroma and the transparent cornea is formed. Very recent fate mapping studies in mouse have revealed that in addition to neural crest cells, head mesoderm contributes to corneal endothelial and stromal layers and trabecular meshwork. Thus, the cornea has three tissue origins: mesodermal and neural crest cells form the mesothelium and the substantia propria, whereas the outer layer of the cornea, called the **anterior epithelium**, is derived from the overlying surface ectoderm.

Formation of Pupillary Membrane

By the 9th week, the mesenchyme overlying the lens splits into two layers that enclose a new cavity called

17

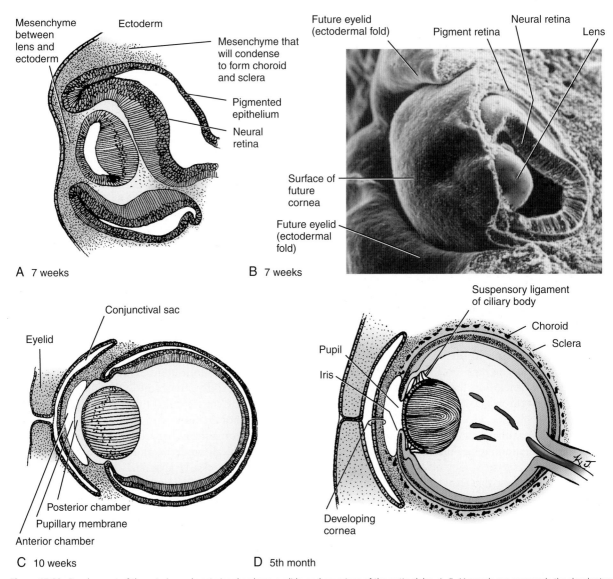

Figure 17-22. Development of the anterior and posterior chambers, eyelids, and coverings of the optic globe. *A, B,* Mesenchyme surrounds the developing eyeball (optic globe) between the 5th and 7th weeks to form the choroid and sclera. *C, D,* Vacuolization within this mesenchyme in the 7th week forms the anterior chamber. Shortly thereafter, vacuolization in the layer of mesenchyme immediately anterior to the lens forms the posterior chamber. The pupillary membrane, which initially separates the anterior and posterior chambers, breaks down in early fetal life. The upper and lower eyelids form as folds of surface ectoderm. They fuse together by the end of the 8th week and separate again between the 5th and 7th months.

the **anterior chamber of the eye** (see Fig. 17-22C). The anterior (superficial) wall of this chamber is continuous with the sclera, and the posterior (deep) wall is continuous with the choroid. The thick posterior wall of the anterior chamber rests directly against the lens. The deep layers of this wall subsequently break down by a process of vacuolization to create a new space, the **posterior chamber**, between the lens and the thin remaining layer of the wall (see Fig. 17-22C).

This thin remaining layer, called the **pupillary membrane**, regresses early in the fetal period (between the 6th and 8th month) to form the opening called the **pupil** through which the anterior and posterior chambers communicate. On rare occasions, the pupillary membrane fails to break down completely, leaving strands that traverse the pupil. The posterior chamber eventually expands to underlie the iris and part of the ciliary body (discussed in next paragraph).

Formation of Iris and Ciliary Body

At the end of the 3rd month, the anterior rim of the optic cup expands to form a thin ring that projects between the anterior and posterior chambers and overlaps the lens (see Fig. 17-22*B*). This ring differentiates into the **iris** of the eye. The iris stroma develops from anterior segment mesenchymal tissue of neural crest cell origin. The posterior iris epithelium and the circumferentially arranged smooth muscle bundles of the **pupillary muscles** in the iris originate from the neuroepithelium of the optic cup. These muscles act as a diaphragm, controlling the diameter of the pupil and thus the amount of light that enters the eye.

Just posterior to the developing iris, the optic cup differentiates and folds to form the **ciliary body.** The lens is suspended from the ciliary body by a radial network of elastic fibers called the **suspensory ligament** of the lens (lens zonules). Around the insertions of these fibers, the optic cup epithelia of the ciliary body proliferate to form a ring of highly vascularized, feathery elaborations that are specialized to secrete the aqueous humor of the eye. Neural crest cells that invade the choroid of the ciliary body differentiate to form the smooth muscle bundles of the **ciliary muscle,** which controls the shape and hence the focusing power (accommodation) of the lens. Contraction of this muscle reduces the diameter of the ciliary ring from which the lens is suspended, thus allowing the lens to relax toward its natural spherical shape and providing the greater focusing power needed for near vision.

Formation of Eyelids

By the 6th week, small folds of surface ectoderm with a mesenchymal core appear just cranial and caudal to the developing cornea (see Fig. 17-22). These upper (frontonasal process) and lower (maxillary process) eyelid primordia rapidly grow toward each other, meeting and fusing by the 8th week. The space between the fused eyelids and the cornea is called the **conjunctival sac.** The eyelids separate again between the 5th and 7th months. The eyelid muscles (orbicularis and levator) are derived from mesoderm.

The **lacrimal glands** form from invaginations of the ectoderm at the superolateral angles of the conjunctival sacs but do not mature until about 6 weeks after birth. The tear fluid produced by the glands is excreted into the conjunctival sac, where it lubricates the cornea. Excess tear fluid drains through the **nasolacrimal duct** (discussed in Ch. 16) into the nasal cavity.

IN THE CLINIC

ABNORMALITIES OF EYE

Congenital eye defects can arise at any stage of eye morphogenesis and differentiation. The scope of defects depends on the timing of the embryologic insult. Eye malformations can be widespread or can affect specific regions or specific cell types. Eye defects can be isolated, but are often part of other genetic syndromes. Because of the close relationship between eye and brain development, malformations of the eye often suggest the presence of underlying abnormalities of the brain.

Abnormalities occurring in the very earliest stages of eye development can disrupt formation of the optic field, as in the case of **anophthalmia** in which the eyes are absent. Defects occurring at later stages of development can result in small eyes (**microphthalmia**) or abnormalities of various components of the eye. For example, a **coloboma** results when the optic fissure fails to fuse, leaving a gap in eye structures. A complete coloboma extends throughout the entire eye (from optic nerve to iris), whereas more localized colobomata may occur, as in coloboma of the iris (Fig. 17-23).

Abnormalities of the most anterior eye structures, the eyelids and the sclera, are common. Many types of eyelid anomalies occur. Folds of skin that cover the inner corner (i.e., canthus) of the eye, **epicanthal folds,** are a characteristic feature of **Down syndrome,** but they are also normally present in many ethnic groups. The fissure that separates upper and lower eyelids (i.e., the palpebral fissure) can fail to form properly, resulting in fusion of the eyelids. In **cryptophthalmos** fusion is complete, whereas in **blepharophimosis** the lids are partially fused. Other anomalies of the eyelids include **ptosis** (drooping eyelids) and **epicanthus inversus** (folds curving down and laterally from the inner canthus). Mutation of the forkhead gene *FOXL2* results in a syndrome characterized by blepharophimosis, ptosis, and epicanthus inversus. Mutations in another forkhead gene *FOXC2* result in **distichiasis** (an extra row of eyelashes along the eyelid margin) along with lymphedema of the limbs. Tumorous growth of the sclera, called **epibulbar dermoids,** is one of the cardinal findings in **Goldenhar syndrome** (part of the **OAVS spectrum** discussed earlier in the chapter and in Ch. 16). Ocular **telangiectasia** (permanent dilation of capillaries of the sclera) is seen in **ataxia-telangiectasia** (also mentioned in Ch. 9) and is associated with cerebellar degeneration (resulting in ataxia) and immunodeficiency.

17

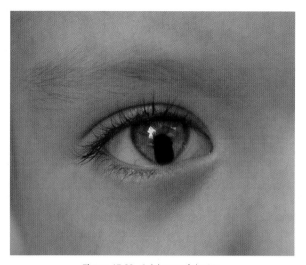

Figure 17-23. Coloboma of the iris.

Strabismus, or misalignment of gaze, can be caused by abnormalities of the extraocular muscles or their innervation. **Duane anomaly** is a rare cause of strabismus characterized by abnormal abduction/adduction, narrowing of the eye fissure, and retraction of the globe with adduction, and it is caused by abnormal development of the **abducens nerve** (cranial nerve VI), which innervates the **lateral rectus** eye muscle. Duane anomaly, accompanied by abnormalities of the hands, heart, and ears, is caused by mutations in the gene encoding the *SAL4* transcription factor. If left untreated, strabismus can lead to **amblyopia**, a permanent loss of vision resulting from changes in the visual cortex. Injury to the lateral rectus muscle and/or its innervation (the abducens nerve) sometimes results from forceps-assisted deliveries. This injury typically resolves itself within a few weeks after birth.

Various defects of the anterior part of the eye can occur. **Anterior segment ocular dysgenesis (ASOD)** involves defects of the cornea, iris, lens, and ciliary body. Similar defects occur in **Axenfeld-Rieger anomaly** and **Peters anomaly,** with the latter also involving **sclerocornea** (corneal clouding). These defects are etiologically related, being caused by an overlapping set of genes (the result, for example, of mutations in the *FOXC1, FOXE3, PITX2/3,* and *PAX6* transcription factors). Given its key role in eye development, mutations in *PAX6* can result in **aniridia** (the absence of the iris, as in **WAGR association**—Wilms' tumor, aniridia, genitourinary anomalies, mental retardation), together with more widespread ocular defects affecting the cornea, lens, retina, and optic nerve. Persistence of the **pupillary membrane** may occur as part of the above

anomalies or may occur as an isolated defect. The presence of nodules on the iris, called **Lisch nodules,** can be a clue to the diagnosis of neurofibromatosis type 1 (discussed in Ch. 10).

Congenital cataracts (lens opacities) can result from genetic or environmental factors. Genetic factors involve a large number of mutations in diverse genes ranging from structural components of the lens, such as mutations in *CRYSTALLIN* or gap junction proteins, to transcription factors such as *MAF* or *HEAT SHOCK TRANSCRIPTION FACTOR 4* (*HSF4*). Cataracts may also develop due to metabolic disorders such as **galactosemia** (a defect in galactose metabolism) or as a result of congenital infections such as **rubella**.

Defects of the **retina** are common. For example, the photoreceptors die in **Leber congenital amaurosis syndrome**, the genetic syndrome affecting the retina most frequently, and in **retinis pigmentosa**. These two syndromes can be the result of mutations in *RPE65*, the enzyme that converts 11-*cis* retinaldehyde to its all-*trans* form following activation of the photoreceptor.

Wnt signaling plays an important role in eye development, including development of the retina. **Norrie disease,** characterized by **retinal dysplasia** and abnormal vascularization (and sensorineural hearing loss), arises from mutations in a novel ligand for the *WNT* pathway, *NORRIN*. Moreover, mutations in the *WNT* (and *NORRIN*) *RECEPTOR FRIZZLED4* cause **familial exudative vitreoretinopathy**, another syndrome characterized in part by incomplete vascularization of the retina (the retinal blood vessels do not reach the periphery of the retina). Abnormal vascularization also occurs in **osteoporosis-pseudoglioma syndrome**, which is the result of a mutation in the *WNT* coreceptor *LRP5*. However, in this case the hyaloid artery persists, rather than regressing as it normally does.

The retina has one of the highest requirements for oxygen in the body, utilizing more oxygen/unit weight than any other tissue. Therefore, the eye is exceptionally sensitive to defects in vascularization. During development, angiogenesis is controlled by local regions of hypoxia generated by the newly differentiated ganglion cells. Hypoxia induces the astrocyte and Müller cells to express the angiogenic factor *Vegf*, promoting further vascularization. Increases in oxygen levels (e.g., during oxygen support for premature babies) prevent angiogenesis. The neovascularization that follows from this can lead to hemorrhage and fibrosis—a condition known as **retinopathy of prematurity,** which is a major cause of infantile blindness.

Hypoplasia of the optic nerve occurs in a wide array of syndromes. In **septo-optic dysplasia** (also called **De Morsier**

syndrome), caused by mutations in the *HESX1* gene, optic nerve hypoplasia occurs in conjunction with pituitary hypoplasia and midline brain abnormalities. Children with this syndrome are short due to growth hormone deficiency. Defects in the dorsal quadrant of the eye result in superior segmental optic nerve hypoplasia with inferior visual defects. This occurs in as many as 9% of children born to diabetic mothers.

Suggested Readings

Ear Development

Alsina B, Giraldez F, Varela-Nieto I. 2003. Growth factors and early development of otic neurons: interactions between intrinsic and extrinsic signals. Curr Top Dev Biol 57:177-206.

Anagnostopoulos AV. 2002. A compendium of mouse knockouts with inner ear defects. Trends Genet 18:499.

Barald KF, Kelley MW. 2004. From placode to polarization: new tunes in inner ear development. Development 131:4119-4130.

Bober E, Rinkwitz S, Herbrand H. 2003. Molecular basis of otic commitment and morphogenesis: a role for homeodomain-containing transcription factors and signaling molecules. Curr Top Dev Biol 57:151-175.

Brown ST, Martin K, Groves AK. 2003. Molecular basis of inner ear induction. Curr Top Dev Biol 57:115-149.

Call LM, Morton CC. 2002. Continuing to break the sound barrier: genes in hearing. Curr Opin Genet Dev 12:343-348.

Dabdoub A, Kelley MW. 2005. Planar cell polarity and a potential role for a Wnt morphogen gradient in stereociliary bundle orientation in the mammalian inner ear. J Neurobiol 64:446-457.

Eatock RA, Hurley KM. 2003. Functional development of hair cells. Curr Top Dev Biol 57:389-448.

Fekete DM, Wu DK. 2002. Revisiting cell fate specification in the inner ear. Curr Opin Neurobiol 12:35-42.

Forge A, Wright T. 2002. The molecular architecture of the inner ear. Br Med Bull 63:5-24.

Fritzsch B, Beisel KW, Hansen LA. 2006. The molecular basis of neurosensory cell formation in ear development: a blueprint for hair cell and sensory neuron regeneration? Bioessays 28:1181-1193.

Fritzsch B, Pauley S, Beisel KW. 2006. Cells, molecules and morphogenesis: the making of the vertebrate ear. Brain Res 1091:151-171.

Frolenkov GI, Belyantseva IA, Friedman TB, Griffith AJ. 2004. Genetic insights into the morphogenesis of inner ear hair cells. Nat Rev Genet 5:489-498.

Gao WQ. 2003. Hair cell development in higher vertebrates. Curr Top Dev Biol 57:293-319.

Kelley MW. 2006. Regulation of cell fate in the sensory epithelia of the inner ear. Nat Rev Neurosci 7:837-849.

Kelley MW. 2006. Hair cell development: commitment through differentiation. Brain Res 1091:172-185.

Lewis J, Davies A. 2002. Planar cell polarity in the inner ear: how do hair cells acquire their oriented structure? J Neurobiol 53:190-201.

Lin HW, Schneider ME, Kachar B. 2005. When size matters: the dynamic regulation of stereocilia lengths. Curr Opin Cell Biol 17:55-61.

Mallo M. 2003. Formation of the outer and middle ear, molecular mechanisms. Curr Top Dev Biol 57:85-113.

Noramly S, Grainger RM. 2002. Determination of the embryonic inner ear. J Neurobiol 53:100-128.

Petit C, Levilliers J, Hardelin JP. 2001. Molecular genetics of hearing loss. Annu Rev Genet 35:589-646.

Quint E, Steel KP. 2003. Use of mouse genetics for studying inner ear development. Curr Top Dev Biol 57:45-83.

Riley BB, Phillips BT. 2003. Ringing in the new ear: resolution of cell interactions in otic development. Dev Biol 261:289-312.

Rinkwitz S, Bober E, Baker R. 2001. Development of the vertebrate inner ear. Ann N Y Acad Sci 942:1-14.

Santos-Sacchi J. 2003. New tunes from Corti's organ: the outer hair cell boogie rules. Curr Opin Neurobiol 13:459-468.

Semple MN, Scott BH. 2003. Cortical mechanisms in hearing. Curr Opin Neurobiol 13:167-173.

Steel KP, Kros CJ. 2001. A genetic approach to understanding auditory function. Nat Genet 27:143-149.

Wangemann P. 2002. K$^+$ cycling and the endocochlear potential. Hear Res 165:1-9.

Wright TJ, Mansour SL. 2003. FGF signaling in ear development and innervation. Curr Top Dev Biol 57:225-259.

Zuo J. 2002. Transgenic and gene targeting studies of hair cell function in mouse inner ear. J Neurobiol 53:286-305.

Eye Development

Amato MA, Boy S, Perron M. 2004. Hedgehog signaling in vertebrate eye development: a growing puzzle. Cell Mol Life Sci 61:899-910.

Ashery-Padan R, Gruss P. 2001. Pax6 lights-up the way for eye development. Curr Opin Cell Biol 13:706-714.

Baker CV, Bronner-Fraser M. 2001. Vertebrate cranial placodes I. Embryonic induction. Dev Biol 232:1-61.

Bharti K, Nguyen MT, Skuntz S, et al. 2006. The other pigment cell: specification and development of the pigmented epithelium of the vertebrate eye. Pigment Cell Res 19:380-394.

Cayouette M, Poggi L, Harris WA. 2006. Lineage in the vertebrate retina. Trends Neurosci 29:563-570.

Chow RL, Altmann CR, Lang RA, Hemmati-Brivanlou A. 1999. Pax6 induces ectopic eyes in a vertebrate. Development 126:4213-4222.

Cvekl A, Tamm ER. 2004. Anterior eye development and ocular mesenchyme: new insights from mouse models and human diseases. Bioessays 26:374-386.

Dalke C, Graw J. 2005. Mouse mutants as models for congenital retinal disorders. Exp Eye Res 81:503-512.

Deeb SS. 2006. Genetics of variation in human color vision and the retinal cone mosaic. Curr Opin Genet Dev 16:301-307.

Donner AL, Lachke SA, Maas RL. 2006. Lens induction in vertebrates: Variations on a conserved theme of signaling events. Semin Cell Dev Biol 17(6):676-678.

Dyer MA, Cepko CL. 2001. Regulating proliferation during retinal development. Nat Rev Neurosci 2:333-342.

Fain GL. 2006. Why photoreceptors die (and why they don't). Bioessays 28:344-354.

Gariano RF, Gardner TW. 2005. Retinal angiogenesis in development and disease. Nature 438:960-966.

Gould DB, Smith RS, John SW. 2004. Anterior segment development relevant to glaucoma. Int J Dev Biol 48:1015-1029.

17

Graw J. 2003. The genetic and molecular basis of congenital eye defects. Nat Rev Genet 4:876-888.

Hatakeyama J, Kageyama R. 2004. Retinal cell fate determination and bHLH factors. Semin Cell Dev Biol 15:83-89.

He S, Dong W, Deng Q, Weng S, Sun W. 2003. Seeing more clearly: recent advances in understanding retinal circuitry. Science 302:408-411.

Kumar JP. 2001. Signaling pathways in Drosophila and vertebrate retinal development. Nat Rev Genet 2:846-857.

Lemke G, Reber M. 2005. Retinotectal mapping: new insights from molecular genetics. Annu Rev Cell Dev Biol 21:551-580.

Levine EM, Green ES. 2004. Cell-intrinsic regulators of proliferation in vertebrate retinal progenitors. Semin Cell Dev Biol 15:63-74.

Livesey FJ, Cepko CL. 2001. Vertebrate neural cell-fate determination: lessons from the retina. Nat Rev Neurosci 2:109-118.

Lovicu FJ, McAvoy JW. 2005. Growth factor regulation of lens development. Dev Biol 280:1-14.

Malicki J. 2004. Cell fate decisions and patterning in the vertebrate retina: the importance of timing, asymmetry, polarity and waves. Curr Opin Neurobiol 14:15-21.

Mann F, Harris WA, Holt CE. 2004. New views on retinal axon development: a navigation guide. Int J Dev Biol 48:957-964.

Martinez-Morales JR, Rodrigo I, Bovolenta P. 2004. Eye development: a view from the retina pigmented epithelium. Bioessays 26:766-777.

McLaughlin T, Hindges R, O'Leary DD. 2003. Regulation of axial patterning of the retina and its topographic mapping in the brain. Curr Opin Neurobiol 13:57-69.

Moshiri A, Close J, Reh TA. 2004. Retinal stem cells and regeneration. Int J Dev Biol 48:1003-1014.

Mu X, Klein WH. 2004. A gene regulatory hierarchy for retinal ganglion cell specification and differentiation. Semin Cell Dev Biol 15:115-123.

Oster SF, Deiner M, Birgbauer E, Sretavan DW. 2004. Ganglion cell axon pathfinding in the retina and optic nerve. Semin Cell Dev Biol 15:125-136.

Peters MA. 2002. Patterning the neural retina. Curr Opin Neurobiol 12:43-48.

Pichaud F, Desplan C. 2002. Pax genes and eye organogenesis. Curr Opin Genet Dev 12:430-434.

Poggi L, Zolessi FR, Harris WA. 2005. Time-lapse analysis of retinal differentiation. Curr Opin Cell Biol 17:676-681.

Russell C. 2003. The roles of Hedgehogs and Fibroblast Growth Factors in eye development and retinal cell rescue. Vision Res 43:899-912.

Saint-Geniez M, D'Amore PA. 2004. Development and pathology of the hyaloid, choroidal and retinal vasculature. Int J Dev Biol 48:1045-1058.

Sernagor E. 2005. Retinal development: second sight comes first. Curr Biol 15:R556-R559.

Stuermer CA, Bastmeyer M. 2000. The retinal axon's pathfinding to the optic disk. Prog Neurobiol 62:197-214.

van Horck FP, Weinl C, Holt CE. 2004. Retinal axon guidance: novel mechanisms for steering. Curr Opin Neurobiol 14:61-66.

Williams SE, Mason CA, Herrera E. 2004. The optic chiasm as a midline choice point. Curr Opin Neurobiol 14:51-60.

Yang XJ. 2004. Roles of cell-extrinsic growth factors in vertebrate eye pattern formation and retinogenesis. Semin Cell Dev Biol 15:91-103.

Development of the Limbs

18

Summary
The upper **limb buds** appear on day 24 as small bulges on the lateral body wall at about the level of C5 to T1. By the end of the 4th week, the upper limb buds have grown to form pronounced structures protruding from the body wall, and the lower limb buds first appear, forming at the level of L1 to L5. Limb morphogenesis takes place from the 4th to the 8th weeks, with the development of the lower limbs lagging slightly behind the development of the upper limbs. Each limb bud consists of a **mesenchymal core** of mesoderm covered by an **epithelial cap** of ectoderm. Along the distal margin of the limb bud, the ectoderm thickens to form an **apical ectodermal ridge**. This structure maintains outgrowth of the limb bud along the **proximal-distal axis**.

By 33 days the **hand plates** are visible at the end of the lengthening upper limb buds, and the lower limb buds have begun to elongate. By the end of the 6th week, the segments of the upper and lower limbs can be distinguished. **Digital rays** appear on the handplates and footplates during the 6th (upper limbs) and 7th (lower limbs) weeks. A process of **programmed cell death** occurs between the rays to free the fingers and toes. By the end of the 8th week, all of the components of the upper and lower limbs are distinct.

The **skeletal elements** of the limbs develop from mesodermal condensations that appear along the long axis of the limb bud during the 5th week. The cartilaginous precursors of the limb bones chondrify within this mesenchymal condensation starting in the 6th week. Ossification of these cartilaginous precursors begins in the 7th to 12th weeks.

The bones, tendons, and other connective tissues of the limbs arise from the lateral plate mesoderm, but the limb muscles and endothelial cells arise in the somitic mesoderm and migrate into the limb buds. In general, the muscles that form on the ventral side of the developing long bones become the flexors and pronators of the upper limbs, and the flexors and adductors of the lower limbs. These muscles are innervated by ventral branches of the ventral primary rami of the spinal nerves. The muscles that form on the dorsal side of the long bones generally become the extensor and supinator muscles of the upper limbs, and the extensor and abductor muscles of the lower limbs. These muscles are innervated by dorsal branches of the ventral primary rami. However, some muscles of the limbs shift their position dramatically during development either by differential growth or by passive displacement during lateral rotation of the upper limb and medial rotation of the lower limb.

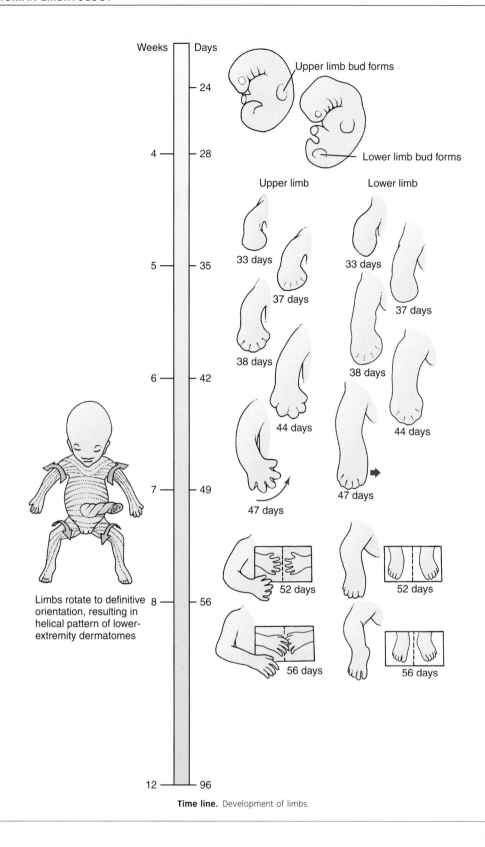

Weeks · Days

24 — Upper limb bud forms

4 — 28 — Lower limb bud forms

Upper limb · Lower limb

33 days · 33 days

37 days · 37 days

38 days · 38 days

5 — 35

6 — 42

44 days · 44 days

47 days · 47 days

7 — 49

52 days · 52 days

Limbs rotate to definitive orientation, resulting in helical pattern of lower-extremity dermatomes

8 — 56

56 days · 56 days

12 — 96

Time line. Development of limbs.

Clinical Taster Freddie Musena M'tile (Musena means friend in Kenyan) was born in 2004 in Kenya with a condition called **tetra-amelia** (absence of all four limbs; Fig. 18-1). Children with birth defects are shunned in some cultures, and Freddie's biologic mother gave him up for adoption, fearing that her husband would kill him. A British charity worker and her Kenyan husband adopted him and brought him to the UK for treatment. The case received notoriety after Freddie was, for a time, denied a British visa. With donations obtained through Thalidomide UK, he was fitted with prosthetic devices to help him sit up, with future plans to fit him with artificial limbs. Sadly, Freddie died of a fungal infection after returning to Africa. By the time of his death, Freddie had become a national symbol in Kenya.

Although the cause of Freddie's birth defects is not certain, his biologic mother took medicine that was believed to have been **thalidomide**. Once banned after causing an estimated 12,000 cases of limb defects like Freddie's in the late 1950s and early 1960s, thalidomide use is on the rise again. Originally prescribed in Europe and the UK to treat morning sickness during pregnancy, thalidomide is now being used to treat leprosy, AIDS, and certain cancers. It is widely available in third-world countries, and Freddie's case helped raise awareness of the risks of thalidomide exposure during pregnancy, especially in countries where literacy rates are low.

The thalidomide epidemic that occurred now almost 50 years ago led to concerns about methods used to validate the safety of new drugs. This resulted in new Food and Drug Administration (FDA) guidelines for drug testing—guidelines that remain in effect today.

Thalidomide is a potent **teratogen** that causes defects at single exposures as low as 100 mg. The exact mechanism by which thalidomide causes amelia (absent limbs) or phocomelia (hands or feet projecting directly from the shoulder or hip, respectively) is unknown. However, the drug's ability to inhibit angiogenesis (blood vessel formation) is a potentially strong mechanism. Disruption of blood supply has long been hypothesized to play a role in similar limb reduction defects.

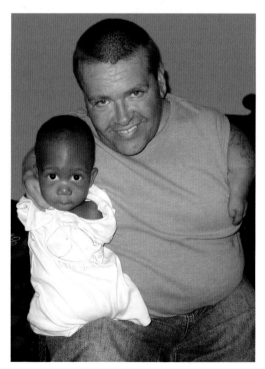

Figure 18-1. Freddie Musena M'tile meets Freddie Astbury, a thalidomide survivor of the original epidemic and President of Thalidomide UK. Freddie Musena M'tile was born in Kenya with tetra-amelia.

Epithelial-Mesenchymal Interactions Control Limb Outgrowth

Limb development takes place over a 5-week period from the 4th to the 8th weeks. The upper limbs develop slightly in advance of the lower limbs, although by the end of the period of limb development, the two limbs are nearly synchronized. Initiation of limb development starts with the proliferation of the somatic lateral plate mesoderm in the limb regions of the lateral body wall (Fig. 18-2). The upper limb bud appears in the lower cervical region at 24 days, and the lower limb bud appears in the lower lumbar region at 28 days. Each limb bud consists of an outer ectodermal cap and an inner mesodermal core.

As each limb bud forms, the ectoderm along the distal tip of the bud is induced by the underlying somatic mesoderm to form a ridge-like thickening called the **apical ectodermal ridge** (AER) (see Fig. 18-2). This structure forms at the dorsal-ventral boundary of the limb bud and plays an essential role in the outgrowth of the limb.

18

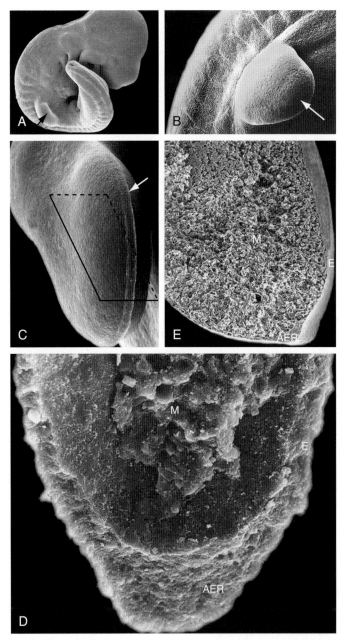

Figure 18-2. Scanning electron micrographs showing limb buds. The limb buds are formed from lateral plate mesoderm. *A*, Embryo with newly formed upper limb bud (arrow). *B*, By day 29, the upper limb bud (arrow) is flattened. *C*, Day 32, limb bud showing the apical ectodermal ridge (arrow) as a thickened crest of ectoderm at the distal edge of the growing upper limb bud. Rectangle indicates plane of sectioning shown in *E*. *D*, Limb bud ectoderm (*E*) removed to show its internal face and attached mesenchymal core (*M*); note the thickened apical ectodermal ridge (AER). *E*, Limb bud sectioned at the level indicated by the rectangle in *C*, showing the inner mesenchymal core (M), the outer ectodermal cap (E), and the thickened apical ectodermal ridge (AER).

PATTERNING OF LIMB BUD

Formation of the limb bud is initiated by signals from the **intermediate mesoderm**. Once the limb bud has formed, it differentiates with respect to three axes (Fig. 18-3). The **proximal-distal axis** runs from the shoulder or hip to the fingers or toes and consists of the **stylopod** (humerus or femur), **zeugopod** (radius and ulna or tibia and fibula), and **autopod** (the carpals and metacarpals or tarsal and metatarsals and the phalanges). Along the **cranial-caudal axis** (often called the anterior-posterior axis), the thumb is the most cranial digit, whereas the little finger is the most caudal digit. Along the **dorsal-ventral axis**, the knuckle side of the hand or top side of the foot is dorsal, whereas the palm or sole of the hand or foot, respectively, is ventral. The limb bud develops from an initially homogeneous cell population; thus, a cell in the limb bud must respond appropriately to its position relative to all three axes. Several questions arise such as: How does one part of the limb bud form the shoulder and another the forearm? How does one digital ray in the hand plate form an index finger and another the thumb? How do dorsal and ventral sides of the limb become differentiated from each other? Significant advances have been made toward answering these questions. We now know the key players that pattern the limb bud, and we can link these key players to mutations that cause human birth defects. The following paragraphs of this "In the Research Lab" discuss development of the limb along the proximal-distal axis, including the initiation of limb outgrowth. Development along the other two axes is discussed in the subsequent "In the Research Lab."

GROWTH AND PATTERNING ALONG PROXIMAL-DISTAL AXIS

Classical embryologic experiments have shown that **proximal-distal outgrowth** is controlled by the apical ectodermal ridge (AER). Removal of the AER results in the arrest of limb development, with the degree of development being determined by the stage of development at which the AER was removed (Fig. 18-4). For example, in the chick, removal at stage 20 of development results in the formation of a limb truncated at the elbow joint, whereas removal slightly later at stage 24 leads to a limb lacking just the digits. Furthermore, in chick *wingless* and mouse *limb deformity* mutants, in which the AER develops initially but is not maintained, the limbs are truncated. Initiation of limb development without further maintenance occurs naturally in some species of snakes, whales, and dolphins. In these species, small hindlimb buds initially form. However, they do not develop, as the AER either does not form or is not maintained.

Several members of the *Fgf* family are expressed in the AER (*Fgf4, 8, 9,* and *17*). These factors are key regulators of limb outgrowth (Fig. 18-5). Beads soaked in *Fgfs* and transplanted to the tip of a limb bud following AER removal can proxy for the AER and maintain limb outgrowth. Moreover, there is redundancy in their function such that several different *Fgfs* can proxy for the AER and for each other. For example, limbs lacking *Fgf4, 9,* or *17* are normal. Gene inactivation of *Fgf8* in mice results in the formation of a much smaller limb bud, affecting growth of all of the limb segments. In these limbs, *Fgf8* function is rescued by *Fgf4*, as gene inactivation of both *Fgf8* and *Fgf4* results in increased apoptosis of the limb mesenchymal cells and completely abolishes limb outgrowth.

Fgf signaling, in conjunction with expression of T-box genes and Retinoic acid signaling, is essential for the *initiation* of limb development. Strikingly, application of an *Fgf*-soaked bead into the interlimb flank of an early chick embryo induces the formation of an extra limb (Fig. 18-6). At the forelimb level, *Tbx5* induces *Fgf10* expression in the presumptive forelimb mesenchyme. *Fgf10* signaling in the mesoderm then induces *Wnt3a* (in the chick) in the overlying ectoderm. *Wnt3a* in turn induces *Fgf8* in the presumptive AER, which maintains *Fgf10* expression in the underlying mesenchyme and establishes a feedback loop between *Fgf8* and *Fgf10* to maintain limb outgrowth. The interplay between *Wnt3a* and *Fgf8* continues throughout development of the limb, with the misexpression of *Wnt3a* resulting in the induction of ectopic AER formation. Parallel processes occur in the mouse, where *Wnt/β-Catenin* signaling is required for both AER formation and maintenance.

How patterning is specified along the proximal-distal axis is still uncertain. One model to explain this patterning is called the **progress zone model**. The **progress zone** is a narrow zone of mesenchyme about 300 μm in width underlying the AER, where cells are thought to acquire **positional information** that will inform them of their final **positional address** along the proximal-distal axis (Fig. 18-7). Cells that exit the progress zone after a short residence are destined to form proximal structures such as the humerus. Cells with the longest residence in the progress zone become the most distal structures, that is, the phalanges. How cells actually acquire positional information during residence in the progress zone is unknown. However, a timing mechanism in which a cell counts the number of mitotic divisions was proposed in the late 1970s. Initial evidence for this model included the AER removal experiments discussed above—earlier removal affects the

18

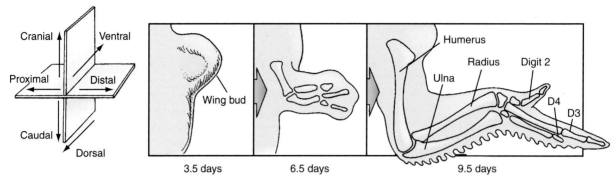

Figure 18-3. The limb buds of birds and other vertebrates (right panels) grow with respect to three axes of symmetry (left drawing): cranial-caudal, dorsal-ventral, and proximal-distal.

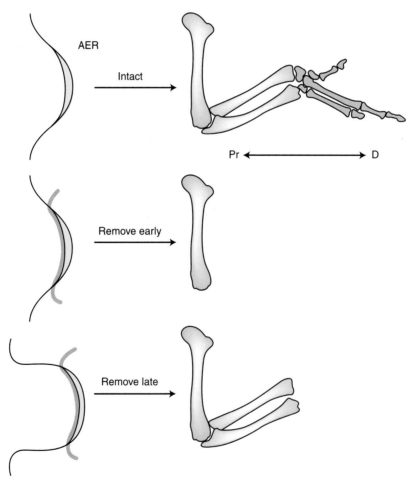

Figure 18-4. Skeletal development along the proximal (Pr)-distal (D) axis following removal of the apical ectodermal ridge (AER) at different stages of development.

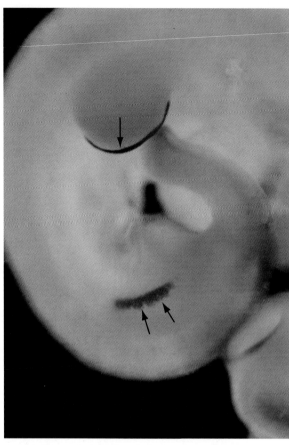

Figure 18-5. In situ hybridization showing that mRNA transcripts for *Fibroblast growth factor 8* are expressed in the ectoderm prior to limb bud outgrowth (two arrows mark expression in the hindlimb region near the bottom of the photograph) and then become discretely contained within the apical ectodermal ridge (single arrow) during later development. (The development of the forelimb bud is advanced with respect to that of the hindlimb bud.)

development of the majority of skeletal elements, whereas later removal only affects more distal structures (see Fig. 18-4).

However, it was later argued that cell death could account for these differences, leading to another model to explain proximal-distal patterning called the **early specification model** (see Fig. 18-7). For example, removal of the AER early in development results in cell death encompassing the autopod and zeugopod progenitors, whereas removal of the AER later in development results in

cell death now restricted to the domain of the presumptive autopod. The alternative model is also, in part, based on fate mapping studies, which have shown that progenitors of the stylopod, zeugopod, and autopod are already localized into discrete regions along the proximal-distal axis in the early limb bud. Therefore, labeling the progress zone early during limb development does not label all limb structures, as would be expected from the progress zone model, but only labels the digits, consistent with the early specification model. In the early specification model, *Fgf* signaling from the AER is required for the prespecified limb segments to develop and expand.

Regardless of which model is correct, insight into the molecular mechanisms that regulate growth of each region of the limb bud has been obtained. As described in Chapters 5 and 16, 4 clusters of *Hox* genes are sequentially activated in vertebrates (including humans) following the 3' to 5' sequence along the DNA of the four respective chromosomes. Moreover, the most 5' members of the *Hoxd* and *Hoxa* clusters (9 to 13) are coordinately expressed in nested cranial-caudal and proximal-distal domains within the growing limb bud (Fig. 18-8). This temporal and nested expression is known as **temporal and spatial colinearity**. Ultimately, the expression of each of the 5' *Hoxd* genes (along with those of the *Hoxa* group) can be correlated with development of specific skeletal elements of upper and lower limb segments. For example, in the forelimb, *Hoxd9* is expressed within the segment forming the scapula; *Hoxd9* and *Hoxd10* within the arm (containing the humerus); *Hoxd9*, *Hoxd10*, and *Hoxd11* within the forearm and proximal wrist (containing ulna, radius, and proximal carpals); *Hoxd9*, *Hoxd10*, *Hoxd11*, and *Hoxd12* within the distal wrist (containing distal carpals); and *Hoxd9*, *Hoxd10*, *Hoxd11*, *Hoxd12*, and *Hoxd13* within the hand and fingers (containing metacarpals and phalanges; Fig. 18-9). These genes are required for growth of the different regions of the limb bud.

The requirement for *Hox* genes in regional growth of the limb bud is directly shown by the knockouts of multiple paralogs of *Hox* genes. For example, in forelimbs lacking *Hoxa11* and *Hoxd11* genes, the radius and ulna are completely lacking (Fig. 18-10). Analysis of these mutants has shown that there is reduced *Fgf* signaling, resulting in smaller skeletal condensations and delayed chondrocyte differentiation. Once these cartilaginous elements have formed, there is also a growth plate defect that significantly contributes to the hypoplasia/aplasia of these elements at birth.

18

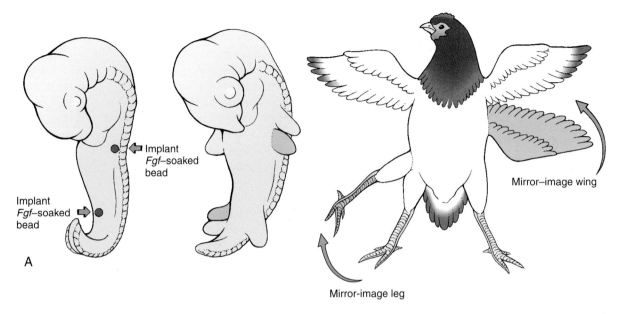

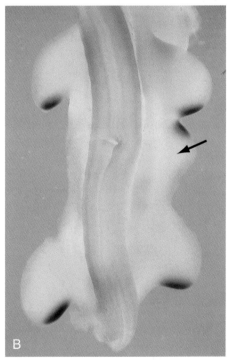

Figure 18-6. *Fgf*–soaked beads induce supernumerary limbs. *A*, Schematic drawing of the experimental procedure and results. *B*, Whole mount in situ hybridization shows *Shh* expression in the zone of polarization activity in each limb bud (two wing buds, two leg buds, and a supernumerary bud) of a chick embryo 48 hours after application of an *Fgf* bead. Arrow marks the induced supernumerary limb.

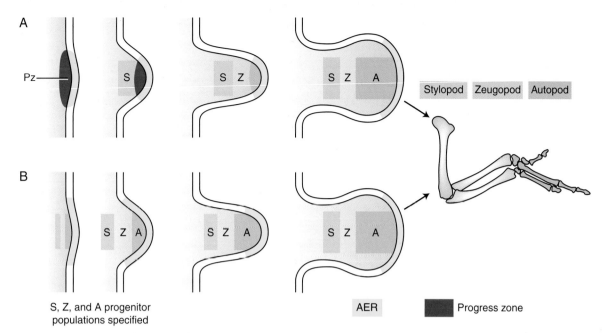

Pz

S

S Z

S Z A

Stylopod | Zeugopod | Autopod

S Z A

S Z A

S Z A

S, Z, and A progenitor
populations specified

AER

Progress zone

Figure 18-7. Two models used to explain patterning along the proximal-distal axis. *A*, Progress zone model; *B*, Early specification model.

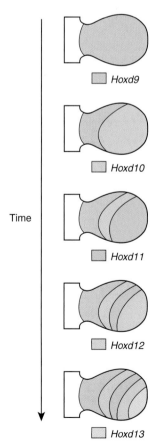

Hoxd9

Hoxd10

Time

Hoxd11

Hoxd12

Hoxd13

Figure 18-8. Progressive expression of *Hoxd* paralogs over time and space.

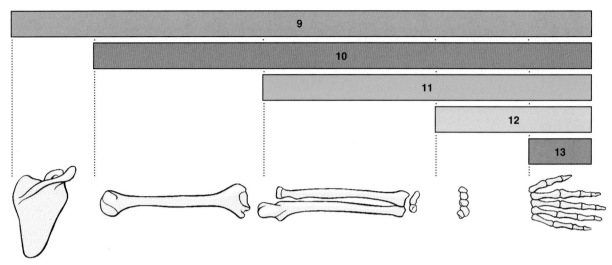

Figure 18-9. *Hoxd* gene expression patterns in relation to definitive segments of the upper limb.

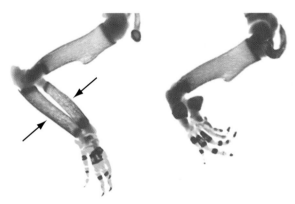

Figure 18-10. Aplasia of the radius and ulna (zeugopod) following gene inactivation of the *Hox11* paralogs. Left, wild-type mouse (arrows mark zeugopod); right, mutant mouse (i.e., forelimb lacks *Hoxa11* and *d11* expression).

Morphogenesis of Limb Bud

Once the AER has been established, the limb continues to grow with development occurring predominantly along the proximal-distal axis. Proliferation and growth is also slightly higher on the dorsal side of the limb bud, resulting in a ventral curvature of the developing limbs. Later development takes place as follows (Fig. 18-11).

Day 33. In the upper limb, the **hand plate, forearm, arm,** and **shoulder** regions can be distinguished. In the lower limb, a somewhat rounded cranial part can be distinguished from a more tapering caudal part. The distal tip of the tapering caudal part will form the foot.

Day 37. In the hand plate of the upper limb, a central **carpal region** is surrounded by a thinner crescentic rim, the **digital plate**, which will form the fingers. In the lower limb, the **thigh, leg,** and **foot** have become distinct.

Day 38. Finger rays (more generally, **digital rays**) are visible as radial thickenings in the digital plate of the upper limb. The tips of the finger rays project slightly, producing a crenulated rim on the digital plate. A process of **programmed cell death** in the **necrotic zones** between the digital rays will gradually sculpt the digital rays out of the digital plate by removing intervening tissue. This will free the fingers and toes. Although by tradition the term *necrotic* is used, the cells in these areas actually die by **apoptosis**, not necrosis. The lower limb bud has increased in length, and a clearly defined **footplate** has formed on the distal end of the bud.

Day 44. In the upper limb, the distal margin of the digital plate is deeply notched and the grooves between the finger rays are deeper. The bend where the elbow will form along the proximal-distal axis is becoming defined. **Toe rays** are visible in the digital plate of the foot, but the rim of the plate is not yet crenulated.

Day 47. The entire upper limb has undergone **ventral flexion** (Fig. 18-12*A*; see Fig. 18-11). The lower limb has also begun to flex toward the midline. The toe rays are more prominent, although the margin of the digital plate is still smooth (see Fig. 18-11).

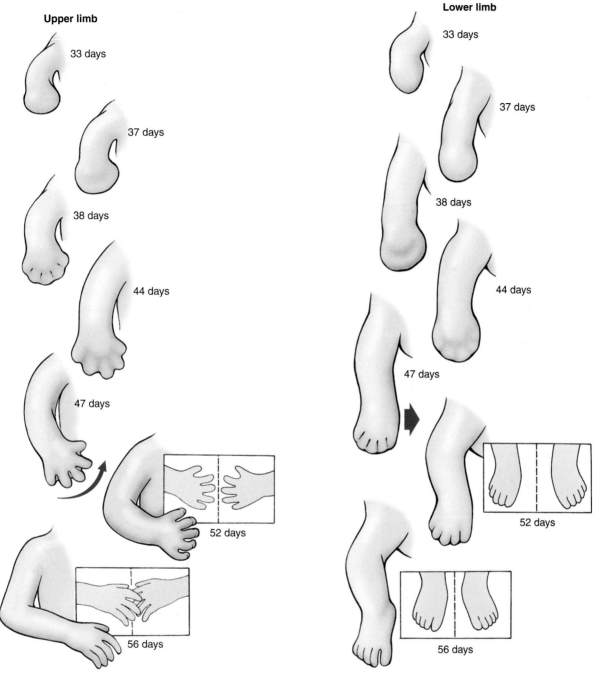

Figure 18-11. Development of the upper and lower limb buds occurs between the 5th and 8th weeks. Every stage in the development of the lower limb bud takes place later than in the upper limb bud.

18

Day 52. The upper limbs are bent at the elbows, and the fingers have developed distal swellings called **tactile pads** (Fig. 18-12*B*; see Fig. 18-11). The hands are slightly flexed at the wrists and meet at the midline in front of the cardiac eminence. The legs are longer, and the feet have begun to approach each other at the midline. The rim of the digital plate is notched.

Day 56. All regions of the arms and legs are well defined, including the tactile pads on the toes (Fig. 18-12*C*). The fingers of the two hands overlap at the midline.

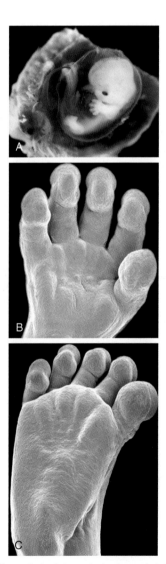

Figure 18-12. Human limbs during early development. *A*, By 7 weeks, the digits are clearly visible in both upper and lower extremities. *B, C,* Scanning electron micrograph showing the tactile pads in the hands and feet, respectively, of human embryos.

IN THE RESEARCH LAB

SPECIFICATION OF CRANIAL-CAUDAL AXIS

The cranial-caudal (anterior-posterior) axis is determined by signals from a small region of mesenchyme in the caudal part of the limb bud known as the **zone of polarizing activity** (ZPA). Transplantation of the ZPA to the cranial portion of the limb bud induces mirror-image digit duplications (Fig. 18-13). Classic experiments originally showed that the number of ZPA cells transplanted or the length of exposure of the cranial limb bud cells to the ZPA signal determined the cranial-caudal identity of the digits that formed. If more ZPA cells were transplanted or cells were exposed for a longer time, the resulting ectopic digits would have a more caudal identity. This suggested that a **morphogen** is produced by the ZPA that diffuses across the cranial-caudal axis. A high dose of the morphogen would induce the caudal digits, whereas progressively lower concentrations would induce the more cranial digits.

In support of the morphogen model, *Sonic hedgehog* (*Shh*) is expressed in the ZPA (Fig. 18-14*A*), and ectopic expression of *Shh* at the cranial side of the limb bud induces digit duplications. Retinoic acid (RA) signaling is also strongest in the caudal limb bud, and ectopic application of RA at the cranial side of the limb bud can also induce *Shh* expression and digit duplications. However, genetic fate mapping of the ZPA cells and their descendents, as well as genetic fate mapping of the cells that receive the *Shh* signal, has challenged a simple diffusion morphogen model. These studies have shown that patterning of the digits is achieved by a combination of diffusion of a morphogen and the duration of exposure to *Shh* signaling. Specifically, the fate map of the ZPA cells showed that 1) these cells sweep cranially from the ZPA (and the source of *Shh*), ultimately contributing to digits 3 to 5; and 2) *all* cells in digits 4 and 5 are derived from the ZPA, but cells in digit 3 arise from both ZPA and non–ZPA descendents. By labeling the ZPA cells at different stages of development, it was found that digit 5 arises from the ZPA after the development of digit 4; that is, because the ZPA is the source of *Shh* signaling, digit 5 is exposed to *Shh* signaling for the longest period of time (Fig. 18-14*B, C*).

In the converse experiment, the fate of the cells receiving a *Shh* signal (that is, cells expressing *Gli1*, a transcriptional target of *Shh*) was determined. In this case it was found that digits 2 to 5 have responded to *Shh* signaling at some point during their development. Combining these data, the current model proposes that the most cranial digit develops independently of *Shh* signaling (Fig. 18-14*D*); this is consistent with the formation of one

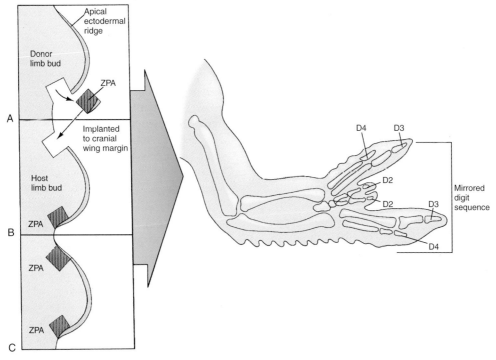

Figure 18-13. Transplantation of the zone of polarizing activity (ZPA) of one limb bud to the cranial edge of another induces mirror-image polydactyly.

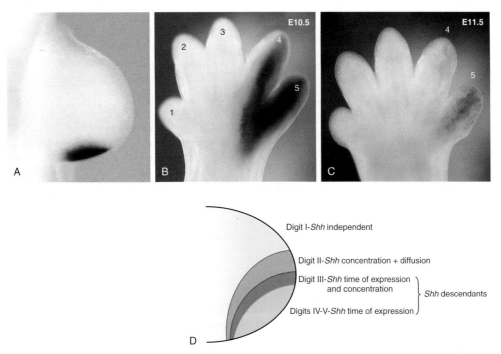

Figure 18-14. Cranial-caudal patterning of the limb bud. *A,* Expression of *Shh* in the zone of polarizing activity (ZPA) of the limb bud of a mouse embryo. *B, C,* Fate maps of ZPA descendents when labeled at E10.5 and E11.5, respectively. Cells formerly in the ZPA express a reporter gene, allowing them to be traced over time. *D,* Model for explaining *Shh*-mediated cranial-caudal patterning of the digits.

digit (presumably digit 1) in the *Shh* mutant hindlimb (Fig. 18-15*B*). Digit 2 depends on diffusion of *Shh* for its development (as it does not arise from the ZPA), whereas digits 3 to 5 arise from the *Shh*-expressing cells themselves (see Fig. 18-14*B, C*). The cells that stay in the ZPA the longest form the most caudal digit 5. This model is also consistent with the limb phenotype of the *dispatched 1* mouse mutant. *Dispatched 1* is required for *Shh* movement/signaling in non-*Shh* expressing cells; in this mutant, digit 2 does not form.

Shh also regulates outgrowth of the limb bud by maintaining *Fgf* expression in the AER. *Fgfs* in turn maintain *Shh* expression in the ZPA and *Hoxd11-13* expression in the limb mesenchyme. Therefore, in the *Shh* mutant, as in the *Fgf8* mutant, the limb bud is severely truncated, but in this case most of the distal structures are absent (Fig. 18-15*A, B*). *Shh* maintains the expression of *Fgfs* in the AER via the expression of *Gremlin*, a secreted *Bmp* antagonist that blocks the repressive actions of *Bmps* on AER function (Fig. 18-15*E*). In *Gremlin* mouse mutants, *Fgf4* and *8* expression is either absent or reduced, respectively, again resulting in limb truncations.

The limb bud is prepatterned across the cranial-caudal axis prior to the expression of *Shh*. *Gli3* and the *Aristaless-like 4* paired-type homeodomain protein *Alx4* function in the cranial mesenchyme to restrict the expression of *Hand2* to the caudal mesenchyme prior to *Shh* expression (Fig. 18-15*D*). *Shh* expression is then activated in the caudal mesenchyme by the combined action of Retinoic acid, *Hand2*, 5′ *Hox* genes, and *Fgf* signaling (see Fig. 18-15*E*). The *Strong's luxoid* mutant, which is characterized by polydactyly, results from mutations in *Alx4*. In this mutant, the prepatterning that normally restricts *Hand2* to the caudal limb bud does not occur. Consequently, an ectopic domain of *Shh* expression forms in the cranial mesenchyme (Fig. 18-16). Ectopic *Shh* or *Ihh* expression in the cranial limb bud has also been observed in other polydactylous mutants, including the *hemimelic extra toes* (*Xt*; discussed in the following paragraph), *recombination-induced mutant 4*, *sasquatch*, and *doublefoot* mouse mutants.

Shh signaling is mediated by *Gli3*. In the absence of *Shh*, *Gli3* is processed to its shorter form, which acts as a potent transcriptional repressor (*Gli3R*; *R* indicates the repressor form). In the presence of *Shh* signaling, this processing is prevented and now the full-length *Gli3* protein acts as a weak transcriptional activator. *Gli3* is mutated in the *Xt* mouse mutant, which exhibits hemimelia and polydactyly with between 6 to 11 morphologically indistinguishable digits (see Fig. 18-15*C*). As *Gli3* function, which normally restricts *Shh* expression to the caudal mesenchyme, is

absent, *Shh* is ectopically expressed in the cranial mesenchyme. However, unlike the polydactylous mutants discussed above, polydactyly is not the result of excess *Shh* signaling because the compound *Shh/Xt* mutants have the same phenotype as *Xt* mutants. Instead, polydactyly in the *Xt* mutant results from extended domains of *Hox* gene and *Gremlin* expression in the cranial mesenchyme, which are normally repressed by Gli3R. The double compound mutant shows that the failure of limb outgrowth in the *Shh* null mutant is due to ectopic *Gli3R* in the caudal mesenchyme. Therefore, in the absence of both functional *Shh* and *Gli3*, outgrowth can occur and the limb forms, but the digits are not patterned.

SPECIFICATION OF DORSAL-VENTRAL AXIS

The third axis of the limb, the dorsal-ventral axis, is first regulated by signals from the mesenchyme and then from the ectoderm. If just the ectodermal covering of the limb bud is surgically rotated 180 degrees with respect to the mesenchyme, the dorsal-ventral polarity of the skeletal elements that are subsequently formed is reversed. *Wnt7a*, which is expressed in the dorsal ectoderm, is one regulator of dorsal-ventral patterning. In the *Wnt7a* knockout mouse, the paws are ventralized with foot pads forming on the dorsal surface. *Wnt7a* activity is mediated by the *Lmx1b* homeobox gene, which is expressed in the dorsal mesenchyme. *Lmx1b*-mutant mouse limbs lack dorsal structures, whereas ectopic expression of *Lmx1b* in chick limb buds is able to dorsalize the limb. Mutation of *LMX1B* in humans leads to **nail-patella syndrome** (see Table 18-2), indicating that *dorsal* structures in the limb are mainly affected when this gene is not functional. *Wnt7a* also regulates *Shh* expression. Hence, in *Wnt7a* knockout mice, in addition to dorsal-ventral defects, there are abnormalities in limb outgrowth and the development of the caudal digits. The homeobox transcription factor *Engrailed 1* is expressed in the ventral ectoderm and prevents the expression of *Wnt7a*. In the *Engrailed 1* null mouse, *Wnt7a* is ectopically expressed in the ventral ectoderm, and the ventral limb bud is dorsalized. *Bmp* signaling in the ventral ectoderm induces both *Engrailed 1* expression and the initial expression of *Fgf8* in the AER. This is in contrast to a later role in limb development for *Bmps*, which is to inhibit AER function.

CESSATION OF LIMB OUTGROWTH AND MORPHOGENESIS OF AUTOPOD

Once the digital rays have started to form, the identity of each digit is ultimately determined by signals from each region of adjacent caudal interdigital mesenchyme. If this mesenchyme is removed, the immediately cranial digit will

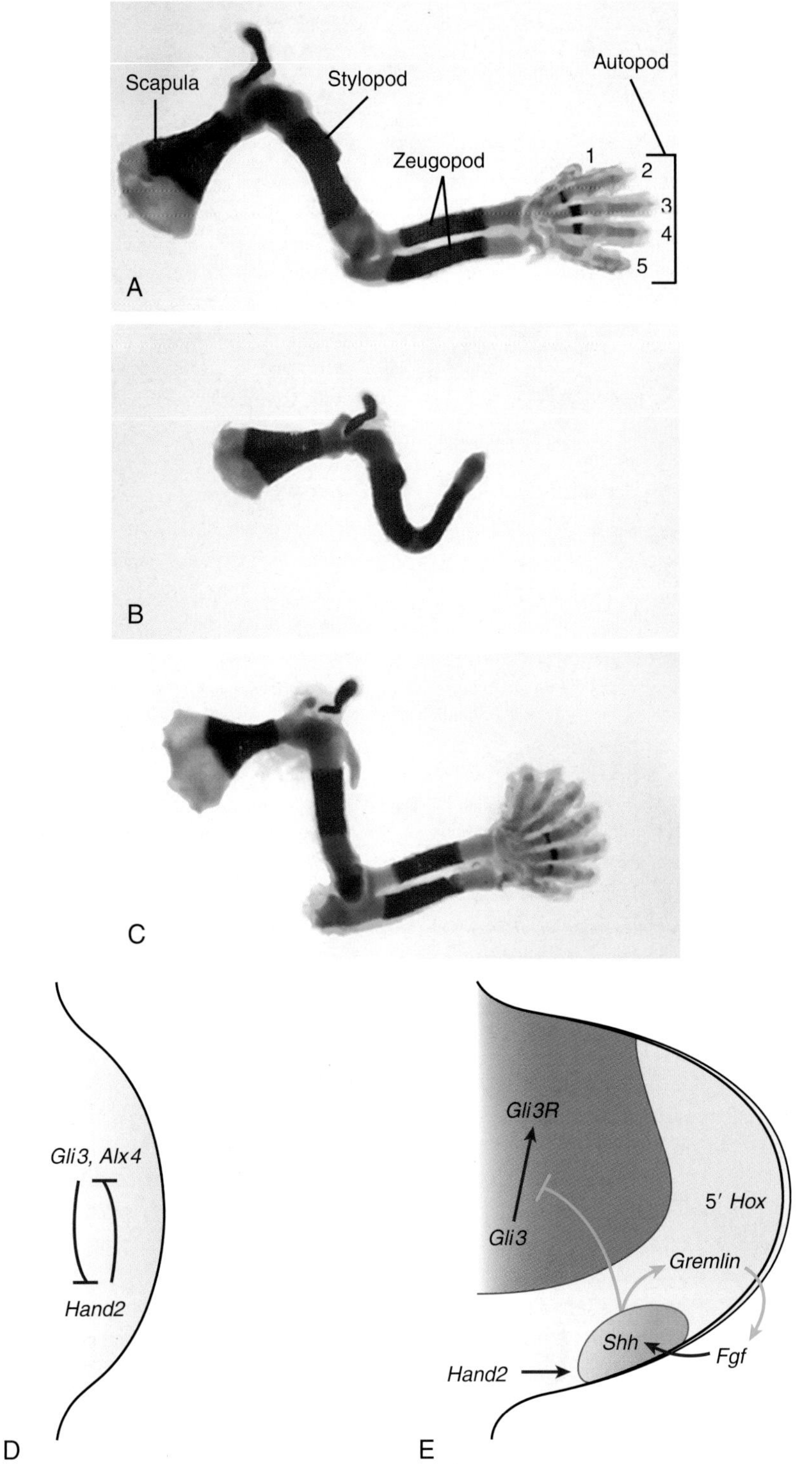

Figure 18-15. Roles for *Shh* signaling in the mouse forelimb. *A-C,* Skeletal structures in limbs of wild-type, *Shh* mutant, and *Gli3 Xt* mutant mice. *B* and *C* illustrate that *Shh* signaling is required for both outgrowth and cranial-caudal patterning. *D, E,* Schemes showing signaling interactions during limb development prior to and after the onset of *Shh* signaling, respectively.

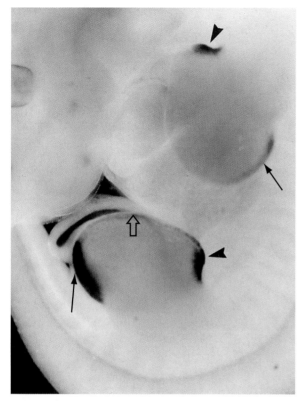

Figure 18-16. Gene expression in the *Strong's luxoid* mouse mutant limb labeled with double probes for *Shh* and *Fgf4*. In situ hybridization showing *Shh* mRNA in its normal location in the zone of polarizing activity (arrows) in both the forelimb and hindlimb buds, and at an ectopic cranial location in each bud (arrowheads). Due to the ectopic expression of *Shh*, *Fgf4*, which is normally restricted to the caudal AER is now extended throughout the craniocaudal extent of the AER (open arrow).

be cranialized. For example, removal of the interdigital mesenchyme between digits 3 and 4 will result in the morphologic transformation of digit 3 to one with the identity of digit 2. Furthermore, bisection of developing digit 3 with the insertion of a piece of foil to prevent healing results in the formation of an ectopic digit: the caudal digit has the original identity (in this case, digit 3), whereas the digit arising from the cranial part of the bisected digit has the characteristics of digit 2. A gradient of *Bmp* signaling, with highest levels caudally, has been implicated in this specification, and application of a bead soaked in the *Bmp* antagonist *Noggin* can cranialize a digit.

Patterning and the formation of additional structures stops when the caudal limb cells can no longer express *Gremlin* in response to *Shh*. This happens because cells that express or have expressed *Shh* (i.e. those of the ZPA) are unable to express *Gremlin*. Therefore, as the ZPA derivatives sweep cranially during development, the signaling loop

between *Shh* and *Fgfs* breaks down. This is because *Gremlin* which normally antagonizes the *Bmp* repression of *Fgf* expression in the AER is lost. However, maintenance of *Fgf* expression, for example by placing *Shh* beads into the interdigital mesenchyme or misexpressing a *Bmp* antagonist in the AER, prolongs limb outgrowth and can increase the number of phalanges that form.

Finally, the interdigital mesenchyme is removed by **programmed cell death**, thereby freeing the digits and allowing the mobility required to carry out their specialized tasks. This removal does not occur in the duck foot, which is specialized for swimming, and also does not occur in **soft-tissue syndactyly**, which is a frequent clinical observation. Members of the *Bmp* family, *Bmp2, 4,* and *7*, regulate interdigital cell death. Manipulation that increases *Bmp* activity leads to increased cell death in the interdigital necrotic zone (INZ), whereas decreasing *Bmp* activity by expressing dominant negative *Bmp* receptors prevents INZ cell death and leads to digital webbing. *Bmps* mediate interdigital cell death by signaling to the AER to decrease the expression of the cell survival factors, *Fgf4* and *8*. Therefore, excess *Fgf* signaling can result in syndactyly. This is seen in **Pfeiffer, Apert,** and **Jackson-Weiss syndromes**, which are due to constitutive activation of the *FGF8* receptor, *FGFR2*. Other regions of programmed cell death are found within the AER, in the mesenchyme at the cranial and caudal limit of the AER, and in the mesenchyme between the radius and ulna or between the fibula and tibia. The developmental function of these areas of cell death is less clear, although the regions at the edges of the AER may determine the AER length and hence digit number.

IN THE CLINIC

CONGENITAL ANOMALIES OF LIMBS

Humans exhibit a wide variety of limb defects. In general, these fall into four categories. In **reduction defects**, part of the limb is missing, a condition called **meromelia** (Fig. 18-17A), or an entire limb is missing, a condition called **amelia** (Fig. 18-17B). In **duplication defects**, supernumerary limb elements are present. Examples include **polydactyly** (i.e., the presence of entire extra digits; Fig. 18-17C), and **triphalangeal thumb** in which a third phalange is present rather than just the normal two (Fig. 18-17D). In **dysplasias**, there can be fusion of limb parts such as in **syndactyly** (i.e., fusion of digits; Fig. 18-17E), or **disproportionate growth**, in which a part of the limb is abnormally larger, smaller, longer, or shorter. In **deformations**, physical forces, for

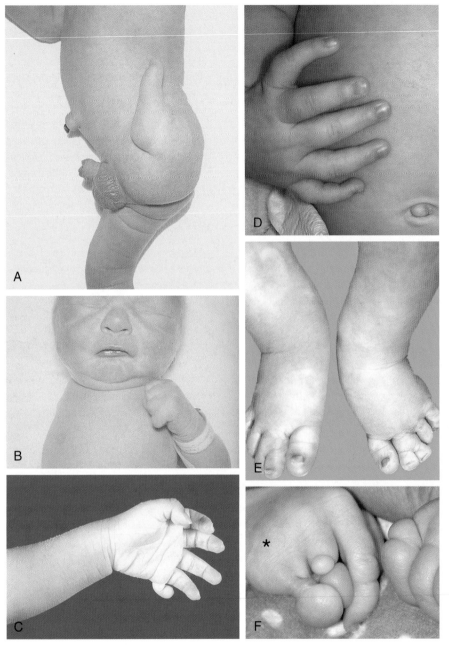

Figure 18-17. Limb defects in humans. *A*, Meromelia. In this example, the distal end of the infant's left lower limb has not completely formed. *B*, Amelia. In this example, the infant's entire right upper limb failed to form. *C*, Postaxial polydactyly (in this case, six digits). *D*, Right hand of an infant with a triphalangeal thumb (three phalanges in digit 1, rather than the normal two). *E*, Feet of an infant showing syndactyly; the bony elements of toes 2 and 3 are also fused. *F*, Hand of an infant with amniotic band–associated terminal limb defects. Note on the right hand, syndactyly (asterisk) proximal to the constriction and swelling distal to the constriction.

example, from **amniotic bands**, damage developing limbs (Fig. 18-17*F*). Table 18-1 lists a number of terms in common use to describe limb defects.

In addition to clinically significant defects of the limbs such as those just described, minor anomalies (variations of normal) are relatively common. Although a single **transverse palmar crease** (Fig. 18-18*A*) is often seen in infants with **trisomy 21 (Down syndrome)**, it is also found in 4% of normal newborns. Cutaneous syndactyly between toes 2 and 3 is considered a normal variant if the fusion extends less than one third the length of the toes (Fig. 18-18*B*).

Genetic Causes of Limb Anomalies

A variety of specific gene mutations causing limb anomalies have been characterized in humans (Table 18-2). The generation of animal models has highlighted the conservation of signaling pathways across species. For example, mutations in *Wnt3* (a member of the Drosophila *Wingless* family) have been linked to **tetra-amelia** in humans and other vertebrates, reflecting the requirement for *Wnt* signaling in limb bud initiation and outgrowth. Polydactyly occurs in **Greig cephalopolysyndactyly, Pallister-Hall**, and **post-axial polydactyly type A**, all due to mutations in *Gli3*, a component of *Shh* signaling pathway. The Greig cephalopolysyndactyly syndrome is due to loss of function of one copy of *GLI3* (i.e., haploinsufficiency), whereas in

Pallister-Hall, mutant GLI3 proteins are thought to retain some *GLI3* repressor activity. Ectopic activation or deletion of the normal *SHH* expression domain in humans also affects limb development. A 450 bp highly conserved **ZPA regulatory sequence** (ZRS) regulates *Shh* expression in the ZPA. Mutations in the ZRS sequence have been identified in the polydactylous mouse mutants *hx* and *m100081*, and in both of these mutants, *Shh* is ectopically expressed in the cranial limb mesenchyme. Similar ZRS mutations have been identified in humans with preaxial duplications, ranging from the mildest phenotype of a **triphalangeal thumb** to more severe phenotypes of up to several additional digits (**polydactyly**) on the hands and/or feet (an example of such a severe duplication in humans, although of unknown genetic cause, is shown in Fig. 18-19). A large 5 to 6 kb deletion in the *LMBR1* gene, which is adjacent to the *SHH* gene, has also been linked to **acheiropodia**, a severe defect that includes the absence of the hands and feet. It is very likely that this phenotype is the result of disruption of regulatory elements that control expression of *SHH* in the caudal limb bud.

Mutations in the transcription factor *TP73L* (also known as *P63*) result in **split-hand/split-foot type 4 syndome** Fig. 18-20*A*). These mutations can lead as well to **ectrodactyly-ectodermal dysplasia-clefting (EEC) syndrome**, which is in part also characterized by a split-hand and split-foot anomaly

Table 18-1 Some Common Terms for Limb Malformations

Term	Definition
Acheiropodia	Absence of the hands and feet
Adactyly	Absence of all the digits on a limb
Amelia, ectromelia	Absence of one or more limbs
Arachnodactyly	Elongated digits
Brachydactyly	Shortened digits
Camptodactyly	Flexion contracture of a finger (often fourth or fifth), which cannot be fully extended
Clinodactyly	Curving of fifth finger toward the fourth
Ectrodactyly	Longitudinal divisions of the autopod into two parts, often with absence of central digits (also called split-hand or split-foot malformation)
Meromelia	Absence of part of a limb
Mesomelia	Shortened zeugopod
Oligodactyly	Absence of any number of fingers or toes
Phocomelia	Absence of proximal limb structures
Polydactyly	Presence of extra digits or parts of digits
Rhizomelia	Shortened stylopod
Syndactyly	Fusion of digits
Synostosis	Fusion of bones or intervening soft tissue
Triphalangeal thumb	A thumb with 3 rather than 2 phalanges

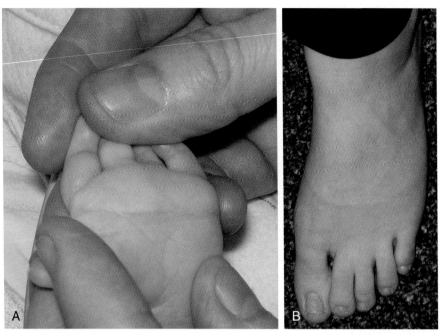

Figure 18-18. *A*, Single transverse palmar crease can occur in individuals with certain syndromes or can be a normal variant. *B*, Cutaneous syndactyly of toes 2 and 3, without the fusion of bony elements. This case would be considered a normal variant because cutaneous fusion extends less than one third of the length of the toes. Compare this case to that shown in Figure 18-17*E*.

Table 18-2 Examples of Human Mutations Affecting Limb Development

Gene	Human Syndrome	Effect on Limbs
ATPSK2	Spondyloepimetaphyseal dysplasia	Bowed long bones, brachydactyly, enlarged knee joints, joint degeneration
BBS1 (10 others)	Bardet-Biedl	Postaxial polydactyly, brachydactyly
EVC	Ellis-van Creveld	Short limbs, post-axial polydactyly
FANCA (10 others)	Fanconi anemia	Radial/thumb aplasia/hypoplasia, preaxial polydactyly
FGFR1, FGFR2	Pfeiffer	Broad digit 1, brachydactyly, syndactyly
FGFR2	Apert	Syndactyly (synostotic or cutaneous) broad thumbs
FGFR2	Jackson-Weiss	2-3 toe syndactyly, broad halluces
FGFR3	Achondroplasia/hypochondroplasia	Brachydactyly, rhizomelia
GL13	Greig cephalopolysyndactyly Pallister-Hall	Postaxial (hands) or preaxial (feet) polydactyly, syndactyly, broad digit 1 Post-axial polydactyly, syndactyly
GPC3	Simpson-Golabi-Behmel	Brachydactyly, post-axial polydactyly
HOXA13	Hand-foot-genital	Short thumbs, short/absent halluces, carpal fusions, delayed ossification
HOXD11	Radioulnar synostois with amegakaryocytic thrombocytopenia	Proximal fusion of radius and ulna
HOXD13	Synpolydactyly Brachydactyly type D and E	Syndactyly (synostotic), polydactyly (4th and 5th digits), ectrodactyly Brachydactyly

Continued

18

Table 18-2 Examples of Human Mutations Affecting Limb Development—cont'd

Gene	Human Syndrome	Effect on Limbs
LMX1B	Nail-patella syndrome	Hypoplasia/aplasia of the patella, dysplastic nails, club foot
NIPBL	Cornelia de Lange	Small hands/feet, ectrodactyly, syndactyly, meromelia/amelia
OFD1	Oral-facial-digital type 1	Brachydactyly, syndactyly, polydactyly (pre- or postaxial)
TP73L (P63)	Ectrodactyly	Split-hand/Split-foot malformation, syndactyly
ROR2	Robinow Brachydactyly type B1	Mesomelia, small hands, broad thumb, dysplastic nails Brachydactyly
SALL1	Townes-Brocks	Preaxial polydactyly, bifid or finger-like thumb
SHH	Preaxial polydactyly Acheiropodia	Polydactyly Absence of hands/feet
SHOX	Léri-Weill dyschondrosteosis Langer mesomelic dysplasia	Mesomelia, brachydactyly Mesomelia, limb bowing, fibular hypoplasia
SOX9	Campomelic dysplasia	Bowed long bones, club foot
TBX3	Ulnar-mammary	Ulnar hypoplasia/aplasia, absent 3rd, 4th, or 5th digits, postaxial polydactyly
TBX5	Holt-Oram	Absent, bifid, or finger-like thumb, ectrodactyly, meromelia
TWIST	Saethre-Chotzen	Brachydactyly, syndactyly (soft tissue), bifid phalanges

See www.ncbi.nlm.nih.gov/entrez/query.fcgi?db=OMIM for further details of the syndromes.

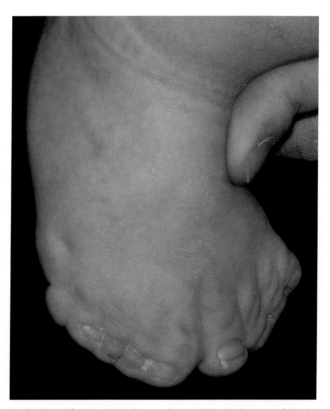

Figure 18-19. Foot of a child with mirror hands and feet (Laurin-Sandrow syndrome). Although the cause of the duplication is unknown in this syndrome, based on experiments in animal models it is likely to involve ectopic *SHH* signaling in the cranial limb bud mesenchyme.

(a condition referred to as **ectrodactyly**). In the *p63* mouse mutants, the AER does not form appropriately and there is decreased *Fgf8* signaling, providing a potential mechanism as the AER (or part of the AER) may degenerate prematurely. A split-hand or split-foot anomaly is also seen in the mouse *Dlx5/6* double mutants. *Dlx5* and *Dlx6* are expressed in the AER. In the mouse *Dlx5/6* double mutants, analysis of AER markers clearly shows that the AER degenerates centrally, providing a mechanism for the loss of the central digits (Fig. 18-20*B*, *C*).

Reflecting their key roles in limb outgrowth, mutations in the *Hox* gene family have been identified in human syndromes. Mutation in *HOXD13* results in **synpolydactyly and brachydactyly types D** and **E** (Fig. 18-21), whereas mutation in *HOXA13* results in **hand-foot-genital syndrome**. *HOXD11* mutations result in defects in more proximal limb structures in **radioulnar synostosis** (a partial or full fusion of the radius and ulnar with one another) with **amegakaryocytic thrombocytopenia syndrome**.

Mutations in three members of the T-box family of transcription factors have been shown to cause limb malformations. Mutation in *TBX3* results in the autosomal dominant disorder **ulnar-mammary syndrome**. In this syndrome, the caudal side of the limb is affected, with reduction or complete loss of the ulna and posterior digits, as well as mammary gland defects. This phenotype is recapitulated in the *Tbx3* mutant mouse, where analysis of the limb buds has shown that *Shh* is not expressed,

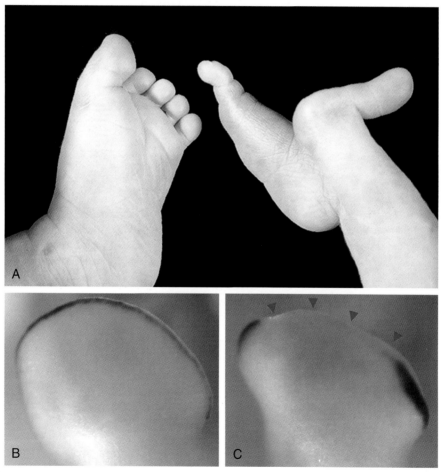

Figure 18-20. Split-foot anomaly. *A*, Photograph showing a child with a unilateral split-foot anomaly. *B*, *C*, *Fgf8* expression in a wild-type mouse limb bud and in the *Dlx5/6* double mutant limb bud. Note the absence of *Fgf8* expression in the central region of the apical ectodermal ridge (AER). Failure of this portion of the AER to develop properly likely explains split-hand and split-foot anomalies, such as shown in part *A*.

18

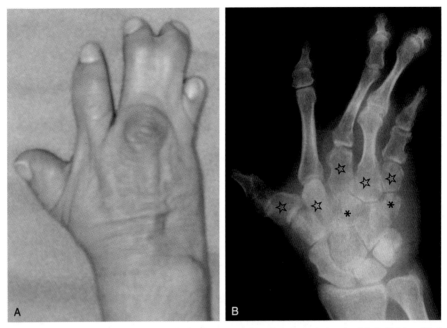

Figure 18-21. Hand, *A*, and radiograph, *B*, of a homozygous individual with a *HOXD13* mutation. Note syndactyly of digits III, IV, and V, their single knuckle, the transformation of metacarpals I, II, III, and V to short carpal-like bones (stars), two additional carpal bones (asterisks), and short second phalanges. The radius, ulna, and proximal carpal bones appear normal.

explaining the loss of caudal limb structures. *Tbx4* and *Tbx5* expression is restricted to the hindlimb and forelimb, respectively, and this is reflected in the human syndromes resulting from mutation in these genes. Mutation in *TBX4* causes **small patella syndrome**, whereas mutation in *TBX5* results in **Holt-Oram syndrome**, which affects the forelimb (but not hindlimb) and heart (see Table 18-2).

The **craniosynostosis syndromes**, **Apert** and **Pfeiffer** (discussed in Chs. 5 and 16), which result from mutations in *FGF RECEPTORS*, are also associated with limb defects. These include syndactyly and broad, short thumbs and big toes.

Another classical multiple malformation syndrome associated with limb anomalies is **Cornelia de Lange syndrome** (CdLS), first described in 1933. Most patients with this syndrome have upper limb anomalies ranging from small hands to severe limb reduction defects (Fig. 18-22). It was recently discovered that 50% of CdLS patients have mutations in the *NIPBL* gene (ortholog of the Drosophila *Nipped-B–like* gene), which encodes a protein called *Delangin*. The function of this protein is unclear, but it seems to regulate the activity of other genes involved in development via its role in regulating chromatin organization.

Nongenetic Causes of Limb Defects

As with other regions of the body, genetic mutations and environmental causes can result in abnormalities. A variety of drugs and environmental **teratogens** have been shown to cause limb defects in experimental animals. Some of these agents are also associated with limb defects in humans. Not surprisingly, agents that influence general cell metabolism or cell proliferation are likely to cause limb defects if administered during the period of limb morphogenesis. Such agents include chemotherapeutic agents like **5'-fluoro-2-deoxyuridine**, an inhibitor of thymidylate synthetase, and **acetazolamide**, a carbonic anhydrase inhibitor used for treatment of glaucoma.

Other drugs that induce limb malformations in laboratory animals and humans are the anticonvulsants **valproic acid** and **phenytoin**, the anticoagulant **warfarin**, and (as discussed in the "Clinical Taster" for this chapter) the antileprosy, anticancer drug **thalidomide**. Nontherapeutic drugs that can induce limb malformations include **alcohol** and **cocaine**. Children with **fetal alcohol syndrome** can have hypoplasia of the distal digits, joint contractures, and radial limb defects. Cocaine abuse in pregnancy is associated with limb reduction defects.

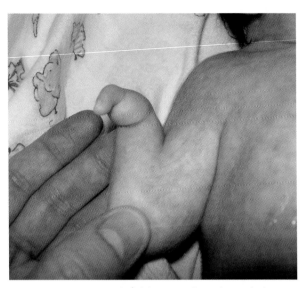

Figure 18-22. Severe upper limb defect in an infant with Cornelia de Lange syndrome. The autopod terminates in a single digit (monodactyly).

Fetal-maternal environmental factors associated with limb defects include **gestational diabetes, congenital varicella infection**, and **hyperthermia**. Limb defects can also result from physical factors. For example, a constricted uterine environment caused by **oligohydramnios** (insufficient amniotic fluid) or reduced fetal movement can result in **club foot deformity (talipes equinovarus**; Fig. 18-23), and early **chorionic villus sampling** has been linked to an increased frequency of limb malformations. Vascular compromise in the fetus, due to vessel malformation or clots, has been proposed to be the cause of unilateral limb anomalies seen in **Poland anomaly**.

Tissue Origins of Limb Structures

Quail-chick transplantation chimeras (discussed in Ch. 5) have been used to study the cell populations that give rise to the various elements of the limbs. These studies have demonstrated that the lateral plate mesoderm gives rise to the **bones, ligaments, tendons**, and **dermis** of the limbs. In contrast, the limb **musculature** and **endothelial cells** migrate into the developing limb bud from the somites (discussed in Ch. 8), and the **melanocytes** and **Schwann cells** of the limb are derived from migrating neural crest cells (as occurs elsewhere in the body; discussed in Ch. 4).

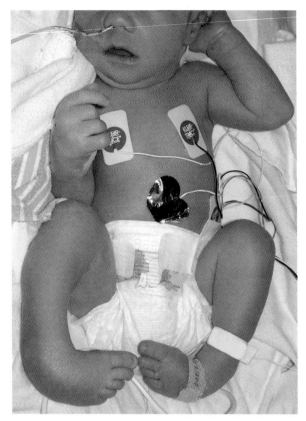

Figure 18-23. Newborn infant with bilateral talipes equinovarus deformity (club foot).

Differentiation of Limb Bones

With the exception of the clavicle, which is in part a membrane bone, the limb skeletal elements form by endochondral ossification (discussed in Ch. 8). The mesenchyme of the limb buds first begins to condense in the 5th week. In general, the bones of the upper limb form slightly earlier than their counterparts in the lower limb. The proximal elements (i.e., the femur and humerus in the stylopod) differentiate first and the distal elements (i.e., the digits in the autopod) differentiate last.

By the end of the 5th week, the mesenchymal condensation that will give rise to the proximal limb skeleton (the scapula and humerus in the upper limb; the pelvic bones and femur in the lower limb) are distinct. By the early 6th week, the mesenchymal anlagen of the distal limb skeleton is distinct in the upper and lower limbs, and chondrification commences in the

18

humerus, ulna, and radius. By the end of the 6th week, the carpal and metacarpal elements also begin to chondrify. In the lower limb, the femur, the tibia, and (to a lesser extent) the fibula begin to chondrify by the middle of the 6th week, and the tarsals and metatarsals begin to chondrify near the end of the 6th week. By the early 7th week, all the skeletal elements of the upper limb except the distal phalanges of the second to fifth digits are undergoing chondrification. By the end of the 7th week, the distal phalanges of the hand have begun to chondrify, and chondrification is also underway in all the elements of the lower limb except the distal row of phalanges. The distal phalanges of the toes do not chondrify until the 8th week.

The primary ossification centers of most of the limb bones appear in weeks 7 to 12. By the early 7th week, ossification has commenced in the clavicle, followed by the humerus, radius, and ulna at the end of the 7th week. Ossification begins in the femur and tibia in the 8th week. During the 9th week, the scapula and ilium begin to ossify, followed in the next 3 weeks by the metacarpals, metatarsals, distal phalanges, proximal phalanges, and finally the middle phalanges. The ischium and pubis begin to ossify in the 15th and 20th weeks, respectively, and ossification of the calcaneus finally begins at about 16 weeks. Some of the smaller carpal and tarsal bones do not start ossification until early childhood.

Synovial joints (discussed in Ch. 8) separate most of the skeletal elements. **Synchondroidal or fibrous joints**, such as those connecting the bones of the pelvis, also develop from interzones between forming bony elements, but the interzone mesenchyme simply differentiates into a single layer of fibrocartilage.

Innervation of Developing Limb Bud

As described in Chapter 10, each spinal nerve splits into main branches, the dorsal and ventral rami, shortly after it exits the spinal cord. The limb muscles are innervated by branches of the ventral rami of spinal nerves C5 through T1 (for the upper limb) and L4 through S3 (for the lower limb). Muscles originating in the dorsal muscle mass are served by *dorsal* branches of these ventral rami (arising from the LMCl neurons; discussed in the following "In the Research Lab"), whereas muscles originating in the ventral muscle mass are served by *ventral* branches

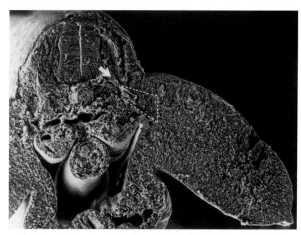

Figure 18-24. Scanning electron micrograph of a transversely sectioned embryo showing axons (arrow) entering the base of the limb bud (dotted area).

of the ventral rami (arising from the LMCm neurons; discussed in the following "In the Research Lab"). Thus, the innervation of a muscle shows whether it originated in the dorsal or the ventral muscle mass.

As illustrated in Figure 18-24, the motor axons that innervate the limbs perform an intricate feat of pathfinding to reach their target muscles. This is not dependent on muscles, as axons migrate almost normally in limbs lacking muscles. The ventral ramus axons destined for the limbs apparently travel to the base of the limb bud by growing along **permissive pathways**. The **growth cones** of these axons avoid or are unable to penetrate regions of dense mesenchyme or mesenchyme-containing *Glycosaminoglycans*. The axons heading for the lower limb are thus deflected around the developing pelvic anlagen. In both the upper and lower limb buds, the axons from the nerves cranial to the limb bud grow toward the craniodorsal side of the limb bud, whereas the axons from the nerves caudal to the limb bud grow toward the ventrocaudal side of the limb bud (Fig. 18-25).

Once the motor axons arrive at the base of the limb bud, they mix in a specific pattern to form the **brachial plexus** of the upper limb and the **lumbosacral plexus** of the lower limb. This zone thus constitutes a **decision-making region** for the axons (discussed in the following "In the Research Lab").

Once the axons have sorted out in the plexus, the growth cones continue into the limb bud, presumably traveling along permissive pathways that lead in the general direction of the appropriate muscle

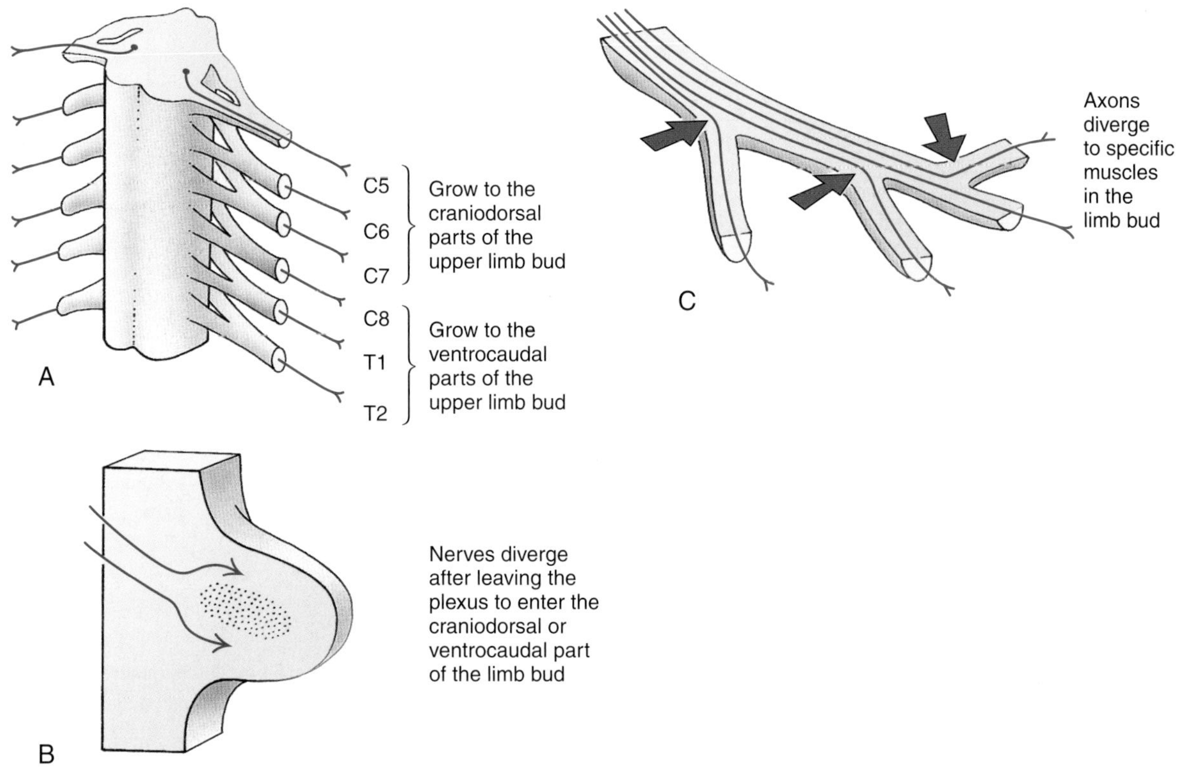

Figure 18-25. Growth of spinal nerve axons into the limb buds. *A, B,* Axons grow into the limb buds along permissive pathways. As the axons of the various spinal nerves mingle at the base of the limb buds to form the brachial and lumbosacral plexuses, each axon must "decide" whether to grow into the dorsal or ventral muscle mass. Factors that may play a role in directing axon growth include areas of dense mesenchyme or *Glycosaminoglycan*-containing mesenchyme, which are avoided by outgrowing axons. *C,* Once the axons grow into the bud, decision points (arrows) under the control of "local factors" may regulate the invasion of specific muscle anlagen by specific axons.

compartment. Axons from the dorsal divisions of the plexuses tend to grow into the dorsal side of the limb bud and thus innervate mainly extensors, supinators, and abductor muscles; axons from the ventral divisions of the plexus grow into the ventral side of the limb bud and thus innervate mainly flexors, pronators, and adductor muscles. Over the very last part of an axon's path, axonal pathfinding is probably regulated by cues produced by the muscle itself. Similarly, local differences in cell surface molecules among muscle fibers most likely direct the final branching and distribution of axons within specific muscles.

As mentioned earlier in the chapter (see Fig. 18-11), the upper and lower limb buds rotate from their original orientation: basically, from a coronal orientation to a parasagittal orientation. Subsequently (between the 6th and 8th weeks), they also rotate around their long axis. The upper limb rotates *laterally* so that the elbow points caudally and the original ventral surface of the limb bud becomes the cranial surface of the limb. The lower limb rotates *medially* so that the knee points cranially and the original ventral surface of the limb bud becomes the caudal surface of the limb. As shown in Figure 18-26, this rotation causes the originally straight segmental pattern of lower limb innervation to twist into a spiral. The rotation of the upper limb is less extreme than that of the lower limb and is accomplished partly through the caudal migration of the shoulder girdle. Moreover, some of the dermatomes in the upper limb bud exhibit overgrowth and come to dominate the limb surface.

18

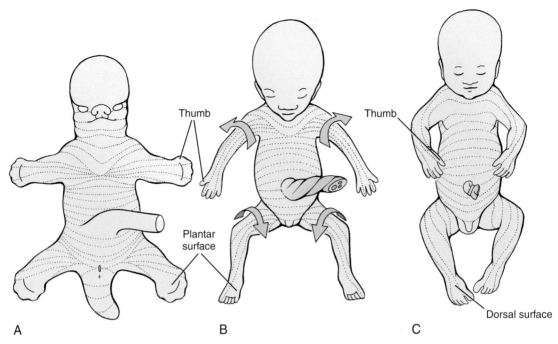

Figure 18-26. Rotation of the limbs. The dramatic medial rotation of the lower limbs during the 6th to 8th weeks causes the mature dermatomes to spiral down the limb. The configuration of the upper limb dermatomes is partially modified by more limited lateral rotation of the upper limb during the same period.

IN THE RESEARCH LAB

SPECIFICATION AND PROJECTION OF LIMB MOTOR AXONS

A number of factors are thought to control axonal specification, migration, and projection including the *Lim* and *Hox* homeobox proteins, *Eph/Ephrin* signaling, *ET-S* transcription factors, and cell adhesion molecules such as type II *Cadherins* and *NCam*. The motor neurons that innervate the limb bud form in the **lateral medial columns** (LMC) within the neural tube in response to retinoic acid signaling from the paraxial mesoderm. The LMC has two columns composed of LMCm (medial) and LMCl (lateral) neurons, which are distinguished by the differential expression of *Lim* homeobox proteins, and project to the ventral and dorsal limb mesenchyme, respectively. LMCm neurons are *Isl1* and *Isl2* positive, whereas LMCl neurons express *Lim1* and *Isl2*. Transplantation studies have shown that the axons have a remarkable ability to reach their appropriate targets. Thus, if the neural tube is shifted slightly along its cranial-caudal axis, the axons will still be able to project properly, being guided by a combination of local repulsive/attractive and chemoattractive cues.

The LMCm and LMCl axons migrate along a common pathway to the plexus, where they pause and change their nearest neighbors: this resting period and the timing of subsequent ingrowth into the limb bud is determined by signals from the limb mesenchyme such as *Ephrin* and *Semaphorin 3A*. At the junction of *Lbx1*-expressing and nonexpressing mesenchyme (*Lbx1* is an ortholog of the Drosophila *Lady bird late* gene, a homeobox gene), a decision is made as to whether to enter the dorsal and ventral limb mesenchyme (Fig. 18-27A). LMCl neurons require *Lim1* and its downstream target, *EphA4*, to project appropriately into the dorsal mesenchyme. The *EphA4* axons avoid the ventral mesenchyme, which expresses high levels of *EphrinA2* and *Ephrin A5*. In the absence of *Lim1* the LMCl neurons project randomly (Fig. 18-27B). Likewise, in *EphA4* mutant mice, the LMCl neurons project abnormally but in this case they all enter the ventral limb mesenchyme (Fig. 18-27C). In the converse situation, ectopic misexpression of *EphA4* results in the LMCm neurons projecting dorsally. Similar repulsive interactions "force/guide" the LMCm neurons to enter the ventral mesenchyme: a subset of LMCm neurons express the secreted *Semphorin* coreceptor *Neuropilin 2* and avoid the *Semaphorin 3F*-expressing dorsal mesenchyme. Loss of function of *Lmx1b*, which controls dorsal-ventral limb identity (discussed in the preceding "In the Research Lab"), results in the random projection of both LMCm and LMCl neurons (Fig. 18-27D).

EphA4 together with EphrinB3 signaling is also required for the development of the central pattern generators in the ventromedial region of the spinal cord that control coordination of limb movement. This provides an additional explanation for the inability of EphA4 or EphrinB3 mouse mutants to alternate their leg movements during walking.

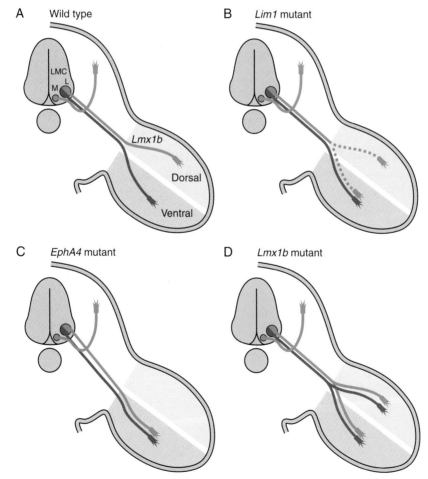

Figure 18-27. LMCm and LMCl axonal projections in the developing limb as seen in transverse section. A, Wild-type mouse. B-D, Lim1, EphA4, and Lmx1b mutant mice, respectively. The green projection innervates muscles (not shown) adjacent to the vertebral column and derived from the corresponding segmental somatic myotoms.

18

Suggested Readings

Cai J, Jabs EW. 2005. A twisted hand: bHLH protein phosphorylation and dimerization regulate limb development. Bioessays 27:1102-1106.

Capdevila J, Izpisua Belmonte JC. 2001. Patterning mechanisms controlling vertebrate limb development. Annu Rev Cell Dev Biol 17:87-132.

Dudley AT, Tabin CJ. 2000. Constructive antagonism in limb development. Curr Opin Genet Dev 10:387-392.

Freitas R, Cohn MJ. 2006. Genomic regulation of Hox collinearity. Dev Cell 10:8-9.

Goodman FR. 2002. Limb malformations and the human HOX genes. Am J Med Genet 112:256-265.

Hill RE, Heaney SJ, Lettice LA. 2003. Sonic hedgehog: restricted expression and limb dysmorphologies. J Anat 202:13-20.

Holmes LB. 2002. Teratogen-induced limb defects. Am J Med Genet 112:297-303.

King M, Arnold JS, Shanske A, Morrow BE. 2006. T-genes and limb bud development. Am J Med Genet A 140:1407-1413.

Kmita M, Duboule D. 2003. Organizing axes in time and space; 25 years of colinear tinkering. Science 301:331-333.

Kraus P, Lufkin T. 2006. Dlx homeobox gene control of mammalian limb and craniofacial development. Am J Med Genet A 140:1366-1374.

Krull CE, Koblar SA. 2000. Motor axon pathfinding in the peripheral nervous system. Brain Res Bull 53:479-487.

Landmesser LT. 2001. The acquisition of motoneuron subtype identity and motor circuit formation. Int J Dev Neurosci 19:175-182.

Lettice LA, Hill RE. 2005. Preaxial polydactyly: a model for defective long-range regulation in congenital abnormalities. Curr Opin Genet Dev 15:294-300.

Mariani FV, Martin GR. 2003. Deciphering skeletal patterning: clues from the limb. Nature 423:319-325.

Martin G. 2001. Making a vertebrate limb: new players enter from the wings. Bioessays 23:865-868.

Morasso MI, Radoja N. 2005. Dlx genes, p63, and ectodermal dysplasias. Birth Defects Res C Embryo Today 75:163-171.

Niswander L. 2002. Interplay between the molecular signals that control vertebrate limb development. Int J Dev Biol 46:877-881.

Niswander L. 2003. Pattern formation: old models out on a limb. Nat Rev Genet 4:133-143.

Panman L, Zeller R. 2003. Patterning the limb before and after SHH signaling. J Anat 202:3-12.

Robert B, Lallemand Y. 2006. Anteroposterior patterning in the limb and digit specification: contribution of mouse genetics. Dev Dyn 235:2337-2352.

Sanz-Ezquerro JJ, Tickle C. 2001. "Fingering" the vertebrate limb. Differentiation 69:91-99.

Sanz-Ezquerro JJ, Tickle C. 2003. Digital development and morphogenesis. J Anat 202:51-58.

Sharma K, Belmonte JC. 2001. Development of the limb neuromuscular system. Curr Opin Cell Biol 13:204-210.

Shirasaki R, Pfaff SL. 2002. Transcriptional codes and the control of neuronal identity. Annu Rev Neurosci 25:251-281.

Sifakis S, Basel D, Ianakiev P, et al. 2001. Distal limb malformations: underlying mechanisms and clinical associations. Clin Genet 60:165-172.

Tabin C, Wolpert L. 2007. Rethinking the proximodistal axis of the vertebrate limb in the molecular era. Genes Dev 21:1433-1442.

Talamillo A, Bastida MF, Fernandez-Teran M, Ros MA. 2005. The developing limb and the control of the number of digits. Clin Genet 67:143-153.

Tickle C. 2002. Molecular basis of vertebrate limb patterning. Am J Med Genet 112:250-255.

Tickle C. 2003. Patterning systems—from one end of the limb to the other. Dev Cell 4:449-458.

Tickle C. 2004. The contribution of chicken embryology to the understanding of vertebrate limb development. Mech Dev 121:1019-1029.

Tickle C. 2006. Making digit patterns in the vertebrate limb. Nat Rev Mol Cell Biol 7:45-53.

Tickle C, Munsterberg A. 2001. Vertebrate limb development—the early stages in chick and mouse. Curr Opin Genet Dev 11:476-481.

Wilkie AO. 2003. Why study human limb malformations? J Anat 202:27-35.

Wilkie AO, Patey SJ, Kan SH, et al. 2002. FGFs, their receptors, and human limb malformations: clinical and molecular correlations. Am J Med Genet 112:266-278.

Yang Y. 2003. Wnts and wing: Wnt signaling in vertebrate limb development and musculoskeletal morphogenesis. Birth Defects Res C Embryo Today 69:305-317.

Credits

Cover photo. Courtesy of Dr. Robert E. Waterman and the University of New Mexico, Albuquerque.

Figure Intro-1. Adapted from Gasser RF. 1975. Atlas of Human Embryos. Harper and Row, New York.

Figure Intro-2. Photo courtesy of the Progeria Research Foundation and the child's parents.

Figure Intro-4. Adapted from Moore KL and Persaud TVN. 2003. The Developing Human. Clinically Oriented Embryology. Seventh Edition. Saunders, Philadelphia.

Table Intro-1. Columns 1 through 5 from O'Rahilly R, Müller F. 1987. Developmental Stages in Human Embryos. Carnegie Institute, Washington, D.C., Publ. No. 637.

Figure 1-1 *C.* Courtesy of Drs. Peter Nichol and A. Shaaban.

Figure 1-4. Inset photo in *B* courtesy of Dr. Daniel S. Friend. *C,* Courtesy of Drs. Gary Schatten and Calvin Simerly.

Figure 1-7. *A,* From Phillips DM, Shalgi R. 1980. Surface architecture of the mouse and hamster zona pellucida and oocyte. J Ultrastruct Res 72:1-12. *B,* Courtesy of Dr. David M. Phillips.

Figures 1-8 *B,* **9, 10.** Courtesy of Dr. Arthur Brothman.

Figure 1-11. Courtesy of Dr. Arthur Brothman. Adapted from Morelli SH, Deubler DA, Brothman LJ, Carey JC, Brothman AR. 1999. Partial trisomy 17p by spectral karyotyping. Clin Genet 55:372-375.

Figure 1-12. *B,* Courtesy of Drs. Gary Schatten and Calvin Simerly.

Figure 1-14. *B,C,* Courtesy of Dr. David M. Phillips.

Figure 1-15. Courtesy of Drs. Gary Schatten and Calvin Simerly.

Figure 1-16. From Boatman DE. 1987. In vitro growth of nonhuman primate pre- and peri-implantation embryos. In Bavister BD (ed): The Mammalian Preimplantation Embryo. Plenum, New York. Photos courtesy of Drs. Barry Bavister and D.E. Boatman.

Figure 1-17. From Nikas G, Asangla A, Winston RML, Handyside AH. 1996. Compaction and surface polarity in the human embryo in vitro. Biol Reprod 55:32-37. Photos courtesy of Dr. G. Nikas.

Figure 1-19. Courtesy of Dr. I. Santiago Alvarez.

Figure 1-20. Courtesy of Dr. Michael J. Tucker, Georgia Reproductive Specialists.

Figure 1-21. Courtesy of Dr. I. Santiago Alvarez.

Figure 2-7. From the Digitally Reproduced Embryonic Morphology (DREM) project, courtesy of Dr. Ray Gasser.

Figure 2-9. Courtesy of Dr. Tariq Siddiqi.

Figure 2-12. Adapted from Reik W, Walter J. 2001. Genomic imprinting: parental influence on the genome. Nat Rev Genet 2:21-32.

Figure 3-3. From Sulik K, Dehart, DB, Inagaki, T, Carson, JL, Vrablic, T, Gesteland, K and Schoenwolf GC. 1994. Morphogenesis of the murine node and notochordal plate. Dev Dyn 201:260-278.

Figure 3-4. *A,* Adapted from Yost HJ. 2003. Left-right asymmetry: nodal cilia make and catch a wave. Curr Biol 13:R808-809. *B,* Adapted from McGrath J, Somlo S, Makova S, Tian X, Brueckner M. 2003. Two populations of node monocilia initiate left-right asymmetry in the mouse. Cell 114:61-73.

Figure 3-5. *A,* Courtesy of N. Hirokawa. *A, B,* Adapted from Tanaka Y, Okada Y, Hirokawa N. 2005. FGF-induced vesicular release of Sonic hedgehog and retinoic acid in leftward nodal flow is critical for left-right determination. Nature 435:172-177.

Figure 3-6. *C,* From Schoenwolf, GC. 2001. Laboratory Studies of Vertebrate and Invertebrate Embryos. Guide and Atlas of Descriptive and Experimental Development. Eighth Edition. Prentice Hall, New Jersey.

Figure 3-8. From Tamarin A. 1983. Stage 9 macaque embryos studied by electron microscopy. J Anat 137:765-779.

Figure 3-13. From Schoenwolf, GC. 2001. Laboratory Studies of Vertebrate and Invertebrate Embryos. Guide and Atlas of Descriptive and Experimental Development. Eighth Edition. Prentice Hall, New Jersey.

Figure 3-16. Courtesy of Dr. Olivier Pourquie. *A-F,* Adapted from McGrew MJ, Dale JK, Fraboulet S, Pourquie O. 1998. The lunatic fringe gene is a target of the molecular clock linked to somite segmentation in avian embryos. Curr Biol 8:979-982. *G-J,* Adapted from Dubrulle J, McGrew MJ, Pourquie O. 2001. FGF signaling controls somite boundary position and regulates segmentation clock control of spatiotemporal Hox gene activation. Cell 106:219-232.

Figure 3-17. Adapted from Pourquie O. 2004. The chick embryo: a leading model in somitogenesis studies. Mech Dev 121: 1069-1079.

Figure 3-18. Adapted from Reuters.

Figure 3-19. Adapted from Smith, JL, Schoenwolf GC. 1998. Getting organized: New insights into the organizer of higher vertebrates. Curr Topics Dev Biol 40:79-110.

Figure 3-21. From Tamarin A. 1983. Stage 9 macaque embryos studied by electron microscopy. J Anat 137:765-779.

Figure 3-22. From the Digitally Reproduced Embryonic Morphology (DREM) project, courtesy of Dr. Ray Gasser.

Figure 3-23. *A,* Courtesy of Dr. Doug Melton. *B,* From Steinbeisser H, De Robertis EM, Ku M, Kessler DS, Melton DA. 1993.

Xenopus axis formation: induction of goosecoid by injected X-wnt-8 and activin mRNAs. Development 118:499-507.

Figure 3-24. *A,* Courtesy of Dr. Mahua Mukhopadhyay; From Mukhopadhyay M, Shtrom S, Rodriguez-Esteban C, Chen L, Tsukui T, Gomer L, Dorward DW, Glinka A, Grinberg A, Huang SP, Niehrs C, Belmonte JC, Westphal H. 2001. Dickkopf1 is required for embryonic head induction and limb morphogenesis in the mouse. Dev Cell 1:423-434. *B,* Courtesy of William Shawlot; From Shawlot W, Behringer RR. 1995. Requirement for Lim1 in head-organizer function. Nature 374:425-430.

Figure 4-2. Courtesy of Dr. Arnold Tamarin.

Figure 4-3. *A,* Courtesy of Drs. Peter Nichol and A. Shaaban. *B,* Courtesy of Dr. Earl Downey.

Figure 4-4. *B,* Courtesy of Dr. Kohei Shiota. From Yamada S, Uwabe, C, Nakatsu-Komatsu T, Minekura Y, Iwakura M, Motoki T, Nishimiya K, Iiyama M, Kakusho K, Minoh M, Mizuta S, Matsuda T, Matsuda Y, Haishi T, Kose K, Fujii S, Shiota K. 2006. Graphics and movie illustrations of human prenatal development and their application to embryological education based on the human embryo specimens in the Kyoto collection. Dev Dyn, 235:468-477. *C,* Adapted from Schoenwolf, GC. 2001. Laboratory Studies of Vertebrate and Invertebrate Embryos. Guide and Atlas of Descriptive and Experimental Development. Eighth Edition. Prentice Hall, New Jersey. Courtesy of Dr. Robert E. Waterman.

Figure 4-5. Adapted from Schoenwolf, GC. 2001. Laboratory Studies of Vertebrate and Invertebrate Embryos. Guide and Atlas of Descriptive and Experimental Development. Eighth Edition. Prentice Hall, New Jersey. Colas JF, Schoenwolf GC. 2001. Towards a cellular and molecular understanding of neurulation. Dev Dyn 221:117-145.

Figure 4-7. Courtesy of Dr. Amel Gritli-Linde.

Figures 4-8, 4-9, 4-10. Courtesy of Dr. John Kestle.

Figure 4-11. *A,* Courtesy of Dr. John Carey. *B, C,* Courtesy of Dr. John Kestle.

Figure 4-14. From Schoenwolf, GC. 2001. Laboratory Studies of Vertebrate and Invertebrate Embryos. Guide and Atlas of Descriptive and Experimental Development. Eighth Edition. Prentice Hall, New Jersey. Colas JF, Schoenwolf GC. 2001. Towards a cellular and molecular understanding of neurulation. Dev Dyn 221:117-145.

Figure 4-15. Photo courtesy of Drs. Antone Jacobson and Patrick Tam.

Figure 4-19. Redrawn from the data of D'Amico-Martel A, Noden DM. 1983. Contributions of placodal and neural crest cells to avian cranial peripheral ganglia. Am. J. Anat. 166:445-468. Adapted from Baker C. 2005 Neural crest and cranial ectodermal placodes. In: Developmental Neurobiology, 4th Ed., Rao MS and Jacobson M., Eds. Kluwer Academic/Plenum Publishers, New York.

Figure 4-21. Adapted from Farlie PG, McKeown SJ, Newgreen DF. 2004. The neural crest: basic biology and clinical relationships in the craniofacial and enteric nervous systems. Birth Defects Res C Embryo Today 72:173-189.

Figure 4-23. Adapted from Schoenwolf, GC. 2001. Laboratory Studies of Vertebrate and Invertebrate Embryos. Guide and Atlas of Descriptive and Experimental Development. Eighth Edition. Prentice Hall, New Jersey.

Figure 4-24. Adapted from Brand-Saberi B, Christ B. 2000. Evolution and development of distinct cell lineages derived from somites. Curr Top Dev Biol 48:1-42. Courtesy of Dr. Heinz Jacob.

Figure 5-1. *A,* Courtesy of Dr. Max Muenke. Adapted from El-Jaick KB, Powers SE, Bartholin L, Myers KR, Hahn J, Orioli IM, Ouspenskaia M, Lacbawan F, Roessler E, Wotton D, Muenke M. 2006. Functional analysis of mutations in TGIF associated with holoprosencephaly. Mol Genet Metab 90:97-111. *B,* Courtesy of Dr. Leslie Biesecker. Adapted from Biesecker LG. 2005. Mapping phenotypes to language: a proposal to organize and standardize the clinical descriptions of malformations. Clin Genet 68:320-326.

Figure 5-2. Courtesy of Dr. Susan Lewin and the child's family.

Figure 5-3. Courtesy of Dr. Roger A. Fleischman.

Figures 5-4–5-7. Adapted from Wolpert L. 2002. Principles of Development. New York: Oxford University Press.

Figure 5-8. *A, B,* Courtesy of Drs. Sophie Creuzet and Nichole Le Douarin. Adapted from Le Douarin NM. 2004. The avian embryo as a model to study the development of the neural crest: a long and still ongoing story. Mech Dev 121:1089-1102.

Figures 5-9, 5-10. Adapted from Wolpert L. 2002. Principles of Development. New York: Oxford University Press.

Figure 5-11. Adapted from Schoenwolf GC. 2001. Cutting, pasting and painting: experimental embryology and neural development. Nat Rev Neurosci 2:763-771.

Figure 5-12. Adapted from Schoenwolf GC. 2001. Cutting, pasting and painting: experimental embryology and neural development. Nat Rev Neurosci 2:763-771.

Figures 5-13, 5-14. Adapted from Schoenwolf, GC. 2001. Laboratory Studies of Vertebrate and Invertebrate Embryos. Guide and Atlas of Descriptive and Experimental Development. Eighth Edition. Prentice Hall, New Jersey.

Figure 5-15. Adapted from Schoenwolf GC. 2001. Cutting, pasting and painting: experimental embryology and neural development. Nat Rev Neurosci 2:763-771.

Figures 5-16, 5-17. Adapted from Nagy A, Gertsenstein M, Vintersten K, Behringer R. 2003. Manipulating the Mouse Embryo. A Laboratory Manual. Cold Spring Harbor, New York.

Figures 5-18, 5-19. Adapted from Wolpert L. 2002. Principles of Development. New York: Oxford University Press.

Figure 5-20. Adapted from Krumlauf R. 1993. *Hox* genes and pattern formation in the branchial region of the vertebrate head. Trends Genet 9:106-112.

Figure 5-21. Adapted from Kalthoff K. 2001. Analysis of Biological Development. McGraw-Hill Higher Education, New York.

Figure 5-22. Adapted from Logan CY, Nusse R. 2004. The Wnt signaling pathway in development and disease. Annu Rev Cell Dev Biol 20:781-810.

Figure 5-23. Adapted from McMahon AP, Ingham PW, Tabin CJ. 2003. Developmental roles and clinical significance of hedgehog signaling. Curr Top Dev Biol 53:1-114.

Figure 5-24. Adapted from Massague J, Chen YG. 2000. Controlling TGF-beta signaling. Genes Dev 14:627-644.

Figure 5-25. Adapted from Wolpert L. 2002. Principles of Development. Oxford University Press, New York.

Figures 5-26, 5-27. Adapted from Gilbert SF. 2006. Developmental Biology. Eighth Edition. Sinauer Associates, Inc, Sunderland, Massachusetts.

Figure 5-28. Adapted from Maden M. 2002. Retinoid signalling in the development of the central nervous system. Nat Rev Neurosci 3:843-853.

Figure 6-1. Courtesy of Dr. Robert E. Waterman and the University of New Mexico School of Medicine, Albuquerque.

Figure 6-3. Adapted from Benirschke K. 1998. Remarkable placenta. Clin Anat 11:194-205.

Figure 6-4. From Castellucci M, Scheper M, Scheffen I, Celona A, Kaufmann P. 1990. The development of the human placental villous tree. Anat Embryol (Berl) 181:117-128.

Figure 6-7. *A, B,* Courtesy of Dr. Janice L.B. Byrne

Figure 6-9. *A, B,* Courtesy of Dr. Peter Nichol and A. Shaaban.

Figure 6-11. Courtesy of Babies First Ultrasound, San Diego, California; www.bfiultrasound.com/default.html.

Figure 6-12. Courtesy of Dr. Gregorio Acacio, Hospital Israelita Albert Einstein, Sao Paulo, Brazil.

Figures 6-13, 6-14. Adapted from Jorde LB, Carey JC, Bamshad MJ, White RL. 2006. Medical Genetics. Third Edition, Updated Edition. Mosby, St. Louis.

Figure 6-15. Adapted from Harrison MR, Adzick NS, Longaker MT, Goldberg JD, Rosen MA, Filly RA, Evans MI, Golbus MS. 1990. Successful repair in utero of a fetal diaphragmatic hernia after removal of herniated viscera from the left thorax. N Engl J Med 322:1582-1584.

Figure 6-16. From Jones HW, Scott WW. 1958. Hermaphroditism, Genital Anomalies and Related Endocrine Disorders. Williams and Wilkins, Baltimore.

Table 6-1. Adapted from BabyCenter at http://www.babycenter.com/general/pregnancy/1290794.html.

Figure 7-1. Courtesy of Dr. Alan Rope.

Figure 7-2. Adapted from Holbrook KA, Dale BA, Smith LT, Foster CA, Williams ML, Hoff MS, Dabelsteen E, Bauer EA. 1987. Markers of adult skin expressed in the skin of the first trimester fetus. Curr Probl Dermatol 16:94-108.

Figure 7-3. Adapted from Foster CA, Bertram JF, Holbrook KA.1988. Morphometric and statistical analyses describing the in utero growth of human epidermis. Anat Rec 222: 201-206.

Figure 7-4. Adapted from Wilson A, Radtke F. 2006. Multiple functions of Notch signaling in self-renewing organs and cancer. FEBS Lett 580:2860-2868.

Figure 7-5. Courtesy of Dr. Alea Mills. Adapted from Keyes WM, Wu Y, Vogel H, Guo X, Lowe SW, Mills AA. 2005. p63 deficiency activates a program of cellular senescence and leads to accelerated aging. Genes Dev 19:1986-1999.

Figure 7-6. Courtesy of Drs. John Harper and Alan Irvine. Adapted from Irvine AD, Christiano AM. 2001. Hair on a gene string: recent advances in understanding the molecular genetics of hair loss. Clin Exp Dermatol 26:59-71.

Figure 7-7. *A,* Adapted from Holbrook KA. 1988. Structural abnormalities of the epidermally derived appendages in skin from patients with ectodermal dysplasia: insight into developmental errors. Birth Defects Orig Artic Ser 24:15-44. *B,* Adapted from Foster CA, Holbrook KA. 1989. Ontogeny of Langerhans cells in human embryonic and fetal skin: cell densities and phenotypic expression relative to epidermal growth. Am J Anat 184: 157-164.

Figure 7-8. Adapted from Williams PL, Warwick R, Dyson M, Bannister LH. 1989. Gray's Anatomy. Churchill Livingstone, Edinburgh.

Figure 7-9. Courtesy of Dr. Irma Thesleff. Adapted from Mikkola ML, Thesleff I. 2003. Ectodysplasin signaling in development. Cytokine Growth Factor Rev 14:211-224.

Figure 7-10. Adapted from Holbrook KA. 1988. Structural abnormalities of the epidermally derived appendages in skin from patients with ectodermal dysplasia: insight into developmental errors. Birth Defects Orig Artic Ser 24:15-44.

Figure 7-11. Adapted from Fuchs E, Raghavan S. 2002. Getting under the skin of epidermal morphogenesis. Nat Rev Genet 3:199 209.

Figure 7-12. *A,* Courtesy of Dr. Irma Thesleff. Adapted from Pispa J, Thesleff I. 2003. Mechanisms of ectodermal organogenesis. Dev Biol 262:195-205. *B-D,* Courtesy of Drs. Elaine Fuchs and Ramanuj DasGupta. Adapted from DasGupta R, Fuchs E. 1999. Multiple roles for activated LEF/TCF transcription complexes during hair follicle development and differentiation. Development 126:4557-4568.

Figure 7-15. *A-C,* Adapted from Holbrook KA. 1988. Structural abnormalities of the epidermally derived appendages in skin from patients with ectodermal dysplasia: insight into developmental errors. Birth Defects Orig Artic Ser 24:15-44. *D, E,* Courtesy of Dr. Alexandra L. Joyner. Adapted from Guo Q, Loomis C, Joyner AL. 2003. Fate map of mouse ventral limb ectoderm and the apical ectodermal ridge. Dev Biol 264:166-178.

Figure 7-17. Courtesy of Drs. YiPing Chen and Yanding Zhang. Adapted from Zhang YD, Chen Z, Song YQ, Liu C, Chen YP. 2005. Making a tooth: growth factors, transcription factors, and stem cells. Cell Res 15:301-316.

Figure 8-1. Courtesy of Dr. Lynn Jorde. From Jorde LB, Carey JC, Bamshad MJ, White RL. 2006. Medical Genetics. Third Edition, Updated Edition. Mosby, St. Louis.

Figure 8-2. Courtesy of Dr. Michael Owen. Adapted from Otto F, Thornell AP, Crompton T, Denzel A, Gilmour KC, Rosewell IR, Stamp GW, Beddington RS, Mundlos S, Olsen BR, Selby PB, Owen MJ. 1997. Cbfa1, a candidate gene for cleidocranial dysplasia syndrome, is essential for osteoblast differentiation and bone development. Cell 89:765-771.

Figure 8-3. *A,* Adapted from Buckingham M, Bajard L, Chang T, Daubas P, Hadchouel J, Meilhac S, Montarras D, Rocancourt D, Relaix F. 2003. The formation of skeletal muscle: from somite to limb. J Anat 202:59-68. *B,* Adapted from Schoenwolf, GC. 2001. Laboratory Studies of Vertebrate and Invertebrate Embryos. Guide and Atlas of Descriptive and Experimental Development. Eighth Edition. Prentice Hall, New Jersey. *C,* Adapted from Adapted from Brand-Saberi B, Christ B. 2000. Evolution and development of distinct cell lineages derived from somites. Curr Top Dev Biol 48:1-42. Courtesy of Dr. Heinz Jacob.

Figure 8-6. Courtesy of Drs. Cathy Krull and Marianne Bronner-Fraser. Adapted from Krull CE, Lansford R, Gale NW, Collazo A, Marcelle C, Yancopoulos GD, Fraser SE, Bronner-Fraser M. 1997. Interactions of Eph-related receptors and ligands confer rostrocaudal pattern to trunk neural crest migration. Curr Biol 7:571-580.

Figure 8-10. Adapted from Hunt P, Krumlauf R. 1992. Hox codes and positional specification in vertebrate embryonic axes. Annu Rev Cell Biol 8:227-256.

Figure 8-11. *A,* Courtesy of Dr. Mario Capecchi. Adapted from Wellik DM, Capecchi MR. 2003. Hox10 and Hox11 genes are required to globally pattern the mammalian skeleton. Science 301:363-367. *B,* Courtesy of Dr. Moises Mallo. Adapted from Carapuco M, Novoa A, Bobola N, Mallo M. 2005. Hox genes specify vertebral types in the presomitic mesoderm. Genes Dev 19:2116-2121.

Figure 8-12. Adapted from Conlon RA. 1995. Retinoic acid and pattern formation in vertebrates. Trends Genet 11:314-319. P. 316, Fig. 2. Lohnes D. 2003. The Cdx1 homeodomain protein: an integrator of posterior signaling in the mouse. Bioessays 25:971-980.

Figure 8-13. *A,* Courtesy of Dr. Peter D. Turnpenny. Adapted from Whittock NV, Sparrow DB, Wouters MA, Sillence D, Ellard S, Dunwoodie SL, Turnpenny PD. 2004. Mutated MESP2 causes spondylocostal dysostosis in humans. Am J Hum Genet 74:1249-1254. *B, C,* Courtesy of Drs. Ian Krantz and Kenro Kusumi. Adapted from Pourquie O, Kusumi K. 2001. When body segmentation goes wrong. Clin Genet 60:409-416.

Figure 8-15. Adapted from Buckingham M. 2006. Myogenic progenitor cells and skeletal myogenesis in vertebrates. Curr Opin Genet Dev 16:525-532.

Figure 8-16. *A, B,* Adapted from Kronenberg HM. 2003. Developmental regulation of the growth plate. Nature 423: 332-336. *B,* Also adapted from Hartmann C, Tabin CJ. 2000. Dual roles of Wnt signaling during chondrogenesis in the chicken limb. Development 127:3141-3159.

Figure 8-18. Adapted from Francis-West PH, Abdelfattah A, Chen P, Allen C, Parish J, Ladher R, Allen S, MacPherson S, Luyten FP, Archer CW. 1999. Mechanisms of GDF-5 action during skeletal development. Development 126:1305-1315.

Figure 8-19. Courtesy of Drs. Frank Luyten and J. Terrig Thomas. Adapted from Thomas JT, Kilpatrick MW, Lin K, Erlacher L, Lembessis P, Costa T, Tsipouras P, Luyten FP. 1997. Disruption of human limb morphogenesis by a dominant negative mutation in CDMP1. Nat Genet 17:58-64.

Figure 8-20. Courtesy of Dr. Bjorn Olsen. Adapted from Zelzer E, Olsen BR. 2003. The genetic basis for skeletal diseases. Nature 423:343-348.

Figure 8-22. Adapted from Chevallier A, Kieny M, Mauger A. 1977. Limb-somite relationship: origin of the limb musculature. J Embryol Exp Morphol 41:245-258.

Figure 8-23. *A,* Courtesy of Dr. C. Birchmeier. Adapted from Brohmann H, Jagla K, Birchmeier C. 2000. The role of Lbx1 in migration of muscle precursor cells. Development 127:437-445. *B,* Adapted from Buckingham M, Bajard L, Chang T, Daubas P, Hadchouel J, Meilhac S, Montarras D, Rocancourt D, Relaix F. 2003. The formation of skeletal muscle: from somite to limb. J Anat 202:59-68.

Table 8-1. Data from Crafts RC. 1985. A Textbook of Human Anatomy. Third Ed. Churchill Livingstone, New York.

Figure 9-2. *A, B,* Adapted from Kiecker C, Lumsden A. 2005. Compartments and their boundaries in vertebrate brain development. Nat Rev Neurosci 6:553-564. *C,* Adapted from Rowitch DH. 2004. Glial specification in the vertebrate neural tube. Nat Rev Neurosci 5:409-419.

Figure 9-3. *A,* Adapted from Rakic P. 1982. Early developmental events: cell lineages, acquisition of neuronal positions, and areal and laminar development. Neurosci Res Prog Bull 20:439-451. *B,* Courtesy of Dr. Kathryn Tosney.

Figure 9-5. Adapted from Williams PL, Warwick R, Dyson M, Bannister LH. 1989. Gray's Anatomy. Churchill Livingstone, Edinburgh.

Figure 9-10. *D,* Courtesy of Dr. Alexandra Joyner.

Figure 9-12. Courtesy of Children's Hospital Medical Center, Cincinnati, OH.

Figure 9-16. Adapted from Roberts A, Taylor JSH. 1983. A study of the growth cones of developing embryonic sensory neurites. J Embryol Exp Morphol 75:31-47.

Figure 9-18. Adapted from Lambot MA, Depasse F, Noel JC, Vanderhaeghen P. 2005. Mapping labels in the human developing visual system and the evolution of binocular vision. J Neurosci 25:7232-7237.

Figure 9-19. From Colello RJ, Guillery RW. 1990. The early development of retinal ganglion cells with uncrossed axons in the mouse: retinal position and axomal course. Development 108:515-523.

Figure 9-20. Adapted from McLaughlin T, Hindges R, O'Leary DD. 2003. Regulation of axial patterning of the retina and its topographic mapping in the brain. Curr Opin Neurobiol 13:57-69.

Figure 9-21. *G,* Courtesy of Dr. Arnold Tamarin.

Figure 9-24. Courtesy of Dr. Andrew Lumsden.

Figure 9-27. Adapted from Bond J, Roberts E, Mochida GH, Hampshire DJ, Scott S, Askham JM, Springell K, Mahadevan M, Crow YJ, Markham AF, Walsh CA, Woods CG. 2002. ASPM is a major determinant of cerebral cortical size. Nat Genet 32:316-320.

Figure 10-1. *A, B,* From Bonkowsky JL, Johnson J, Carey JC, Smith AG, Swoboda KJ. 2003. An infant with primary tooth loss and palmar hyperkeratosis: a novel mutation in the NTRK1 gene causing congenital insensitivity to pain with anhidrosis. Pediatrics 112:e237-241. Courtesy of Dr. Josh Bonkowsky.

Figure 10-2. Courtesy of Dr. Maya Sieber-Blum.

Figure 10-3. Courtesy of Dr. Carol Erickson.

Figure 10-5. *B,* Courtesy of Drs. James Weston and Michael Marusich.

Figure 10-6. Courtesy of Teri Belecky-Adams and Dr. Linda Parysek.

Figure 10-12. From Bridgman PC, Dailey ME. 1989. The organization of myosin and actin in rapid frozen nerve growth cones. J Cell Biol 108:95-109.

Figure 11-2. Courtesy of Dr. Kurt Albertine.

Figure 11-5. Modified from Peters K, Werner S, Liao X, Wert S, Whitsett J, Williams L. 1994. Targeted expression of a dominant negative FGF receptor blocks branching morphogenesis and epithelial differentiation of the mouse lung. EMBO J 13:3296-3301.

Figure 11-13. Courtesy of Children's Hospital Medical Center, Cincinnati, OH.

Table 11-1. Adapted from Langston C, Kida K, Reed M, Thurlbeck WM. 1984. Human lung growth in late gestation in the neonate. Am Rev Respir Dis 129:607-613.

Figure 12-1. Adapted from Brand T. 2003. Heart development: molecular insights into cardiac specification and early morphogenesis. Dev Biol 258:1-19.

Figure 12-2. Adapted from Ladd AN, Yatskievych TA, Antin PB. 1998. Regulation of avian cardiac myogenesis by activin/TGFbeta and bone morphogenetic proteins. Dev Biol 204:407-419.

Figure 12-3. Adapted from Marvin MJ, DiRocco G, Gardiner A, Bush SM, Lassar, AB. 2001. Genes Dev 15:316-327.

Figure 12-4. *A,* Adapted from Markwald RR, Eisenberg C, Eisenberg L, Trusk T, Sugi Y. 1996. Epithelial-mesenchymal transformation in early avian heart develoment. Acta Anat 156:173-186. *D,* Adapted from Hurle JM, Icardo JM, Ojeda JL. 1980.

Compositional and structural heterogeneity of the cardiac jelly of the chick embryo tubular heart: a TEM, SEM and histochemical study. J Embryol Exp Morphol 56:211-223.

Figure 12-5. Adapted from Coffin JD, Poole TJ. 1988. Embryonic vascular development: immunohistochemical identification of the origin and subsequent morphogenesis of the major vessel primordia in quail embryos. Development 102:735-748.

Figures 12-7, 12-9. Photos adapted from Kaufman MH. 1981. The role of embryology in teratological research, with particular reference to the development of the neural tube and the heart. J Reprod Fertil 62:607-623.

Figure 12-11. Adapted from Buckingham M, Meilhac S, Zaffran S. 2005. Building the mammalian heart from two sources of myocardial cells. Nature Rev Genet 6:826-835.

Figure 12-12. Adapted from van den Hoff M, Kruithof BPT, Moorman AFM. 2004. Making more heart muscle. BioEssays 26:248-261.

Figures 12-13, 12-14. From Manner J. 2000. Cardiac looping in the chick embryo: a morphological review with special reference to terminology and biomechanical aspects of the looping process. Anat Rec 259:248-262.

Figure 12-15 B. Courtesy of Children's Hospital Medical Center, Cincinnati, OH.

Figure 12-17. A-C, Drawn from data in Yutzey KE, Rhee JT, Bader D. 1994. Expression of the atrial-specific myosin heavy chain AMHC1 and the establishment of anteroposterior polarity in the developing chicken heart. Development 120:871-883. D-E, Drawn from data in Christoffels VM, Habets PE, Franco D, Campione M, de Jong F, Lamers WH, Bao ZZ, Palmer S, Biben C, Harvey RP, Moorman AF. 2000. Chamber formation and morphogenesis in the developing mammalian heart. Dev Biol 223:266-278.

Figure 12-22. Adapted from Mjaatvedt CH, Markwald RR. 1989. Induction of an epithelial-mesenchymal transition by an in vivo adheron-like complex. Dev Biol 136:118-128.

Figure 12-23. Courtesy of Dr. Ray Runyan. From Person AD, Klewer SE, Runyan RB. 2005. Cell biology of cardiac cushion development. Int Rev Cytol 243: 287-335.

Figure 12-24. B, C, Adapted from Icardo JM. 1988. Heart anatomy and developmental biology. Experientia 44:910-919.

Figure 12-25. B, Adapted from Hendrix MJC, Morse DE. 1977. Atrial septation. I. Scanning electron microscopy in the chick. Dev Biol 57:345-363.

Figure 12-28. Adapted from Mjaatvedt C, Yamamura H, Wessels A, Ramsdell A, Turner D, Markwald RR. 1999. Mechanisms of segmentation, septation, and remodeling of the tubular heart: endocardial cushion fate and cardiac looping. In Harvey RP, Rosenthal N [eds]: Heart Development. Academic Press, New York, NY.

Figure 12-30. Adapted from Mikawa, T. 1999. Cardiac lineages. In Harvey RP, Rosenthal N [eds]: Heart Development. Academic Press, New York, NY.

Figure 12-32. Courtesy of Dr. Ray Runyan. From Person AD, Klewer SE, Runyan RB. 2005. Cell biology of cardiac cushion development. Int Rev Cytol 243: 287-335.

Figure 12-33. Adapted from Steding G, Seidl W. 1980. Contribution to the development of the heart. Part I. Normal development. Thorac Cardiovasc Surg 28:386-409.

Figure 12-34. A, Adapted from Hurle JM, Colvee E, Blanco AM. 1980. Development of mouse semilunar valves. Anat Embryol 160:83-91.

Figure 12-35. From Anderson RH, Webb S, Brown NA, Lamers W, Moorman A. 2006. Development of the heart: (3) Formation of the ventricular outflow tracts, arterial valves, and intrapericardial arterial trunks. Heart 89:1110-1118.

Figure 12-36. Adapted from Kirby ML. 1988. Role of extracardiac factors in heart development. Experientia 44:944-951.

Figure 12-37. Courtesy of Dr. Mark Majesky. From Majesky MW 2004. Development of the coronary vessels. Cur Topics Dev Biol 62:225-259.

Figure 12-38. Photo courtesy of Children's Hospital Medical Center, Cincinnati, OH.

Figure 12-39. Adapted from Pexieder T. 1978. Development of the outflow tract of the embryonic heart. Birth Defects XIV:29-68.

Figure 12-40. B, Photo courtesy of Dr. Margaret Kirby and the Medical College of Georgia, Augusta. D, Photo courtesy of Children's Hospital Medical Center, Cincinnati, OH.

Figure 12-41. B, Photo courtesy of Children's Hospital Medical Center, Cincinnati, OH.

Figure 13-1. A, B, Adapted from Eichmann A, Yuan L, Moyon D, Lenoble F, Pardanaud L, Breant C. 2005. Vascular development: from precursor cells to branched arterial and venous networks. Int J Dev Biol 49:259-267.

Figures 13-2, 13-3. Adapted from Tavian M, Peault B. 2005. Embryonic development of the human hematopoietic system. Int J Dev Biol 49:243-250.

Figure 13-4. A, Adapted from Ody C, Vaigot P. Quéué, P, Imhof BA, Corbel C. 1999. Glycoprotein IIb-IIIa is expressed on avian multilineage hematopoietic progenitor cells. Blood 93:2898-2906. B, Adapted from Corbel C., Salaün J. 2002. AlphaIIb integrin expression during development of the murine hematopoietic system. Dev Biol 243:301-311. C, Adapted from Emmel VE. 1916. The cell clusters in the dorsal aorta of mammalian embryos. Am J Anat 19:5141-5146. D, Adapted from Dieterlen-Lievre F, Le Douarin NM. 2004. From the hemangioblast to self-tolerance: a series of innovations gained from studies on the avian embryo. Mech Dev 121:1117-1128.

Figure 13-6. Adapted from Pardanaud L, Luton D, Prigent M, Bourcheix LM, Catala M, Dieterlen-Lievre F. 1996. Two distinct endothelial lineages in ontogeny, one of them related to hemo-poiesis. Development 122:1363-1371.

Figure 13-7. A, From Effmann E. 1982. Development of the right and left pulmonary arteries: a microangiographic study in the mouse. Invest Radiol 17:529-538. B, C, Courtesy of Dr. Anne Moon, University of Utah. D, Adapted from Coffin D, Poole TJ. 1988. Embryonic vascular development: immunohistochemical identification of the origin and subsequent morphogenesis of the major vessel primordia of quail embryos. Development 102:735-748. E, Adapted from Bockman DE, Redmond ME, Kirby ML. 1989. Alteration of early vascular development after ablation of cranial neural crest. Anat Rec 225:209-217. F, From Hirakow R, Hiruma T. 1981. Scanning electron microscopic study in the development of primitive blood vessels in chick embryos at the early somite stage. Anat Embryol 163:299-306.

Figure 13-8. Adapted from Smith BR. 2001. Magnetic resonance microscopy in cardiac development. Microsc Res Tech 52: 323-330.

Figure 13-10. A, From Kurz H, Burri PH, Djonov VG. 2003. News Physiol Sci 18:65-70. B, Adapted from Burri PH, Hlushchuk R,

Djonov V. 2004. Intussusceptive angiogenesis: its emergence, its characteristics, and its significance. Dev Dyn 231:474-488.

Figure 13-11. From Burri PH, Hlushchuk R, Djonov V. 2004. Intussusceptive angiogenesis: its emergence, its characteristics, and its significance. Dev Dyn 231:474-488.

Figure 13-12. Adapted from Dor Y, Porat R, Keshet E. 2001. Vascular endothelial growth factor and vascular adjustments to perturbations in oxygen homeostasis. Am J Physiol Cell Physiol 280:C1367-1374.

Figure 13-13. Adapted from Rossant J, Howard L. 2002. Signaling pathways in vascular development. Annu Rev Cell Dev Biol 18:541-573.

Figure 13-14. *A, B,* Adapted from Bruckner AL, Frieden IJ. 2003. Hemangiomas of infancy. J Am Acad Dermatol 48:477-493.

Figure 13-18. Adapted from Bockman DE, Redmond ME, Kirby ML. 1989. Alteration of early vascular development after ablation of cranial neural crest. Anat Rec 225:209-217.

Figure 13-26. *A,* Adapted from Carlson BM. 1999. Human Embryology and Developmental Biology, second edition, Mosby, Inc., St. Louis, MO. *B,* Adapted from Langman's Medical Embryology, 7th edition by T.W. Sadler, 1995, Williams and Wilkins, Baltimore, MD.

Figure 13-27. *D,* Courtesy of Children's Hospital Medical Center, Cincinnati, OH.

Figure 13-32. Adapted from Eichmann A, Yuan L, Moyon D, Lenoble F, Pardanaud L, Breant C. 2005. Vascular development: from precursor cells to branched arterial and venous networks. Int J Dev Biol 49:259-267.

Figure 14-5. Adapted from Wells JM, Melton DA. 1999. Vertebrate endoderm development. Annu Rev Cell Dev Biol 15:393-410.

Figure 14-6. Adapted from Roberts DJ. 2000. Molecular mechanisms of development of the gastrointestinal tract. Dev Dyn 219: 109-120.

Figure 14-10. From Madsen OD, Serup P, Jensen J, Petersen HV, Heller RS. 2001. An historical and phylogenetic perspective on islet development. In: Habener JF, Hussain MA, editors. Molecular basis of pancreas development and function. Kluwer Academic Press, Norvell, MA. p 1–17; reproduced in Jensen J. 2004. Gene regulatory factors in pancreatic development. Dev Dyn 229:176-200.

Figure 14-11. Adapted from Jensen J. 2004. Gene regulatory factors in pancreatic development. Dev Dyn 229:176-200.

Figure 14-13. Adapted from Wilson ME, Scheel D, German MS. 2003. Gene expression cascades in pancreatic development. Mech Dev 120:65-80.

Figure 14-21. Drawings adapted from those provided courtesy of Children's Hospital Medical Center, Cincinnati, OH.

Figure 14-23. Adapted from Radtke F, Clevers H. 2005. Self-renewal and cancer of the gut: two sides of a coin. Science 307:1904-1909.

Figure 14-24. Adapted from Batlle E, Henderson JT, Beghtel H, van den Born MM, Sancho E, Huls G, Meeldijk J, Robertson J, van de Wetering M, Pawson T, Clevers H. 2002. Beta-catenin and TCF mediate cell positioning in the intestinal epithelium by controlling the expression of EphB/ephrinB. Cell 111:251-263.

Figure 14-25. Adapted from Yang Q, Bermingham NA, Finegold MJ, Zoghbi HY. 2001. Requirement of Math1 for secretory cell lineage commitment in the mouse intestine. Science 294:2155-2158.

Figure 14-26. Adapted from Logan CY, Nusse R. 2004. The *Wnt* signaling pathway in development and disease. Annu Rev Cell Dev Biol 20:781-810.

Figure 14-27. Adapted from Sukegawa A, Narita T, Kameda T, Saitoh K, Nohno T, Iba H, Yasugi S, Fukuda K. 2000. The concentric structure of the developing gut is regulated by Sonic hedgehog derived from endodermal epithelium. Development 127:1971-1980.

Figure 14-28. Adapted from Le Douarin NM. 2004. The avian embryo as a model to study the development of the neural crest: a long and still ongoing story. Mech Dev 121:1089-1102.

Figure 14-29. Courtesy of Children's Hospital Medical Center, Cincinnati, OH.

Figure 14-31. Courtesy of Dr. Rutger-Jan Nievelstein. Adapted from Nievelstein RA, van der Werff JF, Verbeek FJ, Valk J, Vermeij-Keers C. 1998. Normal and abnormal embryonic development of the anorectum in human embryos. Teratology 57:70-78.

Figure 15-3. Courtesy of Dr. Thomas J. Poole.

Figures 15-8, 15-9. Adapted from Dressler G. 2002. Tubulogenesis in the developing mammalian kidney. Trends Cell Biol 12:390-395.

Figure 15-15. Adapted from Brauer PR. 2003. Human Embryology: The Ultimate USMLE Step 1 Review, Hanley & Belfus, Inc. (an imprint of Elsevier), Philadelphia.

Figure 15-17. From Evan AP, Gattone VC II, Blomgren PM. 1984. Application of scanning electron microscopy to kidney development and nephron maturation. Scanning Electron Microsc 1:455-473.

Figure 15-22. From Miller A, Hong MK, Hutson JM. 2004. The broad ligament: a review of its anatomy and development in different species and hormonal environments. Clin Anat 17:244-251.

Figures 15-24, 15-25. Adapted from Wilhelm D, Koopman P. 2006. The makings of maleness: towards an integrated view of male sexual development. Nat Rev Genet 7:620-631.

Figure 15-27. Adapted from Ludbrook LM, Harley VR. 2004. Sex determination: a 'window' of DAX1 activity. Trends Endocrinol Metab 15:116-121.

Figure 15-29. From Brauer PR. 2003. Human Embryology: The Ultimate USMLE Step 1 Review, Hanley & Belfus, Inc. (an imprint of Elsevier), Philadelphia.

Figure 15-30. *B, C,* Courtesy of Dr. Rutger-Jan Nievelstein. From Nievelstein RA, van der Werff JF, Verbeek FJ, Valk J, Vermeij-Keers C. 1998. Normal and abnormal embryonic development of the anorectum in human embryos. Teratology 57:70-78.

Figure 15-31. *B,* Adapted from Yamada G, Satoh Y, Baskin LS, Cunha GR. 2003. Cellular and molecular mechanisms of development of the external genitalia. Differentiation 71:445-460.

Figure 15-32. Adapted from Wilhelm D, Koopman P. 2006. The makings of maleness: towards an integrated view of male sexual development. Nat Rev Genet 7:620-631.

Figure 15-33. Courtesy of Dr. G. Yamada.

Figure 15-34. Adapted from Brauer PR. 2003. Human Embryology: The Ultimate USMLE Step 1 Review, Hanley & Belfus, Inc. (an imprint of Elsevier), Philadelphia.

Figure 15-36. *D,* Courtesy of Children's Hospital Medical Center, Cincinnati, OH.

Figure 15-38. *A-C,* Adapted from Brauer, PR. 2003. Human Embryology: The Ultimate USMLE Step 1 Review, Hanley & Belfus, Inc. (an imprint of Elsevier), Philadelphia.

Figure 15-39. *D,* Courtesy of Children's Hospital Medical Center, Cincinnati, OH.

Figure 15-40. *A,* From Warkany J. 1971. Congenital Malformations. Notes and Comments. Year Book Medical Pubs, Inc, Chicago. *B-D,* From Jones HW, Scott WW. 1958. Hermaphroditism, Genital Anomalies and Related Endocrine Disorders. Williams and Wilkins, Baltimore.

Figure 16-1. Courtesy of Dr. Alan Rope.

Figure 16-5. Courtesy of Children's Hospital Medical Center, Cincinnati, OH.

Figure 16-6. *A,* Courtesy of Dr. David Billmire. *B, C,* Adapted from Morriss-Kay GM, Wilkie AO. 2005. Growth of the normal skull vault and its alteration in craniosynostosis: insights from human genetics and experimental studies. J Anat 207:637-653.

Figure 16-7. *A-C,* Courtesy of Dr. Arnold Tamarin. **E,** Courtesy of Dr. Robert E. Waterman.

Figure 16-12. *A,* Adapted from Lumsden A, Keynes R. 1989. Segmental patterns of neuronal development in the chick hindbrain. Nature 337:424-428. *B,* Adapted from Kontges G, Lumsden A. 1996. Rhombencephalic neural crest segmentation is preserved throughout craniofacial ontogeny. Development 122:3229-3242.

Figure 16-13. *A,* Courtesy of Dr. Abigail Tucker. *B,* Courtesy of Dr. Moises Mallo. Adapted from Bobola N, Carapuco M, Ohnemus S, Kanzler B, Leibbrandt A, Neubuser A, Drouin J, Mallo M. 2003. Mesenchymal patterning by Hoxa2 requires blocking Fgf-dependent activation of Ptx1. Development 130:3403-3414.

Figure 16-14. *A,* Courtesy of Drs. Susan Reijntjes and Malcolm Maden. Adapted from Reijntjes S, Gale E, Maden M. 2004. Generating gradients of retinoic acid in the chick embryo: Cyp26C1 expression and a comparative analysis of the Cyp26 enzymes. Dev Dyn 230:509-517. *B,* Adapted from Mark M, Ghyselinck NB, Chambon P. 2004. Retinoic acid signalling in the development of branchial arches. Curr Opin Genet Dev 14:591-598.

Figure 16-15. *A, B,* Courtesy of Dr. Arnold Tamarin.

Figure 16-16. *A, C,* Courtesy of Dr. Arnold Tamarin.

Figure 16-17. *A, B,* Adapted from Tucker AS, Lumsden A. 2004. Neural crest cells provide species-specific patterning information in the developing branchial skeleton. Evol Dev 6:32-40. Courtesy of Dr. Abigail Tucker. *C,* Adapted from Eames BF, Schneider RA. 2005. Quail-duck chimeras reveal spatiotemporal plasticity in molecular and histogenic programs of cranial feather development. Development 132:1499-1509. Courtesy of Dr. Richard Schneider.

Figure 16-18. Adapted from Depew MJ, Lufkin T, Rubenstein JL. 2002. Specification of jaw subdivisions by Dlx genes. Science 298:381-385. Courtesy of Dr. Michael Depew.

Figure 16-19. *D,* Courtesy of Dr. Arnold Tamarin.

Figure 16-20. *B,* Courtesy of Dr. Arnold Tamarin.

Figure 16-21. *D,* Courtesy of Children's Hospital Medical Center, Cincinnati, OH.

Figure 16-25. *C,* Courtesy of Dr. Arnold Tamarin.

Figure 16-29. Courtesy of Irving D, Willhite C, Burk D. 1986. Morphogenesis of isotretinoin-induced microcephaly and micrognathia studied by scanning electron microscopy. Teratology 34:141-153.

Figure 17-1. *A,* Courtesy of the family. *B,* Courtesy of Drs. Nancy Bonini and Derek Lessing.

Figure 17-2. *A,* Courtesy of Dr. Robert E. Waterman. *B, G,* Adapted from Kikuchi T, Tonosaki A, Takasaka T. 1988. Development of apical-surface structures of mouse otic placode. Acta Otolaryngol 106:200-207.

Figure 17-4. Courtesy of Dr. Doris K. Wu. Adapted from Morsli H, Choo D, Ryan A, Johnson R, Wu DK. 1998. Development of the mouse inner ear and origin of its sensory organs. J Neurosci 18:3327-3335.

Figure 17-5. *A,* Courtesy of Dr. Suzanne L. Mansour and C. Albert Noyes. *B,* Adapted from Kelley MW. 2006. Regulation of cell fate in the sensory epithelia of the inner ear. Nat Rev Neurosci 7:837-849.

Figure 17-6. Adapted from Riccomagno MM, Takada S, Epstein DJ. 2005. Wnt-dependent regulation of inner ear morphogenesis is balanced by the opposing and supporting roles of Shh. Genes Dev 19:1612-1623.

Figure 17-7. Adapted from Fritzsch B, Beisel K. 1998. Development and maintenance of ear innervation and function: lessons from mutations in mouse and man. Am J Hum Genet 63:1263-1270.

Figure 17-8. *A, B,* Adapted from Barald KF, Kelley MW. 2004. From placode to polarization: new tunes in inner ear development. Development 131:4119-4130. *C,* Adapted from Frolenkov GI, Belyantseva IA, Friedman TB, Griffith AJ. 2004. Genetic insights into the morphogenesis of inner ear hair cells. Nat Rev Genet 5:489-498. *D,* Adapted from Kelley MW. 2006. Regulation of cell fate in the sensory epithelia of the inner ear. Nat Rev Neurosci 7:837-849.

Figure 17-10. Adapted from Kelley MW. 2006. Regulation of cell fate in the sensory epithelia of the inner ear. Nat Rev Neurosci 7:837-849.

Figure 17-11. *A,* Courtesy of Dr. Gregory Frolenkov. Adapted from Frolenkov GI, Belyantseva IA, Friedman TB, Griffith AJ. 2004. Genetic insights into the morphogenesis of inner ear hair cells. Nat Rev Genet 5:489-498. *B, C,* Courtesy of Dr. Jenny Murdoch. Adapted from Curtin JA, Quint E, Tsipouri V, Arkell RM, Cattanach B, Copp AJ, Henderson DJ, Spurr N, Stanier P, Fisher EM, Nolan PM, Steel KP, Brown SD, Gray IC, Murdoch JN. 2003. Mutation of Celsr1 disrupts planar polarity of inner ear hair cells and causes severe neural tube defects in the mouse. Curr Biol 13:1129-1133.

Figure 17-12. Adapted from Dahlen RT, Harnsberger HR, Gray SD, Shelton C, Allen R, Parkin JL, Scalzo D. 1997. Overlapping thin-section fast spin-echo MR of the large vestibular aqueduct syndrome. AJNR Am J Neuroradiol 18:67-75.

Figure 17-13. Adapted from Steel KP, Kros CJ. 2001. A genetic approach to understanding auditory function. Nat Genet 27:143-149.

Figure 17-14. *A,* Courtesy of Dr. Arnold Tamarin.

Figure 17-15. *A-D, F,* Courtesy of Dr. Roger E. Stevenson. Adapted from Carey JC 2006. Ear. In: Human Malformations and Related Anomalies, Second Edition, Stevenson RE, Hall, JG (ed). Pp. 327-371. Oxford University Press, London. *E,* Courtesy of Dr. John C. Carey and Meg Weist. Adapted from Kumar S, Marres HA, Cremers CW, Kimberling WJ. 1998. Autosomal-dominant branchio-otic (BO) syndrome is not allelic to the branchio-oto-renal (BOR) gene at 8q13. Am J Med Genet 76:395-401.

Figure 17-16. *A, B,* Courtesy of Dr. Robert E. Waterman. *C,* Adapted from Morriss-Kay GM. 1981. Growth and development of pattern in the cranial neural epithelium of rat embryos during neurulation. J Embryol Exp Morphol 65 Suppl:225-241. *F,* Adapted from Garcia-Porrero JA, Colvee E, Ojeda JL. 1987. Retinal cell death occurs in the absence of retinal disc invagination: experimental evidence in papaverine-treated chicken embryos. Anat Rec 217:395-401. *H,* Adapted from Morse DE, McCann PS. 1984. Neuroectoderm of the early embryonic rat eye. Scanning electron microscopy. Invest Ophthalmol Vis Sci 25:899-907.

Figure 17-18. *A, B,* Courtesy of Dr. Arnold Tamarin.

Figure 17-21. *A, B,* Courtesy of Dr. Sabine Fuhrmann. *C,* Adapted from Martinez-Morales JR, Rodrigo I, Bovolenta P. 2004. Eye development: a view from the retina pigmented epithelium. Bioessays 26:766-777. *D,* Adapted from Ashery-Padan R, Gruss P. 2001. Pax6 lights-up the way for eye development. Curr Opin Cell Biol 13:706-714.

Figure 17-23. Adapted from Traboulsi EI 2006. Eye. In: Human Malformations and Related Anomalies, Second Edition, Stevenson RE, Hall, JG, Ed., Pp. 297-325. Oxford University Press, London.

Figure 18-1. Courtesy of Freddie Astbury. Modified from Thalidomide UK (www.thalidomideuk.com).

Figure 18-2. *A,* Courtesy of Dr. Robert E. Waterman. *B-D,* Adapted from Kelley RO. 1985. Early development of the vertebrate limb: an introduction to morphogenetic tissue interactions using scanning electron microscopy. Scan Electron Microsc 1985:827-836.

Figure 18-3. Adapted from Alberts B, Johnson A, Lewis J, Raff M, Roberts K, Walter P. 2002. Molecular Biology of the Cell. Fourth Edition. Garland Science, New York.

Figure 18-4. Adapted from Mariani FV, Martin GR. 2003. Deciphering skeletal patterning: clues from the limb. Nature 423:319-325.

Figure 18-5. Courtesy of Drs. Sheila Bell and W. Scott.

Figure 18-6. *B,* Courtesy of Dr. Martin J. Cohn. Adapted from Cohn MJ, Izpisua-Belmonte JC, Abud H, Heath JK, Tickle C. 1995. Fibroblast growth factors induce additional limb development from the flank of chick embryos. Cell 80:739-746.

Figure 18-7. Adapted from Mariani FV, Martin GR. 2003. Deciphering skeletal patterning: clues from the limb. Nature 423:319-325.

Figure 18-8. Adapted from Izpisua-Belmonte JC, Duboule D. 1992. Homeobox genes and pattern formation in the vertebrate limb. Dev Biol 152:26-36.

Figure 18-9. Adapted from Davis AP, Witte DP, Hsieh-Li HM, Potter SS, Capecchi MR. 1995. Absence of radius and ulna in mice lacking hoxa-11 and hoxd-11. Nature 375:791-795.

Figure 18-10. Courtesy of Dr. Mario Capecchi. Adapted from Wellik DM, Capecchi MR. 2003. Hox10 and Hox11 genes are required to globally pattern the mammalian skeleton. Science 301:363-367.

Figure 18-12. *A,* Courtesy of Dr. Arnold Tamarin. *B, C,* Courtesy of Dr. Robert E. Waterman.

Figure 18-13. Adapted from Alberts B, Johnson A, Lewis J, Raff M, Roberts K, Walter P. 2002. Molecular Biology of the Cell. Fourth Edition. Garland Science, New York.

Figure 18-14. A, Courtesy of Dr. Rolf Zeller. Adapted from Panman L, Zeller R. 2003. Patterning the limb before and after SHH signalling. J Anat 202:3-12. **B, C,** Courtesy of Dr. Cliff Tabin. Adapted from Harfe BD, Scherz PJ, Nissim S, Tian H, McMahon AP, Tabin CJ. 2004. Evidence for an expansion-based temporal Shh gradient in specifying vertebrate digit identities. Cell 118:517-528.

Figure 18-15. Courtesy of Dr. Rolf Zeller. Adapted from te Welscher P, Zuniga A, Kuijper S, Drenth T, Goedemans HJ, Meijlink F, Zeller R. 2002. Progression of vertebrate limb development through SHH-mediated counteraction of GLI3. Science 298:827-830.

Figure 18-16. Adapted from Chan DC, Laufer E, Tabin C, Leder P. 1995. Polydactylous limbs in Strong's Luxoid mice result from ectopic polarizing activity. Development 121:1971-1978.

Figure 18-17. *A-C, E,* Courtesy of Children's Hospital Medical Center, Cincinnati, OH. *D,* Courtesy of Dr. David Vischokil. *F,* Courtesy of Dr. John C. Carey.

Figure 18-18, 19. Courtesy of Dr. Irene Hung.

Figure 18-20. *A,* Courtesy of Children's Hospital Medical Center, Cincinnati, OH. *B, C,* Courtesy of Dr. Thomas Lufkin. Adapted from Kraus P, Lufkin T. 2006. Dlx homeobox gene control of mammalian limb and craniofacial development. Am J Med Genet A 140:1366-1374.

Figure 18-21. Courtesy of Muragaki Y, Mundlos S, Upton J, Olsen BR. 1996. Altered growth and branching patterns in synpolydactyly caused by mutations in HOXD13. Science 272:548-551.

Figures 18-22, 18-23. Courtesy of Dr. Irene Hung.

Figure 18-24. Adapted from Tosney KW, Landmesser LT. 1985. Development of the major pathways for neurite outgrowth in the chick hindlimb. Dev Biol 109:193-214.

Figure 18-25. Adapted from Tosney KW, Landmesser LT. 1984. Pattern and specificity of axonal outgrowth following varying degrees of chick limb bud ablation. J Neurosci 4:2518-2527.

Figure 18-27. *A, B, D,* Adapted from Kania A, Johnson RL, Jessell TM. 2000. Coordinate roles for LIM homeobox genes in directing the dorsoventral trajectory of motor axons in the vertebrate limb. Cell 102:161-173. *C,* Adapted from Shirasaki R, Pfaff SL. 2002. Transcriptional codes and the control of neuronal identity. Annu Rev Neurosci 25:251-281.

Index